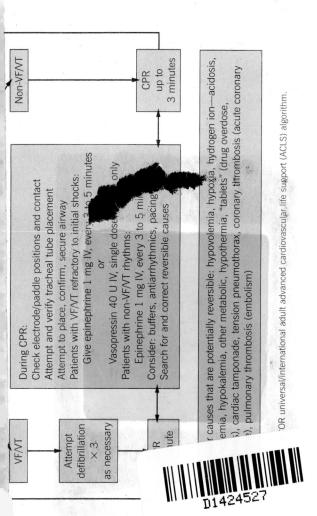

Non-VF/VT

VF/VT

Attempt defibrillation
×3
as necessary

CPR
up to
3 minutes

During CPR:
Check electrode/paddle positions and contact
Attempt and verify tracheal tube placement
Attempt to place, confirm, secure airway
Patients with VF/VT refractory to initial shocks:
 Give epinephrine 1 mg IV, every 3 to 5 minutes
 or
 Vasopressin 40 U IV, single dose   only
Patients with non-VF/VT rhythms:
 Epinephrine 1 mg IV, every 3 to 5 min
Consider: buffers, antiarrhythmics, pacing
Search for and correct reversible causes

... causes that are potentially reversible: hypovolemia, hypoxia, hydrogen ion—acidosis,
...emia, hypokalemia, other metabolic, hypothermia, "tablets" (drug overdose,
...s), cardiac tamponade, tension pneumothorax, coronary thrombosis (acute coronary
...e), pulmonary thrombosis (embolism)

...OR universal/international adult advanced cardiovascular life support (ACLS) algorithm.

Barcode ... next page

D1424527

Books ar

THE OSLER
MEDICAL
HANDBOOK

THE OSLER MEDICAL HANDBOOK

The Osler Medical Service
The Johns Hopkins Hospital

EDITORS

Alan Cheng, MD
Fellow, Cardiovascular Disease
Division of Cardiovascular Disease
Department of Medicine
Johns Hopkins University School of Medicine
Baltimore, Maryland

Aimee Zaas, MD
Fellow, Infectious Diseases
Division of Infectious Diseases and International Health
Department of Internal Medicine
Duke University Medical Center
Durham, North Carolina

with 197 illustrations and 30 color plates

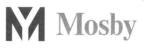

Mosby

An Affiliate of Elsevier Science

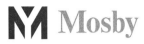

An Affiliate of Elsevier Science

The Curtis Center
Independence Square West
Philadelphia, Pennsylvania 19106

THE OSLER MEDICAL HANDBOOK ISBN 0-323-01930-7
Copyright © 2003, The Johns Hopkins University. All rights reserved.

Inside cover illustrations from Hazinski MF, Cummins RO, Field JM, editors.
*2000 Handbook of emergency cardiovascular care for healthcare
providers.* Dallas: American Heart Association; 2000.

NOTICE

Medicine is an ever-changing field. Standard safety precautions must
be followed, but as new research and clinical experience broaden our
knowledge, changes in treatment and drug therapy may become necessary or appropriate. Readers are advised to check the most current
product information provided by the manufacturer of each drug to be
administered to verify the recommended dose, the method and duration
of administration, and contraindications. It is the responsibility of the
licensed prescriber, relying on experience and knowledge of the patient,
to determine dosages and the best treatment for each individual patient.
Neither the publisher nor the editors assume any liability for any injury
and/or damage to persons or property arising from this publication.

International Standard Book Number 0-323-01930-7

Acquisitions Editor: Dolores Meloni
Developmental Editor: Rebecca Gruliow
Publishing Services Manager: Patricia Tannian
Designer: Gail Morey Hudson

Printed in United States of America

Last digit is the print number: 9 8 7 6 5 4 3 2 1

To our parents
Mr. and Mrs. Jensen and Rosita Cheng
and
Dr. Morton Kirsch and Ms. Sharon Kirsch
Whose unfailing love and support throughout our lives
have inspired us to be the best we can be

To our families
Dr. Tong-Yi Yao
My best friend and lifelong companion,
who has provided me with her love, support, and patience
through both thick and thin

Alex Cheng and Andy Cheng
Daily reminders of how truly blessed I am

Dr. David Zaas
Whose love, support, and help make my achievements
worthwhile and possible

To our mentors
Dr. Charles Wiener
Director of the Osler Medical Housestaff
and
Dr. Myron Weisfeldt
Sir William Osler Professor of Medicine and Physician-in-Chief
The Johns Hopkins Hospital

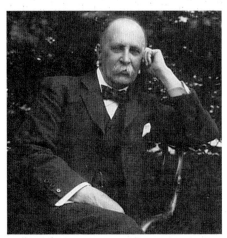

Sir William Osler—*1849-1919*

Nearly a century after his death, Sir William Osler is still probably the most famous and oft-quoted physician in North America and in Europe. Over the course of his professional life at McGill University, the University of Pennsylvania, Johns Hopkins University, and Oxford University, he placed an indelible stamp on medical practice and teaching that persists to this day.

William Osler came to Johns Hopkins in 1889 as the first chief physician of the new Hospital and School of Medicine. He wanted to create a hospital and school that would be "a place of refuge for the sick and poor of the city—a place where the best that is known is taught to a group of the best students—a place where new thought is materialized in research—a school where men are encouraged to base the art upon the science of medicine—a fountain to which teachers in every subject would come for inspiration—a place with a hearty welcome to every practitioner who seeks help—a consulting center for the whole country in cases of obscurity." The spirit of dedication to patient care, teaching, and research that was instilled by Osler and his colleagues remains the mission of the Johns Hopkins Hospital and the School of Medicine.

It was during Osler's time at Johns Hopkins (1889-1905) that he wrote *Principles and Practice of Medicine*. Osler was a renowned author even before he took on the task of singlehandedly writing a state-of-the-art, comprehensive textbook of medicine. His book was "designed for the use of practitioners and students of medicine" and was the first modern textbook that took a scientific approach to the diagnosis and practice of medicine. *Principles and Practice of Medicine,* first published in 1892, was a worldwide success and greatly enhanced the professional stature of physicians because it rooted medicine in science and in rigorous observation. The explosion of medical publishing over the past 100 years can be traced to the publication of this remarkable book.

Another of Osler's legacies is the Osler Medical Housestaff and the Osler Medical Service at the Johns Hopkins Hospital. Although in Osler's day medical training commonly included a period of residency, he was among the first to appoint residents to his own service based on their intellectual prowess as well as their personal characteristics. He valued collegial interactions and believed strongly that because the attending physician and resident would have frequent intense contact, they should have similar values and goals for improving health, understanding medicine, and communicating with patients. He led and taught by example, advising his students to "care more particularly for the individual patient, than for the special features of the disease" and frequently reminding them that "medicine is learned by the bedside and not in the classroom." These principles remain the foundation on which clinical education and housestaff training are based at Johns Hopkins. Osler did not minimize the value of scholarship and reading. His scholastic expectations for physicians and trainees were extremely high. He expected doctors to read about their cases and to have a current understanding of pathophysiology: "It is astonishing with how little reading a doctor can practice medicine, but it is not astonishing how badly he may do it."

It is in the spirit of professionalism, scholarship, and collegiality that this book was written. In 1998, as interns on the Janeway Firm of the Osler Medical Service, Alan Cheng and Aimee Zaas decided that the Osler Medical Housestaff, in conjunction with faculty, should write a book focusing on evidence-guided approaches to the care of patients admitted to a general medical service. This book would be modeled on the highly successful *Harriet Lane Handbook* written by the Johns Hopkins Pediatrics Housestaff. Over the past 5 years Alan and Aimee have driven the creation of *The Osler Medical Handbook*. They and their colleagues on the housestaff have spent innumerable hours reading, writing, and editing. We offer this book to our medical colleagues on behalf of the past, present, and future Johns Hopkins housestaff in the spirit of a love for patient care and a dedication to scholarship.

As the current Program Director of the Osler Medical Housestaff, I have immeasurable pride in our housestaff, who daily perpetuate the values that William Osler lived and taught at Johns Hopkins. We hope that this book, which is also "designed for the use of practitioners and students of medicine," is as useful and as successful as was his.

Charles Wiener, MD

Director, Osler Medical Housestaff
The Johns Hopkins Hospital
Vice Chairman, Department of Medicine
Johns Hopkins School of Medicine

Foreword

Medical residencies as we now know them began at The Johns Hopkins Hospital in the 1890s. There were residency physicians in a literal sense—physicians who resided in hospitals—before The Johns Hopkins Hospital opened in 1889. The graduated residency program, however, was initiated at Hopkins by William Osler, the first physician-in-chief. The system included interns, junior and senior assistant residents, and a chief resident, called the resident physician, who had a long tenure. During his 16 years (1889-1905) at Hopkins, Osler had only five resident physicians.

From the beginning, major responsibility for the care of the patients was given to the resident staff. The graduated residency made this possible, with juniors learning from their seniors. It may not be facetious to suggest that the traditionally strong and independent character of the Osler Medical Service's residency program can be traced in part to the hot Baltimore summers. By the end of June most faculty had departed for cooler climates.

I was a member of the Osler Housestaff as an intern for 15 months (April 1946 to June 1947) and a junior assistant resident from 1947 to 1948. After a 2-year interlude in cardiovascular research, I returned to the Osler Medical Service as senior assistant resident from 1950 to 1951 and then resident physician from 1951 to 1952.

When I was the resident physician, the Osler Housestaff worked in the Osler Building. The patients were the responsibility of the resident staff, with the ultimate responsibility resting with the physician-in-chief. There were four general medical wards and no specialty wards; two additional wards were devoted to patients with infectious diseases requiring isolation and a metabolic research unit. Each of the four general medical units had accommodations for 29 patients and was staffed by two or three interns and a junior or senior assistant resident. Patients had long hospital stays, and most of the residency experience was with inpatients. Both interns and assistant residents "covered" the Emergency Department (then called the "Accident Room"), however. Admissions to the Osler Service from the clinic or Emergency Department were determined by the senior residents, who rotated through the duty of admitting officer.

Each of the four major general medical units was the base for instruction for five or six fourth-year medical students. (Third-year medicine was taught in the outpatient clinics.) These medical students played a major role in patient care. In turn, the housestaff played a major role in the clinical education of the students. The only remuneration the assistant residents received for teaching was a paltry $200 a year, although room, board, and laundry were provided. Interns received no stipend. Each unit had a visiting physician whose role was advisory and pedagogical; he or she was not an attending physician in the sense of physician-of-record. Medical students spent 8 weeks in their senior year on one unit. Interns and junior assistant residents rotated monthly, whereas senior residents stayed with the student group for their entire 8 weeks.

The resident physician made rounds on each unit in the morning and more extensive rounds in the evening. After the morning tour through the Osler Building, the resident physician reported to the physician-in-chief. He or she had an opportunity to keep in touch with the patients passing through the clinic and was available for consultation on particular problems. In addition, the resident physician played a major role in consultations on the residency services in other departments, such as surgery, ophthalmology, gynecology, and psychiatry. Resident's rounds at 5 PM Monday through Friday were a major teaching event during which housestaff presented their most instructive or puzzling patients and thereby taught one another.

In the pyramidal system, each echelon learned from the more experienced. The unit's visiting physician made rounds with the students and resident staff for 2 hours three mornings a week. By hearing from the students (or sometimes the intern) about particular patients, the visiting physician maintained some familiarity with the patients on the unit. By rotation through the four teaching units the physician-in-chief made rounds for 2 hours three mornings a week, during which students usually presented two patients for detailed discussion. He was available at other times to consult on difficult problems.

I became director of the Department of Medicine in 1973, 21 years after I completed my residency. The Osler residency program had changed and was now overseen by two chief residents. The residency group was no longer a close-knit cadre whose members became well known to one another and to the chief resident, who could foster their development as physicians. The situation was less satisfactory, with fewer opportunities for juniors to learn from seniors and all to learn from one another.

Changes in medicine at that time included an increased awareness of the importance of outpatient experience in the training of physicians. Economic pressures were reducing the length of hospital stays. Public programs for support of medical care, such as Medicare, which was instituted in 1964, demanded clearer definition of the physician-of-record. By long tradition, on the Osler Service the intern was the primary physician for the patients in his or her care. The intern was assisted by the medical student assigned to each patient, was supervised by the assistant resident(s) assigned to the ward, and received advice from the visiting physician. It was the intern who wrote medication and other orders for the patient. However, an intern or an assistant resident would not be acceptable as a physician-of-record. Designating the visiting physician as physician-of-record for patients on units that traditionally constitute the ward service was considered undesirable because this would erode the independence of the housestaff, which had been so important in their training.

These considerations led to the creation of the Osler Firm System in 1975. The system split the housestaff into four units, or firms (a term used for units in British teaching hospitals), each headed by an assistant chief of service (ACS). The ACS was physician-of-record for the patients in the firm.

Each firm had one of the original Osler wards as a home base and also had responsibility for part of the Private Service.

It was originally planned that the ACS position would be a 2-year job, in imitation of the long-tenured chief residents of Osler's time. Two new ACSs would be appointed each year, giving useful overlap. However, the job was found to be too grueling and to require the ACS to be away too long from subspecialty training and research for a 2-year tenure to be acceptable.

Today the Osler Firm System is an established institution that has adapted well to socioeconomic change while preserving its advantages for clinical learning. It provides the camaraderie and collegiality that have been so important in the teaching of interns and junior residents by senior residents. The Firm System has been able to accommodate the shift toward greater involvement of physicians-in-training in ambulatory medicine.

This book has grown out of the Osler tradition of giving housestaff a pivotal role in educating colleagues and peers. Each chapter was written by a member of the Osler housestaff with direct supervision of a member of the Johns Hopkins faculty. Despite revolutionary changes in medicine and the U.S. health care system, we hold true to the core values Osler taught by precept and example, namely, that it is our mission to improve the health of our patients and as physicians to strive consistently to improve our knowledge and experience. The Osler housestaff offers *The Osler Medical Handbook* in that spirit.

Victor A. McKusick, MD
Former William Osler Professor and
Director, Department of Medicine,
Johns Hopkins University, and
Physician-in-Chief,
The Johns Hopkins Hospital (1973-1985)

Preface

Sir William Osler was one of the greatest physicians in history, and his legacy at Johns Hopkins continues today in the strong emphasis on patient care, research, and teaching. Osler was a brilliant teacher and scholar whose life was devoted to investigation. Although he *discovered* little, he is regarded as a pioneer of medicine because of his ability to observe and his belief that medicine must rest on the discoveries of science. In addition to being a master clinician, Osler was a supreme humanist who tirelessly displayed compassion for his patients, students, and colleagues. His charisma and enthusiasm for the advancement of medicine remain unparalleled.

It is against this backdrop that the Osler Medical Housestaff was formed and continues to advance the teachings and principles of its founder. Our training program instilled in us a strong sense of responsibility for our patients and emphasized the importance of the medical house officer. As our understanding of disease pathogenesis grew, however, we found it difficult to keep up with the advances of science and constantly emerging discoveries in therapeutics while maintaining our clinical responsibilities. Simply getting together with fellow residents and informally discussing interesting cases proved to be a highly effective way of educating one another and advancing patient care. During one of these gatherings we discussed ways of presenting the information in a user-friendly format that would perpetuate our interests in teaching and learning. The result is *The Osler Medical Handbook*.

Each disease-based chapter is designed to address diagnoses commonly encountered at the Johns Hopkins Hospital. In most chapters the format includes the subheadings Fast Facts, Epidemiology, Clinical Presentation, Diagnostics, Management, Pearls and Pitfalls, and References. Diagnostic and therapeutic algorithms are provided throughout the book, as are differential diagnoses for diseases with presentations similar to the main disease being discussed. The Pearls and Pitfalls section at the end of each chapter highlights clinical pearls, addresses concerns relating to comorbidities, gives tips for avoidance of error, and mentions populations or groups of individuals at particular risk for death and disease. Despite every effort made to provide evidence-based management recommendations, there were occasions where data were lacking or inconclusive. In these situations recommendations are made based on currently accepted standards of practice or expert opinion of the faculty advisor. In an effort to help the reader identify what types of references are being cited, a "strength of evidence" scale from "a" to "d" has been incorporated for each reference listed. Category **"a"** describes articles that are randomized, placebo-controlled, double-blind studies; category **"b"** describes articles that are prospective trials, retrospective trials, case reports, or basic science reports; category **"c"** describes articles that are review papers or metaanalyses; category **"d"** describes articles that are guidelines or position papers from authoritative medical associations (e.g., American College of Cardiology, American College of Physicians), editorials, or expert opinion.

The development of *The Osler Medical Handbook,* like all multidisciplinary endeavors, was a team effort and epitomized the spirit of collegiality that defines the Osler Medical Service. The foundations of this book rest solely on the Osler Medical Housestaff, who not only spent countless hours managing some of the sickest patients in our community, but worked tirelessly in preparing the manuscript. We owe a debt of gratitude to each of them and their faculty advisors.

Resident	Chapter Number	Faculty Advisor
Moeen Abedin, MD	7	Hugh Calkins, MD
Gregory B. Ang, MD	28	Mark Donowitz, MD, Cynthia L. Sears, MD
Hossein Ardehali, MD, PhD	5, 48	Ch. 5, Stephen C. Achuff, MD; Ch. 48, Eric Nuermberger, MD
Susan Arnold, PharmD	Formulary	
Kenneth Bilchick, MD	13	Ronald Berger, MD, PhD
Jeffrey Brewer, PharmD	Formulary	
Cynthia Brown, MD	55	Gail V. Berkenblit, MD, PhD
Hetty Carraway, MD	32	Michael Streiff, MD
Kerri L. Cavanaugh, MD	30, 54	Ch. 30, Mary L. Harris, MD; Ch. 54, Derek M. Fine, MD
Matthews Chacko, MD	8	Edward Kasper, MD
Hunter C. Champion, MD, PhD	16, 17, 18, 66	Ch. 16, Mark Linzer, MD; Ch. 17, Albert L. Hyman, MD*; Ch. 18, Stephen C. Achuff, MD; Ch. 66, Sean P. Gaine, MD, PhD†
Katherine Chang, MD	46	Anne Rompalo, MD, ScM
Tze-Ming (Benson) Chen, MD	2	Henry E. Fessler, MD
Alan Cheng, MD	1, 3, 9, 13, 43, 44	Ch. 3, D. William Schlott, MD; Ch. 9, Roger Blumenthal, MD; Ch. 13, Ronald Berger, MD, PhD; Ch. 43, John Bartlett, MD; Ch. 44, Paul Auwaerter, MD
Patty P. Chi, MD	53	Derek M. Fine, MD
Rachel Y. Chong, MD	29	Mary L. Harris, MD
Sharon A. Chung, MD	11	Michael J. Klag, MD
Gregory O. Clark, MD	22	Christopher D. Saudek, MD
Amanda M. Clark, RN, BSN, CWCN	20	
John Clarke, MD	49	David Thomas, MD
Megan E. Bowles Clowse, MD, MPH	71	Alan Matsumoto, MD
Keliegh S. Culpepper, MD	19	Susan Laman, MD, MPH
Chrishonda M. Curry	Rapid References	
Rachel Damico, MD, PhD	42	John Mann, MD
J. Lucian Davis, Jr., MD	68	Landon S. King, MD
Sanjay Desai, MD	14	Gary Gerstenblith, MD
Luis Diaz, MD	34	Lawrence Gardner, MD
Kerry Dunbar, MD	62	Albert J. Polito, MD

continued

continued

Philip Seo, MD	70	
Assil Saleh, MD	21	Paul W. Ladenson, MD
Anastasio Saliaris, MD	24	Francis Giardiello, MD
Abe Shaikh	Rapid References	
Patrick R. Sosnay, MD	47	Sara Cosgrove, MD
Nimalie D. Stone, MD, PhD	38	Justin McArthur, MBBS, MPH
Dechen P. Surkhang, RD, LD	57	Tricia Brusco, MS, RD, LD
Sabrina M. Tom, MD	15	J.G.N. Garcia, MD
Jean S. Wang, MD	31	David M. Cromwell, MD
David Wang, MD	36	Carole Miller, MD
Richard Waters, MD	6	Mark Kelemen, MD
Amy C. Weintrob, MD	37	Charles B. Hicks, MD§
Carolyn Wong Simpkins, MD, PhD	69	Philip L. Smith, MD
Eric H. Yang, MD	5, 16, 17, 18	Ch. 5, Stephen C. Achuff, MD; Ch. 16, Mark Linzer, MD¶; Ch. 17, Albert L. Hyman, MD*; Ch. 18, Stephen C. Achuff, MD
David Zaas, MD	59, 64	Ch. 59, Robert Wise, MD; Ch. 64, David Pearse, MD
Aimee Zaas, MD	1, 40, 43, 44	Ch. 40, Stuart C. Ray, MD; Ch. 43, John Bartlett, MD; Ch. 44, Paul Auwaerter, MD
David A. Zidar, MD	41	Stuart C. Ray, MD

*Division of Cardiology, Tulane University School of Medicine, New Orleans, La.

†Department of Respiratory Medicine, Misericordiae Hospital, Dublin, Ireland.

‡University of Pennsylvania, Gastroenterology Division, Philadelphia, Pa.

§Duke University Medical Center, Durham, N.C.

¶General Internal Medicine, University of Wisconsin Hospital and Clinics, Madison, Wisc.

Editing the information and applying it to clinical practice were integral parts of the production of this book. We thank the following individuals who served in this capacity.

Resident Reviewers	Medical Student Reviewers
Megan E. Bowles Clowse, MD	Shin Lin
Rachel Damico, MD, PhD	Atif Qasim
J. Lucian Davis, Jr., MD	Byron Hing Lung Lee
David N. Hager, MD	Alex Sun Huang
Anna Hemnes, MD	Homaa Ahmad
Rosalyn Juergens, MD	
Michael J. McWilliams, MD	
E. Ann Misch, MD	
Sarah B. Noonberg, MD, PhD	
Phil Nivatpumin, MD	
Geoffrey C. Nguyen, MD	
Vandana R. Long, MD	
Micol Rothman, MD	
Philip Seo, MD	
Patrick R. Sosnay, MD	

Our staunchest advocate has been Dr. Charles Wiener, whose constant leadership and enthusiasm have encouraged us to strive for excellence in all we do. Without his help this book would not have been possible. We also extend our heartfelt appreciation to Drs. John Bartlett, Stuart Ray, Kristin Thomas, David B. Hellmann, and Myron Weisfeldt, the current Sir William Osler Professor of Medicine and Physician-in-Chief of The Johns Hopkins Hospital, for their valuable encouragement throughout the production of this book. Early support from Shannon Lewis and MaryEllen Hagerty is also greatly appreciated.

To Dolores Meloni, Rebecca Gruliow, Patricia Tannian, and countless behind-the-scenes staff members at Elsevier Science, including Maria Lorusso and Andrea Bucci, we extend our appreciation for your guidance and help every step of the way. To Julie Gottlieb and Patricia Friend, we thank you for your support and help in making this possible.

We are honored to have worked with so many members of the Osler Medical Housestaff. On their behalf, we present this book and hope that it will continue to serve its purpose—to improve on the practice of medicine for the benefit of all as Sir William Osler envisioned many years ago.

Alan Cheng
Aimee Zaas

Contents

Hematology and Oncology

HIV-Related Infectious Diseases

Infectious Diseases

Color plates follow p. 326

PART I

Acute Care of the Adult Patient

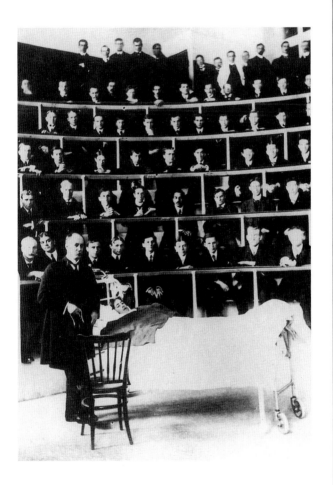

Cardiopulmonary Resuscitation and Advanced Cardiac Life Support

The following pages introduce the latest Advanced Cardiac Life Support (ACLS) guidelines for management of cardiac arrest and certain dysrhythmias. These guidelines represent the consensus recommendations from the International Guidelines 2000 Conference on CPR and Emergency Cardiovascular Care, as well as recommendations from the 1999 Evidence Evaluation Conference and the 1999 consensus recommendations of the American College of Cardiology/American Heart Association Task Force on Practice Guidelines. The algorithms selected for this handbook include those used most commonly in inpatient practice.

The ABCs of basic life support still apply when using advanced cardiac life support.

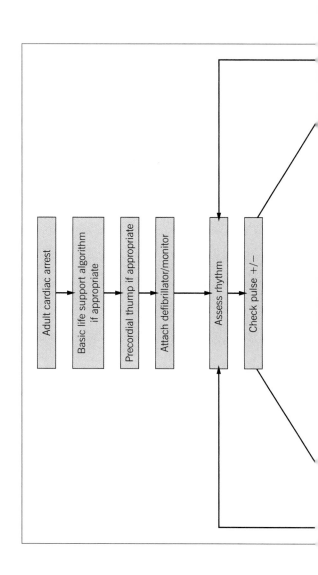

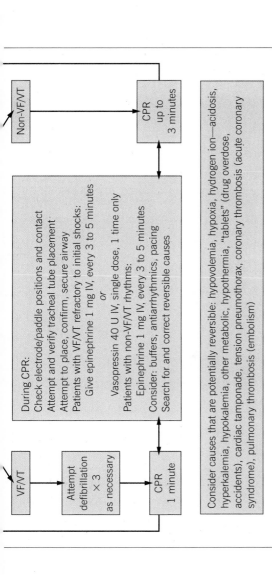

FIG. 1-1

ILCOR universal/international adult advanced cardiovascular life support (ACLS) algorithm. *CPR*, Cardiopulmonary resuscitation; *VF*, ventricular fibrillation; *VT*, ventricular tachycardia. (From Hazinski MF, Cummins RO, Field JM, editors. *2000 Handbook of emergency cardiovascular care for healthcare providers*. Dallas: American Heart Association; 2000.)

CARDIOPULMONARY RESUSCITATION AND ACLS

1

Contents of figure:

Non-VF/VT

VF/VT

Attempt defibrillation × 3 as necessary

CPR 1 minute

CPR up to 3 minutes

During CPR:
Check electrode/paddle positions and contact
Attempt and verify tracheal tube placement
Attempt to place, confirm, secure airway
Patients with VF/VT refractory to initial shocks:
Give epinephrine 1 mg IV, every 3 to 5 minutes
or
Vasopressin 40 U IV, single dose, 1 time only
Patients with non-VF/VT rhythms:
Epinephrine 1 mg IV, every 3 to 5 minutes
Consider: buffers, antiarrhythmics, pacing
Search for and correct reversible causes

Consider causes that are potentially reversible: hypovolemia, hypoxia, hydrogen ion—acidosis, hyperkalemia, hypokalemia, other metabolic, hypothermia, "tablets" (drug overdose, accidents), cardiac tamponade, tension pneumothorax, coronary thrombosis (acute coronary syndrome), pulmonary thrombosis (embolism)

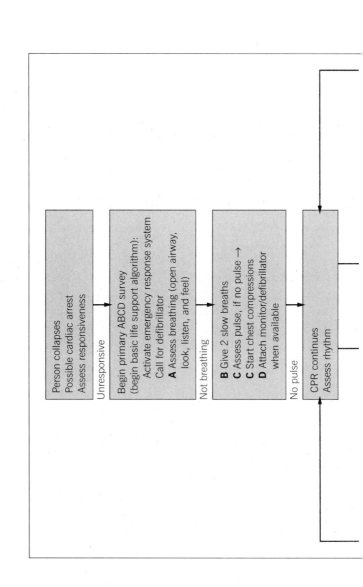

Person collapses
Possible cardiac arrest
Assess responsiveness

Unresponsive

Begin primary ABCD survey
(begin basic life support algorithm):
Activate emergency response system
Call for defibrillator
A Assess breathing (open airway,
look, listen, and feel)

Not breathing

B Give 2 slow breaths
C Assess pulse, if no pulse →
C Start chest compressions
D Attach monitor/defibrillator
when available

No pulse

CPR continues
Assess rhythm

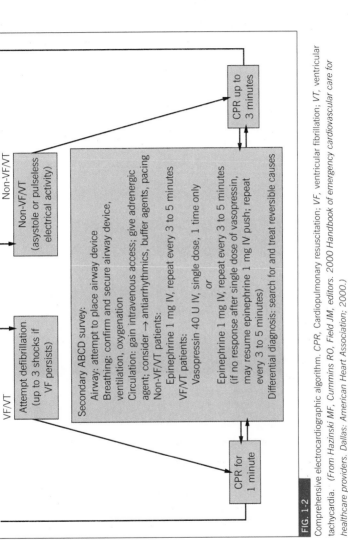

FIG. 1-2

Comprehensive electrocardiographic algorithm. *CPR,* Cardiopulmonary resuscitation; *VF,* ventricular fibrillation; *VT,* ventricular tachycardia. *(From Hazinski MF, Cummins RO, Field JM, editors. 2000 Handbook of emergency cardiovascular care for healthcare providers. Dallas: American Heart Association; 2000.)*

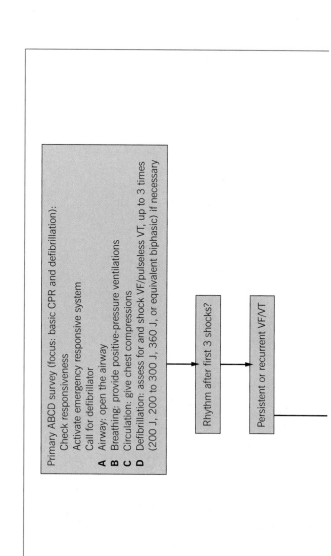

Primary ABCD survey (focus: basic CPR and defibrillation):

Check responsiveness

Activate emergency responsive system

Call for defibrillator

A Airway: open the airway

B Breathing: provide positive-pressure ventilations

C Circulation: give chest compressions

D Defibrillation: assess for and shock VF/pulseless VT, up to 3 times (200 J, 200 to 300 J, 360 J, or equivalent biphasic) if necessary

Rhythm after first 3 shocks?

Persistent or recurrent VF/VT

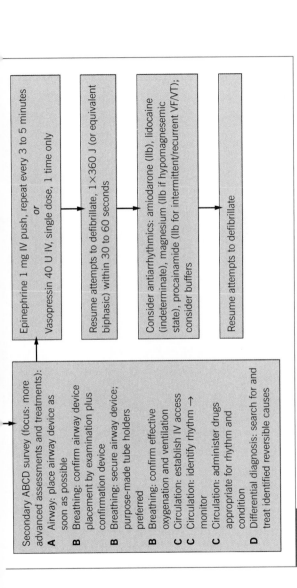

FIG. 1-3

Ventricular fibrillation/pulseless ventricular tachycardia algorithm. *VF,* ventricular fibrillation; *VT,* ventricular tachycardia. (From Hazinski MF, Cummins RO, Field JM, editors. *2000 Handbook of emergency cardiovascular care for healthcare providers.* Dallas: American Heart Association; 2000.)

Secondary ABCD survey (focus: more advanced assessments and treatments):

A Airway: place airway device as soon as possible

B Breathing: confirm airway device placement by examination plus confirmation device

B Breathing: secure airway device; purpose-made tube holders preferred

B Breathing: confirm effective oxygenation and ventilation

C Circulation: establish IV access

C Circulation: identify rhythm → monitor

C Circulation: administer drugs appropriate for rhythm and condition

D Differential diagnosis: search for and treat identified reversible causes

Epinephrine 1 mg IV push, repeat every 3 to 5 minutes
or
Vasopressin 40 U IV, single dose, 1 time only

Resume attempts to defibrillate, 1×360 J (or equivalent biphasic) within 30 to 60 seconds

Consider antiarrhythmics: amiodarone (IIb), lidocaine (indeterminate), magnesium (IIb if hypomagnesemic state), procainamide (IIb for intermittent/recurrent VF/VT); consider buffers

Resume attempts to defibrillate

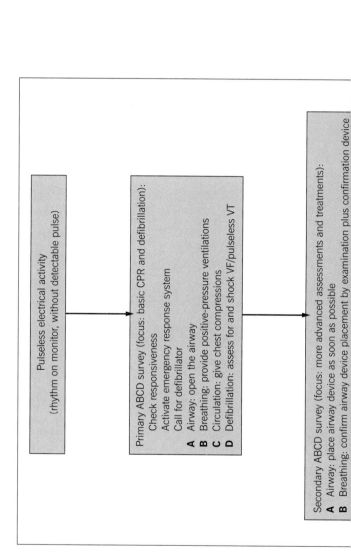

Pulseless electrical activity
(rhythm on monitor, without detectable pulse)

Primary ABCD survey (focus: basic CPR and defibrillation):
  Check responsiveness
  Activate emergency response system
  Call for defibrillator
  A Airway: open the airway
  B Breathing: provide positive-pressure ventilations
  C Circulation: give chest compressions
  D Defibrillation: assess for and shock VF/pulseless VT

Secondary ABCD survey (focus: more advanced assessments and treatments):
  A Airway: place airway device as soon as possible
  B Breathing: confirm airway device placement by examination plus confirmation device

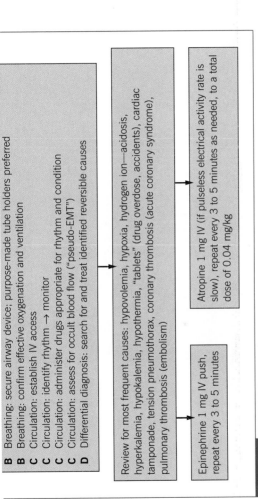

- **B** Breathing: secure airway device; purpose-made tube holders preferred
- **B** Breathing: confirm effective oxygenation and ventilation
- **C** Circulation: establish IV access
- **C** Circulation: identify rhythm → monitor
- **C** Circulation: administer drugs appropriate for rhythm and condition
- **C** Circulation: assess for occult blood flow ("pseudo-EMT")
- **D** Differential diagnosis: search for and treat identified reversible causes

Review for most frequent causes: hypovolemia, hypoxia, hydrogen ion—acidosis, hyperkalemia, hypokalemia, hypothermia, "tablets" (drug overdose, accidents), cardiac tamponade, tension pneumothorax, coronary thrombosis (acute coronary syndrome), pulmonary thrombosis (embolism)

Epinephrine 1 mg IV push, repeat every 3 to 5 minutes

Atropine 1 mg IV (if pulseless electrical activity rate is slow), repeat every 3 to 5 minutes as needed, to a total dose of 0.04 mg/kg

FIG. 1-4

Pulseless electrical activity algorithm. *EMT*, Electromechanical dissociation; *VF*, ventricular fibrillation; *VT*, ventricular tachycardia. *(From Hazinski MF, Cummins RO, Field JM, editors. 2000 Handbook of emergency cardiovascular care for healthcare providers. Dallas: American Heart Association; 2000.)*

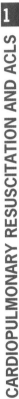

CARDIOPULMONARY RESUSCITATION AND ACLS

1

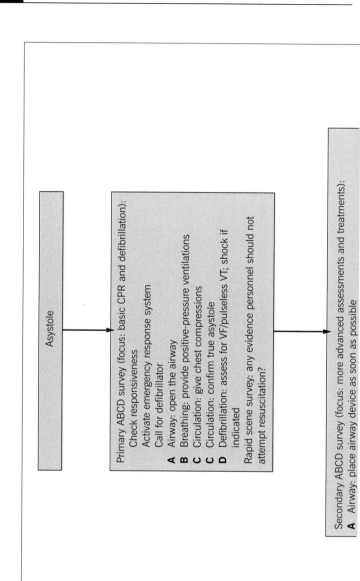

Asystole

Primary ABCD survey (focus: basic CPR and defibrillation):
  Check responsiveness
  Activate emergency response system
  Call for defibrillator
  A Airway: open the airway
  B Breathing: provide positive-pressure ventilations
  C Circulation: give chest compressions
  C Circulation: confirm true asystole
  D Defibrillation: assess for VF/pulseless VT; shock if
     indicated
  Rapid scene survey: any evidence personnel should not
  attempt resuscitation?

Secondary ABCD survey (focus: more advanced assessments and treatments):
  A Airway: place airway device as soon as possible

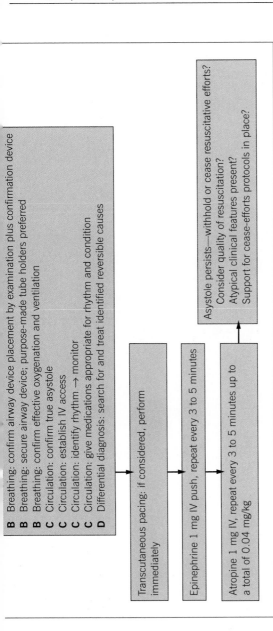

B Breathing: confirm airway device placement by examination plus confirmation device
B Breathing: secure airway device; purpose-made tube holders preferred
B Breathing: confirm effective oxygenation and ventilation
C Circulation: confirm true asystole
C Circulation: establish IV access
C Circulation: identify rhythm → monitor
C Circulation: give medications appropriate for rhythm and condition
D Differential diagnosis: search for and treat identified reversible causes

Transcutaneous pacing: if considered, perform immediately

Epinephrine 1 mg IV push, repeat every 3 to 5 minutes

Atropine 1 mg IV, repeat every 3 to 5 minutes up to a total of 0.04 mg/kg

Asystole persists—withhold or cease resuscitative efforts?
Consider quality of resuscitation?
Atypical clinical features present?
Support for cease-efforts protocols in place?

FIG. 1-5

Asystole: the silent heart rhythm. *VF,* ventricular fibrillation; *VT,* ventricular tachycardia. *(From Hazinski MF, Cummins RO, Field JM, editors. 2000 Handbook of emergency cardiovascular care for healthcare providers. Dallas: American Heart Association; 2000.)*

CARDIOPULMONARY RESUSCITATION AND ACLS **1**

Bradycardia

Slow (absolute bradycardia=rate <60 beats/min)

or

Relatively slow (rate less than expected relative to underlying condition or cause)

Primary ABCD survey:
  Assess ABCs
  Secure airway noninvasively
  Ensure monitor/defibrillator is available
Secondary ABCD survey:
  Assess secondary ABCs (invasive airway management needed?)
  Oxygen–IV access–monitor–fluids
  Vital signs, pulse oximeter, monitor blood pressure
  Obtain and review 12-lead electrocardiogram
  Obtain and review portable chest x-ray
  Problem-focused history
  Problem-focused physical examination
  Consider causes (differential diagnoses)

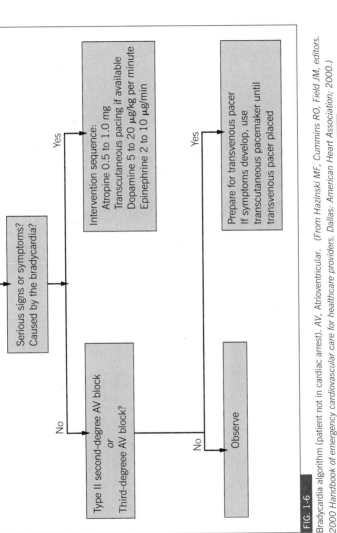

FIG. 1-6

Bradycardia algorithm (patient not in cardiac arrest). AV, Atrioventricular. (From Hazinski MF, Cummins RO, Field JM, editors. 2000 Handbook of emergency cardiovascular care for healthcare providers. Dallas: American Heart Association; 2000.)

CARDIOPULMONARY RESUSCITATION AND ACLS 1

Text within figure:

Serious signs or symptoms?
Caused by the bradycardia?

Yes →

Intervention sequence:
Atropine 0.5 to 1.0 mg
Transcutaneous pacing if available
Dopamine 5 to 20 μg/kg per minute
Epinephrine 2 to 10 μg/min

No →

Type II second-degree AV block
or
Third-degreee AV block?

Yes →

Prepare for transvenous pacer
If symptoms develop, use
transcutaneous pacemaker until
transvenous pacer placed

No →

Observe

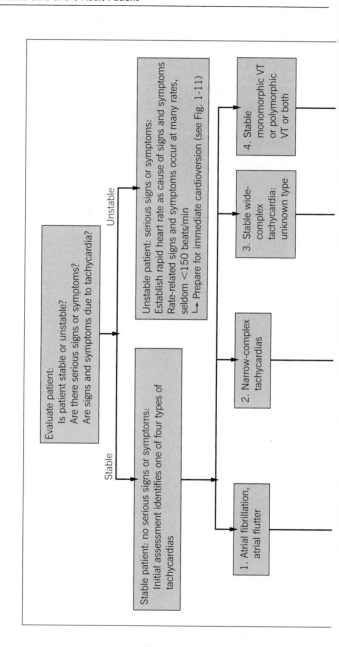

Evaluate patient:
Is patient stable or unstable?
Are there serious signs or symptoms?
Are signs and symptoms due to tachycardia?

Stable

Unstable

Stable patient: no serious signs or symptoms:
Initial assessment identifies one of four types of tachycardias

Unstable patient: serious signs or symptoms:
Establish rapid heart rate as cause of signs and symptoms
Rate-related signs and symptoms occur at many rates,
seldom <150 beats/min
└─ Prepare for immediate cardioversion (see Fig. 1-11)

1. Atrial fibrillation,
atrial flutter

2. Narrow-complex
tachycardias

3. Stable wide-
complex
tachycardia:
unknown type

4. Stable
monomorphic VT
or polymorphic
VT or both

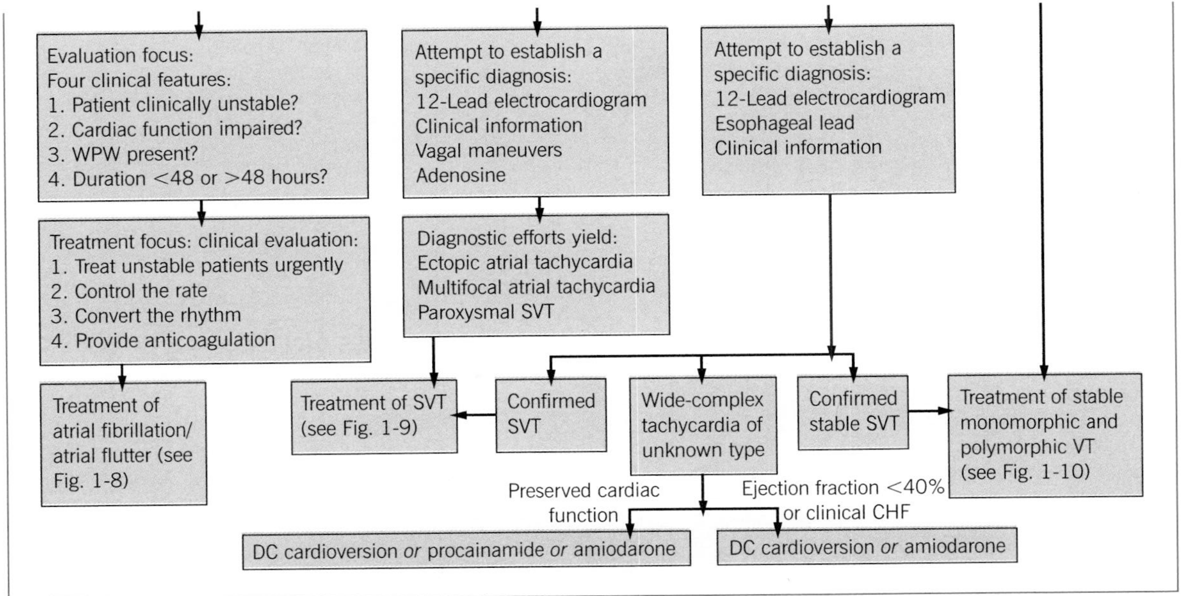
Evaluation focus:
Four clinical features:
1. Patient clinically unstable?
2. Cardiac function impaired?
3. WPW present?
4. Duration <48 or >48 hours?
Attempt to establish a specific diagnosis:
12-Lead electrocardiogram
Clinical information
Vagal maneuvers
Adenosine
Attempt to establish a specific diagnosis:
12-Lead electrocardiogram
Esophageal lead
Clinical information
Treatment focus: clinical evaluation:
1. Treat unstable patients urgently
2. Control the rate
3. Convert the rhythm
4. Provide anticoagulation
Diagnostic efforts yield:
Ectopic atrial tachycardia
Multifocal atrial tachycardia
Paroxysmal SVT
Treatment of atrial fibrillation/atrial flutter (see Fig. 1-8)
Treatment of SVT (see Fig. 1-9)
Confirmed SVT
Wide-complex tachycardia of unknown type
Confirmed stable SVT
Treatment of stable monomorphic and polymorphic VT (see Fig. 1-10)
Preserved cardiac function
Ejection fraction <40% or clinical CHF
DC cardioversion or procainamide or amiodarone
DC cardioversion or amiodarone

FIG. 1-7

Tachycardia overview algorithm. *CHF,* Congestive heart failure; *SVT,* supraventricular tachycardia; *VT,* ventricular tachycardia; *WPW,* Wolff-Parkinson-White syndrome. *(From Hazinski MF, Cummins RO, Field JM, editors. 2000 Handbook of emergency cardiovascular care for healthcare providers. Dallas: American Heart Association; 2000.)*

Atrial Fibrillation/ Atrial Flutter with: Normal Heart Impaired Heart WPW	1. Control Rate		2. Convert Rhythm	
	Heart Function Preserved	Impaired Heart Ejection Fraction <40% or CHF	Duration <48 Hours	Duration >48 Hours or Unknown
Normal cardiac function	Note: If AF >48 hours' duration, use agents to convert rhythm with extreme caution in patients not receiving adequate anticoagulation because of possible embolic complications. Use only one of the following agents (see note below): Calcium channel blockers (class I) β-Blockers (class I) For additional drugs that are class IIb recommendations, see Guidelines or	(Does not apply)	Consider: DC cardioversion Use only one of the following agents (see note below): Amiodarone (class IIa) Ibutilide (class IIa) Flecainide (class IIa) Propafenone (class IIa) Procainamide (class IIa) For additional drugs that are class IIb recommendations, see Guidelines or ACLS text	NO DC cardioversion! Note: Conversion of AF to normal sinus rhythm with drugs or shock may cause embolization of atrial thrombi unless patient has adequate anticoagulation. Use antiarrhythmic agents with extreme caution if AF >48 hours' duration (see note above). or Delayed cardioversion: Anticoagulation × 3 weeks at proper levels Cardioversion then Anticoagulation × 4 weeks more

	ACLS text			
Impaired heart (ejection fraction <40% or CHF)	(Does not apply)	Note: If AF >48 hours' duration, use agents to convert rhythm with extreme caution in patients not receiving adequate anticoagulation because of possible embolic complications. Use only one of the following agents (see note below): Digoxin (class IIb) Diltiazem (class IIb) Amiodarone (class IIb)	Consider DC cardioversion *or* Amiodarone (class IIb)	*or* Early cardioversion: Begin IV heparin at once Transesophageal echocardiogram to exclude atrial clot *then* Cardioversion within 24 hours *then* Anticoagulation as described above, followed by DC cardioversion

Note: Occasionally two of the named antiarrhythmic agents may be used, but use of these agents in combination may have proarrhythmic potential. The classes listed represent the class of recommendation rather than the Vaughn-Williams classification of antiarrhythmics.

FIG. 1-8
Tachycardia: atrial fibrillation and fluttter, control rate and rhythm. *AF,* Atrial fibrillation; *WPW,* Wolff-Parkinson-White syndrome. *(From Hazinski MF, Cummins RO, Field JM, editors. 2000 Handbook of emergency cardiovascular care for healthcare providers. Dallas: American Heart Association; 2000.)*

Atrial Fibrillation/ Atrial Flutter with: Normal Heart Impaired Heart WPW	1. Control Rate		2. Convert Rhythm	
	Heart Function Preserved	Impaired Heart Ejection Fraction <40% or CHF	Duration <48 Hours	Duration >48 Hours or Unknown
WPW	Note: If AF >48 hours' duration, use agents to convert rhythm with extreme caution in patients not receiving adequate anticoagulation because of possible embolic complications. DC cardioversion *or* Primary antiarrhythmic agents: Use only one of the following agents (see note below): Amiodarone (class IIb) Flecainide (class IIb)	Note: If AF >48 hours' duration, use agents to convert rhythm with extreme caution in patients not receiving adequate anticoagulation because of possible embolic complications. DC cardioversion *or* Amiodarone (class IIb)	DC cardioversion *or* Primary antiarrhythmic agents: Use only one of the following agents (see note below): Amiodarone (class IIb) Flecainide (class IIb) Procainamide (class IIb) Propafenone (class IIb) Sotalol (class IIb) Class III (can be	Anticoagulation as described above, followed by DC cardioversion

Procainamide
(class IIb)
Propafenone (class IIb)

Class III (can be harmful)
Adenosine
β-Blockers
Calcium blockers
Digoxin

harmful)
Adenosine
β-Blockers
Calcium blockers
Digoxin

Note: Occasionally two of the named antiarrhythmic agents may be used, but use of these agents in combination may have proarrhythmic potential. The classes listed represent the class of recommendation rather than the Vaughn-Williams classification of antiarrhythmics.

FIG. 1-8

Tachycardia: atrial fibrillation and fluttter, control rate and rhythm. *AF*, Atrial fibrillation; *WPW*, Wolff-Parkinson-White syndrome. *(From Hazinski MF, Cummins RO, Field JM, editors. 2000 Handbook of emergency cardiovascular care for healthcare providers. Dallas: American Heart Association; 2000.)*

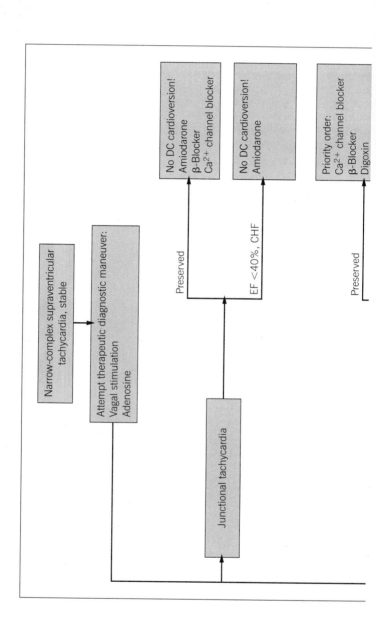

Narrow-complex supraventricular tachycardia, stable

Attempt therapeutic diagnostic maneuver:
Vagal stimulation
Adenosine

Preserved

No DC cardioversion!
Amiodarone
β-Blocker
Ca²⁺ channel blocker

EF <40%, CHF

No DC cardioversion!
Amiodarone

Junctional tachycardia

Preserved

Priority order:
Ca²⁺ channel blocker
β-Blocker
Digoxin

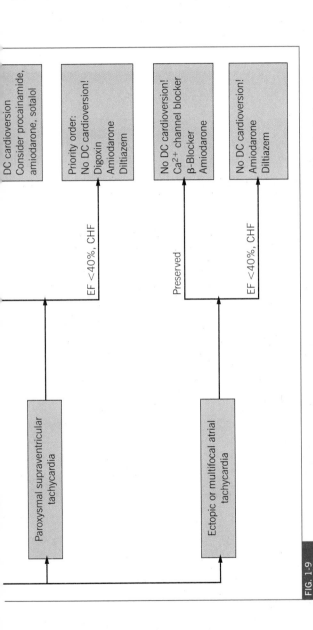

FIG. 1-9

Narrow-complex tachycardia. *EF,* Ejection fraction. *(From Hazinski MF, Cummins RO, Field JM, editors. 2000 Handbook of emergency cardiovascular care for healthcare providers. Dallas: American Heart Association; 2000.)*

CARDIOPULMONARY RESUSCITATION AND ACLS 1

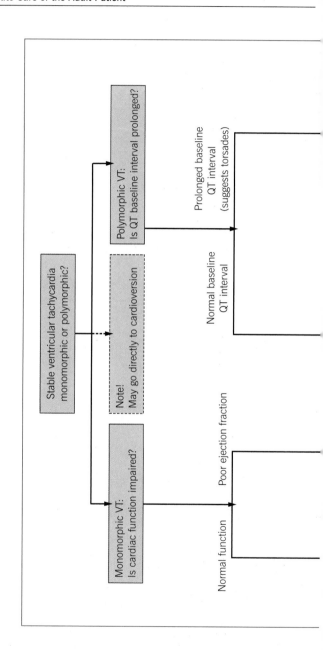

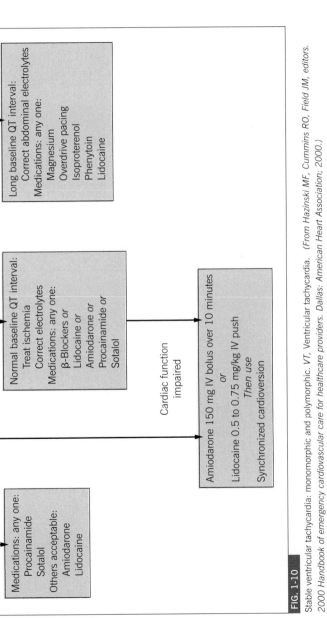

FIG. 1-10

Stable ventricular tachycardia: monomorphic and polymorphic. *VT,* Ventricular tachycardia. *(From Hazinski MF, Cummins RO, Field JM, editors. 2000 Handbook of emergency cardiovascular care for healthcare providers. Dallas: American Heart Association; 2000.)*

CARDIOPULMONARY RESUSCITATION AND ACLS

1

Long baseline QT interval:
Correct abdominal electrolytes
Medications: any one:
Magnesium
Overdrive pacing
Isoproterenol
Phenytoin
Lidocaine

Normal baseline QT interval:
Treat ischemia
Correct electrolytes
Medications: any one:
β-Blockers *or*
Lidocaine *or*
Amiodarone or
Procainamide *or*
Sotalol

Cardiac function impaired

Amiodarone 150 mg IV bolus over 10 minutes
or
Lidocaine 0.5 to 0.75 mg/kg IV push
Then use
Synchronized cardioversion

Medications: any one:
Procainamide
Sotalol
Others acceptable:
Amiodarone
Lidocaine

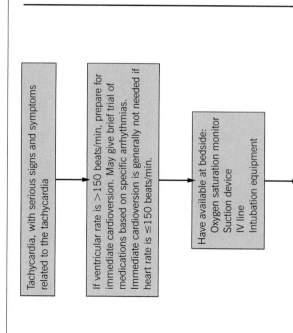

Tachycardia, with serious signs and symptoms related to the tachycardia

If ventricular rate is >150 beats/min, prepare for immediate cardioversion. May give brief trial of medications based on specific arrhythmias. Immediate cardioversion is generally not needed if heart rate is ≤150 beats/min.

Have available at bedside:
Oxygen saturation monitor
Suction device
IV line
Intubation equipment

Premedicate whenever possible

Steps for Synchronized Cardioversion

1. Consider sedation.
2. Turn on defibrillator (monophasic or biphasic).
3. Attach monitor leads to the patient ("white to right, red to ribs, what's left over to the left shoulder") and ensure proper display of the patient's rhythm.
4. Engage the synchronization mode by pressing the "sync" control button.
5. Look for markers on R waves indicating sync mode.
6. If necessary, adjust monitor gain until sync markers occur with each R wave.
7. Select appropriate energy level.
8. Position conductor pads on patient (or apply gel to paddles).
9. Position paddles on patient (sternum-apex).
10. Announce to team members:
    "Charging defibrillator—stand clear!"
11. Press "charge" button on apex paddle (right hand).
12. When the defibrillator is charged, begin the final clearing chant. State firmly in a forceful voice:

    "I am going to shock on three. One, I'm

clear. (Check to make sure you are clear of contact with the patient, the stretcher, and the equipment.)

"Two, you are clear." (Make a visual check to ensure that no one continues to touch the patient or stretcher. In particular, do not forget about the person providing ventilations. That person's hands should not be touching the ventilatory adjuncts, including the tracheal tube!)

"Three, everybody's clear." (Check yourself one more time before pressing the "shock" buttons.)

13. Apply 25 lb pressure on both paddles.
14. Press the "discharge" buttons simultaneously.
15. Check the monitor. If tachycardia persists, increase the joules according to the electrical cardioversion algorithm.
16. Reset the sync mode after each synchronized cardioversion because most defibrillators default back to unsynchronized mode. This default allows an immediate defibrillation if the cardioversion produces ventricular fibrillation.

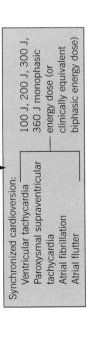

Synchronized cardioversion:

Ventricular tachycardia	100 J, 200 J, 300 J,
Paroxysmal supraventricular tachycardia	360 J monophasic
Atrial fibrillation	energy dose (or
Atrial flutter	clinically equivalent
	biphasic energy dose)

Notes:

1. Effective regimens have included a sedative (e.g., diazepam, midazolam, barbiturates, etomidate, ketamine, methohexital) with or without an analgesic agent (e.g., fentanyl, morphine, meperidine). Many experts recommend anesthesia if service is readily available.
2. Both monophasic and biphasic waveforms are acceptable if documented as clinically equivalent to reports of monophasic shock success.
3. Note possible need to resynchronize after each cardioversion.
4. If delays in synchronization occur and clinical condition is critical, go immediately to unsynchronized shocks.
5. Treat polymorphic ventricular tachycardia (irregular form and rate) like ventricular fibrillation: see Fig. 1-7.
6. Paroxysmal supraventricular tachycardia and atrial flutter often repond to lower energy levels (start with 50 J).

FIG. 1-11

Electrical cardioversion algorithm. *(From Hazinski MF, Cummins RO, Field JM, editors. 2000 Handbook of emergency cardiovascular care for healthcare providers. Dallas: American Heart Association; 2000.)*

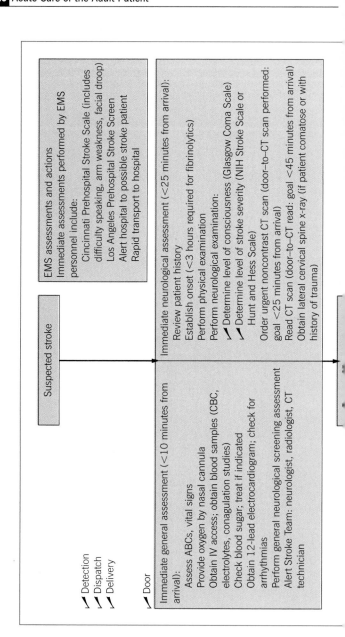

Detection
Dispatch
Delivery

Suspected stroke

EMS assessments and actions
Immediate assessments performed by EMS personnel include:
  Cincinnati Prehospital Stroke Scale (includes difficulty speaking, arm weakness, facial droop)
  Los Angeles Prehospital Stroke Screen
  Alert hospital to possible stroke patient
  Rapid transport to hospital

Door

Immediate general assessment (<10 minutes from arrival):
  Assess ABCs, vital signs
  Provide oxygen by nasal cannula
  Obtain IV access; obtain blood samples (CBC, electrolytes, conagulation studies)
  Check blood sugar; treat if indicated
  Obtain 12-lead electrocardiogram; check for arrhythmias
  Perform general neurological screening assessment
  Alert Stroke Team: neurologist, radiologist, CT technician

Immediate neurological assessment (<25 minutes from arrival):
  Review patient history
  Establish onset (<3 hours required for fibrinolytics)
  Perform physical examination
  Perform neurological examination:
  ✓ Determine level of consciousness (Glasgow Coma Scale)
  ✓ Determine level of stroke severity (NIH Stroke Scale or Hunt and Hess Scale)
  Order urgent noncontrast CT scan (door-to-CT scan performed: goal <25 minutes from arrival)
  Read CT scan (door-to-CT read: goal <45 minutes from arrival)
  Obtain lateral cervical spine x-ray (if patient comatose or with history of trauma)

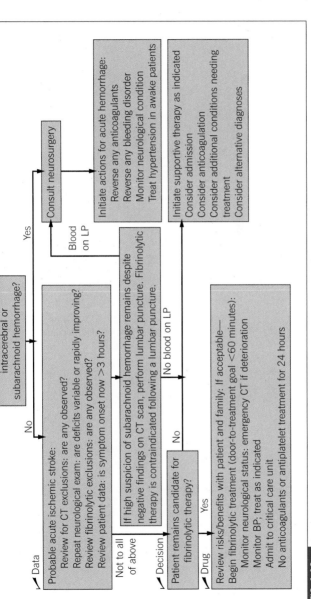

FIG. 1-12

Algorithm for suspected stroke. *CT,* Computed tomography; *EMS,* emergency medical services; *LP,* lumbar puncture. *(From Hazinski MF, Cummins RO, Field JM, editors. 2000 Handbook of emergency cardiovascular care for healthcare providers. Dallas: American Heart Association; 2000.)*

Procedures

Tze-Ming (Benson) Chen, MD, and Henry E. Fessler, MD

Knee Arthrocentesis[1,2]

A. INDICATIONS
1. Evaluation of a joint effusion.
2. Draining of a joint effusion or hemarthrosis.
3. Injection of medications.

B. CONTRAINDICATIONS
1. Infection of the overlying skin or soft tissue.
2. Coagulopathy or anticoagulation therapy.
3. Unstable joint from trauma.

C. EQUIPMENT
1. Fenestrated sterile drape.
2. Sterile gloves.
3. Povidone-iodine (Betadine) solution.
4. Sterile 4 × 4 gauze.
5. Towels.
6. Lidocaine 1%.
7. Needles.
   a. 25-gauge × 5/8-inch.
   b. 22-gauge × 1 1/2-inch.
   c. 20-gauge × 1 1/2-inch.
   d. 18-gauge × 1 1/2-inch.
8. Syringes.
   a. 3-mL.
   b. 5-mL.
   c. 10-mL.
   d. 30-mL.
9. Sterile specimen tubes.
10. Band-Aid.

D. TECHNIQUE: ANTEROMEDIAL APPROACH
1. Place the patient in the supine position, and flex the patient's knee approximately 160 degrees to open the joint space. Insert towels beneath the knee to support the leg.
2. Identify the medial edge of the patella, and perform sterile preparation of the area with Betadine. Drape accordingly.
3. Apply local anesthesia with 1% lidocaine using the 25-gauge needle attached to a 5-mL syringe. Always draw back on the syringe to ensure that the needle bevel is not within a blood vessel before injecting lidocaine. Start with a subcutaneous injection until a wheal is formed. Then insert the needle toward the inferior aspect of the patella, infiltrating the tissue with lidocaine (Fig. 2-1).
4. Exchange the 25-gauge needle for a 22-gauge needle, and continue

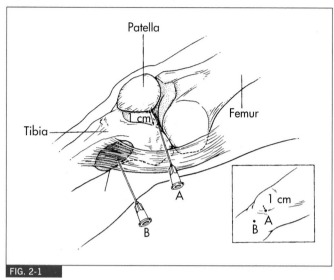

FIG. 2-1

Arthrocentesis—medical approach. The needle *(A)* is inserted 1 cm below the patella, parallel to the plane of the table. See text for details. *(From Salm TJV, Cutler BS, Wheeler HB, editors. Atlas of bedside procedures. Boston: Little, Brown; 1979.)*

anesthetizing the soft tissue until the periosteum of the patella is reached. Anesthetize this area well because it is very sensitive. Withdraw the anesthesia needle.

5. Insert the 18-gauge needle attached to a 10 mL syringe, and guide it to the inferior aspect of the patella.
6. After making contact with the patella, march the needle until it is just inferior to the patella.
7. Advance the needle into the joint space while gently aspirating back until joint fluid is obtained.
8. Withdraw the needle after aspiration of the joint fluid.
9. Hold pressure over the insertion site until bleeding has stopped.
10. Apply the Band-Aid over the insertion site.
11. Send aspirated fluid for cell count and differential, glucose, Gram's stain and culture, and crystalline examination under polarized light.

E. COMPLICATIONS
1. Pain.
2. Infection.
3. Bleeding.
4. Hemarthrosis.
5. Tendon rupture.

Lumbar Puncture[2-4]

A. INDICATIONS
1. Assess for the possibility of infectious meningitis or encephalitis.
2. Assess for the possibility of a subarachnoid hemorrhage.[5,6]
3. Assess for the possibility of meningeal carcinomatosis, tertiary syphilis.
4. Administer intrathecal medication.
5. Measure cerebrospinal fluid (CSF) pressure.

B. CONTRAINDICATIONS
1. Infection involving the path of the spinal needle (e.g., cellulitis, epidural abscess).
2. Increased intracranial pressure.
3. Bleeding diathesis or anticoagulant therapy.

C. EQUIPMENT
1. Fenestrated sterile drape.
2. 1% Lidocaine, 5 mL.
3. Sterile gloves.
4. Betadine solution.
5. Sterile 4 × 4 gauze.
6. Towels.
7. Three-way stopcock.
8. Needles.
   a. 25-gauge × ⅝-inch.
   b. 22-gauge × 1½-inch.
9. Spinal needle with stylet.
   a. 20-gauge × 3½-inch.
10. Syringe, 3-mL.
11. Four sterile specimen tubes.
12. Band-Aid.

D. TECHNIQUE
1. Place the patient in the lateral decubitus position with a pillow to keep the head in line with the spinous processes, or seat the patient upright on the edge of the bed leaning forward over a bedside table (Fig. 2-2).
2. Find the superior edge of the iliac crests, and imagine a line across the back connecting these landmarks. The intersection of this line with the spinous processes localizes the L4-5 area.
3. Palpate the space between the L4-5 spinous processes to identify the spinal needle insertion site.
4. Perform sterile preparation of the insertion site with Betadine.
5. Apply local anesthesia with 1% lidocaine using the 25-gauge needle. Always draw back on the syringe to ensure that the needle bevel is not within a blood vessel before injecting lidocaine. Start with a subcutaneous injection until a wheal is formed. Then insert the needle along the sagittal plane that includes the spinous processes, angled toward the umbilicus (Fig. 2-3).

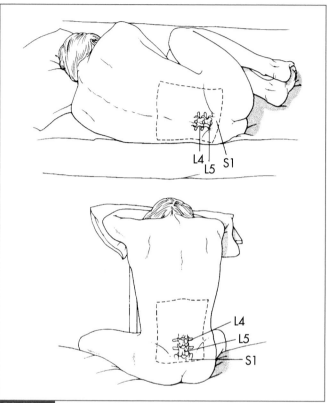

Lumbar puncture—proper positioning. The patient is placed either in a lateral decubitus position *(above)* or sitting upright with the back slightly flexed forward *(below)*. An imaginary line drawn between the two superior iliac crests approximates the L4-L5 intervertebral space. The patient should be prepped and draped to include the area in the dotted box. See text for details. *(From Salm TJV, Cutler BS, Wheeler HB, editors. Atlas of bedside procedures. Boston: Little, Brown; 1979.)*

6. Exchange the 25-gauge needle for a 22-gauge needle, and continue anesthetizing the soft tissue until the periosteum of the vertebrae is reached. Anesthetize this area well because it is very sensitive. Withdraw the anesthesia needle.
7. Insert the 20-gauge spinal needle (with the stylet inserted) along the previously described sagittal plane, angled toward the umbilicus.
8. Advance the needle until a slight sudden yielding of the needle is noticed.
9. Withdraw the stylet to collect the CSF.

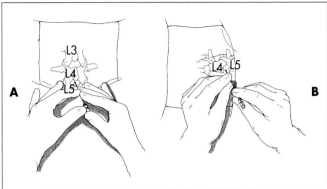

FIG. 2-3

Lumbar puncture—techniques in needle insertion. The needle should be advanced slowly with the bevel in the 12 o'clock position. **A,** Both hands are used to hold the needle. The ring fingers are positioned against the patient's back to help guide the needle into the intervertebral space. **B,** Another approach requires one hand pressed against the patient's back and the other slowly advancing the needle into the intervertebral space. See text for details. *(From Salm TJV, Cutler BS, Wheeler HB, editors. Atlas of bedside procedures. Boston: Little, Brown; 1979.)*

10. If, while advancing the needle, you encounter a bony process, withdraw the needle until the tip is about 1 mm below the skin surface and then reinsert the needle after redirecting it a few degrees in the cephalad direction.
11. If bone is encountered at a shallower level, redirect the needle as described in step 10, but caudally.
12. After collecting a sufficient amount of CSF, reinsert the stylet and then withdraw the spinal needle.
13. Hold pressure until visible bleeding has stopped.
14. Place a Band-Aid over the insertion site.

E. COMPLICATIONS
  1. **Herniation syndrome:** High risk with supratentorial mass lesions.
  2. **Infection:** Possible increase in risk of meningitis if the patient is bacteremic.[7,8]
  3. **Subdural or epidural hematoma.**
  4. **Post–lumbar puncture headache.**
  a. Incidence.
     (1) One in nine lumbar punctures performed with a 26-gauge spinal needle.[9]
     (2) One in three lumbar punctures performed with a 22-gauge spinal needle.[9]
     (3) Between 5% and 30% of lumbar punctures.

b. Timing: May start within minutes or up to 48 hours after completion of the lumbar puncture and may last a day to 2 weeks.

c. Risk factors: Younger patients, females, prior lumbar puncture headache history.

5. **Minor backache:** Occurs in 90% of cases.

6. **Implantation of epidermoid tumors:** Occurs years after the procedure and is associated with the use of needles without stylets.[3]

7. **Aspiration of nerve roots:** Occurs with the use of needles without stylets.[3]

8. **Disk herniation:** Possible if the needle is advanced beyond the subarachnoid space into the anulus fibrosus.[1]

Paracentesis[2,10,11]

A. INDICATIONS
1. Therapeutic.
a. To relieve cardiopulmonary and gastrointestinal complications of tense ascites.
2. Diagnostic.
a. To rule out spontaneous bacterial peritonitis.
b. To determine cause of ascites of unclear etiology.

B. CONTRAINDICATIONS
1. **Coagulopathy:** One study of paracentesis and thoracentesis demonstrated that among 608 patients, 71% of whom were coagulopathic, transfusion was provided in less than 0.2% (1 patient), but 3.1% had a decrease in hemoglobin level of ≥ 2 g/dL.[12]
2. **Pregnancy, second- or third-trimester:** Recommend ultrasound guidance to avoid uterine laceration and perforation.
3. **Multiple previous abdominal surgeries:** Avoid inserting the needle into areas of the abdominal wall with prior surgical scars because of the high likelihood of bowel adherent to the peritoneum in these areas.
4. Infection of overlying skin or soft tissue.
5. Acute abdomen.
6. Bowel obstruction unless bowel distention has been ruled out radiographically.

C. EQUIPMENT
1. Fenestrated sterile drape.
2. 1% Lidocaine.
3. Sterile gloves.
4. Betadine solution.
5. Sterile 4 × 4 gauze.
6. Needles.
a. 25-gauge × ⅝-inch.
b. 22-gauge × 1½-inch.
c. 20-gauge × 1½-inch.
d. 18-gauge × 1½-inch.

   e. Caldwell paracentesis needle.
7. **Syringes.**
   a. 3-mL.
   b. 20-mL.
8. **Sterile specimen tubes.**
9. **Vacutainer bottles.**
10. **High-pressure tubing line.**
11. **Band-Aid.**

D. TECHNIQUE

1. **Infraumbilical approach.**
   a. Place the patient in the lateral decubitus position.
   b. Percuss the abdominal wall to determine where dullness is present.
   c. The insertion site for a paracentesis is 3 to 4 cm below the umbilicus
      in the abdominal midline perpendicular to the skin (Fig. 2-4).
   d. Perform sterile preparation of the insertion site with Betadine, and
      provide local anesthesia with 1% lidocaine, using a 25-gauge needle.

2

PROCEDURES

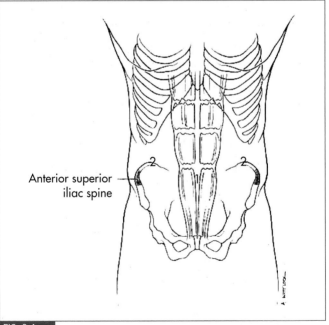

Anterior superior
iliac spine

FIG. 2-4

Paracentesis—anterior abdominal anatomy. The anterior superior iliac crests *(2)* are
noted as landmarks. The point of insertion for an infraumbilical approach is highlighted
(1). See text for details. *(From Roberts JR, Hedges JR. Clinical procedures in
emergency medicine, 3rd ed. Philadelphia: WB Saunders; 1998.)*

e. With the 20-mL syringe attached, insert an 18- to 20-gauge needle for a diagnostic paracentesis or a 16- to 18-gauge Caldwell needle for a therapeutic paracentesis, pulling back on the syringe plunger gently as the needle is slowly advanced.

f. Continue with step no. 3 detailed below for therapeutic paracentesis. Continue with step no. 4 detailed below for diagnostic paracentesis.

2. **Lower quadrant approach.**

a. Place the patient in the supine position.

b. Examine the abdominal wall to assess for the presence of hepatosplenomegaly. If either organ is enlarged, the paracentesis insertion site should be on the opposite side of the organomegaly. If both hepatomegaly and splenomegaly are present, use the infraumbilical approach or obtain an ultrasound-guided mark.

c. Percuss the abdominal wall to determine the level of dullness.

d. The insertion site is along the anterior axillary line lateral to the rectus sheath, halfway between the umbilicus and the anterior superior iliac spine or 1 to 2 cm below the level of percussed dullness (Fig. 2-4.)

e. Perform sterile preparation of the insertion site with Betadine, and apply local anesthesia with 1% lidocaine, using a 25-gauge needle.

f. With the 20-mL syringe attached, insert an 18- to 20-gauge needle for a diagnostic paracentesis or a 16- to 18-gauge Caldwell needle for a therapeutic paracentesis, pulling back on the syringe plunger gently as the needle is slowly advanced.

3. Remove the Caldwell needle stylet and attach the high-pressure tubing line to a Vacutainer bottle for a therapeutic paracentesis.

4. If the ascitic fluid flow slows or ceases, stop the suction, readjust the catheter by tilting the tip inferiorly, and reapply the suction. If this is unsuccessful, advance or withdraw the catheter slowly 0.5 to 1 cm at a time.

5. Once the procedure has been completed, remove the catheter and immediately cover the insertion site with gauze and hold pressure until visible bleeding ceases.

6. Place a Band-Aid over the insertion site.

E. **COMPLICATIONS**[13]

1. Pneumoperitoneum.
2. Peritonitis.
3. Perforated bladder.
4. Perforated bowel.
5. Intraabdominal hemorrhage.
6. Abdominal wall hematoma.
7. Persistent fluid leak.
8. Infection.
9. Renal insufficiency (controversial). There is some evidence of a renoprotective effect of IV albumin administered after paracentesis.[14-17] Use of 8 g of IV albumin per liter of ascites removed is recommended.[1]

Thoracentesis[1,18]

A. INDICATIONS
1. Evaluation of a pleural effusion of unknown etiology.
2. Therapeutic drainage of a pleural effusion.

B. CONTRAINDICATIONS
1. Severe contralateral lung impairment.
2. Bleeding diathesis or anticoagulant therapy.
3. Positive-pressure ventilation.

C. EQUIPMENT
1. Fenestrated sterile drape.
2. 1% Lidocaine.
3. Sterile gloves.
4. Betadine solution.
5. Sterile 4 × 4 gauze.
6. Needles.
   a. 25-gauge × ⅝-inch.
   b. 22-gauge × 1½-inch.
   c. 20-gauge × 1½-inch.
   d. 18-gauge × 2½-inch introducer needle.
   e. 17-gauge × 6-inch thoracentesis needle with a 14-gauge Teflon catheter.
7. Syringes.
   a. 3-mL.
   b. Two 20-mL.
8. Single-lumen central line kit.
9. Three-way stopcock.
10. Two-way valve.
11. Sterile specimen tubes.
12. Vacutainer bottles.
13. High-pressure tubing line.
14. Band-Aid.

D. TECHNIQUE
1. Review chest radiograph of patient in the erect and lateral decubitus positions, and confirm location of the pleural effusion.
2. Place the patient in a sitting position over the edge of the bed, leaning over a bedside table (Fig. 2-5).
3. Percuss out the effusion by noting the superior edge of dullness on the posterior aspect of the chest wall.
4. Confirm by auscultation, listening for diminished breath sounds.
5. Provide local anesthesia with 1% lidocaine, using the 25-gauge needle attached to a 3-mL syringe. Always draw back on the syringe to ensure that the needle bevel is not within a blood vessel before injecting lidocaine. Start with a subcutaneous injection until a wheal is formed. Then insert the needle aiming for the middle of the rib just below the superior edge of percussed dullness in the posterior axillary line.

2

PROCEDURES

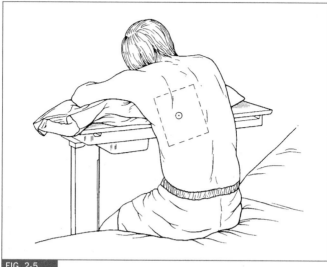

FIG. 2-5

Thoracentesis—proper positioning. The patient is positioned as shown leaning forward against a pillow on a bedside table. Examination of the back should be performed to ensure that the anticipated entry site is dull to percussion before the patient is prepped and draped. After adequate local anesthesia the needle should be inserted into the intercostal space over the superior aspect of the rib to avoid the vascular-nerve bundle. See text for details. *(From Salm TJV, Cutler BS, Wheeler HB, editors. Atlas of bedside procedures. Boston: Little, Brown; 1979.)*

6. Exchange the 25-gauge for the 22-gauge needle and continue anesthetizing until you reach the periosteum of the rib. Anesthetize this area well because it is very sensitive.
7. Once the needle has come in contact with the rib, march the needle superiorly over the edge of the rib, gently withdrawing on the syringe plunger and anesthetizing the area well (Fig. 2-6).
8. When the needle enters the pleural space, the syringe will fill with pleural fluid. At that time, remove the anesthesia needle and insert the 18-gauge needle for a diagnostic thoracentesis or the 17-gauge needle for a therapeutic thoracentesis attached to the 20-mL syringe into the pleural space, following the same path as the anesthesia needle.
9. Once the needle has reentered the pleural space, fill the 20-mL syringe.
10. Diagnostic thoracentesis.
  a. Insert the 18-gauge introducer attached to the 20-mL syringe into the pleural space following the same path as the anesthesia needle,

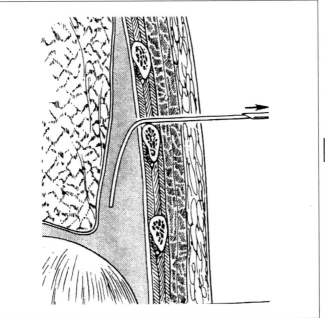

FIG. 2-6

Thoracentesis—path of needle into pleural space. *(From Kassirer J, ed. Current therapy in adult medicine, 4th ed. St Louis: Mosby; 1998.)*

       withdrawing gently on the syringe plunger as the needle is advanced.

  b. Once the needle enters the pleural space, fill the syringe and remove the needle.

11. **Therapeutic thoracentesis.**
  a. Using a single-lumen catheter.
    (1) Insert the 18-gauge introducer attached to the 20-mL syringe into the pleural space following the same path as the anesthesia needle, withdrawing gently on the syringe plunger.
    (2) Once the needle has entered the pleural space, have the patient perform a Valsalva maneuver to increase the intrapleural pressure. This will decrease the likelihood that a pneumothorax will develop while the syringe is being disconnected from the needle.
    (3) Disconnect the syringe from the needle, and cover the hub of the needle with your fingertip.
    (4) Pass half of the guidewire from the central line kit into the pleural space through the 18-gauge needle.

      (5) Remove the 18-gauge needle.

      (6) Advance the single-lumen catheter over the wire, remove the wire, leaving the thoracentesis catheter in the pleural space, and cover the hub with your fingertip.

      (7) Continue with step c or d.

  b. Using a standard thoracentesis needle.

      (1) Insert the 17-gauge thoracentesis needle (with overlying Teflon catheter) attached to the 20-mL syringe into the pleural space following the same path as the anesthesia needle, withdrawing gently on the syringe plunger as the needle is advanced.

      (2) Once the needle has entered the pleural space, have the patient perform a Valsalva maneuver to increase the intrapleural pressure. This will decrease the likelihood that a pneumothorax will develop while the syringe is being disconnected from the needle.

      (3) Advance the 14-gauge Teflon catheter over the needle into the pleural space. Once the catheter is in place, remove the 17-gauge needle.

      (4) Continue with step c or d.

  c. Using a three-way stopcock.

      (1) Attach one port of the stopcock to the hub of the single-lumen catheter or 14-gauge Teflon catheter, and turn the valve of the stopcock to seal off this port.

      (2) Attach the high-pressure tubing line to another port of the stopcock.

      (3) Attach the high-pressure tubing line to the Vacutainer.

  d. Using a two-way valve.

      (1) Attach the inflow port of the one-way valve to the hub of the single-lumen catheter or 14-gauge Teflon catheter.

      (2) Attach a 20-mL syringe to the outflow port of the one-way valve.

      (3) Attach a high-pressure tubing line to the drainage port of the one-way valve.

      (4) Connect the high-pressure tubing to a collection bottle.

      (5) Drain the pleural fluid by pulling on the syringe plunger, and then push the plunger to flush the fluid through the valve into the collection bottle.

  e. After removing the desired amount of fluid, withdraw the single-lumen catheter while the patient performs a Valsalva maneuver.

12. Hold pressure over the insertion site until no bleeding is visible.

13. Place a Band-Aid over the insertion site.

14. Obtain a chest radiograph to assess for the presence or absence of a pneumothorax.

E. COMPLICATIONS

  1. **Bleeding:** Chest wall hematoma or hemothorax.

  2. **Pneumothorax.**

  3. **Infection.**

  4. **Hepatic or splenic laceration or puncture.**

Radial Arterial Line[1,19]

A. INDICATIONS
1. Continuous arterial blood pressure monitoring.
2. Frequent arterial blood sampling.

B. CONTRAINDICATIONS
1. Infection of the overlying tissue.
2. Inadequate collateral arterial supply.
3. Coagulopathy.

C. EQUIPMENT
1. Fenestrated drape.
2. 1% Lidocaine.
3. Sterile gloves.
4. Betadine solution.
5. Sterile 4 × 4 gauze.
6. Needles.
a. 25-gauge × ⅝-inch.
7. Syringes.
a. 3-mL.
8. Angiocatheter, 20-gauge × 1-inch.
9. Radial artery catheterization kit: 20-gauge × 1¾-inch cannula over a 22-gauge introducer needle with a spring-wire guide.
10. Arterial pressure transducer.
11. Pressure tubing.
12. Band-Aid.

D. TECHNIQUE
1. Allen test.
a. Occlude the radial and ulnar arteries by applying pressure with your thumbs.
b. Have the patient make a tight fist with that hand and then relax.
c. After observing the blanching of the hand, release one artery and watch for normalization of the hand color.
d. Repeat, except release the other artery.
e. If both arteries provide adequate perfusion of the hand, release of each artery should result in normal hand color within 3 to 5 seconds.
f. If inadequate perfusion is demonstrated, do not cannulate either artery.
2. Place the patient in the supine position, abduct the arm, supinate the forearm, and hyperextend the hand.
3. Place padding beneath the hand to help maintain this position (Fig. 2-7).
4. Palpate the radial artery with two fingertips placed 2 cm apart.
5. Perform sterile preparation of the insertion site with Betadine, and apply local anesthesia with 1% lidocaine, using a 25-gauge needle.
6. Delineate a line between the fingertips, and insert the angiocatheter along this line at a 45-degree angle from the skin into the radial artery.

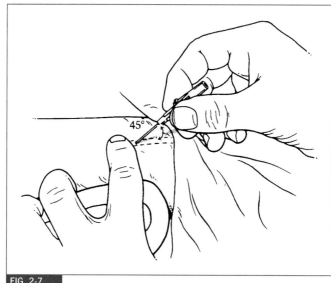

FIG. 2-7

Arterial line insertion. The patient's arm is properly supinated and the wrist hyper-extended. The angiocatheter is inserted at a 45-degree angle. *(From Salm TJV, Cutler BS, Wheeler HB, editors. Atlas of bedside procedures. Boston: Little, Brown; 1979.)*

7. **Using the transfixing technique (Fig. 2-8).**
   a. Once you see a flash of bright red-blood in the needle hub, advance the whole apparatus until the artery has been transfixed.
   b. Withdraw the needle, and leave the cannula in place.
   c. Pull back on the cannula until pulsatile blood flow is noted out of the cannula hub, confirming arterial placement.
   d. Advance the cannula until the hub is flush with the skin.
8. **Using an alternative transfixing technique (Fig. 2-9).**
   a. Once you see a flash of blood in the needle hub, advance the whole apparatus 1 to 2 mm into the artery.
   b. Advance the cannula over the needle into the artery until the cannula hub is flush with the skin, and remove the needle.
   c. Confirm arterial placement with presence of pulsatile blood flow out of the cannula hub.
9. **Using a radial artery catheterization kit.**
   a. Once a flash of blood is seen in the needle hub, advance the guide wire into the artery.
   b. Advance the cannula over the wire into the artery.
   c. Withdraw the needle and attached wire, and confirm arterial placement with the presence of pulsatile blood flow out of the cannula hub.

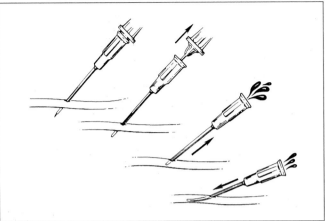

FIG. 2-8

Arterial line insertion—transfixing technique. The angiocatheter is inserted at a 45-degree angle and advanced until a flash of blood is seen. The needle is carefully removed while the cannula is slowly advanced. See text for details. *(From Salm TJV, Cutler BS, Wheeler HB, editors. Atlas of bedside procedures. Boston: Little, Brown; 1979.)*

2

PROCEDURES

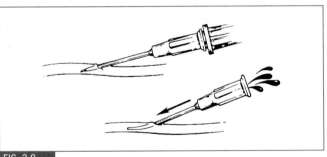

FIG. 2-9

Arterial line insertion—alternate transfixing technique. See text for details. *(From Salm TJV, Cutler BS, Wheeler HB, editors. Atlas of bedside procedures. Boston: Little, Brown; 1979.)*

10. Attach the pressure transducer, and suture the line in place.
11. Confirm placement with the pressure wave on the cardiac monitor.
12. Apply a sterile dressing over the insertion site and the cannula.

E. COMPLICATIONS
1. Bleeding.
2. Infection.
3. Hand ischemia.
4. Retrograde air embolism.

Central Line Placement[20-22]

A. INDICATIONS
1. Securing of intravenous access for medications and blood products.
2. Phlebotomy.
3. Central venous pressure monitoring.

B. CONTRAINDICATIONS
1. Infection of the area overlying the target vessel.
2. Thrombosis of the target vessel.
3. **Coagulopathy:** Avoid subclavian vein attempts, given the difficulty of compressing blood vessels in this area.
4. **Inferior vena cava filter:** Relative contraindication for femoral vein approaches. If necessary, use only single-lumen catheters because the guidewire for this device is the shortest available.
5. **Respiratory distress or impending respiratory failure:** Avoid the subclavian approach if a pneumothorax is likely to be fatal.

C. EQUIPMENT
1. Sterile gown.
2. Sterile cap.
3. Surgical mask with eye shield.
4. Sterile fenestrated drape.
5. Sterile towels.
6. 1% Lidocaine.
7. Sterile gloves.
8. Betadine solution.
9. Sterile 4 × 4 gauze.
10. Needles.
    a. 25-gauge × 5/8-inch.
    b. 22-gauge × 1½-inch.
    c. 18-gauge × 2½-inch introducer needle.
11. Syringes.
    a. 3-mL.
    b. Two 10-mL.
12. Scalpel.
13. Skin dilator.
14. Injectable saline, 30 mL.
15. Single-, double-, or triple-lumen catheter with associated guidewires.

16. Needleless or needle-adapted hub caps, number appropriate for the particular catheter.
17. 3-0 skin suture.
18. Suture scissors.
19. Povidone-iodine ointment.

D. TECHNIQUE

1. Place the patient in the supine position. Examine the patient to determine the most appropriate location for the line.

a. Internal jugular vein site.
   (1) Turn the patient's head so that the chin is directed away from the target vessel.
   (2) Place the patient in a 15- to 20-degree Trendelenburg position.
   (3) Identify the triangle formed by the anterior and posterior bellies of the sternocleidomastoid muscle and the clavicle.
   (4) The insertion site is near the apex of this triangle, just lateral to the palpable pulsation of the carotid artery.
   (5) Perform sterile preparation of the insertion site with Betadine, and apply local anesthesia with 1% lidocaine, using a 25-gauge needle and the 10-mL syringe.
   (6) Palpate the carotid artery in the triangle, and retract it medially.
   (7) Insert the 25-gauge needle at a 45-degree angle to the skin into the triangle apex just lateral to the carotid pulsation, with the bevel in the 12 o'clock position, advancing toward the ipsilateral nipple.
   (8) Pull back on the syringe plunger gently while advancing the needle, and infiltrate the tissue with lidocaine.
   (9) Exchange the 25-gauge needle for a 22-gauge needle and continue to advance the needle as described in step (7).
   (10) The internal jugular vein should be entered within a depth of approximately 3 cm (may be deeper with more obese patients).
   (11) If it is not, withdraw the needle to just beneath the skin surface and redirect the needle laterally.
   (12) Once the 22-gauge needle is in the internal jugular vein, maintain its position and take the 18-gauge needle attached to a 10-mL syringe and insert it following the path of the 22-gauge needle.
   (13) Once the 18-gauge needle has entered the internal jugular vein, withdraw the 22-gauge needle.
   (14) Continue with step d.

b. Subclavian vein site.
   (1) Turn the patient's head away from the target vessel (Fig. 2-10).
   (2) Place the patient in a 15- to 20-degree Trendelenburg position.
   (3) Identify the lateral margin of the posterior belly of the sternocleidomastoid muscle as it inserts onto the clavicle.
   (4) The insertion site is 1 cm inferior and 1 cm lateral to the inferior aspect of the clavicle bone, just below the insertion site of the posterior belly of the sternocleidomastoid muscle.

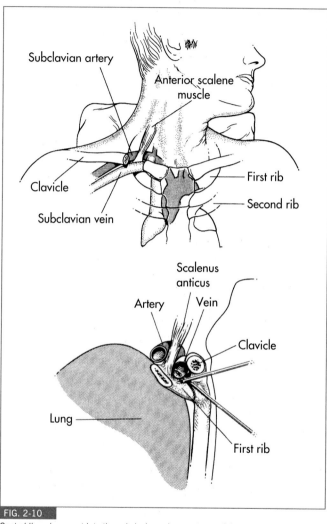

FIG. 2-10

Central line placement into the subclavian vein—anatomy of the upper chest. See text for details. *(From Salm TJV, Cutler BS, Wheeler HB, editors. Atlas of bedside procedures. Boston: Little, Brown; 1979.)*

Cont'd

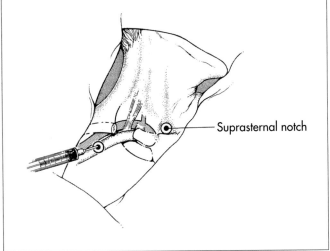

Suprasternal notch

FIG. 2-10—cont'd

(5) Perform sterile preparation of the insertion site with Betadine, and apply local anesthesia with 1% lidocaine, using a 25-gauge needle attached to a 10-mL syringe.
(6) Insert the 25-gauge needle almost parallel to the skin, with the bevel in the 12 o'clock position, aiming for the clavicle.
(7) Pull back on the syringe plunger gently while advancing the needle, and infiltrate the tissue with lidocaine.
(8) Exchange the 25-gauge needle for a 22-gauge needle and continue to advance the needle as described in step (6).
(9) Advance the needle until it hits the clavicle. Anesthetize the periosteum well because it is very sensitive.
(10) Pass the needle underneath the clavicle toward the suprasternal notch, parallel to the patient's back.
(11) Remove the 22-gauge needle. Using the 18-gauge needle attached to a 10-mL syringe, advance the needle toward the subclavian vein following the path of the 22-gauge needle. Draw back on the syringe as you are advancing.
(12) Once the 18-gauge needle has entered the subclavian vein, continue with step d.
c. Femoral vein site.
(1) Identify the pulsation of the femoral artery.
(2) The insertion site is just medial to the femoral artery pulsation and 1 cm inferior to the inguinal ligament.
(3) Prepare the insertion site sterilely with Betadine, and apply local

        anesthesia with 1% lidocaine using a 25-gauge needle attached to a 10-mL syringe.

    (4) Insert the 25-gauge needle with the bevel in the 12 o'clock position at a 45- to 60-degree angle, aiming just medial to the femoral artery pulsation.

    (5) Pull back on the syringe plunger gently while advancing the needle, and infiltrate the tissue with lidocaine.

    (6) Once the hub of the 25-gauge needle has been reached, change to the 22-gauge needle and continue to advance the needle as described in step (4).

    (7) If the femoral vein is not cannulated within a depth of 4 cm, withdraw the needle to just beneath the skin surface and redirect the needle medially. The depth may vary depending on the patient's body habitus.

d. When the needle enters a blood vessel, attempt to confirm that the needle is in the vein by detaching the syringe from the needle and observing the color of the blood and the absence of pulsatile flow.

e. If the vein has been cannulated, insert the curved end of the guidewire through the needle and advance it gently. To prevent embolization, do not insert more than one half of the length of the guidewire.

f. If you feel resistance to the insertion of the guidewire, withdraw the wire, rotate the 16-gauge needle to change the bevel position, and reinsert the wire gently.

g. If the patient is receiving cardiac monitoring and an arrhythmia develops after the wire has been inserted, pull back on the wire and wait for resolution of the abnormal rhythm. If the abnormal rhythm persists, institute appropriate advanced cardiac life support (ACLS).

h. Once the guidewire has been inserted, withdraw the needle.

i. Make a 2-mm nick in the skin at the wire entry site with the scalpel, and withdraw the blade.

j. Place the dilator over the guidewire, insert the dilator to a depth of 1 cm while turning the instrument, and then withdraw it.

k. Insert the proximal end of the guidewire into the tip of the central venous catheter, and pull back the wire until the wire tip protrudes from the proximal lumen of the catheter. *Always maintain a grasp of a section of the guidewire to prevent its embolization.*

l. While grasping the proximal end of the guidewire tip, insert the catheter into the insertion site over the guidewire, using a twisting motion.

m. Insert the catheter to a depth of 15 cm for a right-sided internal vein jugular placement, to 17 cm for a left-sided internal-jugular vein placement, to 15 cm for a right-sided subclavian vein placement, to 17 cm for a left-sided subclavian vein placement, and to the catheter hub with a femoral vein placement.

n. Withdraw the guidewire, and check for blood return in all catheter ports. Flush all ports with saline, and suture the line in place.

o. Apply the povidone-iodine ointment to the insertion site, and apply a sterile dressing.

p. For internal jugular and subclavian vein placements, obtain a chest radiograph to check for line position and assess for pneumothorax and hemothorax.

E. COMPLICATIONS

1. Pain.
2. Infection.
3. Bleeding.
4. Arterial or venous laceration.
5. Arterial cannulation.
6. Pneumothorax.
7. Hemothorax
8. Cardiac arrhythmia.

PEARLS AND PITFALLS

- Knee arthrocentesis.
  - Obtain signed informed consent before performing any elective procedure.
  - Consider orthopedic consultation for septic joints.
  - Radiographic imaging of the joint before arthrocentesis is not routinely indicated unless trauma is suspected.
  - Gout is composed of monosodium urate crystals while pseudogout crystals are composed of calcium pyrophosphate. Urate crystals are needle shaped and negatively birefringent and appear yellow when the crystals are parallel to the beam of polarized light (blue when they are perpendicular). Pseudogout crystals are rhomboid shaped and are positively birefringent when viewed with polarized light. See Chapter 71 for details.
- Lumbar puncture (Table 2-1).
  - Obtain signed informed consent before performing any elective procedures.
  - Suggested treatment for post–lumbar puncture headaches.
    - Prone positioning for 3 hours after the procedure.[23]
    - Caffeine sodium benzoate 500 mg in 2 mL of normal saline IV push.[24]
    - Aminophylline 5 to 6 mg IV over 20 minutes.[25] (Original study was performed in patients with hypertensive headaches.)
    - Blood patch for a prolonged low-pressure headache after conservative therapy has failed. The patch is less effective if the headache has been present for more than 2 weeks. It has a failure rate of 15% to 20%.[2,26] The theory underlying the effectiveness of this technique is that post–lumbar puncture headaches are caused by a leakage of CSF from a persistent dural perforation with a resultant decrease in CSF pressure. Infiltrating the tissue surrounding this perforation with 10 to 15 mL of autologous blood will theoretically

TABLE 2-1

CEREBROSPINAL FLUID ABNORMALITIES IN VARIOUS CENTRAL NERVOUS SYSTEM CONDITIONS

	Appearance	Glucose (mg/dL)	Protein (mg/dL)	Cell Count (cells/mm³) and Cell Type	Pressure (mm Hg)
Normal	Clear	50-80	20-45	<6 Lymphocytes	100-200
Acute bacterial meningitis	Cloudy	↓↓	↑↑	↑↑ PMNs	↑↑
Aseptic (viral) meningitis	Clear/cloudy	N	↑	↑, Usually mononuclear cells May be PMNs in early stages	N/↑
Hemorrhage	Bloody/xanthochromic	N/↓	↑	↑↑ RBCs	↑
Neoplasm	Clear/xanthochromic	N/↓	N/↑	N/↑ Lymphocytes	↑↑
Tuberculous meningitis	Cloudy	↓	↑	↑ PMNs (early) ↑ Lymphocytes (later)	↑
Fungal meningitis	Clear/cloudy	↓	↑	↑ Monocytes	↑
Neurosyphilis	Clear/cloudy	N	↑	↑ Monocytes	N/↑
Guillain-Barré syndrome	Clear/cloudy	N	↑↑	N/↑ Lymphocytes	N

From Ferri FF: Practical guide to the care of the medical patient, 5th ed. St Louis: Mosby; 2001.

↑, Increased; ↑↑, markedly increased; ↓, decreased; ↓↓, markedly decreased; N, normal; PMNs, polymorphonucleocytes; RBCs, red blood cells.

tamponade the CSF leakage. This procedure is performed mainly by anesthesiologists.

- Cerebrospinal fluid abnormalities in various central nervous system conditions are detailed in Table 2-1.
- Computed tomography (CT) imaging of the head before a lumbar puncture has been advocated in the past because of concerns about post–lumbar puncture brainstem herniation. A recent study aimed to identify clinical predictors for an abnormal CT scan of the head in adults with suspected meningitis.[27] The clinical features were age greater than 60 years, immunocompromise, history of central nervous system disease, history of seizures within the week before presentation, abnormal level of consciousness, and abnormal neurological examination. If none of these features were present, it was unlikely that the CT scan was abnormal (97% negative predictive value).
- Paracentesis.
  - Obtain a signed informed consent before performing any elective procedure.
  - Avoid inserting the needle into the rectus muscles because this is where the epigastric arteries run.
  - Persistent ascitic fluid leak is common and can be minimized by use of a Z-track approach. (This is performed by retracting the skin 2 to 3 cm caudally, inserting the needle slowly, and releasing the skin after the needle has entered the peritoneal space.)
  - Calculate the serum-ascites albumin gradient (serum albumin/ascites albumin) to aid in determining the cause of ascites (Table 2-2).

TABLE 2-2

CLASSIFICATION OF TYPES OF ASCITES ACCORDING TO LEVEL OF SERUM/ASCITES ALBUMIN GRADIENT

High Gradient (≥ 1.1 g/dL)	Low Gradient (<1.1 g/dL)
Cirrhosis	Peritoneal carcinomatosis
Alcoholic hepatitis	Peritoneal tuberculosis
Cardiac failure	Pancreatic ascites
Massive liver metastases	Biliary ascites
Fulminant hepatic failure	Nephrotic syndrome
Budd-Chiari syndrome	Serositis
Portal vein thrombosis	Bowel obstruction or infarction
Venoocclusive disease	
Fatty liver of pregnancy	
Myxedema	
"Mixed" ascites*	

Modified from Runyon BA: *N Engl J Med* 1994; 330:339. In Ferri FF: *Practical guide to the care of the medical patient*, 5th ed. St Louis: Mosby; 2001.

*Found in patients with portal hypertension and another cause of ascites formation (e.g., cirrhosis plus peritoneal tuberculosis). The portal pressure remains elevated in such patients, and the serum/ascites albumin gradient is high.

TABLE 2-3

EVALUATION OF PLEURAL EFFUSIONS

Test	Exudate	Transudate
Fluid LDH	>200 IU/dL	<200 IU/dL
Fluid protein	>3 g	<3 g
Fluid/serum LDH ratio	>0.6 IU/dL	<0.6 IU/dL
Fluid/serum protein ratio	>0.5 IU/dL	<0.5 IU/dL
Specific gravity	>1.016 IU/dL	<1.016 IU/dL
Appearance	Cloudy	Clear, thin
	Viscous	Nonclotting

From Ferri FF. Practical guide to the care of the medical patient, 5th ed. St Louis: Mosby; 2001.
LDH, Lactate dehydrogenase.

- Thoracentesis.
  - Obtain signed informed consent before performing any elective procedure.
  - When performing a therapeutic thoracentesis, aim to remove no more than 1 L of fluid to avoid the possibility of reexpansion pulmonary edema.
  - Criteria for a transudative and exudative pleural effusion are listed in Table 2-3.
  - Causes of transudative pleural effusions include congestive heart failure, pericardial disease, hepatic hydrothorax, nephrotic syndrome, peritoneal dialysis, myxedema, bone marrow transplantation, and Fontan's procedure.
  - Causes of exudative pleural effusions include parapneumonic effusions or empyema, tuberculous pleuritis, actinomycosis, nocardiosis, fungal diseases of the pleura, viral infections, parasitic diseases, esophageal perforation, pancreatitis, diaphragmatic hernia, abdominal surgery, liver transplantation, lung transplantation, Dressler's syndrome, rheumatoid arthritis, lupus pleuritis, uremia, Meigs' syndrome, asbestos exposure, pulmonary embolism, and sarcoidosis.
  - Box 2-1 provides a list of factors suggesting the need for an invasive approach to parapneumonic effusion.
- Radial arterial line.
  - Obtain signed informed consent before performing any elective procedure.
  - Appropriate hyperextension of the hand will minimize inadvertent artery movement during the procedure.
- Central line placement.
  - Obtain signed informed consent before any elective procedure.
  - The location of the line affects the risk of infection. Femoral lines have the highest incidence of infection.
  - See Chapter 40 for details on management of line infections.

BOX 2-1

FACTORS SUGGESTING THAT A MORE INVASIVE APPROACH WILL BE NECESSARY FOR THE RESOLUTION OF A PARAPNEUMONIC EFFUSION

Thick pus is present in the pleural space

Pleural fluid Gram's stain is positive

Pleural fluid glucose level is <60 mg/dL

Pleural fluid culture is positive

Pleural fluid lactate dehydrogenase level is greater than three times upper normal limit for serum

Pleural fluid is loculated

From Murray JF, Nadel JA. Textbook of respiratory medicine, 3rd ed. Philadelphia: WB Saunders; 2001.

2

PROCEDURES

- Rotate the bevel to the 3 o'clock position to facilitate passage of the wire into the superior vena cava (Fig. 2-11).
- If in doubt as to whether the line is in the artery or the vein, consider sending a sample of blood for arterial blood gas analysis.
- If the femoral artery is cannulated, remove the catheter promptly and apply direct pressure for at least 15 minutes at the point in which the artery is cannulated. Confirm that the lower extremity appears well perfused.
- If the carotid artery is cannulated, consider surgical consultation before removing the catheter.

REFERENCES

[d] 1. Haist SA, Robbins JB, Gomella LG. Internal medicine on call, 2nd ed. Stamford, Conn: Appleton & Lange; 1997.

[d] 2. Roberts JR, Hedges, JR. Clinical procedures in emergency medicine, 3rd ed. Philadelphia: WB Saunders; 1998.

[d] 3. Davidson RI. Lumbar puncture. In Salm TJV, Cutler BS, Wheeler HB, editors. Atlas of bedside procedures. Boston: Little, Brown; 1979.

[b] 4. Adams HP et al. CT and clinical correlations in recent aneurysmal subarachnoid hemorrhage: a preliminary report of the Cooperative Aneurysm Study. Neurology 1983; 33:981.

[b] 5. Hayward RD, O'Reilly GVA. Intracerebral haemorrhage: accuracy of computerized transverse axial scanning in predicting underlying aetiology. Lancet 1976; 1:1.

[b] 6. Petersdorf RG, Swarner DR, Garcia M. Studies on the pathogenesis of meningitis. II. Development of meningitis during pneumococcal bacteremia. J Clin Invest 1962; 41:320.

[b] 7. Teele DW et al. Meningitis after lumbar puncture in children with bacteremia. N Engl J Med 1981; 305:1079.

[a] 8. Tourtellotte WW et al. A randomized double-blind clinical trial comparing the 22- versus 26-gauge needle in the production of the post–lumbar puncture syndrome in normal individuals. Headache 1972; 12:73.

[b] 9. Brocker RJ. Technique to avoid spinal-tap headache. JAMA 1958; 168:261.

[d] 10. Silva WE. Diagnostic paracentesis and lavage. In Salm TJV, Cutler BS, Wheeler HB, editors. Atlas of bedside procedures. Boston: Little, Brown; 1979.

[c] 11. McVay PA, Toy PTCY. Lack of increased bleeding after paracentesis and thoracentesis in patients with mild coagulation abnormalities. Transfusion 1991; 31:164.

[b] 12. Runyon BA. Paracentesis of ascitic fluid: a safe procedure. Arch Intern Med 1986; 146:2259.

[b] 13. Planas R et al. Dextran-70 versus albumin as plasma expanders in cirrhotic patients with tense ascites treated with total paracentesis: results of a randomized study. Gastroenterology 1990; 99:1736.

[b] 14. Altman C et al. Randomized comparative multicenter study of hydroxyethyl starch versus albumin as a plasma expander in cirrhotic patients with tense ascites treated with paracentesis. Eur J Gastroenterol 1998; 10:5.

[d] 15. Wilkinson SP. Treatment options for cirrhotic ascites. Eur J Gastroenterol 1998; 10:1.

[b] 16. Wong PY, Carroll RE, Lipinski TL, et al. Studies on the renin-angiotensin-aldosterone system in patients with cirrhosis and ascites: effect of saline and albumin infusion. Gastroenterology 1979; 77:1171.

[c] 17. Vermeulen LC Jr et al. A paradigm for consensus: the University Hospital Consortium guidelines for the use of albumin, nonprotein colloid, and crystalloid solutions. Arch Intern Med 1995; 155:373.

[d] 18. Alm TJV. Thoracentesis. In Salm TJV, Cutler BS, Wheeler HB, editors. Atlas of bedside procedures. Boston: Little, Brown; 1979.

[d] 19. Salm TJV. Arterial cannula insertion, percutaneous. In Salm TJV, Cutler BS, Wheeler HB, editors. Atlas of bedside procedures. Boston: Little, Brown; 1979.

[d] 20. Salm TJV. Subclavian vein cannulation. In Salm TJV, Cutler BS, Wheeler HB, editors. Atlas of bedside procedures. Boston: Little, Brown; 1979.

[d] 21. Salm TJV. Internal jugular vein cannulation. In Salm TJV, Cutler BS, Wheeler HB, editors. Atlas of bedside procedures. Boston: Little, Brown; 1979.

[d] 22. Akins CM. Aspiration and injection of joints, bursae, and tendons. In Salm TJV, Cutler BS, Wheeler HB, editors. Atlas of bedside procedures. Boston: Little, Brown; 1979.

[c] 23. Sechzer PH, Abel L. Post–spinal anesthesia headache treated with caffeine: evaluation with demand method. I. Curr Ther Res 1978; 24:307.

[c] 24. Moyer JH et al. The effect of theophylline with ethylenediamine (aminophylline) and caffeine on cerebral hemodynamics and cerebrospinal fluid pressure in patients with hypertensive headaches. Am J Med Sci 1952; 224:377.

[c] 25. Bradsky JB. Epidural blood patch: a safe effective treatment for post–lumbar puncture headaches. West J Med 1978; 129:85.

[c] 26. Olsen KS. Epidural blood patch in the treatment of post-lumbar headache. Pain 1987; 30:293.

[b] 27. Hasbun R et al. Computed tomography of the head before lumbar puncture in adults with suspected meningitis. N Engl J Med 2001; 345:1727.

Care of the Hospitalized Patient

Alan Cheng, MD, and D. William Schlott, MD

In recent years, greater emphasis has been placed on the unique requirements for care of the hospitalized patient. Although patients receive inherent benefits from treatment in a supervised, monitored hospital setting, they are at risk for complications related to hospitalization. This chapter highlights the problems most commonly encountered by house officers and provides guidelines to ensure the appropriate response.

Fever

3

I. DIAGNOSTICS

1. Normal body temperature varies by as much as 1° F with the nadir around 6 AM and the acme between 4 and 6 PM. Fever is defined as an elevation of normal body temperature above 38° C (100.6° F). Because fever can be a sign of an important or even life-threatening problem and can lead to malaise, increased insensible fluid loss, delirium, and even convulsions, rapid identification of the underlying cause is important.

2. Historically, fever patterns have provided clues to the underlying etiology (Table 3-1), but in general they tend to be nonspecific. Infection is the most immediate concern but by no means the only possibility (Box 3-1). Careful, thorough clinical evaluation with particular attention to potential sources of infection is the essential initial step. Any site in which a catheter or tube has been inserted should be inspected for erythema or tenderness. The skin should be carefully inspected for signs that may indicate a local or systemic infection or a drug reaction.

TABLE 3-1
FEVER PATTERNS AS DIAGNOSTIC CLUES

Fever Pattern	Cause
Alternate-day fever	*Plasmodium vivax, P. ovale*
Fever every third day	*P. malariae*
Relapsing fever: daily for 3-6 days; fever-free interval for about 1 week supervenes	*Borrelia* species, rat-bite fever *(Streptococcus moniliformis, Spirillum minus)*
Continuous "undulating fever"	Brucellosis, typhoid
Periodic pyrexia (Pel-Ebstein phenomenon) with variable cycles	Hodgkin's disease

From Goldman L, Bennett JC. Cecil textbook of medicine, 21st ed. Philadelphia: WB Saunders; 2000.

BOX 3-1

CAUSES OF FEVER OF UNKNOWN ORIGIN

INFECTIONS

Abscesses: hepatic, subhepatic, gallbladder, subphrenic, splenic, periappendiceal, perinephric, pelvic, and other sites

Granulomatous: extrapulmonary and miliary tuberculosis, atypical mycobacterial infection, fungal infection

Intravascular: catheter-related endocarditis, meningococcemia, gonococcemia, *Listeria, Brucella,* rat-bite fever, relapsing fever

Viral, rickettsial, and chlamydial: infectious mononucleosis, cytomegalovirus, human immunodeficiency virus, hepatitis, Q fever, psittacosis

Parasitic: extraintestinal amebiasis, malaria, toxoplasmosis

NONINFECTIOUS INFLAMMATORY DISORDERS

Collagen-vascular disease: rheumatic fever, systemic lupus erythematosus, rheumatoid arthritis (particularly Still's disease), vasculitis (all types)

Granulomatous: sarcoidosis, granulomatous hepatitis, Crohn's disease

Tissue injury: pulmonary emboli, sickle cell disease, hemolytic anemia

NEOPLASTIC DISEASES

Lymphoma/leukemia: Hodgkin's disease and non-Hodgkin's lymphoma, acute leukemia, myelodysplastic syndrome

Carcinoma: kidney, pancreas, liver, gastrointestinal tract, lung, especially when metastatic

Atrial myxomas

Central nervous system tumors

DRUG FEVERS

Sulfonamides, penicillins, thiouracils, barbiturates, quinidine, laxatives (especially with phenolphthalein)

FACTITIOUS ILLNESSES

Injections of toxic material, manipulation or exchange of thermometers

OTHER CAUSES

Familial Mediterranean fever, Fabry's disease, cyclic neutropenia

From Goldman L, Bennett JC. Cecil textbook of medicine, 21st ed. Philadelphia: WB Saunders; 2000.

II. MANAGEMENT

1. If possible, all catheters should be removed (and replaced, if necessary) and sent for microbiological analysis. Two sets of blood cultures, a urinalysis, and a chest radiograph should be obtained as part of the investigation for infection.

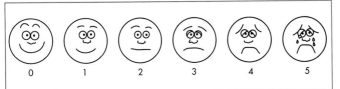

FIG. 3-1

Pain scale. *(From Wong D et al: Essentials of pediatric nursing, 6th ed. St Louis: Mosby; 2000.)*

2. Whether the physician should treat the fever is still debated. Although experimental data support the notion that elevated temperatures enhance host defense mechanisms, little clinical evidence has demonstrated that patients with temperatures as high as 105° F have improved outcomes when antipyretics are used. Temperatures greater than 105° F, however, may be life threatening and warrant prompt antipyretic therapy. Regardless of the actual temperature, the physician may consider treatment of febrile individuals who appear ill or are particularly sensitive to minor changes in metabolic catabolism or oxygen consumption (e.g., cardiopulmonary disease, severe anemia).
3. Acetaminophen (325-650 mg PO or PR q4h) remains the mainstay of therapy because of its antipyretic and analgesic properties. It does not have an antiinflammatory or antiplatelet effect. Ibuprofen (200-800 mg PO tid or qid) and naproxen (250-500 mg PO bid) may be more effective owing to their antiinflammatory properties. Ketorolac (15-30 mg IV or IM q6h) can also be considered, especially for patients who cannot tolerate adequate enteral intake. Increased risk of bleeding has been reported when ketorolac was used for more than 5 days.
4. Although effective, use of corticosteroids is not recommended for routine treatment of fever unless it clearly has a noninfectious origin or may be the result of acute adrenal insufficiency.

Pain

I. DIAGNOSTICS

1. The presentation of acute pain in a hospitalized patient may be a symptom of a known disease, may indicate a recurrence of a preexisting problem, may be caused by a new disorder, or may be a complication of a procedure or treatment the patient has received. New pain complaints must be thoroughly evaluated to properly identify the underlying etiology and to guide appropriate treatment. In light of the subjective nature of pain, quantifying its severity (Fig. 3-1) can be helpful in monitoring the response to treatment.

3

CARE OF THE HOSPITALIZED PATIENT

I. MANAGEMENT

See section in Chapter 33.

Insomnia

I. DIAGNOSTICS

1. Acute insomnia is common in hospitalized patients and frequently results from anxiety, medical illness, or simply being in the hospital environment. Management of chronic insomnia is not addressed in this section. The reader is referred to recent reviews on this subject.[1]

II. MANAGEMENT

1. The cornerstone of treatment of insomnia rests on enforcing good sleep hygiene practices, which is a significant challenge with hospitalized patients.[2] Hence, short-term management of acute insomnia in inpatients centers on pharmacotherapy. Minimizing side effects and maximizing sleep time are the goals of treatment. Diphenhydramine (25-50 mg PO qhs) and chloral hydrate (1-2 g PO qhs) are safe sedatives with minimal side effects and are commonly used initially. Chloral hydrate has been shown to cause gastrointestinal irritation and should not be given to patients with significant hepatic or renal disease. It has also been reported to increase the anticoagulant effect of warfarin. Diphenhydramine and chloral hydrate may be less effective in the elderly population and may cause an increase in anticholinergic-mediated side effects.

2. For elderly patients or younger individuals who fail to respond to either of these agents, short- to intermediate-acting benzodiazepine or selective benzodiazepine agonists (e.g., zolpidem, zaleplon, zopiclone) are appropriate options (Table 3-2). Longer-acting agents tend to worsen insomnia by promoting daytime somnolence and subsequent alterations in sleep-wake cycles. Tolerance develops, and withdrawal symptoms may occur after as little as 2 weeks of therapy. Therefore tapering the dose by approximately 25% to 30% per week at the time of discharge is prudent. Routine use of other psychotropic agents (e.g., selective serotonin reuptake inhibitors, tricyclic antidepressants) that may also cause sedation is not recommended for treatment of acute, isolated insomnia. It is important to remember that sedatives and hypnotics, especially in the elderly, commonly cause delirium and increase the risk of falls. Often the best treatment of insomnia is not medication but efforts to provide a quiet environment and minimize nighttime interruptions for vital sign assessment and medication administration.

Delirium

See Chapter 55.

TABLE 3-2

DRUGS FOR ANXIETY AND PANIC

Drug	Trade Name	Initial Dose	Target Dose Range	Side Effects	Comments
SEDATIVE HYPNOTICS					
Chloral hydrate	Noctel	500 mg	500-1000 mg	Sedation; overdose risk	Seldom appropriate
Meprobamate	Miltown	200 mg tid	1200-1600 mg		
ANTIHISTAMINES					
Diphenhydramine	Benadryl	25 mg PO qhs	50 mg	Dry mouth; mental confusion	Most useful at bedtime for associated sleep disturbance
Hydroxyzine	Atarax	0.5 mg PO			
BENZODIAZEPINES					
Lorazepam	Ativan	0.5 mg PO	2-10 mg, tid doses		Also effective for generalized anxiety
Diazepam	Valium	5 mg PO	5-10 mg bid	Addictive	Abuse potential in many
Triazolam	Halcion	0.125 mg	0.25-0.5 mg hs		
Chlordiazepoxide	Librium	5 mg bid	10-30 mg		
Temazepam	Restoril	7.5 mg hs	15-30 mg		
Alprazolam	Xanax	0.25 mg bid	2-8 mg/day	Ataxia, drowsiness	
Clorazepate	Tranxene	7.5 mg hs	15-60 mg/day		Abuse potential
Flurazepam	Dalmane	15 mg hs	30-60 mg	Ataxia, drowsiness	
Oxazepam	Serax	10 mg bid	60-120 mg/day		Long duration of action permits once daily dose
Clonazepam	Klonopin	0.25 mg qd	1-3 mg/day	Sedation, ataxia	
Buspirone	Buspar	5 mg bid	20-30 mg/day	Nervousness, headache	No dependence with prolonged use
Zolpidem	Ambien	10 mg hs	10 mg hs	Habituation, drowsiness	Most useful on an as-needed basis

From Goldman L, Bennett JC. Cecil textbook of medicine, 21st ed. Philadelphia: WB Saunders; 2000.

CARE OF THE HOSPITALIZED PATIENT

3

Prophylaxis for Gastrointestinal Ulceration

I. DIAGNOSTICS

1. Hospitalized patients at highest risk for acute gastrointestinal ulceration include those in the intensive care unit setting who have either a coagulopathy or respiratory failure requiring mechanical ventilation.[3] The incidence of this complication among patients who are neither critically ill nor restricted from oral intake is low.
2. Unless the patient was taking gastrointestinal prophylaxis before hospitalization, use of agents such as H_2-blockers or proton pump inhibitors for the prevention of stress ulcers is not routinely indicated.

II. MANAGEMENT

1. Critically ill patients with coagulopathy or receiving mechanical ventilation benefit from gastrointestinal prophylaxis with H_2-receptor antagonists (ranitidine 50 mg IV q8h), sucralfate 1000 mg PO q6h, or proton pump inhibitors (omeprazole 10 mg PO bid). The reduction of gastric acidity has been thought to be a risk factor for nosocomial pneumonias, particularly in patients receiving mechanical ventilation. This is the reason sucralfate had been recommended as a first-line agent in the past. However, more recent studies do not substantiate this belief. Furthermore, these studies suggest that ranitidine or a proton pump inhibitor may be more effective in ulcer prevention than sucralfate.[4]

Prophylaxis for Deep Venous Thrombosis

I. DIAGNOSTICS

1. Venous thromboembolism occurs commonly in hospitalized patients and requires heightened awareness and preventive measures.
2. Risk factors for deep venous thrombosis (DVT) in hospitalized patients include age over 40 years; more than 4 days of bed rest; paralysis; prior history of DVT; acute stroke; obesity; malignancy; major abdominal, lower extremity, or pelvic surgery; pregnancy (particularly in the third trimester and immediate postpartum period); acute trauma; femoral vein catheters; nephrotic syndrome; inflammatory bowel disease; estrogen therapy; and hypercoagulable states (e.g., factor V Leiden, prothrombin gene mutations).[5]
3. Physical examination findings such as edema, Homans' sign (calf pain with passive foot dorsiflexion), Bancroft's sign (pain when the soleus muscle is squeezed), and Louvel's sign (pain with coughing) are neither sensitive nor specific individually, but if they occur in combination, they are highly suggestive of a DVT.

II. MANAGEMENT

1. Anticoagulation is commonly used to prevent DVT, although its effectiveness has been the subject of debate (see Chapter 64 for treat-

ment of DVT and pulmonary embolisms). Patients with medical illnesses or undergoing general surgery are commonly treated with unfractionated heparin 5000 U SQ q12h in the absence of contraindications. This may induce immune-mediated thrombocytopenia or dramatically increase the activated partial thromboplastin time (aPTT) in a patient with malnourishment or liver disease. Therefore periodic measurement of the aPTT and platelet count is prudent. Enoxaparin 40 mg SQ qd has also been used in this patient population.[6]

2. Patients undergoing orthopedic surgery are at higher risk for DVTs. Enoxaparin 30 mg SQ q12h or 40 mg SQ qd beginning 12 to 24 hours before surgery or warfarin 5 mg PO qd in the immediate postoperative state is a common prophylactic measure.

3. Patients with contraindications to heparin-related products can be treated with the newer direct thrombin inhibitors.

4. Patients with contraindications to anticoagulation may benefit from elastic stockings and sequential compression devices. The use of these modalities on the upper extremities may also be effective in preventing DVTs in the lower extremities.

5. No consensus has been reached on the most effective duration of treatment, although many suggest that once a patient is fully ambulatory, prophylactic treatment can be discontinued.

Malnutrition

See Chapter 57.

REFERENCES

[c] 1. Barthlen GM. Sleep disorders: obstructive sleep apnea syndrome, restless leg syndrome, and insomnia in geriatric patients. Geriatrics 2002; 57:34.

[c] 2. Lenhart SE et al. Treatment of insomnia in hospitalized patients. Ann Pharmacother 2001; 35:1449.

[c] 3. Cook DJ et al. Stress ulcer prophylaxis in critically ill patients: resolving discordant meta-analyses. JAMA 1996; 275:308.

[a] 4. Cook D et al. A comparison of sucralfate and ranitidine for the prevention of upper gastrointestinal bleeding in patients requiring mechanical ventilation. N Engl J Med 1998; 338:791.

[c] 5. Clagett GP et al. Prevention of venous thromboembolism. Chest 1998; 114:531S.

[a] 6. Samama MM et al. A comparison of enoxaparin with placebo for the prevention of venous thromboembolism in acutely ill medical patients. N Engl J Med 1999; 341:793.

3

CARE OF THE HOSPITALIZED PATIENT

PART II

Diagnostic and Therapeutic Information

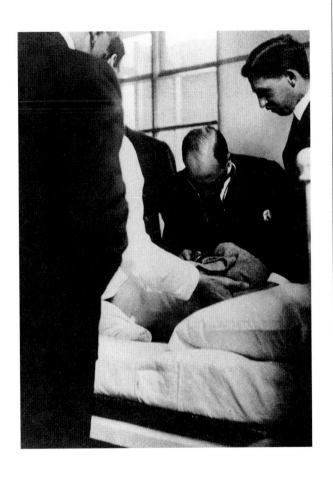

Chest Pain in the Emergency Department

Paul R. Forfia, MD, R. Chris Jones, MD, Michael Londner, MD, and Steven P. Schulman, MD

FAST FACTS

- Chest pain is the most common complaint in the emergency department in patients over the age of 45.
- Acute coronary syndrome (ACS) is diagnosed in 20% of patients with chest pain in the emergency department.
- The initial or primary survey should include assessment of the airway, breathing, circulation, and disability (ABCD) of the patient, along with the 12-lead electrocardiogram (ECG).
- The purpose of immediate review of the 12-lead ECG is to identify patients with an ST elevation myocardial infarction (MI) so that reperfusion strategies may begin immediately.
- By far the most common and most challenging subgroup of patients is those who have chest pain without ST elevation, and a careful secondary assessment is mandatory to differentiate cardiac from noncardiac causes.
- Patients with suspected ACS are a heterogeneous group. Risk stratification is essential to dictate proper management.
- Patients with intermediate or high clinical probability for pulmonary embolism should be given anticoagulants during the diagnostic workup.
- Aortic dissection should be considered for all patients with chest pain in the emergency department, both because of its inherent risks and because therapies such as thrombolytic agents and heparin may lead to catastrophic consequences if wrongfully implemented.
- Over 90% of patients with acute aortic dissection complain of chest, back, or abdominal pain, with abrupt onset and extreme intensity as the key features.
- Secondary spontaneous pneumothorax is often associated with a greater degree of cardiopulmonary embarrassment than occurs with primary spontaneous pneumothorax.
- Over 50% of cases of esophageal rupture are iatrogenic in origin.

I. EPIDEMIOLOGY

1. Nontraumatic chest pain accounts for approximately 5 million visits to the emergency department in the United States annually and is the most common complaint in the emergency department among patients over the age of 45.[1] The differential diagnosis is vast, as are the

prognostic implications, varying from the benign to the life threatening (Box 4-1).

A. APPROACH TO THE PATIENT

1. To establish the most likely origin of the patient's chest discomfort complaints, the physician should first consider all morbid causes

---

BOX 4-1

DIFFERENTIAL DIAGNOSIS OF CHEST PAIN

CARDIAC

ST elevation myocardial infarction

Non–ST elevation myocardial infarction or unstable angina

Aortic valve disease

Myocarditis

NONCARDIAC

Pulmonary embolism

Aortic dissection

Spontaneous pneumothorax

Ruptured esophagus

Pericarditis

Pneumonia

Pleuritis

Esophageal reflux and spasm

Pancreatitis

Costochondritis (Tietze's syndrome)

Nerve root and spinal pain

Herpes zoster

Mondor's disease

Breast cancer or infection

Intercostal myositis or cramp

Shoulder disorders

Cervical disk disease

Thoracic outlet syndrome

Thyroiditis

Tabes dorsalis

Mediastinitis

Primary pulmonary hypertension

Sinus of Valsalva aneurysmal rupture

Mallory-Weiss tear

Zenker's diverticulum

Plummer-Vinson syndrome

Peptic ulcer disease, nonulcer dyspepsia

Biliary diseases

Subphrenic abscesses

Splenic infarct

Psychogenic or hyperventilatory syndrome

of chest pain, such as an acute MI, unstable angina, pulmonary embolism, aortic dissection, pneumothorax, and esophageal rupture. All patients with chest discomfort at presentation should undergo an evaluation that begins with a 12-lead ECG and a focused history and physical examination.[2] Continuous ECG monitoring should be initiated and intravenous access obtained. Blood pressures should be measured in both arms. If based on this initial primary survey[3] the patient has neither a resuscitative requirement nor evidence of an ST segment elevation MI, attention should then be directed to obtaining a more detailed history and performing a physical examination with particular attention focused on the description of the discomfort and an assessment of cardiac risk factors (Fig. 4-1). A history of recent cocaine ingestion is relevant because young, otherwise healthy patients have an estimated 24-fold increased risk of MI within 24 hours of ingestion.[4]

2. On physical examination, signs of cardiopulmonary embarrassment should be sought, including the presence of jugular venous distention, a left parasternal lift, gallop rhythms, and rales. The 12-lead ECG should be reviewed in conjunction with the primary survey, with particular emphasis on identifying an ST segment elevation or a new left bundle branch block (LBBB). The presence of ST segment elevation in this context is virtually diagnostic of an ST elevation MI and identifies a well-defined, high-risk group of patients who should be evaluated by a cardiologist as soon as possible. The remaining patients (without ST elevation or new LBBB) represent the majority of those with chest discomfort whose initial presentation is often nonspecific with regard to an etiology. It is to this population that the secondary survey applies most directly. In the secondary survey the physician obtains more information from the patient regarding the history, physical examination, and diagnostic tests. Patients whose chest pain is suspected to be of cardiac origin or to reflect an ACS should be risk stratified to direct proper management. However, risk stratification should not be limited to ACS, since a wide spectrum of risk exists within the noncardiac, morbid causes of chest discomfort. After establishment of a diagnosis, disease-specific management should begin.

3. The remainder of the discussion focuses on the morbid causes of chest pain, including ACS, aortic dissection, pulmonary embolism, pneumothorax, and esophageal rupture. Each diagnostic possibility is discussed with regard to epidemiology, clinical presentation, diagnosis, and management. The goal of the discussion is to review the salient features of each process so that, when confronted with the complaint of chest pain, the physician can identify high-risk patients and implement the appropriate diagnostic and therapeutic plan efficiently and consistently.

4

CHEST PAIN IN THE EMERGENCY DEPARTMENT

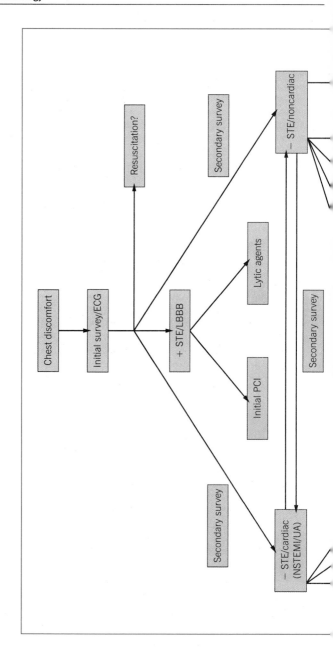

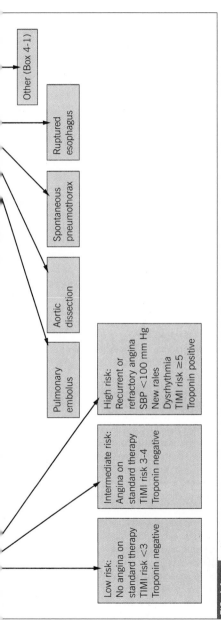

Other (Box 4-1)

Ruptured esophagus

Spontaneous pneumothorax

Aortic dissection

Pulmonary embolus

High risk:
Recurrent or refractory angina
SBP <100 mm Hg
New rales
Dysrhythmia
TIMI risk ≥5
Troponin positive

Intermediate risk:
Angina on standard therapy
TIMI risk 3-4
Troponin negative

Low risk:
No angina on standard therapy
TIMI risk <3
Troponin negative

FIG. 4-1

Approach to chest discomfort. *ECG,* Electrocardiogram; *PCI,* percutaneous coronary intervention; *STE,* ST elevation; *LBBB,* left bundle branch block; *NSTEMI,* non–ST elevation myocardial infarction; *SBP,* systolic blood pressure; *TIMI,* thrombolysis in myocardial infarction; *UA,* urinalysis.

CHEST PAIN IN THE EMERGENCY DEPARTMENT

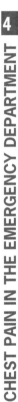

4

Acute Coronary Syndromes

I. EPIDEMIOLOGY

1. ACS is divided into ST segment elevation myocardial infarction (ST elevation MI), non–ST segment elevation myocardial infarction (non–ST elevation MI), and unstable angina. The latter two are known collectively as the non–ST elevation acute coronary syndromes (see Chapter 5). This classification schema has replaced the traditional division of patients with an ACS into Q wave, non–Q wave MI, or unstable angina. The diagnosis of an ST elevation MI is made through a combination of clinical and ECG features, whereas the differentiation of the non–ST elevation syndromes (MI versus unstable angina) is based on the presence or absence of elevated cardiac specific biomarkers such as troponins or creatine phosphokinase (CPK). Taken together, these syndromes account for an estimated 20% of all chest discomfort complaints annually in U.S. emergency departments, representing by far the most common morbid cause of chest discomfort and the leading cause of death in the United States.[1]

2. Atherosclerosis is present in almost all cases of ACS. Thus the traditional risk factors for coronary artery disease can be applied as risk factors for an ACS. The major risk factors include, in no particular order, age 45 years or older in men or 55 years or older in women, active cigarette smoking, hypertension, hyperlipidemia, and diabetes mellitus. In addition, family history is an independent risk factor for coronary artery disease, with risk directly proportional to the number, and inversely proportional to the age, of primary relatives affected.[5,6] More recently, hyperhomocysteinemia and elevated serum C-reactive protein levels have been linked to coronary artery disease (see Chapter 9).[7,8]

3. Unstable angina, non–ST elevation MI, and ST elevation MI represent part of the continuum from transient severe myocardial ischemia to sustained ischemia with resultant myocardial necrosis. Autopsy and angiographic data suggest that unstable angina and non–ST elevation MI result from severe, transient, platelet-rich occlusion of the culprit coronary artery with eventual spontaneous reperfusion, whereas ST elevation MI is due to severe, sustained, fibrin-rich occlusion. In each case the inciting event is coronary artery plaque rupture, with subsequent platelet activation and superimposed thrombus generation.[9] The extent of myocardial necrosis reflects the balance between the severity and duration of myocardial ischemia and the extent and compromise of preexisting collateral circulation. Despite sharing a common pathophysiology, however, these conditions have different clinical manifestations and treatment, accounting for the variable prognoses among patients with ACS. In general, patients with ST elevation MI have a 30-day mortality of approximately 9% to 12% in the reperfusion era, whereas estimates for patients with non–ST elevation MI

and unstable angina are estimated to be 6% and 3%, respectively. However, clinical, ECG, and laboratory features define a wide range of clinical risk within each division of ACS. Thus a high-risk patient with unstable angina has short- and long-term outcomes similar to those of a patient with a low-risk ST elevation MI.[9,10]

II. CLINICAL PRESENTATION

1. No process is more closely associated with the complaint of chest discomfort than the acute coronary syndromes. The presentation of these syndromes can be quite heterogeneous (Box 4-2).
2. The typical quality of ischemic pain is pressure, tightness, aching, or squeezing. The term "sharp" is used frequently, often in reference to intensity rather than quality of the pain. The discomfort is usually substernal but may be localized to the left or right precordium. As with any visceral pain, radiation is common, classically to the inner aspect of the left arm. Radiation to the neck, jaw, right arm, or both arms has also been described. In fact, right arm and bilateral arm radiation may be a more specific indicator of ischemic pain than left arm radiation.[11] On occasion the sites of radiation are the source of the primary

---

BOX 4-2

PRESENTATION OF ACUTE CORONARY SYNDROMES

Typical Symptoms with Acute Coronary Syndrome

<65 years
Male
Current smoker
Hyperlipidemia
ST segment elevation

Atypical Symptoms with Acute Coronary Syndrome

>75 years
Prior heart failure
Prior stroke
Diabetes
Female
Nonwhite racial or ethnic group
No ST segment elevation

Atypical Symptoms Without Acute Coronary Syndrome

Positional symptoms
Pleuritic symptoms
Pain described as sharp or stabbing
Pain reducible by palpation
Absence of typical risk factors for coronary artery disease

complaint. Timing is variable, although the incidence of an ACS is highest between 6 and 11 AM, mimicking the diurnal variations in sympathetic nervous system activity.[12] Ischemic chest discomfort most commonly lasts minutes (not seconds or hours), but protracted pain should not rule out ACS because patients often delay seeking treatment. In contrast to patients with stable angina, those with ischemic pain characteristically report chest discomfort at rest or with minimal exertion. In addition, chest pain that is similar to or more prolonged or severe than a patient's prior angina predicts a fourfold increased risk of a major cardiovascular event, which is nearly as predictive as new ST depression or T wave inversion in the context of chest discomfort.[13] Patients may report relief after sublingual administration of nitroglycerin or occasionally after taking antacids, belching, or vomiting. None of these features are reliable, however, and they should not be used to discriminate cardiac from noncardiac syndromes.[14] Associated symptoms include dyspnea, nausea, vomiting, diaphoresis, fatigue, weakness, and a sense of apprehension. As shown in Box 4-2, atypical presentations are more likely to be associated with, in descending order, prior heart failure, prior stroke, older age (>75 years), diabetes, female sex, and nonwhite racial or ethnic group.[15] This was illustrated in a prospective registry of almost 400,000 patients, which showed that overall one third of patients with an MI did not complain of chest discomfort. Furthermore, those with three or more of the above characteristics did not have chest discomfort in 50% of cases, and patients with none of the characteristics were free of chest pain in only 17% of cases. Those without chest discomfort most often reported dyspnea as their primary complaint. Interestingly, a similar patient profile is evident among patients who have an MI without characteristic ECG changes and among those who have an MI and are mistakenly discharged from the emergency department.[16,17] Atypical features not consistent with an ACS include the combination of sharp, pleuritic, and positional discomfort, which is quite reliable in identifying patients at very low risk for an acute MI.[11]

3. The physical examination is often overlooked but is useful for risk stratification and may help in the diagnosis of an acute MI. In a seminal article by Killip and Kimball, patients with an acute MI had in-hospital mortality rates of 6% with no rales, 17% with rales, and 81% with rales and hypotension.[18] More recently, Goldman and associates showed that the presence of systolic blood pressure less than 100 mm Hg and rales above the bases predicted a twofold to threefold increased risk of serious arrhythmia, pump failure, and recurrent ischemia.[13] In the context of a suspected ACS, other findings that support a diagnosis of ischemia are the appearance or accentuation of an S_3 or S_4 gallop, a sustained apical impulse, or a left parasternal lift caused by ischemic postcapillary pulmonary hypertension. Mechanical complications of ischemia such as papillary mus-

cle ischemia or rupture classically lead to a new or worsening murmur of mitral regurgitation, and a murmur heard over the left lower sternal border suggests acute ventricular septal defect in a patient with right ventricular failure. Jugular venous distention can be seen in patients with ischemia-induced left ventricular failure, right ventricular infarction, or pericardial tamponade caused by myocardial rupture.

III. DIAGNOSTICS

A. ELECTROCARDIOGRAM

1. Along with chest discomfort, the diagnosis of an ACS relies on coincident ECG changes and elevations in cardiac markers. The ECG remains the cornerstone of diagnosis in an ACS, and its findings are the basis for urgent coronary revascularization. In addition, the ECG is a powerful prognostic indicator in patients with ACS. In the setting of myocardial ischemia the ECG may show ST segment elevations, ST segment depressions, and T wave inversions. ST elevations consistent with acute transmural myocardial ischemia are defined as ST segment elevation of >1 mm in the limb leads or >2 mm in the precordial leads of at least two anatomically contiguous leads. Other processes that can produce ST elevations include benign early repolarization, acute pericarditis, left ventricular aneurysm, LBBB, and ventricularly paced rhythm.[19] Benign early repolarization produces diffuse ST elevations and is not associated with reciprocal ST depressions. ST depression is defined as >1 mm of ST depression, and T wave inversion as >1 mm of symmetrical T wave inversion in at least two contiguous leads. In a recent analysis of the ECG findings of almost 400,000 patients with an acute MI, the ECG showed 57% diagnostic sensitivity when characteristic ST segment elevation or depression was present, and an additional 35% of patients showed nonspecific ST segment or T wave changes. Approximately 7% of patients with an MI had a normal ECG.[20] Elevation of the ST segment is 90% specific for acute MI, and ST depression and T wave inversion predict MI in approximately 48% and 31% of cases, respectively.[20,21] Of patients with unstable angina/non–ST elevation MI, approximately 50% have ST depression or T wave inversion on serial ECGs. The presence of ST or T wave changes and their degree of interval change in patients with suspected ACS serve as powerful predictors of subsequent MI and predict an increase in short- and long-term adverse cardiovascular events. Additional adverse prognostic ECG findings include extremes of heart rate, increasing QRS duration, new bundle branch block, left anterior and posterior fascicular block, and the presence of atrial fibrillation.[22,23]

B. CARDIAC BIOMARKERS

1. The cardiac markers used most frequently in the diagnosis and risk stratification of patients with an ACS are CPK and CPK-MB and the cardiac troponins (troponin I and T). The troponins are the most sensitive and specific biomarkers of cardiac injury and provide key

information in the risk stratification of patients with unstable angina/non–ST elevation MI. For example, Hamm and associates showed that elevations of troponin T or I were 98% to 100% sensitive in the diagnosis of MI when levels were measured more than 6 hours after onset of symptoms, whereas normal troponin levels more than 6 hours after symptom onset were associated with a remarkably low risk of an adverse cardiovascular event at 30 days' follow-up.[24] In addition, numerous studies have shown that troponin elevation in the setting of unstable angina/non–ST elevation MI defines a high-risk population and that these patients derive the greatest benefit from glycoprotein IIb/IIIa inhibitors and an early invasive strategy.[25-27] The probable reason is that troponin elevation results from myocardial necrosis at the microvascular level caused by distal embolization of unstable plaque material. In contrast, CPK and the relatively cardiac-specific CPK-MB are only 90% sensitive for an MI and lack cardiac specificity in the event of concomitant skeletal muscle injury (e.g., in rhabdomyolysis and after cardiopulmonary resuscitation or electrical cardioversion). In addition, CPK-MB and troponin T lose cardiac specificity in renal failure. In contrast, troponin I has been shown in a small prospective study to be a specific marker of myocardial injury in patients with renal disease.[28] Clinicians should be cautious about dismissing an elevated troponin T level in patients with renal insufficiency, however, because troponin T remains a powerful predictor of adverse cardiovascular events in this population.[29] CPK, CPK-MB, and troponin levels rise approximately 4 to 6 hours after symptom onset and return to baseline 48 to 72 hours after symptom onset for CPK and CPK-MB and 10 to 14 days after symptom onset for troponins. Thus CPK and CPK-MB are useful in the timing of cardiovascular events because the characteristic rising and falling pattern of these markers indicates a relatively recent or recurrent event (Fig. 5-2).

IV. MANAGEMENT

1. The management of an ACS is contingent on the presence or absence of persistent, characteristic ST segment elevations (or new LBBB) on the ECG. Patients with ST elevation MI are eligible for reperfusion therapy, either by thrombolysis or by primary angioplasty. If both are available, primary angioplasty is preferred, based on higher success in achieving patency of the infarct-related artery, lower incidence of recurrent ischemia, better preservation of ventricular function, and lower short- and long-term mortality. Primary angioplasty is not appropriate, however, if the patient is a candidate for thrombolytic agents and percutaneous intervention may be delayed for more than an hour.[30] Candidates for thrombolysis should be carefully evaluated for potential contraindications, optimally with use of a bedside checklist. Thrombolysis should be initiated within 30 minutes of arrival in the emergency department. Patients, regardless of reperfusion strat-

egy, should receive 160 to 325 mg of aspirin, to be chewed and swallowed in the emergency department. In this setting, invasive procedures such as arterial lines should be minimized and if central venous access is needed, a compressible site should be used. Foley catheter trauma is common and can lead to significant genitourinary bleeding, particularly in elderly men. This same principle applies to patients receiving other antithrombotic and antiplatelet agents. Alternative antiplatelet therapies for those who cannot tolerate aspirin include clopridogrel (preferred) and ticlopidine. Intravenous β-blockade with metoprolol or atenolol should be initiated with a target heart rate of less than 70 beats/min, followed by oral β-blockade. Full-dose heparin is indicated for all patients who will undergo angioplasty, whereas only those receiving the fibrin-specific lytic agents (t-PA and reteplase, not streptokinase or urokinase) should be given heparin. IV administration of nitroglycerin and morphine sulfate is appropriate in the hemodynamically stable patient, with the goal of alleviating chest pain and pulmonary congestion.

2. The treatment strategies in unstable angina/non–ST elevation MI are much more heterogeneous and depend heavily on patient risk, which is typically graded as low, intermediate, or high. The most commonly used and best validated means of risk stratification is the calculated TIMI risk score.[25,31] The TIMI risk score comprises seven historical, clinical, and diagnostic features, each assigned a value of 1 point. These features are age 65 or older, prior coronary stenosis of greater than 50%, three or more cardiac risk factors, elevated levels of cardiac markers, ST deviation, chest pain more than twice in the prior 24 hours, and aspirin use within 7 days before symptom onset (Box 5-1). Regardless of clinical risk, patients with unstable angina/non–ST elevation MI should receive aspirin, β-blockade, nitroglycerin, and morphine in the same fashion as those with ST elevation MI. Patients with low-risk unstable angina/non–ST elevation MI must be hemodynamically stable, show no signs of cardiopulmonary embarrassment caused by ischemia (i.e., rales, new mitral regurgitation, dysrhythmias), often have only nonspecific ECG changes, do not have troponin elevations at initial examination, and, in keeping, have a TIMI risk score of less than 3. These patients are managed with the standard therapies listed previously and become candidates for heparin and glycoprotein IIb/IIIa inhibitors as their clinical risk increases from low to intermediate and from intermediate to high, respectively. Intermediate-risk patients also demonstrate hemodynamic stability but may have chest pain unabated by standard therapies or have more pronounced ECG changes (i.e., dynamic T wave inversions). Furthermore, intermediate-risk patients initially are troponin negative and have a TIMI risk score of 3 to 4. High-risk unstable angina/non–ST elevation MI is defined as hemodynamic instability at any TIMI risk score, initial troponin positivity, or TIMI risk greater than 4. High-risk

patients should be treated with heparin (preferably low molecular weight), and glycoprotein IIb/IIIa inhibitors should be considered for adjunctive medical therapy (tirofiban or eftifibatide) or if therapeutic catheterization is imminent (abciximab). High-risk patients with unstable angina/non–ST elevation MI treated with these therapies have had significantly lower short- and long-term rates of death and MI than those not receiving such therapies. In addition, these patients have been shown to receive additional benefit from an early invasive strategy (percutaneous revascularization or coronary artery bypass grafting) within 48 hours of hospitalization.[30,31] Additional features associated with high risk include ST deviation greater than 2 mm, heart failure, and recurrent or refractory ischemia. These patients will probably also benefit from IIb/IIIa inhibitors and an early invasive strategy.[32,33] All these treatment strategies are designed for patients with an ACS caused by an unstable plaque. This contrasts sharply with demand ischemia, which is common and often caused by anemia, or extremes of heart rate or blood pressure in the setting of a fixed atherosclerotic plaque. These patients may not benefit from the therapeutic approaches described (and may be harmed) and require correction of the underlying cause for proper management.

Pulmonary Embolism (see Chapter 64)

I. EPIDEMIOLOGY

1. The second most common cause of serious chest pain is pulmonary embolism, which accounts for an estimated 2% of all chest pain complaints in the emergency department. This is probably an underestimate, given the often subtle clinical presentation of pulmonary embolism. Despite efforts by investigators to improve the diagnosis of pulmonary embolism, its prevalence at autopsy has remained unchanged (12% to 15%) over the past 30 years.[34]

2. In approximately 95% of cases of pulmonary embolism the source of the embolus is deep venous thrombosis (DVT), usually in the iliac, femoral, or popliteal venous system. Primary pulmonary artery thrombosis is uncommon and is seen primarily in patients with preexisting severe pulmonary hypertension or hypercoagulability. Thus in the majority of cases the risk factors for pulmonary embolism are shared with DVT. The three major factors that predispose to venous thrombosis are, in descending order, stasis or immobility, vessel damage, and hypercoagulability.[34,35] Other important risk factors to consider are age over 60 years, obesity, malignancy, cigarette smoking, pregnancy, oral contraceptive use, and hormone replacement therapy. Occasionally, thromboembolism may herald an occult malignancy.

3. The pathophysiology of pulmonary embolism is dictated by mechanical obstruction of the pulmonary vasculature, as well as pulmonary vaso-

constriction and bronchoconstriction by paracrine mediators such as serotonin and thromboxane released from the resident thrombus. Reduction in pulmonary vascular surface area and pulmonary vasoconstriction serve to increase pulmonary vascular resistance and thus right ventricular afterload. The absolute increase and the rate of rise of right ventricular afterload can result in right ventricular failure. If left inadequately treated, this can lead to systemic hypotension, shock, and death. In addition, patients may become markedly hypoxemic owing to alterations in regional ventilation-perfusion relationships. In untreated persons mortality approaches 30%. With treatment, mortality is reduced to 17% at 3 months, with most patients dying during the initial hospitalization.[36]

II. CLINICAL PRESENTATION

1. Approximately 70% of patients with a pulmonary embolism complain of chest discomfort. Pleuritic chest discomfort occurs much more often than angina-like pain. Anginal pain is typically nonradiating and is more often associated with central, massive pulmonary embolism, whereas pleuritic pain typically heralds a smaller, more peripheral pulmonary embolism. Dyspnea is still the most common complaint, present in over 80% of patients with pulmonary embolism. Over 90% of patients report dyspnea, tachypnea, or pleuritic pain. Other important symptoms include hemoptysis, cough, palpitations, apprehension, and syncope. Syncope is clearly more prevalent in patients with massive pulmonary embolism.[35,37]

2. On physical examination the most common sign is tachypnea, present in 70% to 80% of patients with pulmonary embolism. Tachycardia is present in 30% to 50% of patients and is more prevalent among those with massive pulmonary embolism and hypotension at initial examination. Pulse oximetry has a limited role in the diagnosis of pulmonary embolism, reflecting the fact that 30% to 40% of patients have a Po_2 greater than 70 mm Hg at presentation. Thus a normal Spo_2 should not decrease the clinical suspicion for pulmonary embolism.[37] Other findings include accentuation of the pulmonic component of S_2, a left parasternal lift, and an S_4 heard best at the left lower sternal border. Inspection of the neck veins may reveal an elevated jugular venous pressure, at times accompanied by an exaggerated v wave caused by tricuspid insufficiency. Consistent with right ventricular strain, these findings often herald the presence of a larger pulmonary embolism. Physical findings suggesting DVT are uncommon, as illustrated by the presence of Homans' sign in only 4% of patients.[35,37]

III. DIAGNOSTICS

1. Useful diagnostic modalities include an ECG, chest radiography, arterial blood gas analysis, D-dimer assay, ventilation-perfusion

scanning, venous ultrasonography, pulmonary angiography, and computed tomographic (CT) angiography.

A. ELECTROCARDIOGRAM AND CHEST RADIOGRAPH

1. The ECG and chest radiograph are abnormal in 70% to 80% of patients with confirmed pulmonary embolism, but no specific abnormality has proved sensitive or specific in the diagnosis of pulmonary embolism.[35,37] The commonly cited Hampton's hump and Westermark's sign have been shown in prospective studies to have virtually no utility in the diagnosis of pulmonary embolism. The most common ECG findings are nonspecific ST and T wave abnormalities and sinus tachycardia, seen in approximately 50% and 30% of patients, respectively. Purported classic findings such as right axis deviation, right bundle branch block, an $S_IQ_{III}T_{III}$ pattern, and atrial fibrillation each occur in less than 5% of cases. The chest radiograph shows nonspecific, often subtle findings such as atelectasis or pleural effusion (usually unilateral) in up to 70% of cases. It is, however, the relative lack of radiographic evidence of airspace disease that is characteristic of pulmonary embolism and should raise the clinician's suspicion when the patient has hypoxemia or other findings that suggest pulmonary embolism. As mentioned previously, pulse oximetry alone is not sufficient for establishing or excluding pulmonary embolism. The alveolar-arterial gradient is normal in less than 10% of patients, however, which reflects the ability of many patients with a pulmonary embolism to maintain their oxygenation, although at the expense of increased alveolar ventilation and hypocapnia. Severe hypoxemia should raise the suspicion of a massive pulmonary embolism.

B. D-DIMER ASSAY

1. The D-dimer assay is a relatively novel serological test used in the diagnosis of a DVT or pulmonary embolism. It measures the amount of fibrin degradation product resulting from activation of the coagulation and fibrinolytic processes. Two major assays have been well validated, the enzyme-linked immunosorbent assay (ELISA) (negative result is <500 pg/L) and the SimpliRED agglutination test. In two separate prospective trials the predictive value of a negative D-dimer by ELISA or agglutination assay exceeded 98% for excluding pulmonary embolism.[39,40] Furthermore, when a negative D-dimer assay was combined with an arterial P_{O_2} greater than 80 mm Hg, the predictive value increased to 100%. Thus some investigators have proposed that a low clinical probability plus a negative D-dimer assay is sufficient to exclude pulmonary embolism. However, in populations with a high likelihood of thromboembolism, the D-dimer may be inadequate in excluding the diagnosis, since one study showed a negative predictive value of less than 80% in 121 patients with cancer and suspected pulmonary embolism.[41] The specificity of a positive D-dimer assay for pulmonary embolism is less than 30% and thus is not use-

ful in establishing a diagnosis of pulmonary embolism.[39] Two recent studies have demonstrated serum troponin elevations in 30% to 40% of patients with pulmonary embolism, with a correlation between troponin positivity and size of the perfusion abnormality on ventilation-perfusion ($\dot{V}/\dot{Q}$) scan, as well as an increase in in-hospital mortality.[42,43]

C. VENTILATION-PERFUSION SCAN

1. The ventilation-perfusion scan is the most frequently used and well validated of the imaging modalities for pulmonary embolism.[44] The Prospective Investigation of Pulmonary Embolism Diagnosis (PIOPED) study tested the sensitivity of the $\dot{V}/\dot{Q}$ scan in patients with low, intermediate, and high clinical probability of a pulmonary embolism. This study showed that patients with intermediate to high clinical probability and a high-probability scan had an 86% to 95% likelihood of a pulmonary embolism, whereas those with a low clinical probability and a normal or low-probability scan had a 2% to 4% risk of a pulmonary embolism. In contrast, patients with intermediate clinical probability and a normal or low-probability scan still had a 6% to 15% likelihood of a pulmonary embolism. Thus careful assessment of clinical probability is essential because it can markedly affect the posttest probability of the $\dot{V}/\dot{Q}$ scan. Ultrasound examination of the lower extremities is necessary to raise or lower the probability of pulmonary embolism in the majority of patients for whom a diagnosis of pulmonary embolism has not been ruled in or out after a $\dot{V}/\dot{Q}$ scan. Presence of DVT mandates treatment for presumed pulmonary embolism, whereas a negative result may not sufficiently exclude thromboembolism. In selected cases patients are referred for pulmonary angiography as the final diagnostic step. Evidence suggests, however, that when intermediate scan results are coupled with a negative ultrasound examination and a negative D-dimer assay, pulmonary embolism can be excluded without angiography.[45]

D. COMPUTED TOMOGRAPHY

1. Spiral CT has an increasing role in the diagnosis of a pulmonary embolism. Spiral CT is approximately 70% sensitive and 90% specific for a pulmonary embolism, although the examiner's experience seems to affect the number of false positive results. Its advantages are specificity, convenience, and the ability to diagnose other intrathoracic abnormalities. Its limitations are its lack of high-quality prospective clinical validation, suboptimal visualization of subsegmental pulmonary vessels, and relative contraindication for patients with renal insufficiency.[46] Nevertheless, in a recent retrospective cohort study of 993 patients with suspected pulmonary embolism and negative findings on spiral CT, the 3-month cumulative incidence of a DVT or pulmonary embolism was 0.5%; fatal pulmonary embolisms occurred in 0.3% of patients.[47] Prospective validation of CT angiography in the diagnosis of pulmonary embolism is ongoing.

IV. MANAGEMENT

1. The mainstay of therapy in acute pulmonary embolism is heparin. In the absence of absolute contraindications, such as active gastrointestinal or intracranial bleeding, patients with intermediate or high clinical probability of pulmonary embolism should begin anticoagulation with heparin during the diagnostic workup. According to a weight-based nomogram, patients should be given a bolus of unfractionated heparin, followed by a continuous infusion with a goal activated partial thromboplastin time (aPTT) ratio between 1.5 and 2.5 (standard bolus 60 to 80 U/kg, and infusion 14 to 18 U/kg). As an alternative, patients can be treated with fractionated, or low molecular weight, heparin, which has been shown to be as safe and effective as unfractionated heparin in the treatment of acute pulmonary embolism.[48] In the event of massive pulmonary embolism, defined as pulmonary embolism in the presence of hypotension or severe hypoxemia, thrombolytic therapy should be considered. In such a case an emergency pulmonary consultation should be obtained to guide therapy.

Aortic Dissection

I. EPIDEMIOLOGY

1. Aortic dissection is a relatively uncommon but frequently fatal cause of chest pain in the emergency department. In a recent large prospective study, aortic dissection was present in 0.3% of patients with acute chest pain, outweighed by ACS approximately 80:1.[49] Nevertheless, acute aortic dissection, defined as a separation of the intimal and medial layers of the aorta, is the most common aortic surgical emergency, surpassing ruptured abdominal aortic aneurysm. The majority of patients with this condition have an intimal flap identified on imaging, surgery, or autopsy. The remainder may have dissection caused by hemorrhage into the media from the vasa vasorum. The typical patient is a 60- to 80-year-old man with a history of hypertension.[50] Other predisposing factors, especially in younger patients, include connective tissue disorders (Marfan's syndrome, Ehlers-Danlos syndrome, and cystic medial necrosis), coarctation of the aorta, bicuspid aortic valve, and Turner's syndrome. Half of all aortic dissections in women under the age of 40 occur during pregnancy. Iatrogenic causes are occasionally reported, usually a complication of left-sided cardiac catheterization or aortic cannulation during cardiac surgery. Aortic dissection has also been reported among weight lifters during weight lifting. In addition, acute dissection of the aorta has been reported in young patients who use cocaine, particularly crack cocaine.[51] The original classification system by DeBakey was denoted as type I (ascending and descending aortic involvement), type II (ascending aorta only), and type III (descending aorta only). Today the more commonly used Stanford classification divides aortic

dissection into types A and B. Type A dissections involve the ascending aorta, and all others are type B. An aortic dissection is described as acute if symptoms are present for less than 2 weeks; otherwise, it is chronic (Table 4-1 and Fig. 4-2).

2. As mentioned previously, the inciting event in aortic dissection is a tear in the aortic intima. This usually occurs approximately 2 cm superior to the aortic valve on the right lateral wall of the ascending aorta, the point of maximal shear stress. The pathophysiological process of dissection is primarily the passage of blood into the false lumen under arterial pressure, followed by propagation of the dissection proximally or distally or both. Proximal extension can lead to cardiac tamponade, dissection into coronary ostia with resultant myocardial ischemia, or acute aortic insufficiency. Distal extension may cause occlusion of branch vessels with resultant end-organ ischemia, as well as aortic rupture and exsanguination. Patient outcome is variable, depending on the type of dissection and the treatment used. For example, in-hospital mortality for patients with type A dissection who receive surgery is approximately 25%, versus 60% in patients not receiving surgery. In contrast, patients with type B dissection treated medically have a 10% in-hospital mortality as compared with 33% for those who undergo surgery.[50]

II. CLINICAL PRESENTATION

1. In aortic dissection the classic presentation is chest pain that is described as tearing or ripping and radiating to the back. However, data from the International Registry of Acute Aortic Dissection (IRAD) show that the presentation is much more diverse.[49] Overall, pain in

TABLE 4-1

CLASSIFICATION SYSTEMS COMMONLY USED TO DESCRIBE AORTIC DISSECTION

Type	Site of Origin and Extent of Aortic Involvement
DEBAKEY	
Type I	Originates in the ascending aorta; propagates at least to the aortic arch and often beyond it distally
Type II	Originates in and is confined to the ascending aorta
Type III	Originates in the descending aorta and extends distally down the aorta or, rarely, retrograde into the aortic arch and ascending aorta
STANFORD	
Type A	All dissections involving the ascending aorta, regardless of the site of origin
Type B	All dissections not involving the ascending aorta
DESCRIPTIVE	
Proximal	Includes DeBakey types I and II or Stanford type A
Distal	Includes DeBakey type III or Stanford type B

Data from Braunwald E: Heart disease: a textbook of cardiovascular medicine, 5th ed. Philadelphia: WB Saunders; 1996.

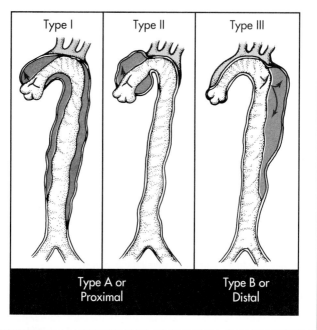

FIG. 4-2

Commonly used classification systems for aortic dissection (see Table 4-1). *(From Braunwald E et al. Heart disease, 6th ed. Philadelphia: WB Saunders; 2001.)*

the chest, back, or abdomen was present in over 95% of patients. Chest pain was present in only 73% of patients with dissection. Anterior pain was more likely in type A dissection, and back pain and abdominal pain were more common in type B dissection. Regardless of the location of pain, 90% of patients described it as abrupt in onset, severe, or the worst pain they ever experienced. Surprisingly, only 50% of patients reported ripping or tearing pain, with no difference between type A and B dissection. Although present in less than 10% of patients, syncope was more often associated with type A dissection than type B.

2. The most common physical finding in acute dissection is hypertension, which is present in 50% of all patients and up to 70% of those with type B dissection. The murmur of aortic insufficiency is present in up to 30% of patients with dissection and is more common with involvement of the ascending aorta. This murmur is often heard best not

at the left lower sternal border (as noted when aortic insufficiency is due to primary valvular disease) but at the right upper sternal border. Proximal extension of a type A dissection may lead to coronary artery occlusion and thus signs of myocardial ischemia or to rupture into the pericardium and cardiac tamponade. Rupture into a hemithorax, most often the left, may produce signs of a pleural effusion. Indications of aortic branch vessel occlusion, such as a focal neurological deficit, a blood pressure differential in the upper extremities, signs of bowel ischemia, and lower limb pulse deficits, should be sought and can reveal the extent and location of the dissection along the length of the aorta.

III. DIAGNOSTICS
A. ELECTROCARDIOGRAM AND CHEST RADIOGRAPHS

1. Diagnostic evaluation of aortic dissection begins with analysis of the chest radiograph and ECG and ends with a transesophageal echocardiogram, spiral CT, magnetic resonance angiography, or magnetic resonance imaging (MRI). The chest radiograph and ECG, as in pulmonary embolism, are abnormal in the vast majority of patients with aortic dissection, but no single finding reliably establishes the diagnosis. The most common chest radiograph abnormality is widening of the mediastinum or an abnormal aortic contour. Although these findings are seen in other common conditions (e.g., hypertension, atherosclerotic disease, valvular disease), a recent study of patients with suspected aortic dissection showed that the combination of mediastinal widening or abnormal aortic contour on the chest radiograph in the setting of characteristic symptoms of aortic dissection or blood pressure differentials had a diagnostic sensitivity of 83% and 100%, respectively, for the presence of aortic dissection.[52] Unilateral left pleural effusion may represent underlying hemothorax. The 12-lead ECG shows nonspecific ST and T wave abnormalities in up to 50% of patients. At presentation 3% to 4% of patients with type A dissection have ST elevation, typically in the inferior leads as a consequence of right coronary artery ostial occlusion. Thus, as shown in Box 4-1, aortic dissection should be considered whenever a patient is seen for acute chest pain, since dissection is an absolute contraindication to virtually all other therapies for acute chest pain in the emergency department.

B. TRANSESOPHAGEAL ECHOCARDIOGRAPHY, COMPUTED TOMOGRAPHY SCANS, AND MAGNETIC RESONANCE IMAGING

1. Transesophageal echocardiography, spiral CT scan, and MRI all have greater than 90% sensitivity and specificity in detecting an aortic dissection. However, each has its limitations and advantages (Table 4-2). Transesophageal echocardiography (TEE) is rapid, portable, and highly sensitive and specific, and it does not interfere with pa-

TABLE 4-2

DIAGNOSTIC PERFORMANCE OF IMAGING MODALITIES IN THE EVALUATION OF SUSPECTED AORTIC DISSECTION

Diagnostic Performance	Angiography	Computed Tomography	Magnetic Resonance Imaging	TEE
Sensitivity	++	++	+++	+++
Specificity	+++	+++	+++	++/+++
Site of intimal tear	++	+	+++	++
Presence of thrombus	+++	++	+++	+
Presence of aortic insufficiency	+++	−	+	+++
Pericardial effusion	−	++	+++	+++
Branch vessel involvement	+++	+	++	+
Coronary artery involvement	++	−	−	++

Data from Cigarroa JE et al. N Engl J Med 1993; 328:35.
+++, Excellent; ++, good; +, fair; −, not detected; *TEE*, transesophageal echocardiography.

tient monitoring and resuscitation. Thus TEE is the imaging modality of choice in patients with suspected aortic dissection and hemodynamic instability. Disadvantages include the need for endoesophageal intubation and the dependence on a highly trained operator to obtain and interpret the images. Because of its availability and rapidity, spiral CT is often the first imaging modality used for patients with suspected aortic dissection. In addition to its practical advantages, spiral CT can be used to identify pleural and pericardial effusions and to visualize the aorta and its branch vessels along its entire length. Drawbacks include the need for IV contrast material and the potential interruption of patient monitoring. MRI is currently the most accurate noninvasive imaging modality for patients with suspected aortic dissection. Because of the need for prolonged scanning and patient inaccessibility, however, MRI is not recommended for unstable patients. Currently the optimal role for MRI is in the stable patient with type B dissection, who is being followed with serial MRI evaluation to document progression of the dissection.

C. CARDIAC BIOMARKERS

1. A recently developed assay of circulating smooth muscle myosin heavy-chain protein allows the serological detection of damaged aortic medial smooth muscle during acute dissection.[53] When used in more than 200 patients with suspected acute dissection, the assay had a sensitivity of 91% and a specificity of 98%. At present this assay is not routinely available, but in the future it may prove valuable in the initial assessment of patients with chest pain by allowing physicians to determine whether aortic dissection is a possibility in patients about to undergo therapies contraindicated in acute dissection.

IV. MANAGEMENT

1. Management of acute aortic dissection requires initial medical stabilization and emergency cardiology and cardiothoracic surgery consultation. The goal of medical management is the rapid lowering of left ventricular contractility and arterial blood pressure. This decreases the stress imposed on the aortic defect, which in turn reduces the likelihood of propagation or rupture of the dissection. Initial treatment is intravenous β-blockade, usually with labetalol or the short-acting agent esmolol (Table 5-4). Once the heart rate is reduced to 50 to 60 beats/min, if the systolic blood pressure remains above 100 mm Hg, IV sodium nitroprusside should be added. An arterial cannula should be inserted for continuous pressure monitoring, and urine output and mentation should be monitored to gauge the limits of blood pressure reduction. In general, patients with acute type A dissection obtain the maximal reduction in mortality from emergency surgical intervention, whereas patients with type B dissection are often managed more successfully with blood pressure control and serial imaging of the aorta.

Spontaneous Pneumothorax

I. EPIDEMIOLOGY

1. The classic presentation of spontaneous pneumothorax (not caused by iatrogenic, traumatic, or another precipitating factor) is chest pain associated with dyspnea. Primary spontaneous pneumothorax (PPTX) occurs in patients with no clinically apparent lung disease, whereas secondary spontaneous pneumothorax (SPTX) is a complication of preexisting lung disease. They have a similar incidence, approximately 6 cases per 100,000 men per year and 2 cases per 100,000 women per year.[54] Primary spontaneous pneumothorax typically occurs in males between the ages of 10 and 30 years and is rare after the age of 40. The patient is typically tall and thin, although no clear relation between body habitus and underlying pathophysiology has been shown. As mentioned previously, PPTX derives its name from the absence of clinical lung disease; however, thoracotomy or CT scanning shows that 80% to 100% of patients have subpleural bullae. An estimated 90% of patients are active cigarette smokers, and those who smoke more than one pack per day increase their risk of PPTX by 70- to 100-fold.[55] Secondary spontaneous pneumothorax usually occurs in patients over the age of 60, in parallel with the peak rate of chronic lung disease in the general population. The most common predisposing condition is chronic obstructive pulmonary disease; patients with an FEV_1 less than 1 L are at greatest risk. Other important predisposing conditions include *Pneumocystis carinii* pneumonia (PCP), interstitial lung diseases such as pulmonary sarcoidosis, connective tissue disease, and underlying lung cancer. The outcome of patients with PPTX and SPTX is quite different. In general, patients with PPTX have a benign clinical course, with an estimated case-fatality rate of 0.1%. Those with larger pneumothoraces or tension pneumothorax have greater cardiopulmonary embarrassment and represent a high-risk subset of patients with PPTX. In comparison, those with SPTX have a 20-fold increased risk of death, with an estimated 2% case-fatality rate. These patients are much more likely to have hypotension and significant hypoxemia at presentation. At particularly high risk are patients with SPTX and underlying PCP, as shown by an in-hospital mortality rate of 25% and a median survival of 3 months.[56]

II. CLINICAL PRESENTATION

1. The vast majority of patients with spontaneous pneumothorax have ipsilateral pleuritic chest pain or acute dyspnea that is abrupt in onset. Pleuritic pain may be more prevalent in primary than in secondary PTX. Dyspnea, which varies from mild to severe in primary PTX, is typically severe in secondary PTX. Symptoms associated with PPTX often resolve within 24 hours, even if untreated. This contrasts with the progressive nature of SPTX.

2. The physical findings in PPTX are variable and depend on the size of the pneumothorax. Patients with a PPTX occupying less than 15% of the hemithorax may have a normal physical examination. The most common features in these patients are tachycardia and tachypnea. Hypoxemia, found on either pulse oximetry or an arterial blood gas analysis, is uncommon because most patients have enough alveolar reserve to preserve oxygenation. An abnormal A-a gradient is more common and is often due largely to hypocapnia as a result of a rise in alveolar ventilation. As the size of the pneumothorax increases, the expected signs emerge, such as diminished breath sounds, decreased fremitus, and hyperresonance to percussion on the involved side. In contrast, patients with SPTX typically have hypoxemia and hypercapnia at presentation, reflecting both increased shunt and dead space physiology. The typical percussive and auscultatory findings are less reliable, especially in patients with severe chronic obstructive pulmonary disease. In either case hypotension with diminished breath sounds heralds tension pneumothorax, which warrants emergency attention.

III. DIAGNOSTICS

1. The diagnosis of pneumothorax is confirmed by the identification of a thin visceral pleural line that is displaced from the chest wall on a standard chest radiograph. In patients with severe emphysema and bullous disease the diseased areas of lung, or bullae, are hyperlucent and collapse to a lesser degree than normal areas of lung, making the pleural line more difficult to visualize. With a pneumothorax the pleural line runs parallel to and is convex toward the lateral chest wall, as opposed to the concave orientation of bullae. Any uncertainty about the diagnosis can be settled by a noncontrast CT scan of the chest. Arterial blood gas analysis may reveal hypoxemia, with accompanying respiratory alkalosis and acidosis in PPTX and SPTX, respectively.

IV. MANAGEMENT

1. Management of PTX should focus initially on evacuation of air from the pleural space, then on prevention of recurrence. Current therapeutic options include observation, supplemental oxygen, simple aspiration, tube thoracostomy, pleurodesis, thoracoscopy, and thoracotomy. No hard evidence has been presented to support many of these therapies and their indications, although expert consensus dictates that the size and type of the PTX, severity of the clinical presentation, and persistence of an air leak determine which approaches are used.[57] In the event of tension pneumothorax, emergency decompression is warranted, with insertion of an 18-gauge angiocatheter into the second intercostal space at the midclavicular line or into the fourth intercostal space at the anterior axillary line. Primary spontaneous pneumothorax occupying less than 15% of the

4

CHEST PAIN IN THE EMERGENCY DEPARTMENT

volume of the hemithorax can be treated with observation and supplemental oxygen. Supplemental oxygen creates a nitrogen diffusion gradient from the pleural space into pulmonary capillaries that accelerates the resorption of air from the pleural space by fourfold to sixfold. If the PPTX is greater than 15% of hemithorax volume, simple aspiration or tube thoracostomy is indicated. For simple aspiration a standard central venous catheter (or catheter from a thoracentesis kit) is inserted into the pleural space and the pleural air is evacuated manually, usually via a 60-mL syringe. Once the space is evacuated, as indicated by the inability to withdraw further air into the syringe, the catheter is clamped and a chest radiograph is obtained in 4 to 6 hours. The absence of PTX on follow-up chest radiograph equates to successful management, and in most circumstances these patients can be discharged with close outpatient follow-up. Alternatively, tube thoracostomy can be used to manage PPTX of greater than 15%, although most experts believe that this should be reserved for patients in whom aspiration is unsuccessful or who have recurrent PPTX. In contrast, chest tube insertion is recommended as the initial therapy for all patients with SPTX because of the risk of respiratory decline in these patients. In both PPTX and SPTX, routine application of suction to the chest tube is not necessary or appropriate, although it is indicated if a PTX fails to resolve when the chest tube is connected to water-seal drainage or to a one-way Heimlich valve. Recurrence can be prevented by chemical pleurodesis or surgery, with the particular approach tailored to the type of pneumothorax and its likelihood of recurrence. Special emphasis is placed on secondary prevention in patients with SPTX because of the seriousness of primary and recurrent events.

Esophageal Rupture

I. EPIDEMIOLOGY

1. Esophageal rupture is the least common cause of morbid chest pain. Esophageal rupture may be divided into spontaneous (Boerhaave's syndrome) and nonspontaneous causes. Although this condition is probably underreported, an estimated 300 cases have been reported worldwide, over half of which are iatrogenic in origin. Spontaneous or out-of-hospital perforations result from barogenic esophageal injury that has led to a transmural tear of the esophagus. This usually occurs at the left posterolateral wall of the esophagus, 2 to 3 cm superior to the gastroesophageal junction (weakest point of esophagus).

2. Esophageal rupture classically occurs in the midst of retching or vomiting, and the cause is postulated to be muscular incoordination that leads to failure of cricopharyngeus relaxation and critical elevations in intraesophageal pressure. Spontaneous rupture typically occurs in men over 50 years of age with a history of excessive dietary and alco-

hol intake. Occasionally patients have an underlying esophageal defect such as Barrett's esophagitis or, in immunocompromised patients, infectious ulcers. The nonspontaneous, or in-hospital, causes of esophageal rupture include medical instrumentation and paraesophageal surgery.

3. Iatrogenic cases of esophageal perforation are by far the most common. In both spontaneous and nonspontaneous cases the most powerful predictor of outcome is time between rupture and the diagnosis and definitive management. The overall mortality rate is 35%, but fatality rates increase to 50% if surgery is delayed more than 24 hours and to 90% if it is delayed more than 48 hours.[58]

II. CLINICAL PRESENTATION

1. Ruptured esophagus is almost always accompanied by chest discomfort, typically retrosternal and severe. Many patients report epigastric pain as well. In cases of out-of-hospital rupture the majority report a recent history of retching or vomiting, quite distinct from iatrogenic esophageal injury. Pain may radiate to the back or left shoulder and is often exacerbated by swallowing. Because of potential communication between the esophagus and the pleural cavity, patients may report a cough, or a cough precipitated by swallowing. Furthermore, patients may present with frank dyspnea or shock, especially if the presentation has been delayed more than 24 hours. Unfortunately, the physical examination is usually not helpful, especially if the patient is early in the course of the condition. Subcutaneous emphysema is an important finding, although present in only 30% of patients, and completes the Mackler triad (subcutaneous emphysema, vomiting, and lower thoracic pain). Signs of a pleural effusion may be present, usually on the left. At presentation patients may have abdominal rigidity or may have pneumoperitoneum caused by transdiaphragmatic rupture of the esophagus. Signs of clinical instability such as hypotension, tachycardia, and fever may reflect underlying sepsis and are more common in patients examined at least 24 hours after onset of rupture.

III. DIAGNOSTICS

A. CHEST RADIOGRAPHS, COMPUTED TOMOGRAPHY, AND ESOPHAGOGRAMS

1. A ruptured esophagus almost always produces abnormalities on routine chest radiographs. The most common finding is mediastinal air, at times accompanied by free peritoneal air, depending on whether the rupture has crossed the diaphragm. The presence of pneumopericardium is strongly suggestive of esophageal rupture and in combination with pneumomediastinum or pneumoperitoneum is virtually diagnostic. Unilateral left pleural effusion is commonly seen on radiographs. For practical reasons the next test ordered is often thoracic CT, which shows mediastinal air in virtually all cases. However, a

4

CHEST PAIN IN THE EMERGENCY DEPARTMENT

Gastrografin esophagogram is required for diagnostic confirmation and for precise localization of the tear so that a surgical approach can be determined. The use of barium is warranted only if the results of a water-soluble contrast study are negative and improved definition is sought. Laboratory findings are nonspecific, although presence of leukocytosis with a left shift is not uncommon. In addition, up to half of patients have a hematocrit value exceeding 50%, reflecting hemoconcentration caused by extracellular volume loss into pleural and tissue spaces. Pleural fluid analysis often reveals a pH less than 6 and an elevated amylase content.

IV. MANAGEMENT

1. Timely surgical intervention is crucial in the management of ruptured esophagus. The goals of surgery are primary repair of the esophagus, mediastinal débridement, and pleural drainage. Broad-spectrum intravenous antibiotics should be started as soon as the diagnosis is suspected. Aggressive volume resuscitation and vasopressor use may be warranted for a patient with severe systemic infection, especially when the treatment is being initiated more than 24 hours from onset.

PEARLS & PITFALLS

- Patients with chest discomfort should be evaluated first for the possibility of an ST elevation MI, aortic dissection, pulmonary embolus, or esophageal rupture.
- Blood pressure should be measured in both arms in the evaluation of patients with chest discomfort.

REFERENCES

[c] 1. Burt CW. Summary statistics for acute cardiac ischemia and chest pain visits to United States EDs, 1995-1996. Am J Emerg Med 1999; 17:552.

[c] 2. Hlatky MA. Evaluation of chest pain in the emergency department. N Engl J Med 1997; 337:1687.

[c] 3. Essentials of ACLS. In Cummins RO, editor. Advanced cardiac life support. Dallas: American Heart Association; 1997.

[b] 4. Weber JE, Hollander JE. Cocaine-associated chest pain: how common is myocardial infarction? Acad Emerg Med 2000; 7:873.

[c] 5. Wilson PW. Established risk factors and coronary artery disease: the Framingham Study. Am J Hypertens 1994; 7:7S.

[b] 6. Roncaglioni MC et al. Role of family history in patients with myocardial infarction: an Italian case-control study. GISSI-EFIRM Investigators. Circulation 1992; 85(6): 2065.

[b] 7. Ridker PM et al. C-reactive protein adds to the predictive value of total and HDL cholesterol in determining risk of first myocardial infarction. Circulation 1998; 97(20):2007.

[b] 8. Stampfer MJ et al. A prospective study of plasma homocysteine and risk of myocardial infarction in US physicians. JAMA 1992; 268(7):877.

[c] 9. Yeghiazarians Y et al. Unstable angina pectoris. N Engl J Med 2000; 342(2):101.

[c] 10. Popma JJ et al. Use of coronary revascularization in patients with unstable and non–ST segment elevation acute myocardial infarction. Am J Cardiol 2001; 88:25K.

[c] 11. Panju AA et al. Is this patient having a myocardial infarction? JAMA 1998; 280:1256.

[c] 12. Cohen MC et al. Meta-analysis of the morning excess of acute myocardial infarction and sudden cardiac death. Am J Cardiol 1997; 79:1512.

[a] 13. Goldman L et al. Prediction of the need for intensive care in patients who come to emergency departments with acute chest pain. N Engl J Med 1996; 334:1498.

[b] 14. Castrina FP. Unexplained noncardiac chest pain. Ann Intern Med 1997; 126:663.

[b] 15. Canto JG et al. Prevalence, clinical characteristics, and mortality among patients with myocardial infarction presenting without chest pain. JAMA 2000; 283:3223.

[b] 16. Welch RD et al. Prognostic value of a normal or nonspecific initial electrocardiogram in acute myocardial infarction. JAMA 2001; 286:1977.

[b] 17. Pope JH et al. Missed diagnoses of acute cardiac ischemia in the emergency department. N Engl J Med 2001; 342:1163.

[a] 18. Killip T, Kimball JT. Treatment of myocardial infarction in a coronary care unit. Am J Cardiol 1967; 20:457.

[c] 19. Brady WJ et al. Electrocardiographic manifestations: benign early repolarization. J Emerg Med 1999; 17(3):473.

[b] 20. Hathaway WR et al. Prognostic significance of the initial electrocardiogram in patients with acute myocardial infarction. JAMA 1998; 279:387.

[b] 21. Savonitto S et al. Prognostic value of the admission electrocardiogram in acute coronary syndromes. JAMA 1999; 281:707.

[b] 22. Kaul P et al. Prognostic value of ST segment depression in acute coronary syndromes. J Am Coll Cardiol 2001; 38(1):64.

[b] 23. Go AS et al. Bundle-branch block and in-hospital mortality in acute myocardial infarction. Ann Intern Med 1998; 129:690.

[b] 24. Hamm CW et al. Emergency room triage of patients with acute chest pain by means of rapid testing for cardiac troponin T or troponin I. N Engl J Med 1997; 337:1648.

[c] 25. Fleming SM, Daly KM. Cardiac troponins in suspected acute coronary syndrome: a meta-analysis of published trials. Cardiology 2001; 95:66.

[b] 26. Antman EM et al. Cardiac-specific troponin I levels predict the risk of mortality in patients with acute coronary syndromes. N Engl J Med 1996; 335:1342.

[a] 27. Cannon CP et al. Comparison of early invasive and conservative strategies in patients with unstable coronary syndromes treated with the glycoprotein IIb/IIIa inhibitor tirofiban. N Engl J Med 2001; 344:1879.

[b] 28. Martin GS et al. Cardiac troponin I accurately predicts myocardial injury in renal failure. Nephrol Dial Transplant 1998; 13:1709.

[b] 29. Aviles RJ et al. Troponin T levels in patients with acute coronary syndromes, with or without renal dysfunction. N Engl J Med 2002; 346:2047.

[b] 30. 1999 Update: ACC/AHA guidelines for the management of patients with acute myocardial infarction: executive summary and recommendations. Circulation 1999; 100:1016.

[d] 31. Antman EM et al. The TIMI risk score for unstable angina/non–ST elevation MI. JAMA 284:835.

[b] 32. ACC/AHA guidelines for the management of patients with unstable angina and non–ST elevation myocardial infarction: executive summary and recommendations. Circulation 2000; 102:1193.

[d] 33. Boersma E et al. Platelet glycoprotein IIb/IIIa inhibitors in acute coronary syndromes: a meta-analysis of all major randomized clinical trials. Lancet 2002; 359:189.

[c] 34. Goldhaber SZ. Pulmonary embolism. N Engl J Med 1998; 339:93.

[c] 35. Stein PD et al. Clinical, laboratory, roentgenographic, and electrocardiographic findings in patients with acute pulmonary embolism and no pre-existing cardiac or pulmonary disease. Chest 1991; 100:598.

[b] 36. Goldhaber SZ et al. Acute pulmonary embolism: clinical outcomes in the International Cooperative Pulmonary Embolism Registry (ICOPER). Lancet 1999; 353:1386.

[b] 37. Stein PD et al. History and physical examination in acute pulmonary embolism in patients without preexisting cardiac or pulmonary disease. Am J Cardiol 1981; 47:218.

[b] 38. Rodger MA et al. Diagnostic value of arterial blood gas measurement in suspected pulmonary embolism. Am J Respir Crit Care Med 2000; 162:2105.

[b] 39. Egermayer P et al. Usefulness of D-dimer, blood gas, and respiratory rate measurements for excluding pulmonary embolism. Thorax 1998; 53:830.

[b] 40. Perrier A et al. D-dimer testing for suspected pulmonary embolism in outpatients. Am J Respir Crit Care Med 1997; 156:492.

4

CHEST PAIN IN THE EMERGENCY DEPARTMENT

[b] 41. Lee AT et al. Clinical utility of a rapid whole-blood D-dimer assay in patients with cancer who present with suspected acute deep venous thrombosis. Ann Intern Med 1999; 131(6):417.

[b] 42. Giannitsis E et al. Independent prognostic value of cardiac troponin T in patients with confirmed pulmonary embolism. Circulation 2000; 102:211.

[b] 43. Meyer T et al. Cardiac troponin I elevation in acute pulmonary embolism is associated with right ventricular dysfunction. J Am Coll Cardiol 2000; 36(5):1632.

[a] 44. PIOPED Investigators. Value of the ventilation/perfusion scan in acute pulmonary embolism: results of the Prospective Investigation of Pulmonary Embolism Diagnosis (PIOPED). JAMA 1990; 263:2753.

[b] 45. Perrier A et al. Contribution of D-dimer plasma measurement and lower limb venous ultrasound to the diagnosis of pulmonary embolism. Am Heart J 1994;127(3):624.

[b] 46. Ryu JH et al. Diagnosis of pulmonary embolism with use of computed tomographic angiography. Mayo Clin Proc 2001; 76(1):59.

[b] 47. Swensen SJ et al. Outcomes after withholding anticoagulation from patients with suspected acute pulmonary embolism and negative computed tomographic findings: a cohort study. Mayo Clin Proc 2002; 77:130.

[d] 48. Hyers TM et al. Antithrombotic therapy for venous thromboembolic disease. Chest 2001;119:176S.

[c] 49. Dmowski AT et al. Aortic dissection. Am J Emerg Med 1999;17:372.

[b] 50. Hagan PG et al. The International Registry of Acute Aortic Dissection (IRAD). JAMA 2000; 283(7):897.

[b] 51. Hsue PY et al. Acute aortic dissection related to crack cocaine. Circulation 2002; 105:1592.

[b] 52. von Kodolitsch et al. Clinical prediction of acute aortic dissection. Arch Intern Med 2000; 160:2977.

[b] 53. Suzuki T et al. Diagnostic implications of elevated levels of smooth-muscle myosin heavy-chain protein in acute aortic dissection. Ann Intern Med 2000; 133(7):537.

[c] 54. Sahn SA, Heffner JE. Spontaneous pneumothorax. N Engl J Med 2000; 342(12):868.

[b] 55. Bense L et al. Smoking and the increased risk of contracting spontaneous pneumothorax. Chest 1987; 92(6):1009.

[c] 56. Trachiotis GD et al. Management of AIDS-related pneumothorax. Ann Thorac Surg 1996; 62:1608.

[c] 57. Baumann MH et al. Management of spontaneous pneumothorax: an American College of Chest Physicians Delphi Consensus Statement. Chest 2001; 119:590.

[c] 58. Pate JW et al. Spontaneous rupture of the esophagus: a 30-year experience. Ann Thorac Surg 1989; 47:689.

Acute Coronary Syndromes: Non–ST Elevation

Eric H. Yang, MD, Hossein Ardehali, MD, PhD, and Stephen C. Achuff, MD

FAST FACTS

- Acute coronary syndrome (ACS) is the current term used to describe patients with signs and symptoms compatible with acute, nonexertional myocardial ischemia. In the past, these individuals were described with terms such as unstable angina and Q wave or non–Q wave myocardial infarctions (see Chapter 4).
- Individuals with ACS are further classified as having ST-segment elevation ACS or non-ST-segment elevation ACS.
- Risk stratification is the most important task in the management of patients with non–ST elevation ACS.
- Use of glycoprotein IIb/IIIa inhibitors is recommended only for high- and intermediate-risk patients.
- Aggressive risk factor modification and secondary prevention with medical and nonmedical therapy should be applied to all patients in the post-ACS state.

I. EPIDEMIOLOGY

1. Cardiovascular disease is the leading cause of death in the United States and abroad. In 1997 alone, over 5 million Americans were evaluated in emergency departments for complaints of chest pain and approximately 15% of these individuals demonstrated evidence of a myocardial infarction.
2. With a greater understanding of the pathophysiology of cardiac chest discomfort in recent years, the term "acute coronary syndrome (ACS)" has been adopted to include patients with signs and symptoms consistent with acute, nonexertional myocardial ischemia. This revised term illustrates that most episodes of myocardial ischemia are initiated by an unstable ruptured plaque and replaces prior "labels" used in this condition such as unstable angina and Q wave or non–Q wave myocardial infarction (MI).
3. The management of patients with ACS varies depending on the electrocardiogram (ECG). Patients with ST elevations (previously referred to as Q wave MI) demonstrate evidence of transmural myocardial injury and are at particularly high risk of 30-day death and morbidity. These individuals are treated aggressively (see Chapter 6). Individuals without ST elevations (includes those previously noted as non–Q wave MI or unstable angina) are thought to have nontransmural myocardial injury and are at lower risk of 30-day

mortality. Treatment of these patients is individualized based on risk stratification.

4. The approach to the management of non–ST elevation ACS is shown in Fig. 5-1. The diagnosis and management of non–ST elevation ACS are the focus of this chapter.

II. CLINICAL PRESENTATION

1. A careful history is the most important tool for diagnosing ACS. Specific factors that suggest ACS rather than stable angina include the following (Table 5-1).

2. **Quality and frequency of chest discomfort:** Chest discomfort that is more severe than the patient's "usual chest pain" or is occurring more frequently suggests ACS. Some patients with ACS have frequent and repetitive chest pain that becomes more severe with each episode.

3. **Rest pain:** Chest discomfort that usually has occurred only with exertion but now occurs at rest or with minimal activity is suggestive of an ACS.

4. **Duration of chest pain:** Stable angina rarely causes chest discomfort lasting longer than 10 to 15 minutes. Therefore chest pain that lasts longer is more likely to be ACS.

5. **Prior cardiac history:** Patients with a recent myocardial infarction or coronary intervention (either percutaneous or surgical) who develop chest pain within 2 months of the initial event have ACS until proven otherwise.

6. **Associated symptoms:** Diaphoresis, shortness of breath, palpitations, or nausea usually accompanies chest pain caused by an ACS.

III. DIAGNOSTICS

1. All patients being evaluated for an ACS should be placed on a cardiac monitor and have a 12-lead ECG performed as soon as possible. ECG should be repetitively obtained with changes in complaints of chest discomfort. Blood work should also be sent for a comprehensive metabolic panel, troponin level, fractionated creatine kinases (CK), complete blood count, and prothrombin and activated partial thromboplastin times. A chest radiograph, urinalysis, and careful physical examination including assessment of the blood pressure in both arms should also be performed. Risk stratification of the patient should then be employed.

A. ELECTROCARDIOGRAM

1. Patients with non–ST segment elevation ACS may initially have a normal ECG or nonspecific ST-T wave changes. Although a normal ECG cannot be used to exclude this diagnosis, ST segment depressions of greater than 1 mm in two or more contiguous limb leads (or >2 mm in two or more contiguous precordial leads) are considered to be a predictor of an increased risk for adverse cardiac events.

2. A 12-lead ECG should be obtained immediately or within 10 minutes of presentation for every patient with signs and symptoms suggestive

TABLE 5-1
LIKELIHOOD THAT SIGNS AND SYMPTOMS REPRESENT AN ACUTE CORONARY SYNDROME RESULTING FROM CORONARY ARTERY DISEASE

Feature	High Likelihood (Any of the Following)	Intermediate Likelihood (Absence of High-Likelihood Features and Presence of Any of the Following)	Low Likelihood (Absence of High- or Intermediate-Likelihood Features but May Have Any of the Following)
History	Chest or left arm pain or discomfort as chief symptom reproducing prior documented angina; known history of coronary artery disease, including myocardial infarction	Chest or left arm pain or discomfort as chief symptom; age >70 years; male sex; diabetes mellitus	Probable ischemic symptoms in absence of any of the intermediate-likelihood characteristics; recent cocaine use
Examination	Transient MR, hypotension, diaphoresis, pulmonary edema, or rales	Extracardiac vascular disease	Chest discomfort reproduced by palpation
ECG	New, or presumably new, transient ST segment deviation (≥0.05 mV) or T wave inversion (≥0.2 mV) with symptoms	Fixed Q waves; abnormal ST segments or T waves not documented to be new	T wave flattening or inversion in leads with dominant R waves; normal ECG
Cardiac markers	Elevated cardiac TnI, TnT, or CK-MB	Normal	Normal

From Braunwald E et al. Unstable angina: diagnosis and management. Rockville, Md: Agency for Health Care Policy and Research and the National Heart, Lung and Blood Institute, U.S. Public Health Service, U.S. Department of Health and Human Services; 1994; AHCPR Pub No 94-0602.
CK-MB, Creatine kinase, myocardial bound; *ECG*, electrocardiogram; *TnI*, troponin I; *TnT*, troponin T.

ACUTE CORONARY SYNDROMES: NON–ST ELEVATION 5

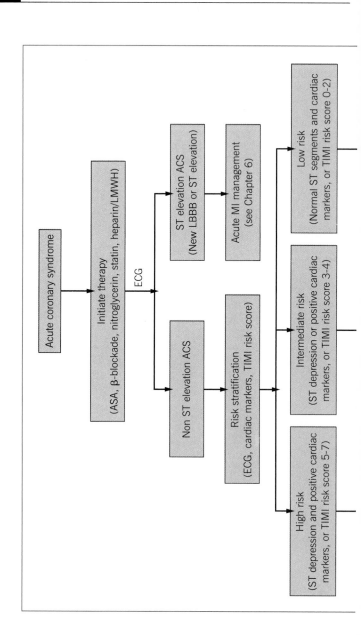

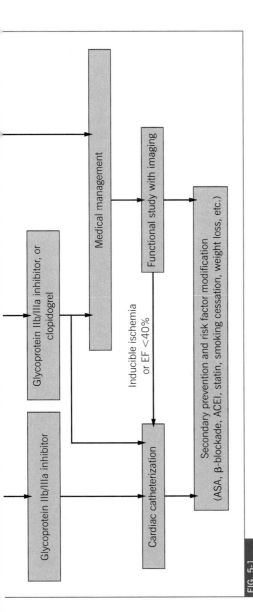

FIG. 5-1

Management of acute coronary syndrome. The TIMI risk score calculation appears in Box 5-1. Abciximab should not be used for patients who are not expected to undergo immediate catheterization. *ASA,* Aspirin; *ACEI,* ACE inhibitor; *ECG,* electrocardiogram; *EF,* ejection fraction; *LBBB,* left bundle branch block; *LMWH,* low molecular weight heparin.

ACUTE CORONARY SYNDROMES: NON–ST ELEVATION 5

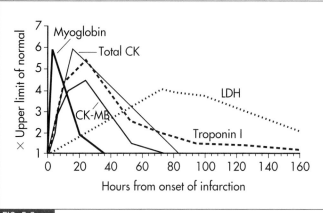

FIG. 5-2

Time course of elevations of serum markers after acute myocardial infarction (AMI). This figure summarizes the relative timing, rate of rise, peak values, and duration of elevation above the upper limit of normal for multiple serum markers after AMI. Although traditionally total creatine kinase (CK), myocardial bound creatine kinase (CK-MB), and lactic dehydrogenase (LDH) (with isoenzymes) are measured, the relatively slow rate of rise above normal for CK and the potential confusion with noncardiac sources of enzyme release for both total CK and LDH have inspired the search for additional serum markers. The smaller molecule myoglobin is released quickly from infarcted myocardium but is not cardiac specific. Therefore elevations of myoglobin that may be detected quite early after the onset of infarction require confirmation with a more cardiac-specific marker such as CK-MB or troponin I. Troponin I (and troponin T; not shown) rises more slowly than myoglobin and may be useful for diagnosis of infarction even up to 3 to 4 days after the event. Assays for cardiac-specific troponin I and troponin T using monoclonal antibodies are now available. *(From Antman EM. General hospital management. In Julian DG, Braunwald E, eds. Management of acute myocardial infarction. London: WB Saunders; 1994.)*

of myocardial ischemia. Obtaining a previous ECG (if available) for comparison is desirable. In patients with active chest discomfort, repeating the ECG once the discomfort has resolved may also be helpful in looking for the presence of dynamic ST-T wave changes.

B. CARDIAC BIOMARKERS

1. Biomarkers for cardiac necrosis are helpful in risk stratification and further categorization ischemia or myocardial infarction in patients with non–ST segment elevation ACS. Because all biomarkers are delayed in reaching elevated levels from the time of injury, individuals with non–ST segment elevation ACS may have normal values at presentation (Fig. 5-2 and Table 5-2). The traditional markers have

TABLE 5-2
MOLECULAR MARKERS USED OR PROPOSED FOR USE IN THE DIAGNOSIS OF ACUTE MYOCARDIAL INFARCTION

Marker	Molecular Weight (daltons)	Range of Times to Initial Elevation (hr)	Mean Time to Peak Elevations (Nonthrombolysis)	Time to Return to Normal Range	Most Common Sampling Schedule
Hfabp	14,000-15,000	1.5	5-10 hr	24 hr	On presentation, then 4 hr later
Myoglobin	17,800	1-4	6-7 hr	24 hr	Frequent; 1-2 hr after CP
MLC	19,000-27,000	6-12	2-4 days	6-12 days	Once at least 12 hr after CP
cTnI	23,500	3-12	24 hr	5-10 days	Once at least 12 hr after CP
cTnT	33,000	3-12	12 hr-2 days	5-14 days	Once at least 12 hr after CP
MB-CK	86,000	3-12	24 hr	48-72 hr	Every 12 hr × 3*
MM-CK tissue isoform	86,000	1-6	12 hr	38 hr	60-90 min after CP
MB-CK tissue isoform	86,000	2-6	18 hr	Unknown	60-90 min after CP
Enolase	90,000	6-10	24 hr	48 hr	Every 12 hr × 3
LD	135,000	10	24-48 hr	10-14 days	Once at least 24 hr after CP
MHC	400,000	48	5-6 days	14 days	Once at least 2 days after CP

Modified from Adams J III, Abendschein D, Jaffe A. Circulation 1993; 88:750. In Braunwald E: Heart disease: a textbook of cardiovascular medicine, 5th ed. Philadelphia: WB Saunders; 1996.
CP, Chest pain; *cTnI*, cardiac troponin I; *cTnT*, cardiac troponin T; *Hfabp*, heart fatty acid binding proteins; *LD*, lactate dehydrogenase; *MB-CK*, MB isoenzyme of creatine kinase; *MHC*, myosin heavy chain; *MLC*, myosin light chain; *MM-CK*, MM isoenzyme of creatine kinase.
*Increased sensitivity can be achieved with sampling every 6 or 8 hours.

ACUTE CORONARY SYNDROMES: NON–ST ELEVATION 5

included CK, troponins, and myoglobin. Based on current guidelines the cardiac-specific troponins such as troponin T and troponin I are the preferred markers. Troponin T is typically detectable in the serum within 3 to 4 hours after myocardial injury has occurred and remains elevated for about 7 to 10 days. Although this protein is cardiac specific, levels can also be elevated in the setting of renal dysfunction. Troponin I is typically released into the circulation within 4 to 6 hours from the time of injury, and the level stays elevated for 7 to 10 days as well. These levels are less likely to be elevated in the setting of renal dysfunction. It is recommended that blood be drawn immediately at the time of presentation and a repeat level obtained 8 hours after presentation.

2. CK exists in three isoforms, of which CK-MB is the cardiac-specific component. Although once thought to be the gold standard for determining the presence of myocardial necrosis and infarction, CK-MB can be significantly affected by a number of conditions such as trauma, surgery, rhabdomyolysis, sepsis, or renal dysfunction. CK-MB levels typically are elevated approximately 3 to 6 hours from the time of myocardial injury, peaking at 12 to 24 hours and returning to normal levels within 2 to 3 days. Traditionally, CK-MB levels are measured immediately at the time of presentation and repeated at 6 hours and 12 hours from the time of presentation.

3. Myoglobin is a highly sensitive marker of muscle damage. Levels begin to increase within 1 to 2 hours from the time of myocardial injury, making it the first protein to be released into the circulation. Unfortunately, the specificity is low because myoglobin can be elevated in other conditions such as skeletal muscle injury, trauma, intramuscular injections, alcohol abuse, hypothermia or hyperthermia, and renal dysfunction.

C. RISK STRATIFICATION

1. Risk stratification is an integral component in the management of patients with non–ST segment elevation ACS. Stratification is essential because not all patients with ACS are equally likely to have adverse cardiac events. Therapy must therefore be tailored based on the risk of adverse outcomes. As shown in Fig. 5-1, patients are classified as being at high risk, intermediate risk, or low risk. The following two clinical tools can help the clinician decide how to risk stratify patients.

a. Electrocardiogram and cardiac biomarkers: As stated previously, ST segment depression and elevated cardiac biomarkers are associated with a higher risk of adverse outcomes. Patients with both ST segment depression and elevated markers are considered to be at high risk. Those with only one of the two factors are classified as being at intermediate risk, and those with neither of the factors can be considered to be at low risk. A list of additional factors the American Heart Association has adopted in assisting with risk stratification is provided in Table 5-3.

TABLE 5-3

SHORT-TERM RISK OF DEATH OR NONFATAL MYOCARDIAL INFARCTION IN PATIENTS WITH UNSTABLE ANGINA

Feature	High Likelihood (At Least One of the Following Features Must Be Present)	Intermediate Likelihood (No High-Risk Feature But Must Have One of the Following)	Low Likelihood (No High- or Intermediate-Risk Feature but May Have Any of the Following)
History	Accelerating tempo of ischemic symptoms in preceding 48 hr	Prior MI, peripheral or cerebrovascular disease, or CABG; prior aspirin use	New-onset or progressive CCS class III or IV angina for past 2 wk without prolonged (>20 min) rest pain but with moderate or high likelihood of CAD (see Table 5-1)
Character of pain	Prolonged ongoing (>20 min) rest pain	Prolonged (>20 min) rest angina, now re-solved, with moderate or high likelihood of CAD; rest angina (<20 min) or relieved with rest or sublingual NTG	
Clinical findings	Pulmonary edema, most likely due to isch-emia; new or worsening MR murmur; S₃ or new or worsening rales; hypotension, bradycardia, tachycardia; age >75 yr	Age >70 yr	
ECG	Angina at rest with transient ST segment changes >0.05 mV; bundle branch block, new or presumed new; sustained ventricular tachycardia	T wave inversions >0.2 mV; pathological Q waves	Normal or unchanged ECG during an episode of chest discomfort
Cardiac markers	Elevated cardiac TnI, TnT, or CK-MB	Slightly elevated (e.g., TnT >0.01 but <0.1 ng/mL)	Normal

Modified from AHCPR Clinical Practice Guideline No. 10. Unstable Angina: Diagnosis and Management. Rockville, Md: Agency for Health Care Policy and Research and the National Heart, Lung and Blood Institute, U.S. Public Health Service, U.S. Department of Health and Human Services; 1994; AHCPR Pub No 94-0602.

CABG, Coronary artery bypass grafting; *CAD*, coronary artery disease; *CCS*, Canadian Cardiovascular Society; *CK-MB*, creatine kinase, myocardial bound; *ECG*, electrocardiogram; *NTG*, nitroglycerin; *TnI*, troponin I; *TnT*, troponin T.

ACUTE CORONARY SYNDROMES: NON–ST ELEVATION | 5

BOX 5-1

TIMI RISK FACTOR SCORE

RISK FACTORS

1. Age >65 years
2. Three or more risk factors for coronary artery disease
3. Prior coronary stenosis ≥50%
4. Two or more anginal events in past 24 hours
5. Aspirin use in past 7 days
6. ST segment changes
7. Positive cardiac markers

RISK OF ADVERSE CARDIAC EVENT*

Number of Risk Factors	Risk (%)
0-1	4.7
2	8.3
3	13.2
4	19.9
5	26.2
6-7	41.0

*Defined as myocardial infarction, cardiac-related death, or persistent ischemia. Low risk = score 0-2; intermediate risk = score 3-4; high risk = score 5-7.

b. TIMI risk score: ECG and cardiac biomarkers are helpful objective measures of adverse outcomes, but they do not consider important subjective markers that are also associated with adverse outcomes. The TIMI risk factor score was developed to help clinicians predict the probability of adverse cardiac outcomes in patients with non–ST elevation ACS.[1] The seven factors and the likelihood of an adverse cardiac event (myocardial infarction, cardiac death, or persistent ischemia) appear in Box 5-1. Patients with a score of less than 3 are at low risk, those with a score of 3 or 4 are at intermediate risk, and those with a score of 5 or higher are considered at high risk.

IV. MANAGEMENT

1. The management of patients with non–ST elevation ACS is shown in Fig. 5-1 and is based on risk stratification. All patients are initially treated with aspirin, β-blockers, nitrates, and heparin unless contrain-dications exist. Once these therapies are initiated, the first decision is whether or not the patient should receive a glycoprotein IIb/IIIa in-hibitor. The next decision is whether the patient should undergo an early invasive or a noninvasive management strategy.

2. If the noninvasive management strategy is chosen and there is no evidence of myocardial necrosis (elevation in cardiac biomarkers) after 6 to 12 hours from the time chest discomfort began, a noninvasive

TABLE 5-4			
PROPERTIES OF β-BLOCKERS IN CLINICAL USE			
Drug	Selectivity	Partial Agonist Activity	Usual Dose for Angina
Propranolol	None	No	20-80 mg bid
Metoprolol	β_1	No	50-200 mg bid
Atenolol	β_1	No	50-200 mg/day
Nadolol	None	No	40-80 mg/day
Timolol	None	No	10 mg bid
Acebutolol	β_1	Yes	200-600 mg bid
Betaxolol	β_1	No	10-20 mg/day
Bisoprolol	β_1	No	10 mg/day
Esmolol (intravenous)	β_1	No	50-300 $\mu g \cdot kg^{-1} \cdot min^{-1}$
Labetalol*	None	Yes	200-600 mg bid
Pindolol	None	Yes	2.5-7.5 mg tid

Modified from Gibbons RJ et al. J Am Coll Cardiol 1999; 33:2092. In Hazinski MF, Cummins RO, Field JM, eds. 2000 Handbook of emergency cardiovascular care for health care providers. Dallas: American Heart Association; 2000.
*Labetalol is a combined α- and β-blocker.

stress test to investigate the presence of inducible ischemia is a reasonable approach. Depending on the results of this test, consideration can then be given to cardiac catheterization. For patients who demonstrate evidence of myocardial necrosis on routine assessment of the patient's cardiac biomarkers, most cardiologists would recommend subsequent evaluation by cardiac catheterization.

3. **Aspirin:** Platelet aggregation plays an important role in the pathophysiology of ACS. Plaque rupture initiates the clotting cascade, which stimulates platelet aggregation. Thromboxane is a mediator that helps activate platelets. The synthesis of thromboxane is inhibited by aspirin. Aspirin should be given as soon as possible in the emergency department. The dose can be either four 81-mg tablets or one 325-mg tablet. The pills should be crushed, and enteric-coated pills should not be used. Patients with an aspirin allergy can be given clopidogrel (see later discussion). Ticlopidine should not be used in place of clopidogrel because it has a slow onset of action.

4. **β-Blockers** (Table 5-4): β-Blockers help to reduce myocardial oxygen demand by exerting negative inotropic and chronotropic effects. They also offer protection against cardiac arrhythmias. Metoprolol is usually the drug of choice because of its β_1-selective activity. It is initially given as an IV bolus of 5 mg. If tolerated, the 5-mg dose is repeated at 10-minute intervals for a maximum dose of 15 mg. The patient is then started on orally administered metoprolol. The goal mean arterial pressure (MAP) is 60 to 70 mm Hg with a heart rate of about 60 beats/min. If these hemodynamic goals are not tolerated, the lowest possible MAP and pulse should be obtained. Patients with proven adverse

TABLE 5-5			
NITROGLYCERIN AND NITRATES IN ANGINA			
Compound	Route	Dose/Dosage	Duration of Effect
Nitroglycerin	Sublingual tablets	0.3-0.6 mg up to 1.5 mg	1-7 min
	Spray	0.4 mg as needed	Similar to sublingual tablets
	Transdermal	0.2-0.8 mg/hr q12h	8-12 hr during intermittent therapy
	Intravenous	5-200 mg/min	Tolerance in 7-8 hr
Isosorbide dinitrate	Oral	5-80 mg bid or tid	Up to 8 hr
	Oral, slow release	40 mg qd or bid	Up to 8 hr
Isosorbide mononitrate	Oral	20 mg bid	12-24 hr
	Oral, slow release	60-240 mg once daily	
Pentaerythritol tetranitrate	Sublingual	10 mg as needed	Not known
Erythritol tetranitrate	Sublingual	5-10 mg as needed	Not known
	Oral	10-30 mg tid	Not known

Modified from Gibbons RJ et al. J Am Coll Cardiol 1999; 33:2092. In Hazinski MF, Cummins RO, Field JM, eds. 2000 Handbook of emergency cardiovascular care for health care providers. Dallas: American Heart Association; 2000.

reactions to β-blockers or those at high risk for adverse reactions can be given diltiazem or verapamil.

5. **Nitrates (Table 5-5):** Nitrates reduce myocardial oxygen demand by reducing preload. They also enhance coronary vasodilatation, resulting in improved blood flow. Sublingual nitroglycerin tablets or spray should be used initially if the patient is not hypotensive and has no other contraindications to these agents, such as use of sildenafil in the previous 24 hours. If the patient's chest discomfort does not resolve after three 0.4-mg nitroglycerin tablets with each given 5 minutes apart, the physician should consider initiating an intravenous nitroglycerin drip. After initiation at 10 μg/min the drip should be titrated upward by 10 μg every 3 to 5 minutes until the patient's discomfort resolves or the mean arterial blood pressure drops below 25% of initial values in an initially hypertensive patient (or the systolic blood pressure drops below 110 mm Hg in a previously normotensive patient). Once a steady dose of intravenous nitroglycerin has been achieved, the medication can be continued for up to 2 to 4 weeks, usually without concern for increasing methemoglobin levels.[2] Common side effects include hypotension and headaches. A reflex tachycardia can also occur in patients not given β-blockers or other negative chronotropic therapy.

6. **Heparin.**

a. Plaque rupture exposes tissue factor, which initiates the clotting cascade. Anticoagulation with heparin is therefore important in the management of chest pain. Patients with coronary pain other than stable angina should receive anticoagulation with heparin unless a major contraindication exists. Two forms of heparin can be used: unfractionated heparin and low molecular weight heparin. Patients with a history of heparin-induced thrombocytopenia who need anticoagulation can be given lepirudin, a direct thrombin inhibitor administered as a bolus of 0.4 mg/kg followed by an infusion of 0.15 mg/kg/hr with a goal-activated partial thromboplastin time (aPTT) of 1.5 to 2.5 times the upper limit of normal.

b. Unfractionated heparin is initiated as an IV bolus followed by a continuous infusion. The American Heart Association recommends a weight-based dosage regimen consisting of a bolus of 60 to 70 U/kg (maximum 5000 U) followed by a maintenance dose of 12 to 15 U/kg/hr. The aPTT should be measured 6 hours after every dose adjustment. The drip should be adjusted to reach a goal aPTT ratio of 2 to 2.5 times the upper limit of normal. Patients who receive glycoprotein IIb/IIIa inhibitors should be maintained with a heparin drip having a lower aPTT goal (1.8 to 2 times the upper end of normal) to minimize the risk of bleeding.

c. In recent years the use of low molecular weight heparins in clinical situations has been increasing. Enoxaparin at a dose of 1 mg/kg bid subcutaneously has been shown to be as effective as unfractionated heparin in ACS.[3,4] Like the other low molecular weight heparins, enoxaparin is easy to use, quickly reaches a therapeutic level, and does not require frequent aPTT assays. Enoxaparin, however, has a long half-life, and its therapeutic effect cannot be quickly reversed. Therefore enoxaparin may not be the best choice in patients who will undergo emergency cardiac catheterization or who may require quick reversal of anticoagulation. Limited data are available regarding the use of low molecular weight heparin in conjunction with the glycoprotein IIb/IIIa inhibitors. Caution should be exercised when using these medications in patients with renal failure or obesity (weight >120 kg).

7. **Glycoprotein IIb/IIIa receptor inhibitors:** The final pathway in platelet activation is expression of the glycoprotein IIb/IIIa receptor, which allows platelets to bind to fibrinogen and von Willebrand factor. Three glycoprotein IIb/IIIa inhibitors are used in the United States: abciximab, a monoclonal antibody against the IIb/IIIa receptor; tirofiban, a nonpeptide inhibitor; and eptifibatide, a cyclic peptide inhibitor. Several studies have shown the clinical efficacy of eptifibatide and tirofiban in the setting of ACS.[5-7] Subgroup analysis of the data in these studies has revealed that the greatest clinical benefit occurs in high- and intermediate-risk patients. Results from a large-scale randomized trial suggest that abciximab should not be given to patients with an ACS who are not expected to undergo early revascularization with percutaneous coronary intervention.[8] These patients should be given either tirofiban or eptifibatide.

5

ACUTE CORONARY SYNDROMES: NON–ST ELEVATION

8. **Early percutaneous coronary revascularization:** Since the pathophysiology of an ACS involves platelet aggregation and clot formation, early use of percutaneous coronary intervention is a potential therapy to prevent total occlusion and progression toward transmural myocardial injury. Two large-scale, randomized, prospective studies have shown clinical benefit of the use of an early invasive strategy in conjunction with aggressive medical management.[9,10] Subgroup analysis of these two studies has shown that high- and intermediate-risk patients benefit the most from an early invasive strategy. Low-risk patients with abnormal systolic function (ejection fraction <40%) have also been shown to benefit from revascularization. The American Heart Association guidelines on non–ST elevation ACS recommend that these patients undergo cardiac catheterization on a nonemergency basis.[11] An early noninvasive strategy followed by a stress test with imaging can be used as an alternative approach in patients at intermediate risk. Thrombolytics have not been shown to be effective in the management of non–ST elevation ACS.

9. **Stress test with imaging:** Patients with an ACS who are treated with a noninvasive strategy and do not demonstrate evidence of myocardial necrosis after careful laboratory evaluation should undergo inpatient stress testing with imaging. For patients who demonstrate evidence of myocardial necrosis, most cardiologists would recommend initial evaluation with a cardiac catheterization.

10. **Early use of HMG-CoA reductase inhibitors:** These agents, known simply as the "statins," offer therapeutic benefits in addition to their lipid-lowering activity. The statins have been shown to have antiplatelet as well as antioxidant activity, which makes them potentially useful for the acute management of patients with ACS. One prospective randomized trial, as well as a retrospective trial, has shown that these agents offer some benefit in the acute management of ACS.[12,13] Although further studies are needed, use of statins in the acute management of ACS may offer protection against adverse cardiac events and should be considered.

11. **Clopidogrel:** Thienopyridines are agents that inhibit the adenosine diphosphate–mediated activation of platelets. Clopidogrel, unlike the other thienopyridine ticlopidine, has a quick onset of action with immediate platelet inhibition. The use of clopidogrel in non–ST elevation ACS was assessed in a large-scale randomized trial involving 12,000 patients with an ACS who would not be undergoing emergency cardiac catheterization.[14] Patients treated with clopidogrel (300 mg PO loading dose followed by 75 mg PO qd) in addition to aspirin had a 20% relative risk reduction in major adverse cardiac events. Clopidogrel use also resulted in more bleeding complications.

   At this time the role of clopidogrel in the acute management of non–ST elevation ACS is unclear. This uncertainty centers on whether clopidogrel should be used in place of or in conjunction with the more potent glycoprotein IIb/IIIa inhibitors. We believe that clopidogrel should be used as an alternative to glycoprotein IIb/IIIa inhibitors in patients not undergoing cardiac catheterization. Further studies comparing clopidogrel alone or in conjunction with the IIb/IIIa inhibitors in high- and intermediate-risk patients are needed to clarify the role of clopidogrel.

12. **Post–acute coronary syndrome treatment:** The management of an ACS should be aggressive in both the acute and the post-ACS setting. Once stabilized, patients with an ACS should undergo risk factor modification followed by the initiation of medications for secondary prevention (see Chapter 9). Risk factor modification should include aggressive smoking cessation and dietary counseling. Patients should be encouraged to increase the amount of weekly exercise and to undergo weight loss if needed. Diabetic patients should maintain tight glucose control. Secondary prevention medications, including angiotensin-converting enzyme inhibitors, β-blockers, aspirin, and lipid-lowering agents, should be initiated. Patients who underwent stent placement should be given a 30-day course of clopidogrel.

PEARLS AND PITFALLS

- Non–ST elevation ACS encompasses the two prior terms "unstable angina" and "non–Q wave MI."
- Patients with an ACS at presentation should be questioned about a history of cocaine or sildenafil use.
- For patients with heparin allergies or heparin-induced thrombocytopenia who need anticoagulation, lepirudin or another type of direct thrombin inhibitor should be initiated.
- β_1-Selective β-blockers can be safely used in patients with a history of mild to moderate obstructive pulmonary disease.[15]

REFERENCES

[b] 1. Antman E et al. The TIMI risk score for unstable angina/non-ST elevation MI: a method for prognostication and therapeutic decision making. JAMA 2000; 284:835.

[d] 2. ACC/AHA 2002 guideline update for the management of patients with unstable angina and non–ST-segment elevation myocardial infarction. www.americanheart.org.

[d] 3. Antman E et al. Enoxaparin prevents death and cardiac ischemic events in unstable angina/non–Q wave myocardial infarction. Circulation 1999; 100:1593.

[a] 4. Cohen M et al. A comparison of low–molecular weight heparin with unfractionated heparin for unstable coronary disease. N Engl J Med 1997; 337:447.

[a] 5. Platelet Receptor Inhibition in Ischemic Syndrome Management (PRISM) Study Investigators: A comparison of aspirin plus tirofiban with aspirin plus heparin for unstable angina. N Engl J Med 1998; 338:1498.

[a] 6. PRISM-PLUS Investigators. Inhibition of the platelet glycoprotein IIb/IIIa receptor with tirofiban in unstable angina and non-Q-wave myocardial infarction. N Engl J Med 1998, 338:1488.

[a] 7. PURSUIT Investigators. Inhibition of platelet glycoprotein IIb/IIIa with eftifibatide in patients with acute coronary syndromes. N Engl J Med 1998, 339:436.

[a] 8. Simoons M. Effect of glycoprotein IIb/IIIa receptor blocker abciximab on outcome in patients with acute coronary syndromes without early coronary revascularisation: the GUSTO IV-ACS randomised trial. Lancet 2001; 357; 9272:1915.

[a] 9. Fragmin and Fast Revascularisation During Instability in Coronary Artery Disease (FRISC II) Investigators. Invasive compared with non-invasive treatment in unstable coronary-artery disease: FRISC II prospective randomised multicentre study. Lancet 1999; 354:708.

[a] 10. Cannon C et al. Tactics—TIMI 18. N Engl J Med 2001; 344:1879.

[c] 11. ACC/AHA guidelines for the management of patients with unstable angina and non–ST-segment elevation myocardial infarction: executive summary and recommendations: a report of the American College of Cardiology/American Heart Association Task Force on Practice Guideline Committee on the Management of Patients with Unstable Angina. Circulation 2000; 102:1193.

[a] 12. Schwartz G et al. Effects of atorvastatin on early recurrent ischemic events in acute coronary syndromes: the MIRACL study. JAMA 2001; 285:1711.

[b] 13. Stenestrand U et al. Early statin treatment following acute myocardial infarction and 1 year survival. JAMA 2001; 285:430.

[a] 14. Mehta S et al. The clopidogrel in unstable angina to prevent recurrent events (CURE) trial. N Engl J Med 2001; 345:494.

[c] 15. Salpeter SR et al. Cardioselective β-blockers in patients with reactive airway disease: a meta-analysis. Ann Intern Med 2002; 137:715.

Acute Coronary Syndromes: ST Elevation

James O. Mudd, MD, Richard Waters, MD, and Mark Kelemen, MD

6

FAST FACTS

- The electrocardiographic (ECG) diagnosis of ST elevation acute coronary syndrome (ACS) is defined by greater than 1 mm of ST elevation in two limb leads, greater than 2 mm of ST elevation in two precordial leads, or a new or presumed new left bundle branch block (LBBB).
- Time is of great consequence once a diagnosis of ST elevation ACS is made, and obtaining prompt reperfusion of the infarct-related artery (IRA) is essential.
- Current treatment recommendations for ST elevation ACS include thrombolytic therapy within 30 minutes or percutaneous coronary intervention (PCI) within 90 minutes.
- Primary PCI is associated with less bleeding and more favorable outcomes than thrombolytic therapy when performed in high-volume, skilled centers.
- Use of glycoprotein IIb/IIIa receptor antagonists with primary PCI appears to reduce the need for repeat revascularization procedures.

I. EPIDEMIOLOGY

1. Acute myocardial infarction (AMI) affects approximately 800,000 individuals annually in the United States. Unfortunately, over 200,000 people will die without receiving medical evaluation. This fact underscores the need for ongoing public education efforts and improved triage systems to enable more thorough and efficient delivery of potentially life-saving therapy.

II. CLINICAL PRESENTATION

1. The most important tools in the diagnosis of an ACS are the history, physical examination, and ECG. The cardinal symptom of myocardial infarction is retrosternal or left-sided chest pain, typically described as severe, crushing, or constricting. It is commonly associated with dyspnea (40%) or diaphoresis (25%) and can radiate to the neck, jaw, left shoulder, and upper arm. The pain is gradual in onset, and the peak intensity may not occur for several minutes. The duration of chest discomfort in acute infarction is usually longer than 30 minutes and may last hours. Elderly patients often have atypical presenting features. See Chapters 4 and 5 for details.

III. DIAGNOSTICS

1. The ECG helps differentiate ST elevation ACS from non–ST elevation ACS. Making this distinction is vital because treatment differs considerably between the two syndromes.

2. The current ECG criteria for the diagnosis of ST elevation ACS require greater than 1 mm ST elevation in two or more anatomically contiguous limb leads, greater than 2 mm ST elevation in two or more anatomically contiguous precordial leads, or a new or presumed new LBBB.

3. Careful serial ECG analysis is essential because a suspected non–ST elevation ACS may evolve into an ST elevation ACS.

4. When the ECG meets ST-elevation ACS criteria, the patient becomes eligible for acute reperfusion therapy. The current recommendations are to administer thrombolytic therapy within 30 minutes or perform PCI within 90 minutes of diagnosis.

IV. MANAGEMENT

A. RISK STRATIFICATION

1. As with all forms of ACS, immediate risk stratification is crucial in patient management.

2. A classification scheme, developed in the late 1960s by Killip and Kimble, is based on the link between heart failure and patient outcome.[1] This early risk stratification guide consisted of four classes: class I, no signs of heart failure; class II, rales, S_3 gallop, and jugular venous distention; class III, severe heart failure with frank pulmonary edema; and class IV, cardiogenic shock with systolic blood pressure less than 90 mm Hg. Many studies have validated the Killip classification with short- and long-term mortality after myocardial infarction (MI).

3. The Thrombolysis in Myocardial Infarction (TIMI) study group developed and validated a simple bedside prediction and stratification tool for patients with ST elevation ACS (Table 6-1).[2] The TIMI risk score assigns points for clinical risk indicators based on patient history, physical examination, and features of presentation. This scoring system has been validated by use of the 84,029 patients in the National Registry of Myocardial Infarction (NRMI) 3 database and reveals a graded increased risk in 30-day mortality ranging from 1.1% to 30.0% for scores ranging from 0 to >8, respectively (Fig. 6-1).[3]

B. THROMBOLYTICS VERSUS PRIMARY PERCUTANEOUS INTERVENTION

1. As discussed in Chapters 4 and 5, patients should be treated with an antiischemic drug regimen of aspirin, β-blockers, nitroglycerin, HMG-CoA reductase inhibitors, and unfractionated heparin or low molecular weight heparin in a timely manner after an ACS is suspected. Once a diagnosis of an ST elevation ACS has been made, patients become eligible for acute reperfusion therapy with either thrombolytic agents or

TABLE 6-1

CHARACTERISTICS OF THE TIMI RISK SCORE FOR ST ELEVATION MYOCARDIAL INFARCTION

Clinical Risk Indicators	Points
HISTORY	
≥75 years of age	3
65-74 years of age	2
History of diabetes, hypertension, or angina	1
EXAMINATION	
Systolic blood pressure <100 mm Hg	3
Heart rate >100 beats/min	2
Killip class II-IV	2
Weight <67 kg	1
PRESENTATION	
Anterior ST elevation or left bundle branch block	1
Time to reperfusion therapy >4 hr	1
TOTAL POSSIBLE POINTS	14

Data from Morrow DA et al: JAMA 2001; 286:1356.

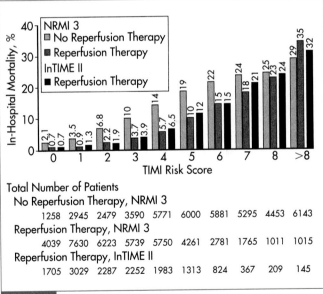

FIG. 6-1

Prediction of in-hospital mortality with TIMI risk score for ST elevation myocardial infarction. *NRMI 3,* National Registry of Myocardial Infarction 3. Data for the Intravenous nPA for Treatment of Infarcting Myocardium Early (InTime II) trial are from Morrow DA et al: Circulation 2000; 102:2031. *(From Morrow DA et al: JAMA 2001; 286: 1356.)*

primary PCI. One of the major goals of acute reperfusion therapy is the early restoration of flow in the IRA. Restoration of flow to the IRA has been described angiographically using the TIMI grading system: grade 0, complete occlusion of the IRA; grade 1, some flow beyond the obstruction but none distally; grade 2, reperfusion of the entire IRA but slower flow than normal; grade 3, normal flow through the IRA.[4] Acute reperfusion therapy aims to achieve TIMI grade 3 flow in the IRA.

2. Thrombolytic therapy is based on understanding of the pathophysiology of an ACS (see Chapter 4). Acute thrombotic occlusion of an epicardial coronary artery results from the rupture of an atherosclerotic plaque. This in turn promotes formation of an occlusive platelet- and fibrin-rich thrombus. Currently available thrombolytic (fibrinolytic) agents act by directly or indirectly activating plasminogen, a fibrinolytic proenzyme, which when converted to plasmin has broad proteolytic properties that enhance thrombus dissolution. Thrombolytic therapy has been studied extensively, and the beneficial effects in individuals with ST-elevation ACS are widely known and appreciated. Numerous large randomized controlled trials have demonstrated relative mortality benefits on the order of 20%.

a. ISIS-2 was one of the first large-scale, placebo-controlled, randomized trials comparing thrombolytic therapy to placebo. This trial demonstrated that streptokinase reduced 30-day mortality from 12% to 9.2% ($p < .00001$). This study also demonstrated the synergistic benefits between antiplatelet and thrombolytic agents, since 30-day mortality was reduced to a greater extent with the combination of aspirin and streptokinase (13.2% versus 8.0%, $p < .0001$) than with aspirin alone (11.8% versus 9.4%, $p < .00001$).[5] Subsequent long-term data from the ISIS trial confirmed that the mortality benefit with streptokinase persisted for at least 10 years.[6]

b. Similar trials with other thrombolytic agents have shown complementary findings, and a systematic overview of all trials in which more than 1000 patients were randomized to thrombolytic agents or placebo ($n = 58,600$) reported a significant 30-day mortality reduction with thrombolytic therapy (11.5% versus 9.6%).[7] Currently available thrombolytic regimens are listed in Table 6-2.[8] Given data from the GUSTO-I trial, accelerated tissue plasminogen activator (tPa) offers a higher mortality benefit when compared with streptokinase in patients with the following features: less than 75 years old, anterior wall myocardial infarction, and presentation within 4 hours of symptom onset.[9] Accelerated tPa should be administered with heparin and aspirin.

c. Reduction in the time from symptom onset to thrombolytic therapy has been shown to correlate with decreased mortality. The greatest benefit is achieved when treatment can be given within 3 hours of symptom onset, although benefit can be seen up to 12 hours.[10] Of note, the

TABLE 6-2					
COMPARISON OF CURRENTLY AVAILABLE THROMBOLYTIC AGENTS*					
	Streptokinase	tPA	rPA	Anistreplase	TNK-tPa
Half-life (hr)	25	4-8	15	70-120	20-24
Dose	1.5 million units over 30-60 min	†	Two 10-unit injections 30 min apart	30 units over 5 min	‡
Fibrin specificity	No	Yes	Yes	No	Yes
Cost ($)	543	2750	2750	2836	2750
Heparin therapy	SQ or IV	IV	IV	SQ or IV	IV

Modified from Wright RS, Kopecky SL, Reeder GS. Mayo Clin Proc 2000; 75:1185.

IV, Intravenously; *SQ*, subcutaneously.

*Patency rates reported only as the sum of TIMI 2 plus TIMI 3 flow in two studies.

†Dosage of tPa: 15 mg IV bolus, followed by a 30-minute infusion of 0.75 mg/kg (not to exceed 50 mg), followed by a 60-minute infusion of 0.5 mg/kg (not to exceed 35 mg) for a total dose of ≤100 mg administered over 90 minutes.

‡Dosage of TNK-tPA: single bolus administration. For body weight <60 kg, 30 mg; 60-70 kg, 35 mg; 70-80 kg, 40 mg; 80-90 kg, 45 mg; >90 kg, 50 mg. All doses administered over 5 seconds.

average time from symptom onset to arrival in the hospital remains 2.7 hours, despite the public health messages geared to getting patients to come in quickly when they have chest pain.

d. Before thrombolytic agents are administered, patients must be screened for potential contraindications because of the increased risk of intracranial hemorrhage and bleeding (Box 6-1).

e. Once an agent has been chosen (Table 6-2) and administered, an assessment of thrombolytic response is vital in predicting the likelihood of restored IRA flow. Despite the challenge inherent in this task, efficacy of thrombolysis can be assessed with continuous electrocardiographic (ECG) monitoring. In general, patients with complete resolution of ST segment elevation at 90 minutes have a 93% likelihood of IRA patency and a nearly 80% probability of TIMI 3 flow.[11] Continued analysis of bedside ECGs during thrombolysis can help identify patients in need of rescue PCI. Individuals (approximately 20% to 30% of those receiving thrombolytic agents) who do not have complete resolution of chest discomfort or at least a 50% reduction in the degree of ST elevation within 60 minutes from the time of thrombolytic administration should be referred for immediate PCI.[12]

f. Current recommendations of the American College of Cardiology (ACC) and American Heart Association (AHA) for thrombolytic therapy are shown in Box 6-2 (updates can be obtained at www.acc.org).[13]

3. Primary angioplasty has emerged as an alternative, and perhaps preferable, form of acute reperfusion therapy for ST elevation ACS. However, this strategy depends on the constant availability of the

---

BOX 6-1

CONTRAINDICATIONS AND CAUTIONS FOR THROMBOLYTIC USE IN ACUTE MYOCARDIAL INFARCTION

CONTRAINDICATIONS

Previous hemorrhagic stroke at any time; other strokes or cerebrovascular events within 1 year

Known intracranial neoplasm

Active internal bleeding (e.g., gastrointestinal), not including menses

Suspected aortic dissection

CAUTIONS OR RELATIVE CONTRAINDICATIONS

Severe or uncontrolled hypertension on presentation (>180/110 mm Hg)

History of prior cerebrovascular accident or known intracerebral pathological condition not covered in contraindications

Current use of anticoagulants in therapeutic doses (INR ≥2-3) or known bleeding diathesis

Recent trauma (within 2-4 weeks), including head trauma or traumatic or prolonged (>10 minutes) cardiopulmonary resuscitation or major surgery (<3 weeks)

Noncompressible vascular punctures

Internal bleeding within 2-4 weeks

For streptokinase or anistreplase: prior exposure (especially within 5 days to 2 years) or prior allergic reaction

Pregnancy

Active peptic ulcer

Age >75 years

History of proliferative retinopathy

Data from TIMI Study Group. N Engl J Med 1985; 312:932.
INR, International normalized ratio.

cardiac catheterization laboratory and well-trained interventional cardiologists. Therefore, in many hospitals across the United States, thrombolytic therapy is the only option for acute reperfusion. In randomized controlled trials, primary PCI offers better TIMI 3 flow rates, more sustained IRA patency, and less hemorrhagic complications than thrombolytic therapy.[14]

a. A metaanalysis combining the results of all published thrombolytic and PCI comparison trials reported a significantly lower rate of 30-day mortality with PCI (4.4% versus 6.5%, $p = .02$), as well as a significantly lower rate of the combined endpoint of death or reinfarction (7.2% versus 11.9%, $p < .001$).[15]

b. Long-term outcome data also favor PCI reperfusion. Primary PCI has been shown to provide a significant reduction in mortality over streptokinase at 5 years (13.4% versus 23.9%, $p = .01$).[16] Elderly patients (>60 years of age) with ST elevation ACS appear to benefit selectively from primary PCI, since this group had the greatest relative reduction

---

BOX 6-2

RECOMMENDATIONS OF THE AMERICAN COLLEGE OF CARDIOLOGY AND AMERICAN HEART ASSOCIATION FOR THROMBOLYTIC THERAPY

CLASS I*

1. ST elevation (>0.1 mm in two or more contiguous leads), time to therapy 12 hours or less, age <75 years
2. Bundle branch block (obscuring ST segment analysis) and history suggesting acute myocardial infarction

CLASS IIa

1. ST elevation, age 75 years or older

CLASS IIb

1. ST elevation, time to therapy >12 to 24 hours
2. Blood pressure on presentation >180 mm Hg systolic or >100 mm Hg diastolic, or both, associated with high-risk myocardial infarction

CLASS III

1. ST elevation, time to therapy >24 hours, ischemic pain resolved

Data from Ryan TJ et al. ACC/AHA guidelines for management of patients with acute myocardial infarction. 1999 Update: a report of the American College of Cardiology/American Heart Association Task Force on Practice Guidelines (Committee on Management of Acute Myocardial Infarction). Available at www.acc.org.
*ACC/AHA classification:
Class I: Conditions for which there is evidence or general agreement that a given procedure or treatment is beneficial, useful, and effective.
Class II: Conditions for which there is conflicting evidence or a divergence of opinion about the usefulness or efficacy of a procedure or treatment.
　Class IIa: Weight of evidence or opinion is in favor of usefulness or efficacy.
　Class IIb: Usefulness or efficacy is less well established by evidence or opinion.
Class III: Conditions for which there is evidence or general agreement that a procedure or treatment is not useful or effective and in some cases may be harmful.

in death or nonfatal reinfarction with primary PCI versus thrombolytic agents in the metaanalysis.[15] Thus primary PCI appears to significantly reduce mortality for patients with ST elevation ACS at presentation and may have a greater benefit in high-risk patients.

c. Primary PCI may also be preferable for patients with cardiogenic shock from ST elevation ACS. Traditionally these patients have undergone medical stabilization before revascularization. In the SHOCK randomized trial 302 patients with cardiogenic shock were assigned to a strategy of "initial medical stabilization (which included thrombolysis and intraaortic counterpulsation) and subsequent revascularization" or "early revascularization with either angioplasty or coronary artery bypass grafting." One-year survival was 46.7% in the early revascularization group compared with 33.6% in the medical stabilization group.[17]

d. Unlike thrombolytic therapy, primary PCI requires the rapid, continuously available response of a skilled catheterization laboratory staff. Furthermore, observational analyses have demonstrated that hospitals with low primary PCI volume do not have improved outcomes with primary PCI when compared with thrombolytic agents. Finally, primary PCI must be performed in a timely manner (door-to-balloon time ≤90 minutes) to maximize myocardial salvage and positively influence clinical outcomes. Thus primary PCI has emerged as the preferred reperfusion strategy for ST elevation ACS at high-volume, tertiary hospitals, but thrombolytic therapy remains the more widely used reperfusion strategy because it is rapidly available at all hospitals.

e. Current ACC/AHA recommendations for primary PCI are summarized in Box 6-3.

4. **The role of glycoprotein (GP) IIb/IIIa receptor inhibitor use in ST elevation ACS is still being defined. Many believe that a combination approach with thrombolytic therapy will provide more complete macrovascular and microvascular reperfusion than thrombolytic monotherapy. Several small trials evaluating a combined full- or low-dose thrombolytic agent with GP IIb/IIIa receptor inhibition have suggested improvements in endpoints such as early angiographic IRA patency, IRA reocclusion, and ST segment resolution.[18-20]**

a. Larger trials, such as ASSENT 3 (tenecteplase plus abciximab)[21] and GUSTO V (reteplase plus abciximab)[22] have demonstrated fewer reinfarctions with combined therapy, although no additional mortality benefit has been demonstrated. In addition, there is some concern about an increased propensity for bleeding complications, including an unacceptably high rate of intracranial hemorrhage, particularly in the elderly. Thus the clinical results with combination pharmacological reperfusion therapy do not justify routine clinical use at this point, and further study of optimal dosage regimens is needed to target improved efficacy and safety.

b. When coupled with primary PCI, GP IIb/IIIa receptor inhibition reduces the composite endpoint of death, myocardial infarction, and the need for urgent revascularization. The benefits of GP IIb/IIIa receptor inhibitors for patients undergoing primary PCI were first noted in a small subgroup analysis from the EPIC trial, which compared the GP IIb/IIIa receptor inhibitor abciximab to placebo in patients undergoing high-risk PCI. Patients (n = 45) with ST elevation ACS treated with abciximab had a large reduction in death, reinfarction, or repeat revascularization at 30 days (4.5% versus 26.1%, $p = .06$).[23] Subsequently the ADMIRAL trial (n = 300) demonstrated a significant reduction in death, reinfarction, or urgent need for repeat revascularization with abciximab in patients undergoing PCI for ST elevation ACS (6.0% versus 14.6%, $p = .01$).[24] The largest study of GP IIb/IIIa receptor inhibitors during primary PCI, CADILLAC, enrolled 2082 patients with ST elevation ACS and demonstrated a significant benefit when abciximab was used with PCI (with or without stenting). Major adverse events occurred in 20% of

---

BOX 6-3

RECOMMENDATIONS FOR PRIMARY PERCUTANEOUS TRANSLUMINAL CORONARY ANGIOPLASTY

CLASS I

1. As an alternative to thrombolytic therapy in patients with AMI and ST segment elevation or new or presumed new LBBB who can undergo angioplasty of the infarct-related artery within 12 hours of onset of symptoms or >12 hours if ischemic symptoms persist, if performed in a timely fashion by persons skilled in the procedure and supported by experienced personnel in an appropriate laboratory environment

2. In patients who are within 36 hours of an acute ST elevation/Q wave or new LBBB MI who are in cardiogenic shock, are <75 years of age, and can undergo revascularization within 18 hours of onset of shock

CLASS IIa

1. As a reperfusion strategy in candidates for reperfusion who have contraindication to thrombolytic therapy

CLASS IIb

1. In patients with AMI who do not have ST elevation but who have reduced (less than TIMI grade 2) flow in the infarct-related artery and in whom angioplasty can be performed within 12 hours of onset of symptoms

CLASS III

This classification applies to patients with AMI in the following circumstances:

1. Patient can undergo elective angioplasty of the non-infarct-related artery at the time of AMI.

2. Patient is >12 hours after the onset of symptoms and has no evidence of myocardial ischemia.

3. Patient has received fibrinolytic therapy and has no symptoms of myocardial ischemia.

4. Patient is eligible for thrombolysis and is undergoing primary angioplasty performed by a low-volume operator in a laboratory without surgical capability.

AMI, Acute myocardial infarction; *LBBB,* left bundle branch block; *MI,* myocardial infarction.

patients in the primary PCI group, 16.5% with primary PCI plus abciximab, 11.5% with stenting alone, and 10.2% with stenting plus abciximab ($p < .001$). The majority of benefit seen with abciximab plus stenting, however, was related to a reduced risk of repeat revascularization procedures.[25] Nonetheless, as interventional techniques evolve, GP IIb/IIIa receptor inhibitors continue to demonstrate consistent benefits for patients treated with PCI reperfusion.

5. Most in hospital mortality related to ST elevation ACS is caused by acute circulatory failure from mechanical complications (Table 6-3). Acute cardiogenic shock is usually the final result and is often due to

TABLE 6-3			

COMPLICATIONS OF MYOCARDIAL INFARCTION

	Prevalence (%)	Time to Onset After MI	Percent of MI-Associated Mortality
Papillary rupture causing severe mitral regurgitation		2-7 days	5
Left ventricular rupture		5-14 days	10
Acute ventricular septal defect	2		5
Severe left ventricular dysfunction and shock	7	Anytime	80

MI, Myocardial infarction.

severe mitral regurgitation from a ruptured papillary muscle, left ventricular free wall rupture, acute ventricular septal defect, hemodynamically significant right ventricular infarction, or severe left ventricular pump failure.[26] Prompt evaluation with bedside echocardiography in the setting of circulatory collapse will help the clinician make the diagnosis, and a referral for prompt surgical correction can be made if necessary.

6. Although not a direct complication of AMI, reperfusion arrhythmias are commonly seen after successful restoration of blood flow. In addition to premature ventricular contractions, nonsustained ventricular tachycardia, accelerated idioventricular rhythm, and heart block, some patients with inferior infarcts may have sinus bradycardia and transient hypotension (Bezold-Jarisch reflex).

PEARLS AND PITFALLS

• Rapid triage, patient assessment including the 12-lead ECG, and risk stratification optimize the time to reperfusion, which confers a direct mortality benefit.

• Primary PCI with stenting has a more favorable outcome than thrombolysis when available in experienced centers for an acute MI.

• Door–to–balloon inflation times less than 90 minutes result in better clinical outcomes.

• If PCI is not available on site, consideration should be given to prompt patient transfer to a center equipped to perform primary PCI. Morbidity and mortality benefits are still seen up to 3 hours from the time of symptom onset.

• A right-sided ECG should be considered for a patient with ST elevations in the inferior leads. ST elevations seen in V_4 of the right-sided leads suggest a right ventricular infarction.

REFERENCES

[b] 1. Killip T, Kimball JT. Treatment of myocardial infarction in a coronary care unit. Am J Cardiol 1967; 20:457.

[b] 2. Morrow DA et al. TIMI risk score for ST-elevation myocardial infarction: a convenient, bedside, clinical score for risk assessment at presentation; an InTIME II trial substudy. Circulation 2000; 102:2031.

[b] 3. Morrow DA et al. Application of the TIMI risk score for ST-elevation MI in the National Registry of Myocardial Infarction 3. JAMA 2001; 286:1356.

[a] 4. TIMI Study Group. The thrombolysis in myocardial in myocardial infarction (TIMI) trial: phase I findings. N Engl J Med 1985; 312:932.

[a] 5. ISIS-2 (Second International Study of Infarct Survival) Collaborative Group. Randomised trial of intravenous streptokinase, oral aspirin, both, or neither among 171,817 cases of suspected acute myocardial infarction: ISIS-2. Lancet 1988; 2:349.

[b] 6. Baigent C et al. ISIS-2: 10 year survival among patients with suspected acute myocardial infarction in randomised comparison of intravenous streptokinase, oral aspirin, both, or neither. Br Med J 1998; 316:1337.

[c] 7. Indications for fibrinolytic therapy in suspected acute myocardial infarction: collaborative overview of early mortality and major morbidity results from all randomized trials of more than 1000 patients. Fibrinolytic Therapy Trialists' (FTT) Collaborative Group. Lancet 1994; 343:311.

[c] 8. Wright RS et al. Update on intravenous fibrinolytic therapy for acute myocardial infarction. Mayo Clin Proc 2000; 75:1185.

[a] 9. GUSTO Investigators. An international randomized trial comparing four thrombolytic strategies for acute myocardial infarction. N Engl J Med 1993; 329:673.

[a] 10. Gruppo Italiano per lo Studio della Streptochiniasi nell'Infarto Miocardico (GISSI). Effectiveness of intravenous thrombolytic treatment in acute myocardial infarction. Lancet 1986; 1:397.

[c] 11. de Lemos JA, Braunwald E. ST segment resolution as a tool for assessing the efficacy of reperfusion therapy. J Am Coll Cardiol 2001; 38:1283.

[b] 12. Fernandez AR et al. ST segment tracking for rapid determination of patency of the infarct-related artery in acute myocardial infarction. J Am Coll Cardiol 1995; 26:675.

[d] 13. Ryan TJ et al. ACC/AHA guidelines for management of patients with acute myocardial infarction. 1999 Update: a report of the American College of Cardiology/American Heart Association Task Force on Practice Guidelines (Committee on Management of Acute Myocardial Infarction). Available at www.acc.org. Accessed on December 24, 2002.

[a] 14. Global Use of Strategies to Open Occluded Coronary Arteries in Acute Coronary Syndromes (GUSTO IIb) Angioplasty Substudy Investigators. A clinical trial comparing primary coronary angioplasty with tissue plasminogen activator for acute myocardial infarction. N Engl J Med 1997; 336:1621.

[c] 15. Weaver WD et al. Comparison of primary coronary angioplasty and intravenous thrombolytic therapy for acute myocardial infarction: a quantitative review. JAMA 1997; 278:2093.

[b] 16. Zijlstra F et al. Long-term benefit of primary angioplasty as compared to thrombolytic therapy for acute myocardial infarction. N Engl J Med 1999; 341:1431.

[b] 17. Hochman JS et al. One-year survival following early revascularization for cardiogenic shock. JAMA 2001; 285:190.

[b] 18. Kleiman NS et al. Profound inhibition of platelet aggregation with monoclonal antibody 7E3 Fab after thrombolytic therapy: results of the thrombolysis and angioplasty in myocardial infarction (TAMI)-8 pilot study. J Am Coll Cardiol 1993; 22:381.

[b] 19. de Lemos J et al. Abciximab improves both epicardial flow and myocardial reperfusion in ST-elevation myocardial infarction: observations from the TIMI 14 trial. Circulation 2000; 101:239.

[b] 20. Strategies for Patency Enhancement in the Emergency Department (SPEED) Group. Trial of abciximab with and without low dose reteplase for acute myocardial infarction. Circulation 2000; 100:2788.

[a] 21. ASSENT-3 Investigators. Efficacy and safety of tenecteplase in combination with enoxaparin, abciximab, or unfractionated heparin: the ASSENT 3 randomised trial in acute myocardial infarction. Lancet 2001; 358:605.

[a] 22. GUSTO-V Investigators. Reperfusion therapy for acute myocardial infarction with fibrinolytic therapy or combination reduced fibrinolytic therapy and platelet glycoprotein IIb/IIIa inhibition: the GUSTO-V randomised trial. Lancet 2001; 357:1905.

[b] 23. Lefkovitz J et al. Effects of platelet glycoprotein IIb/IIIa receptor blockade by a chimeric monoclonal antibody (abciximab) on acute and six-month outcomes after percutaneous transluminal coronary angioplasty for acute myocardial infarction. EPIC Investigators. Am J Cardiol 1996; 77:1045.

[b] 24. Montalescot G et al. Abciximab before direct angioplasty and stenting in myocardial infarction regarding acute and long-term follow-up. N Engl J Med 2001; 344:1895.

[a] 25. Stone GW et al. Comparison of angioplasty with stenting, with or without abciximab, in acute myocardial infarction. N Engl J Med 2002; 346:957.

[b] 26. Reeder GS. Identification and treatment of complications of myocardial infarction. Mayo Clin Proc 1995; 70:880.

Atrial Fibrillation

Moen Abedin, MD, and Hugh Calkins, MD

FAST FACTS

- Atrial fibrillation is the most common chronic rhythm disorder.
- The mechanism is uncertain but may be due to rapid firing of arrhythmogenic foci in the pulmonary veins or micro reentry within the atria.
- Initial evaluation of atrial fibrillation should include the following:
  - Assessment of hemodynamic stability.
  - Determination of duration of atrial fibrillation (important to decide need for anticoagulation).
  - Presence of preexisting cardiac disease including risk factors for systemic emboli.
- Three major issues to consider in management of atrial fibrillation:
  - Establishment of ventricular rate control.
  - Anticoagulation for prevention of systemic emboli.
  - Consideration for cardioversion and maintenance of sinus rhythm.

I. EPIDEMIOLOGY

1. Most common chronic rhythm disorder, affecting 5% of adults over age 65.[1]
2. The presence of atrial fibrillation doubles the risk of cardiovascular mortality in patients with other cardiovascular disease.[2]
3. Three main groups of patients.
   a. Paroxysmal atrial fibrillation: Atrial fibrillation that starts and stops spontaneously.
   b. Persistent atrial fibrillation: Atrial fibrillation that requires electrical or pharmacological cardioversion to terminate an episode.
   c. Chronic atrial fibrillation: Atrial fibrillation that persists despite therapy or based on a decision not to attempt to restore and maintain sinus rhythm.
4. Lone atrial fibrillation can be paroxysmal, persistent, or chronic. Lone atrial fibrillation is defined as atrial fibrillation occurring in patients less than 65 years of age and not associated with any other cardiovascular disease.

II. CLINICAL PRESENTATION

A. SYMPTOMS

1. Most common symptoms are nonspecific and include fatigue, reduced exercise tolerance, and dyspnea.[3]
2. Among patients hospitalized for atrial fibrillation, only 26% complained of palpitations.[4]

BOX 7-1
SECONDARY CAUSES OF ATRIAL FIBRILLATION
CONDITIONS THAT INCREASE ATRIAL SIZE
Hypertensive heart disease (most common associated condition)*
Congestive heart failure (left ventricular systolic dysfunction)
Atrial septal defect
Valvular heart disease
Acute pulmonary emboli
CONDITIONS THAT INCREASE ATRIAL IRRITABILITY
Myocarditis
Thyrotoxicosis
Post cardiac surgery
Theophylline
Binge alcohol consumption
Hyperadrenergic states (i.e., postoperative state, sepsis)

*Data from Kannel WB et al. N Engl J Med 1982; 306:1018.

3. Tachycardia can exacerbate other cardiac conditions such as coronary artery disease or congestive heart failure (CHF).[5]
4. Ambulatory monitoring of patients with atrial fibrillation reveals that most episodes of atrial fibrillation are asymptomatic.[3]

B. PATHOPHYSIOLOGY

1. Multiple migrating reentrant microwavelets lead to a loss of coordinated atrial contraction, sometimes arising as a result of rapid repetitive activation of ectopic foci in the pulmonary veins.
2. These wavelets rarely complete a circuit because of variation in conduction and refractoriness across the atrium, known as spatial heterogeneity.
3. Factors that affect spatial heterogeneity, by affecting conduction (inflammation or fibrosis) or refractoriness (thyrotoxicosis) or both (ischemia and age), can contribute to the generation of microwavelets responsible for atrial fibrillation.[5]
4. Many cases of lone atrial fibrillation originate from a focus of premature atrial contractions in one or more of the pulmonary veins, which results in micro reentry at the local level, leading to overall chaotic atrial contraction.[3]
5. Consider secondary causes of atrial fibrillation when making the initial evaluation. These are listed in Box 7-1.

III. DIAGNOSTICS

1. Irregularly irregular rate on cardiac auscultation is consistent with but not diagnostic of atrial fibrillation. Other conditions, such as sinus rhythm with frequent supraventricular or ventricular ectopic beats, sinus arrhythmia, or multifocal atrial tachycardia, can cause irregularly

irregular pulse. An electrocardiogram is necessary to confirm the diagnosis.

2. The key electrocardiographic diagnostic findings of atrial fibrillation are a narrow QRS with irregularly irregular QRS complexes and the absence of P waves. The QRS complex may be wide if there is aberrant conduction in the His-Purkinje system, as occurs in patients with preexisting bundle branch block.

3. Potential pitfalls.
   a. Sometimes F waves (fibrillatory waves) mimic P waves.
   b. Extremely rapid ventricular response can appear to be regular.
   c. Aberrant ventricular conduction with rapid ventricular response can result in a wide complex tachycardia. It is important to differentiate this situation from ventricular tachycardia, which has significantly different clinical implications.[6]
      (1) Ventricular tachycardia is usually regular (<28% variation in cycle length).
      (2) Rapid atrial fibrillation with aberrant conduction should have a QRS morphology with a typical right or left bundle branch block pattern.
      (3) If a wide complex tachycardia does not resemble a typical right or left bunch branch block, it is more likely to be ventricular tachycardia.
      (4) R:S ratio >1 in lead V_1 with R:S ratio <1 in V_6 is consistent with ventricular tachycardia.
      (5) Ventricular tachycardia is by far the most common cause of a wide complex tachycardia, regardless of hemodynamic tolerance.

IV. MANAGEMENT

See Fig. 7-1 for overview.

1. Determine if the patient is hemodynamically stable with acceptable blood pressure and is free of symptoms related to hypoperfusion, such as dizziness, neurological signs, or renal failure. If this is the case, proceed to DC cardioversion immediately.

2. Control the ventricular rate. The goal is to have a ventricular response between 80 and 100 beats/min (see Table 7-1).
   a. β-Blockers are the most effective drugs for rate control and should be used unless contraindications exist. The presence of Wolff-Parkinson-White syndrome is a contraindication to β-blocker therapy because slowing AV node conduction can lead to ventricular fibrillation from rapid conduction via the accessory pathway. Catheter ablation should be recommended for patients with atrial fibrillation in the setting of Wolff-Parkinson-White syndrome. β-Blockers that can be used include the following.
      (1) Esmolol.
      (2) Metoprolol.
      (3) Atenolol.
      (4) Propranolol.

7

ATRIAL FIBRILLATION

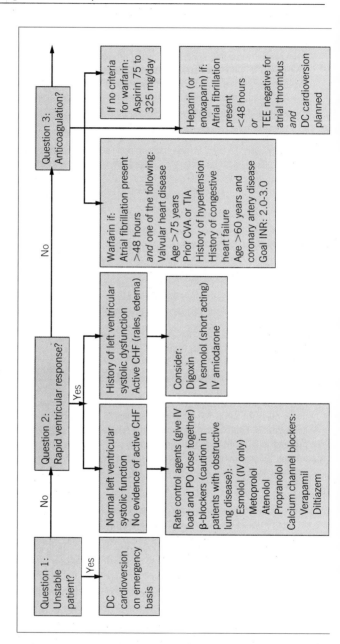

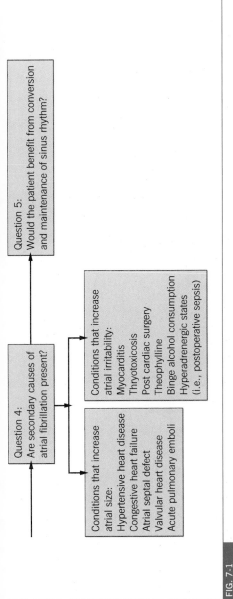

FIG. 7-1

Acute management of atrial fibrillation.

ATRIAL FIBRILLATION 7

TABLE 7-1

RATE CONTROL AGENTS

Drug	Starting Dose	Maximum Dose	Comments
β-BLOCKERS			
			Do not attempt in patients with Wolff-Parkinson-White syndrome
Esmolol	IV: 500 µg/kg/min over 1 minute; increase by 50 µg/kg/min every 4 minutes; new bolus of 500 µg/kg every 4 minutes	200 µg/kg/min	Effects wear off rapidly (within minutes) with drug discontinuation; because of rapid reversal, useful in patients with reactive airway disease whose tolerance of β-blockers is unknown
Metoprolol	IV: load 5 mg over 1 minute, repeat twice at 5-minute intervals PO: start 50 mg bid	PO: 450 mg/day	Metabolized by liver; available in once a day extended release formulation (Toprol XL)
Atenolol	IV: 5 mg over 5 minutes, repeat after 10 minutes PO: start 50 mg qd	PO: 200 mg/day	Excreted by kidney
Propranolol	IV: 1-3 mg at 1 mg/min; can repeat after 2 minutes, then every 4 hours PO: start 10 mg tid or qid	PO: 640 mg/day	Metabolized by liver; available in once a day extended release formulation (Inderal LA)
CALCIUM CHANNEL BLOCKERS			
			Do not attempt in patients with Wolff-Parkinson-White syndrome
Verapamil	IV: 2.5-10 mg over 2 minutes, can repeat 5-10 mg after 15-30 minutes PO: 80-120 mg tid or qid	IV: 20 mg PO: 480 mg/day	Requires dose adjustment for renal and hepatic insufficiency; consider starting bowel regimen; several once a day preparations available
Diltiazem	IV: 20 mg over 2 minutes bolus, 5-15 mg/hr drip for 24 hours PO: start 30 mg qid	PO: 360 mg	Hepatic metabolism and excretion; several once a day preparations available

OTHER			
Digoxin	IV: 0.5-1.0 mg, 50% initially, then 25% 6 to 12 hours later twice PO: load 0.75-1.25 mg, then 0.05-0.25 mg/day	Check levels and electrocardiogram	Primary metabolism via kidney; therapeutic level 0.8-2.0 ng/mL (stay at lower end of therapeutic range for women and the elderly)
Amiodarone	IV: 150 mg IV bolus over 10 minutes, then 1 mg/min for 6 hours, then 0.5 mg/min for 18 hours PO: 800-1600 mg qd for 1-3 weeks for load, divided bid or tid, maintenance at 200-400 mg/day		Monitor for thyroid, hepatic, and thyroid toxicity; amiodarone should *not* be used as the first agent for rate control in the ambulatory setting; IV amiodarone can be helpful as a second-line rate control agent in hospitalized patients

ATRIAL FIBRILLATION

7

b. Calcium channel blockers are also effective for rate control, but less effective than β-blockers. For resistant patients, these drugs can be used in combination.
   (1) Verapamil.
   (2) Diltiazem.
c. Antiarrhythmics: Amiodarone has multiple antiarrhythmic effects that make it an excellent drug for rate control. Despite this, amiodarone has many side effects and should not be used for long-term rate control of atrial fibrillation. Amiodarone should be considered in the acute setting for patients with rapid ventricular response despite β-blocker or calcium channel blocker therapy. Because amiodarone may cause conversion to sinus rhythm, consideration must be given to the risk of thromboembolism.
d. Digoxin: This is the least effective drug for rate control of atrial fibrillation. Digoxin is not useful in situations where there is increased sympathetic tone or decreased vagal input (i.e., during exercise); therefore it is not useful in providing rate control in physically active patients whose primary problem is tachycardia with exercise.[7]
e. Clinical variables influence which agent is used.
   (1) Obstructive lung disease. Calcium channel blockers are preferred because β-blockers may exacerbate asthma or chronic obstructive pulmonary disease (particularly in patients who have wheezing on pulmonary auscultation). Esmolol is a reasonable β-blocker to try as well because its effects resolve rapidly after discontinuation of the infusion.
   (2) CHF. Negative inotropes, including β-blockers and calcium channel blockers, may exacerbate CHF and should be used with caution. A short-acting β-blocker (esmolol) can be considered in the acute setting. Digoxin is commonly used along with β-blocker therapy for rate control of atrial fibrillation in patients with CHF.
   (3) Hypotension. Rapid ventricular response can shorten left ventricular (LV) filling and cause hypotension, particularly in patients with structural heart disease and diastolic dysfunction. Slowing the ventricular response may improve hemodynamics by improving LV filling. Use of short-acting esmolol or IV amiodarone can be considered for these patients.
   (4) Acute atrial fibrillation (i.e., in postoperative, septic, or other critically ill patients) commonly converts to sinus rhythm with establishment of rate control and treatment of the underlying condition.

3. Assess the need and safety of anticoagulation based on the duration of atrial fibrillation and the patient's comorbidities.
a. Why?
   (1) Based on Framingham data, atrial fibrillation increases the risk of stroke fivefold, independent of associated CHF and coronary artery disease. Overall incidence is 5% per year.[8]

    (2) Independent risk factors associated with recurrent transient ischemic attack (TIA) or cerebral ischemia were derived from a study by the European Atrial Fibrillation Trial Study Group of 375 patients with nonrheumatic atrial fibrillation.[9] These include the following.

      (a) Previous thromboembolism.

      (b) Ischemic heart disease.

      (c) Cardiomegaly on chest radiography.

      (d) Systolic blood pressure greater than 160 mm Hg.

      (e) Atrial fibrillation for more than 1 year.

      (f) Evidence of ischemic event on brain computed tomography.

      (g) Spontaneous echo contrast in left atrial appendage seen on transesophageal echocardiography (TEE).

b. Who?

    (1) Patients with atrial fibrillation and the following comorbidities should receive anticoagulation (warfarin) if no contraindications exist, targeting the international normalized ratio (INR) between 2.0 and 3.0.[10]

      (a) Valvular heart disease, most importantly mitral stenosis.

      (b) Age greater than 75 years.

      (c) History of prior TIA or stroke.

      (d) History of hypertension, particularly if systolic blood pressure exceeds 160 mm Hg.

      (e) CHF.

      (f) Diabetes (if age >60 years).

      (g) Coronary artery disease (if age >60 years).

      NOTE: (b), (c), and (d) were identified in analysis of patients who had sustained a stroke while being treated with aspirin in the Stroke Prevention in Atrial Fibrillation (SPAF) trials.[11]

    (2) Patients between the ages 65 and 75 without any of the above may benefit more from warfarin than aspirin if no contraindications to anticoagulation exist.

    (3) In patients less than 65 years old and without any of the above comorbidities, aspirin alone is generally sufficient.

c. Evidence (Table 7-2).

    (1) Benefit of anticoagulation versus placebo: SPAF trial.[12]

      (a) The first SPAF study involved 1330 patients who had had atrial fibrillation within the previous 12 months. Patients were randomly assigned to receive aspirin, warfarin, or placebo. The primary endpoint was ischemic stroke and peripheral emboli, for which patients were assessed every 3 months over 2 years. The incidence of events for warfarin versus placebo was 2.3% per year versus 7.4% per year. For aspirin versus placebo the event rates were 3.6% per year versus 6.3% per year. This study supports the conclusion that aspirin or warfarin significantly reduces events when compared with placebo. It is important to

7

ATRIAL FIBRILLATION

TABLE 7-2

IMPORTANT ANTICOAGULATION TRIALS IN ATRIAL FIBRILLATION

Trial	n	Patient Characteristics	Notable Exclusions	Treatment	Primary Endpoint	Results (event rates, percent per year)	Conclusions
AFASAK[13]	1007	Median age 75, 50% CHF	Stroke within 1 month; BP >180/100 mm Hg	Warfarin versus aspirin or placebo	Thromboembolism	Warfarin versus aspirin/placebo, 2% versus 5.5%; no significant difference in mortality	Warfarin superior to aspirin in this population
BAATAF[14]	420	Median age 68, 25% CHF	Stroke within 6 months; severe CHF	Warfarin versus placebo	Thromboembolism	Warfarin versus placebo, 0.4% versus 2.98%; statistically higher mortality in control group (RR 0.38, 95% CI 0.17-0.82)	Warfarin superior to placebo in this population
SPAF-I[12]	1330	Average age 67, 20% CHF	Class IV CHF; stroke within 2 years	Warfarin or aspirin versus placebo	Ischemic stroke and peripheral emboli	Warfarin versus placebo, 2.3% versus 7.4%; aspirin versus placebo, 3.6% versus 6.3%	Anticoagulation superior in population that includes modest CHF and hypertension (not meant to compare aspirin to warfarin)

| SPAF-II[15] | 1100 | Age 75 and below with hypertension, CHF, or previous thromboembolism | same as SPAF-I | Warfarin versus aspirin 325 mg | same as SPAF-I | Warfarin versus aspirin, 1.5% versus 2.9%; bleeding: 1.7% versus 0.9% | Additional risk reduction of warfarin comes with comparable increased risk of bleeding in high-risk patients younger than 75 |
| | | Above age 75 with hypertension, CHF, or previous thromboembolism | | | | Warfarin versus aspirin, 4.2% versus 7.2%; bleeding: 4.3% versus 1.6%; NOTE: For the overall study population, there was no signifi-cant difference in events | Warfarin provides acceptable thromboembolic risk reduction in patients older than 75 |

cont'd

All of these trials excluded patients with rheumatic heart disease or prosthetic heart valves who should receive anticoagulation.
BP, Blood pressure; *CHF*, congestive heart failure.

ATRIAL FIBRILLATION

7

TABLE 7-2
IMPORTANT ANTICOAGULATION TRIALS IN ATRIAL FIBRILLATION—cont'd

Trial	n	Patient Characteristics	Notable Exclusions	Treatment	Primary Endpoint	Results (event rates, percent per year)	Conclusions
SPAF-III[16]	892	Mean age 67	CHF, previous thromboemboli, female over age 75, systolic blood pressure greater than 160 mm Hg	Aspirin 325 mg (observational study)	Same as SPAF-I	2.2% (3.6% in patients with hypertension versus 1.1% if no hypertension); bleeding rate overall 0.5%	Low-risk patients (no history of thromboemboli or CHF) with no prior hypertension can receive adequate prophylaxis with aspirin; warfarin can be considered for low-risk patients with history of hypertension

All of these trials excluded patients with rheumatic heart disease or prosthetic heart valves who should receive anticoagulation.
BP, Blood pressure; *CHF,* congestive heart failure.

note that SPAF is not a comparison of aspirin with warfarin. Retrospective analysis suggested a lack of benefit of anticoagulation for patients younger than 60 years.

(2) Benefit of warfarin over aspirin: AFASAK, BAATAF, and SPAF II trials.

(a) The Atrial Fibrillation, Aspirin, Anticoagulation (AFASAK) trial enrolled 1007 patients with atrial fibrillation.[13] The patients were randomly assigned to receive warfarin (INR 2.8-4.2; open label), aspirin 75 mg, or placebo. The primary endpoint of the study was thromboembolic events with a secondary endpoint of mortality. The study was terminated early because of a substantial reduction in thromboembolic events with warfarin versus aspirin or placebo (2% per year versus 5.5% per year). No significant difference in mortality was found. The bleeding rates observed in the study were 6% per year with warfarin and 1% per year with aspirin or placebo. This study supported the conclusion that warfarin is superior to aspirin and placebo in preventing thromboembolic events among a largely elderly population.

(b) The Boston Area Anticoagulation Trial for Atrial Fibrillation (BAATAF) study enrolled 420 patients with atrial fibrillation noted on two separate occasions who were randomly assigned to receive warfarin, with an INR goal between 1.5 and 2.7 (open label) versus control (no placebo, but aspirin was allowed).[14] The study's primary endpoint was a combination of ischemic stroke and peripheral embolic events. After a mean follow-up of 2.2 years, the study was terminated prematurely because of a significant reduction in events in the group treated with warfarin (0.4% per year versus 2.98% per year in the control group, an overall 86% decrease). Increased mortality was noted in the control group (RR 0.38, 95% CI 0.17- 0.82, $p = .005$). No significant difference in bleeding events was found. BAATAF supports the conclusion that warfarin is superior to placebo in reducing thromboembolic events and mortality.

(c) The SPAF-II trial[15] included 419 new patients plus 681 patients from SPAF-I, with a prespecified analysis of anticoagulation in patients above 75 years of age.[13] This open label trial assigned patients to aspirin 325 mg versus warfarin with a goal prothrombin time ratio between 1.3 and 1.8 (corresponding to an INR of 2.0-4.5). Assessments were performed every 3 months for the combined primary endpoint of ischemic stroke and peripheral emboli. The incidence of the primary event was 2.7% per year for the aspirin group versus 1.9% per year for the warfarin group (not statistically significant). Among patients with risk factors for thromboembolic events (hypertension, CHF, or prior thromboembolic event), patients younger than 75 years had

7

ATRIAL FIBRILLATION

event rates of 2.9% per year versus 1.5% year for aspirin and warfarin, respectively. High-risk patients above 75 years of age had event rates of 7.2% per year versus 4.2% year (aspirin versus warfarin). The risk of bleeding for aspirin versus warfarin was 1.6% per year versus 4.3% per year in patients over 75 years and 0.9% per year versus 1.7% per year in those younger than 75. In conclusion, SPAF-II demonstrated higher event rates in high-risk patients over 75 years old. Although event rates were reduced with warfarin anticoagulation, an increased risk for bleeding was noted.

(3) Aspirin in low-risk patients: SPAF-III trial.[16]

(a) This study included 892 patients who had had atrial fibrillation within the previous 6 months and excluded patients with current hypertension or left ventricular dysfunction. All patients received 325 mg aspirin daily with a follow-up period of 2 years. The primary endpoints included TIA, stroke, and peripheral embolus. The overall event rate was 2.2% per year. The event rate was 3.6% per year for patients with any history of hypertension versus 1.1% per year for patients with no history of hypertension ($p <.001$). The aspirin-associated bleeding rate was 0.5% per year. SPAF-III supports the use of aspirin for thromboembolic prophylaxis in low-risk patients and suggests that patients with prior hypertension may be at sufficient risk to justify anticoagulation with warfarin.

4. **Conversion and maintenance of sinus rhythm.**

a. The issue of treating patients with atrial fibrillation with rate control agents versus using antiarrhythmic drugs to maintain sinus rhythm has been addressed by two recent clinical trials: AFFIRM[17] and RACE.[18]

(1) The Atrial Fibrillation Follow-up Investigation of Rhythm Management (AFFIRM) included 4060 patients over the age of 65 with atrial fibrillation. In this randomized trial, patients were assigned to a strategy of rate control with β-blockers and calcium channel blockers, targeted to a goal resting heart rate of 80 beats/min or to rhythm control with use of antiarrhythmic drugs. Average follow-up was 3.5 years; sinus rhythm was maintained in 63% of patients in the rhythm control group at 5 years, compared with 35% in the rate control group. Chronic anticoagulation was recommended for all patients in the rate control group (on average, 85% were taking warfarin) and was left to the discretion of the treating physician in the rhythm control group (on average, 70% were taking warfarin). There was a nonsignificant trend toward higher total mortality in the rhythm control group, the study's primary endpoint. Prespecified subgroup analysis demonstrated a statistically significant mortality benefit with rate control for patients above the age of 65. No significant difference was found in the incidence of

stroke (roughly 1% per year); the majority (73%) of ischemic strokes occurred in patients who had discontinued warfarin or had an INR below 2.0. These findings support the recommendation that anticoagulation be continued in patients even if atrial fibrillation is successfully suppressed. AFFIRM demonstrated that a rhythm control strategy for recurrent atrial fibrillation had no advantage and suggests that a rate control strategy may be superior in patients above the age of 65. The patients enrolled in this study were minimally symptomatic, however, and the results do not necessarily apply to patients with highly symptomatic atrial fibrillation.

(2) In the Rate Control Versus Electrical Cardioversion for Persistent Atrial Fibrillation (RACE) trial, 522 patients with persistent atrial fibrillation of less than 1 year's duration were randomly assigned to rate control with digitalis, calcium channel blockers, or β-blockers or DC cardioversion (without antiarrhythmic drugs) followed by initiation of sotalol. Patients with recurrence of atrial fibrillation during treatment with sotalol were subsequently treated with flecainide. Individuals who failed to maintain sinus rhythm with flecainide therapy were then treated with amiodarone. Mean follow-up was 2.3 years. At the study's end, 39% of patients in the rhythm control group were in sinus rhythm, compared with 10% in the rate control group. The primary endpoint of the study was a composite of death from cardiovascular causes, heart failure, thromboembolic events, bleeding, need for pacemaker, or adverse drug effects. The incidence of the primary endpoint was higher in the rhythm control group (23% versus 17%), but this difference was not statistically significant. In the rhythm control group the incidence of each component of the primary endpoint did not differ significantly based on the presence of sinus rhythm. A post hoc analysis demonstrated significantly higher incidence of the primary endpoint with rhythm control in women and hypertensive patients. No significant difference in cardiovascular death or thromboembolic events was noted, but 83% of all thromboembolic events occurred in patients who had discontinued warfarin or had an INR below 2.0. In conclusion, the study demonstrated no significant advantage to a rhythm control strategy for the management of persistent atrial fibrillation.

(3) Taken together, these studies indicate that a strategy of rhythm control has no significant mortality benefit over rate control with anticoagulation among elderly patients with minimally symptomatic atrial fibrillation. These trials were more about the ineffectiveness of antiarrhythmic therapy in the prevention of atrial fibrillation than about rate versus rhythm control strategies. Practice guidelines have not yet been revised to account for the trial results, but we offer these recommendations.

7

ATRIAL FIBRILLATION

        (a) A rate control strategy is an acceptable approach to management of patients with atrial fibrillation, particularly if they are asymptomatic and elderly.

        (b) Rhythm control should be reserved for patients with symptomatic atrial fibrillation. This strategy should also be considered for minimally symptomatic young patients with atrial fibrillation.

  b. Anticoagulation for conversion to sinus rhythm.

    (1) When it is clear that atrial fibrillation is less than 48 hours in duration, cardioversion can be attempted without delay. The presence of atrial fibrillation for more than 48 hours necessitates 3 to 4 weeks of therapeutic anticoagulation before attempted conversion, unless a clot can be ruled out in the left atrium and its appendage by transesophageal echocardiography (TEE). Regardless of whether TEE is performed, systemic anticoagulation is required for 3 weeks after cardioversion in all patients with atrial fibrillation or more than 48 hours' duration. Evidence supporting this approach comes from the Assessment of Cardioversion Using Transesophageal Echocardiography (ACUTE) trial.[19]

    (2) The ACUTE trial included 1222 patients with atrial fibrillation who were recommended for DC cardioversion and met criteria for long-term anticoagulation. They were randomly assigned to TEE followed by DC cardioversion (if no intracardiac clot was found) versus conventional therapy, which consisted of 3 weeks of anticoagulation before DC cardioversion. It is important to note that all patients had therapeutic anticoagulation before TEE (activated partial thromboplastin time 1.5- 2.5 times normal or an INR of 2.0-3.0). All subjects (TEE group and conventional therapy group) received therapeutic anticoagulation for 4 weeks after cardioversion. Patients with atrial flutter but no history of atrial fibrillation and hemodynamic instability were excluded. At 8 weeks from the time of enrollment there was no significant difference in the primary endpoints of cerebrovascular accident, TIA, and peripheral embolus. However, significantly fewer bleeding events were noted in the TEE group.

    (3) The risk of thromboembolic events is higher in the 3 to 4 weeks immediately after conversion to sinus rhythm. This is believed to be due to atrial stunning, a term describing the observation of reduced atrial systolic function after conversion to sinus rhythm. Atrial stunning can allow relative stasis of blood within the atrium, potentially resulting in thrombus formation. Patients should receive anticoagulation with warfarin for 3 weeks after conversion to sinus rhythm even if they are in a low-risk category for thromboembolic events. Patients who have the indications for chronic anticoagulation with warfarin mentioned above (valvular heart disease, age over 75 years, prior thromboembolic event, hypertension, heart failure, coronary artery disease, or diabetes over age 60) should receive long-term anticoagulation after cardioversion.

c. DC cardioversion.
   (1) Emergency electrical cardioversion is indicated if the patient is hemodynamically unstable as a result of tachycardia.
   (2) Rectilinear biphasic defibrillation: A biphasic defibrillation modulates internal impedance of the defibrillator to maintain constant current delivery during shock. Biphasic defibrillation allows a similar current delivery (which is the most important variable for achieving cardioversion) with lower energy. An early nonrandomized biphasic defibrillator trial[20] demonstrated a first shock conversion rate of 68% with biphasic and 21% with monophasic defibrillation. The BiCard study included 203 patients in a randomized, double-blind control trial.[21] Patients were assigned at random to monophasic or biphasic defibrillation. The biphasic defibrillation group demonstrated a 60% conversion to sinus rhythm after delivery of the first shock, compared with 22% in the monophasic defibrillation group. No significant difference in conversion rates between the two groups was found at the end of the protocol. The incidence of dermal injury was 17% with biphasic and 41% with monophasic defibrillation, with significantly lower energy used and fewer shocks in the biphasic group.
   (3) Cardioversion can be performed either with a standard monophasic defibrillator or with a new defibrillator capable of delivering biphasic waveforms. If a standard defibrillator fails, cardioversion should be repeated with a biphasic defibrillator.
d. Chemical cardioversion.
   (1) Ibutilide is a class III antiarrhythmic used to facilitate DC cardioversion, particularly when DC cardioversion is initially unsuccessful. Ibutilide can be used only for patients with documented normal left ventricular systolic function because of the risk of inducing ventricular tachycardia and torsades de pointes. Patients also require at least 4 hours of ECG monitoring after cardioversion to monitor for arrhythmias. In the Ibutilide Trial 100 patients with at least 6 hours of atrial fibrillation were randomly assigned to receive 1 mg IV Ibutilide over 10 minutes before conventional defibrillation (sequence: 50, 100, 200, 300, 360 J) or to receive shock alone.[22] Ten patients in the Ibutilide group converted with Ibutilide alone; the remaining 40 patients converted with an average of 166 ± 80 J. In the conventional shock group, 36 patients (72%) were converted with an average energy of 228 ± 93 J. Of 14 patients who did not convert initially, all had successful DC cardioversion after receiving Ibutilide. No ventricular arrhythmias occurred with Ibutilide in patients with normal LV function (two events occurred in patients with abnormal LV function). Ibutilide should not be administered to patients at increased risk for ventricular arrhythmias, including those with prolonged QT, depressed left ventricular

7

ATRIAL FIBRILLATION

function (ejection fraction <0.30), hypokalemia, or hypomagnesemia.

(2) Dofetilide: See discussion in next section.

e. Maintenance of sinus rhythm.

  (1) General points.

    (a) The evidence from AFFIRM and RACE shows no significant difference in mortality between a strategy of rate control for atrial fibrillation and the use of rhythm control with antiarrhythmic drug (AAD) therapy. As noted above, antiarrhythmic therapy is indicated for patients with significant symptoms from atrial fibrillation. Rate control alone should be the primary strategy for management of minimally symptomatic patients, particularly if they are elderly.

    (b) For moderate to severe left ventricular systolic dysfunction the agent of choice available in the United States is amiodarone. Dofetilide can be used as well, but its use is tightly regulated in the United States and it can be prescribed only by physicians certified in its use. All other antiarrhythmic drugs are relatively contraindicated in patients with LV dysfunction because of the potential for proarrhythmia.

    (c) For ischemic heart disease with preserved LV systolic function, sotalol may be particularly useful because of its β-blocker effect.

  (2) Overview of antiarrhythmic drugs (organized by class).

    (a) Class IA agents (quinidine, procainamide, disopyramide) are rarely if ever used for treatment of atrial fibrillation in the United States. Among these drugs, disopyramide is the most commonly used, particularly in patients suspected of having atrial fibrillation precipitated by increased vagal tone.

    (b) Class IC agents used in atrial fibrillation include flecainide and propafenone, reserved for patients without ischemic heart disease. These agents can be administered daily for maintenance of sinus rhythm. They can also be used as needed for acute conversion in patients with intermittent symptomatic paroxysmal atrial fibrillation—a "pill in the pocket" approach.

     i. Flecainide can be given as a 300-mg oral dose.

     ii. A 600-mg oral dose of propafenone results in conversion within 4 hours in 70% to 80% of patients.[7]

     iii. When a "pill in the pocket" approach is considered, it should be tried first while the patient is being monitored. A β-blocker or calcium channel blocker should be administered 30 to 60 minutes before administration of the antiarrhythmic agent.

     iv. Treatment of lone atrial fibrillation with class IC agents can result in conversion to atrial flutter because of these drugs' effects on the atrial refractory period and conduction velocity. The reported incidence of this phenomenon varies widely in the literature, from 3.5% to 20% of patients whose lone atrial fibrillation is treated with class IC drugs. This "class IC atrial flutter" can be treated with ablation of the right atrial isthmus followed by continuation of the antiarrhythmic drug. A study of 13 patients with class IC flutter demonstrated complete relief of symptoms in 9 patients and overall clinical improvement in 11 patients, suggesting clinical validity of this approach in these patients.[23]

(c) Class III agents include amiodarone, sotalol, and dofetilide.

   i. Amiodarone has multiple adverse reactions; patients receiving amiodarone need monitoring of pulmonary function tests (carbon monoxide diffusion in lung), thyroid function, and liver function. Despite the absence of a U.S. Food and Drug Administration indication for use of amiodarone in atrial fibrillation, this drug is by far the most commonly prescribed antiarrhythmic agent for this purpose. Amiodarone can be initiated on an outpatient basis, usually at 400 mg/day for a month initially, decreasing thereafter to 200 mg/day.

   ii. Evidence supporting the efficacy of amiodarone comes from the Canadian Trial of Atrial Fibrillation (CTAF).[24] CTAF was a randomized, open label study of amiodarone versus sotalol or propafenone for maintenance of sinus rhythm in 403 patients with paroxysmal atrial fibrillation. The trial excluded patients with heart failure and renal insufficiency. The 201 patients in the amiodarone group received 10 mg/kg/day for 14 days, followed by cardioversion, 300 mg/day for 4 weeks, and maintenance with 200 mg/day thereafter. The sotalol group included 101 patients, most given 160 mg bid. The dose was reduced to 80 mg tid for a creatinine level greater than 1.5 mg/dL and to 80 mg bid in women over age 70 with creatinine levels above 1.2 mg/dL. The propafenone group included 101 patients who received 300 mg qid, which was reduced to 150 mg tid for patients over 70 years or weighing under 70 kg. A significant reduction in atrial fibrillation (35% versus 63%) was seen in patients treated with amiodarone when compared with those receiving sotalol or propafenone. At 1-year follow-up, 69% of patients treated with amiodarone were in sinus rhythm, compared with 39% of patients treated with sotalol or propafenone. Amiodarone was associated with a higher rate of discontinuation resulting from side effects, but the difference was not statistically significant. No significant difference in total mortality was found between the groups.

   iii. Dofetilide requires in-hospital initiation for observation for arrhythmias. Safety of dofetilide in patients with heart failure is supported by the Danish Investigations of Arrhythmia and Mortality on Dofetilide in Congestive Heart Failure

7

ATRIAL FIBRILLATION

(DIAMOND-CHF)[25] study, a double-blind, placebo-controlled trial of 1518 patients with LV ejection fractions below 35%. The dofetilide dose was 500 µg bid; this was adjusted to 250 µg bid for patients with creatinine clearances between 40 and 60 mL/min and 250 µg qd with creatinine clearances between 20 and 40 mL/min. Patients with creatinine clearance less than 20mL/min were excluded. No significant difference in total mortality, the primary endpoint of the study, was found. Retrospective analysis of the results demonstrated that 12% of patients with atrial fibrillation in the treatment group had conversion to sinus rhythm, compared with 1% in the placebo group, and that the treatment group had a significant reduction in the subsequent development of atrial fibrillation.

iv. Sotalol. Because of the potential for arrhythmias, sotalol should not be given to patients with renal dysfunction, se-vere LV hypertrophy, prolonged QT intervals, bradycardia, or electrolyte abnormalities. Nodally active agents should be stopped or decreased before initiation of sotalol because of the risk of bradycardia from β-blocking effects that occur at a dosage of 40 mg bid. The class III antiarrhythmic effect (action potential prolongation) appears at 120 to 160 mg bid. Suggested sotalol loading is noted below (in-hospital ad-ministration to observe for arrhythmias, bradycardia, and prolonged QT with a daily ECG). Sotalol should not be given to patients with significant renal insufficiency.[7]

(1) First dose is 80 mg tid for 1 day.

(2) Then 120 mg bid on second day.

(3) Then 160 mg bid on third day.

(4) Discharge on 120 mg bid, with increase to 160 mg bid if needed.

f. Options for persistent symptomatic atrial fibrillation other than rate control, cardioversion, and maintenance of sinus rhythm.

(1) Atrioventricular node ablation with permanent pacemaker implantation is an option for management of patients who have paroxysmal or persistent atrial fibrillation with rapid ventricular response and cannot tolerate rate control or rhythm control agents. This situation often occurs in patients with LV dysfunction because they cannot tolerate the negative inotropic effects of the doses of antinodal agents necessary to achieve rate control. It also occurs in patients who have recurrent symptomatic atrial fibrillation despite antiarrhythmic drug therapy. The relative safety of this approach was demonstrated in a retrospective study of the Mayo Clinic experience of atrioventricular node ablation with pacemaker implantation. Review of the records of 350 patients who underwent the procedure

from July 1990 to December 1998 uncovered a total of 50 deaths during an average follow-up of 36 ± 26 months.[26] The overall survival of patients undergoing atrioventricular node ablation and pacemaker insertion was the same as a matched group of patients treated with antiarrhythmic drugs. Despite the ease and high efficacy of this approach, it is rarely performed because it does not eliminate atrial fibrillation or the need for anticoagulation, it renders the patient pacemaker dependent, and it causes ventricular dyssynchrony. Atrioventricular node ablation should rarely if ever be performed on young patients with atrial fibrillation

(2) Pulmonary vein radiofrequency ablation: This procedure is typically reserved for patients with lone or paroxysmal atrial fibrillation who have failed one or more trials of antiarrhythmic therapy. Recent studies have reported that atrial fibrillation can be cured with catheter ablation techniques that target arrhythmogenic foci in the pulmonary veins. The best results of this procedure (up to 85% success rate)[27] have been achieved in patients with lone atrial fibrillation. Lower success rates (50%-70%) have been reported in other subsets of patients with atrial fibrillation. Potential complications of the procedure include pulmonary vein stenosis, stroke, and pericardial tamponade. The techniques for ablation of atrial fibrillation are evolving rapidly and probably will improve over the next 3 to 5 years.

(3) Atrial defibrillator: This device, implanted like a permanent pacemaker, can sense atrial fibrillation and produce cardioversion to sinus rhythm with minimal discomfort. It can be set for cardioversion of the patient on detection of atrial fibrillation or on the patient's or physician's command. It has been typically implanted after the failure of antiarrhythmic drug therapy in patients with symptomatic paroxysmal atrial fibrillation.[28] Atrial defibrillators have not gained widespread acceptance because of the pain associated with the shock therapy.

(4) Maze procedure: This procedure is occasionally performed in conjunction with cardiac surgery for other indications. Criss-crossing scars are placed in the atria in an attempt to prevent micro reentry that leads to atrial fibrillation. Success rates are approximately 80% to 90%. A percutaneous, catheter-based version of the procedure is also possible but is time intensive and associated with high recurrence rates of atrial fibrillation; therefore it is not part of routine clinical practice.

PEARLS AND PITFALLS

- In the management of atrial fibrillation, these issues must addressed:
  - Emergency cardioversion of patients who are unstable.
  - Control of rapid ventricular response.
  - Reduction of thromboembolic events with anticoagulation.
  - Evaluation and treatment of conditions that may cause atrial fibrillation.

7

ATRIAL FIBRILLATION

- Consideration of conversion to sinus rhythm.
- In the outpatient setting.
  - Not all patients require inpatient hospitalization on diagnosis.
  - Indications for hospital admission.
    - Extremely rapid ventricular response (>150 beats/min).
    - Angina.
    - Evidence of CHF (dyspnea, rales, elevated jugular venous pressure, peripheral edema).
    - Relative hypotension.
    - Syncope or presyncope.
    - Neurological complaints.
  - Stable patients can be started on a rate control agent and monitored for a few hours to ensure that the ventricular rate remains controlled. Anticoagulation with warfarin can be started. Close outpatient follow-up is essential. Anticoagulation on an outpatient basis should not be attempted if the patient will not be available for close follow-up. The outpatient evaluation should include arrangements for echocardiography.
    - Immediate anticoagulation with unfractionated heparin or low molecular weight heparin is not necessary. The annual risk of thromboembolic events in high-risk patients is 5% to 7%, making the daily risk 0.02%, which is relatively low for the few days it takes to achieve a therapeutic INR. Warfarin-induced protein C and S inhibition, which occurs earlier than inhibition of the coagulation system, is a theoretical concern for a possible prothrombotic state in the first few days of warfarin initiation without heparin coverage; however, there is no clinical evidence demonstrating increased thrombotic events after initiation of warfarin without heparin.
- In the ICU setting.
  - Atrial fibrillation often occurs in critically ill patients because of increased sympathetic tone.
  - Secondary causes, including pulmonary emboli, should be considered.
  - Initiation of anticoagulation is indicated within 48 hours of onset of atrial fibrillation, particularly if cardioversion is being planned.
  - Rapid ventricular response in patients with structural heart disease can contribute to hypotension by shortening LV diastolic filling. Control of rapid ventricular response can improve blood pressure. A trial of short-acting esmolol may be warranted in these patients. In the ICU setting, administration of amiodarone may also be considered. DC cardioversion should be considered for unstable patients.
- Best method for DC cardioversion.
  - A short-acting (5-10 minutes) general anesthetic with monitoring by qualified personnel is needed.
  - Be sure the patient has had therapeutic anticoagulation for 3 to 4 weeks (INR >2.0, checked at least biweekly) or therapeutic

anticoagulation since a TEE that has demonstrated no evidence of an intracardiac clot.

- Electrode pads should be placed in an anteroposterior orientation (front at T4 level just left of the sternum, back at same level).
- The initial setting is 100 J in the biphasic mode, or 200 J in the monophasic mode, with the defibrillator set in sync mode.
- With use of a nonconducting material (e.g., a folded dry towel), 5 to 10 pounds of gentle pressure should be placed on the pads to improve contact.
- If 100 J is unsuccessful, increase to 150 J, then 200 J.
- ECG monitoring is needed during the procedure to assess efficacy.
- The patches should be removed while the patient is still under anesthesia, to minimize discomfort.
- The patient should be observed for maintenance of sinus rhythm and recovery for a few hours after the procedure.
- Continuation of anticoagulation after cardioversion is essential if the duration of atrial fibrillation has been more than 48 hours.
- Atrial flutter.[29]
  - Mechanism. Atrial flutter is a supraventricular tachycardia frequently found in association with atrial fibrillation. It is, however, an entity distinct from atrial fibrillation. Atrial flutter is the result of macro reentry involving the entire atrium in the circuit. The typical atrial flutter circuit moves counterclockwise through the right atrium when the heart is viewed from the apex. Establishment of the reentrant circuit in typical atrial flutter relies on conduction through the isthmus, or the area between the tricuspid annulus, the inferior vena cava, and the coronary sinus. Atypical atrial flutter, which involves other parts of the atria in the reentrant circuit, can also be found.
  - Presentation and diagnosis. Atrial flutter often has the same symptoms as atrial fibrillation. The atrial rate is typically between 250 and 350 beats/min, with resultant 2:1 or 4:1 atrioventricular conduction block. Diagnosis is based on the 12-lead ECG. The blocked flutter waves may not be readily apparent on 12-lead ECG because they may be masked by the QRS complex. The presence of a regular, narrow complex tachycardia at 150 beats/min should raise suspicion for the presence of atrial flutter and prompt a close comparison of the ECG with a prior sinus rhythm ECG to look for blocked flutter waves.
  - Management.
    - Acute management of atrial flutter does not differ significantly from that of atrial fibrillation. Patients with hemodynamic compromise should undergo emergency cardioversion. Stable patients can be treated acutely with β-blockers or calcium channel blockers for rate control.
    - Atrial flutter can be cured with radiofrequency catheter ablation. The ablation creates a scar that interrupts the macro reentrant circuit, preventing the propagation of the tachycardia. The procedure is

effective, particularly in patients who do not have concomitant atrial fibrillation.

- For patients with recurrent, symptomatic atrial flutter, first-line therapy should be ablation rather than antiarrhythmic drug therapy. In a randomized study 61 patients with atrial flutter were assigned to primary treatment with catheter ablation or antiarrhythmic drug (AAD) therapy. At the end of 1 year, atrial flutter had recurred in 6% of the ablation group and 93% of the AAD group; atrial fibrillation occurred in 29% of the ablation group and 60% of the AAD group. Hospitalizations were also less frequent in the patients treated primarily with ablation (22% versus 63%).[30]

- The risk of thromboembolic events from atrial flutter is essentially the same as with atrial fibrillation. Therefore the recommendations for anticoagulation with atrial flutter are the same as with atrial fibrillation. No clinical studies of anticoagulation specifically in patients with atrial flutter are available.

REFERENCES

[c] 1. Abedin Z, Conner R. Interpretation of cardiac arrhythmias: self assessment approach. Norwell, Mass: Kluwer; 2000.

[c] 2. Kannel WB et al. Epidemiologic features of chronic atrial fibrillation. N Engl J Med 1982; 306:1018.

[c] 3. Falk RH. Medical progress: atrial fibrillation. N Engl J Med 2001; 344:1067.

[b] 4. Lip GYH, Tean KN, Dunn FG. Treatment of atrial fibrillation in a district general hospital. Br Heart J 1994; 71:92.

[c] 5. Narayan SM, Cain ME, Smith JM. Atrial fibrillation. Lancet 1997; 350:943.

[c] 6. Gupta AK, Thakur RK. Wide QRS tachycardia. Med Clin North Am 2001; 85:245.

[c] 7. Reiffel JA. Drug choices in the treatment of atrial fibrillation. Am J Cardiol 2000; 85:2D.

[b] 8. Wolf PA et al. Duration of atrial fibrillation and the imminence of stroke: the Framingham study. Stroke 1983; 14:664.

[b] 9. Van Latum JC et al. Predictors of major vascular event in patient with a transient ischemic attack or minor ischemic stroke with non rheumatic atrial fibrillation. European Atrial Fibrillation Trial (EAFT) Study Group. Stroke 1995; 25:801.

[d] 10. ACC/AHA/ESC guidelines for the management of patients with atrial fibrillation—executive summary. Circulation 2001; 104:2118.

[b] 11. Hart RG et al. Factors associated with ischemic stroke during aspiring therapy in atrial fibrillation: analysis of 2012 participants in the SPAF I-III clinical trials. Stroke 1999; 30:1223.

[a] 12. Stroke Prevention in Atrial Fibrillation Investigators. Stroke Prevention in Atrial Fibrillation study: final results. Circulation 1991; 84:527.

[a] 13. Peterson P et al. Placebo-controlled randomized trial of warfarin and aspirin for prevention of thromboembolic complications in chronic atrial fibrillation: the Copenhagen AFASAK study. Lancet 1989; 28:175.

[a] 14. Boston Area Anticoagulation Trial for Atrial Fibrillation Investigators. The effect of low dose warfarin on the risk of stroke in patients with nonrheumatic atrial fibrillation. N Engl J Med 1990; 323:1505.

[a] 15. Stroke Prevention in Atrial Fibrillation Investigators. Warfarin versus aspirin for prevention of thromboembolism in atrial fibrillation: SPAF II Study. Lancet 1994; 343:687.

[b] 16. SPAF III Writing Committee for the Stroke Prevention in Atrial Fibrillation Investigators. Patients with nonvalvular atrial fibrillation at low risk of stroke during treatment with aspirin: SPAF III study. JAMA 1998; 279:1273.

[a] 17. Atrial Fibrillation Follow-up Investigation of Rhythm Management (AFFIRM) Investigators. A comparison of rate control with rhythm control in patients with atrial fibrillation. N Engl J Med 2002; 347:1825.

[a] 18. vanGelder I et al. A comparison of rate control and rhythm control in patients with recurrent persistent atrial fibrillation. N Engl J Med 2002; 347:1834.

[a] 19. Klein AL et al. Use of transesophageal echocardiography to guide cardioversion in patients with atrial fibrillation. N Engl J Med 2001; 344:1411.

[b] 20. Mittal S et al. Transthoracic cardioversion of atrial fibrillation: comparison of rectilinear biphasic versus damped sine wave monophasic shocks. Circulation 2000; 101:282.

[a] 21. Page RL et al. Biphasic versus monophasic shock waveform for conversion of atrial fibrillation: the results of an international randomized, double-blind multicenter trial. J Am Coll Cardiol 2002; 39:1956.

[a] 22. Oral H et al. Facilitating transthoracic cardioversion of atrial fibrillation with ibutilide pretreatment. N Engl J Med 1999; 340:1849.

[c] 23. Nabar A et al. Radiofrequency ablation of "Class IC atrial flutter" in patients with resistant atrial fibrillation. Am J Cardiol 1999; 83:785.

[a] 24. Roy D et al. Amiodarone to prevent recurrence of atrial fibrillation. N Engl J Med 2000; 342:913.

[a] 25. Torp-Pedersen C et al. Dofetilide in patients with congestive heart failure and left ventricular dysfunction. N Engl J Med 1999; 341:857.

[b] 26. Ozcan C et al. Long-term survival after ablation of the atrioventricular node and implantation of permanent pacemaker in patients with atrial fibrillation. N Engl J Med 2001; 344:1043.

[c] 27. Chen SA et al. Initiation of atrial fibrillation by ectopic beats originating from the pulmonary veins: electrophysiological characteristics, pharmacological responses and effects of radiofrequency ablation. Circulation 1999; 100:1879.

[b] 28. Wellens HJ et al. Atrioverter: an implantable device for the treatment of atrial fibrillation. Circulation 1998; 98:1651.

[c] 29. Wellens HJJ. Contemporary management of atrial flutter. Circulation 2002; 106:649.

[b] 30. Natale A et al. Prospective randomized comparison of antiarrhythmic therapy versus first-line radiofrequency ablation in patients with atrial flutter. J Am Coll Cardiol 2000; 35:1898.

7

ATRIAL FIBRILLATION

Heart Failure

Michael Field, MD, Matthews Chacko, MD, and Edward Kasper, MD

FAST FACTS

- The most common causes of heart failure (HF) in the United States are ischemic heart disease, hypertension, valvular heart disease, and idiopathic dilated cardiomyopathy.
- HF can result from either systolic dysfunction (impaired contraction) or diastolic dysfunction (impaired relaxation).
- Patients can be classified into four hemodynamic subsets based on whether they have pulmonary congestion (wet or dry) and whether they have low perfusion (cold or warm).
- Initial management must involve identification and correction of precipitating causes.
- Diuretics are the cornerstone of therapy for decompensated failure. Their use is indicated for patients with symptomatic HF even after edema has been resolved. The dose and type of diuretic drug may change according to fluid status, but the diuretic will generally be needed indefinitely.
- Angiotensin-converting enzyme (ACE) inhibitors are indicated for all patients with left ventricular systolic dysfunction regardless of symptoms. They reduce symptoms and improve survival. They have added benefit at higher doses and should be titrated to the maximum tolerated dose. They are superior to hydralazine and isosorbide dinitrate.
- Digoxin improves symptoms and decreases hospitalizations for HF but does not affect mortality.
- β-Blockers improve survival and reduce symptoms in patients with New York Heart Association (NYHA) class II to IV HF. Usually the ACE inhibitor dose is adjusted first and the β-blocker is then carefully titrated on an outpatient basis. β-Blockade is not initiated in acute decompensated HF.
- Spironolactone decreases mortality among select patients with NYHA class III or IV symptoms.

I. EPIDEMIOLOGY

1. HF results from the heart's inability to meet the metabolic needs of the tissues or to respond to elevations in cardiac filling pressures.
2. The cardinal manifestations of this syndrome are dyspnea on exertion and orthopnea (resulting from elevated filling pressures) and fatigue (resulting from decreased cardiac output).
3. The term "heart failure" should not be used interchangeably with

"cardiomyopathy," which denotes heart muscle disease. The causes of cardiomyopathy are listed in Box 8-1.

4. HF may result from systolic dysfunction (impaired contraction) or diastolic dysfunction (impaired relaxation and filling). Causes of systolic dysfunction include coronary artery disease (about 60% of cases), hypertension, valvular disease, myocardial toxins, myocarditis, and idiopathic dilated cardiomyopathy.

5. Diastolic dysfunction is diagnosed in patients with clinical evidence of increased filling pressures but normal ejection fraction (EF >50%). Causes of diastolic dysfunction include restrictive cardiomyopathy

---

BOX 8-1

CAUSES OF CARDIOMYOPATHY

Ischemic

Carcinoid

Connective tissue disorders: lupus, polyarteritis nodosa, rheumatoid arthritis, scleroderma, granulomatous disease, dermatomyositis

Endocrine and metabolic: thyrotoxicosis, hypothyroidism, pheochromocytoma, diabetes, myxedema, uremia, acromegaly, hypocalcemia, hypophosphatemia, porphyria, gout

Fabry's disease

Gaucher's disease

Glycogen-storage diseases

Hematologic: polycythemia vera, sickle cell disease, leukemia, Loeffler's disease

Hypertensive disease

Idiopathic and familial

Infectious and inflammatory: Coxsackie B, human immunodeficiency virus, Chagas' disease, Lyme disease, adenovirus, cytomegalovirus, HIV

Infiltrative disorders: amyloid, hemochromatosis, sarcoid

Medications and toxins: alcohol, cocaine, catecholamines, anthracyclines (doxorubicin), irradiation, cyclophosphamide, bleomycin, 5-fluorouracil, carbon monoxide, lithium, chloroquine, arsenic, cobalt, antimony, snake venom, methysergide, lead, antidepressants, disopyramide, phosphorus poisoning, sulfa-drug hypersensitivity

Muscular dystrophies: Duchenne, Becker-type, facioscapulohumeral, limb-girdle, and myotonic

Nutritional deficiencies: kwashiorkor, selenium, beri-beri (thiamine), carnitine deficiency

Pericardial diseases (pseudocardiomyopathy)

Peripartum

Refsum's disease

Sleep apnea

Tachycardia-induced cardiomyopathy

Transplant rejection

Valvular disease

Whipple's disease

and disorders that lead to left ventricular hypertrophy (LVH), such as hypertension, aortic stenosis, and hypertrophic cardiomyopathy. About 50% of HF cases are due primarily to diastolic dysfunction.[1-3] In most patients evidence of systolic and diastolic dysfunction coexists, and clinical manifestations are similar for both types.

II. CLINICAL PRESENTATION

1. Dyspnea is the most common clinical complaint in HF. A differential diagnosis for dyspnea is included in Box 8-2.
2. The signs and symptoms of HF include pulmonary rales, pleural effusions, S_3 gallop sounds, pulsus alternans, electrical alternans, Cheyne-Stokes respirations, low-grade fevers, accentuation of P_2, and other signs of right-sided failure such as edema, congestive hepatomegaly, jugular venous distention, hepatojugular reflux, and ascites.

BOX 8-2

DIFFERENTIAL DIAGNOSIS FOR DYSPNEA

Airway obstruction
Anemia
Anxiety
Asthma
Bronchopulmonary malignancy
Chest trauma causing pulmonary contusion or flail chest
Chronic obstructive pulmonary disease
Congestive heart failure
Cystic fibrosis
Fever
Guillain-Barré disease
Hyperthyroidism
Increased intracranial pressure
Interstitial lung disease
Metabolic acidosis
Myasthenia gravis
Myocardial ischemia
Obesity
Pericardial effusion with or without tamponade
Phrenic nerve dysfunction
Pleurisy
Pneumonia
Pneumothorax with or without tamponade
Pulmonary embolus
Pulmonary hypertension
Salicylate overdose
Shock
Tracheobronchitis

8

HEART FAILURE

Low perfusion at rest?	Congestion at rest?	No	Yes
	No	Warm and dry	Warm and wet
	Yes	Cold and dry	Cold and wet

FIG. 8-1

Assessment of hemodynamic profile. *(Modified from Nohria A, Lewis E, Stevenson L. JAMA 2002; 287:628.)*

BOX 8-3

NEW YORK HEART ASSOCIATION CLASSIFICATION

Class I	Symptoms of heart failure only at levels that would limit normal individuals
Class II	Symptoms of heart failure with ordinary exertion
Class III	Symptoms of heart failure on less than ordinary exertion
Class IV	Symptoms of heart failure at rest

3. Laboratory findings may include proteinuria, mild elevations in blood urea nitrogen and creatinine levels, and relatively normal electrolyte panels. Depending on an individual's medication regimen, alterations in sodium and potassium levels are not uncommon. Liver function tests can be mildly elevated because of hepatic congestion, and depending on the chronicity of HF, signs of hepatic synthetic dysfunction (e.g., low albumin) may also be seen.
4. One approach to using clinical findings to help guide management is to divide patients into two basic hemodynamic subsets: those caused by congestion from elevated filling pressures and fluid retention (wet versus dry) and those caused by poor perfusion from decreased cardiac output (cold versus warm). Based on these criteria a patient can be placed into one of the four hemodynamic profiles illustrated in Fig. 8-1. Severity of symptoms is quantified according to the NYHA classification shown in Box 8-3.

A. EVIDENCE OF CONGESTION

1. **Symptoms:** Elevated left-sided filling pressures cause dyspnea early in exertion, orthopnea (shortness of breath or coughing while lying flat), and paroxysmal nocturnal dyspnea. Elevated right-sided filling pressures

BOX 8-4

CLINICAL FINDINGS IN HEART FAILURE BY SUBSET

EVIDENCE OF CONGESTION

Orthopnea

High jugular venous pressure

Abdominojugular reflux

Increasing S_3

Loud P_2

Rales

Edema

Ascites

EVIDENCE OF LOW PERFUSION

Fatigue

Somnolence, obtundation

Narrow pulse pressure

Pulsus alternans

Cool forearms and legs

Angiotensin-converting enzyme inhibitor–related hypotension

Declining serum sodium

Worsening renal function

Data from Nohria A, Lewis E, Stevenson L. JAMA 2002; 287:628.

result in dependent edema, anorexia, and abdominal bloating or fullness.

2. **Signs:** The most useful sign is an elevated jugular venous pressure. Rales are present in acute pulmonary congestion but most often are absent in patients with chronically elevated filling pressures because of compensation by pulmonary lymphatics.[4] Abdominojugular reflux, new or increasing S_3, loud P_2, peripheral edema, and ascites may indicate congestion and fluid overload (Box 8-4).

B. EVIDENCE OF LOW PERFUSION

1. **Symptoms:** Findings are nonspecific and include fatigue, weakness, difficulty concentrating, and somnolence.

2. **Signs:** A narrow pulse pressure, often defined as a proportional pulse pressure (PPP) less than 25%, correlates with low cardiac output [PPP = (SBP-DBP)/SBP]. Other signs include low volume pulses, pulsus alternans, cool forearms and legs, poor renal function, low serum sodium level, and ACE inhibitor–related hypotension (Box 8-4).

C. EXAMINATION FOR EVIDENCE OF SYSTOLIC OR DIASTOLIC DYSFUNCTION

In addition to the preceding classification by hemodynamic subset, the physician should distinguish at initial evaluation whether the patient has HF caused primarily by systolic or diastolic dysfunction, since this will guide management. Quick bedside echocardiography can provide valuable information. In addition, aspects of the patient's history and physical examination can often lead to the correct diagnosis.

1. **Systolic dysfunction:** Findings that are helpful in identifying patients with EF less than 40% are cardiomegaly on chest radiograph, redistribution on chest radiograph (increased vascular markings in upper lung zones), anterior Q waves, LBBB, and abnormal apical impulses. Also suggestive are a pulse greater than 100 beats/min and decreased PPP.[5]

2. **Diastolic dysfunction:** Presence of hypertension during the HF episode (systolic blood pressure >160 beats/min or diastolic >100 beats/min) is suggestive of diastolic dysfunction. Less useful findings, but still suggestive of diastolic dysfunction, include obesity, older age, absence of history of myocardial infarction (MI), and absence of tachycardia. A normal heart size on a chest radiograph is helpful if present, but many patients with diastolic dysfunction have cardiomegaly reflecting cardiac hypertrophy.[5] Electrocardiographic (ECG) evidence of LVH, history of hypertension, female sex, and presence of S_4 may be helpful if taken together.

III. DIAGNOSTICS

A. ECHOCARDIOGRAPHY

1. Transthoracic echocardiography should be performed in all patients with new-onset HF and provides information about ventricular size as well as systolic and diastolic function.

2. Other important findings include evidence of valvular disease, focal wall motion abnormalities, estimation of pulmonary pressures, evidence of pericardial thickening (constrictive pericarditis), and infiltration of the myocardium (glistening appearance in amyloidosis).

3. Diastolic filling properties can be estimated by examination of the Doppler flow pattern across the mitral valve as a function of time.

B. LABORATORY TESTS

1. A complete blood count, comprehensive metabolic panel, urinalysis, creatine kinase with isoenzymes, thyroid-stimulating hormone, and liver function panel should be sent for all patients with acute HF.

2. At the patient's first presentation for HF, assays for ferritin, total iron-binding capacity, antinuclear antibody, rheumatoid factor, urinary metanephrines, human immunodeficiency virus antibody, and serum and urine protein electrophoresis may be helpful to determine an etiology.

C. ELECTROCARDIOGRAPHY

1. An ECG should be obtained for all patients at the time of presentation to assess for evidence of myocardial ischemia, Q waves, LBBB, left ventricular hypertrophy, right ventricular hypertrophy, low voltage (consider amyloidosis, effusion), or biatrial enlargement.

D. CHEST RADIOGRAPHY

1. Radiographic findings depend on the degree of HF and may include cardiomegaly, diffuse bilateral infiltrates extending from the hila, and

Kerley B lines. Pleural effusions may indicate chronic left ventricular failure.

2. The absence of pulmonary vascular congestion is not unusual if the patient has primarily right ventricular failure or if long-term adaptation to left ventricular failure has occurred, even in the presence of high left-sided filling pressures.

E. CARDIAC CATHETERIZATION

1. Left-sided heart catheterization with coronary angiography is indicated for virtually all patients with a new-onset HF in the absence of contraindications to rule out an ischemic etiology.

2. Right-sided heart catheterization may provide additional useful information about cardiac output and intracardiac and pulmonary artery pressures.

F. ENDOMYOCARDIAL BIOPSY

1. Endomyocardial biopsy may be performed on patients in whom an inflammatory or infiltrative disorder of the heart is suspected.[6]

G. EXERCISE TESTING

1. Exercise testing can be used to detect ischemic heart disease and provides an estimation of functional capacity for risk stratification and prognosis.

2. Measurement of maximal oxygen uptake (Vo_{2max}) is an objective index of functional severity and is the best index of prognosis in patients with symptomatic HF. It can be used to determine the necessity and timing of cardiac transplantation.

3. A simpler test used in practice, which correlates with Vo_{2max}, is the 6-minute walk test (distance the patient can walk in 6 minutes).

IV. MANAGEMENT

A. ACUTE HEART FAILURE

1. **Identification and correction of the precipitating cause:** A systematic search for precipitating causes must be performed in every patient with new-onset or worsening HF. Box 8-5 lists possible precipitating causes.

BOX 8-5

PRECIPITATING CAUSES OF HEART FAILURE

Ischemia and myocardial infarction

Infection

Arrhythmia

Systemic hypertension

Noncompliance with medication

Sodium and fluid indiscretion

Excessive alcohol intake

Pulmonary embolism

Thyrotoxicosis

High output (thyrotoxicosis, arteriovenous fistula, pregnancy, anemia)

Myocarditis

8

HEART FAILURE

> **BOX 8-6**
>
> **FUROSEMIDE DOSAGE AND EXPECTED RESPONSE**
>
> Generally, IV administration of furosemide is twice as potent as oral administration.
>
> Patients admitted to the hospital with heart failure should receive IV diuresis to overcome poor absorption caused by gastrointestinal tract edema.
>
> Typically the starting IV dose is equivalent to the patient's home oral dose (i.e., a patient taking furosemide 40 mg PO qd should receive 20 mg IV).
>
> If response (100-200 mL urine output) does not occur in 30 minutes to 1 hour, the diagnosis of decompensated congestive heart failure should be reassessed. If the diagnosis is correct, the furosemide dose should be doubled and this algorithm repeated.
>
> Indwelling urinary catheters can help in gauging urine output.
>
> Furosemide has a diuretic effect for 6 hours. After this the kidneys are highly sodium avid and diuresis will lose its effect if the patient is not on a low-sodium diet as well.

Once considered, therapy should be directed to an underlying cause (if identified and treatable) and standard HF therapy initiated based on one of four hemodynamic profiles (Fig. 8-1).

2. **Hemodynamic profiles.**

a. Wet and warm: This is the most common subgroup of patients admitted with HF. Patients have congestion resulting from elevated filling pressures and volume overload that can be relieved with intravenous loop diuretics (Box 8-6) or the more recently available brain natriuretic peptide analog, nesiritide. In addition, they may benefit from intravenous or oral vasodilators such as nitroglycerin. Positive inotropic agents are often unnecessary and may be detrimental.

b. Wet and cold: Patients with congestion and critically limited hypo-perfusion often must be "warmed up" before they can be "dried out."[7] Perfusion may be improved through the use of vasodilators alone. However, these patients may have therapy-limiting hypotension, which often necessitates circulatory support in the form of inotropic agents such as dopamine, milrinone, or dobutamine. In cases not responsive to inotropes, mechanical circulatory support such as a left ventricular assist device may be necessary, often as a lifesaving measure until heart transplantation.

c. Dry and warm: This hemodynamic profile represents compensated HF, and many patients with this form do not require inpatient management. Efforts should be aimed at maintaining stable volume status and preventing disease progression as outlined later in the chapter.

d. Dry and cold: This small subgroup of patients has a low cardiac output and evidence of poor perfusion but no clinical evidence of elevated filling pressures. Little data exist to guide therapy. Patients may respond to inotropes, although transiently, but long-term use has produced adverse effects. Careful management with ACE inhibitors, β-blockers, and digoxin may in time lead to improvement. Some patients have unrecognized congestion and may benefit from diuresis.

3. **Diuretics.**

a. Loop diuretics: Loop diuretics, such as furosemide, are the cornerstone of therapy in acute decompensated HF. Furosemide produces both acute venodilation and a powerful diuretic effect, which reduces preload and decreases pulmonary congestion. In acute HF, patients who have been on an oral regimen of loop diuretics should be switched to intravenous therapy to maximize bioavailability. Patients with renal insufficiency require higher doses of loop diuretics. Some patients respond better to a continuous infusion than to intermittent doses (Box 8-6). Markers of adequate diuresis include resolution of dyspnea, decrease in jugular venous pressure, decrease in intensity of S_3, elevation of serum creatinine level, and attainment of dry weight. Side effects of loop diuretics include hypokalemia, hypomagnesemia, hyponatremia or hypernatremia, volume depletion, renal failure, ototoxicity, and drug reactions (related to the sulfa group).

b. Thiazide diuretics: Adding a thiazide diuretic such as chlorothiazide may potentiate the effect of loop diuretics by preventing distal tubular reabsorption of sodium.

4. **Vasodilators.**

a. ACE inhibitors: ACE inhibitors are begun at low doses with short-acting agents such as captopril and are titrated while the blood pressure response, symptoms, and serum potassium and creatinine levels are monitored. Once short-acting agents are tolerated, transition to long-acting agents can occur before discharge. About 10% to 30% of patients with advanced HF cannot tolerate ACE inhibitors because of the hypotension or renal dysfunction associated with these agents.[7]

b. Nitrates: The pharmacological action of organic nitrates such as nitroglycerin is vasodilation, particularly of the systemic veins, resulting in decreased preload. Nitrates have a role in the management of acute pulmonary edema and HF in the setting of hypertension or angina. Contraindications include severe aortic stenosis and concurrent sildenafil use.

c. Hydralazine: Hydralazine is a potent short-acting arterial vasodilator that can be used alone or in combination with nitrates for rapid afterload reduction. It is often considered as an alternative to ACE inhibitors and angiotensin II receptor blockers (ARBs) in patients with acute renal failure and other conditions in which ACE inhibitors are contraindicated.

d. Nitroprusside: Nitroprusside is a potent intravenous arterial vasodilator that may be warranted if further vasodilation and afterload reduction are needed. Adverse effects include thiocyanate toxicity, particularly in patients with hepatic dysfunction or renal failure, and coronary steal phenomenon in patients with ischemic heart disease.

e. Nesiritide: Nesiritide, or recombinant B–type natriuretic peptide (BNP), produces hemodynamic improvement and relieves symptoms in patients with decompensated HF through a vasodilator and natriuretic effect.[8] The most common adverse effect is hypotension. Until more data are available, nesiritide should probably be reserved for patients who do not respond to standard HF therapies and should be used in consultation with a cardiologist.

5. **Inotropes:** Potentially appropriate uses of inotropes include the temporary treatment of diuretic-refractory acute HF (i.e., cold and wet) and a bridge to definitive treatment such as revascularization or cardiac transplantation. Inotropes may also be appropriate as a palliative measure in patients with truly end-stage HF. The routine use of inotropes as HF therapy is not indicated in either acute or chronic HF.[10] Optimization may require invasive hemodynamic monitoring with a pulmonary artery catheter.

a. Dopamine: Dopamine is an endogenous catecholamine that has distinct cardiovascular effects at escalating doses. Low-dose dopamine (1-3 μg/kg/min) acting through dopaminergic receptors leads to increases in renal blood flow and natriuresis. Intermediate doses (2-10 μg/kg/min) result in predominant β-adrenergic receptor stimulation, which increases cardiac output by augmentation of contractility and heart rate. Higher doses (10-20 μg/kg/min) result in significant α-adrenergic stimulation that increases afterload and may be detrimental in HF. Dopamine should be used primarily for stabilization of hypotensive patients. Tachycardia may be an undesirable side effect, particularly in those with ischemic heart disease or diastolic dysfunction. Low-dose dopamine in critically ill patients has not been shown to improve diuresis and does not provide renal protection in patients with renal dysfunction.[9]

b. Dobutamine: Dobutamine is a β-adrenergic agonist with a predominant hemodynamic effect of direct inotropic stimulation with reflex arterial vasodilation, resulting in afterload reduction and augmentation of cardiac output. It may cause hypotension, precipitate ventricular arrhythmias, and worsen ischemic heart disease by increasing myocardial oxygen demand. Some patients with chronic refractory HF require intermittent outpatient infusions. Dobutamine tolerance has been described, and some studies have indicated an increased mortality among patients treated with continuous dobutamine.[11]

c. Milrinone: Milrinone, a phosphodiesterase inhibitor, increases contractility and produces vasodilation by increasing intracellular cyclic adenosine monophosphate. As with dobutamine, hypotension and arrhythmias may occur. Long-term use has been shown to increase mortality.[12]

6. **Supplemental oxygen:** Supplemental oxygen is indicated primarily for patients with arterial desaturation. If patients with HF require substantial amounts of oxygen, coexisting pulmonary disease, pulmonary embolism, or pneumonia should be considered. Patients with acute pulmonary edema may require mechanical ventilation.

7. **Morphine:** Morphine is a μ-opioid receptor agonist with both vascular

and central effects. Morphine (2-4 mg IV) may provide symptomatic relief in acute pulmonary edema through venodilation and decreased perception of dyspnea. Side effects may include hypotension, somnolence, and respiratory depression, particularly in the elderly or patients with coexisting pulmonary disease.

B. CHRONIC HEART FAILURE

Long-term HF therapy for systolic and diastolic dysfunction is discussed separately.

1. **Systolic dysfunction.**

a. Staging: HF can be viewed as a continuum of stages progressing from asymptomatic to advanced disease. Fig. 8-2 considers four stages in the evolution of HF with examples and appropriate therapy.[13]

   (1) Stage A: Patients at high risk for left ventricular dysfunction.

   (a) Many conditions that are associated with risk of HF can be identified early, before the development of structural heart disease. These include hypertension, coronary artery disease, diabetes mellitus, and presence of cardiotoxins. Modification of these risk factors can often reduce the risk of HF.

   (b) Interventions include controlling hypertension and hyperlipidemia, discouraging smoking, excessive alcohol intake, and illicit drug use, and encouraging exercise and weight loss. ACE inhibitors are indicated for patients with atherosclerotic vascular disease (MI, cerebrovascular accident, peripheral vascular disease) or diabetes with associated risk factors.[14]

   (2) Stage B: Patients with left ventricular dysfunction in whom symptoms have not developed.

   (a) Asymptomatic patients who have had a prior MI or evidence of LVH, left ventricular dysfunction, or valvular disease are at very high risk for HF.

   (b) In addition to the recommendations listed under stage A, all patients with systolic dysfunction, regardless of symptoms, should receive ACE inhibitors. ACE inhibitors and β-blockers are indicated for patients with a history of MI regardless of the ejection fraction. β-Blockers may be used for patients with asymptomatic systolic dysfunction, although evidence supporting their use for this population is not as strong as it is for symptomatic patients with systolic dysfunction. Valvular repair or replacement should be performed according to published guidelines.[15]

   (3) Stage C: Patients with left ventricular dysfunction with current or prior symptoms.

   (a) General measures: Readmission for HF occurs at a high rate (30%-50%) within 6 months after discharge. A number of criteria should be met before discharge, including transition to oral medications for 24 hours, achievement of dry weight, stable or improving renal function, and ambulation with decreased

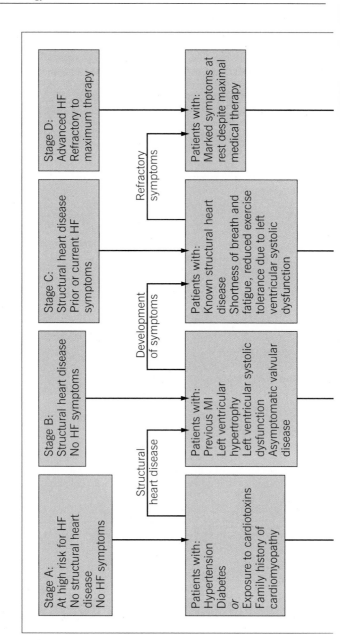

Stage A:
At high risk for HF
No structural heart disease
No HF symptoms

→ Patients with:
Hypertension
Diabetes
or
Exposure to cardiotoxins
Family history of cardiomyopathy

Structural heart disease

Stage B:
Structural heart disease
No HF symptoms

→ Patients with:
Previous MI
Left ventricular hypertrophy
Left ventricular systolic dysfunction
Asymptomatic valvular disease

Development of symptoms

Stage C:
Structural heart disease
Prior or current HF symptoms

→ Patients with:
Known structural heart disease
Shortness of breath and fatigue, reduced exercise tolerance due to left ventricular systolic dysfunction

Refractory symptoms

Stage D:
Advanced HF
Refractory to maximum therapy

→ Patients with:
Marked symptoms at rest despite maximal medical therapy

FIG. 8-2

Stages in the evolution of heart failure and recommended therapy by stage. *ACE,* Angiotensin-converting enzyme; *EF,* ejection fraction; *HF,* heart failure; *HTN,* hypertension; *MI,* myocardial infarction.

Therapy:
Treat hypertension
Treat lipid disorders
Stop smoking
Avoid alcohol
ACE inhibitors in patients with vascular disease, diabetes, or HTN and cardiovascular risk factors

Therapy:
Stage A measures *and*
ACE inhibitors if history of MI or reduced EF
β-Blockers if history of MI or reduced EF
Valve surgery if indicated

Therapy:
Stage A measures *and*
Diuretics
ACE inhibitors
β-Blockers
Digoxin
Salt restriction
± Spironolactone

Therapy:
Stage A, B, and C measures *and*
Mechanical assist devices
Heart transplantation
Continuous (not intermittent) IV infusions for palliation
Hospice care

dyspnea and without symptomatic hypotension. During the hospitalization patients should receive education about sodium and fluid restriction and recommendations for exercise. Patients should monitor their weight at home and may benefit from a sliding scale diuretic regimen. Vaccination for pneumococcal infection and influenza is recommended. Use of nonsteroidal antiinflammatory drugs for patients with advanced HF should be avoided because they may lead to fluid retention and worsen the HF. Recommendations listed under stage A and B apply as well.

(b) Vasodilators.

   i. ACE inhibitors.

      (1) ACE inhibitors are indicated for all patients with systolic dysfunction, regardless of symptoms. Success of ACE inhibitors in improving survival, relieving symptoms, preventing hospitalization, and halting the progression of left ventricular remodeling has been documented in numerous clinical trials.[16,17] They may have added benefit at higher doses,[18] and attempts should be made to achieve the target doses reported in the major clinical trials (lisinopril 20-40 mg/day, enalapril 10 mg bid, or captopril 50 mg tid).

      (2) It should be emphasized that the benefit of ACE inhibitors in HF is independent of the ability to lower blood pressure and the relative absence of hypertension is not relevant in the decision to begin therapy. Cough and angioedema are the adverse effects most commonly associated with ACE inhibitors. Contraindications include symptomatic hypotension, acute renal failure, bilateral renal artery stenosis, hyperkalemia, and pregnancy. Reports of adverse events or contraindications should be scrutinized so that patients are not incorrectly excluded from receiving this important class of medications.

  ii. ARBs: ARBs should be used in place of ACE inhibitors when the latter cause angioedema or cough. However, as with ACE inhibitors, ARBs should not be used in the presence of acute renal failure or hyperkalemia and may produce symptomatic hypotension. Studies directly comparing ARBs and ACE inhibitors have shown no greater survival with use of ARBs.[19,20] Given the greater experience with ACE inhibitors, they should be used as first-line agents and ARBs should be reserved for patients who cannot tolerate ACE inhibitors.

  iii. Nitrates and hydralazine: Isosorbide dinitrate (40 mg qid) combined with hydralazine (75 mg qid) has been shown to improve survival in chronic HF.[21] Although inferior to ACE inhibitors, this combination should be considered for patients who cannot tolerate ACE inhibitors and ARBs for any of the aforementioned reasons.[22] A "nitrate-free" interval should be allowed to prevent the development of nitrate tolerance in patients on long-term therapy.

(c) β-Blockers: Several β-blockers have been shown to reduce mortality in patients with symptomatic HF and systolic dysfunction.[23-25] All stable, euvolemic patients with NYHA class II to IV HF resulting from left ventricular dysfunction should receive a β-blocker unless they cannot tolerate β-blockers or have a contraindication. Usually an ACE inhibitor is titrated first and the β-blocker in then added in the outpatient setting. Metoprolol extended release (Toprol XL) can be initiated at 25 mg PO qd (12.5 mg PO qd in NYHA class IV) and titrated slowly (monthly) to a maximum dose of 200 PO qd. Carvedilol is begun at 3.125 mg PO bid and titrated to a maximum dose of 25 to 50 mg PO bid. Bisoprolol is begun at a dose of 1.25 PO qd and titrated to 10 mg PO qd. Contraindications to β-blockade include acute decompensated HF, symptomatic bradycardia, advanced heart block, and severe bronchospastic disease. Although many patients take atenolol, no studies evaluating the use of atenolol in CHF have been presented.

(d) Diuretics.

   i. Loop diuretics: In addition to their role in acute management of HF, loop diuretics such as furosemide have a central role in long-term management to attenuate progressive volume overload caused by compensatory sodium avidity. Therefore diuretics are indicated for patients with symptomatic HF even after they have been rendered free of edema. The dose and type of diuretic drug may change according to fluid status, but generally a diuretic will be needed indefinitely.

   ii. Spironolactone: Spironolactone, a potassium-sparing diuretic, has been shown to decrease both mortality and rehospitalization by one third in patients with primarily NYHA class III to IV HF.[26] Spironolactone is given as a once daily dose of 25 mg. Patients, especially those who have unstable renal function and are taking high doses of ACE inhibitors, are at increased risk of hyperkalemia. Patients should have serum creatinine levels that are stable and less than 2 mg/dL, receive frequent electrolyte monitoring, and discontinue potassium supplementation. Gynecomastia is a troubling side effect in about 10% of male patients.

(e) Digoxin: Digoxin is a glycoside shown to improve symptoms and prevent hospitalization in patients with systolic dysfunction.[27] It is indicated for patients with HF symptoms despite optimal therapy with ACE inhibitors and diuretics or for patients with coexisting atrial fibrillation. Toxic effects of digoxin are more likely to occur in patients with renal insufficiency, electrolyte abnormalities (potassium and magnesium), advanced age, and coadministration of certain drugs (amiodarone, quinidine, verapamil, propafenone). Manifestations include confusion, nonspecific gastrointestinal complaints, vision and color disturbances, and many types of arrhythmias (heart block, tachycardias).

(f) Warfarin sodium: Anticoagulation with warfarin sodium (Coumadin) is warranted for patients with concomitant atrial fibrillation, visible thrombus on echocardiogram, or a previous cardioembolic event. Anticoagulation should be considered for patients with a very low EF (<25%), with a goal international normalized ratio (INR) of 2.0 to 3.0. However, few studies are available to support its routine use for HF.[28]

(g) Exercise: A prescription for exercise for those with HF may improve functional capacity and quality of life and prevent death from cardiovascular disease.[29]

(4) Stage D: Patients with refractory end-stage heart failure.

(a) Recommendations include meticulous control of fluid retention with diuretics. ACE inhibitors and β-blockers are beneficial. However, this group of patients is at particular risk of developing hypotension and renal failure with ACE inhibitors and worsening HF with β-blockers.

(b) Cardiac transplantation should be considered in eligible patients.

(c) Left ventricular assist devices provide hemodynamic support for patients awaiting heart transplantation and may be beneficial even for patients who are not candidates for heart transplant.[30]

(d) Continuous intravenous inotropic infusions and hospice may be used for palliative measures in patients with truly end-stage HF.

2. **Diastolic dysfunction (Fig. 8-3):** In contrast to the treatment of systolic dysfunction, few clinical trials are available to guide management of HF caused by diastolic dysfunction. Based on pathophysiology, four management principles may be followed.[13]

a. Control of blood pressure: β-Blockers, ACE inhibitors, ARBs, or calcium channel blockers may be used to control systolic and diastolic blood pressure according to published guidelines. Few trials exist to define optimal management.

b. Control of tachycardia: Patients with atrial fibrillation require rate control and may benefit from a trial of cardioversion.

c. Diuretics to control pulmonary congestion and edema: Patients may have rales and evidence of volume overload (elevated neck veins and peripheral edema). Loop diuretics such as furosemide will decrease filling pressures and relieve pulmonary congestion. Care must be taken with diuresis because patients with diastolic HF are sensitive to preload reduction and hypertension or prerenal azotemia may develop.

d. Assessment and control of ischemia: Revascularization should be considered for patients with evidence of ischemia.

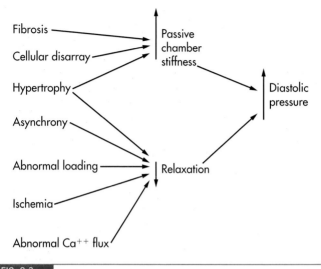

FIG. 8-3

Factors responsible for diastolic dysfunction and increased left ventricular diastolic pressure. *(From Gaasch WH, Izzi G. Clinical diagnosis and management of left ventricular diastolic function. In Hori M et al, eds. Cardiac mechanics and function in the normal and diseased heart. New York: Springer-Verlag; 1989.)*

8

HEART FAILURE

REFERENCES

[b] 1. Vasan RS et al. Congestive heart failure in subjects with normal versus reduced left ventricular ejection fraction: prevalence and mortality in a population-based cohort. J Am Coll Cardiol 1999; 33 (7):1948.

[b] 2. Vasan R, Benjamin E, Levy D. Prevalence, clinical features and prognosis of diastolic heart failure: an epidemiologic perspective. J Am Coll Cardiol 1995; 26 (7):1565.

[b] 3. Senni M et al. Congestive heart failure in the community: a study of all incident cases in Olmstead County, Minnesota in 1991. Circulation 1998; 98:2282.

[d] 4. Stevenson L, Perloff J. The limited reliability of physical signs for estimating hemodynamics in chronic heart failure. JAMA 1989; 261:884.

[c] 5. Badgett R, Lucey C, Mulrow C. Can the clinical examination diagnose left-sided heart failure in adults? JAMA 1997; 277:1712.

[c] 6. Wu L, Lapeyre A, Cooper L. Current role of endomyocardial biopsy in the management of dilated cardiomyopathy and myocarditis. Mayo Clin Proc 2001; 76:1030.

[c] 7. Nohria A, Lewis E, Stevenson L. Medical management of advanced heart failure. JAMA 2002; 287:628.

[a] 8. Colucci W et al. Intravenous nesiritide, a natriuretic peptide, in the treatment of decompensated congestive heart failure. N Engl J Med 2000; 343:246.

[a] 9. Australian and New Zealand Intensive Care Society Clinical Trials Group. Low-dose dopamine in patients with early renal dysfunction: a placebo-controlled randomized trial. Lancet 2000; 356:2139.

[c] 10. Felker G et al. Inotropic therapy for heart failure: an evidence-based approach. Am Heart J 2001; 142:393.

[b] 11. Dies F et al. Intermittent dobutamine in ambulatory outpatients with chronic cardiac failure. Circulation 1986; 74(suppl II): II-39.

[a] 12. Packer M et al: The effect of carvedilol on morbidity and mortality in chronic heart failure. U.S. Carvedilol Heart Failure Study Group. N Engl J Med 1996; 334:1349.

[d] 13. Hunt S et al. ACC/AHA guidelines for the evaluation and management of chronic heart failure in the adult. J Am Coll Cardiol 2001; 38:2101.

[a] 14. Heart Outcomes Prevention Evaluation (HOPE) Investigators. Effects of an angiotensin-converting enzyme inhibitor, ramipril, on cardiovascular events in high risk patients. N Engl J Med 2000; 342:145.

[d] 15. Bonow RO et al. ACC/AHA guidelines for the management of patients with valvular heart disease: a report of the American College of Cardiology/American Heart Association Task Force on Practice Guidelines (Committee on Management of Patients with Valvular Heart Disease). J Am Coll Cardiol 1998; 32:1486.

[a] 16. CONSENSUS Trial Study Group. Effects of enalapril on mortality in severe congestive heart failure: results of the Cooperative North Scandinavian Enalapril Survival Study. N Engl J Med 1987; 316:1429.

[a] 17. SOLVD Investigators. Effect of enalapril on survival in patients with reduced left ventricular ejection fractions and congestive heart failure. N Engl J Med 1991; 325:293.

[a] 18. Packer M et al. Comparative effects of low and high doses of the angiotensin-converting enzyme inhibitor, lisinopril, on morbidity and mortality in chronic heart failure. ATLAS Study Group. Circulation 1999; 100:2312.

[a] 19. Pitt B et al. Randomized trial of losartan versus captopril in patients over 65 with heart failure. Evaluation of Losartan in the Elderly (ELITE) Study Investigators. Lancet 1997; 349:747.

[a] 20. Pitt B et al. Effect of losartan compared with captopril on mortality in patients with symptomatic heart failure: randomised trial—the Losartan Heart Failure Survival Study ELITE II. Lancet 2000; 6(355):1582.

[a] 21. Cohn JN et al. The effect of vasodilator therapy on mortality in chronic congestive heart failure: the results of the VA Cooperative Study. VA Cooperative Study Group. N Engl J Med 1986; 314:1547.

[a] 22. Cohn JN et al. A comparison of enalapril with hydralazine–isosorbide dinitrate in the treatment of chronic congestive heart failure. N Engl J Med 1991; 325(5):303.

[a] 23. MERIT-HF Study Group. Effect of metoprolol CR/XL in chronic heart failure: metoprolol CR/XL randomized intervention trial in congestive heart failure. Lancet 1999; 353:2001.

[a] 24. Packer M et al. Effect of carvedilol on survival in severe chronic heart failure. N Engl J Med 2001; 344:1651.

[a] 25. CIBIS-II Investigators and Committees. The Cardiac Insufficiency Bisoprolol Study II: a randomized trial. Lancet 1999; 353:9.

[a] 26. RALES Investigators. Effectiveness of spironolactone added to an angiotensin-converting enzyme inhibitor and a loop diuretic for severe chronic congestive heart failure (the Randomized Aldactone Evaluation Study). Am J Cardiol 1996; 78:902.

[a] 27. Digitalis Investigators Group Study (DIG). The effect of digoxin on mortality and morbidity in patients with heart failure. N Engl J Med 1997; 336:525.

[d] 28. Graham SP. To anticoagulate or not to anticoagulate patients with cardiomyopathy. Cardiol Clin 2001; 19(4):605.

[a] 29. Belardinelli R et al. Randomized controlled trial of long-term moderate exercise training in chronic heart failure: effects on functional capacity, quality of life, and clinical outcomes. Circulation 1999; 99:1173.

[a] 30. Rose E et al. Long-term use of a left ventricular assist device for end-stage heart failure. Randomized Evaluation of Mechanical Assistance for the Treatment of Congestive Heart Failure (REMATCH) Study Group. N Engl J Med 2001; 345:1435.

Primary and Secondary Prevention of Coronary Artery Disease

Alan Cheng, MD, and Roger Blumenthal, MD

Fast Facts

- Every person admitted to the hospital should be evaluated for his or her risk of cardiovascular disease.

I. EPIDEMIOLOGY

1. Despite significant improvements in the management of cardiovascular disease (CVD), it has remained the leading cause of morbidity and mortality in the United States. Over the past 20 years, compelling evidence has emerged to implicate a number of major and minor risk factors that play a role in the development of CVD (Fig. 9-1). Addressing each and every risk factor in every person is logistically challenging and may be unnecessary. Hence, efforts toward reducing a person's risk for CVD should be tailored to his or her overall risk profile.

2. One approach targets the major independent risk factors (Tables 9-1 and 9-2).[1-16] These include age, male gender, postmenopausal state, family history of premature atherosclerosis, hypertension, hyperlipidemia, diabetes mellitus, obesity, cigarette smoking, and physical inactivity. Based on recommendations from the Joint National Committee, the American Heart Association, the American College of Cardiology, and the National Cholesterol Education Program, optimal goals for each modifiable risk factor have been established to enable assessment of each patient's risk of CVD.

II. MAJOR MODIFIABLE RISK FACTORS

A. TOBACCO USE

1. Cigarette use remains a major public health issue, with 25% to 30% of Americans actively smoking. Passive smoke exposure[15] and cigar smoking[16] have also been causally linked to CVD development. The mechanisms by which these events occur are probably related to increased levels of oxidized low-density lipoprotein cholesterol and direct toxic effects of carbon monoxide and nicotine on endothelial cells.[17-19] Surprisingly, despite these findings, clinical studies show that within 3 years of smoking cessation the risk that CVD will develop declines dramatically to nearly that of a nonsmoker.[20,21] This finding is even more striking in individuals with known CVD. Patients who

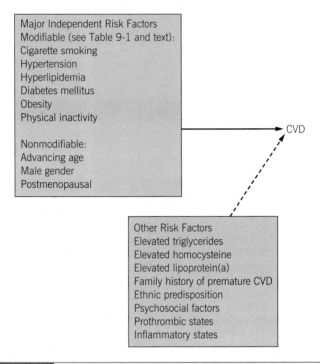

FIG. 9-1

Risk factors for cardiovascular disease (CVD). Major risk factors, as recognized by the American Heart Association, have been demonstrated to contribute independently to CVD. Other risk factors have also been described, but their role in pathogenesis of CVD is less clear. Some have been suggested to independently impart an increased risk for CVD, whereas others have been shown to accentuate known independent risk factors (see Tables 9-1 and 9-2). The Framingham Study investigators did not consider a family history of premature CVD to be an independent risk factor for CVD, but investigators from the National Cholesterol Education Program do.

    participated in the Coronary Artery Surgery Study reduced their risk of a second coronary event by 50% if they stopped smoking,[22] which emphasizes that continued cigarette smoking is the most powerful risk factor predictive of future need for coronary revascularization.[23]

2. Despite the publicity surrounding smoking cessation, its long-term success remains poor. Patients' concerns regarding intense nicotine craving, heightened anxiety, and increased weight gain are typically blamed. Large clinical trials have demonstrated reasonable efficacy

TABLE 9-1

MODIFIABLE MAJOR INDEPENDENT RISK FACTORS FOR
CARDIOVASCULAR DISEASE

Factor	Increased Risk States
Cigarette smoking	Smoking to any degree increases risk of CVD; exposure to passive smoke also increases risk[15]; cigar smoking contributes to a lesser degree[16]
Hypertension	Blood pressures >140/90 mm Hg
LDL-C	LDL-C >130 mg/dL for patients with established CVD or type 2 diabetes and LDL-C >160 mg/dL for others
HDL-C	HDL-C <40 mg/dL in men and <50 mg/dL in women
Diabetes mellitus	Fasting blood sugar level >125 mg/dL or HgbA$_1$C >7%
Obesity	Body mass index >30 kg/m^2; waist circumference >102 cm (40 inches) in men or >88 cm (35 inches) in women
Physical inactivity	Sedentary lifestyle before and after initial myocardial infarction

Data from Cheng A et al. Clin Cardiol 2002; 25:205.
All patients should be screened, counseled, and treated for these risk factors when appropriate.
Modified from the National Cholesterol Education Program Report and the American Heart
Association. Refer to text for details and references.
CVD, Cardiovascular disease; HDL-C, high-density lipoprotein; HgbA$_1$C, glycosylated hemoglobin;
LDL-C, low-density lipoprotein cholesterol.

from the use of nicotine replacement therapy or bupropion 150 mg PO bid.[24] A more recent study has suggested greater long-term efficacy (to levels as high as 35%) with minimal weight gain when nicotine replacement with bupropion was prescribed.[25] Caution should be exercised when prescribing bupropion for patients with a history of a seizure disorder, psychiatric illness, or bulimia because it can lower the seizure threshold. Bupropion occasionally exacerbates sleeplessness, so the second dose is typically given in the late afternoon to avoid insomnia.

B. HYPERTENSION

1. Hypertension is the most prevalent medical condition in the United States. An estimated 50 million Americans are affected. By impairing endothelial cell function and promoting left ventricular hypertrophy, hypertension plays a significant role in CVD development.[26] Based on the Sixth Report of the Joint National Committee (JNC VI) on high blood pressure, hypertension is defined as a systolic blood pressure greater than 140 mm Hg and a diastolic blood pressure greater than 90 mm Hg.[27] This report, derived from available clinical evidence (Table 9-3[28-36]) and expert opinion, recommends treatment for hypertension based on an individual's risk for CVD.

2. Three categories were developed (Table 9-4). Risk group A includes individuals with no clinical evidence of CVD, risk group B comprises patients with other known major risk factors for CVD except diabetes mellitus, and risk group C includes individuals with diabetes mellitus, end-organ disease (e.g., renal failure), or known CVD. Although all

TABLE 9-2

OTHER RISK FACTORS FOR CARDIOVASCULAR DISEASE

Factor	Risk
Hypertriglyceridemia	Based on guidelines of the National Cholesterol Education Program, triglyceride levels are classified into four categories: <150 mg/dL (desirable), 150-200 (borderline high), 200-500 (high), >500 (very high). Individuals with CVD or diabetes should be treated to reach a goal of <150 mg/dL. The VA-HIT study demonstrated a mortality benefit with gemfibrozil, but whether this was due to an increase in HDL-C, a decrease in triglycerides, or both remains unclear.
Hyperhomocysteinemia	Homocysteine levels >24 µM have been demonstrated to be a risk factor for CVD development.[1] Other studies have demonstrated that folic acid supplementation (1 mg qd) can reduce homocysteine levels,[2] but none to date demonstrate a mortality benefit with folate therapy.
Elevated Lp(a) level	Lp(a) is LDL-C with the addition of an apolipoprotein(a) moiety. Elevated levels (>30 mg/dL) have been associated with increased CVD risk.[3] Since there is no reliable intervention to lower Lp(a) levels other than niacin, many have recommended that with elevated Lp(a) levels, target LDL-C level should be <80 mg/dL.[4]
Family history of CVD	A family history of premature CVD exists if CVD occurs in first-degree relatives (<55 years old for men and <65 years old for women).[5]
Ethnic predisposition	South Asians (Indians and Pakistanis) have a twofold greater risk of CVD compared with whites, even when major risk factors are matched.[6] Hispanic-Americans have a risk comparable to that of whites,[7] and Asian-Americans have lower risk.
Psychosocial factors	Early observational studies have demonstrated an association between type A personality traits and increased CVD risk.[8] Subsequent studies (MRFIT, Framingham) did not validate these findings. More recent studies have shown some association of increased CVD risk with depression, social isolation, passive-submissive personalities, and hostility.[9,10]
Prothrombotic states	Elevated levels of fibrinogen,[11] PAI-1, factor VIII, and von Willebrand factor[12] have been associated with increased CVD risk.
Inflammatory states	Elevated C-reactive protein levels, leukocyte counts, and prooxidant states have been associated with increased CVD risk.[13] These findings may in part explain the mortality benefits of aspirin beyond its ability to inhibit platelet aggregation. Infections have been implicated,[14] although their role remains uncertain.

Data from Cheng A et al. Clin Cardiol 2002; 25:205.

Whether the factors in this table have an independent effect on CVD risk is unclear, but all have been demonstrated to impart some risk. Routine measurement of these factors is not recommended, however.

CVD, Cardiovascular disease; *HDL-C,* high-density lipoprotein cholesterol; *LDL-C,* low-density lipoprotein cholesterol; *Lp(a),* lipoprotein(a) cholesterol; *PAI-1,* plasminogen activator inhibitor-1.

individuals are encouraged to exercise, lose weight, and modify their diet, the timing of initiating pharmacotherapy varies. The guidelines are described in Table 9-4.

3. When pharmacotherapy is advised, the use of diuretics or β-blockers as first-line agents is appropriate regardless of risk group status. Concerns about depression, fatigue, and sexual dysfunction from the use of β-blockers are derived from older studies with higher doses of nonselective adrenergic blocking agents.[37]

4. Certain populations may benefit from more specific agents. The HOPE trial demonstrated that in individuals 55 years old or greater with known CVD or diabetes plus one additional CVD risk factor, the use of angiotensin-converting enzyme (ACE) inhibitors (specifically ramipril) may impart a mortality benefit.[38] Angiotensin receptor blockers (ARBs) may also be beneficial in situations where ACE inhibitors are poorly tolerated. These agents, specifically losartan, were recently found to confer greater reductions in CVD morbidity and mortality when compared with the use of atenolol for patients with hypertension, diabetes, and left ventricular hypertrophy.[39] Patients without CVD but at high risk for CVD (10-year CVD risk of ≥6% based on the Framingham Risk Score, described later) may also benefit from antiplatelet therapy (e.g., aspirin, clopidogrel) once their blood pressure is controlled.[40,41]

C. HYPERLIPIDEMIA

1. It is estimated that more than 40 million Americans have total cholesterol levels above 220 mg/dL.[42] Early clinical studies found significant reductions in CVD-related mortality when levels of total cholesterol and low-density lipoprotein cholesterol (LDL-C) were lowered or high-density lipoprotein cholesterol (HDL-C) levels were raised in populations with or without known CVD (Table 9-5).[43-51] The National Cholesterol Education Program recently published its latest guidelines on the management of hyperlipidemia in adults, which provide recommendations on the time to initiate dietary modification and drug treatment as primary and secondary CVD prevention.[52] As in their previous report, the diagnosis and treatment of hypercholesterolemia are based on a patient's additional CVD risk factors. Patients are categorized based on the number of additional risk factors present (Table 9-6, Figs. 9-2 and 9-3).

D. DIABETES

1. An estimated 16.7 million Americans have diabetes mellitus, making this a major public health problem.[53] Diabetic patients have a two to four times greater risk of symptomatic CVD than nondiabetic persons matched for the same level of total cholesterol.[54] The reason for this increased risk is unclear, since the severity of hyperglycemia is not directly related to an increased risk of CVD development.[55] Nevertheless, the American Diabetes Association (ADA) recommends tight glucose control in an effort to mitigate the microvascular complications of this disease. Using the glycosylated hemoglobin

TABLE 9-3
SELECT TRIALS ASSESSING THE EFFICACY OF VARIOUS ANTIHYPERTENSIVE MEDICATIONS

Study	Year	Design and Number of Subjects	Age (yr)	Findings
MAPHY[28]	1988	PRO n = 3234	40-64	Do β-blockers or thiazides have a role in CVD primary prevention? Men with HTN were treated with metoprolol or thiazides. Regardless of the drug, patients with lower blood pressures had lower CVD mortality. The reduction was greatest in those treated with β-blockers.
SHEP[29]	1991	PPRDB n = 4763	>59	Do blood pressure medications reduce stroke risk in patients with systolic HTN? Men and women with no CVD were treated with atenolol and chlorthalidone to assess the risk of stroke and CVD (secondary endpoint). All treated had a 36% stroke reduction and a 27% decrease in nonfatal MI and CVD death compared with placebo at 5 years' follow-up.
STOP-HTN[30]	1991	PPRDB n = 1600	70-84	Does treating HTN in the elderly reduce stroke risk and CVD death? Men and women without a history of MI or stroke in the year before enrollment were treated with various blood pressure medications. At 2 years' follow-up, a 47% stroke reduction and a 70% CVD death reduction were observed in those treated.
MRC[31]	1992	PPRSB n = 4400	65-74	Does treatment with diuretics or β-blockers reduce stroke risk, CVD, and death in hypertensive patients? Men and women without a history of MI or stroke in the 3 months before enrollment were treated with blood pressure medications or placebo. After 6 years treated patients had 19% fewer CVD events. Effect was greatest with diuretics compared with β-blockers.
VA Coop Study[32]	1993	PPRDB n = 1292	≥21	Do age and race affect blood pressure medication efficacy? Men were treated with one of six blood pressure medications or placebo for 1 year. This study demonstrated that for hypertension control, diltiazem is best for young or old African-Americans, captopril appeared best for young Caucasians, and atenolol was best for older Caucasians. No CVD death endpoints were addressed.

Study	Year	Design	Age	n	Description
Syst-Eur[33]	1997	PPRDB	≥60	n = 4695	Does treating isolated systolic HTN reduce the incidence of stroke and MI in the elderly? Men and women with HTN and no history of MI within 1 year of enrollment were treated for 2 years with nitrendipine ± enalapril and HCTZ if necessary or placebo. Treated patients had 31% fewer CVD endpoints and a 42% reduction in strokes.
HOT[34]	1998	PPRDB (partially open study)	50-80	n = 18,790	Does more aggressive HTN control decrease CVD morbidity and mortality? Does aspirin therapy in individuals with HTN decrease CVD events? Men and women with HTN and no history of CVD were treated in a five-step approach with felodipine, ACE inhibitors, β-blockers, or HCTZ to three targets for diastolic blood pressure (<90, <85, or <80 mm Hg) to assess whether tighter BP control improved CVD endpoints. The study was also designed to assess whether low-dose aspirin in HTN improved CVD outcomes. After 2 years greatest benefit was obtained when diastolic blood pressure = 82.6 mm Hg. Diabetic patients had a mortality reduction when diastolic blood pressure was <80 mm Hg; nondiabetics had no mortality benefit but had improved quality of life[35] with diastolic blood pressure <80 mm Hg. Aspirin use resulted in a 15% reduction in MI without an increased stroke risk.
CAPPP[36]	1999	PRO	25-66	n = 10,985	Is captopril better than other blood pressure medications at lowering CVD morbidity and mortality? Men and women with HTN and with or without CVD were treated for 6 years with captopril, metoprolol or atenolol, or HCTZ to assess whether captopril improves CVD morbidity and mortality. Captopril showed a trend toward lower CVD mortality compared with the other medications, but this was counterbalanced by an increase in stroke incidence. The CVD nonfatal events were similar between captopril and other medications.

ACE, Angiotensin-converting enzyme; *CVD*, cardiovascular disease; *HCTZ*, hydrochlorothiazide; *HTN*, hypertension; *MI*, myocardial infarction; *PPRDB*, prospective, placebo-controlled, randomized, double-blind study; *PPRSB*, prospective, placebo-controlled, randomized, single-blind study; *PRO*, prospective, randomized open study.

PREVENTION OF CORONARY ARTERY DISEASE 9

TABLE 9-4

GUIDELINES FOR THE MANAGEMENT OF HYPERTENSION

Risk Group	Description	Blood Pressure at Which to Initiate Medications	Target Blood Pressure (mm Hg)
A	No CVD and no additional CVD risk factors	>160/100 mm Hg or failure to achieve target blood pressure after 3-6 months of lifestyle changes	<140/90
B	No CVD, but other CVD risk factors present except diabetes mellitus	>160/100 mm Hg or failure to achieve target blood pressure after 3-6 months of lifestyle changes	<140/90
C	History of CVD or diabetes	>130/85 mm Hg for diabetics >140/90 mm Hg or failure to achieve target blood pressure after 3-6 months of lifestyle changes for patients with CVD	<130/85 (non-diabetic patients) <130/80 (diabetic patients) <125/75 (diabetic patients with >1 g proteinuria/day)

(HgbA$_1$C) level as a marker of long-term glucose control, the ADA recommends a target goal of less than 7%. More recent studies suggest that even lower levels of HgbA$_1$C (approximately 6%) may be better.[56]

2. Since tight glycemic control has little effect in reducing CVD risk, the ADA also recommends aggressive treatment of hypertension and hyperlipidemia if present. For diabetic patients the target LDL-C level is less than 100 mg/dL and the HDL-C goal is greater than 45 mg/dL. Goal triglyceride level is less than 150 mg/dL. Blood pressure should also be tightly controlled with a goal of less than 130/80 mm Hg. The goal is less than 125/75 mm Hg for individuals with urine protein levels greater than 1 g in a 24-hour period.[34] Specific agents have been shown to improve cardiovascular outcomes in diabetic patients and should be used as appropriate. The use of ACE inhibitors, specifically ramipril, was found to significantly reduce the composite endpoint of death, heart attacks, and cerebrovascular accidents in diabetic patients 55 years old and older.[57] The ADA also recommends low-dose aspirin (81 mg PO qd) as a primary preventive strategy.

E. OBESITY AND PHYSICAL INACTIVITY

1. According to recent guidelines, approximately 50% of Americans are overweight or obese.[58] Based on an ideal body mass index (BMI) of less than 25 kg/m^2, patients with BMIs between 25 and 30 kg/m^2 are considered overweight, those between 30 and 40 kg/m^2 are considered obese, and those greater than 40 kg/m^2 are considered morbidly obese. Whether obesity is an "independent" risk factor for CVD remains unclear, but compelling observations from a large clinical

Text continued on p. 179

TABLE 9-5

SELECT PROSPECTIVE TRIALS ASSESSING THE EFFICACY OF LIPID-LOWERING MEDICATIONS

Study	Year	Medication	Subjects	Age (years)	LDL-C Reduction (%)	HDL-C Increase (%)	Follow-Up (years)	CVD Decrease (%)	Mortality Decrease (%)
PRIMARY PREVENTION									
LRC-CPPT[44]	1984	Cholestyramine	3806 men	35-59	20	0	7.4	19	7
Helsinki Heart Study[45]	1987	Gemfibrozil	4081 men	40-55	8	10	5	34	0
WOSCOPS[46]	1998	Pravastatin	6595 men	45-64	26	5	4.9	31	22
AFCAPS/TexCAPS[47]	1998	Lovastatin	6605 (997 women)	45-73	26	5	5.2	37	0
SECONDARY PREVENTION									
4S[48]	1994	Simvastatin	4444 (827 women)	35-70	36	7	5.4	34	30
CARE[49]	1995	Pravastatin	4159 (576 women)	21-75	28	5	5	24	9
LIPID[50]	1998	Pravastatin	9014 (1508 women)	31-75	25	5	6.1	24	22
VA-HIT[51]	1999	Gemfibrozil	2531 men	64 (mean)	0	7.5	5.1	22	22
HPS[52]	2002	Simvastatin	20,536 (5082 women)	40-80	40	8	5	25	13
TNT	2004	Atorvastatin	8600 goal				5		
SEARCH	2004	Simvastatin	12,000 goal				5		

9

PREVENTION OF CORONARY ARTERY DISEASE

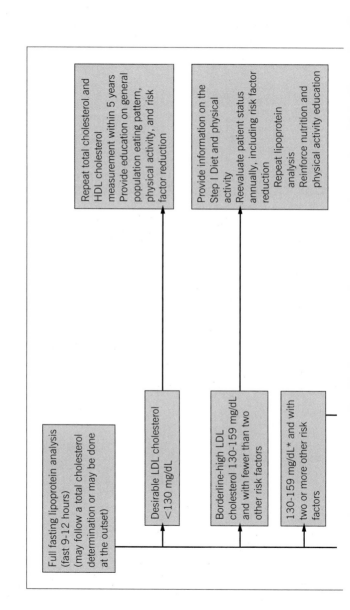

Full fasting lipoprotein analysis (fast 9-12 hours) (may follow a total cholesterol determination or may be done at the outset)

Desirable LDL cholesterol <130 mg/dL

→ Repeat total cholesterol and HDL cholesterol measurement within 5 years Provide education on general population eating pattern, physical activity, and risk factor reduction

Borderline-high LDL cholesterol 130-159 mg/dL and with fewer than two other risk factors

130-159 mg/dL * and with two or more other risk factors

→ Provide information on the Step I Diet and physical activity Reevaluate patient status annually, including risk factor reduction Repeat lipoprotein analysis Reinforce nutrition and physical activity education

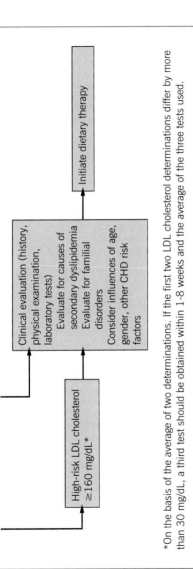

FIG. 9-2

Primary prevention classification by low-density lipoprotein cholesterol. In patients without coronary artery disease or other atherosclerotic disease who have low high-density lipoprotein cholesterol, borderline-high total cholesterol in the presence of two or more risk factors, or high total cholesterol, full fasting lipoprotein analysis is required to determine low-density lipoprotein cholesterol level. *CHD,* Coronary heart disease; *HDL,* high-density lipoprotein; *LDL,* low-density lipoprotein. *(Data from National Cholesterol Education Program. JAMA 1993; 269:3015; and Circulation 1994; 89:1329.)*

PREVENTION OF CORONARY ARTERY DISEASE 9

Text within figure:

High-risk LDL cholesterol ≥160 mg/dL*

Clinical evaluation (history, physical examination, laboratory tests)
Evaluate for causes of secondary dyslipidemia
Evaluate for familial disorders
Consider influences of age, gender, other CHD risk factors

Initiate dietary therapy

*On the basis of the average of two determinations. If the first two LDL cholesterol determinations differ by more than 30 mg/dL, a third test should be obtained within 1-8 weeks and the average of the three tests used.

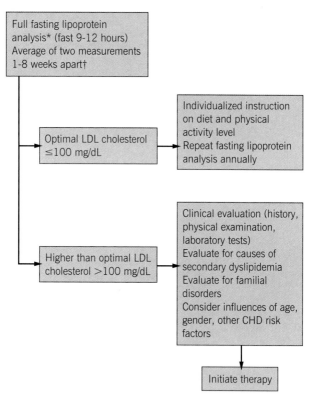

Full fasting lipoprotein analysis* (fast 9-12 hours) Average of two measurements 1-8 weeks apart†

Optimal LDL cholesterol ≤100 mg/dL

Individualized instruction on diet and physical activity level Repeat fasting lipoprotein analysis annually

Higher than optimal LDL cholesterol >100 mg/dL

Clinical evaluation (history, physical examination, laboratory tests) Evaluate for causes of secondary dyslipidemia Evaluate for familial disorders Consider influences of age, gender, other CHD risk factors

Initiate therapy

*Lipoprotein analysis should be performed when the patient is not in the recovery phase from an acute coronary or other medical event that would lower his or her usual LDL cholesterol level.
†If the first two LDL cholesterol determinations differ by more than 30 mg/dL, a third test should be obtained within 1-8 weeks and the average of the three tests used.

FIG. 9-3

Secondary prevention classification by low-density lipoprotein cholesterol. In patients with coronary artery disease or other atherosclerotic disease, initial assessment for dyslipidemia is by the fasting lipoprotein analysis to determine low-density lipoprotein cholesterol level. *CHD,* Coronary heart disease; *LDL,* low-density lipoprotein. *(Data from National Cholesterol Education Program. JAMA 1993; 269:3015; and Circulation 1994; 89:1329.)*

TABLE 9-6

NATIONAL CHOLESTEROL EDUCATION PROGRAM GUIDELINES ON THE
MANAGEMENT OF HYPERLIPIDEMIA

Risk Group	Description	LDL-C (mg/dL) at Which to Initiate Lifestyle Changes	LDL-C (mg/dL) at Which to Initiate Medications	Target LDL-C (mg/dL)
1	No CVD and no or one additional CVD risk factor	>160	>190	<160
2	No CVD and more than one additional CVD risk factor present except diabetes mellitus	>130	>160	<130
3	History of CVD or diabetes	>100	>100	<100

study in women have led to recommendations for weight loss to achieve a BMI below 25 kg/m^2.[59]

2. Physical inactivity has been shown to increase a person's risk for CVD. Furthermore, many clinical trials have established reductions in CVD with mild to moderate exercise.[60] Current recommendations are that all patients without known CVD engage in moderate-intensity exercise for 20 to 30 minutes a day on most if not all days of the week. Patients with a history of CVD often undergo a symptom-limited stress test approximately 4 to 12 weeks after a CVD event. An exercise program should then be instituted with the supervision of a cardiologist or a cardiac rehabilitation specialist.

F. **ASSESSING A PERSON'S RISK FOR CARDIOVASCULAR DISEASE**

1. Devising a strategy to address an individual's global risk for CVD can be challenging. Multiple "small" risk factors may confer greater risk for CVD than a single "large" risk factor. The Framingham Risk Score was developed to give the health care provider a way of estimating a patient's global risk for CVD (Fig. 9-4).[61] This information does not provide target goals but does allow the identification of specific risk factors that may need further modification.

PEARLS AND PITFALLS

- Assess the risk of CVD in every individual who is hospitalized, and exercise primary prevention whenever possible.
- Elderly patients should be treated as aggressively as younger patients to prevent CVD.

9

PREVENTION OF CORONARY ARTERY DISEASE

Age Points

	20-34 Yr	35-39 Yr	40-44 Yr	45-49 Yr	50-54 Yr	55-59 Yr	60-64 Yr	65-69 Yr	70-74 Yr	75-79 Yr
Male	-9	-4	0	3	6	8	10	11	12	13
Female	-7	-3	0	3	6	8	10	12	14	16

Total-C Points

Total-C (mg/dL)	20-39 Yr Male	20-39 Yr Female	40-49 Yr Male	40-49 Yr Female	50-59 Yr Male	50-59 Yr Female	60-69 Yr Male	60-69 Yr Female	70-79 Yr Male	70-79 Yr Female
<160	0	0	0	0	0	0	0	0	0	0
160-199	4	4	3	3	2	2	1	1	0	1
200-239	7	8	5	6	3	4	1	2	0	1
240-279	9	11	6	8	4	5	2	3	1	2
≥280	11	13	8	10	5	7	3	4	1	2

Smoking Points

Smoking Status	20-39 Yr Male	20-39 Yr Female	40-49 Yr Male	40-49 Yr Female	50-59 Yr Male	50-59 Yr Female	60-69 Yr Male	60-69 Yr Female	70-79 Yr Male	70-79 Yr Female
Nonsmoker	0	0	0	0	0	0	0	0	0	0
Smoker	8	9	5	7	3	4	1	2	1	1

HDL-C Points

HDL-C	≥60 mg/dL	50-59 mg/dL	40-49 mg/dL	<40 mg/dL
Male	-1	0	1	2
Female	-1	0	1	2

Cumulative Risk Points

Systolic BP	<120 mm Hg	120-129 mm Hg	130-139 mm Hg	140-159 mm Hg	≥160 mm Hg	BP Points
Untreated male	0	0	1	1	2	
Treated male	0	1	2	2	3	

Note: Chart adapted from ATP III executive summary.

Total Points ————

Final Point Assessment Scale

Males

Point total	<0	0	1	2	3	4	5	6	7	8	9	10	11	12	13	14	15	16	≥17
10-year risk, %	<1	1	1	1	1	1	2	2	3	4	5	6	8	10	12	16	20	25	≥30

Females

Point total	<9	9	10	11	12	13	14	15	16	17	18	19	20	21	22	23	24	≥25	≥30
10-year risk, %	<1	1	1	1	1	2	2	3	4	5	6	8	11	14	17	22	24	27	≥30

FIG. 9-4

Framingham risk assessment system for calculating 10-year risk. *BP,* Blood pressure; *HDL-C,* high-density lipoprotein cholesterol; *LDL,* low-density lipoprotein; *TGs,* triglycerides; *total-C,* total cholesterol; *VLDL,* very low-density lipoprotein. *(From National Cholesterol Education Program Expert Panel. JAMA 2001; 285:2486.)*

cont'd

PREVENTION OF CORONARY ARTERY DISEASE 9

Risk Assessment Screening

Physicians are advised to check *all* lipid parameters at the initial screening—including total C, LDL, HDL, and TGs. (Previously, initial screening checked only total C and HDL.)

As part of dietary changes to lower LDL, physicians are now encouraged to recommend plant stanols/sterols and foods with viscous (soluble) fiber to their patients.

Stanols/sterols are found in certain margarine products and salad dressings.

Sources of soluble fiber include legumes, cereal grains, beans, and many fruits and vegetables.

For people with TG ≥200 mg/dL, physicians are advised to treat both LDL and non-HDL cholesterol (a new parameter obtained by combining LDL + VLDL [very low density lipids]).

For postmenopausal women with hyperlipidemia, the guidelines now recommend statin therapy as an alternative to hormone replacement therapy, because of recent clinical findings.

FIG. 9-4 —cont'd

Framingham risk assessment system for calculating 10-year risk. *BP,* Blood pressure; *HDL-C,* high-density lipoprotein cholesterol; *LDL,* low-density lipoprotein; *TGs,* triglycerides; *total-C,* total cholesterol; *VLDL,* very low-density lipoprotein. *(From National Cholesterol Education Program Expert Panel. JAMA 2001; 285:2486.)*

REFERENCES

[c] 1. Clarke R, Stansbie D. Assessment of homocysteine as a cardiovascular risk factor in clinical practice. Ann Clin Biochem 2001; 38:624.

[b] 2. Jacques PF et al. The effect of folic acid fortification on plasma folate and total homocysteine concentrations. N Engl J Med 1999; 340:1449.

[b] 3. Bostom AG et al. Elevated plasma lipoprotein(a) and coronary heart disease in men 55 years old and younger: a prospective study. JAMA 1996; 276:544.

[a] 4. Maher VM et al. Effects of lowering elevated LDL cholesterol on the cardiovascular risk of lipoprotein(a). JAMA 1995; 274:1771.

[b] 5. Colditz GA et al. A prospective study of parental history of MI and coronary artery disease in men. Am J Cardiol 1991; 67:933.

[b] 6. Williams R, Bhopal R, Hunt K. Coronary risk in a British Punjabi population: a comparative profile of non-biochemical factors. Int J Epidemiol 1994; 23:28.

[b] 7. Goff DC et al. Greater case-fatality after myocardial infarction among Mexican Americans and women than among non-Hispanic whites and men: the Corpus Christi heart project. Am J Epidemiol 1994; 139:474.

[b] 8. Rosenman RH et al. Coronary heart disease in the Western Collaborative Group Study: final follow-up experience of 8½ years. JAMA 1975; 233:872.

[b] 9. Jiang W et al. Mental stress-induced myocardial ischemia and cardiac events. JAMA 1996; 275:1651.

[b] 10. Schulz R et al. Association between depression and mortality in older adults: the cardiovascular health study. Arch Intern Med 2000; 160:1761.

[c] 11. Danesh J et al. Association of fibrinogen, C-reactive protein, albumin or leukocyte count with coronary heart disease. JAMA 1998; 279:1477.

[b] 12. Folsom AR et al. Prospective study of hemostatic factors and incidence of coronary heart disease: atherosclerosis risk in communities (ARIC). Circulation 1997; 96:1102.

[b] 13. Koenig W et al. C-reactive protein, a sensitive marker of inflammation, predicts future risk of coronary heart disease in initially healthy middle-aged men: results from the MONICA Augsburg cohort study, 1984-1992. Circulation 1999; 99:237.

[b] 14. Ridker PM et al. Prospective study of Chlamydia pneumoniae IgG seropositivity and risks of future MI. Circulation 1999; 99:1161.

[b] 15. He J et al. Passive smoking and the risk of coronary heart disease—a meta-analysis of epidemiologic studies. N Engl J Med 1999; 340:920.

[b] 16. Iribarren C et al. Effect of cigar smoking on the risk of cardiovascular disease, chronic obstructive pulmonary disease and cancer in men. N Engl J Med 1999; 340:1773.

[b] 17. Frei B et al. Gas phase oxidants of cigarette smoke induced lipid peroxidation and changes in lipoprotein properties in human blood plasma: protective effects of ascorbic acid. Biochem J 1991; 277:133.

[b] 18. Rival J, Riddle JM, Stein PD. Effects of chronic smoking on platelet function. Thromb Res 1987; 45:75.

[b] 19. Folsom AR et al. Population correlates of plasma fibrinogen and factor VII, putative cardiovascular risk factors. Atherosclerosis 1991; 91:191.

[b] 20. Rosenberg L et al. The risk of myocardial infarction after quitting smoking in men under 55 years of age. N Engl J Med 1985; 313:1511.

[b] 21. Kawachi I et al. Smoking cessation and time course of decreased risks of coronary heart disease in middle-aged women. Arch Intern Med 1994; 154:169.

[b] 22. Hermanson B et al. Beneficial six-year outcome of smoking cessation in older men and women with coronary heart disease: results from the CASS registry. N Engl J Med 1988; 319:1365.

[b] 23. Cameron A, Davis K, Rogers W. Recurrence of angina after coronary artery bypass surgery: predictors and prognosis (CASS Registry). J Am Coll Cardiol 1995; 26:895.

[a] 24. Hurt RD et al. A comparison of sustained-release bupropion and placebo for smoking cessation. N Engl J Med 1997; 337:1195.

[a] 25. Jorenby DE et al. A controlled trial of sustained-release bupropion, a nicotine patch, or both for smoking cessation. N Engl J Med 1999; 340:685.

[b] 26. van den Hoogen PC et al. The relation between blood pressure and mortality due to coronary heart disease among men in different parts of the world. N Engl J Med 2000; 342:1.

9

PREVENTION OF CORONARY ARTERY DISEASE

[d] 27. JNC VI. The sixth report of the Joint National Committee on Prevention, Detection, Evaluation and Treatment of High Blood Pressure. Arch Intern Med 1997; 157:2413.

[b] 28. Metoprolol Atherosclerosis Prevention in Hypertension (MAPHY) Investigators. Primary prevention with metoprolol in patients with hypertension: mortality results from the MAPHY study. JAMA 1988; 259:1976.

[a] 29. SHEP Cooperative Research Group. Prevention of stroke by antihypertensive drug treatment in older persons with isolated systolic hypertension: final results of the Systolic Hypertension in the Elderly Program (SHEP). JAMA 1991; 265:3255.

[a] 30. Dahlof B et al. Swedish trial in old patients with hypertension (STOP-HTN): morbidity and mortality in the STOP-HTN. Lancet 1991; 338:1281.

[a] 31. Medical Research Council (MRC) Working Party. MRC trial of treatment of hypertension in older adults: principal results. BMJ 1992; 304:405.

[a] 32. Materson BJ et al. Single-drug therapy for hypertension in men: a comparison of 6 antihypertensive agents with placebo; VA cooperative study. N Engl J Med 1993; 328:914.

[a] 33. Staessen JA et al. Randomised double-blind comparison of placebo and active treatment for older patients with isolated systolic hypertension (Syst-Eur). Lancet 1997; 350:757.

[a] 34. Hansson L et al. Effects of intensive blood pressure lowering and low dose aspirin in patients with hypertension: principal results of the Hypertension Optimal Treatment Randomized Trial (HOT). Lancet 1998; 351:1755.

[a] 35. Wiklund I et al. Does lowering the blood pressure improve the mood? Quality-of-life results from the Hypertension Optimal Treatment (HOT) study. Blood Press 1997; 6:357.

[b] 36. Hansson L et al. Effect of angiotensin-converting-enzyme inhibition compared with conventional therapy on cardiovascular morbidity and mortality in hypertension: the Captopril Prevention Project (CAPPP) randomised trial. Lancet 1999; 353:611.

[c] 37. Ko DT et al. β-Blocker therapy and symptoms of depression, fatigue and sexual dysfunction. JAMA 2002; 288:351.

[a] 38. Heart Outcomes Prevention Evaluation (HOPE) Study Investigators. Effects of an angiotensin-converting-enzyme inhibitor, ramipril, on cardiovascular events in high-risk patients. N Engl J Med 2000; 342:145.

[a] 39. Lindholm LH et al. Cardiovascular morbidity and mortality in patients with diabetes in the Losartan Intervention for Endpoint Reduction in Hypertension study (LIFE): a randomised trial against atenolol. Lancet 2002; 359: 1004.

[b] 40. Meade TW, Brennan PJ. Determination of who may derive most benefit from aspirin in primary prevention: subgroup results from a randomised controlled trial. Br Med J 2000; 321:13.

[c] 41. Lauer MS. Aspirin for primary prevention of coronary events. N Engl J Med 2002; 346:1468.

[d] 42. American Heart Association. 2000 Heart and stroke statistical update. Proceedings of the Annual American Heart Association Meeting in Dallas, Texas, 1999.

[d] 43. National Cholesterol Education Program Expert Panel. Executive summary of the third report of the NCEP expert panel on detection, evaluation and treatment of high blood cholesterol in adults. JAMA 2001; 285:2486.

[a] 44. Lipid Research Clinics Group. Lipid Research Clinics coronary primary prevention trial results. JAMA 1984; 251:351.

[a] 45. Frick MH et al. Helsinki Heart Study: primary prevention trial with gemfibrozil in middle-aged men with dyslipidemia. N Engl J Med 1987; 317:1237.

[a] 46. Shepherd J et al. Prevention of coronary heart disease with pravastatin in men with hypercholesterolemia. West of Scotland Coronary Prevention Study Group (WOSCOPS). N Engl J Med 1995; 333:1301.

[a] 47. Downs JR et al. Primary prevention of acute coronary events with lovastatin in men and women with average cholesterol levels. Air Force/Texas Coronary Atherosclerosis Prevention Study Research Group (AFCAPS/TexCAPS). JAMA 1998; 279:1615.

[a] 48. Scandinavian Simvastatin Survival Study Group. Randomized trial of cholesterol lowering in 4,444 patients with coronary artery disease: the Scandinavian Simvastatin Survival Study (4S). Lancet 1994; 344:1383.

[a] 49. Sacks FM et al. The effect of pravastatin on coronary events after myocardial infarction in patients with average cholesterol levels. The Cholesterol and Recurrent Events (CARE) trial. N Engl J Med 1996; 335:1001.

[a] 50. Long-Term Intervention with Pravastatin in Ischemic Disease (LIPID) Study Group. Prevention of cardiovascular events and death with pravastatin in patients with coronary heart disease and a broad range of initial cholesterol levels. N Engl J Med 1998; 339:1349.

[a] 51. Rubins HB et al. Gemfibrozil for the secondary prevention of coronary heart disease in men with low levels of high-density lipoprotein cholesterol. Veterans Affairs HDL Cholesterol Intervention Trial (VA-HIT) Study Group. N Engl J Med 1999; 341:410.

[a] 52. MRC/BHF Heart Protection Study of cholesterol lowering with simvastatin in 20,536 high-risk individuals: a randomised placebo-controlled trial. Heart Protection Study Collaborative Group. Lancet 2002; 360:7.

[d] 53. American Diabetes Association. Standards of medical care for patients with diabetes mellitus. Diabetes Care 2000; 23:S32.

[d] 54. Grundy SM et al. Diabetes and cardiovascular disease. Circulation 1999; 100:1134.

[b] 55. Wilson WF, Cupples AD, Kannel WB. Is hyperglycemia associated with cardiovascular disease? Am Heart J 1991; 2:586.

[b] 56. Stratton IM et al. Association of glycaemia with macrovascular and microvascular complications of type 2 diabetes: prospective observational study. Br Med J 2000; 321:405.

[a] 57. HOPE Study Investigators. Effects of ramipril on cardiovascular and microvascular outcomes in people with diabetes mellitus. Lancet 2000; 355:253.

[c] 58. Willett WC, Dietz WH, Colditz GA. Guidelines for healthy weight. N Engl J Med 1999; 341:427.

[b] 59. Willett WC et al. Weight, weight change and coronary heart diseases in women: risk within the "normal" weight range. JAMA 1995; 273:461.

[d] 60. Fletcher G et al. Statement on exercise: benefits and recommendations for physical activity programs for all Americans. Circulation 1996; 94:857.

[b] 61. Wilson PW et al. Prediction of coronary heart disease using risk factor categories. Circulation 1998; 97:1837.

9

PREVENTION OF CORONARY ARTERY DISEASE

Electrocardiogram Analysis

David Kuperman, MD, Joseph Rahman, MD, and Kevin Donahue, MD

FAST FACTS

- Analysis of the electrocardiogram (ECG) should always begin with determination of the rate, rhythm, axis, and intervals.
- The physician should verify that the ECG being examined belongs to the correct patient.
- An old ECG should be obtained if available.

10

I. INTRODUCTION

1. The electrocardiogram (ECG) is one of the most frequently ordered diagnostic tests in clinical medicine. The ECG provides information about the heart's structure, past cardiac events, and most important, what is happening at the time of examination. The usefulness of the ECG is determined by the knowledge and skill of the person reading it. In this chapter we recommend a systematic approach to ECG reading that emphasizes accurate and practical clinical information.

2. The heart is an electrical as well as a mechanical organ. An ECG is a test that examines the electrical impulse originating within the heart. This impulse is created by a process called depolarization. In the normal heart, the impulse develops in the sinoatrial (SA) node in the right atrium. It travels through the atria to the atrioventricular (AV) node and then through the bundle of His to the ventricles. A recharging process called repolarization follows the depolarization, thus completing a cycle of electrical activity that leads to myocardial contraction.

3. The electrical impulse originating from the SA node is detected by sensors called leads. The impulse is then graphically depicted on a tracing. If the depolarization is moving toward a lead, the line on the ECG tracing will be deflected upward, producing a positive wave. If the impulse is moving away from a given lead, the line on the tracing is deflected downward, producing a negative wave. The height or depth of the wave is related to the magnitude of the impulse; that is, large electrical charges create large waves.

4. The waves seen on the tracing are named P, Q, R, S, and T (Fig. 10-1). The P wave is formed by the depolarization of the atrium. The electrical impulse in the ventricles creates the QRS complex. The R wave is the first positive deflection of the QRS complex. The Q wave is a negative wave that precedes the positive R wave. If a negative wave follows the R wave, it is called an S wave. Ventricular repolarization establishes the T wave. Other waves such as the U wave may be created by special circumstances.

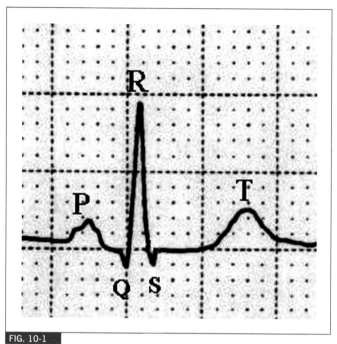

FIG. 10-1

P, Q, R, S, and T waves. *(From Braunwald E, Zipes DP, Libby P. Heart disease: a textbook of cardiovascular medicine. 6th ed. Philadelphia: WB Saunders; 2001.)*

5. Just as important as the waves themselves are the spaces between them called intervals. The important intervals are the PR, QT, width of the QRS complex, and the ST segment. The PR interval is measured from the beginning of the P wave to the onset of the QRS complex. The QT interval starts with the QRS complex and ends at the termination of the T wave. The width of the QRS complex is measured from the beginning of the complex to its completion. The ST segment commences with the end of the QRS complex and ends with the start of the T wave. The point where the ST segment begins is called the J point. Changes in the duration of these intervals can often suggest pathological conditions.

6. The standard placement of the leads is shown in Fig. 10-2.[1] Leads I, II, and III are called the limb leads. Leads aVF, aVL, and aVR are the unipolar leads. Leads V_1 through V_6 are the precordial leads. Additional leads are sometimes necessary in certain clinical situation. The most commonly used additional lead is a right-sided V_4, which is placed at the fifth rib space at the right midclavicular line.

7. The physician should be familiar with certain important standards when evaluating an ECG. Each small box is 1 mm^2 and equivalent to 0.04 second. Each large box is 5 mm^2 and equivalent to 0.2 second. Usually 10 mm in height is equal to 1 mV. The standard criteria for height are determined by examining the lefthand side of the tracing. A standard 1-mV square wave is found at this location. It should be 10 mm tall.

8. ECGs must be reviewed in a systematic manner so that no useful information is overlooked. One way to assess ECGs is to evaluate the tracing in a definitive sequence: rate, rhythm, intervals, axis, hypertrophy, and waveform.

II. RATE

1. Rate is defined as the frequency of a given waveform. Most commonly the frequency of R waves is measured to assess rate. In a normal sinus rhythm the rate of any of the component waves can be used to assess the overall rate. However, in cases of atrioventricular disassociation, the rates of P waves may not have a one-to-one correlation with the R waves (e.g., second- or third-degree atrioventricular block). In these cases, knowing the rate of each individual wave may be useful.

2. Regular rates can be easily estimated by counting the number of big boxes (e.g., five small boxes) between successive waves and dividing this number into 300. For example, if there are four big boxes between consecutive R waves, the rate is 300 divided by 4, which is 75. For irregular rhythms or very slow rates, a rhythm strip is useful. The strip has small hatch marks (on either the very top or bottom of the ECG) that are spaced by 3 seconds. By counting the number of waves over a 6-second period and multiplying by 10, the examiner can determine an overall rate.

III. RHYTHM

1. Rhythm is the pattern of waveforms. The rhythm is determined by where the depolarization begins. The depolarization can begin at the SA node, the atria, the AV node, or the ventricles (Tables 10-1 to 10-4, Fig. 10-3).

IV. INTERVALS

1. Alterations in the PR, width of the QRS, and QT are shown in Tables 10-5 to 10-7 and Figs. 10-4 and 10-5.

V. AXIS

1. The electrical axis is an estimate of the overall direction of the impulse as it passes through the heart. The axis can give information that hints at alteration in the conduction system of the heart. These alterations may be due to bundle branch blocks, myocardial infarctions, or

Text continued on p. 201

10

ELECTROCARDIOGRAM ANALYSIS

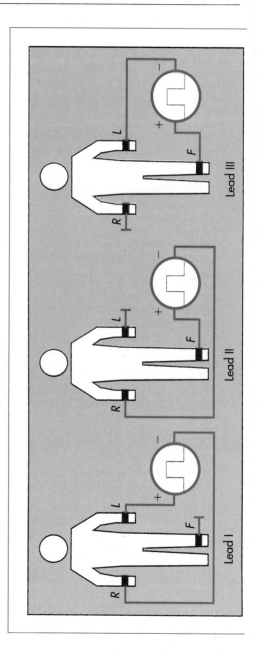

Lead I

Lead II

Lead III

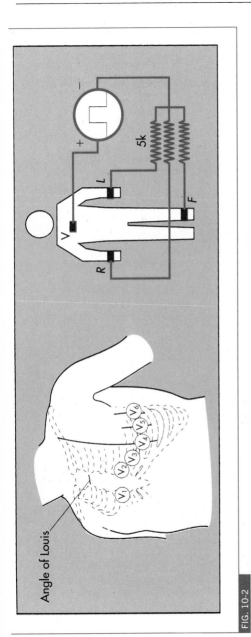

FIG. 10-2

Normal lead placement. *(From Braunwald E, Zipes DP, Libby P. Heart disease: a textbook of cardiovascular medicine. 6th ed. Philadelphia: WB Saunders; 2001.)*

TABLE 10-1
SINOATRIAL NODE RHYTHMS

Rhythm	Morphological Criteria	Rate (beats/min)	Example
Normal sinus rhythm	P wave followed by QRS complex (1:1 association); P wave upright in I, II	60-100; <60 is sinus bradycardia, >100 is sinus tachycardia	
Sinus arrhythmia	Sinus rhythm with phasic changes in PP interval (resulting from respiration)	60-100	
Sinus pause or arrest	Sinus rhythm with PP interval greater than 1.6-2.0 seconds		

TABLE 10-2
ATRIAL RHYTHMS

Name of Rhythm	Morphological Criteria	Rate (beats/min)	Example
Wandering atrial pacemaker/multifocal atrial tachycardia	P waves with three or more morphologies	If <100, wandering atrial pacemaker; if >100, multifocal atrial tachycardia.	
Atrial flutter	Rapid regular atrial waves (characteristic flutter waves); rate of 150 beats/min is highly suggestive	Atrial rate 240-340 and ventricular rate variable depending on ratio of conducted beats (classically, 2:1 ratio, giving rate of 150 beats/min)	
Atrial fibrillation	P waves absent; totally irregular and chaotic leading to a wavy baseline before QRS	Any rate can be present; if >100, called atrial fibrillation with rapid ventricular response	
Premature atrial contraction	P wave different from the other P waves; occurs earlier than would be expected; QRS narrow	N/A	

ELECTROCARDIOGRAM ANALYSIS 10

TABLE 10-3

ATRIOVENTRICULAR JUNCTIONAL RHYTHMS

Rhythm	Morphological Criteria	Rate (beats/min)	Example
AV junctional escape complexes and rhythms	Normal QRS morphology, unless aberrant or preexisting interventricular conduction defect; no preceding P wave; occurs when intrinsic sinoatrial node activity fails; rate is regular	40-60 (if >60, accelerated AV junctional rhythm)	
AV nodal reentrant tachycardia	Characterized by narrow complex tachycardia, often with sudden onset and termination	150-250	

AV, Atrioventricular.

TABLE 10-4
VENTRICULAR RHYTHMS

Rhythm	Morphological Criteria	Rate (beats/min)	Example
Ventricular escape beat or rhythm	Wide, notched, or slurred QRS complex (QRS almost always >0.12 second); not preceded by P wave	30-40 (if rate 60-110, called accelerated idioventricular rhythm)	
Ventricular tachycardia	Rapid succession of three or more premature ventricular beats; AV dissociation common; abrupt onset and conclusion	>100	
Ventricular fibrillation	Extremely rapid, irregular ventricular rhythm; absence of identifiable P waves, QRS complexes, or T waves	N/A	
Premature ventricular contraction	Wide QRS complex occurring earlier than expected; must be fewer than three in a row	N/A	

ELECTROCARDIOGRAM ANALYSIS 10

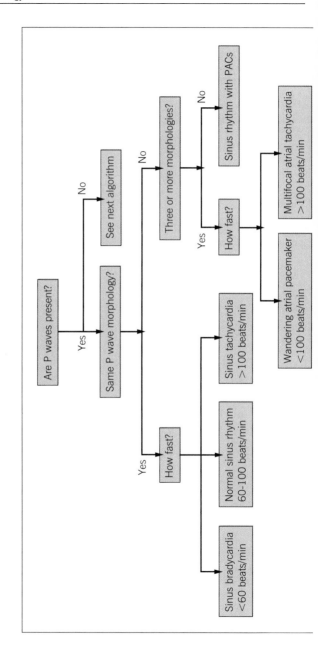

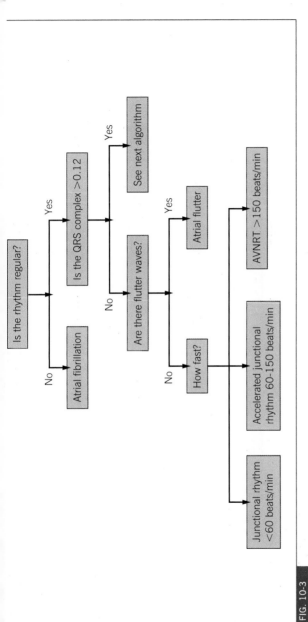

cont'd

FIG. 10-3
Rhythm determination.

ELECTROCARDIOGRAM ANALYSIS

10

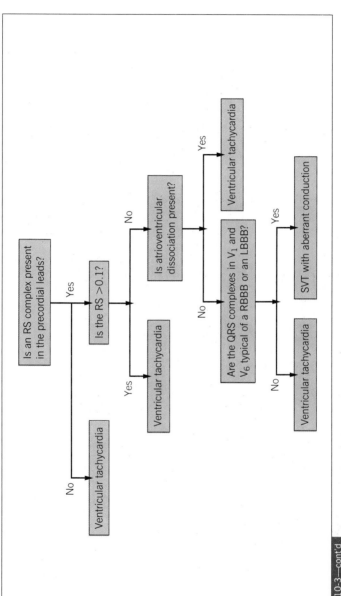

FIG. 10-3—cont'd

TABLE 10-5
ATRIOVENTRICULAR CONDUCTION ABNORMALITIES

Rhythm	Morphological Criteria	Example
First-degree AV block	PR interval ≥0.2 second; each P wave followed by a QRS complex	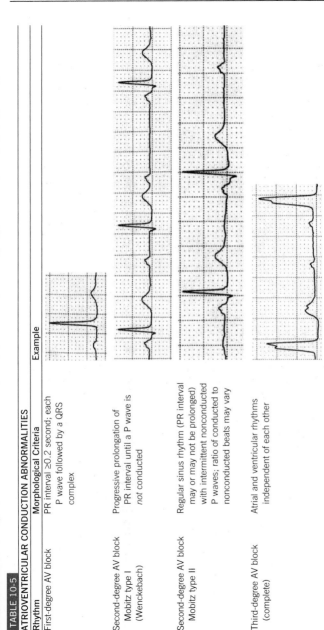
Second-degree AV block Mobitz type I (Wenckebach)	Progressive prolongation of PR interval until a P wave is *not* conducted	
Second-degree AV block Mobitz type II	Regular sinus rhythm (PR interval may or may not be prolonged) with intermittent nonconducted P waves; ratio of conducted to nonconducted beats may vary	
Third-degree AV block (complete)	Atrial and ventricular rhythms independent of each other	

AV, Atrioventricular.

10

ELECTROCARDIOGRAM ANALYSIS

TABLE 10-6
INTRAVENTRICULAR CONDUCTION ABNORMALITIES

Conduction Abnormality	Morphological Criteria	Example
Right bundle branch block	Prolonged QRS duration (>0.12 second); rsR' in V_1 and V_2 and wide slurred S waves in I, V_5, and V_6	
Left bundle branch block	Prolonged QRS duration (≥0.12 second); broad monophasic R waves in lead I, V_5, V_6; delayed onset of intrinsicoid deflection in leads I, V_5, V_6	
Left anterior fascicular block	Left axis deviation (axis between −45° and −90°); qR in lead I and rS in lead III; normal or slightly prolonged QRS duration (0.08-0.10 second)	
Left posterior fascicular block	Right axis deviation with mean QRS axis between +100° and +180°; deep S wave in lead I; Q wave in lead III; normal or slightly prolonged QRS duration (0.08-0.10 second)	

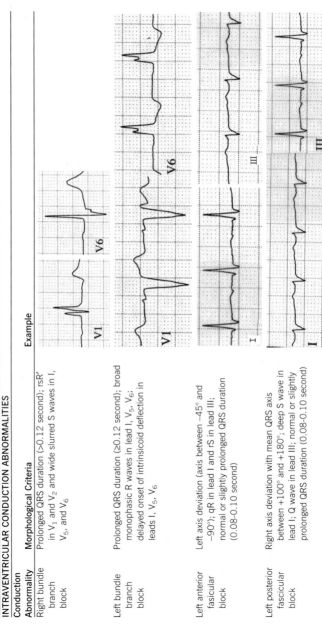

TABLE 10-7

PROLONGED QT INTERVAL

Abnormality	Morphological Criteria	Associated Conditions
Prolonged QT Interval	QTc = QT interval divided by square root of RR interval; QTc ≥0.46 second	Drugs (quinidine, procainamide, disopyramide, amiodarone, sotalol, lithium); hypomagnesemia; hypocalcemia; myocarditis; intracranial hemorrhage; mitral valve prolapse; hypothyroidism; hypothermia; long QT syndrome (familial)

enlargement of ventricles. In the normal heart the impulse begins in the right atrium and travels toward the left ventricle. It should therefore move from right to left and from superior to inferior. Lead I, which is located on the patient's left, and aVF, which is located inferiorly, should therefore have positive deflections. If lead I is negative and aVF positive, right axis deviation is present. If lead I is positive and aVF negative, left axis deviation is present. If both are negative, the patient has extreme axis deviation and whether right or left axis deviation exists cannot be determined.

2. Exact measurement of the axis is also possible. This may be important for determining certain conduction abnormalities such as hemifasicular blocks or right ventricular hypertrophy. Several methods exist for determining the exact measurement of the axis. The simplest way is to look at the axis measured by the ECG machine. This is usually reliable.

VI. CHAMBER ENLARGEMENT AND HYPERTROPHY

1. The ECG can provide a great deal of information about the relative sizes of the heart chambers. Most of this data is derived from measurements of the magnitude of the waves.

A. ATRIAL ENLARGEMENT

1. Table 10-8 outlines criteria for atrial enlargement.

B. RIGHT VENTRICULAR HYPERTROPHY

1. The criteria for right ventricular hypertrophy are found in Table 10-9. Before making the diagnosis of RVH, the physician must remember that certain pathological entitities may have findings similar to those in RVH. Old posterior wall myocardial infarction, Wolff-Parkinson-White syndrome, hypertrophic cardiomyopathy (septal hypertrophy), and right bundle branch block may mimic RVH. Additional clues may be necessary to determine the presence of RVH, such as right axis deviation, right atrial enlargement, or right-sided strain.

C. LEFT VENTRICULAR HYPERTROPHY

1. Many criteria are used to determine the presence of left ventricular hypertrophy. Some of these are listed in Table 10-10.

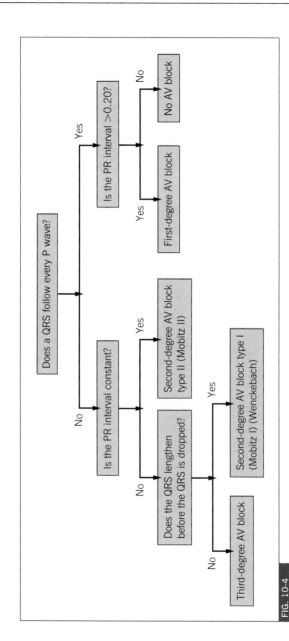

FIG. 10-4

Atrioventricular block.

TABLE 10-8

ATRIAL ENLARGEMENT

Abnormality	Morphological Criteria	Example
Right atrial abnormality	Upright P wave >2.5 mm in leads II, III, and aVF *or* >1.5 mm in leads V_1 or V_2	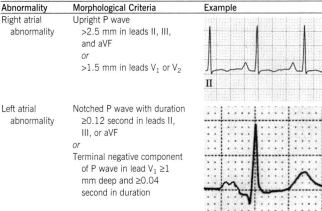
Left atrial abnormality	Notched P wave with duration ≥0.12 second in leads II, III, or aVF *or* Terminal negative component of P wave in lead V_1 ≥1 mm deep and ≥0.04 second in duration	

TABLE 10-9

RIGHT VENTRICULAR HYPERTROPHY

Abnormality	Morphological Criteria
Right ventricular hypertrophy	Right axis deviation ≥+100° R wave in V_1 ≥7 mm *or* R wave in V_1 + S wave in V_5 or V_6 >10.5 mm

10

ELECTROCARDIOGRAM ANALYSIS

VII. WAVEFORMS

1. The shape of the waves can yield valuable information. It shows ischemia, irritation of the heart, alterations in conduction pathways, and other metabolic changes.

A. ISCHEMIC CHANGES

1. The ECG is one of the most useful diagnostic tools in the evaluation of suspected acute coronary syndromes. In fact, the ECG can give clues to the extent, localization, and duration (i.e., old versus new) of myocardial ischemia and infarction. Ischemia induces stereotypical, time-dependent changes to the QRS complex, ST segment, and T waves as a reflection of changes to the electrical properties of the myocardium. The earliest changes seen in acute ischemia are changes to the ST segment (i.e., depression or elevation) and hyperacute T waves. ST segment elevation and depression are classically thought to represent transmural (i.e., full thickness) and subendocardial (i.e., partial thickness) ischemia, respectively. However, this distinction has

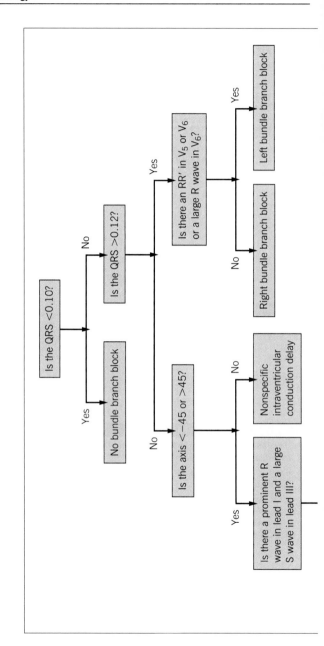

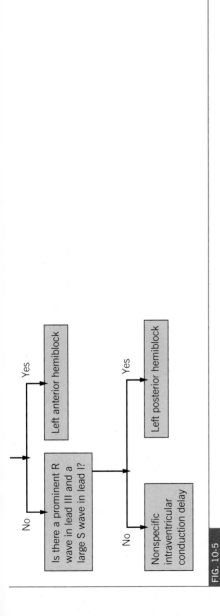

FIG. 10-5

Ventricular conduction delay.

10

ELECTROCARDIOGRAM ANALYSIS

TABLE 10-10	
LEFT VENTRICULAR HYPERTROPHY	
Abnormality	Morphological Criteria
Left ventricular hypertrophy	Cornell criteria
	R wave in aVL + S wave in V_3 >24 mm in males
	R wave in aVL + S wave in V_3 >20 mm in females
	Other criteria
	R wave in aVL ≥12 mm
	R wave in V_5 or V_6 + S wave in V_1 >35 mm
	Maximum R wave + S wave in precordial leads >45 mm
	R in aVF >20 mm
	R in aVR >14 mm
	R in V_5 or V_6 >26 mm

clinical utility only in distinguishing patients who are candidates for reperfusion therapy (with thrombolytics). Please refer to Chapters 5 and 6. ST segment elevation is also more useful (than depression) in depicting the exact geographical, and hence vascular, territory involved in an ischemic insult. In addition, ST segment depression can often represent so-called reciprocal changes when they occur in an ECG distribution opposite or adjacent to the ischemic territory. For instance, acute inferior wall ischemia is reflected by ST segment elevations in leads II, III, and aVF, and reciprocal ST segment depression in leads I and AVL. Finally, the amplitude of the ST deviation, as well as the number of contiguous leads involved, correlates with the magnitude of the ischemic event.

2. Although ST segment elevations are the earliest signs of acute myocardial injury, within several hours to days the ST segment begins to flatten and pathological Q waves (1 mm wide or one third of the R wave amplitude) and T wave inversions develop. Reversible ischemia can occur in a syndrome known as Prinzmetal's variant angina, in which transient ST elevation occurs as a result of coronary vasospasm.

3. Table 10-11 outlines waveform abnormalities associated with ischemia.

4. Table 10-12 outlines ECG changes found in acute myocardial infarction.

B. PERICARDITIS

1. Inflammation of the pericardial sac that contains the heart is associated with characteristic ECG findings. Classically, diffuse ST segment elevation (flat or slightly concave with the middle sagging downward) is seen. This may be accompanied by PR segment depression.

C. WOLFF-PARKINSON-WHITE SYNDROME

1. WPW syndrome is an electrical conduction abnormality. It occurs when electrical impulses bypass the AV node, through so-called

TABLE 10-11		
WAVEFORM ABNORMALITIES OF ISCHEMIA		
Abnormality	Morphological Criteria	Example
ST segment elevation	Elevation of the ST segment ≥1 mm	
ST segment depression	Depression of the ST segment ≥1 mm	
T wave inversions	T wave with its greatest amplitude in the direction opposite to the greatest amplitude of the QRS complex	
Wellens T waves	Deep symmetrical T wave inversions associated with proximal left anterior descending artery lesions or increased intracerebral pressure	

accessory pathways, and cause premature excitation of the ventricle. The premature excitation leads to the formation of a delta wave, a slow upward deflection that leads into the QRS complex. This wave can misleadingly shorten the PR interval and concomitantly lengthen the QRS complex. WPW is important to identify because patients are at risk for life-threatening paroxysmal tachycardia by two major mechanisms: a supraventricular tachycardia (e.g, atrial fibrillation) that can be rapidly conducted to the ventricles without the normal conduction impedance at the AV node or a reentry circuit that develops between the atria and ventricle, so that each ventricular impulse is immediately transmitted back to the atria, leading to rapid reentrant tachycardia.

D. METABOLIC ALTERATIONS

1. Changes in the metabolic environment of the heart can alter waveform. The most important of these are hyperkalemia, hypokalemia, hypercalcemia, hypocalcemia, and hypothermia (Tables 10-13 and 10-14).

TABLE 10-12

ELECTROCARDIOGRAPHIC CHANGES OF ACUTE MYOCARDIAL INFARCTION

Electrocardiographic Findings	Region of Cardiac Ischemia	Anatomy of Lesion	30-Day Mortality Rate (%)	1-Year Mortality Rate (%)
ST ↑ V_{1-6}, I, aVL, and fasicular or bundle branch block	Anterior-lateral plus septum	Proximal LAD (proximal to first septal perforator)	19.6	25.6
ST ↑ V_{1-6}, I, aVL	Anterior-lateral	Proximal LAD (proximal to large diagonal but distal to first perforator)	9.2	12.4
ST ↑ V_{5-6}, I, aVL	Lateral	Distal LAD or large diagonal	6.8	10.2
ST ↑ II, III, aVF, and V_{5-6}	Inferior-lateral	Proximal RCA or left circumflex	6.4	8.4
ST ↑ II, III, aVF, and R>S in V_1 and V_2	Inferior-posterior			
ST ↑ II, III, aVF only	Inferior	Distal RCA or left circumflex (depending on coronary anatomy)	4.5	6.7

Modified from Topol EJ, Van de Werf FJ. Acute myocardial infarction: early diagnosis and management. In Topol EJ, ed. Textbook of cardiovascular medicine. New York: Lippincott-Raven; 1998.

All patients received reperfusion therapy (mortality data from GUSTO I).

LAD, Left anterior descending artery; *RCA,* right circumflex artery.

TABLE 10-13

WAVEFORM ABNORMALITIES ASSOCIATED WITH METABOLIC ALTERATIONS

Abnormality	Effects on Electrocardiogram
Hyperkalemia	Peaked T waves (earliest change); widening of the PR interval; widening of the QRS interval; ventricular fibrillation (late finding)
Hypokalemia	Flat or inverted T waves; U waves; slight ST depression; larger P wave; longer PR; longer QTc; premature beats; tachyarrhythmias
Hypercalcemia	Shortened QTc; increased amplitude of QRS complex (extreme cases only); biphasic T waves (extreme cases only); creation of a new wave at the J point in the same direction as the QRS complex (Osborne wave) (extreme cases only)
Hypocalcemia	Prolonged QTc; T wave inversion
Hypothermia	Creation of a new wave at the J point in the same direction as the QRS complex (Osborne wave); amplitude often correlates with degree of hypothermia

10

ELECTROCARDIOGRAM ANALYSIS

PEARLS AND PITFALLS

- Always obtain an old ECG for comparison.
- Check the name on the ECG (make sure it belongs to your patient).
- Always check the voltage standard before making measurements of wave amplitude.
- If evidence of inferior ischemia is seen, obtain a right-sided ECG.
- Compare the ECGs with and without chest pain (and before and after sublingual administration of nitroglycerin).
- Obtain a rhythm strip when evaluating an arrhythmia, since a 12-lead ECG may not be sufficient.
- When in doubt, repeat the ECG and check lead placements.
- Use calipers to analyze arrhythmias—they make it much easier.
- Diffuse ST elevation and PR interval depression are characteristic of pericarditis.
- A normal ECG does not exclude ischemia.
- The most common ECG finding in acute pulmonary embolus is sinus tachycardia (S waves in lead I, Q waves in lead III, and inverted T waves in lead III are neither sensitive nor specific for a pulmonary embolus).
- R waves in lead V_1 should suggest one of the following: right bundle branch block, right ventricular hypertrophy, old posterior MI, WPW, Duchenne's muscular dystrophy, or lead placement error.
- Limb lead reversal (reversal of right and left arm leads) results in inversion of the normal upright P-QRS-T complex in leads I and aVL. In addition, abrupt changes in R wave progression across the precordial leads suggest precordial lead reversal.
- Parkinson's tremor can simulate atrial flutter with a rate of near 300 per minute, whereas an essential tremor is typically faster at 500 per minute.

TABLE 10-14

OTHER WAVEFORM ALTERATIONS

Abnormality	Morphological Criteria	Example
J point elevation	Elevation of initiation of ST segment	
Wolff-Parkinson-White syndrome	Delta wave leading to shortened PR interval and widened QRS complex	
Peaked T waves	T wave >6 mm in limb leads *or* T wave >10 mm in precordial leads	
Pericarditis	Diffuse ST elevations and PR interval depressions	
Digitalis effect	"Coved" ST segment depression; flat T waves; decreased QTc interval	

- The intervals and axis measurements made by the ECG machine are usually reliable, but the "diagnosis" is often wrong.
- Not all ST segment elevation is due to an MI. Pericarditis or J point elevation may also cause ST elevation.
- Look for patterns of waveform changes to make the diagnosis.
- When a regular junctional tachycardia develops in a patient who is taking digoxin and has a history of atrial fibrillation, the possibility of digoxin toxicity should be considered. Digitalis toxicity does not necessarily correlate with the serum level. Look at the patient and the ECG to determine toxicity. Serious manifestations of digitalis toxicity include bradycardia, ventricular tachycardia, and ventricular fibrillation.

10

ELECTROCARDIOGRAM ANALYSIS

Hypertensive Urgency and Emergency

Edward C. Hsiao, MD, PhD, Sharon A. Chung, MD, and Michael J. Klag, MD, MPH

FAST FACTS

- When examining a hypertensive patient, the physician should always assess for end organ damage. The most commonly affected organs are the brain, heart, kidneys, and eyes.
- Hypertensive urgency is defined as a systolic pressure greater than 180 mm Hg or a diastolic pressure greater than 130 mm Hg, but with no evident end organ damage. Blood pressure may be reduced to 160/110 mm Hg over 24 hours.
- Hypertensive emergency may occur at any blood pressure but involves damage to at least one organ system. Mean arterial blood pressure should be reduced by at most 25% in the first 2 hours, and then to a blood pressure of 160/110 mm Hg within the first 6 hours of treatment.
- The long-term goal blood pressure should be determined by the patient's clinical findings and risk factors. Blood pressure should be controlled to below 140/90 mm Hg for patients with uncomplicated hypertension, 130/80 mm Hg for patients with diabetes, or 125/75 mm Hg for patients with renal insufficiency and proteinuria (>1 g/24 hr).[1]
- Patients who are hypertensive because of an acute stroke or an acute coronary event may require a higher blood pressure to maintain adequate organ perfusion.

I. EPIDEMIOLOGY

1. See Table 11-1 for the Joint National Committee VI classification of hypertension in adults older than 18 years.[1]
2. According to the National Health and Nutrition Examination Survey (NHANES III) data,[2] 24% of the adult American population, or approximately 43 million people, have stage 1, 2, or 3 hypertension. Approximately 30% of these people are unaware of their hypertension, and 58% of those who are treated continue to have uncontrolled hypertension.
3. Hypertensive urgencies and emergencies may occur at any age and may be the patient's initial presentation of hypertension. Many cases, however, are the result of inadequate control of known existing hypertension.[3] Major risk factors include dyslipidemia, diabetes mellitus, age greater than 60 years, male gender, postmenopausal

TABLE 11-1

CLASSIFICATION OF HYPERTENSION IN ADULTS OLDER THAN 18 YEARS

Hypertensive Category	Blood Pressure (mm Hg)	
	Systolic	Diastolic
Optimal	<120	<80
Normal	120-129	80-84
High normal	130-139	85-89
Stage 1 (mild) hypertension	140-159	90-99
Stage 2 (moderate) hypertension	160-179	100-109
Stage 3 (severe) hypertension	>180	>110
Hypertensive urgency (no evident organ damage)	Usually >180	Usually >130
Hypertensive emergency (rapid increase in blood pressure or evidence of acute organ injury)	Usually >210	Usually >130

status, and family history (early hypertension in women <65 or men <55 years of age). Other important factors include obesity, sedentary lifestyle, nutritional factors, and alcohol use.

4. The main goal of treatment for hypertension and hypertensive crises is to reduce cardiovascular disease and organ injury. Early diagnosis and control of elevated blood pressure decrease morbidity and mortality from cardiovascular disease, coronary artery disease, and other causes, even in young patients.[4] Recent trials, including the Hypertension Optimal Treatment (HOT) trial,[5] indicate that long-term aggressive control of hypertension using multiple medications decreases the incidence of cardiovascular events.

II. CLINICAL PRESENTATION

1. The initial evaluation of any patient with suspected hypertensive urgency or emergency should focus on determining whether acute organ damage is present and whether rapid control of the blood pressure is needed (i.e., whether an inpatient or intensive care unit admission is appropriate). Boxes 11-1 and 11-2 list key aspects of the history, physical examination, and laboratory assessment of the hypertensive patient. In addition, the evaluation should attempt to determine whether the elevated blood pressure is acute or chronic. Acute elevations in blood pressure may be associated with pressure-dependent organ perfusion and should be managed with caution.

2. The four organs most commonly involved in hypertensive emergency are the heart, brain, kidneys, and eyes (Box 11-3). All hypertensive patients should undergo a thorough workup to identify signs and symptoms of secondary hypertension (Box 11-4).

3. The cause of hypertension may be difficult to separate from the sequelae of hypertension. For example, patients with acute renal

disease, acute stroke, or acute coronary artery ischemia may need to have the underlying process addressed to control the blood pressure. As always, appropriate evaluation and treatment should be guided by the patient's clinical picture.

III. MANAGEMENT

1. Fig. 11-1 presents an algorithm for triage of the hypertensive patient. In all cases treatment of the patient should be guided by the clinical presentation.
2. When treating hypertensive urgency or emergency, the health practitioner must remember the following caveats.
   a. The initial antihypertensive regimen should be chosen based on the patient's clinical presentation, the target organs that are affected, and other comorbidities that may be present.
   b. Treatment should always involve controlled blood pressure regulation. Short-acting calcium channel blockers that cannot be titrated should be avoided. These include orally and sublingually administered forms of nifedipine because they are associated with increased mortality from acute myocardial infarction.[6]
   c. Use of multiple classes of medications, including diuretics, is often needed for optimal blood pressure control.
   d. Management of hypertensive urgencies and emergencies should not rely on nonpharmacological interventions alone. However, it is important to encourage patients to make healthy lifestyle choices.
   e. A secondary cause of hypertension is present in up to 5% of hypertensive patients and possibly in a much higher percentage of persons with hypertensive urgency or emergency. After blood pressure has been controlled in patients with hypertensive urgency or emergency, workup for causes of secondary hypertension should be pursued (Box 11-4).

A. HYPERTENSIVE EMERGENCY

1. The immediate treatment goal for a patient with hypertensive emergency is to reduce end organ damage through controlled blood pressure management. The mean arterial blood pressure should be reduced by no more than 25% within 2 hours using intravenous and oral therapy (Tables 11-2 and 11-3) and then to a blood pressure of 160/110 mm Hg within the first 6 hours of treatment.[1,3,7]
2. The patient should be admitted to an intensive care unit if acute organ damage is present or ongoing (e.g., hypertensive encephalopathy, myocardial infarction, acute stroke). In most cases of hypertensive emergency, parenteral medications should be used to decrease blood pressure in a rapid and controlled manner. An arterial line and continuous blood pressure monitoring are usually necessary for titration of parenteral medications.
3. Rapid decrease in blood pressure may cause vasospasm, leading to

BOX 11-1

KEY ASPECTS OF THE HISTORY AND PHYSICAL EXAMINATION OF THE HYPERTENSIVE PATIENT

HISTORY

Hypertension History
Last known normal blood pressure
Prior diagnosis and treatments
Dietary and social factors

Cardiac History
Previous heart attacks, angina, arrhythmias
Symptoms of dyspnea, chest pain, claudication
Flank pain, back pain

Neurological History
History of prior strokes, neurological dysfunction
Visual changes, blurriness, loss of visual fields
Headache, nausea and vomiting

Renal History
Foamy urine or history of proteinuria
History of renal disease
Changes in urinary frequency or urine color

Endocrine History
Diabetes
Thyroid dysfunction
Cushing's syndrome

Family History
Early hypertension in family members
Cerebrovascular and cardiovascular disease
Diabetes, pheochromocytoma

Social History
Smoking, alcohol, illicit drugs (especially cocaine, stimulants), noncompliance

Medications
Steroids, estrogens, sympathomimetics
Nutritional supplements (e.g., ephedra, mah huang)

Other Comorbidities
Organ transplant (especially cardiac or renal)
Current pregnancy (eclampsia or preeclampsia)

hypoperfusion of organs and thereby to secondary organ damage, including new or worsened acute stroke and acute renal failure. This type of disordered autoregulation may limit how fast blood pressure can be reduced.

4. Once a patient with hypertensive emergency has been stabilized, a transition to oral antihypertensive medications should be made based on the patient's risk factors and comorbidities.

BOX 11-1—cont'd

KEY ASPECTS OF THE HISTORY AND PHYSICAL EXAMINATION OF THE
HYPERTENSIVE PATIENT

PHYSICAL EXAMINATION

Vital Signs
Blood pressure
Pulse rate
Weight, body habitus, buffalo hump, moon facies

Cardiovascular
Enlarged heart
Presence of S_3 or S_4 heart sounds
Bounding or asymmetrical pulses
Arrhythmias

Neck
Enlarged thyroid
Carotid pulses
Jugular venous distention

Pulmonary
Signs of left ventricular dysfunction (crackles, rhonchi)

Renal
Presence of renal bruit or abdominal masses

Neurological
Abnormal examination (evidence of stroke)

Ophthalmological
Funduscopic examination (papilledema, hemorrhage)
Exophthalmia
Lid lag

Extremities
Diminished or delayed pulses
Edema
Acromegaly

B. **HYPERTENSIVE URGENCY**
1. The treatment goal of a patient with hypertensive urgency is to minimize the risk of potential end organ injury. Blood pressure should be reduced to 160/110 mm Hg during the first 24 hours using oral therapy (Table 11-4) and then to normal blood pressure ranges as tolerated. Patients should be monitored closely for secondary organ damage from hypoperfusion or disordered autoregulation. Development of these complications may require additional monitoring or admission to an intensive care unit.
2. Patients with long-standing, stable hypertension without end organ involvement may be considered for outpatient management. As always, close follow-up of these patients is important. Patients who

---

BOX 11-2

LABORATORY ASSESSMENT OF THE HYPERTENSIVE PATIENT

INITIAL EVALUATION

Electrocardiogram

Hematocrit, white blood cell count

Basic chemistries (sodium, potassium, glucose, blood urea nitrogen, serum creatinine)

Urinalysis with microscopic examination

Chest radiograph (if heart failure or aortic dissection is suspected)

Thyroid-stimulating hormone

Head computed tomographic scan (if neurological findings are abnormal)

OTHER EVALUATION, ONCE PATIENT IS STABLE

Echocardiogram (for left ventricular dysfunction, valve abnormalities)

Lipid profile (preferably fasting)

Thyroid function studies

Renal artery imaging (if renal stenosis is suspected)

Other evaluations as guided by clinical presentation

---

may not be reliable or are at risk for worsening sequelae from their hypertensive urgency should be treated in an inpatient setting. Most medications may be titrated upward rapidly over 6 to 12 hours to achieve optimal blood pressure control.

3. After stabilization of the patient's hypertensive urgency or emergency, the long-term blood pressure goal should be determined by the patient's risk factors. The treatment goal should be less than 140/90 mm Hg for patients with uncomplicated hypertension, less than 130/80 mm Hg for patients with diabetes, and less than 125/75 mm Hg for patients with renal insufficiency and proteinuria (>1 g/24 hr).[1]

PEARLS AND PITFALLS

- Antihypertensive treatment should be individualized based on concomitant conditions. Some medications may worsen a patient's preexisting condition, whereas others may help treat coexisting disease.[1,7-10] Some common considerations are listed in Table 11-5. Other considerations may be appropriate, depending on the patient's clinical situation.

- Hypertension in the setting of an acute stroke or in the immediate poststroke period should be managed under close monitoring because neurological status may be worsened by even small changes in blood pressure.[11,12] There is some suggestion that ACE inhibitors may decrease death rates from stroke.[13]

- Use of nitroglycerin drips should be avoided in the acute management of patients with hypertensive emergencies because this may worsen their

---

BOX 11-3

COMMON SIGNS OF TARGET ORGAN INVOLVEMENT IN SEVERE HYPERTENSION

CARDIOVASCULAR

Myocardial infarction

Angina

Aortic dissection

Aneurysmal dilatation of large vessels

Left ventricular failure

Congestive heart failure

Left ventricular hypertrophy

Bleeding at vascular suture lines

Failure of vascular surgery or graft

RENAL

Hematuria

Proteinuria

Acute renal failure

CENTRAL NERVOUS SYSTEM

Cerebral edema

Altered mental status

Intracerebral or subarachnoid bleeding

Stroke or transient ischemic attack

OPHTHALMOLOGICAL

Retinal hemorrhages or exudates

Papilledema

Arteriovenous nicking

---

neurological status owing to an imbalance of cerebral arterial and venous dilatation. Nitroprusside, labetalol, or ACE inhibitors should be considered instead.

- ACE inhibitors delay progression of renal disease in diabetic patients[14] and those with chronic renal insufficiency.[15] However, ACE inhibitors may worsen renal function in the setting of bilateral renal artery stenosis, dehydration, or acute renal failure.
- In the setting of a myocardial infarction, β-blockers[16] and ACE inhibitors[13,17] have been shown to decrease morbidity and mortality.
- Although α_1-agonists are beneficial in some patients, particularly those with benign prostatic hypertrophy, monotherapy with α_1-antagonists may be associated with increased morbidity and mortality from congestive heart failure with long-term use.[18] These drugs include doxazosin, prazosin, and terazosin.

Text continued on p. 227

11

HYPERTENSIVE URGENCY AND EMERGENCY

BOX 11-4

POTENTIAL CAUSES OF HYPERTENSIVE URGENCY AND EMERGENCY

NEUROLOGICAL

Intracranial hemorrhage
Stroke or transient ischemic attack
Head injury or brain tumor
Seizure, especially postictal state
Encephalitis
Cerebral vasculitis
Acute anxiety

CARDIOVASCULAR

Essential hypertension
Myocardial infarction
Acute left ventricular failure
Vasculitis
Coarctation of the aorta
Aortic dissection
Volume overload (including pulmonary edema)

ENDOCRINE

Hyperthyroidism
Hypercalcemia
Hyperparathyroidism
Mineralocorticoid or glucocorticoid excess
Pheochromocytoma
Acute intermittent porphyria

RENAL

Renal artery stenosis
Renal parenchymal disease, including vasculitis, acute glomerulonephritis,
   hemolytic-uremic syndrome
Uremia, especially in setting of volume overload
Erythropoietin use, particularly in setting of hyperviscosity syndrome
Chronic lead intoxication

PREGNANCY

Eclampsia or preeclampsia

PHARMACOLOGICAL AND MISCELLANEOUS

Drug ingestions, including cocaine, amphetamines
Monoamine oxidase inhibitor interactions
Cyclosporine
Clonidine withdrawal and rebound hypertension
Noncompliance with outpatient medications
Steroids, including synthetic corticosteroids, mineralocorticoids, exogenous steroids
   (e.g., licorice)
Anesthetics, including ketamine
Sympathomimetics, including decongestants, antiemetics, yohimbine, sildenafil

TABLE 11-2
PARENTERAL VASODILATORS FOR USE IN HYPERTENSIVE CONTROL

Agent	Drug Type	Starting Dose/ Maximum Dose	Onset/Duration of Activity	Side Effects and Contraindications
Sodium nitroprusside	Direct peripheral vasodilator	0.25-10 µg/kg/min IV infusion	Immediate/2-3 min	Twitching, nausea, vomiting; monitor for thiocyanate toxicity, methemoglobinemia
Labetalol	α_1- and β-adrenergic antagonist	20-80 mg IV bolus q10 min, then 0.5-2 mg/ min IV infusion	5-10 min/2-6 hr	Bronchoconstriction, heart block, bradycardia
Nitroglycerin	Venous and arterial dilator	5-100 µg/min IV infusion	2-5 min/5-10 min	Headache, tachycardia, vomiting, worsening of neurological status
Hydralazine	Direct peripheral vasodilator	10-20 mg IV bolus or 10-40 mg IM, q4-6h	10-30 min/1-4 hr	Tachycardia, nausea, vomiting, headache, angina
Nicardipine	Calcium channel blocker (arteriolar dilator)	5-15 mg/hr IV infusion	1-5 min/15-30 min; effects may linger for 12 hr at high doses	Tachycardia, nausea, vomiting, headache, increased intracranial pressures
Verapamil	Calcium channel blocker	5-10 mg IV bolus, then 3-25 mg/hr IV infusion	1-5 min/30-60 min	Bradycardia, heart block (especially when used with digitalis or β-blockers)
Enalaprilat	Angiotensin-converting enzyme inhibitor	0.625-1.25 mg IV bolus q6h	15-60 min/12-24 hr	Renal failure in patients with renal artery stenosis

HYPERTENSIVE URGENCY AND EMERGENCY 11

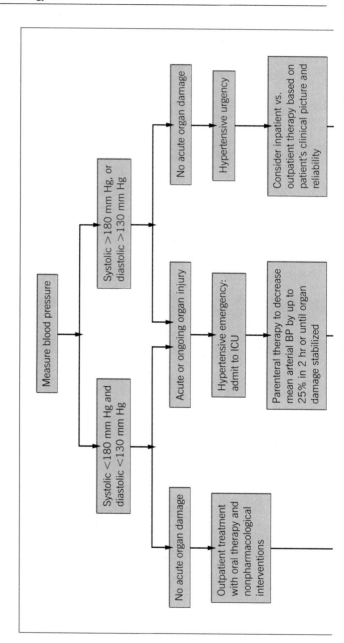

Measure blood pressure

Systolic <180 mm Hg and diastolic <130 mm Hg

Systolic >180 mm Hg, or diastolic >130 mm Hg

No acute organ damage

Outpatient treatment with oral therapy and nonpharmacological interventions

Acute or ongoing organ injury

Hypertensive emergency: admit to ICU

Parenteral therapy to decrease mean arterial BP by up to 25% in 2 hr or until organ damage stabilized

No acute organ damage

Hypertensive urgency

Consider inpatient vs. outpatient therapy based on patient's clinical picture and reliability

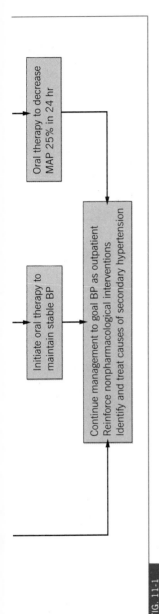

FIG. 11-1

Approach to the hypertensive patient. *BP,* Blood pressure; *ICU,* intensive care unit.

Boxes:
- Initiate oral therapy to maintain stable BP
- Oral therapy to decrease MAP 25% in 24 hr
- Continue management to goal BP as outpatient
- Reinforce nonpharmacological interventions
- Identify and treat causes of secondary hypertension

11

HYPERTENSIVE URGENCY AND EMERGENCY

TABLE 11-3

PARENTERAL ADRENERGIC INHIBITORS FOR USE IN HYPERTENSIVE CONTROL

Agent	Drug Type	Starting Dose/ Maximum Dose	Onset/Duration of Activity	Side Effects and Contraindications
Metoprolol	β-Blocker	5-15 mg IV bolus q30 min	1 hr/3-6 hr	Bronchoconstriction, heart block, bradycardia
Esmolol	β-Blocker	500 μg/kg IV bolus, then 25-100 μg/kg/min IV infusion	1-5 min/15-30 min	Bronchoconstriction, heart block, bradycardia
Phentolamine	α_1-Adrenergic antagonist	5-15 mg IV or IM bolus	1-2 min/10-30 min	Tachycardia, hypotension
Fenoldopam	Dopamine D1 and α_2-agonist	0.025-1.6 μg/kg/min IV infusion; do not give as bolus	5-15 min/1-4 hr	Headache, flushing, nausea, vomiting

TABLE 11-4
ORAL AGENTS COMMONLY USED FOR HYPERTENSIVE CONTROL

Agent	Drug Type	Starting Dose/ Maximum Dose	Onset/Duration of Activity	Side Effects and Contraindications
Labetalol	α- and β-adrenergic blocker	100/1200 mg PO bid	30 min–2 hr/2–12 hr	Bronchoconstriction, heart block, bradycardia
Metoprolol	β-Blocker	50/200 mg PO bid	1 hr/3–6 hr	Bronchoconstriction, heart block, bradycardia
Captopril	Angiotensin-converting enzyme inhibitor	6.25/150 mg PO tid	15–30 min/2–6 hr	Hyperkalemia; may worsen renal function
Clonidine	α_2-Agonist	0.1/1.2 mg PO bid	30–60 min/8–16 hr	Useful in cocaine-related hypertension; may cause rebound hypertension
Methyldopa	α_2-Agonist	250/1500 mg PO bid	3–6 hr/24–48 hr	Hepatitis, cirrhosis; interacts with monoamine oxidase inhibitors
Nifedipine SR	Calcium channel blocker	30/120 mg PO qd	30 min/12–24 hr	May worsen liver function, congestive heart failure, aortic stenosis
Hydralazine	Direct vasodilator	10/100 mg PO qid	1 hr/3–8 hr	Headache, tachycardia, palpitations, edema
Minoxidil	Direct vasodilator	5/100 mg PO qd	30–60 min/10–12 hr	May worsen acute myocardial infarction, pericardial effusions

11

HYPERTENSIVE URGENCY AND EMERGENCY

SPECIAL CIRCUMSTANCES THAT MAY AFFECT THE CHOICE OF
ANTIHYPERTENSIVE AGENTS

Condition	Useful Agents	Agents to Use with Caution
CARDIOPULMONARY DISEASE		
After myocardial infarction	β-Blockers, ACE inhibitors	Direct vasodilators (may worsen coronary insufficiency)
Congestive heart failure (systolic dysfunction)	ACE inhibitors, diuretics; β-blockers (when not in pulmonary edema)	β-Blockers, calcium channel antagonists
Hypertrophic cardiomyopathy (diastolic dysfunction)	β-Blockers, calcium channel blockers	Diuretics, ACE inhibitors, direct vasodilators
Bradycardia, heart block		β-Blockers, calcium channel antagonists
Tachyarrhythmias	β-Blockers (intrinsic antiarrhythmic effect), verapamil	
Peripheral vascular disease		β-Blockers (may decrease peripheral perfusion)
Angina	β-Blockers, calcium antagonists (decrease cardiac O_2 requirement); nitroglycerin (relaxes coronary vessels)	Direct vasodilators (decreased afterload may decrease coronary perfusion pressures)
Aortic dissection	Nitroprusside, β-blockers	Drugs that increase cardiac output (increased shear stress)
Obstructive lung disease	Calcium channel blockers (may help relax airways)	β-Blockers (may induce chronic obstructive pulmonary disease or asthma flare)
RENAL DISEASE		
Bilateral renal artery stenosis		ACE inhibitors, angiotensin receptor blockers (may worsen renal function)
Chronic renal insufficiency	ACE inhibitors (serum creatinine <2.5 mg/dL), loop diuretics, calcium antagonists	ACE inhibitors, angiotensin receptor blockers (may worsen renal function)
Renal transplants		ACE inhibitors (may worsen renal function)

TABLE 11-5

SPECIAL CIRCUMSTANCES THAT MAY AFFECT THE CHOICE OF
ANTIHYPERTENSIVE AGENTS—cont'd

Condition	Useful Agents	Agents to Use with Caution
CENTRAL NERVOUS SYSTEM		
Migraine headaches	β-Blockers, calcium antagonists (may help relieve migraine symptoms)	
Stroke or transient ischemic attack	ACE inhibitors (may allow reestablishment of central nervous system autoregulation)	Vasodilators (may increase intracranial pressure)
OTHER CONDITIONS		
Diabetes	ACE inhibitors (delay renal failure; decrease proteinuria)	
Pregnancy (preeclampsia, eclampsia)	Methyldopa, hydralazine; β-blockers with caution (possible association with low birth weight)	ACE inhibitors, angiotensin receptor blockers (may cause renal agenesis); diuretics
Gout		Diuretics (may worsen joint pain or precipitate gout flare)
Cocaine use	Labetalol; clonidine	Selective β-blockers (unopposed cocaine-induced α-agonism)
Gastrointestinal bleeding	Nonselective β-blockers (lower portal blood pressure)	β-Blockers (may mask signs of acute bleeding)
Pheochromocytoma	Combined α- and β-blockade	Selective β-blockers (unopposed α-agonism)
Benign prostatic hypertrophy	α_1-Antagonist	

ACE, Angiotensin-converting enzyme.

- Endocrine disorders (Cushing's syndrome, hypoaldosteronism) should be considered when patients who are not otherwise being treated with diuretics or ACE inhibitors have elevated blood pressure and electrolyte abnormalities.
- Renal artery stenosis should be considered when the presentation is hypertension and flash pulmonary edema without evidence of systolic heart failure.
- Caution is needed in restarting an outpatient antihypertensive regimen for patients with hypertensive urgency or emergency, particularly patients noncompliant with medication. These patients may not have been taking all of their prescribed medications and may be at risk for iatrogenic hypotension.

- Useful websites include the National Heart, Lung and Blood Institute: www.nhlbi.nih.gov; American Heart Association: www.americanheart.org; and MICROMEDEX Healthcare Series: www.micromedex.com.

REFERENCES

[d] 1. The sixth report of the Joint National Committee on prevention, detection, evaluation, and treatment of high blood pressure. Arch Intern Med 1997; 157(21):2413.

[b] 2. Burt VL et al. Prevalence of hypertension in the US adult population: results from the Third National Health and Nutrition Examination Survey, 1988-1991. Hypertension 1995; 25(3):305.

[c] 3. Kaplan NM. Management of hypertensive emergencies. Lancet 1994; 344(8933):1335.

[b] 4. Miura K et al. Relationship of blood pressure to 25-year mortality due to coronary heart disease, cardiovascular diseases, and all causes in young adult men: the Chicago Heart Association Detection Project in Industry. Arch Intern Med 2001; 161(12):1501.

[a] 5. Hansson LA et al. Effects of intensive blood-pressure lowering and low-dose aspirin in patients with hypertension: principal results of the Hypertension Optimal Treatment (HOT) randomised trial. HOT Study Group. Lancet 1998; 351(9118):1755.

[b] 6. Psaty BM et al. The risk of myocardial infarction associated with antihypertensive drug therapies. JAMA 1995; 274(8):620.

[c] 7. Kaplan NM. Hypertensive crises. In Clinical hypertension. Baltimore: Williams & Wilkins; 1998.

[d] 8. Moser M. National recommendations for the pharmacological treatment of hypertension: should they be revised? Arch Intern Med 1999; 159(13):1403.

[d] 9. Basile JN. Hypertension 2001: how will JNC VII be different from JNC VI? South Med J 2001; 94(9):889.

[d] 10. Kaplan NM. Management of hypertension in patients with type 2 diabetes mellitus: guidelines based on current evidence. Ann Intern Med 2001; 135(12):1079.

[d] 11. Adams HP et al. Guidelines for the management of patients with acute ischemic stroke: a statement for healthcare professionals from a special writing group of the Stroke Council, American Heart Association. Stroke 1994; 25(9):1901.

[c] 12. Tietjen CS et al. Treatment modalities for hypertensive patients with intracranial pathology: options and risks. Crit Care Med 1996; 24(2):311.

[a] 13. Yusuf SP et al. Effects of an angiotensin-converting-enzyme inhibitor, ramipril, on cardiovascular events in high-risk patients. Heart Outcomes Prevention Evaluation Study Investigators. N Engl J Med 2000; 342(3):145.

[a] 14. Lewis EJ et al. The effect of angiotensin-converting-enzyme inhibition on diabetic nephropathy. The Collaborative Study Group. N Engl J Med 1993; 329(20):1456.

[a] 15. Randomised placebo-controlled trial of effect of ramipril on decline in glomerular filtration rate and risk of terminal renal failure in proteinuric, non-diabetic nephropathy. the GISEN Group (Gruppo Italiano di Studi Epidemiologici in Nefrologia). Lancet 1997; 349(9069):1857.

[b] 16. Gottlieb SS et al. Effect of beta-blockade on mortality among high-risk and low-risk patients after myocardial infarction. N Engl J Med 1998; 339(8):489.

[c] 17. Indications for ACE inhibitors in the early treatment of myocardial infarction: systematic overview of individual data from 100,000 patients in randomized trials. ACE Inhibitor Myocardial Infarction Collaborative Group. Circulation 1998; 97(22):2202.

[c] 18. Furberg CD et al. Clinical implications of recent findings from the Antihypertensive and Lipid-Lowering Treatment To Prevent Heart Attack Trial (ALLHAT) and other studies of hypertension. Ann Intern Med 2001; 135(12):1074.

Hypotension and Shock

Saptarsi Haldar, MD, and Charles Wiener, MD

FAST FACTS

- Determine the fundamental hemodynamic derangement (cardiogenic, hypovolemic, low systemic vascular resistance [SVR] shock) before initiating therapy.
- If hypotension has a cardiogenic cause, remember to consider extracardiac disease (tamponade, tension pneumothorax, pulmonary embolism).
- If a hypotensive patient has elevated jugular venous pressures and cardiomegaly on chest radiograph, always consider tamponade before assuming cardiomyopathy.
- If hypotension develops in a patient receiving mechanical ventilation, quickly examine for tension pneumothorax or auto positive end-expiratory pressure (PEEP). Start treatment by disconnecting the ventilator and administering intravenous (IV) fluids.
- If hypovolemic, rule out and control active hemorrhage. Patients can lose large volumes of blood in the retroperitoneal space without overt external bleeding.
- In low-SVR states, always begin therapy with an IV volume challenge. Ensure that the patient is not receiving vasoactive medicines such as opiates, benzodiazepines, β-blockers, or calcium channel blockers.
- In decompensated pulmonary hypertension, both IV volume administration and peripheral vasodilators can rapidly accelerate shock when used in the wrong setting.
- For refractory hypotension, consider the following possibilities: an overwhelming systemic inflammatory state, adrenal insufficiency, a mixed physiological condition (e.g., sepsis and congestive heart failure), and neurogenic shock.
- Intubate when mental status is poor, acid-base or metabolic derangements predispose to sudden death even in the presence of intact mentation, or pulmonary edema and related hypoxia or hypoventilation are limiting volume resuscitation.
- A physiological continuum exists from hypotension to shock to irreversible end-organ dysfunction. The goals of therapy are to maintain perfusion of end organs, correct the underlying pathophysiological derangement, and initiate therapy before the development of end-organ dysfunction or an irreversible physiological state.

12

I. CLINICAL PRESENTATION AND DIAGNOSTICS

A. DETERMINANTS OF ORGAN PERFUSION

1. A simplified model of arterial circulation is based on Ohm's law, which states:

$$\text{Perfusion (flow)} = \frac{\text{Driving pressure}}{\text{Resistance}}$$

2. Perfusion represents blood flow to end organs. The driving pressure is the mean pressure in the arteriolar bed created by the ventricular systole coupled to arterial compliance. Resistance is determined by the vasomotor tone of the medium-sized arteriolar bed.

3. Based on the model, shock (inadequate perfusion) can be categorized into three fundamental physiological derangements: (1) disorders of low driving pressure ("pump failure" or cardiogenic shock), (2) disorders of inappropriately low resistance (distributive shock), and (3) hypovolemia (a "short circuit" or "empty tank" manifest as low ventricular end-diastolic pressure [VEDP]).

4. Table 12-1 and Box 12-1 summarize the fundamental physiological derangements that cause shock.

5. A key concept to remember is autoregulation. The arterial supply of each organ bed has the ability to differentially regulate its resistance to maintain constant flow over a range of systemic pressures. Autoregulation allows an organism to selectively perfuse one organ (e.g., the brain) over another organ (e.g., skeletal muscle) during low-pressure states. During chronic hypertensive states certain organ beds adjust their effective flow through autoregulation. Thus a patient who has had a systolic blood pressure of 190 mm Hg for months may be acutely hypoperfusing the brain at a "normal" systolic blood pressure of 120 mm Hg (Fig. 12-1).

B. HISTORY AND PHYSICAL EXAMINATION

1. In many cases the history and the events preceding shock provide the most likely diagnosis (Box 12-2). Certain key physical findings will corroborate the etiology that is suspected on the basis of the history. After vital signs are assessed, the examination should focus on the heart, lungs, and peripheral circulation.

2. The physical examination should be performed rapidly. Vital signs, including gross mental status and oxygenation, should be assessed first. Every aspect of the examination should be directed at answering three basic questions:

a. What is the underlying pathophysiological derangement?

b. Is any immediately reversible condition (e.g., tension pneumothorax) present?

c. Where on the spectrum of shock does the patient lie: compensated, organ dysfunction, or irreversible failure?

3. The strength and waveform of the peripheral pulse can often be used

TABLE 12-1

DIAGNOSIS OF SHOCK ETIOLOGY USING PULMONARY ARTERY
CATHETERIZATION

Diagnosis	PCWP	CO	Comments
Cardiogenic shock caused by myocardial dysfunction	↑↑	↓↓	Usually occurs with evidence of extensive myocardial infarction (40% of LV infarcted), severe cardiomyopathy, or myocarditis
Cardiogenic shock caused by mechanical defect			
Acute ventricular septal defect	↑	LVCO ↓↓ and RVCO > LVCO	Predominant shunt is left to right, pulmonary blood flow is greater than system blood flow: oxygen "step-up" occurs at RV level
Acute mitral regurgitation	↑↑	Forward CO ↓↓	V waves in PCWP tracing
Right ventricular infarction	Normal or ↓	↓↓	Elevated RA and RV filling pressures with low or normal PCWP
Extracardiac obstructive forms of shock			
Pericardial tamponade	↑	↓ or ↓↓	RA mean, RV end-diastolic, and PCWP mean pressures are elevated and within 5 mm Hg of one another
Massive pulmonary embolism	Normal or ↓	↓↓	Usual finding is elevated right-sided pressures
Hypovolemic shock	↓↓	↓↓	
Distributive forms of shock			
Septic shock	↓ or normal	↑ or normal, rarely ↓	
Anaphylactic shock	↓ or normal	↑ or normal	

Data from Parrillo JE, Ayres SM, eds. Major issues in critical care medicine. Baltimore: Williams & Wilkins; 1984.
CO, Cardiac output; *LVCO*, left ventricular cardiac output; *LV*, left ventricular; *PCWP*, pulmonary capillary wedge pressure; *RA*, right arterial; *RV*, right ventricular; *RVCO*, right ventricular cardiac output.

12

HYPOTENSION AND SHOCK

BOX 12-1

DETERMINANTS OF EFFECTIVE TISSUE PERFUSION

Arterial pressure
Cardiac performance
   Cardiac function
     Preload
     Afterload
     Contractility
     Heart rate
   Venous return
Vascular performance
   Distribution of cardiac output
     Extrinsic regulatory systems
       Sympathetic nervous system
       Adrenal hormone release
     Intrinsic regulatory systems
     Anatomical vascular disease
     Exogenous vasoactive agents
   Microvascular function
     Precapillary and postcapillary sphincter function
     Capillary endothelial integrity
     Microvascular obstruction
Cellular function
   Oxygen unloading and diffusion
     Red blood cell 2,3-diphosphoglycerate
     Blood pH
     Temperature
   Cellular energy generation and substrate utilization
     Citric acid (Krebs') cycle
     Oxidative phosphorylation
     Other energy metabolism pathways

Data from Goldman L, Bennett JC. Cecil textbook of medicine, 21st ed. Philadelphia: WB Saunders; 2000.

   to distinguish a bounding hyperdynamic circulation (as seen in compensated sepsis) from a weak, thready pulse (as seen in cardiogenic shock or hypovolemic shock).

4. Next, the neck veins are examined to estimate the central venous pressure (CVP). In severe hypovolemic and septic shock the meniscus is often barely visible, even if the patient is nearly supine. This corresponds to grossly low ventricular filling pressures. In contrast, grossly distended neck veins are a clue to cardiogenic shock. The character of the central venous waveform can offer clues to severe pulmonary hypertension, atrioventricular dissociation (cannon *a* waves), or severe constrictive pericarditis (Kussmaul's sign).

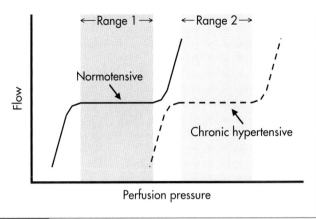

FIG. 12-1

Autoregulation of blood flow in relation to perfusion pressure in normotensive and hypertensive individuals.

5. Lung auscultation should be performed rapidly to assess for the key findings of presence of bilateral breath sounds, amount of air movement, and crackles. Absence of bilateral breath sounds with shock (and possibly elevated neck veins) should immediately raise concern about tension pneumothorax. Signs of hyperinflation, poor air movement, and prolonged expiratory phase should raise concern about auto-PEEP (especially if the patient is receiving mechanical ventilation or has severe obstructive lung disease with bronchospasm). If bilateral breath sounds and good air movement are present, the examiner should listen for crackles. Coarse crackles in a dependent fashion can represent pulmonary edema from cardiogenic shock and high left ventricular (LV) filling pressures. However, similar crackles can be heard in sepsis or systemic inflammatory states with damaged pulmonary microcirculation and alveolar injury (as seen in sepsis with acute respiratory distress syndrome). Suspicion of cardiogenic shock with normal findings on lung examination should raise suspicion of right-sided heart failure and pulmonary embolism.

6. The heart examination should focus on distinguishing a failing heart from a hyperdynamic heart. Palpation of the cardiac impulse can often distinguish an overloaded, decompensated ventricle (heaves, prolonged and diffuse impulse) from a hyperdynamic, compensated ventricle (focused impulse with sharp and dynamic motion). A few things should be rapidly assessed on auscultation. Muffled heart sounds should raise concern for tamponade in the appropriate clinical setting. A new S_3 corroborates the diagnosis of ventricular failure and

---

BOX 12-2

CLASSIFICATION OF SHOCK

HYPOVOLEMIC

Hemorrhagic

Trauma

Gastrointestinal

Retroperitoneal

Fluid Depletion (Nonhemorrhagic)

External fluid loss

    Dehydration

    Vomiting

    Diarrhea

    Polyuria

Interstitial fluid redistribution

    Thermal injury

    Trauma

    Anaphylaxis

Increased Vascular Capacitance (Venodilatation)

Sepsis

Anaphylaxis

Toxins and drugs

CARDIOGENIC

Myopathic

Myocardial infarction

    Left ventricle

    Right ventricle

Myocardial contusion (trauma)

Myocarditis

Cardiomyopathy

Postischemic myocardial stunning

Septic myocardial depression

Pharmacological

    Anthracycline cardiotoxicity

    Calcium channel blockers

Mechanical

Valvular failure (stenotic or regurgitant)

Hypertrophic cardiomyopathy

Ventricular septal defect

Arrhythmic

Bradycardia

Tachycardia

Data from Goldman L, Bennett JC. Cecil textbook of medicine, 21st ed. Philadelphia: WB Saunders; 2000.

BOX 12-2—cont'd

CLASSIFICATION OF SHOCK

EXTRACARDIAC OBSTRUCTIVE

Impaired Diastolic Filling (Decreased Ventricular Preload)

Direct venous obstruction (vena cava)

    Intrathoracic obstructive tumors

Increased intrathoracic pressure

    Tension pneumothorax

    Mechanical ventilation (with excessive pressure or volume depletion)

    Asthma

Decreased cardiac compliance

    Constrictive pericarditis

    Cardiac tamponade

Impaired Systolic Contraction (Increased Ventricular Afterload)

Right ventricle

    Pulmonary embolus (massive)

    Acute pulmonary hypertension

Left ventricle

    Aortic dissection

DISTRIBUTIVE

Septic (bacterial, fungal, viral, rickettsial)

Toxic shock syndrome

Anaphylactic, anaphylactoid

Neurogenic (spinal shock)

Endocrinological

    Adrenal crisis

    Thyroid storm

Toxic (e.g., nitroprusside, bretylium)

12

HYPOTENSION AND SHOCK

cardiogenic shock. A new murmur alerts the physician to decompensated valvular insufficiency or a new mechanical complication such as ventricular septal defect.

7. Once the fundamental physiological insult is defined, the physician should rapidly assess the degree of shock. This can be done by assessing bedside parameters of end-organ perfusion manifested as cool extremities, decreased mental status, or changes in urine output (Table 12-2).

8. Maintaining central nervous system perfusion is the goal of resuscitation, and the adequacy of cerebral perfusion can be evaluated rapidly by assessment of the patient's level of alertness and general cortical function (Glasgow Coma Scale). A rapid assessment of basic brainstem function (pupillary reflex, extraocular movement, and respiratory pattern) should be performed as well. Monitoring of urine

TABLE 12-2

ORGAN SYSTEM DYSFUNCTION IN SHOCK

Organ System	Manifestations
Central nervous system	Encephalopathy (ischemic or septic); cortical necrosis
Heart	Tachycardia; bradycardia; suraventricular tachycardia; ventricular ectopy; myocardial ischemia; myocardial depression
Pulmonary	Acute respiratory failure; adult respiratory distress syndrome
Kidney	Prerenal failure; acute tubular necrosis
Gastrointestinal	Ileus; erosive gastritis; pancreatitis; acalculous cholecystitis; colonic submucosal hemorrhage; transluminal translocation of bacteria and endotoxin
Liver	Ischemic hepatitis; "shock liver"
Hematological	Disseminated intravascular coagulation; dilutional thrombocytopenia
Metabolic	Hyperglycemia; glycogenolysis; gluconeogenesis; hypoglycemia (late); hypertriglyceridemia
Immune system	Gut barrier function depression; cellular immune depression; humoral immune depression

Data from Goldman L, Bennett JC. Cecil textbook of medicine, 21st ed. Philadelphia: WB Saunders; 2000.

output provides a gauge for renal perfusion. The color and temperature of skin and the character of peripheral pulses can be used to gauge the degree of perfusion to distal tissues.

9. Table 12-3 is a guide to key features on examination.

C. LABORATORY TESTS AND IMAGING

1. Laboratory evaluation and imaging should be guided by findings on history and physical examination. Here are a few noteworthy points.

a. If a patient appears septic, culture all possible sites and initiate antibiotic therapy as soon as possible. Ensure adequate volume resuscitation.

b. If cardiogenic shock is present, determine the rhythm, obtain a 12-lead electrocardiogram, and always consider ischemia.

c. Use a chest radiograph and bedside echocardiography for rapid evaluation of suspected pump failure, pneumothorax, and tamponade.

d. Determine the patient's acid-base status, ventilation, and oxygenation by measuring arterial blood gases, serum lactate, and basic electrolytes.

e. If the history is at all ambiguous, order a toxicology screen.

f. Use urine output and levels of blood urea nitrogen, creatinine, and liver enzymes as surrogate markers of end-organ perfusion.

g. If the patient has abdominal pain and signs of sepsis, obtain an abdominal radiograph to rule out obstruction or free air.

h. If coagulopathy is present, consider ischemic liver failure or disseminated intravascular coagulation.

i. Do not send an unstable patient away for a radiological study without carefully weighing the risks, benefits, and alternatives.

II. MANAGEMENT

1. The management of hypotension and shock is aimed at maintaining organ perfusion, (especially to the central nervous system), directing therapy toward the fundamental physiologic derangement, and promptly treating any reversible cause. A basic algorithm is presented in Fig. 12-2. Key guidelines are provided in the following sections.

A. LOW–SYSTEMIC VASCULAR RESISTANCE STATES

1. The fundamental derangement in this condition rests on an uncoupling of the tone and permeability of the resistance vessel bed. In other words, an inciting event causes the blood vessels to have inappropriately low SVR. In addition, systemic inflammation causes the blood vessels to leak intravascular fluid into the interstitial space, making maintenance of perfusion even more difficult. The body compensates by raising cardiac output and selectively shunting flow to the brain at the expense of other organs. If this compensation continues unabated, renal failure, acidosis, and lung injury will ensue, ultimately leading to death.

2. A common scenario is that biochemical mediators initiate a vicious circle of cell injury, systemic inflammation, and vasodilatation that overwhelms the body's compensatory reserve. In the case of bacteremia, one such mediator is lipopolysaccharides. In the case of anaphylaxis it is uncontrolled histamine and mast cell degranulation. In pancreatitis it is the result of protease extravasation into the bloodstream.

3. Therapy should begin with rapid infusion of volume in the form of saline, lactated Ringer's solution, or blood products. Patients should have adequate IV access (e.g., two large-bore [preferably 14-gauge] peripheral IV lines). Anaphylaxis should be recognized immediately with discontinuation of the offending allergen, prompt epinephrine administration, and careful attention to airway patency. Infection should be aggressively sought. Cultures should be obtained from all possible sources that could lead to intravascular seeding. In particular, all indwelling catheters should be cultured (and removed, if they appear infected). Urine, sputum, respiratory secretions, drains, ascites (if present), joints, and skin should be surveyed. A pressure wound can be an occult source in a hospitalized patient.

4. If initial survey for infectious etiologies does not yield an obvious cause, intraabdominal processes such as bowel ischemia or an intraabdominal abscess should be considered. In critically ill patients infections that often "hide" are acalculous cholecystitis, pressure sores, intraabdominal abscesses, and sinusitis. As a rule, empirical IV antibiotics should be administered without delay to provide broad-spectrum coverage against skin, bowel, urinary, and respiratory pathogens.

5. Many conditions can cause systemic inflammation that is similar to bacteremia and sepsis. In these situations an aggressive search for

TABLE 12-3

KEY FINDINGS ON PHYSICAL EXAMINATION

System or Body Area	Finding	Possible Conditions or Action Needed
HEENT	Dry mucous membranes	Dehydration
	Pinpoint pupils	Opiate overdose; pontine injury
	Dilated pupils	Benzodiazepine overdose; midbrain injury
Neck	Elevated JVP	Tamponade physiology; constrictive pericarditis (Kussmaul's sign); ventricular failure
	Flat JVP	Hypovolemia
	Stridor	Airway obstruction; anaphylaxis
Cardiovascular	Bradycardia, tachycardia, irregular	Determine rhythm and prescribe appropriate medication
	Left or right ventricular heave, S_3	Ventricular failure
	Muffled heart sounds	Tamponade
	Delayed carotid upstrokes (pulsus parvus et tardus)	Aortic stenosis
	Pulsus paradoxus	Tamponade physiological state; pulmonary hyperinflation
	New murmurs	Acute valvular lesion; decompensated chronic valvular lesion
Lungs	Tachypnea	Pulmonary embolism; early sepsis
	Kussmaul's breathing	Early sepsis; underlying metabolic acidosis
	Absent breath sounds	Tension pneumothorax, pleural effusion
	Egophony, consolidation	Pneumonia with sepsis; aspiration
	Wheezing	Anaphylaxis; acute asthma with hyperinflation
Abdomen	Tense, distended	Acute condition of the abdomen; perforated viscus; sepsis; ascites; spontaneous bacterial peritonitis; gravid uterus, chorioamnionitis
	High-pitched bowel sounds	Intestinal obstruction
	Grey Turner's or Cullen's sign	Pancreatitis
	Pulsatile mass	Rupture of abdominal aortic aneurysm
Rectal	Bright red blood per rectum, melena	Gastrointestinal hemorrhage
	Diminished tone	Cord injury

TABLE 12-3
KEY FINDINGS ON PHYSICAL EXAMINATION—cont'd

System or Body Area	Finding	Possible Conditions or Action Needed
Extremities	Swollen leg, palpable cord	Deep venous thrombosis leading to pulmonary embolism
	Cool, clammy skin	Shock with compensatory vasoconstriction
	Pulseless extremity	Acute arterial insufficiency
	Peripheral edema	Right heart failure
	Unequal blood pressure in upper extremities	Aortic dissection
	Cellulitis	Toxic shock, gas gangrene, deep infection
	Acute arthritis	Bacteremia, endocarditis
	Groin pain, back pain	Retroperitoneal hemorrhage
Neurological	Agitation, delirium, obtundation	Central nervous system dysfunction from shock; concurrent metabolic derangements
	Meningeal signs	Meningitis
	Focal deficits	Central nervous system infarct or bleeding; spinal cord injury; watershed territorial ischemia
Genitourinary	Anuria	Rule out obstruction
	Oliguria	Diminished renal perfusion

HEENT, Head, eyes, ears, nose, and throat; *JVP,* jugular venous pressure.

infection should still be performed because these entities can often coexist (e.g., pancreatitis and bacteremia from peripancreatic phlegmon). Details of sepsis (see Chapter 45), pancreatitis (see Chapter 26), adult respiratory distress syndrome (see Chapter 68), and the systemic inflammatory states are discussed elsewhere.

6. If parameters of organ perfusion do not respond to volume challenge and antibiotics, an intravenous vasopressor should be administered (Table 12-4). If a central venous catheter is present, measurement of CVP may guide adequacy of volume resuscitation. Because the fundamental derangement is poor systemic resistance, the agent of choice should be a peripheral vasoconstrictor with high α_1-adrenergic activity. Agents commonly used are phenylephrine, norepinephrine, and vasopressin.[1] These agents should be given through a central line with invasive blood pressure monitoring. Because of natural autoregulatory mechanisms, they may worsen renal perfusion and cause ischemia to the extremities. In addition, many of these agents cause supraventricular tachycardias.

B. HYPOVOLEMIA

1. The fundamental insult is loss of cardiac filling. When the body loses intravascular volume, it tries to increase venous tone to augment

Text continued on p. 244

Diagnostic

Initial diagnostic steps:
Directed history and physical examination
Laboratory
  Hemoglobin, WBC, platelets
  PT, PTT
  Arterial blood gases
  Electrolytes: Mg, Ca, PO$_4$
  BUN, creatinine
  Lactate
ECG
Chest radiograph

Shock suspected:
Hypotension
Tachycardia
Peripheral hypoperfusion
Oliguria
Encephalopathy

Diagnosis remains undefined or hemodynamic status requires repeated fluid challenges or vasopressors:
Pulmonary artery catheterization
  Cardiac output
  Oxygen delivery
  Filling pressures
Echocardiography
  Pericardial fluid
  Cardiac function
  Valve or shunt abnormalities

Therapeutic

Initial management steps:
Admit to intensive care unit (ICU)
Venous access (1 or 2 wide-bore catheters)
Central venous catheter
ECG monitoring
Pulse oximetry
Hemodynamic support (MAP <60 mm Hg)
  Fluid challenge
  Vasopressors for severe shock unresponsive to fluids

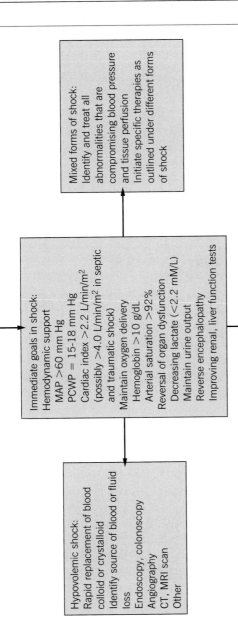

FIG. 12-2

Management of hypotension and shock. *BUN,* Blood urea nitrogen; *CT,* computed tomography; *ECG,* electrocardiogram; *ICU,* intensive care unit; *LV,* left ventricular; *MAP,* Mean arterial pressure; *MRI,* magnetic resonance imaging; *PCWP,* pulmonary capillary wedge pressure; *PT,* prothrombin time; *PTT,* partial thromboplastin time. (*Redrawn from Goldman L, Bennett JC. Cecil textbook of medicine, 21st ed. Philadelphia: WB Saunders; 2000.*) *cont'd*

HYPOTENSION AND SHOCK **12**

Content of figure:

Immediate goals in shock:
Hemodynamic support
MAP >60 mm Hg
PCWP = 15-18 mm Hg
Cardiac index >2.2 L/min/m² (possibly >4.0 L/min/m² in septic and traumatic shock)
Maintain oxygen delivery
Hemoglobin >10 g/dL
Arterial saturation >92%
Reversal of organ dysfunction
Decreasing lactate (<2.2 mM/L)
Maintain urine output
Reverse encephalopathy
Improving renal, liver function tests

Hypovolemic shock:
Rapid replacement of blood colloid or crystalloid
Identify source of blood or fluid loss
Endoscopy, colonoscopy
Angiography
CT, MRI scan
Other

Mixed forms of shock:
Identify and treat all abnormalities that are compromising blood pressure and tissue perfusion
Initiate specific therapies as outlined under different forms of shock

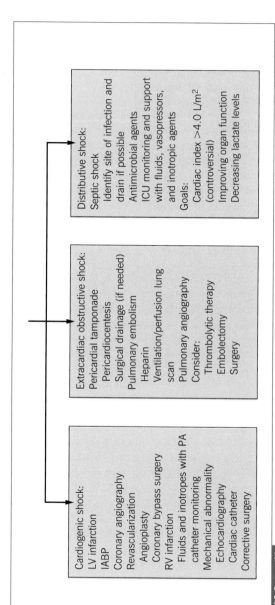

Cardiogenic shock:
LV infarction
IABP
Coronary angiography
Revascularization
Angioplasty
Coronary bypass surgery
RV infarction
Fluids and inotropes with PA
catheter monitoring
Mechanical abnormality
Echocardiography
Cardiac catheter
Corrective surgery

Extracardiac obstructive shock:
Pericardial tamponade
Pericardiocentesis
Surgical drainage (if needed)
Pulmonary embolism
Heparin
Ventilation/perfusion lung
scan
Pulmonary angiography
Consider:
Thrombolytic therapy
Embolectomy
Surgery

Distributive shock:
Septic shock
Identify site of infection and
drain if possible
Antimicrobial agents
ICU monitoring and support
with fluids, vasopressors,
and inotropic agents
Goals:
Cardiac index >4.0 L/m²
(controversial)
Improving organ function
Decreasing lactate levels

FIG. 12-2—cont'd

(Redrawn from Goldman L, Bennett JC. Cecil textbook of medicine, 21st ed. Philadelphia: WB Saunders; 2000.)

TABLE 12-4

RELATIVE POTENCY OF VASOPRESSORS AND INOTROPIC AGENTS IN SHOCK

| Agent | Dosage | Cardiac | | Peripheral Vascular | | |
		Heart Rate	Contractility	Vasoconstriction	Vasodilation	Dopaminergic
Dopamine	1-4 µg/kg/min	1+	1+	0	1+	4+
	4-20 µg/kg/min	2+	2-3+	2-3+	0	2+
Norepinephrine	2-20 µg/min	1+	2+	4+	0	0
Dobutamine	2.5-15 µg/kg/min	1-2+	3-4+	0	2+	0
Isoproterenol	1-5 µg/min	4+	4+	0	4+	0
Epinephrine	1-20 µg/min	4+	4+	4+	3+	0
Phenylephrine	20-200 µg/min	0	0	3+	0	0
Amrinone	0.75 mg/kg bolus; then 5-15 µg/kg/min	1+	3+	0	2+	0
Milrinone	37.5-75 µg/kg bolus; then 0.375-0.75 µg/kg/min	1+	3+	0	2+	0

Data from Parrillo JE, Ayres SM, eds. Major issues in critical care medicine. Baltimore: Williams & Wilkins; 1984.
The 0 to 4+ scoring system is an arbitrary system to allow a judgment of comparative potency among these vasopressor agents.

HYPOTENSION AND SHOCK

12

preload, heart rate and contractility to augment cardiac output, and arteriolar tone to augment systemic pressure. If hypovolemia persists, however, the heart cannot fill in diastole, and eventually cardiac output plummets. Organ ischemia, asystole, pulseless electrical activity (PEA), and eventually death ensue.

2. The physician should search aggressively for evidence of bleeding while simultaneously resuscitating with rapid IV volume. External hemorrhage should be compressed, coagulopathies should be corrected, and endoscopy or arteriography should be performed for gastrointestinal hemorrhage. Initial hematocrits may grossly underestimate the severity of bleeding.[2]

3. Nonhemorrhagic hypovolemia has many causes, including "third spacing." In normal homeostasis a balance between intravascular and extravascular volume exists that is governed by hydrostatic pressure gradient, the oncotic pressure gradient, and the vascular permeability to fluid (Starling forces across the capillary). In some disease states this balance is disrupted: increased hydrostatic pressure (portal hypertension and ascites), increased vascular permeability (e.g., sepsis and systemic inflammation), or low oncotic pressure in the vessel (e.g., hypoalbuminemia). All of these scenarios cause leakage of intravascular fluid into the extravascular space. This creates a disconnect between total body volume and effective circulating volume (i.e., the volume that is sensed by the pressure- and volume-detecting mechanisms). This state is often called "third spacing," referring to leakage of fluid into the extravascular and extracellular compartment. The important concept is that the total body volume may be normal or even grossly elevated, but the effective circulating volume remains low, resulting in hypotension. This situation can be extremely difficult to treat because IV volume therapy is preferentially distributed to the extravascular space, causing anasarca, ascites, or even pulmonary edema with minimal correction of the hypotension. In these situations the physician should maintain intravascular volume as well as possible while treating the underlying distributive defect (hypoalbuminemia, portal hypertension, systemic inflammation). In the case of pulmonary edema, maintenance of oxygenation and ventilation (often requiring intubation) is paramount. Commonly, when the acute illness that causes the "third spacing" resolves, the body reequilibrates the third-spaced fluid into the intravascular space. If necessary, this reequilibration phase can be augmented with diuresis.

4. Proper IV access should be available (either two large-bore peripheral IV lines or a large-bore central venous catheter). Infusion rates through catheters follow the law of laminar flow through rigid cylindrical tubes. This law states that flow is proportional to the cross-sectional radius and inversely proportional to length. Therefore the ideal catheter is large bore and short.

C. CARDIOGENIC SHOCK

1. The primary defect in cardiogenic shock is the inability of the heart to maintain cardiac output (Box 12-3). This is often called "pump failure." Cardiac output is simply the product of stroke volume and heart rate. Therefore cardiogenic shock is caused by disorders that either lower heart rate or lower stroke volume.

2. The disorders that lower heart rate are the bradycardias, and their treatment is delineated in the guidelines for advanced cardiac life support (see Chapter 1). The basic strategy is to define the rhythm, treat the underlying cause of bradycardia (ischemia, drug toxicity, metabolic derangement), and attempt to increase the heart rate by use of chronotropic drugs (atropine and epinephrine) or pacing.

3. Failure of the heart to maintain stroke volume may be due to arrhythmias, myocardial infarction (see Chapter 6), disorders of the myocardial contractility, or mechanical abnormalities of intracardiac or extracardiac structures.

4. The details of arrhythmia management are described in Chapter 1. Arrhythmias can be too slow (bradycardias), too fast (tachycardias), or an absence of coordinated contraction (asystole, PEA, ventricular fibrillation). Tachyarrhythmias depress stroke volume because of supply-demand mismatch and loss of diastasis. Unless the patient has supply-demand mismatch or baseline cardiomyopathy, stroke volume

12

HYPOTENSION AND SHOCK

BOX 12-3

RISK FACTORS AND CARDIOGENIC SHOCK

FACTORS ASSOCIATED WITH DEVELOPMENT OF SHOCK

Older age

Diabetes mellitus

History of prior myocardial infarction, stroke or peripheral vascular disease

Female gender

Reinfarction

Initial ejection fraction <35%

Lack of compensatory hyperkinesis in remote segments

FACTORS ASSOCIATED WITH INCREASED MORTALITY FROM SHOCK

Older age

Prior infarction

Altered sensorium

Peripheral vasoconstriction

Baseline systolic blood pressure

Lower cardiac output

Higher heart rate

Data from Goldman L, Bennett JC. Cecil textbook of medicine, 21st ed. Philadelphia: WB Saunders; 2000.

is usually maintained until heart rate approaches the age-appropriate limit. Therapy is aimed at the underlying mechanism of the tachycardia (reentrant, physiological, automaticity).

5. Disorders of myocardial contractility are diseases in which myocyte contraction and relaxation are depressed. Immediate recognition of ischemia is of paramount importance. If ischemia is present, prompt reperfusion and correction of supply-demand mismatch are essential. Myocardial infarctions with cardiogenic shock (Killip class IV) are discussed in Chapter 6 and detailed in Fig. 12-3, but several points are worth restating here. (1) The physician should always consider right ventricular (RV) infarction. (2) Intraaortic balloon counterpulsation (IABP) reduces supply-demand mismatch and may have a mortality benefit.[3] (3) Ventricular filling pressures may be high or low and may be extremely difficult to assess without invasive hemodynamic assessment via PA catheterization (see Chapter 15).[4] (4) The physician should always listen for a holosystolic murmur and consider ischemic mitral regurgitation or ventricular septal defect (see Table 6-3).

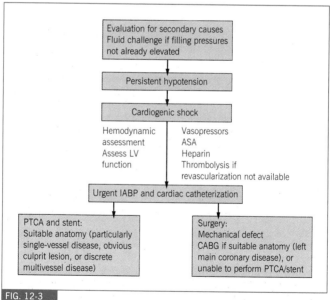

FIG. 12-3

Acute myocardial infarction with hypotension: an aggressive approach. *ASA,* Acetylsalicylic acid; *CABG,* coronary artery bypass grafting; *IABP,* intraaortic balloon pumping; *LV,* left ventricular; *PTCA,* percutaneous transluminal coronary angioplasty. *(Redrawn from Goldman L, Bennett JC. Cecil textbook of medicine, 21st ed. Philadelphia: WB Saunders; 2000.)*

6. Mechanical abnormalities causing hypotension can be due to intracardiac and extracardiac structures. The intracardiac causes are native valvular catastrophes (acute aortic insufficiency or mitral regurgitation), prosthetic valvular catastrophes (thrombosed prosthesis or acute perivalvular leak), or myocardial catastrophes (acute ventricular septal defect, free wall rupture). Some possible clinical scenarios are acute aortic insufficiency in aortic dissection, rupture of the mitral valve chordae with flail leaflet and acute mitral regurgitation, and ischemic ventricular septal defect complicating a myocardial infarction. The patient may die without emergency surgical repair or hemodynamic support. Diagnosis should be based on physical examination and confirmed by rapid bedside echocardiography.

7. Extracardiac causes of cardiogenic shock should be considered because many of them can be rapidly diagnosed and treated. Although the pathophysiology of each entity differs slightly, they all reduce stroke volume by impairing ventricular filling.

8. Tension pneumothorax and hyperinflation should be considered first. In these disorders intrathoracic pressure is abnormally raised to the point at which venous return to the right side of the heart becomes impaired. Hypotension is often rapid and dramatic. These should always be the first diagnoses considered if the patient is receiving positive-pressure ventilation (the scenario in which these disorders are most likely to be encountered by the medical house officer). Ventilator-associated lung injury can create a tension pneumothorax. Patients with obstructive lung disease (especially those who have severe bronchospasm and require prolonged expiratory time) are highly susceptible to breath stacking, hyperinflation, and a tensionlike physiological state. In all cases the patient should be promptly disconnected from the ventilator. The patient should be allowed to self-equilibrate to safer intrathoracic pressures with adjunctive bag-mask ventilation if necessary. True tension pneumothorax should be decompressed on an emergency basis by insertion of a large-bore needle into the affected side at the second intercostal space along the midclavicular line.

a. Pericardial tamponade and severe constrictive pericarditis impair filling by neutralizing the intracardiac pressure gradient and thereby impairing flow between chambers. Diagnosis of tamponade should be made by examination of neck veins and cardiac auscultation. If time permits, rapid bedside echocardiography should be performed. Emergency pericardial drainage should not be delayed. Constrictive pericarditis is less an emergency and may be much harder to diagnose. Diagnosis must often be confirmed by invasive hemodynamic monitoring. Therapy is surgical stripping of the pericardium.

b. Massive pulmonary embolism can cause acute uncompensated RV failure that severely impairs LV filling (see Chapter 64). Thrombolytic therapy and surgical thrombectomy remain controversial therapeutic options.[5]

12

HYPOTENSION AND SHOCK

c. Decompensated pulmonary hypertension results in increased pulmonary resistance beyond the pumping capability of the RV. Although this is a progressive and insidious process, small perturbations in ventricular filling pressures and systemic resistance can greatly alter stroke volume. When dealing with this condition, the physician should be cautious with use of IV fluid resuscitation, diuretics, and all vasoactive medications. Based on a very narrow Starling curve therapeutic window (Fig. 12-4), small perturbations in systemic resistance or volume status can significantly alter the systemic mean pressure.

PEARLS AND PITFALLS

- If pulmonary hypertension is known to be present, think of where the RV and LV lie on their Starling curves in all situations. Volume challenge and vasoactive medicines can make hypertensive patients hypotensive. In contrast, diuresis can augment systemic perfusion.
- Patients who have large myocardial infarctions and are in cardiogenic shock might be expected to have high end-diastolic pressures. In up to 25% of Killip class IV myocardial infarctions, however, patients have low filling pressures and require volume. Thus PA catheterization should be considered.
- Positive-pressure ventilation can have a dose-dependent effect on cardiac output.
- The five main causes of refractory hypotension are inadequate volume resuscitation, adrenal insufficiency, vasoactive drug toxicity, neurogenic shock, and mixed states.

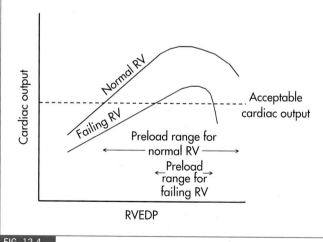

FIG. 12-4

Right ventricular Starling curve. *RV,* Right ventricle; *RVEDP,* right ventricular end-diastolic pressure.

- Septic patients commonly have impressive volume deficits, often ranging from 5 to 10 L. Volume resuscitation must be performed aggressively with isotonic solution via adequate intravenous access. Serial measurement of CVP can help guide adequacy of volume resuscitation. Often, aggressive volume administration can be limited by "third spacing" and pulmonary capillary leakage if systemic inflammation or hypoalbuminemia exists. In this case intubation and mechanical ventilation may be required for continued volume resuscitation.

- Any patient receiving long-term steroid therapy should be assumed to be adrenally insufficient, and "stress-dose" steroids should be instituted without delay. Bacteremia, coagulopathy, and acquired immunodeficiency syndrome are conditions that commonly predispose patients to adrenal hemorrhage and adrenalitis.

- The medicine list should be carefully reviewed to look for any agents that could be exacerbating the hypotension (e.g., β-blockers, calcium channel blockers, opiates, benzodiazepines).

- The thoracic spinal cord has sympathetic efferents that can augment chronotropy, inotropy, and vasomotor tone. Any disorder that interrupts this spinal sympathetic drive should be considered. Examples are high spinal anesthesia and spinal cord trauma, malignancy, ischemia, or infection at a thoracic level.

- Organs that usually compensate may themselves be diseased, creating a "mixed state." One common example is the patient who has concomitant heart failure and sepsis and cannot maintain compensatory elevated cardiac output. A second is the patient with sepsis and hypovolemia, as often occurs with variceal bleeding. These situations can be extremely difficult to treat and often require invasive hemodynamic measurements via a pulmonary artery catheter and arterial line.

REFERENCES

[c] 1. Holmes CL et al. Physiology of vasopressin relevant to management of septic shock. Chest 2001; 120(3):989.

[b] 2. Ebert RV et al. Response of normal subjects to acute blood loss. Arch Intern Med 1941; 68:687.

[b] 3. Ferguson JJ 3rd et al. The current practice of intra-aortic balloon counterpulsation: results from the Benchmark Registry. J Am Coll Cardiol 2001; 38(5):1456.

[b] 4. Zion MM et al. Use of pulmonary artery catheters in patients with acute myocardial infarction: analysis of experience in 5,841 patients in the SPRINT Registry. SPRINT Study Group. Chest 1990; 98(6):1331.

[a] 5. Arcasoy S, Kreit J. Thrombolytic therapy of pulmonary embolism: a comprehensive review of current evidence. Chest 1999; 115:1695.

12

HYPOTENSION AND SHOCK

Pacemakers and Defibrillators

Kenneth Bilchick, MD, Alan Cheng, MD, and Ronald Berger, MD, PhD

FAST FACTS

- Permanent pacemaker systems typically consist of a pulse generator with pacing leads in the right atrium, right ventricle, or both.
- The most common general indication for permanent pacing is symptomatic bradycardia.
- The pacing modes are designated by three- or four-letter codes specifying (in the following order) the chamber paced ("A" for atrium, "V" for ventricle, "D" for both, or "O" for neither), the chamber sensed ("A," "V," "D," or "O" as above), the action taken by the pacemaker ("I" for inhibit, "T" for trigger, or "D" for dual response), and whether or not rate-responsive pacing is present ("R" if present).
- Implantable cardioverter defibrillators (ICDs) detect ventricular tachycardia or fibrillation based primarily on the ventricular rate (not the QRS width) and may deliver an electrical charge (1-36 J) or initiate rapid pacing to terminate these rhythms.
- The 2002 ACC/AHA/NASPE Guideline Update includes important new indications for pacemakers and ICDs for patients with chronic heart failure.

13

I. EPIDEMIOLOGY

1. Pacemakers were introduced in the 1950s for use in patients with pathological conditions of the sinus node, atrioventricular (AV) node, or His-Purkinje system. Since that time they have been refined to allow more complex programming. In addition, periprocedural morbidity has been significantly reduced. As a result, the number of devices implanted has steadily increased, with approximately 153,000 new pacemakers implanted in the United States in 1997 alone.[1]
2. Pacemaker systems consist of a pulse generator (typically the size of a half dollar coin with batteries lasting approximately 5 years) placed subcutaneously in the shoulder area and connected to one or two pacing leads positioned in the right atrium or right ventricle or both. This configuration allows the pacemaker to sense intrinsic cardiac electrical activity and if necessary to initiate myocardial depolarization by delivering a small amount of pacing current. Implantation usually takes about 2 hours and is performed by a surgeon or a cardiologist with the patient under conscious sedation and local anesthesia. Given the myriad programmable settings, an understanding of the available modes is important for the medical practitioner.

II. COMMON PACING MODES

1. Pacing modes are usually described by codes consisting of three or four letters. The first letter refers to the chambers paced: "A" for atrium, "V" for ventricle, "D" for both, and "O" for neither (pacing is turned off). The second letter refers to the chambers sensed, using the same abbreviations as for pacing ("O" denotes that sensing is turned off and asynchronous pacing would occur). The third letter refers to the action taken by the pacemaker in response to a sensed signal and may be one of the following: "I" (inhibit), "T" (trigger), or "D" (dual response of inhibiting or triggering for dual-chamber devices). If a fourth letter is used, it is usually "R," which refers to rate-responsive pacing. Rate-responsive devices contain a crystal capable of adjusting the rate in response to temperature, minute ventilation, oxygen saturation, vibration, and other variables. This facilitates appropriate adjustments in heart rate based on an individual's physical activity. Dual-chamber pacing is often referred to as physiological pacing.

2. **DDD(R) mode:** The DDD(R) mode is a two-lead system that paces and senses both chambers with the ability to inhibit or trigger an artificial cardiac depolarization in response to a sensed signal. For example, if an intrinsic atrial beat is sensed within a programmed heart rate threshold (typically 60 beats/min), the pacer will not trigger an artificial atrial beat (atrial pacing is inhibited). If the intrinsic atrial rate is slower than the programmed rate, the atrial lead will trigger an artificial atrial depolarization. As the atrial beat travels through the AV conduction system, the ventricular lead will sense whether the intrinsic atrial beat has propagated into the ventricle within a preprogrammed time interval (typically 240 msec). If the ventricular lead senses intrinsic depolarization, it will not trigger an artificial ventricular beat (i.e., ventricular pacing is inhibited). If after the set time interval the ventricular lead does not sense intrinsic depolarization, it will trigger an artificial ventricular beat. This mode is especially useful for patients with AV block, a need for AV synchrony to maximize cardiac output, or a history of pacemaker syndrome.

3. **DDI(R) mode:** The DDI(R) mode is a two-lead system that is capable of pacing and sensing the atrium and ventricle. In response to a sensed signal, the pacemaker will inhibit output of an artificial depolarization. For example, if the intrinsic atrial rate is slower than the programmed rate, the atrial lead will trigger an artificial atrial depolarization. Unlike the DDD mode, DDI will not trigger a ventricular artificial depolarization based on atrial activity. The only scenario in which the ventricular lead will trigger an artificial depolarization is if the intrinsic ventricular rate is below a programmed threshold.

4. **VVI(R) mode:** The VVI(R) mode is a one-lead system that paces and senses only the ventricle. If an intrinsic ventricular signal is detected, the ventricular lead will not trigger an artificial ventricular depolarization. This mode is particularly useful for patients with persistent atrial

arrhythmias such as atrial fibrillation. Unlike the DDI(R) mode, the VVI(R) mode does not pace the atrium if an intrinsic atrial signal is absent. The disadvantage of this mode compared with DDI(R) is AV dyssynchrony with possible compromise of cardiac output as a result of impaired diastolic filling of the left ventricle.

5. **AAI mode:** The AAI mode is a one-lead system that paces and senses only the atrium. If an intrinsic atrial signal is sensed, the pacer will not trigger an artificial atrial depolarization. This mode may be appropriate for chronotropically competent (able to mount an appropriate heart rate response) patients with sinus node dysfunction, such as those with symptomatic bradycardia with intact AV conduction. The disadvantage of this mode is the lack of ventricular pacing should AV block occur. In a selected group of patients who were screened to have intact AV node function, the occurrence of clinically significant AV nodal disease was less than 2% per year.[2]

6. **DOO mode:** In the DOO mode both chambers are paced but not sensed. It may be used as a temporary mode before surgery to prevent an interaction between the electrocautery and pacemaker sensing. Such an interaction could result in significant bradycardia or asystole.

7. **VOO mode:** In the VOO mode the ventricle is paced but not sensed. The indication is same as for DOO.

III. MAJOR INDICATIONS FOR PERMANENT PACING

1. Current indications for permanent pacing are based on the 1998 practice guidelines and the 2002 update to these guidelines devised by the American College of Cardiology (ACC), the American Heart Association (AHA), and the North American Society of Pacing and Electrophysiology (NASPE). The indications follow the standard evidence-based tiered system. A class I indication means that a procedure is generally agreed to be beneficial, while class IIa indications are those for which there is conflicting evidence or divergence of opinion but the weight of evidence is in favor. Class IIb is similar to class IIa except that the efficacy of a procedure is less well established.

2. The major indications for permanent pacing may be divided into two categories based on whether patients have symptoms. As a general rule, patients with symptomatic bradycardia having an irreversible cause should have permanent pacing. In addition, certain patients with asymptomatic bradycardia should have a permanent pacemaker.

a. Symptomatic bradycardia having an irreversible cause.

(1) Carotid sinus hypersensitivity (CSH) (I): Class I if recurrent syncope. A recent randomized study of 175 patients older than 50 years who had a history of falls and CSH and received pacing or no pacing showed that those not paced had a fourfold greater risk of recurrent falls than those in the pacing group.[3]

(2) Sinus node dysfunction (I): Class I with symptomatic bradycardia.

(3) Third-degree AV block (I): Class I with symptomatic bradycardia.

(4) Second-degree AV block (I): There is a class I indication for either type I or type II second-degree AV block accompanied by symptomatic bradycardia.

b. Asymptomatic bradycardia.

(1) Third-degree AV block (I or IIa): There is a class I indication if the ventricular rate is less than 40 beats/min or there is asystole lasting longer than 3 seconds. Otherwise, there is only a class IIa indication for permanent pacing in asymptomatic patients.

(2) Mobitz II second-degree AV block (IIa): There is a class I indication if the QRS is wide; if the QRS is narrow, there is a class IIa indication for permanent pacing.

IV. NOVEL APPLICATIONS OF PERMANENT PACING

A. CARDIAC RESYNCHRONIZATION THERAPY

1. Cardiac resynchronization therapy (CRT) is intended for the patient with a dilated cardiomyopathy and an intraventricular conduction delay. The objective is to correct dyssynchrony by pacing the left ventricle alone or in conjunction with the right ventricle (biventricular). Since the left ventricle must be paced via the coronary sinus, left ventricular pacing is more technically difficult than right ventricular pacing. The Multisite Stimulation in Cardiomyopathy (MUSTIC) study has shown statistically significant improvements in the 6-minute walk and quality of life (but not mortality) with biventricular pacing,[4] and the Multisite InSync Randomized Clinical Evaluation (MIRACLE) has shown improvements in functional class, quality of life, and left ventricular dimensions.[5] It is noteworthy that the COMPANION trial investigating the use of CRT with or without ICDs was terminated in November 2002 because of the achievement of a prospectively identified endpoint of reduced combined mortality and hospitalization in patients receiving CRT combined with ICDs. Based on the 2002 Guideline Update, there is now a class IIa indication for biventricular pacing in patients who have idiopathic dilated or ischemic cardiomyopathy and meet the following criteria: class III or IV heart failure symptoms refractory to medical therapy, QRS width greater than or equal to 130 msec, left ventricular (LV) ejection fraction less than or equal to 35%, and LV end-diastolic diameter greater than 55 mm.

B. HYPERTROPHIC OBSTRUCTIVE CARDIOMYOPATHY

1. The objective of permanent pacing in hypertrophic obstructive cardiomyopathy is to improve outflow obstruction with early stimulation of the right ventricular apex. The pacemaker is programmed to DDD mode with leads in the right atrium and right ventricle. In randomized clinical studies such as the Pacemaker in Cardiomyopathy study[6] and the M-PATHY study,[7] DDD pacing resulted in statistically significant reductions in the left ventricular outflow tract pressure gradient but resulted in only mild improvement in functional status. Myo-

mectomy and septal ablation are other treatment options for hypertrophic obstructive cardiomyopathy.

C. PREVENTION OF ATRIAL FIBRILLATION

1. The objective is to prevent atrial fibrillation in at-risk patients through right or biatrial pacing. Whether biatrial pacing confers an advantage over right atrial pacing is controversial.[8,9] Ongoing studies should help clarify these issues.

V. TIERED THERAPY WITH IMPLANTABLE CARDIAC DEFIBRILLATORS

1. Implantable cardiac defibrillators (ICDs) were introduced in the 1980s as a means of continuously monitoring ventricular rates. When the rate exceeds a programmed threshold, the device assumes that the patient has a malignant ventricular arrhythmia. In this way the ICD's detection of ventricular tachycardia is based primarily on the ventricular rate rather than the width of the QRS complex on the surface electrocardiogram (ECG). Current ICD systems all have VVI pacing capability and may consist of either one or two leads, with the latter configuration designed to allow dual-chamber pacing if necessary.

2. The procedure for implanting an ICD system is not much different from that for implanting a pacemaker. With the patient under conscious sedation and local anesthesia, a cardiologist or surgeon inserts a pulse generator subcutaneously and inferior to the left clavicle. The pulse generator is then connected to the lead(s) in the right ventricle (and right atrium for two-lead systems). When the ICD fires, the circuit consists of a ventricular coil as one pole and the pulse generator or another coil in the right atrium as the other. The pulse generator is typically positioned on the patient's left side, allowing the maximum amount of current to traverse the heart (Fig. 13-1).

3. Since the ICD does not have the ability to distinguish ventricular tachycardia from ventricular fibrillation, therapy is individualized based on ventricular rates. For example, most ICDs are programmed to have one to three zones of therapy. The device delivers the programmed therapy based on the heart rate it detects. Available therapies include VVI pacing, antitachycardia pacing (ATP), and shock delivery. In ATP the device initiates a short burst of rapid ventricular pacing in an effort to interrupt the tachycardia reentry circuit by making the region of pacing temporarily refractory to additional ventricular activation. Shock may be delivered in the form of low-energy cardioversion or defibrillation. Most ICDs are capable of delivering 30 J or more to terminate unstable ventricular tachycardia and ventricular fibrillation.

4. All ICDs can be interrogated noninvasively to obtain the program that describes what the device will do for a given abnormal heart rate. Fig. 13-2 is an example of a summary report that would typically be produced through device interrogation by the cardiologist. The "Detection Criteria" section defines different detection modes based

13

PACEMAKERS AND DEFIBRILLATORS

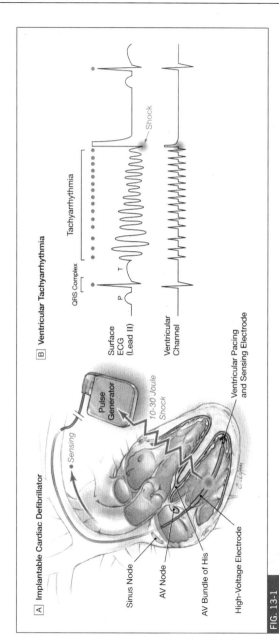

FIG. 13-1

Implantable cardiac defibrillator function. AV, Atrioventricular; ECG, electrocardiogram. *(From Kusumoto FM, Goldschlager N. JAMA 2002; 287 : 1848.)*

on a given heart rate. The "Tachyarrhythmia Therapy" section highlights the specific therapy given for each detection mode. The other sections on the report are beyond the scope of this chapter. Based on this example, if the device were to detect a heart rate of 165 beats/min, the device would enter the "Tach B" mode. According to the program, an ATP burst of eight paced stimuli would be delivered. If the tachycardia persisted at the current rate, another burst would be given (see "Tach B ATP" section). If the patient's tachycardia persisted with the given heart rate zone after two bursts, a final burst of ATP would be delivered. Having completed the ATP algorithm, the device would initiate cardioversion at 27.5 J (i.e., defibrillation) for persistent tachycardia. After an attempt at defibrillation the device would again assess the heart rate to determine whether additional therapy was needed. If the tachycardia persisted, the device would then deliver a charge of 36 J (based on the program). Although the device did not deliver low-energy cardioversion (approximately 1 J) in this example, it could be programmed to do so if desired. If the device had detected a rate less than 160 beats/min at any time during the events described, the algorithm would have been terminated.

VI. MAJOR INDICATIONS FOR IMPLANTABLE CARDIAC DEFIBRILLATORS

1. The indications for ICDs that follow are based on the 1998 ACC/AHA guidelines. (The significance of class I, IIa, and IIb indications is described above.) It should also be noted that in a recently published randomized study, the Multicenter Automatic Defibrillator Implantation Trial (MADIT) II, patients who had prior myocardial infarction and an ejection fraction less than 30% and who received an ICD had a 31% lower mortality after 20 months of follow-up than those given conventional therapy.[10]

a. Cardiac arrest caused by ventricular tachycardia (VT) or ventricular fibrillation (VF) that has an irreversible cause (class I): Mortality benefit has been demonstrated in the Antiarrhythmics Versus Implantable Defibrillator (AVID) trial.[11]

b. Sustained VT in the presence of structural heart disease (class I): A mortality benefit for this indication has also been demonstrated in the AVID trial.[11]

c. Nonsustained VT with coronary disease, prior myocardial infarction, left ventricular dysfunction, and inducible VF or sustained VT on electrophysiological study (EPS) that is not suppressible by class I antiarrhythmic drugs (class I): A mortality benefit has been demonstrated in the Multicenter Automatic Defibrillator Implantation Trial (MADIT-I).[12]

d. Ischemic cardiomyopathy with an ejection fraction less than or equal to 30% at least 1 month after myocardial infarction and 3 months after coronary artery revascularization surgery (class IIa): This new indication is based on the MADIT-II, in which patients with prior

St. Jude Medical

Programmed Parameter Summary

Page 1 of 1

Patient: Demo | Atlas™ DR Model: V-240, Serial: DEMO | Report Date/Time: Jul 29, 2002 1:03 PM

Configuration

Configuration............Defib with Tach A & Tach B | Arrhythmia Sensing............Dual Chamber

Detection Criteria

Fib Detection..........................300 ms/200 bpm
Tach B Detection......375 ms/160 bpm for 12 intervals
Tach A Detection......430 ms/140 bpm for 12 intervals
SVT Upper Limit...............................Same as Fib
Post Fib/Tach B Detection................Same as Tach B

SVT Criteria

V < A Rate Branch
  VT Diagnosis Criteria.................................If Any
  Morphology..........................On (60%, 5 of 8)
  Interval Stability.......On (80 ms), (60 ms), 12 intervals
V = A Rate Branch
  VT Diagnosis Criteria.................................If Any
  Morphology..........................On (60%, 5 of 8)
  Sudden Onset.............................On (100 ms)
  Template......................Active Jul 2, 2002 5:11 AM

MTD...................................30 sec (Tach Therapy)
MTF...........................Same as Tach B for 20 sec

Tachyarrhythmia Therapy

Fib/MTF: [1] Defib	22.5 J	(642 V)
[2] Defib	36.0 J	(801 V)
[3] Defib × 4	36.0 J	(801 V)
Tach B: [1] ATP		
[2] CVRT	27.5 J	(710 V)
[3] CVRT	36.0 J	(801 V)
[4] CVRT × 2	36.0 J	(801 V)
Tach A: [1] Off	Off	
[2] Off	Off	
[3] Off	Off	
[4] Off	Off	

Tach B ATP

Output	7.5 V, 1.0 ms
BCL	85%
Min BCL	200 ms
No. Bursts	3 bursts
Stimuli	8 stimuli (+1 per burst)
Scanning	12 ms
Ramp	On, 8 ms steps

Shock Waveform

Biphasic, Fixed Tilt
RV (+) to SVC/Can (−)
Defib: 65%/65%
CVRT: Same as Defib

Stored EGM

EGM #1	A Sense/Pace, ± 3.6 mV
EGM #2	V Sense/Pace, ± 8.9 mV
Events	Fib, MTD, Tach B, Tach A
Settings	Detection, 16 sec Pre, 1 min Max

FIG. 13-2

Implantable cardiac defibrillator summary report. *(Courtesy Ron Anderson, St. Jude Medical.)*

PACEMAKERS AND DEFIBRILLATORS **13**

myocardial infarction and an ejection fraction less than 30% who received an ICD had a 31% lower mortality after 20 months of follow-up than those given conventional therapy.[10] An important task that lies ahead is to find more specific ways to risk stratify this large population because the economic burden of implanting ICDs in all patients in this group would be considerable.

e. Cardiac arrest presumed to be due to VF when EPS is precluded by other medical conditions (class IIb).

f. Sustained VT in patients awaiting cardiac transplantation (class IIb).

g. Long QT syndrome, hypertrophic cardiomyopathy, and other inherited conditions with a risk for life-threatening ventricular tachyarrhythmias (class IIb).

PEARLS AND PITFALLS

- Characteristic 12-lead ECGs demonstrate a left bundle branch block pattern when the right ventricle is actively paced. A right bundle branch block pattern during ventricular pacing warrants further evaluation of lead positioning.

- Mode switching refers to switching to a mode that is not capable of tracking atrial beats. This is useful in atrial tachyarrhythmias. Examples are switching from DDDR to DDIR or from DDD to VVI. One report of 48 patients with significant histories of supraventricular tachyarrhythmias showed that most preferred mode switching from DDDR to VVIR.[13]

- Not all pacing spikes may be seen on a 12-lead ECG because of sampling intervals. In addition, pacing spikes may be seen in inappropriate places on a cardiac monitor rhythm tracing. This may be a sensitivity artifact of the monitor rather than a sign that the pacemaker is not tracking appropriately. The monitor should be checked to make sure the "pacer" filters are turned off. This will decrease the sensitivity of the monitor and eliminate artifactual pacemaker "spikes."

- Pacing interferes with diagnostic information typically provided by a 12-lead ECG. Of note: placing a magnet over the pacemaker to inhibit pacer activity may not immediately normalize the surface ECG because of T wave memory.

- In patients with bifascicular block (right bundle branch block accompanied by left hemiblock or left bundle branch block alone) and what is sometimes termed "trifascicular" block (bifascicular block and first-degree AV block), permanent pacing is indicated (class I) if type II second-degree AV block, third-degree AV block, or alternating bundle branch block is also present.

- In a patient with syncope and an ECG showing bifascicular or "trifascicular" block but no evidence of advanced AV block, permanent pacing is still indicated (class IIa) as long as other causes (specifically ventricular tachycardia) have been excluded.

- After the acute phase of a myocardial infarction, permanent pacing is indicated (class I) for symptomatic and persistent second- or third-degree AV block. For only transient second- or third-degree AV block, permanent pacing is indicated (class I) if the site of the block is infranodal (suggested by wide QRS, although electrophysiological study may be required). Permanent pacing is usually *not* indicated after myocardial infarction for transient second- or third-degree AV block in the absence of a wide QRS (e.g., with an isolated left anterior fascicular block).

- An asymptomatic sinus pause alone, no matter how long, is not an indication for permanent pacing.
- The length of the pause after carotid sinus massage required for diagnosis of CSH in a patient with recurrent syncope is greater than 3 seconds. Hypotension (>50 mm Hg decrease in blood pressure) after carotid sinus massage will also establish the diagnosis.
- Pacemaker syndrome is caused by the absence of AV synchrony during ventricular pacing, usually resulting in atrial contraction against closed AV valves. Since the atrial contraction may result from retrograde conduction of a ventricular pacing impulse, this syndrome may be more common in patients with sinus node dysfunction and intact AV conduction than in those with AV block. Symptoms of pacemaker syndrome include lightheadedness, weakness, flushing, exercise intolerance, and palpitations. The syndrome may be treated by restoration of AV synchrony with DDD or AAI pacing.
- Having an ICD implanted does not exclude a patient from needing external defibrillation. Since the device assesses the need for therapy based on the heart rate, a patient may have symptomatic ventricular tachycardia that is below the threshold for initiating automated therapy.
- ICDs are not indicated for patients with Wolff-Parkinson-White syndrome, ventricular tachycardia caused by transient or reversible disorders, idiopathic ventricular tachycardia curable by radiofrequency ablation, terminal illnesses, class IV refractory congestive heart failure but not transplant candidate, or significant psychiatric illness aggravated by ICD discharges.
- As demonstrated by the Coronary Artery Bypass Graft (CABG) Patch Trial, prophylactic ICD placement does not provide a mortality benefit even for high-risk patients with left ventricular dysfunction undergoing CABG if they have no history of symptomatic ventricular arrhythmias.[14]

13

PACEMAKERS AND DEFIBRILLATORS

REFERENCES

[b] 1. Bernstein AD, Parsonnet V. Survey of cardiac pacing and implanted defibrillator practice patterns in the United States in 1997. Pacing Clin Electrophysiol 2001; 24:842.

[b] 2. Hayes DL, Furman S. Stability of AV conduction in sick sinus node syndrome patients with implanted atrial pacemakers. Am Heart J 1984; 107:644.

[a] 3. Kenny RA et al. Carotid sinus syndrome: a modifiable risk factor for nonaccidental falls in older adults (SAFE PACE). J Am Coll Cardiol 2001; 38:1491.

[a] 4. Cazeau S et al. Effects of multisite biventricular pacing in patients with heart failure and intraventricular conduction delay. N Engl J Med 2001; 344:873.

[a] 5. Abraham W et al. Cardiac resynchronization in chronic heart failure. N Engl J Med 2002; 346:1845.

[a] 6. Kappenberger L et al. Pacing in hypertrophic obstructive cardiomyopathy: a randomized cross-over study. Eur Heart J 1997; 18:1249.

[b]   7. Maron B et al. Assessment of permanent dual-chamber pacing as a treatment for drug-refractory symptomatic patients with obstructive hypertrophic cardiomyopathy: a randomized, double-blind, crossover study (M-PATHY). Circulation 1999; 99:2927.

[a]   8. Saksena S et al. Prevention of recurrent atrial fibrillation with chronic dual-site right atrial pacing. J Am Coll Cardiol 1996; 28:687.

[a]   9. Levy TS, et al. Evaluation of biatrial pacing, right atrial pacing, and no pacing in patients with drug refractory atrial fibrillation. Am J Cardiol 1999; 84:426.

[a] 10. Moss AJ et al. Prophylactic implantation of a defibrillator in patients with myocardial infarction and reduced ejection fraction. N Engl J Med 2002; 346:877.

[a] 11. A comparison of antiarrhythmic-drug therapy with implantable defibrillators in patients resuscitated from near-fatal ventricular arrhythmias. Antiarrhythmics Versus Implantable Defibrillators (AVID) Investigators. N Engl J Med 1997; 337:1576.

[a] 12. Moss AJ et al. Improved survival with an implanted defibrillator in patients with coronary disease at high risk for ventricular arrhythmia. Multicenter Automatic Defibrillator Implantation Trial Investigators. N Engl J Med 1996; 335:1933.

[a] 13. Kamalvand K et al. Is mode switching beneficial? A randomized study in patients with paroxysmal atrial tachyarrhythmias. J Am Coll Cardiol 1997; 30:496.

[a] 14. Bigger JT. Prophylactic use of implanted cardiac defibrillators in patients at high risk for ventricular arrhythmias after coronary artery bypass graft surgery. Coronary Artery Bypass Graft (CABG) Patch Trial Investigators. N Engl J Med 1997; 337:1569.

Diseases of the Pericardium

Sanjay Desai, MD, and Gary Gerstenblith, MD

FAST FACTS

- Acute inflammation of the pericardium can occur in a vast array of systemic illnesses and is commonly associated with viral infection, uremia, and myocardial infarction.
- Acute pericarditis is a clinical diagnosis that is supported largely by the history, physical examination, and electrocardiography.
- Pericardial disease can compromise cardiac output with either cardiac tamponade or constrictive pericarditis.
- Cardiac tamponade should be suspected when hypotension and elevated jugular venous pressure develop in a patient with recent cardiac surgery, aortic dissection, myocardial infarction, or acute pericarditis. The diagnosis is supported by echocardiographic evidence of effusion and right ventricular (RV) diastolic collapse.
- Constrictive pericarditis may be an indolent disease that is not recognized until significant symptoms of right- and left-sided heart failure develop. This condition must be carefully differentiated from cardiac tamponade and restrictive cardiomyopathy.

I. ANATOMY AND FUNCTION

1. The pericardium is composed of two layers. The outer fibrous layer, which is composed of fibrocollagenous tissues and anchors the pericardium to the great vessels and diaphragm, is the parietal pericardium. The inner serosal layer, formed from interdigitated mesothelial cells and attached to the surface of the heart with connective tissues, is the visceral pericardium. The pericardial sac is primarily a potential space that contains 15 to 35 mL of serous ultrafiltrate from blood plasma.
2. The pericardium serves the heart in several important ways, including the following:
a. A minimal-friction environment within which the heart can contract freely.
b. A structural buttress for the thinner right atrial (RA) and RV chambers.
c. A backstop against acute cardiac cavity dilation. The parietal pericardium is less compliant than myocardium, and the resting RA and RV diastolic pressures reflect its constraint.[1]
d. A barrier to extracardiac inflammation and disease.
e. A circulatory feedback mechanism from its neuroreceptors and chemoreceptors to the heart.

Clinical Syndromes

1. The pericardium can be affected in a vast array of diseases, both primarily and secondarily. The most common clinical manifestation of pericardial involvement is inflammation, causing acute pericarditis. The first section below summarizes the diagnosis, common causes, and treatment of acute pericarditis. The other clinical manifestation of pericardial disease is hemodynamic compromise, resulting from either cardiac tamponade or constrictive pericarditis. The second section below describes diagnosis and management of these syndromes. Last, considerations of pericardial injury in uncommon medical conditions are highlighted.

ACUTE PERICARDITIS

I. EPIDEMIOLOGY

1. Acute inflammation of the pericardium can be an isolated process but more commonly is the result of another systemic condition (Box 14-1).
2. Acute inflammation may or may not be associated with a pericardial effusion.

II. CLINICAL PRESENTATION

1. The most common presentation of acute pericarditis is chest pain.

BOX 14-1

COMMON ETIOLOGIES OF ACUTE PERICARDITIS

Idiopathic (thought to be often viral)
Infection
  Common
    Cardiotropic viruses
    Gram-positive bacteria
    Mycobacterium tuberculosis
  Less common
    Fungi
    Parasites
    Spirochetes
    Rickettsiae
Metabolic
  Renal failure
  Hypothyroidism
Neoplastic
Myocardial infarction
Trauma
Aortic dissection
Esophageal fistula
Drugs and toxins

Although the pain may be difficult to differentiate from that of myocardial ischemia or infarction, it is typically more pleuritic. Often the pain is relieved with sitting up or leaning forward. Associated symptoms may also be nonspecific signs of viral infection or systemic inflammation, commonly including nonproductive cough and fever.

III. DIAGNOSTICS

1. Physical examination.
a. As with many diseases, physical examination is fundamental in the diagnosis of acute pericarditis. The hallmark physical examination finding is auscultation of a pericardial friction rub, heard in approximately 85% of patients with acute pericarditis.[2] The abnormal sound is attributed to the movement of two inflamed surfaces of pericardium against one another. The sound may be generated by movement between the serosal layers, between the parietal layer and the pleura and chest wall structures, or by both processes, depending on the etiology.
b. The friction rub is described as "scratchy" in character and superficial in location. It is heard loudest over the left lower half of the sternum, where the RV is closest to the chest wall. The sound can be easier to detect and differentiated from pleural sounds if the patient suspends respirations. Classically, the rub is triphasic, with an atrial systolic, ventricular systolic, and early diastolic component. The rub is sometimes biphasic, particularly in patients with tachycardia or atrial arrhythmias, because the atrial systolic phase either fuses with the diastolic phase or is absent completely.

2. Electrocardiography
a. Although the pericardium itself has no detectable electrical activity, pericardial inflammation can lead to electrical changes in the epicardial tissue, which are detected by the surface ECG. The ECG changes associated with this epicardial inflammation typically evolve through four phases, which when collectively present are typical for pericarditis (Fig. 14-1).
   (1) Phase I.
      (a) Diffuse ST elevation.
      (b) PR depression in inferolateral leads (II, III, aVF, V_5, V_6).
   (2) Phase II.
      (a) ST and PR segment normalization.
   (3) Phase III.
      (a) Diffuse T wave inversions (occasionally not present).
   (4) Phase IV.
      (a) Resolution of ECG changes.
      (b) Persistence of T wave inversions, indicating "chronic" inflammation.
b. The ECG changes must be differentiated from acute myocardial infarction.[3]

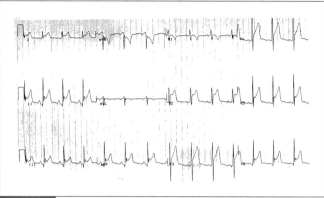

FIG. 14-1

Electrocardiographic changes with acute pericarditis.

   c. Pericarditis typically *does* involve the following:
      (1) ST elevation that is *more* diffuse, concave, less than 5 mm, and without reciprocal changes.
      (2) ST elevation and T wave inversions in temporally *different* phases.
      (3) PR segment deflections.
   d. It *does not* involve:
      (1) Q waves.
      (2) Hyperacute T waves.
      (3) QT prolongation.
   e. The ECG changes must also be differentiated from normal variant early repolarization.[4-6] Pericarditis typically *does* involve the following:
      (1) PR segment deflections.
      (2) J-ST point elevation.
   f. It *does not* involve:
      (1) Tall, peaked T waves.
      (2) Gender or age predilections (early repolarization is most prevalent in males <40 years).
   g. Low ECG voltage and electrical alternans are insensitive indicators of small to moderate pericardial effusion, but when present they are indicative of a large effusion. When they are coupled with sinus tachycardia, pericardial tamponade should be suspected.
  3. Echocardiography can reveal effusions when present and may also illustrate a sunburst pattern in noneffusive pericarditis.
  4. The chest radiograph may show an associated pleural effusion, usually left sided.
  5. Laboratory values that aid the diagnosis are elevated levels of acute-phase reactants and modestly elevated myocardial enzyme levels, reflecting the degree of epicardial inflammation.

IV. MANAGEMENT

1. The differential diagnosis of acute pericarditis is broad and diverse. Although acute inflammation of the pericardium may be unaccompanied by significant effusion, termed dry pericarditis, almost all etiologies can have accompanying effusions. The most common etiological categories are infectious, metabolic, rheumatic, neoplastic, and diseases of contiguous organs, most commonly myocardial infarction.

A. INFECTIOUS PERICARDITIS

1. Viral infections are the most common cause of infectious pericarditis. Cardiotropic viruses are usually implicated, notably Coxsackie virus, influenza virus, human immunodeficiency virus, and the hepatitis A and B viruses. Viral pericarditis is also the presumed cause of most "idiopathic" cases. Clinical presentation is that of a viral syndrome with fever and leukocytosis. The pericardial inflammation usually accompanies a respiratory or gastrointestinal viral disease but may follow the original infection by 1 to 3 weeks.[7] Symptoms usually resolve within 2 weeks, and management should focus on ameliorating the inflammation. Nonsteroidal antiinflammatory drugs (NSAIDs) are the mainstay of therapy. Approximately 50% of patients have recurrence within 8 months, and uncommonly, chronic inflammation develops.

2. Bacterial infections of the pericardium produce more serious conditions. The offending organisms are usually gram-positive pathogens, including staphylococci, streptococci, and pneumococci. Less commonly, and usually in the setting of an immunocompromised state, other organisms such as *Escherichia coli*, *Salmonella*, *Clostridium*, *Neisseria,* and *Mycobacterium tuberculosis* are implicated. Pericardial effusions make the pericardium particularly vulnerable to bacterial infection via hematogenous spread.[8] Similarly, surrounding bacterial infections, such as lobar pneumonia, mediastinitis, and bacterial endocarditis, predispose the pericardium to bacterial invasion. Bacterial pericarditis has an acute presentation, usually with significant fever and pain. An inflammatory, exudative effusion almost always accompanies it. Echocardiography can help identify effusions, and chest x-ray examination may reveal an enlarged cardiac silhouette or in rare cases pneumopericardium caused by a gas-producing organism. Management involves IV antibiotics, which achieve adequate levels in the pericardium.[8] Pericardial drainage, either surgical or catheter guided, is usually necessary to prevent septic loculations or pericardial constriction.

3. *M. tuberculosis* is particularly notable for its predilection for the pericardium. Infection classically evolves through four stages. First, when mycobacterial burden is high, an inflammatory exudate develops. Second, monocytes and foam cells infiltrate the pericardial space and produce a lymphocytic effusion. Third, the effusion is

absorbed, granulomas organize, and fibrosis begins. Fourth, the pericardium undergoes constrictive scarring.[9] The illness usually arises in an indolent fashion, without evidence of extrapericardial tuberculous infection. Typical symptoms of acute pericarditis are more often seen in immunocompromised hosts. Diagnosis is commonly made when hemodynamically significant tamponade or constriction develops, when acute pericarditis is refractory to NSAID treatment, or when specific investigation is prompted by the patient's risk profile. Diagnosis of tuberculous pericarditis, however, can be difficult. Although identification of *M. tuberculosis* in pericardial fluid or tissue biopsy is specific, it is not sensitive and is not helpful when absent. Extrapericardial tuberculosis and positive tuberculin skin tests can help support the diagnosis but are not confirmatory. The optimal test is *M. tuberculosis* DNA identification by polymerase chain reaction amplification in the pericardial fluid, which is 100% sensitive and greater than 70% specific for tuberculous infection.[10,11] Management involves antimycobacterial treatment. Isolates should be tested for sensitivity, and steroids may be used to speed resolution in severe cases.[8,12]

4. Other uncommon infectious causes of acute pericarditis include fungi, parasites, spirochetes, and rickettsial organisms, all of which are more common in immunocompromised hosts or demographically high-risk hosts. The fungi most commonly implicated are *Histoplasma*, *Coccidioides*, *Candida*, *Aspergillus*, and *Actinomyces*.

B. METABOLIC DERANGEMENTS

1. Uremia can cause pericarditis in patients with chronic renal failure, in patients on hemodialysis with inadequate treatment, or less commonly in patients with acute renal failure. No direct correlation exists between the level of uremia and clinical manifestations, but uremia is usually seen in patients with blood urea nitrogen levels above 60 mg/dL. The syndrome can often present with hemorrhagic effusion and can develop into tamponade. The exact pathogenesis of uremic pericarditis remains unclear. It may develop in stable, well-dialyzed patients. Treatment focuses on hemodialysis to correct the uremia and evacuation of the effusion if tamponade develops.

2. Hypothyroidism (see Chapter 23) is also associated with pericarditis. Pericarditis most commonly develops in severely hypothyroid patients with myxedema. The onset is gradual and is primarily an effusive process, with tamponade a concern.[8,13,14] Treatment is aimed at correcting the endocrinopathy.

3. Pericarditis has been observed in other metabolic derangements, notably diabetic ketoacidosis, adrenal failure, gout, and hypercholesterolemia. However, a clear pathogenesis, other than systemic inflammation, has yet to be described in these conditions.[8,14] Management again is focused on treatment of the underlying derangement.

C. RHEUMATIC DISEASES

1. The majority of vasculitides and connective tissue disorders can have associated pericarditis. The same pathological process that leads to blood vessel and tissue inflammation also leads to pericardial inflammation, namely immune complex, complement, and inflammatory cell infiltration of the pericardium.

2. Rheumatoid arthritis is the most commonly implicated rheumatologic disease to involve pericarditis, usually with fibrinous exudates. An autopsy series revealed that almost 50% of patients with rheumatoid arthritis had pericardial involvement.[15] Pericardial inflammation is more common in those with advanced disease and is treated with antiarthritic therapies. Systemic lupus erythematosus (see Chapter 73) is also commonly associated with pericarditis. The pericardial inflammation tends to parallel systemic flares and is often accompanied by large pericardial and pleural effusions.[16,17] Of note, drug-induced lupus can also cause pericarditis. Treatment is targeted at the underlying pathology.

3. Scleroderma, both limited and systemic, can lead to collagen deposition in the pericardium. One series demonstrated effusions in 50% of patients.[8] Since both systemic lupus erythematosus and scleroderma can cause nephropathy, uremic pericarditis must be carefully distinguished from rheumatic pericarditis.

4. Less clinically prevalent associations occur with polymyositis, dermatomyositis, seronegative spondyloarthropathies, mixed connective tissue disease, a collection of systemic vasculitides, Behçet's syndrome, Wegener's granulomatosis, and sarcoidosis.

D. NEOPLASTIC DISEASE

1. Pericardial disease caused by primary pericardial neoplasms is rare. Benign tumors can be found in infants and children, whereas malignant processes typically develop in the third and fourth decades of life.[8] Primary neoplasms of note are mesotheliomas and sarcomas. The presentation is similar to that of acute pericarditis with effusion.

2. Pericardial disease resulting from other malignancies is much more common. Secondary involvement can occur through metastatic disease, usually via pericardial lymphatics, or from direct extension of malignant tissue from breast, lung, or chest wall. Diagnosis can be made with cytological and immunohistochemical analysis of pericardial fluid, or if necessary, with pericardial tissue biopsy. Since malignancies may initially manifest themselves as "idiopathic" pericarditis, a search for systemic neoplasms is warranted in these situations.[18,19]

3. Management of neoplastic pericardial disease requires pericardial drainage, typically with pericardial windows or shunts. Surgical resection is required for recurrent pericardial constriction from the malignancy. Conservative therapy with pericardial sclerosis may be appropriate as palliative treatment in poor surgical candidates.[8]

14

DISEASES OF THE PERICARDIUM

E. MYOCARDIAL INFARCTION

1. Myocardial infarction can be associated with pericarditis, either early (<7 days) or late (weeks to months) after infarction. Almost half of transmural infarctions are associated with early pericarditis. Pericarditis is diagnosed in only a small subset of these patients because the clinical picture is often dominated by the acute myocardial infarction.[4]

2. Early postinfarction pericarditis increases in incidence with infarct size and is a common cause of new chest pain during the first few days after infarction.[8,20,21] Although in-hospital outcomes do not seem to be affected by early postinfarction pericarditis, those occurring 6 months and more after the infarct are associated with poorer outcomes.

3. The inflammation of early pericarditis may cause occlusion of a coronary artery bypass graft. Associated effusions usually develop 1 to 3 days after infarction and often represent hemodynamically insignificant hydropericardium.[8] More severe hemopericardium can develop in the setting of thrombolytic therapy or with ventricular rupture. Diagnosis can be made by auscultation of a pericardial friction rub and the presence of characteristic chest pain symptoms. Pleuritic pain involving the trapezius ridge(s) is highly suggestive of the condition.[8] Recurrent myocardial ischemia, infarction, and pulmonary embolism must be excluded if the diagnosis is uncertain. The condition can be treated safely and effectively with nonantiinflammatory analgesia, such as a mild oral narcotic or acetaminophen.

4. Use of NSAIDs should be avoided in the first 7 to 10 days after infarction because, like corticosteroids, they have been linked to scar thinning, ventricular aneurysm, and free wall rupture. Evidence of early infarction pericarditis is *not* an absolute contraindication to anticoagulation, although anticoagulation should be used with caution in the presence of an effusion because the fluid may represent hemopericardium.

5. Late postinfarction pericarditis is commonly referred to as Dressler syndrome. This syndrome is more common with larger infarcts but can also be associated with nontransmural infarction.[8,22] The syndrome arises between 1 week and several months after infarction and is thought to be immune mediated. Presentation tends to be characteristic for acute pericarditis, and management is focused on antiinflammatory treatment with NSAIDs or with corticosteroids if necessary.

Compressive Syndromes

1. Two pericardial conditions that can significantly compromise hemodynamic function are cardiac tamponade and constrictive pericarditis. Each may be associated with, or be a consequence of, acute pericarditis.

CARDIAC TAMPONADE

I. CLINICAL PRESENTATION

1. Tamponade occurs when excess fluid accumulates in the elastic pericardial sac, raising the intrapericardial pressure to levels that exceed intracardiac pressures. The result is impairment of ventricular filling and thus cardiac output. This can occur acutely, usually after traumatic rupture of cardiac structures or after intervention, or more slowly, usually in conditions more commonly associated with pericarditis. Although the former is a hemodynamic emergency, the latter may have a more subtle presentation with such initial symptoms as dyspnea, lightheadedness and chest pain, before severe hypotension develops.

II. DIAGNOSTICS
A. PHYSICAL EXAMINATION

1. Because tamponade is a clinical diagnosis, a thoughtful physical examination for pertinent findings is crucial. Signs of low cardiac output, including hypotension and compensatory sinus tachycardia, are important. A careful examination of the jugular venous pulse shows an elevated jugular venous pressure, preserved x descent, and a dampened or absent y descent. The y descent reflects passive filling of the ventricle and is absent when pericardial pressure exceeds RV pressure in early diastole. Patients commonly have pulsus paradoxus, an abnormally large decrease (>10 mm Hg) in systolic blood pressure during inspiration. The decreased systolic pressure during normal inspiration seen in tamponade is merely an exaggeration of normal physiology, not a truly paradoxical finding.

2. The pathophysiology of pulsus paradoxus is debated, and various mechanisms are postulated. One likely contributing mechanism is increased ventricular interdependence. Under normal conditions RV diastolic filling is accommodated by expansion of the RV wall into the accommodating pericardial space. With tamponade physiology, however, the high pericardial pressures force RV expansion to be accommodated largely by shift of the interventricular septum into the left ventricle. This septal shift impairs LV diastolic filling, reducing preload and stroke volume. This physiological process occurs throughout the respiratory cycle under tamponade conditions. However, it is exacerbated during inspiration when negative intrathoracic pressure increases venous return from the central veins to the right side of the heart, thereby increasing encumbrance on the left ventricle. Although the mechanism for pulsus paradoxus may be multifactorial, the final common pathway seems to be a decrease in LV stroke volume.

3. Pulsus paradoxus must be measured carefully. It can be palpated as a dampening in the brachial artery pulsation during normal inspiration or

can be determined more precisely with blood pressure measurement. The examiner, using a sphygmomanometer, should take the patient's blood pressure several times to approximate the systolic pressure. Next, as the patient breathes in a normal fashion, the blood pressure cuff should be inflated to a level 10 to 15 mm Hg above the systolic pressure and then very slowly deflated into the systolic range. The examiner should first hear Korotkoff's sounds only during expiration because the inspiratory systolic pressure will be lower. Once the examiner obtains a precise measurement of this pressure, the cuff should be slowly depressurized until Korotkoff's sounds are heard throughout the respiratory cycle. The difference between the two measurements is the pulsus paradoxus. With normal hemodynamics this difference should be negligible, but in severe tamponade it can widen to over 10 mm Hg. It is important to note that pulsus paradoxus also occurs in some nontamponade conditions, notably severe chronic obstructive pulmonary disease, atrial septal defect, and pulmonary embolus.

B. ELECTROCARDIOGRAPHY

1. The changes most commonly seen with tamponade are nonspecific ST segment and T wave changes and changes associated with acute pericarditis. Less commonly, electrical axis alternation can be observed. As fluid occupies the pericardium, the heart effectively operates in a low-viscosity chamber. Therefore, with each contraction, momentum can swing the heart from side to side within the pericardium. This swinging movement can be reflected on the surface electrocardiogram as a shift in electrical axis with each beat (best seen in V_2 to V_4), termed electrical alternans (Fig. 14-2).[8]

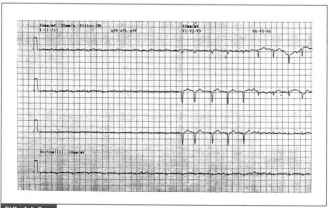

FIG. 14-2

Electrical alternans with cardiac tamponade.

C. ECHOCARDIOGRAPHY

1. Ultrasound examination of the heart can often reveal evidence of tamponade. High pericardial pressures associated with cardiac tamponade mechanically compromise the ventricular chambers. The more compliant RA and RV are particularly affected. This is observed echocardiographically as RA and RV diastolic collapse. Collapse of these chambers may occur with normal hemodynamics in very early diastole, but prolonged diastolic collapse is highly sensitive and specific for high intrapericardial pressure.[8] In addition, dilation of the hepatic veins and inferior vena cava with reduced inspiratory collapse signifies impaired RV filling. However, this is also seen with other causes of impaired RV filling, including restrictive cardiomyopathy and constrictive pericarditis.

III. MANAGEMENT

1. Tamponade, once diagnosed, should be managed with immediate and aggressive volume resuscitation. This crucial intervention increases intracardiac pressures and thus lessens the hemodynamic impact of the pressurized pericardium. Some evidence suggests that pharmacological blood pressure support with agents such as isoproterenol may be an effective temporizing measure.[23]
2. Definitive intervention entails pericardial drainage, optimally performed in a cardiac catheterization laboratory under controlled conditions. An alternative to catheter drainage is open surgery. Although choice of treatment depends largely on the clinical setting, catheter pericardiocentesis has the benefits of simultaneous hemodynamic investigation and less invasiveness, whereas open surgery has the advantages of larger volume evacuation and concomitant pericardial biopsy.
3. If a patient with a large effusion requires defibrillation, the physician must keep in mind that the pericardial fluid will increase the defibrillation threshold.[24]

CONSTRICTIVE PERICARDITIS

I. CLINICAL PRESENTATION

1. Constrictive pericarditis occurs when the pericardial tissue becomes fibrotic and the pericardial space is totally or almost totally obliterated. This can result from a number of pathological processes. This pericardial constriction markedly alters the ventricular pressure-volume relationship, impairing ventricular filling and increasing ventricular interdependence.
2. Well-demonstrated risk factors include a history of cardiac surgery, mediastinal radiation therapy (commonly for Hodgkin's lymphoma), neoplasm, and connective tissue disease with pericardial involvement. A retrospective study of patients who required pericardiectomy for

14

DISEASES OF THE PERICARDIUM

constrictive pericarditis found that 42% of cases were idiopathic and 31% of the patients had received mediastinal radiation therapy a mean of 85 months before presentation. Of the remaining cases, 11% of patients had previous cardiac surgery, 6% had infectious pericarditis, 4% had underlying connective tissue disorders, 3% had neoplasm-associated pericarditis, 2% had uremic pericarditis, and 1% had sarcoidosis.[25]

3. On initial examination patients often complain of chest pain, lower extremity swelling, and increased abdominal girth. Late presentation can involve further symptoms of impaired cardiac output, including dyspnea on exertion, lightheadedness, and fatigue.

III. DIAGNOSTICS

1. On physical examination, signs that mimic right-sided heart failure are helpful, including elevated jugular venous pressure, ascites, and peripheral edema. In hypovolemic patients this elevation may be observed only after vigorous volume repletion. Pulsus paradoxus is less common in constrictive pericarditis than in tamponade, and when present it may indicate an effusive constrictive process. This is perhaps due to limited transmittance of negative intrathoracic pressure to the heart through the scarred and thickened pericardium. In one series from the Mayo Clinic only 19% of patients with constrictive pericarditis had a pulsus paradoxus on presentation.[26] The jugular venous pressure is elevated, with sharp x and y descents. In addition, Kussmaul's sign is a frequent finding. This sign is described as a paradoxical increase in jugular venous pressure during inspiration. In the normal physiological state the negative intrathoracic pressure created with inspiration favors increased venous return into the right side of the heart, thereby decreasing jugular venous pressure. With constriction the ability of the right side of the heart to accommodate increased volume is limited by the pericardium. However, the central veins still fill rapidly as the negative intrathoracic pressure mobilizes venous return from both the caudal and cephalad circulation. This blood volume, once it overcomes the capacity of the right side of the heart, can flow back into the jugular system. Kussmaul observed this retrograde flow in 1863 as a paradoxical increase in jugular venous pressure during inspiration. The phenomenon is more prominently seen in patients with significant edema and ascites in which larger volumes of fluid are mobilized to the central venous system. Other associated signs on physical examination are a third heart sound, heard in almost 50% of patients, and a pericardial friction rub, heard in about 15% of patients.[26]

2. Chest x-ray examination can demonstrate pericardial calcification, which in one series was seen in over 25% of patients with biopsy-proven constrictive pericarditis.[27]

3. Echocardiography may reveal calcified or thickened pericardium. In addition, lack of collapse of the central or hepatic veins and abrupt interventricular septal motion may be present. Doppler study can reveal high early diastolic filling velocities (E wave).

4. Hemodynamic study can be useful in the diagnosis of constrictive pericarditis. Prominent findings are those indicating decreased RV compliance. A characteristic finding is rapid descent followed by rapid increase and subsequent plateauing of RV diastolic pressure, known as the square root sign. This phenomenon is due to rapid RV relaxation, followed by a rapid rise in RV diastolic pressure as the constrained ventricle fills with blood in early diastole. Other findings include elevated RV end-diastolic pressure, prominent x and y descents, and, most important, four-chamber equalization of end-diastolic pressures.

5. Differentiation from cardiac tamponade.

a. It is important to recognize the hemodynamic differences between tamponade and constrictive pericarditis. Tamponade involves decreased ventricular compliance throughout the cardiac cycle as the heart operates in a continuously high-pressure environment. Constrictive pericarditis, however, creates a decreased ventricular compliance only when the cardiac diameter approaches that of the pericardium. This difference affects diastolic venous flow. Specifically, with tamponade, venous return confronts high pressure throughout diastole, producing a single venous return wave as opposed to the normal biphasic return. This can be observed in the jugular veins on physical examination or directly with hemodynamic monitoring. Venous return in restrictive pericarditis, however, is not impeded until RV compliance is decreased, that is, in mid- to late diastole. Therefore the venous return maintains bimodal flow, seen in jugular veins as the x and y descents and directly by hemodynamics. Echocardiography can aid in the differentiation of these entities by showing the presence or absence of an effusion, as well as diastolic RV collapse on two-dimensional images. Loculated effusions may be deceptively absent on echocardiography, however, especially if they develop posteriorly.

6. Differentiation from restrictive cardiomyopathy.

a. Differentiation between constrictive pericarditis and restrictive cardiomyopathy is also important because treatment and outcomes for the two conditions are very different. Restrictive cardiomyopathy is a condition in which the myocardium has intrinsically decreased compliance, often as the result of an infiltrative process such as amyloidosis.

b. The two pathological entities have similar presentations, so differentiation on clinical grounds is often challenging. Both conditions lead to impairment of ventricular filling, thereby producing similar

14

DISEASES OF THE PERICARDIUM

physical examination findings of elevated pressures in the right side of the heart, as well as the typical square root sign seen on right-sided heart catheterization.

c. The overall history and diagnostic evaluation may lead to a collection of findings that together help identify the underlying disease. Clearly a patient history of acute pericarditis or conditions associated with pericarditis favors constriction, just as a history of an infiltrative disease suggests restriction. Physical examination has limited value because the jugular venous dynamics are identical. Electrocardiographic findings of conduction abnormalities, a pseudoinfarct pattern (poor R wave progression without evidence of prior infarct), and diffuse low voltage favor an infiltrative process.

d. Echocardiography is the most reliable method of differentiating constrictive pericarditis from restrictive cardiomyopathy. On the basis of two-dimensional echo and M-mode findings, the two findings most indicative of constrictive pericarditis are abrupt leftward displacement of the ventricular septum during diastole and a thickened pericardium.[28] These findings alone are often insufficient to confidently distinguish the two entities, however, and Doppler analysis is required. In both processes a restrictive Doppler mitral inflow velocity is present, often with an early to late diastolic filling ratio greater than 2. With constriction, however, the respiratory variation is exaggerated in ventricular filling, as demonstrated by a 25% reduction in Doppler mitral inflow velocity with inspiration. This is rarely present in restrictive disease.[29,30]

IV. MANAGEMENT

1. The majority of patients with constrictive pericarditis require surgical pericardiectomy. This treatment, however, is associated with significant morbidity and mortality. Perioperative mortality ranges from 5.6% to 12% across different studies.[25,26,31] Although over 80% of patients become symptom free, long-term survival is still a concern. A series of 135 patients from the Mayo Clinic had a 78% 5-year survival and a 57% 10-year survival. Poor outcomes were associated with older age, with higher New York Heart Association functional class, and particularly with postradiation constriction.[26]

Other Pericardial Injury

1. Pericardial injury can occur as a result of less common conditions as well, including trauma and intervention, aortic dissection, esophageal fistulas, and from drugs and toxins.
2. Trauma and intervention.
a. Penetrating trauma with knives, bullets, and other projectile objects commonly causes pericardial damage. Anterior wounds tend to damage

the pericardium as well as structures of the right side of heart, and posterior wounds often injure the left atrium. Catastrophic tamponade and exsanguination are early and common complications. Minor injuries and contusions may result in inflammatory pericarditis.

b. Cardiac interventions, including surgery, coronary intervention, catheter pericardiocentesis, and central line placement, are also associated with pericardial complications, including tamponade and postintervention constriction. Tamponade after cardiac surgery is a surgical emergency and must be quickly differentiated from other low cardiac output states.[32]

3. **Aortic dissection.**

a. Aortic dissection involving the ascending aorta (type A) may hemorrhage into the pericardium.[8,33] Large-volume ruptures occur, and death most commonly results from cardiac tamponade. Clinical presentation is typical for aortic dissection, with hypotension suggesting tamponade physiology. Aortic dissection is a surgical emergency, and treatment should not be delayed for precise diagnostic studies.

4. **Esophageal fistulas.**

a. Because the pericardium overlies the esophagus, almost any process that compromises the anterior wall of the esophagus can produce esophageal-pericardial fistulas. Causes include previous esophageal surgery or trauma, erosive conditions such as Barrett's esophagus, and neoplasms. Fistulas can vary in size, with smaller fistulas causing inflammatory pericarditis and larger ones creating effusions and possible pneumopyopericardium with tamponade.

5. **Drugs and toxins.**

a. Many treatments for extrapericardial diseases are potential pericardial irritants. Commonly implicated drugs include anthracyclines, amiodarone, procainamide, and hydralazine (as a result of drug-induced lupus), as well as thrombolytics and anticoagulants via secondary hemorrhage. Several toxins are also hazardous to the pericardium, including venom from scorpion fish, talc, silicones, and asbestos. The effects of these chemicals on the pericardium can vary from acute pericardial inflammation to chronic constrictive pericarditis.[8]

PEARLS AND PITFALLS

- Myocardial ischemia must be differentiated from acute pericarditis.
- Evidence of acute pericarditis associated with myocardial infarction is not an absolute contraindication to anticoagulation, but anticoagulation should be performed cautiously in the presence of effusion because the fluid may represent hemopericardium.
- Moderate to large pericardial effusions raise the threshold for defibrillation and cardioversion.
- Cardiac tamponade should be managed with vigorous intravascular volume expansion and pressure support until definitive pericardiocentesis is performed.

14

DISEASES OF THE PERICARDIUM

- Echocardiography or hemodynamic monitoring is usually necessary to make the often difficult distinction between constrictive pericarditis and restrictive cardiomyopathy.

REFERENCES

[c] 1. Spodick DH: Macro- and micro-physiology and anatomy of the pericardium. Am Heart J 1992; 124: 1046.

[b] 2. Zayas R et al. Incidence of specific etiology and role of methods for specific etiologic diagnosis of primary acute pericarditis. Am J Cardiol 1995; 75:378.

[c] 3. Chou TC. Electrocardiography in clinical practice: adult and pediatric, 4th ed. Philadelphia: WB Saunders; 1996.

[c] 4. Spodick DH: Pericardial diseases. In Braunwald E, Zipes DP, Libby P: Heart disease: a textbook of cardiovascular medicine, 6th ed. Philadelphia: WB Saunders; 2001.

[b] 5. Spodick DH: Differential characteristics of the electrocardiogram in early repolarization and acute pericarditis. N Engl J Med 1976; 295:523.

[b] 6. Gintzton LE, Laks M. The differential diagnosis of acute pericarditis from the normal variant: new electrocardiographic criteria. Circulation 1982; 65:1004.

[b] 7. Fujioka S et al: Molecular detection and differentiation of enteroviruses in endomyocardial biopsies and pericardial effusions from dilated cardiomyopathy and myocarditis. Am Heart J 1996; 131:760.

[c] 8. Spodick DH: The pericardium: a comprehensive textbook. New York, Marcel Dekker, 1997.

[b] 9. Tirilomis T, Univerdorben S, von der Emde J: Pericardectomy for chronic constrictive pericarditis. Ann Thorac Surg 1994; 58:1171.

[b] 10. Shah S et al: Rapid diagnosis of tuberculosis in various biopsy and body fluid specimens by the AMPLICOR *Mycobacterium tuberculosis* polymerase chain reaction test. Chest 1998; 113:1190.

[b] 11. Rana BS, Jones RA, Simpson IA: Recurrent pericardial effusion: the value of polymerase chain reaction in the diagnosis of tuberculosis. Heart 1999; 82:246.

[b] 12. Chen WT et al. Clinical response of tuberculosis pericarditis to medical treatment: a retrospective survey. Chin Med J 1996; 58:7.

[c] 13. Spodick DH: Pericarditis in systemic disease. Cardiol Clin 1990; 8:709.

[c] 14. Kabadi UM, Kumer SP: Pericardial effusion in primary hypothyroidism. Am Heart J 1990; 120:1393.

[b] 15. Markiewicz W et al: The acute effect of minocycline on the pericardium: experimental and clinical findings. Chest 1998; 113:861.

[b] 16. Barletta G et al: Cardiac involvement in systemic lupus erythematosus: an echocardiographic score of illness activity. J Am Coll Cardiol 1998; 31:9C.

[b] 17. Leung WH et al: Cardiac abnormalities in systemic lupus erythematosus: a prospective M-mode, cross-sectional and Doppler echocardiographic study. Int J Cardiol 1990; 27:367.

[d] 18. Bardales RH et al: Secondary pericardial malignancies: a critical appraisal of the role of cytology, pericardial biopsy, and DNA ploidy analysis. Am J Pathol 1996; 106:29.

[b] 19. Malamou-Mitsi VD, Zioga AP, Agnantis NJ: Diagnostic accuracy of pericardial fluid cytology: an analysis of 53 specimens from 44 consecutive patients. Diagn Cytopathol 1996; 15:197.

[b] 20. Nagahama Y et al: The role of infarction-associated pericarditis on the occurrence of atrial fibrillation. Eur Heart J 1998; 19:287.

[b] 21. Sugiura T et al: Frequency of pericardial friction rub ("pericarditis") after percutaneous transluminal coronary angioplasty in Q-wave myocardial infarction. Am J Cardiol 1997; 79:362.

[c] 22. Spodick DH: Post-myocardial infarction syndrome (Dressler's syndrome). ACC Curr J Rev 1995; 4:35.

[b] 23. Kerber RE, Gascho JA, Letchfield R. Hemodynamic effects of volume expansion and nitroprusside compared with pericardiocentesis in patients with acute cardiac tamponade. N Engl J Med 1982; 302:929.

[c] 24. Thaker RK et al: Pericardial effusion increases defibrillation energy requirement. PACE 1993; 16:1227.

[c] 25. Cameron J et al. The etiologic spectrum of constrictive pericarditis. Am Heart J 1987; 113:354.

[c] 26. Ling LH et al: Constrictive pericarditis in the modern era: evolving clinical spectrum and impact on outcome after pericardiectomy. Circulation 1999; 100:1380.

[c] 27. Ling LH et al: Calcific constrictive pericarditis: is it still with us? Ann Intern Med 2000; 132:444.

[c] 28. Spodick DH. The normal and diseased pericardium: current concepts of pericardial physiology, diagnosis and treatment. J Am Coll Cardiol 1983; 1:240.

[c] 29. Gillam LD et al. Hydrodynamic compression of the right atrium: a new echocardiographic sign of cardiac tamponade. Circulation 1982; 68:294.

[b] 30. Leimgruber P et al. The hemodynamic derangement associated with right ventricular diastolic collapse in cardiac tamponade: an experimental echocardiographic study. Circulation 1983; 68:612.

[d] 31. DeValeria PA, Baumgartner WA, Casale AS. Current indications, risks, and outcome after pericardiectomy. Ann Thorac Surg 1991; 52:219.

[c] 32. Sabers CJ, Levy NT, Bowen JM: 33-Year-old man with chest pain and fever. Mayo Clin Proc 1999; 74:181.

[c] 33. Harris KM et al: Transesophageal echocardiographic and clinical features of aortic intramural hematoma. J Thorac Cardiovasc Surg 1997; 114:619.

14

DISEASES OF THE PERICARDIUM

Pulmonary Artery Catheters and Intraaortic Balloon Pumps

Sabrina M. Tom, MD, and J.G.N. Garcia, MD

15

Pulmonary Artery Catheters

1. The PAC is a multilumen (usually four) catheter with an inflatable latex balloon at the tip (Fig. 15-1). The PAC is inserted through a vein: internal jugular, subclavian, femoral, or antecubital. The left subclavian and right internal jugular (IJ) veins are the most common sites of insertion.
2. The balloon should not be inflated until the catheter tip is located inside the right atrium approximately 10 to 15 cm from the subclavian or IJ vein.[5,6] At this point the balloon should be inflated 1 to 1.5 cc and smoothly advanced across the tricuspid valve into the right ventricle while the monitor is watched for the appropriate changes in the pressure tracings (Fig. 15-2).[5,6]

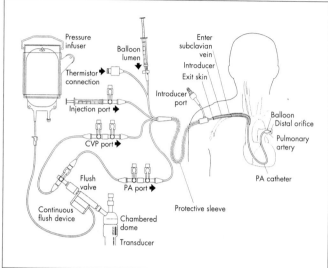

FIG. 15-1

Swan-Ganz pulmonary artery catheter. *CVP,* Central venous pressure; *PA,* pulmonary artery. *(From Mermel L, Maki D. Am J Respir Crit Care Med 1994; 149:1021.)*

3. Once the pulmonary wedge position is reached, the catheter should not be advanced any farther. Generally, the pulmonary artery wedge position should be encountered approximately 50 to 55 cm from the internal jugular vein.[6] The balloon should be inflated whenever the catheter is advanced and deflated whenever it is withdrawn.

I. INDICATIONS FOR USE

1. The PAC provides information regarding a patient's clinical status. This includes cardiac output, hemodynamic status with an estimate of volume status, measurement of pulmonic pressures, and presence of clinically significant shunts.[7] Although it has proved to be a valuable hemodynamic monitoring device, it has not yet been convincingly shown to have a positive effect on mortality.[8-12] Furthermore, an observational study by Connors and associates challenged the safety of the PAC, citing an increase in 30-day mortality associated with catheter use.[8] This article was accompanied by a call for a moratorium on the use of PACs. Since then, the use of PACs has been approached with caution, since physicians cannot deny the importance of this device in certain clinical situations.[13]

2. To date, no large, prospective, randomized controlled studies have been published to demonstrate that use of the PAC improves clinical

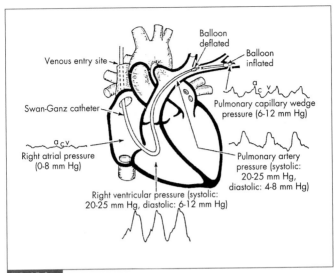

FIG. 15-2

Normal hemodynamic pressure tracings. *(From Amin D, Shah P, Swan H. Disease a Month 1991; 37[8]:518.)*

outcomes. Therefore the indications for use of the PAC developed mainly from the results of retrospective and observational studies combined with clinical expertise in the area of critical care medicine.[14] The PAC should be used when it provides information that will influence treatment decisions; otherwise, the patient may be unnecessarily placed at risk for potential complications of the PAC (which occur in up to 1.5%).[15]

3. Although use of the PAC is controversial, some generally accepted indications are discussed below.

A. COMPLICATED ACUTE MYOCARDIAL INFARCTION

1. Patients with an acute myocardial infarction complicated by cardiogenic shock, mechanical complications (e.g., acute mitral valve regurgitation secondary to papillary muscle rupture, cardiac tamponade, ventricular septal rupture), or right ventricular infarction unresponsive to initial therapy have benefited from the use of a PAC.[5,11,14,15] The PAC can provide crucial hemodynamic information to help guide short-term therapy with vasoactive agents.[16,17]

B. HEART FAILURE

1. When used in patients with severe heart failure and hemodynamic instability, the PAC can aid in determining optimal dosages of diuretics and vasopressors.[14] It can help identify patients who are not responding to the current therapy and may need mechanical support

with intraaortic balloon counterpulsation. In addition, the PAC can verify pericardial tamponade in the absence of definitive echocardiographic or clinical findings.[17]

2. In patients undergoing evaluation for heart transplantation, the PAC is used to determine the extent of pulmonary vascular resistance (PVR) and its reversibility in response to various vasodilators. Patients with high preoperative PVR tend to have a poor outcome.[17]

C. CARDIAC SURGERY

1. The PAC is generally warranted for patients who are undergoing high-risk cardiac surgery. These include patients with known ventricular dysfunction, complex coronary artery or valvular disease, or repeat cardiac surgery. The device can help guide therapy in the perioperative period.

D. SHOCK

1. One of the most common applications of the PAC is the evaluation of shock (see Chapter 12). Distinguishing between cardiogenic, septic, and hypovolemic shock on a clinical basis may be difficult, since all patients in shock are hypotensive. On the basis of the hemodynamic parameters it is possible to differentiate the various states of shock (Table 15-1) and thus deliver the appropriate therapy.[5,16,18]

E. PULMONARY EDEMA

1. The PAC is used to distinguish between cardiogenic and noncardiogenic causes of pulmonary edema.[19] This distinction is important because the treatment of these two conditions is very different. In cardiogenic edema the pulmonary artery wedge pressure (PAWP) is elevated and diuretics with or without vasopressors or inotropic agents are necessary. In noncardiogenic edema the PAWP is relatively normal and treatment consists of supportive care while optimal oxygenation is established. The distinction is exceedingly difficult if based only on the chest radiograph or physical examination of a critically ill patient.[14,16,19-22] In addition, echocardiography is not very sensitive in detecting volume overload. A retrospective observational study of 135 patients with acute lung injury revealed that the use of a PAC was associated with a change in therapeutic management in 78% of patients.[23] An ongoing National Heart Lung Blood Institute–sponsored trial conducted by the ARDS Network should provide valuable information on this issue.

TABLE 15-1

DIFFERENTIATION OF SHOCK STATES USING THE PULMONARY ARTERY CATHETER

Pulmonary Artery Catheter Measurement	Cardiogenic Shock	Septic Shock	Hypovolemic Shock
Central venous pressure	Increased	Decreased	Decreased
Cardiac output	Decreased	Increased	Decreased
Systemic vascular resistance index	Increased	Decreased	Increased

F. PRIMARY PULMONARY HYPERTENSION

1. To establish the diagnosis of primary pulmonary hypertension (PPH), the physician must use a PAC to document the severity of pulmonary vascular resistance (PVR).[17] The PAC is also used to evaluate the acute and chronic response to long-term vasodilator therapy, such as prostacyclin, or to newer therapeutic agents under development.

II. CONTRAINDICATIONS

1. The complications and contraindications for PAC placement are similar to those for central line placement (see Chapter 2). No absolute contraindications to the PAC have been established, but certain risk factors have been reported to increase the likelihood of complications.[6] Patients with known coagulopathies have an increased propensity for excessive bleeding from the procedure. Immunocompromised patients are at increased risk for the development of infection.[24]

III. INTERPRETATION OF PULMONARY ARTERY CATHETER MEASUREMENTS

1. Box 15-1 provides a list of hemodynamic variables and the range of normal values for the PAC.

2. One of the advantages of using a PAC is the ability to evaluate left ventricular end-diastolic pressure (LVEDP), which represents ventricular preload.[5] Generally PAWP is a good estimate of LVEDP. However, this concordance depends on having the catheter tip in the lower lung area, where the pulmonary artery and venous pressures are greater than the alveolar pressures.[5,6] Certain conditions can lead to an overestimation of the LVEDP based on the PAWP. These include mitral stenosis, mitral regurgitation, and pulmonary embolus. Aortic valve regurgitation causes an underestimation of the LVEDP.

BOX 15-1	
PULMONARY ARTERY CATHETER NORMAL VALUES	
MEASURED VALUES	
Central venous pressure (right atrial pressure)	1-6 mm Hg
Mean pulmonary artery pressure	
Systolic	15-30 mm Hg
Diastolic	6-12 mm Hg
Pulmonary artery wedge pressure	6-12 mm Hg
Cardiac output	3.5-7.5 L/min
Mixed venous partial oxygen pressure	70%-75%
DERIVED VALUES	
Cardiac index	2.4-4.0 L/min/m^2
Stroke volume index	40-70 mL/beat/m^2
Systemic vascular resistance	1600-2400 dynes·sec·m^2/cm^5
Pulmonary vascular resistance	200-400 dynes·sec·m^2/cm^5

3. Some clinical situations affect the data obtained by a PAC. The measurements should be obtained at end-expiration to minimize the effects of the respiratory cycle on intrathoracic pressure. The presence of positive end-expiratory pressure (PEEP) can overestimate left atrial pressure, PAWP, and CVP readings.[5,6] CO is measured by the thermodilution method. The accuracy of this value depends on the absence of intrapulmonary and intracardiac shunts.

IV. NONINFECTIOUS COMPLICATIONS

A. COMPLICATIONS ASSOCIATED WITH CATHETER INSERTION

1. Arrhythmias: Premature ventricular contractions (PVCs) are commonly encountered as the catheter migrates through the right side of the heart. Most of these arrhythmias are self-limited, but sustained ventricular tachycardia and ventricular fibrillation are possible.[5,16]

2. Right bundle branch block: This can occur in 3% to 6% of catheterizations.[24] In patients with preexisting left bundle branch block, this complication can lead to complete heart block.[6]

3. Pulmonary artery rupture: This is a rare complication (<1%) that can be caused by balloon overinflation. It is characterized by acute dyspnea, brisk hemoptysis, anxiety, and hypotension.[5,16]

4. Pneumothorax.[16]

5. Carotid or subclavian artery damage.[24]

6. Knotted catheter.

B. COMPLICATIONS DEVELOPING AFTER CATHETER INSERTION

1. Thrombosis: Thrombi can form at the tip of the catheter and serve as a nidus for infection, leading to septic thrombosis or to pulmonary embolization. Heparin-bonded catheters are currently used to decrease the incidence of thrombus formation.

2. Balloon rupture: Overinflation of the balloon can lead to balloon rupture and subsequent air embolism.[5]

3. Hemoptysis: This may be an indication of pulmonary artery rupture caused by balloon perforation after inflation.

V. INFECTIOUS COMPLICATIONS

1. Catheter-related infections (see Chapter 40) are the most common complications of the PAC.[25] The risk of infection increases dramatically with a catheter in place for more than 3 days.[5,24] Patients with bacteremia are susceptible to secondary infective endocarditis (see Chapter 41). Studies have shown an increase in catheter-associated infections with the internal jugular vein site. Coagulase-negative staphylococci (i.e., *S. epidermidis*) and *S. aureus* are the most commonly isolated pathogens in catheter-related bacteremia.[25] As soon as the hemodynamic information derived from the PAC is no longer needed for directing clinical management, the device should be removed to reduce the risk of infection.

VI. FUTURE DIRECTIONS AND STUDIES

1. Because of the need for better data supporting the use of PACs to improve patient outcomes, several clinical trials are under way. The Evaluation Study of Congestive Heart Failure and Pulmonary Artery Catheterization Effectiveness (ESCAPE) trial hopes to recruit 500 hospitalized patients with New York Heart Association class IV congestive heart failure and assign them at random to receive treatment guided by a PAC or clinical assessment alone.[26] The primary endpoint of this study is the number of days of hospitalization in a 6-month follow-up period.

2. In addition, the ARDS Clinical Network is targeting an enrollment of 1000 patients in a multicenter, prospective, randomized, controlled trial comparing the PAC with the central venous catheter for management of acute lung injury and acute respiratory distress syndrome. The primary endpoint of this study is 60-day mortality.

Intraaortic Balloon Pumps

1. The IABP, also known as the intraaortic balloon counterpulsation (IABC), consists of a polyethylene balloon of variable size (34-50 cc) mounted on a catheter. This catheter is connected to a console, which controls the inflation and deflation of the balloon with helium, an inert gas that is rapidly diffusible because of its low density. The catheter is usually inserted through the femoral artery, and the procedure is performed in the operating room, in the cardiac catheterization laboratory, or at the bedside. Fluoroscopy is usually not required.

2. The tip of the catheter is placed in the descending aorta, just distal to the origin of the left subclavian artery. A radiopaque indicator is visible on a chest radiograph.[27]

3. Inflation and deflation of the IABP are synchronized with the cardiac cycle. The IABP is inflated at the onset of diastole, when the aortic valve closes, and remains inflated throughout the diastolic period. This increases perfusion by increasing the peak diastolic pressure (approximately 30%), thus leading to an increase in mean arterial pressure. The higher aortic pressure displaces blood to the peripheral vasculature. In patients with significant myocardial ischemia the coronary artery blood flow is also improved and results in an increase in myocardial perfusion.[3]

4. The IABP deflates at the beginning of systole, when the aortic valve opens. There are two timing options: conventional timing and real timing. In conventional timing the balloon is deflated at the approximate end of diastole, as determined by the operator. This usually correlates with adjusting the pump console to a counterpulsation ratio (the number of balloon inflations per cardiac cycle) of 1:2. Conventional timing is not accurate if the patient has an abnormal cardiac cycle, as in arrhythmias. In real timing, balloon deflation is triggered by the

15

PACs AND INTRAAORTIC BALLOON PUMPS

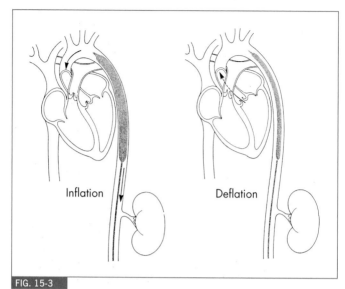

FIG. 15-3

Inflation and deflation of the intraaortic balloon catheter. *(From Quall S, ed. Comprehensive intraaortic balloon counterpulsation, 2nd ed. St Louis: Mosby; 1993.)*

QRS complex, which represents the onset of systole, and is maintained throughout the ejection period. Because the timing is related to the QRS complex, it is not dependent on a regular cardiac cycle.[28] No clear guidelines are available regarding the choice of timing methods (Fig. 15-3). Rapid decrease in intraaortic pressure during balloon deflation reduces the end-diastolic pressure. This translates to lower ventricular afterload, which promotes increased stroke volume, leading to an improvement in CO (up to 20% in patients with cardiogenic shock) (Fig. 15-4).

5. IABP withdrawal is done gradually and can take up to 24 hours. Weaning can be performed by decreasing the counterpulsation ratio (1:2, 1:3, 1:4, etc.) or by slowly reducing the inflation volume to 10% of the initial volume.

I. INDICATIONS FOR USE

1. Adjunctive therapy for high-risk coronary angioplasty (percutaneous transluminal coronary angioplasty).
2. Cardiogenic shock associated with acute myocardial infarction.
3. Myocardial ischemia refractory to maximal medical therapy.
4. Cardiac bypass surgery (perioperative support).
5. Cardiac transplantation (perioperative support).

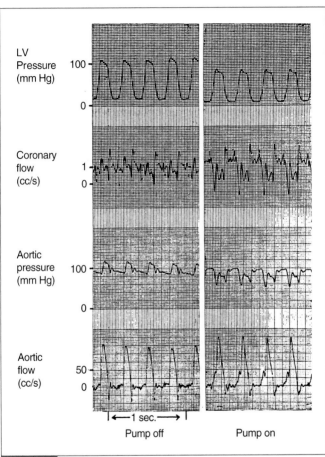

FIG. 15-4

Hemodynamic parameters as measured in canines with heart failure. *(From Unger F, ed. Assisted circulation 3. Berlin: Springer-Verlag; 1989.)*

II. CONTRAINDICATIONS TO USE

1. Severe aortic insufficiency.
2. Abdominal aortic aneurysm.
3. Aortic dissection.
4. Severe bilateral peripheral vascular disease.
5. Bilateral femoral popliteal bypass grafts.
6. Uncontrolled sepsis.

III. COMPLICATIONS

1. The complication most commonly associated with the use of an IABP is limb ischemia. In a series of 733 cases between 1967 and 1982 the most prevalent complication was vascular (9.6% of all insertion attempts).[27] A more recent study of 509 patients treated with an IABP between 1980 and 1994 by Arafa and associates revealed early vascular complications in 56 patients (11%), most of whom had developed unilateral limb ischemia.[4]

2. Other complications include aortic dissection, aortic perforation, hematoma requiring operative correction, and hemorrhage. Risk factors for the development of early vascular complications include peripheral vascular disease, the use of antiplatelet drugs, and duration of IABP use.[4,29]

3. Indwelling catheters are known to increase the risk for bacteremia, sometimes complicated by sepsis. A prospective study of 60 patients with an IABP over a 72-week period by Crystal and associates found that bacteremia developed in 15% and sepsis in 12%.[30] Coagulase-negative *Staphylococcus* was the leading culprit organism isolated in these cases. This brings to light the potential need for antibiotic prophylaxis before IABP insertion.

4. Balloon rupture is a rare complication of IABP use. If this occurs, surgical removal of the balloon may be necessary. If the pump console detects a loss of pressure, it will withdraw the helium from the balloon and turn off the system to prevent helium gas embolization.

PEARLS AND PITFALLS

- To minimize balloon rupture and pulmonary artery rupture, ensure that the balloon is inflated when you advance the PAC and deflated when you withdraw it.
- Beware of inducing complete heart block when advancing the PAC in patients with preexisting LBBB.
- To minimize risk of infection, remove the PAC once necessary information is obtained.
- Check the appropriate positioning of the IABP with a chest radiograph; the tip should be located at the level of the carina.

REFERENCES

[b] 1. Swan H et al. Catheterization of the heart in a man with the use of a flow-directed balloon tipped catheter. N Engl J Med 1973; 283:447.

[c] 2. Unger F, ed. Assisted circulation 3. Heidelberg, Germany: Springer-Verlag; 1989.

[c] 3. Overwalder P. Intra aortic balloon pump (IABP) counterpulsation. Internet J Thorac Cardiovasc Surg 1999; 2: http://www.icaap.org/iuicodeΔ 87.2. 2.2.

[b] 4. Arafa O et al. Vascular complications of the intraaortic balloon pump in patients undergoing open heart operations: 15-year experience. Ann Thorac Surg 1999; 67:645.

[c] 5. Weidemann H, Matthay M, Matthay R. Cardiovascular-pulmonary monitoring in the intensive care unit (part 2). Chest 1984; 85(5):656.

[c] 6. Amin D, Shah P, Swan H. The Swan-Ganz catheter. Dis Mon 1991; 37(8):509.

[c] 7. Hall J, Schmidt G, Wood L, eds. Principles of critical care, 2nd ed. New York: McGraw-Hill; 1998.

[b] 8. Connors A et al. The effectiveness of right heart catheterization in the initial care of critically ill patients. SUPPORT Investigators. JAMA 1996; 276:889.

[b] 9. Afessa B et al. Association of pulmonary artery catheter use with in-hospital mortality. Crit Care Med 2001; 29(6):1145.

[b] 10. Ivanov R, Allen J, Calvin J. The incidence of major morbidity in critically ill patients with pulmonary artery catheters: a meta-analysis. Crit Care Med 2000; 28(3):615.

[c] 11. Cooper A, Doig G, Sibbald W. Pulmonary artery catheters in the critically ill: an overview using the methodology of evidence-based medicine. Crit Care Clin 1996; 12(4):777.

[b] 12. Zion M et al. Use of pulmonary artery catheters in patients with acute myocardial infarction: analysis of experience in 5,841 patients in the SPRINT registry. Chest 1990; 98(6):1331.

[d] 13. Chernow B. Pulmonary artery flotation catheters: a statement by the American College of Chest Physicians and the American Thoracic Society. Chest 1997; 111(2):261.

[d] 14. Pulmonary Artery Catheter Consensus Conference: Consensus statement. Crit Care Med 1997; 25(6):910.

[c] 15. Dalen J. Does pulmonary artery catheterization benefit patients with acute myocardial infarction? Chest 1990; 98(6):1313.

[c] 16. Matthay M, Chatterjee K. Bedside catheterization of the pulmonary artery: risks compared with benefits. Ann Intern Med 1988; 15:826.

[d] 17. Mueller H et al. ACC consensus document: present use of bedside right heart catheterization in patients with cardiac disease. J Am Coll Cardiol 1998; 32(3):840.

[c] 18. Marino P. The ICU book, 2nd ed. Baltimore: Lippincott, Williams & Wilkins, 1998.

[b] 19. Duane P, Colice G. Impact of noninvasive studies to distinguish volume overload from ARDS in acutely ill patients with pulmonary edema: analysis of the medical literature from 1966 to 1998. Chest 2000; 118(6):1709.

[b] 20. Eisenberg P, Jaffe A, Schuster D. Clinical evaluation compared to pulmonary artery catheterization in the hemodynamic assessment of critically ill patients. Crit Care Med 1984; 12(7):549.

[b] 21. Connors A et al. Hemodynamic status in critically ill patients with and without acute heart disease. Chest 1990; 98(5):1200.

[b] 22. Steingrub J et al. Therapeutic impact of pulmonary artery catheterization in a medical/surgical ICU. Chest 1991; 99(6):1451.

[b] 23. Marinelli W et al. Right heart catheterization in acute lung injury: an observational study. Am J Respir Crit Care Med 1999; 160:66.

[c] 24. Sprung C, ed. The pulmonary artery catheter: methodology and clinical applications, 2nd ed. Closter, NJ: Critical Care Research Associates; 1993.

[c] 25. Mermel L, Maki D. Infectious complications of Swan-Ganz pulmonary artery catheters: pathogenesis, epidemiology, prevention, and management. Am J Respir Crit Care Med 1994; 149:1020.

[a] 26. Shah M et al. Evaluation study of congestive heart failure and pulmonary artery catheterization effectiveness (ESCAPE): design and rationale. Am Heart J 2001; 141(4):528.

[c] 27. Kantrowitz A, Cordona R, Freed P. Percutaneous intra-aortic balloon counterpulsation. Crit Care Clin 1992; 8(4):819.

[c] 28. Cadwell C, Quall S. Intra-aortic balloon counterpulsation timing. Am J Crit Care 1996; 5(4):254.

[b] 29. Patel J et al. Prospective evaluation of complications with percutaneous intraaortic balloon counterpulsation. Am J Cardiol 1995; 76:1205.

[b] 30. Crystal E et al. Incidence and clinical significance of bacteremia and sepsis among cardiac patients treated with intra-aortic balloon counterpulsation pump. Am J Cardiol 2000; 86:1281.

15

PACs AND INTRAAORTIC BALLOON PUMPS

Syncope

Eric H. Yang, MD, Hunter C. Champion, MD, PhD, and Mark Linzer, MD

FAST FACTS

- Syncope is a transient loss of consciousness with loss of postural tone and spontaneous recovery.
- Approximately 6% of hospital admissions and 3% of emergency room visits are due to syncope.
- Syncope can be classified as orthostatic hypotension, neurogenic, cardiogenic, neurocardiogenic, and syncope of unknown etiology.
- Neuroimaging and electroencephalography have a low diagnostic yield (<2%) and should be used only when patients have a history suggestive of neurogenic syncope or focal neurological signs on examination.
- All patients with suspected cardiogenic syncope should be evaluated with electrocardiography (ECG), Holter monitor or telemetry, and echocardiography.
- Electrophysiological studies should be reserved for patients with organic heart disease or conduction abnormalities.
- Event monitors should be used if patients have frequent spells (once a week to once every 2 to 3 months) and a negative cardiac workup.
- Tilt table testing should be used for patients with structurally normal hearts and relatively infrequent syncope (more than every 3 months). It should also be used for patients with nondiagnostic loop or Holter monitoring or symptoms suggesting vasovagal syncope but without an obvious precipitating event.

16

I. EPIDEMIOLOGY

1. Syncope is a transient loss of consciousness that is accompanied by loss of postural tone with spontaneous recovery. Approximately 6% of hospital admissions and 3% of emergency room visits are due to syncope.
2. The common causes of syncope are shown in Table 16-1[1] and can be divided into five general categories: orthostatic hypotension, neurogenic, cardiogenic, neurocardiogenic, and syncope of unknown etiology.
3. Orthostatic hypotension accounts for about 8% of syncopal episodes and is due to inadequate intravascular volume. It occurs when a sudden rise from a seated or lying position causes decreased cerebral perfusion and subsequent loss of consciousness. It is considered benign.
4. Neurogenic syncope is loss of consciousness caused by a neurological disorder and is responsible for 10% of syncopal episodes. Common

<table>
<tr><th colspan="2">TABLE 16-1</th><th></th></tr>
<tr><th colspan="3">CAUSES OF SYNCOPE</th></tr>
</table>

Etiology	Characteristics	Prevalence (%)
Orthostatic hypotension	Occurs with standing	8
Neurogenic syncope (migraines, transient ischemic attacks, seizures)	Seizure activity, hemiparesis, visual disturbances, headache	10
Cardiogenic syncope		
Organic heart disease (aortic stenosis, hypertrophic cardiomyopathy, congenital heart disease, myocardial infarction)	Chest pain, exertional syncope, dyspnea	4
Arrhythmias (bradyarrhythmias, tachyarrhythmias)	Sudden syncope without prodrome, subsequent injury	14
Neurocardiogenic syncope		
Vasovagal		18
Situational (cough, micturition, defecation, swallow)		5
Carotid sinus hypersensitivity		1
Syncope of unknown etiology	Negative workup	34

Data from Linzer M et al. Ann Intern Med 1997; 126:989.
Based on five population-based studies in unselected patients with syncope.

neurological diseases associated with syncope are migraines, transient ischemic attacks, and seizures. Syncope may be accompanied by seizure activity, hemiparesis, visual disturbances, or headache.

5. Cardiogenic syncope is due to a pathophysiological cardiovascular condition. The mechanism of syncope results either from organic heart disease or from an arrhythmia. The key feature of cardiogenic syncope is sudden loss of consciousness without a prodrome.

a. Organic heart disease is the cause of 4% of syncopal episodes and includes coronary artery disease, valvular abnormalities, cardiomyopathy, and congenital heart disease.

b. Arrhythmias can be classified as either bradyarrhythmias or tachyarrhythmias and account for 14% of syncopal episodes.

6. Neurocardiogenic syncope accounts for 24% of cases of syncope and is caused by a neurally mediated reflex mechanism known as the Bezold-Jarisch reflex. Inappropriate vasodilation results in an increase in venous pooling and a subsequent decrease in ventricular preload. To maintain cardiac output, the left ventricle contracts vigorously against an underfilled ventricle. This overexertion of the left ventricle is potentially harmful, and the body protects itself through a neurally mediated reflex mechanism. The afferent limb of the reflex begins with C fibers in the left ventricle that detect the sudden increase in pressure. This information is processed in the central nervous system,

and an efferent response is mediated by the vagus nerve. Bradycardia or asystole is induced, which protects against vigorous contraction but also leads to a decrease in cardiac output and the potential for syncope. Included in the category of neurocardiogenic syncope are vasovagal syncope, situational syncope (e.g., cough syncope, micturition syncope), and carotid sinus hypersensitivity.

7. Syncope of unknown etiology is unfortunately the most common type and is responsible for 34% of cases. However, the original epidemiological studies were performed several years ago when current diagnostic tools were not widely used, so the actual portion of patients with unexplained syncope is probably lower.

II. CLINICAL PRESENTATION AND DIAGNOSTICS

1. Diagnosing the cause of syncope can be both costly and frustrating because no gold standard test has been established. Table 16-2 shows the numerous diagnostic tools commonly used in a syncope workup. When deciding which test to order, the physician should remember that a thorough history and physical examination are the best diagnostic tools. The history and physical examination can also guide the clinician in deciding which diagnostic tests to use. A helpful algorithm for diagnosing syncope is shown in Fig. 16-1.

A. HISTORY AND PHYSICAL EXAMINATION

1. The cause of a syncopal episode can be determined in 45% of cases on the basis of the history and physical examination. An important question to ask in the history of present illness is what happened before, during, and after the syncopal episode. Table 16-3 shows the key events and symptoms that are characteristic of the various causes of syncope. It is also important to ask about possible triggers and whether any injury occurred during the event.

2. The past medical history provides insight into the frequency of syncopal episodes and underlying medical conditions predisposing the patient to syncope, and it can help guide the diagnostic tests to order. A thorough review of medications is important, especially in the elderly. The physical examination should include a check for orthostatic blood pressures and a thorough cardiovascular and neurological examination.

B. ELECTROCARDIOGRAPHY

1. Although the 12-lead ECG provides a diagnosis in only 5% of cases, it should be obtained in all cases of syncope. Structural or conduction abnormalities found on a resting ECG help guide more expensive and invasive evaluations for a cardiac etiology.

C. NEUROIMAGING AND ELECTROENCEPHALOGRAPHY

1. Neuroimaging and electroencephalography are extremely low yield (≤2%) when used to find the etiology of a syncopal episode. These modalities are not recommended for patients without a history suggesting neurogenic syncope or focal neurological signs on examination.

TABLE 16-2
DIAGNOSTIC TESTS FOR EVALUATING SYNCOPE

Test	Cost* ($)	Indications for Use	Diagnostic Yield (%)
History and physical examination	160	All patients with syncope	45
Electrocardiogram	90	All patients with syncope	5
Neuroimaging and electroencephalography (EEG)	888 (neuroimaging), 493 (EEG)	Patients with history suggesting neurogenic syncope or focal neurological findings on examination	0-2
Echocardiography	580	Patients with suspected cardiogenic syncope	5-10
Holter monitoring and telemetry	468	Patients with suspected cardiogenic syncope	19
Electrophysiological studies	4678	Patients with organic heart disease or conduction abnormalities	32
Loop recorders	284	Patients with frequent spells and no known structural heart disease; recurrent syncope in those with negative electrophysiological studies	24-47
Tilt table testing	683	Patients with normal hearts and infrequent syncope or those with symptoms suggesting vasovagal syncope but without an obvious precipitating event	?

*Average of cost from University of Wisconsin Hospital, University of Pittsburgh Medical Center, New England Medical Center, and Duke University Medical Center.

D. ECHOCARDIOGRAPHY

1. Transthoracic echocardiography provides a diagnosis for syncope in 5% to 10% of cases. Its cost effectiveness in diagnosing syncope has not been studied. As shown in Fig. 16-1, echocardiography and telemetry or Holter monitoring should be part of the initial workup for all patients with suspected cardiogenic syncope. Patients with abnormalities should then receive further cardiac evaluation.

E. 24-HOUR HOLTER MONITORING AND INPATIENT TELEMETRY

1. Both Holter monitoring and inpatient telemetry can be used to evaluate for rhythm disturbances in patients with suspected cardiogenic syncope. Inpatient telemetry can be used in place of outpatient Holter monitoring. An important point is that the presence of an arrhythmia on monitoring is not diagnostic unless the disturbance reproduces symptoms associated with the patient's syncope. When used for 24 hours, these tests can provide a diagnosis for syncope in 19% of patients. One study evaluating the effect of duration of monitoring on diagnostic yield showed that although 72 hours of monitoring revealed more arrhythmias, the yield for arrhythmias associated with symptoms did not increase.[2] Thus Holter monitoring or inpatient telemetry for 24 hours is recommended for all patients with suspected cardiogenic syncope. Patients with nondiagnostic inpatient telemetry should, in general, *not* be sent home with further Holter monitoring.

F. ELECTROPHYSIOLOGICAL STUDIES

1. Electrophysiological studies are invasive studies that use electrical stimulation and monitoring to discover abnormalities that predispose patients to arrhythmias. These studies are safe but expensive. They have a diagnostic yield of approximately 32%. Patients who do not have organic heart disease and have normal ECGs rarely need electrophysiological studies. They should be reserved for patients who have been shown by echocardiography and telemetry to have organic heart disease or conduction abnormalities.

G. LOOP RECORDERS AND EVENT MONITORS

1. Loop recorders and event monitors consist of two chest ECG leads connected to a small monitor. The monitor constantly records and erases the cardiac rhythm. When the patient has an event, he or she presses a button and the cardiac rhythm occurring before and after the event is recorded on the monitor. The data are then transmitted to a heart station where they are interpreted. The diagnostic yield varies from 24% to 47%. Patients must be able to put the leads on themselves every day and be cognitive enough to activate the memory when an event occurs. Event monitors should be used for patients with frequent spells (once a week to once every 2 to 3 months) and a negative cardiac workup. They should not be used for patients with infrequent syncopal episodes or patients who are incapable of operating the device. Initial studies of implantable event monitors appear

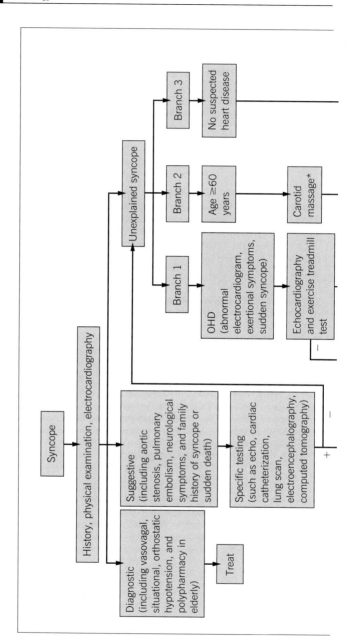

16

SYNCOPE

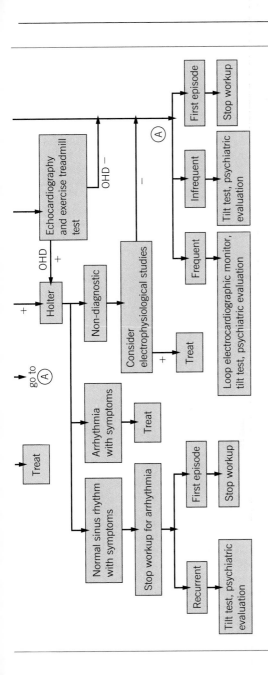

FIG. 16-1

Diagnosis of syncope. *OHD,* Organic heart disease. *(Modified from Linzer M et al. Ann Intern Med 1997; 126:989.)*

TABLE 16-3
CHARACTERISTIC SYNCOPAL SYMPTOMS

Etiology	Symptoms		
	Before Syncope	During Syncope	After Syncope
Orthostatic hypotension	Patient was sitting or lying down	Rising from sitting or lying position; begins feeling lightheaded	No residual effects
Neurogenic syncope	Headache; visual disturbances	Convulsions; seizurelike activity; urinary and fecal incontinence	Residual effects; patient is disoriented after event
Cardiogenic syncope	No prodromal symptoms	Patient has sudden loss of consciousness	No residual effects or injury
Neurocardiogenic syncope	Prodrome with feelings of warmth, nausea; situational trigger present	None	Residual feelings of nausea and warmth

promising.[3] These devices can remain implanted for long periods and do not require daily maintenance.

H. CAROTID SINUS MASSAGE

1. Carotid sinus hypersensitivity is a disease of the elderly and is the cause of syncope in 1% of cases. Patients who are 60 years of age or older and have unexplained syncope should, unless contraindicated, undergo carotid sinus massage as part of their workup.

2. A positive result is defined as symptomatic asystole for 3 or more seconds (cardioinhibitory syncope) or a decrease in systolic blood pressure greater than or equal to 30 mm Hg with a consistent history. Carotid sinus massage should be performed by trained staff and is contraindicated for patients with carotid bruits, history of arrhythmias, recent myocardial infarction, or stroke.

I. TILT TABLE TESTING

1. The tilt table test consists of two phases. In the first, or passive, phase the patient is tilted from a supine position to a 60-degree angle. The patient is left in this position for several minutes in an effort to re-produce syncope or hypotension. If an endpoint (syncope or hypoten-sion) is not reached, the patient is brought back to the supine posi-tion and isoproterenol is infused at 1 μg/min. The patient is then retilted, and the isoproterenol infusion is continued. If an endpoint is not reached, the patient is returned to the supine position and the infusion rate is increased. The patient is then retilted. This protocol is repeated until either an endpoint is obtained or the maximum infusion rate of 3 to 5 μg/min is reached.

2. Before tilt table testing, women of childbearing age should have a preg-nancy test and men older than 45 years of age and women older than 55 years of age should undergo stress testing. The overall sensitivity of tilt table testing ranges between 67% and 83%, and specificity is approximately 75%. Tilt table testing should be used for patients with structurally normal hearts and relatively infrequent syncope (less of-ten than every 3 months). It should also be used for patients with non-diagnostic loop or Holter monitoring or symptoms suggesting vasova-gal syncope but without an obvious precipitating event.

III. MANAGEMENT

1. The first treatment decision is whether or not to admit the patient. Box 16-1 provides some general indications for admission. The next step is to treat the underlying cause of syncope. Fluid rehydration is the treatment of choice for orthostatic hypotension. Use of implantable pacemakers and defibrillators can be considered in cardiogenic syn-cope. A recently published consensus on the treatment of vasova-gal syncope suggests the use of β-blockers for patients who have an increase in heart rate before syncope during tilt table testing. Those with no significant increase in heart rate should be treated with fludrocortisone.[4]

BOX 16-1
CRITERIA FOR ADMISSION
STRONG INDICATION
Cardiogenic syncope

Syncope in patients with heart disease (coronary artery disease, heart failure, electrocardiographic findings (serious bradycardia or tachycardia, increased QT interval, or bundle branch block)

Syncope with accompanying chest pain

Stroke or focal neurological disorder

MODERATE INDICATION
Sudden loss of consciousness resulting in injury

Exertional syncope

Age >70 years

Moderate to severe orthostatic hypotension

Frequent spells

Data from Linzer M et al. Ann Intern Med 1997; 127:76.
Based on six population-based studies of patients with syncope seen in the emergency department.

PEARLS AND PITFALLS
- A history and physical examination can reveal the cause of syncope in approximately 45% of cases.
- Information should be obtained from witnesses of the syncope whenever possible.
- Syncope is not a predictor of increased risk of death unless it is cardiogenic in origin.

REFERENCES
[c] 1. Linzer M et al. Diagnosing syncope. I. Value of history, physical examination, and electrocardiography. Ann Intern Med 1997; 126:989.
[c] 2. Linzer M et al. Diagnosing syncope. II. Unexplained syncope. Ann Intern Med 1997; 127:76.
[c] 3. Calkins H. Pharmacologic approaches to therapy for vasovagal syncope. Am J Cardiol 1999; 84:20Q.
[c] 4. Bloomfield DR et al. Putting it together: a new treatment algorithm for vasovagal syncope and related disorders. Am J Cardiol 1999; 84:33Q.

Valvular Heart Disease

Hunter C. Champion, MD, PhD, Eric H. Yang, MD, and Albert L. Hyman, MD

FAST FACTS

- Mitral stenosis.
  - Symptoms include dyspnea, orthopnea, and paroxysmal nocturnal dyspnea.
  - Symptoms are often precipitated by onset of atrial fibrillation or pregnancy.
  - The physical examination is notable for a prominent mitral first sound, opening snap (usually), and apical diastolic crescendo rumble.
  - Echo-Doppler can be used to confirm the diagnosis and assess the severity by measurement of the mean pressure gradient across the mitral valve.
- Mitral regurgitation.
  - Patients may be asymptomatic for many years (or for life) or may have symptoms consistent with left-sided heart failure.
  - Physical examination reveals a pansystolic murmur at the apex, radiating into the axilla; it is associated with an S_3.
  - Electrocardiography (ECG) reveals left atrial abnormality or atrial fibrillation and left ventricular hypertrophy.
  - The chest radiograph reveals left atrial and ventricular enlargement.
  - Echo-Doppler can be used to confirm the diagnosis and estimate severity.
- Aortic stenosis.
  - Patients are usually asymptomatic until middle or old age. Classic symptoms include angina, exertional syncope, and symptoms of congestive heart failure.
  - Carotid pulses are delayed and diminished.
  - S_2 is soft, absent, or paradoxically split.
  - Harsh systolic murmur can be heard, sometimes with a thrill along the left sternal border and often radiating to the neck. The murmur may be louder at the apex in older patients.
  - ECG usually shows left ventricular hypertrophy; a calcified valve is seen on x-ray examination or fluoroscopy.
  - Echo-Doppler is diagnostic in most cases.
  - Surgery is indicated for all symptomatic patients.
- Aortic regurgitation.
  - Patients are usually asymptomatic until middle age. The presentation may be left-sided heart failure or chest pain.

17

cont'd

Valvular heart disease is a mechanical interruption in the normal function of the heart. Disease can occur in any valve and places a hemodynamic burden on one or both ventricles. It is important for clinicians to recognize valvular heart disease on the basis of the history and physical examination and use appropriate diagnostic tools to further evaluate the extent of the disease. With this information, appropriately guided medical management and either serial follow-up examinations or surgical correction can be achieved (Table 17-1).

Mitral Stenosis

I. EPIDEMIOLOGY

1. Mitral stenosis is usually associated with a history of rheumatic heart disease. The decline in the incidence of rheumatic heart disease has significantly reduced the incidence of mitral stenosis in the developed world.

II. CLINICAL PRESENTATION

A. HISTORY

1. Symptoms typical of left-sided heart failure are observed in patients with mitral valve stenosis. These include dyspnea on exertion, orthopnea, and paroxysms of nocturnal dyspnea. In a minority of patients the presenting symptoms are hemoptysis, hoarseness, and symptoms of right-sided heart failure. Patients with mitral stenosis are often asymptomatic until the onset of atrial fibrillation or pregnancy, when dyspnea and orthopnea are noted.[1-4]
2. The symptoms are caused by increased left atrial pressure and reduced cardiac output as a result of mechanical obstruction of left

ventricular filling. Although the symptoms are those of left ventricular failure, contractility of the left ventricle is usually normal in mitral stenosis. Since the force of providing blood to the left ventricle is transduced to the right ventricle, right ventricular function is compromised first by the afterload imposed on it by high left atrial pressure and then by the development of secondary pulmonary vasoconstriction.[1-5]

B. PHYSICAL EXAMINATION

1. On physical examination, mitral stenosis produces the classic diastolic rumble that follows an opening snap. This is the most common finding in auscultation and can be accentuated with afterload reduction with administration of amyl nitrate. S_1 is characteristically loud because the mitral valve is held open by the transmitral gradient until the force of ventricular systole closes the valve. S_2 is also loud because of an increased P_2 component thought to result from pulmonary hypertension. In severe mitral stenosis with low flow across the mitral valve, the murmur may be soft and difficult to find but the opening snap can usually be heard. These findings are difficult to identify in patients with atrial fibrillation.

2. If the patient has both mitral stenosis and mitral regurgitation, the dominant features may be the systolic murmur of mitral regurgitation with or without a short diastolic murmur and a delayed opening snap. With severe, long-standing disease the presence of a loud P_2 probably indicates that pulmonary hypertension is producing right ventricular overload.[1-4]

III. DIAGNOSTICS

1. Echocardiography is used to assess the degree of mitral stenosis and determine the need for treatment with balloon mitral valvotomy. Planimetric calculation of valve area is performed, and the severity of stenosis can be estimated by measuring the decay of the transvalvular gradient. This "pressure half-time" is based on the principle that as the severity of stenosis worsens, the transmitral flow velocity takes longer to decay. In addition to valve area, left atrial size can be determined. Increased left atrial size denotes an increased likelihood of atrial fibrillation or systemic emboli.

2. Interestingly, atrial myxomas can have physical findings similar to those with mitral stenosis. Use of echocardiography is particularly helpful in these situations.[1-4] Patients who are in sinus rhythm but have had an embolic event should also receive anticoagulation.

IV. MANAGEMENT

1. Mitral stenosis is generally associated with a long asymptomatic phase, followed by subtle limitation of activity. Symptoms are exacerbated by pregnancy and its associated increase in cardiac output. The onset of atrial fibrillation often precipitates more severe

TABLE 17-1

SUMMARY OF SEVERE VALVULAR HEART DISEASE

	Aortic Stenosis	Mitral Stenosis	Mitral Regurgitation	Aortic Regurgitation
Etiology	Idiopathic calcification of a bicuspid or tricuspid valve; congenital; rheumatic	Rheumatic fever; annular calcification	Mitral valve prolapse; ruptured chordae; endocarditis; ischemic papillary muscle dysfunction or rupture; collagen-vascular diseases and syndromes; result of LV myocardial diseases	Annuloaortic ectasia; hypertension; endocarditis; Marfan's syndrome; ankylosing spondylitis; aortic dissection; syphilis; collagen-vascular disease
Pathophysiology	Pressure overload on LV with compensation by LV hypertrophy; as disease advances, reduced coronary flow reserve causes angina; hypertrophy and afterload excess lead to both systolic and diastolic LV dysfunction	Obstruction to LV inflow increases left atrial pressure and limits cardiac output, mimicking LV failure; mitral valve obstruction increases the pressure work of the right ventricle; right ventricular pressure overload is augmented further when pulmonary hypertension develops	Places volume overload on the LV, which responds with eccentric hypertrophy and dilatation, allowing increased ventricular stroke volume; eventually, however, LV dysfunction develops if volume overload is uncorrected	*Chronic:* Total stroke volume causes hyperdynamic circulation, induces systolic hypertension, and thus causes both pressure and volume overload; compensation is by both concentric and eccentric hypertrophy *Acute:* Because cardiac dilation has not developed, hyperdynamic findings are absent; high diastolic LV pressure causes mitral valve preclosure and potentiates LV ischemia and failure

Symptoms	Angina, syncope, heart failure	Dyspnea, orthopnea, PND, hemoptysis, hoarseness, edema, ascites	Dyspnea, orthopnea, PND	Dyspnea, orthopnea, PND, angina, syncope
Signs	Systolic ejection murmur radiating to neck; delayed carotid upstroke; S_4, soft or paradoxical S_2	Diastolic rumble following an opening snap; loud S_1; right ventricular lift; loud P_2	Holosystolic apical murmur radiates to axilla, S_3; displaced PMI	Chronic: Diastolic blowing murmur; hyperdynamic circulation; displaced PMI; Quincke's pulse; DeMusset's sign; etc. Acute: Short diastolic blowing murmur; soft S_1
ECG **Chest radiograph**	LAA; LVH Boot-shaped heart; aortic valve calcification on lateral view	LAA; RVH Straightening of left heart border; double density at right heart border; Kerley B lines; enlarged pulmonary arteries	LAA; LVH Cardiac enlargement	LAA; LVH Chronic: Cardiac enlargement; uncoiling of the aorta Acute: Pulmonary congestion with normal heart size
Echocardiographic changes	Concentric LVH; reduced aortic valve cusp separation; Doppler shows mean gradient ≤50 mm Hg in most severe cases	Restricted mitral leaflet motion; valve area ≤1 cm² in most severe cases; tricuspid Doppler may reveal pulmonary hypertension	LV and left atrial enlargement in chronic severe disease; Doppler: large regurgitant jet	Chronic: LV enlargement; large Doppler jet; PHT <400 msec Acute: small LV; mitral valve preclosure

cont'd

Data from Goldman L, Bennett JC. Cecil textbook of medicine. 21st ed. Philadelphia: WB Saunders; 2000.

AVA, Aortic valve area; *EF*, ejection fraction; *ESD*, end-systolic enlargement; *LAA*, left atrial enlargement; *LV*, left ventricle; *LVEDP*, left ventricular end-diastolic pressure; *LVH*, left ventricular hypertrophy; *MS*, mitral stenosis; *MVA*, mitral valve area; *PHT*, pressure half-time; *PMI*, point of maximal impulse; *PND*, paroxysmal nocturnal dyspnea; *RVH*, right ventricular hypertrophy.

VALVULAR HEART DISEASE 17

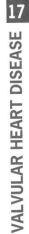

TABLE 17-1

SUMMARY OF SEVERE VALVULAR HEART DISEASE—cont'd

	Aortic Stenosis	Mitral Stenosis	Mitral Regurgitation	Aortic Regurgitation
Catheterization findings	Increased LVEDP; transaortic gradient 50 mm Hg; AVA $\leq$0.7 cm^2 in most severe cases	Elevated pulmonary capillary wedge pressure; transmitral gradient usually >10 mm Hg in severe cases; MVA <1 cm^2	Elevated pulmonary capillary wedge pressure; ventriculography shows regurgitation of dye into left ventricle	Wide pulse pressure; aortography shows regurgitation of dye into LV; usually unnecessary
Medical therapy	Avoid vasodilators; digitalis, diuretics, and nitroglycerin in inoperable cases	Diuretics for mild symptoms; anticoagulation in atrial fibrillation; digitalis, β-blockers, verapamil, or diltiazem for rate control	Vasodilators in acute disease; no proven theory in chronic disease (but vasodilators commonly used)	*Chronic:* Vasodilators in chronic asymptomatic disease with normal left ventricular function *Acute:* Vasodilators
Indications for surgery	Appearance of symptoms in patients with severe disease (see text)	Appearance of more than mild symptoms; development of pulmonary hypertension; appearance of persistent atrial fibrillation	Appearance of symptoms; EF <0.60; ESD $\leq$45 min	*Chronic:* Appearance of symptoms; EF <0.55; ESD $\leq$55 min *Acute:* Even mild heart failure; mitral valve preclosure

Data from Goldman L, Bennett JC. Cecil textbook of medicine, 21st ed. Philadelphia: WB Saunders; 2000.

AVA, Aortic valve area; *EF,* ejection fraction; *ESD,* end-systolic enlargement; *LAA,* left atrial enlargement; *LV,* left ventricle; *LVEDP,* left ventricular end-diastolic pressure; *LVH,* left ventricular hypertrophy; *MS,* mitral stenosis; *MVA,* mitral valve area; *PHT,* pressure half-time; *PMI,* point of maximal impulse; *PND,* paroxysmal nocturnal dyspnea; *RVH,* right ventricular hypertrophy.

symptoms. Conversion to sinus rhythm or ventricular rate control may be required for symptom relief. Conversion to and maintenance of sinus rhythm is most commonly successful when the duration of atrial fibrillation is brief (<12 months) and the left atrium is not severely dilated (diameter <4.5 cm). At the onset of atrial fibrillation the patient should receive warfarin anticoagulation even if sinus rhythm is restored. The reason for this rests in the observation that 20% to 30% of these patients have systemic embolization if untreated. Patients who are in sinus rhythm but have had an embolic event should also receive anticoagulation. For the asymptomatic patient in sinus rhythm, prophylaxis against endocarditis is the only medical therapy indicated. Diuretics are usually effective in lowering left atrial pressure and reducing symptoms in patients with mild symptoms.

2. Indications for treatment of mitral stenosis include New York Heart Association class III or IV heart failure symptoms; a mitral valve area <1.5 cm^2; evidence of pulmonary hypertension (resting pulmonary arterial systolic [PAS] pressure >50 mm Hg or PAS pressure >60 mm Hg with exercise); limitation of activity despite ventricular rate control and medical therapy; and recurrent systemic emboli despite anticoagulation in cases of moderate or severe stenosis.

3. Balloon valvotomy is a treatment option for patients without accompanying mitral regurgitation. Initial success rates of balloon valvotomy are high, especially if valve calcification is not excessive. When balloon valvotomy is not an option, replacement of the valve is indicated. This is usually performed when patients have combined stenosis and insufficiency.[1-4]

Mitral Regurgitation

I. EPIDEMIOLOGY

1. Approximately two thirds of mitral regurgitation cases in the United States result from mitral valve prolapse. Ischemic heart disease is the next most common cause, followed by a number of other causes such as mitral annular disease, dietary medications, endocarditis (see Chapter 41), collagen-vascular disorders, and rheumatic heart disease.[1-6]

II. CLINICAL PRESENTATION

A. HISTORY

1. The clinical presentation of mitral regurgitation depends on the rapidity with which the symptoms develop. Since blood is ejected both into the left atrium and through the aortic valve, the net effect is an increased volume load on the left ventricle. In acute regurgitation, left atrial pressure rises abruptly, which may result in pulmonary edema. However, if the onset is more gradual, the left atrium enlarges

17

VALVULAR HEART DISEASE

progressively but the pressure in the pulmonary veins and capillaries rises only transiently during exertion. Exertional dyspnea and fatigue progress gradually over many years.

2. Like patients with mitral stenosis, those with mitral regurgitation are predisposed to atrial fibrillation. However, this arrhythmia is less likely to provoke acute pulmonary congestion and less than 5% of patients have peripheral arterial emboli. In addition, mitral regurgitation often predisposes to infective endocarditis. These may be presenting conditions in patients with mitral regurgitation.[1-6]

B. PHYSICAL EXAMINATION

1. On physical examination, mitral regurgitation is characterized by a pansystolic murmur maximal at the apex, radiating to the axilla, and a prominent third heart sound. Moreover, a hyperdynamic left ventricular impulse and a brisk carotid upstroke are usually detected. The presence of a third heart sound in mitral regurgitation does not necessarily indicate that the patient has congestive heart failure. This is because the sound is produced when the large volume of blood from the enlarged left atrium rapidly fills the left ventricle.[1-5]

III. DIAGNOSTICS

1. Echocardiography is useful in demonstrating the underlying pathological process (rheumatic, prolapse, flail leaflet), and Doppler techniques provide qualitative and semiquantitative estimates of the degree of mitral regurgitation.

2. Cardiac catheterization allows accurate assessment of regurgitation, left ventricular function, and pulmonary artery pressure. Cardiac catheterization should be used only when there is a potential for surgical intervention and not as a method for longitudinal follow-up.[1-5] Coronary angiography is often indicated to determine the presence of coronary artery disease before valve surgery.

IV. MANAGEMENT

1. Acute mitral regurgitation caused by endocarditis, myocardial infarction, and ruptured chordae tendineae often requires emergency surgery. Some patients can be stabilized with vasodilators or via the use of an intraaortic balloon pump (see Chapter 15), both of which reduce the amount of regurgitant flow by lowering systemic vascular resistance.

2. In chronic mitral regurgitation, surgery is usually necessary when symptoms develop. Because progressive and irreversible deterioration of left ventricular function may occur before the onset of symptoms, however, early operation is indicated even for asymptomatic patients with a declining ejection fraction (<60%) or marked left ventricular dilation (end-systolic left ventricular dimension >45 mm on echocardiography).[1-5]

3. Although vasodilators are successfully used to increase forward output and decrease left ventricular filling pressure in patients with acute mitral regurgitation, there are no data to suggest long-term benefit from their use, especially in asymptomatic patients.[4]

Aortic Stenosis

I. EPIDEMIOLOGY

1. The most common cause of aortic valvular stenosis is the progressive valvular calcification of a congenitally bicuspid valve or a normal valve. In the former group, presentation tends to occur in the fourth or fifth decade of life. In the latter group, the aortic valve becomes sclerotic and, with further calcification, stenotic during the sixth, seventh, or eighth decade of life.

2. Approximately 25% of patients over age 65 and 35% of those over age 70 have echocardiographic evidence of sclerosis, and 2% to 3% of these exhibit hemodynamic evidence of stenosis. Thus aortic stenosis has become the most common surgical valve lesion in developed countries.[1-4,7]

II. CLINICAL PRESENTATION

A. HISTORY

1. Symptoms of failure may have a sudden onset or progress gradually. Angina pectoris frequently occurs in aortic stenosis. Among patients with calcific aortic stenosis, one half of those with angina have significant associated coronary artery disease, in contrast to only one fourth of those without angina.

2. Syncope is typically related to exertion and may be caused by arrhythmias (usually ventricular tachycardia but sometimes sinus bradycardia), hypotension, or decreased cerebral perfusion resulting from increased blood flow to exercising muscle without compensatory increase in cardiac output. Sudden death may occur but is rarely the initial manifestation of aortic stenosis in previously asymptomatic patients.[7]

B. PHYSICAL EXAMINATION

1. In mild or moderate aortic valve stenosis the characteristic sign is a systolic ejection murmur at the aortic area transmitted to the neck and apex that peaks in early systole.

2. In severe cases a palpable left ventricular heave or thrill, a weak to absent A_2, or reversed splitting of the second sound is present. When the valve area is less than 1 cm² (normal, 3-4 cm²), ventricular systole becomes prolonged and the typical carotid pulse pattern of delayed upstroke and low amplitude is present *(parvus et tardus)*. The murmur may disappear over the sternum and then reappear in the apical area, mimicking mitral regurgitation (Gallivardin's phenomenon).[1-4,7]

17

VALVULAR HEART DISEASE

III. DIAGNOSTICS

1. The ECG usually reveals left ventricular hypertrophy or suggestive repolarization changes but may be normal in up to 10% of patients with aortic stenosis.
2. The chest radiograph may show a normal or enlarged cardiac silhouette, calcification of the aortic valve, and dilation and calcification of the ascending aorta.
3. The echocardiogram provides useful data about aortic valve calcification and opening and left ventricular thickness and function, while Doppler can estimate the aortic valve gradient. These data can reliably exclude or diagnose severe stenosis. In patients with moderate obstruction, especially with low cardiac output or concomitant regurgitation, these evaluations may be inaccurate. Echocardiography is also useful in assessing the extent of left ventricular hypertrophy and in estimating left ventricular function.
4. Cardiac catheterization is the definitive diagnostic procedure. The valve gradient is measured and the valve area calculated; a valve area below 0.8 cm^2 indicates severe stenosis. Aortic regurgitation can be quantified by aortic root angiography. Coronary arteriography should be performed in most adults with aortic stenosis to assess for concomitant coronary disease.[1-4]

IV. MANAGEMENT

1. With the exception of prophylaxis against endocarditis (see below), there is no proven medical therapy for aortic stenosis. The only effective relief of this mechanical obstruction to blood flow is aortic valve replacement. After the onset of heart failure, angina, or syncope, the prognosis without surgery is poor (50% 3-year mortality rate). Medical treatment may stabilize patients in heart failure, but surgery is indicated for all symptomatic patients, including those with left ventricular dysfunction, which often improves postoperatively.
2. Asymptomatic patients should be followed with serial echocardiograms to detect declining left ventricular function, very severe left ventricular hypertrophy, and very high gradients (>80 mm Hg) or severely reduced valve areas (<0.7 cm^2).[1-4]
3. The surgical mortality rate for valve replacement is 2% to 5%, but it rises to 10% in persons over the age of 75. Bypass of severe coronary lesions is usually performed at the same time as valve replacement.
4. Anticoagulation with warfarin is required for mechanical prostheses but is not essential with bioprostheses. Although, in the past, bioprosthetic valves have undergone degenerative changes and required replacement within 7 to 10 years (sometimes within 3 years), newer ones may be more durable. In some cases the Ross procedure may be performed. This procedure entails switching the patient's pulmonary valve to the aortic position and placing a bioprosthesis in the pulmonary position. Because bioprostheses do not deteriorate as

fast on the right side of the heart, the Ross procedure has produced good long-term results without anticoagulation.

5. Although percutaneous balloon valvuloplasty can produce short-term reductions in the severity of aortic stenosis, restenosis occurs rapidly in most adults who have calcified valves. Except in adolescents, balloon valvuloplasty should be reserved for patients who are poor candidates for surgery or as an intermediate procedure to stabilize high-risk patients before surgery.[1-4]

Aortic Regurgitation

I. EPIDEMIOLOGY

1. The most common congenital cause of aortic regurgitation is bicuspid aortic valve. Other causes include disorders that affect the valve itself (e.g., infective endocarditis, rheumatic heart disease, dietary medications) and those causing proximal ascending aorta dilatation (e.g., Marfan's syndrome, hypertension-associated ectasia, syphilis, ankylosing spondylitis, and Reiter's syndrome). Causes of acute aortic regurgitation include endocarditis and aortic root dissection.[1-4]

II. CLINICAL PRESENTATION

A. SYMPTOMS

1. The clinical presentation of aortic regurgitation is generally determined by the rapidity with which regurgitation develops. In the case of chronic aortic regurgitation the only sign for many years may be a soft aortic diastolic murmur. As the valve deformity increases, larger amounts of blood are regurgitated, diastolic blood pressures fall, and the left ventricle progressively enlarges. Most patients remain asymptomatic even at this point, and an often prolonged plateau phase, characterized by stable left ventricular dilatation, occurs. Left ventricular failure is a late event and may be sudden in onset. Exertional dyspnea and fatigue are the most common symptoms, but paroxysms of nocturnal dyspnea and pulmonary edema also occur. Angina pectoris or atypical chest pain may or may not be present. Associated coronary artery disease and syncope are less common than in aortic stenosis.[1-4]

B. PHYSICAL EXAMINATION

1. The major physical findings relate to the wide arterial pulse pressure. The pulse has a rapid rise and fall (Corrigan's pulse), with an elevated systolic and a low diastolic pressure. The large stroke volume is responsible for characteristic findings such as Quincke's pulses (subungual capillary pulsations) and Duroziez's sign (diastolic murmur over a partially compressed peripheral artery, commonly the femoral). The apical impulse is prominent, laterally displaced, and usually hyperdynamic and may be sustained. The murmur may be soft and localized. The aortic diastolic murmur is high pitched and decre-

scendo. In advanced aortic regurgitation a middiastolic or late diastolic low-pitched mitral murmur (Austin Flint murmur) may be heard. This occurs because the regurgitant jet partially closes the mitral valve, obstructing mitral flow. Musset's sign (head bobbing) and Hill's sign (systolic blood pressure at least 30 mm Hg higher in the leg than in the arm) may also be seen.[2-4]

2. When aortic regurgitation develops as an acute condition (as in aortic dissection or infective endocarditis), left ventricular failure, manifested primarily as pulmonary edema, may develop rapidly and surgery is urgently required. Patients with acute aortic regurgitation do not have the dilated left ventricle of chronic aortic regurgitation. They also have a shorter diastolic murmur that may be minimal in intensity, and the pulse pressure may not be widened, making clinical diagnosis difficult.[4]

III. DIAGNOSTICS

1. The ECG usually shows moderate to severe left ventricular hypertrophy.
2. Radiographs show cardiomegaly with left ventricular prominence.
3. Echocardiography can demonstrate whether the lesion involves the aortic root or if valvular disease is present. Serial assessments of left ventricular size and function are critical in determining the timing for valve replacement. Doppler techniques can be used to estimate the severity of regurgitation, although "mild" regurgitation is not uncommon and should not be overinterpreted. Scintigraphic studies can be used to quantify left ventricular function and functional reserve during exercise, a useful predictor of prognosis.
4. Cardiac catheterization can help quantify severity and is used to evaluate the coronary and aortic root anatomy preoperatively.

IV. MANAGEMENT

1. Chronic aortic regurgitation can be a long-standing condition, but the prognosis without surgery becomes poor when symptoms occur. Vasodilators, such as hydralazine, nifedipine, and angiotensin-converting enzyme inhibitors, can reduce the severity of regurgitation, and prophylactic treatment may postpone or obviate the need for surgery in asymptomatic patients with severe regurgitation and a dilated left ventricle.
2. Surgery is usually indicated once aortic regurgitation causes symptoms. Surgery is also indicated for patients who have few or no symptoms but have significant left ventricular dysfunction (ejection fraction <45% or 50%) or who exhibit progressive deterioration of left ventricular function, irrespective of symptoms. Although the operative mortality rate is higher when left ventricular function is severely impaired, valve replacement or repair is still indicated, since left ventricular function often improves somewhat and the long-term

prognosis is thereby enhanced. After surgery, left ventricular size usually decreases and left ventricular function improves, except when dysfunction has been a chronic condition.

3. The "55 rule" has been useful in gauging the timing of surgery for aortic regurgitation. Aortic valve surgery should be performed before the ejection fraction falls below 55% or the end-systolic dimension exceeds 55 mm Hg.[4]

Tricuspid Regurgitation

I. EPIDEMIOLOGY

1. The most common cause of tricuspid valve regurgitation is right ventricular overload resulting from left ventricular failure. Tricuspid regurgitation also occurs in association with right ventricular and inferior myocardial infarction. Tricuspid valve endocarditis and resulting regurgitation are common in intravenous drug users. Other causes include pulmonary hypertension, carcinoid syndrome, lupus erythematosus, and myxomatous degeneration of the valve (associated with mitral valve prolapse).

2. Ebstein's anomaly is a congenital defect of the tricuspid valve that often manifests itself in adults as massive right-sided cardiomegaly caused by tricuspid regurgitation.

II. CLINICAL PRESENTATION

1. The symptoms and signs of tricuspid regurgitation are identical to those of right ventricular failure of any cause. Tricuspid regurgitation can be suspected on the basis of an early onset of right-sided heart failure and a harsh systolic murmur along the lower left sternal border that increases in intensity during and just after inspiration (Carvallo's sign). Accentuation of the tricuspid murmur can at times be achieved by pressing down on the liver (Vitum's sign). Both of these signs are neither sensitive nor specific but have been historically used to describe this valvular disorder.

2. Hemodynamic characteristics of tricuspid regurgitation include a prominent regurgitant systolic (v) wave in the right atrium and jugular venous pulse, with a rapid y descent and a small or absent x descent. The regurgitant wave, like the systolic murmur, is increased with inspiration, and its size depends on the size of the right atrium. In tricuspid regurgitation, especially with right ventricular failure, an inspiratory S_3 may be present.

III. DIAGNOSTICS

1. There are no pathognomonic signs of tricuspid regurgitation on the ECG. Associated abnormalities such as atrial enlargement, right ventricular hypertrophy, or right bundle branch block are often seen.

2. The chest radiograph may demonstrate right atrial enlargement, right ventricular enlargement, or pleural effusions.
3. Echocardiography can be used, as in other valvular disorders, to assess the presence and severity of tricuspid regurgitation. Based on this and a modified version of Bernoulli's equation, the right ventricular systolic pressure can be estimated.
4. Cardiac catheterization is rarely needed as part of the diagnostic workup of patients with tricuspid regurgitation.

IV. MANAGEMENT

1. Tricuspid regurgitation resulting from severe mitral valve disease or other left-sided lesions may regress when the underlying disease is corrected. Tricuspid valvular annuloplasty is indicated for patients who require mitral valve surgery and also have severe tricuspid regurgitation and pulmonary hypertension.
2. Surgical valve replacement is most commonly used for patients with severe tricuspid regurgitation and abnormal valve leaflets not amenable to valvuloplasty. Replacement of the tricuspid valve is infrequently performed nowadays.[1,2]

PEARLS AND PITFALLS

- Antibiotic prophylaxis against endocarditis has been used in a number of valvular disease states. The American Heart Association has adopted the following guidelines based on a risk stratification scheme.[8]
  - High-risk individuals requiring prophylaxis are those with prosthetic cardiac valves, including bioprosthetic and homograft valves; previous bacterial endocarditis; complex cyanotic congenital heart disease (e.g., single-ventricle states, transposition of the great arteries, tetralogy of Fallot); or surgically constructed systemic pulmonary shunts or conduits.
  - Moderate-risk individuals requiring prophylaxis include those with most congenital cardiac malformations other than the above; acquired valvular dysfunction (e.g., rheumatic heart disease); hypertrophic cardiomyopathy; and mitral valve prolapse with valvular regurgitation or thickened leaflets.
  - Individuals not recommended for prophylaxis include those with isolated secundum atrial septal defect; surgical repair of atrial septal defect, ventricular septal defect, or patent ductus arteriosus (without residua beyond 6 months); previous coronary artery bypass graft surgery; mitral valve prolapse without valvular regurgitation; physiological, functional, or innocent heart murmurs; previous Kawasaki disease without valvular dysfunction; previous rheumatic fever without valvular dysfunction; and cardiac pacemakers (intravascular and epicardial) and implanted defibrillators.
  - Dental procedures appropriate for prophylaxis are dental extractions; periodontal procedures, including surgery, scaling and root planting, probing, and recall maintenance; dental implant placement and

reimplantation of avulsed teeth; endodontic (root canal) instrumentation or surgery only beyond the apex; subgingival placement of antibiotic fibers or strips; initial placement of orthodontic bands but not brackets; intraligamentary local anesthetic injections; and prophylactic cleaning of teeth or implants when bleeding is anticipated.

- Other procedures appropriate for prophylaxis include tonsillectomy; adenoidectomy; surgical operations that involve respiratory mucosa; bronchoscopy with a rigid bronchoscope; sclerotherapy for esophageal varices; esophageal stricture dilatation; endoscopic retrograde cholangiography with biliary obstruction; surgical operations that involve intestinal mucosa; prostatic surgery; cystoscopy; and urethral dilatation.

- Recommended regimens include amoxicillin 2 g PO 1 hour before the procedure or ampicillin 2 g IV 30 minutes before the procedure. High-risk patients undergoing nondental procedures should be treated with ampicillin and gentamicin. Patients allergic to penicillin can be treated with clindamycin or azithromycin.

REFERENCES

[d] 1. Bonow RO et al. Guidelines for the management of patients with valvular heart disease. Circulation 1998; 98:1949.

[c] 2. Carabello BA, Crawford FA. Valvular heart disease. N Engl J Med 1997; 337:32.

[b] 3. Singh JP et al. Prevalence and clinical determinants of mitral, tricuspid, and aortic regurgitation. Am J Cardiol 1999; 83:897.

[c] 4. Zoghbi WA. Valvular heart disease. Cardiol Clin 1998; 16:3.

[c] 5. Carabello BA. Mitral valve regurgitation. Curr Probl Cardiol 1998; 23:200.

[b] 6. Freed LA et al. Prevalence and clinical outcome of mitral-valve prolapse. N Engl J Med 1999; 341:1

[c] 7. O'Rourke RA. Aortic valve stenosis: a common clinical entity. Curr Probl Cardiol 1998; 23:429.

[d] 8. Dajani AS et al. Prevention of bacterial endocarditis: recommendations by the American Heart Association. Clin Infect Dis 1997; 25:1448.

17

VALVULAR HEART DISEASE

Management of Complications in Patients with Prosthetic Heart Valves

Hunter C. Champion, MD, PhD, Eric H. Yang, MD,
and Stephen C. Achuff, MD

FAST FACTS

- Valve thrombosis.
  - Incidence is approximately 5% per patient-year.
  - Major contributing factors are inadequate anticoagulation therapy and mitral location of the valve.
  - Clinical presentation is notable for evidence of systemic embolism, pulmonary congestion, or poor peripheral perfusion that may manifest as acute hemodynamic decompensation.
  - Physical examination may reveal decreased intensity of opening or closing clicks or presence of a new murmur.
  - Echocardiography may show an increased transvalvular gradient or valvular, and sometimes perivalvular, regurgitation.
- Embolic events.
  - Risk is 1% per patient-year with warfarin therapy.
  - Although associated more often with mechanical valves, embolic events may occur in patients with bioprosthetic valves.
  - The risk is higher with prosthetic valves in the mitral or tricuspid position.
  - Other variables increasing risk include presence of atrial fibrillation, age over 70 years, left atrial enlargement, prior history of thromboembolism, known left atrial thrombus, multiple mechanical valves, caged-ball valves (Starr-Edwards), and low left ventricular ejection fraction.
- Hemorrhage in the setting of anticoagulation.
  - When hemorrhage develops, anticoagulation must be discontinued for the short term and possibly the long term.
  - Consideration should be given to replacement of a mechanical valve with a bioprosthetic valve.
- Structural failure of the prosthetic heart valve.
  - Structural failure is a rare occurrence with mechanical prosthetic valves.
  - A structural defect was found in the Bjork-Shiley convexoconcave single-tilting-disk valve in 1986. Strut fracture resulted in embolization of the disk and acute dyspnea, syncope, severe valvular regurgitation, and even cardiovascular collapse.

18

I. EPIDEMIOLOGY

1. More than 60,000 heart valve replacements are performed in the United States each year.[1-3] The prosthetic valves used in these procedures are either mechanical or bioprosthetic and are associated with a number of complications with which the house officer must be familiar to adequately manage this patient population.

2. Although the complications of the various prosthetic valves are generally similar, these valves differ greatly in their longevity and thrombogenicity. These differences are based largely on their composition and anatomical location.[1-3]

3. Mechanical valves are composed primarily of metal and carbon alloy and, with few exceptions, have a lifespan of at least 20 to 30 years. These mechanical prostheses are classified according to their structure, which includes caged-ball models such as the Starr-Edwards (rarely seen now), the single-tilting-disk valve (e.g., Bjork-Shiley), and the most frequently used bileaflet-tilting-disk model (e.g., St. Jude Medical or the Carbomedics models) (Fig. 18-1).

4. The clinical situation of the patient guides the selection of the model. Generally, mechanical valves are preferred for patients whose life expectancy is greater than 10 to 15 years or who have another indication for long-term anticoagulation (e.g., atrial fibrillation).[1-3]

5. Bioprosthetic valves are divided into heterografts and homografts. Heterografts are composed of porcine valves or bovine pericardium mounted on a metal support structure and include such models as the Hancock, Carpentier-Edwards, Life Sciences–Edwards, and Ionescu-Shiley. Homografts are composed of preserved cadaveric human aortic valves. The advantage of bioprosthetic valves is their low thromboembolic potential, which obviates the need for long-term anticoagulation. The disadvantage is their reduced longevity: 10% to 20% of homografts and 50% of heterograft valves fail within 10 to 15 years

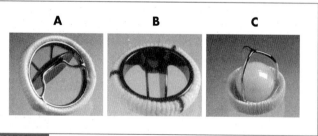

FIG. 18-1

Prosthetic valves. **A,** Bjork-Shiley. **B,** St. Jude's Medical. **C,** Starr-Edwards. *(Courtesy Vincent Gott, MD.)*

of implantation. Bioprosthetic valves are therefore preferred for elderly patients whose life expectancy is less than 10 to 15 years and those for whom long-term anticoagulation therapy would pose considerable difficulty. Since warfarin is associated with teratogenic effects, however, the use of bioprostheses can be considered for women of childbearing age, with the understanding that a second open-chest surgery will be required in the future to replace the bioprosthesis.[1]

II. CLINICAL PRESENTATION AND DIAGNOSTICS

1. To understand the potential complications associated with a prosthetic heart valve, the physician must be able to adequately assess valve function. On physical examination a change in the intensity or quality of the audible sound of the valve or the presence of a new valvular murmur may suggest a potential valve dysfunction. Mechanical valves should produce a crisp sound of opening and closure and differ from bioprosthetic valves, where auscultation should be similar to that of native valves.

2. If prosthetic valve dysfunction is suspected, imaging of the valve should be performed to further assess its function. Two-dimensional transthoracic echocardiography (TTE) with Doppler interrogation is a reliable and inexpensive method for evaluation of prosthetic valves. TTE permits the evaluation of sewing-ring stability, the absence or presence of valvular regurgitation and perivalvular leak, the prosthetic transvalvular gradient, and the motion of bioprosthetic leaflets. Transesophageal echocardiography (TEE) provides better views of the mitral valve than does TTE and should be considered if data obtained by TTE are inadequate.

3. Cinefluoroscopy can be used to assess mechanical valves by observation of the motion of the valve ring but is most useful in detecting the structural integrity of the outlet strut of the Bjork-Shiley tilting-disk valve. Given the significant risk of passing a catheter across a mechanical valve, cinefluoroscopy alone is a preferred method for evaluating valve function.[1]

Valve Thrombosis

I. EPIDEMIOLOGY

1. The risk of valve thrombosis is related to the type and location of the valve. Of the most commonly used mechanical prosthetic valves, the bileaflet-tilting-disk type is the least thrombogenic, followed by the single-tilting-disk and the caged-ball. Of the bioprosthetic valves, heterografts are more thrombogenic than homografts. Mitral valve position of the prosthetic valve is associated with increased incidence of valve thrombosis. With adequate anticoagulation, however, the incidence of valve thrombosis is similar for all valves discussed.[1-3]

18

COMPLICATIONS WITH PROSTHETIC HEART VALVES

II. MANAGEMENT

1. Thrombosis of a prosthetic valve can result in severe hemodynamic compromise. In some cases, however, the onset of symptoms is more gradual (days to weeks). If thrombosis is recognized, treatment depends largely on the size of the thrombus and the hemodynamic stability of the patient. Generally, thrombi that are less than 5 mm in diameter do not obstruct the valve and can be treated with anticoagulation alone. If the thrombus is greater than 5 mm in diameter, however, the risk of complications usually warrants valve replacement or thrombolysis.

2. Because thrombolytic therapy is associated with a high risk of bleeding and embolization ($\leq 20\%$), it is usually considered less optimal than cardiac surgery.

3. For patients with severe hemodynamic compromise, emergency surgery is recommended over thrombolytic therapy, since many valves have pannus formation and tissue ingrowth. The mortality in surgical therapy for valve thrombosis is approximately 15% and usually entails valve replacement rather than thrombectomy because replacement has a lower risk of recurrent thrombosis.[1-3]

Embolic Events

I. EPIDEMIOLOGY

1. Without antithrombotic therapy, the incidence of death or a persistent neurological deficit as a result of embolism is approximately 4% per patient-year in patients with mechanical valves. With antiplatelet therapy alone the risk falls to 2% per patient-year. With warfarin therapy the risk is 1% per patient-year. The majority of embolic events are manifested as embolic strokes, but emboli may also result in renal infarct, bowel infarct, splenic infarct, or lower extremity arterial occlusion. Increased risk of an embolic event is associated with the presence of atrial fibrillation, left atrial enlargement, prior history of thromboembolism, known left atrial thrombus, multiple mechanical valves, caged-ball valves (Starr-Edwards), decreased left ventricular function (ejection fraction <45%), and age over 70 years (Box 18-1).[1,2]

II. MANAGEMENT

1. In patients who have prosthetic heart valves and signs of systemic embolism, the possibility of endocarditis or thrombosis should be considered. Conflicting data are available regarding optimal timing for initiating or continuing anticoagulants when an embolus is the presumed cause of a stroke. Ideally treatment is started early to prevent recurrent emboli, but the early use of heparin (within 72 hours) is associated with an increased chance (15% to 25%) of converting an embolic stroke into a hemorrhagic stroke.

2. Although a case can still be made for immediate use of heparin,

---

BOX 18-1

FACTORS INCREASING THE RISK FOR THROMBOEMBOLIC COMPLICATIONS FROM PROSTHETIC VALVES

Age >70 years
Multiple prosthetic valves
Tricuspid or mitral valve position
Caged-ball valve
History of thromboembolic event
Atrial fibrillation
Left atrial enlargement
Left ventricular systolic dysfunction (ejection fraction <45%)
Known left atrial thrombus

---

the early recurrence of an embolus in patients who have a prosthetic valve and are not taking anticoagulants has not been clearly documented. Generally, if computed tomography of the brain provides no evidence of hemorrhagic conversion of the stroke at 72 hours after the event, heparin is instituted with a goal for the activated partial thromboplastin time of 40 to 50 seconds and is maintained until the international normalized ratio (INR) is therapeutic for the valve position and model. If computed tomography demonstrates significant hemorrhage or if systemic arterial pressure is significantly elevated, antithrombotic therapy should be withheld until the bleeding is treated or has stabilized (7 to 14 days).[1-3]

III. HEMORRHAGE IN THE SETTING OF ANTICOAGULATION

1. The risk of hemorrhage is higher in patients receiving anticoagulation therapy with warfarin or heparin and may be precipitated by trauma. The incidence of intracranial bleeding increases with elevated systemic arterial pressure. When significant bleeding occurs, regardless of the location, antithrombotic therapy should be stopped, and if the patient is at high risk, drug effects should be reversed with fresh frozen plasma in the case of warfarin therapy and with protamine in the case of heparin therapy. If possible, the site of bleeding should be corrected, and antithrombotic therapy restarted as soon as possible.

2. No reliable data are available regarding the time to reinstitute anticoagulation, and decisions should be made on a case-by-case basis. If reanticoagulation is not possible, treatment decisions are difficult. For patients with a mechanical prosthesis or multiple risk factors for thromboemboli, acceptance of intermittent bleeding with acute management of the episodes may be necessary. Some patients with mechanical valves, such as those who have had multiple, large, life- or organ-threatening bleeding episodes, may need replacement of the mechanical valve with a bioprosthetic valve.[1,3]

Structural Failure of the Prosthetic Heart Valve

1. Bioprosthetic valves are more prone to failure, and 50% of heterograft valves and 10% to 20% of homograft valves require replacement within 10 to 15 years.
2. Structural failure of the mechanical prosthetic heart valve is rare but should be considered in the event of a rapid deterioration in hemodynamic stability. A structural defect found in the Bjork-Shiley convexoconcave single-tilting-disk valve in 1986 resulted in its recall. Strut fracture results in embolization of the disk and acute dyspnea, syncope, severe valvular regurgitation, and even cardiovascular collapse.
3. Bioprosthetic valves deteriorate, and about 50% of bioprosthetic valves require replacement within 10 to 15 years of implantation because of failure. The incidence of failure is higher in patients younger than 40 years of age and in patients receiving hemodialysis. Most failures are due to tear or rupture of a valve leaflet that has become calcified and rigid. Symptoms include progressive dyspnea and other symptoms of heart failure. The diagnosis is based on detection of a new murmur during physical examination and is confirmed by echocardiography.[1-3]

Endocarditis

1. Infective endocarditis is discussed in Chapter 41. However, there are a few special considerations for patients with prosthetic valves. Endocarditis occurs at some time in 3% to 6% of patients with prosthetic valves. So-called early endocarditis (occurring less than 60 days after valve replacement) usually results from perioperative bacteremia arising from skin or wound infections. Late prosthetic valve endocarditis (occurring more than 60 days postoperatively) is usually secondary to organisms that cause traditional endocarditis. The risk of endocarditis is similar for mechanical and bioprosthetic valves.
2. In patients who have prosthetic valve endocarditis, fever is the most common symptom. Unexplained fever in a patient with a prosthetic valve should be presumed to be due to endocarditis until proven otherwise. Both transthoracic and transesophageal echocardiography should be performed in patients with suspected prosthetic valve endocarditis.
3. The mortality associated with prosthetic valve endocarditis is 30% to 80% for the early form and 20% to 40% for the late form, and its prevention is imperative. Regular dental care and education concerning antibiotic prophylaxis are essential for patients with prosthetic valves. Careful consideration must be given to replacing a prosthetic valve if blood cultures remain positive while the patient is receiving appropriate therapy.[1,3]

Recommended Antithrombotic Therapy

1. Because of the risk of thromboembolism, patients with mechanical prosthetic valves require long-term anticoagulant therapy, which should be started within 6 to 12 hours after surgery. The degree of anticoagulation depends on the type of prosthetic valve and is summarized in Table 18-1. In patients with a caged-ball valve or more than one mechanical prosthetic valve, the incidence of adverse events is lowest when the INR is kept between 3.0 and 4.5. Adverse events are infrequent when the INR is 2.5 to 3.5 in patients with bileaflet or single-tilting-disk valves.

2. Patients who are more than 70 years old have an increased incidence of bleeding complications when the INR exceeds 3.9, whereas younger patients generally tolerate higher INRs without increased complications. In short, the intensity of anticoagulant therapy should be individualized according to the patient's age, the type and position of the valve, and the number of prosthetic valves.

3. Since patients with heterograft bioprosthetic valves have an increased incidence of thromboembolism during the first 3 months after valve replacement, this patient population should receive low-intensity anticoagulant therapy (target INR, 2.0 to 3.0) during this time.

4. Continued anticoagulant therapy is indicated for patients with atrial fibrillation, left atrial thrombus, previous systemic embolization, or severe left ventricular dysfunction.

5. Good results in minimizing thrombembolic complications have been obtained when lower-dose aspirin (100 mg daily) is combined with warfarin (target INR, 3.0 to 4.5) for patients who have mechanical heart valves or bioprosthetic valves and also have atrial fibrillation or previous systemic embolization.

6. The addition of aspirin to warfarin for patients with prosthetic valves offers additional protection against thromboembolism at the risk of more frequent bleeding complications.[5] Therefore this combination should be reserved for patients with a history or high risk of systemic

TABLE 18-1

SUGGESTED THERAPEUTIC ANTICOAGULATION FOR PATIENTS WITH PROSTHETIC HEART VALVES

Type of Prosthetic Valve	Recommended INR*
Bileaflet disk (St. Jude, Carbomedics)	2.5-3.5
Single tilting disk (Bjork-Shiley)	2.5-3.5
Caged ball (Starr-Edwards)	3.0-4.5
Heterograft bioprosthetic	2.0-3.0 (for first 3 months)
Homograft	Not required

INR, International normalized ratio.

*Target INR is at higher end of recommended range for valves in the mitral position.

embolization (Box 18-1) or with other conditions in which it is indicated, such as coronary artery or peripheral vascular disease.[1-3]

PEARLS AND PITFALLS

- Pregnancy and prosthetic valves.
  - The hemodynamic changes associated with pregnancy are usually well tolerated by women with mechanical valves. What poses a problem is the need for adequate anticoagulation and the hypercoagulable state that occurs in the third trimester and the immediate postpartum period. Treatment with heparin has been tried but has proved to be logistically difficult. Use of warfarin during pregnancy increases the risk of fetal malformation.
  - One alternative explored has been the use of bioprosthetic valves, but this usually necessitates replacement of the valve during the patient's lifetime. Whenever possible, valve replacement should be deferred until after a woman's childbearing years.
  - Management of women who have mechanical valves and subsequently become pregnant remains challenging. The current consensus is to continue warfarin during pregnancy because the risks of thromboembolic complications from inadequate anticoagulation outweigh the risks of impaired fetal development.[6]
- Patients receiving long-term hemodialysis have a high incidence of early bioprosthetic valve failure.

REFERENCES

[c] 1. Vongpatanasin L et al. Prosthetic heart valves. N Engl J Med 1996; 335:407.

[c] 2. McAnulty JH, Rahimtoola SH. Antithrombotic therapy and prosthetic valve disease. In Alexander RW et al, eds. Hurst's the heart, 9th ed. New York: McGraw-Hill; 1999.

[c] 3. Garcia MJ. Prosthetic valve disease. In Topol EJ, ed. Comprehensive cardiovascular medicine. Philadelphia: 1998; Lippincott, Williams & Wilkins.

[d] 4. Fifth ACCP Consensus Conference on Antithrombotic Therapy. Chest 1998; 114:439S.

[a] 5. Meschengieser SS et al. Low intensity oral anticoagulation plus low dose aspirin versus high intensity oral anticoagulation alone: a randomized trial in patients with mechanical prosthetic heart valves. J Thorac Cardiovasc Surg 1997; 113:910.

[b] 6. Sareli P et al. Maternal and fetal sequelae of anticoagulation during pregnancy in patients with mechanical heart valve prostheses. Am J Cardiol 1989; 63:1462.

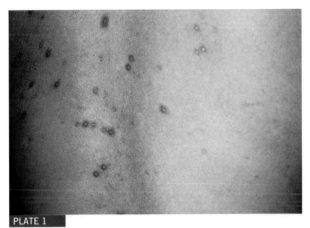

PLATE 1

Prurigo nodules on the back of a patient infected with human immuno-deficiency virus. *(Courtesy David Kouba, MD, PhD.)*

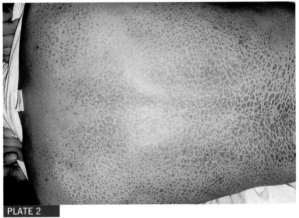

PLATE 2

Ichthyosis. Note the platelike scale characteristic of this condition. This skin finding is more prominent in darker skinned individuals.

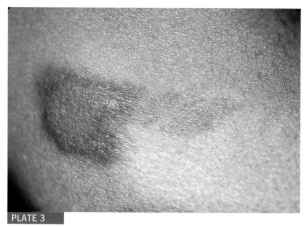

PLATE 3

Kaposi's sarcoma on the leg. The lesion is reddish brown because of its vascular nature and accompanying hemosiderin deposition.

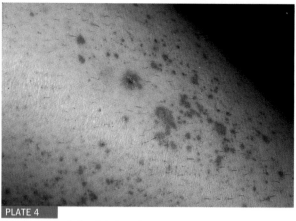

PLATE 4

Palpable purpura is the clinical correlate to small vessel vasculitis. The legs are a common location for this condition.

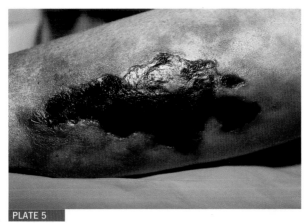

PLATE 5

Calciphylaxis. Angulated black eschar with surrounding livedo. Note the bullous change at the inferior edge of the eschar. Cholesterol emboli may have a similar eschar and often involve the digits.

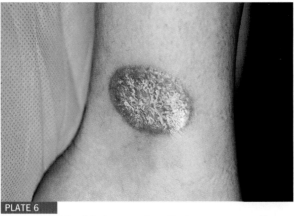

PLATE 6

Necrobiosis lipoidica diabeticorum on the ankle of a young woman with type 1 diabetes. Beneath the scale the skin has a yellowish hue and telangiectasia.

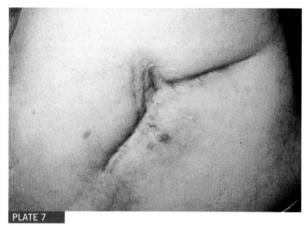

PLATE 7

Colon cancer metastatic to scar. Multiple erythematous nodules are present near the scar. *(Courtesy Ciro Martins, MD.)*

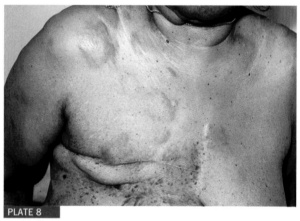

PLATE 8

Metastatic breast carcinoma. *(Courtesy Ciro Martins, MD.)*

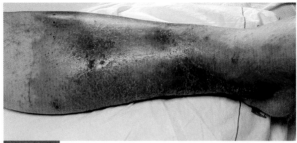

PLATE 9

Stasis dermatitis. Erythema of the lower extremity may mimic cellulitis, but chronic stasis changes (edema, varicosities, speckled brown discoloration of the skin from hemosiderin) are usually present in both lower extremities. *(Courtesy Bernard Cohen, MD, Dermatlas.com.)*

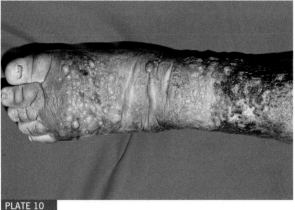

PLATE 10

Lymphedema verrucosa nostra. Diffuse, velvety thickening of the skin with nodules.

PLATE 11

Necrotizing fasciitis in a later stage with skin necrosis. In early stages the patient may have only pain, swelling, and erythema. *(From White G, Cox N. Diseases of the skin: a color atlas and text. London: Mosby; 2000.)*

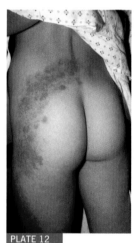

PLATE 12

Herpes zoster. Multiple vesicles are present singly and in clusters in a dermatomal distribution. *(Courtesy Bernard Cohen, MD/Dermatlas.com.)*

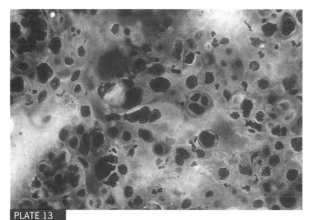

PLATE 13

Tzanck preparation demonstrating multinucleated giant cells in a patient with herpes zoster. Many of the cells with large, deeply purple nuclei are actually multinucleate; their nuclear borders are overlapping, yielding a darker appearance.

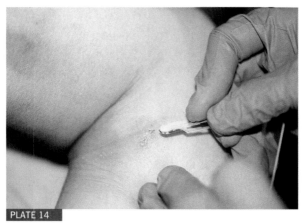

PLATE 14

Tzanck preparation. A no. 15 scalpel blade is used to reflect the blister roof and expose the base of the vesicle.

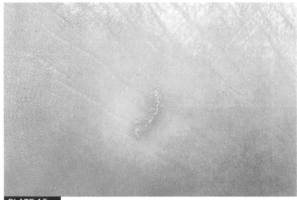

PLATE 15

Scabies burrow. Note the elevated ridge of skin, with mild surrounding erythema. A gray speck (scabies mite) may sometimes be observed at one end of the burrow. *(From White G, Cox N. Diseases of the skin: a color atlas and text. London: Mosby; 2000.)*

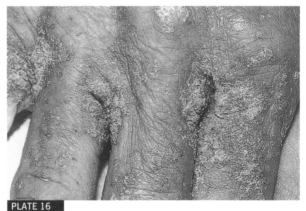

PLATE 16

Crusted scabies. The hyperkeratosis of the skin appears as a fine, sandy thickening, and scrapings demonstrate countless mites. *(From White G, Cox N. Diseases of the skin: a color atlas and text. London: Mosby; 2000.)*

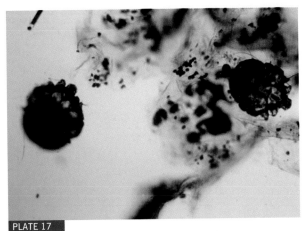

PLATE 17

Scabies scraping. A mite and nearby ovum are demonstrated. *(Courtesy Bernard Cohen, MD/Dermatlas.com.)*

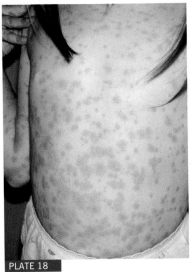

PLATE 18

Morbilliform eruption caused by Augmentin.
(Courtesy Bernard Cohen, MD/Dermatlas.com.)

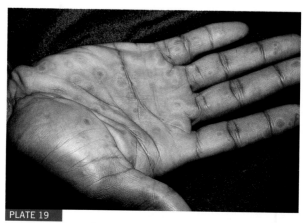

PLATE 19

Erythema multiforme. The classic lesions are erythematous targetoid lesions on the palms and soles. *(From Johns Hopkins Dermatology Residents Teaching Set.)*

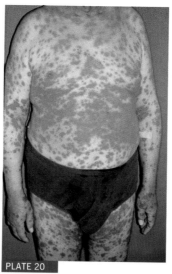

PLATE 20

Erythema multiforme. Diffuse truncal involvement. *(From Johns Hopkins Dermatology Residents Teaching Set.)*

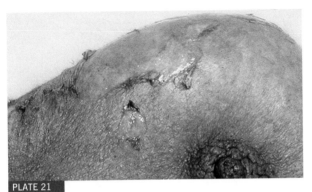

PLATE 21

Toxic epidermal necrolysis. The skin is erythematous and easily denuded.

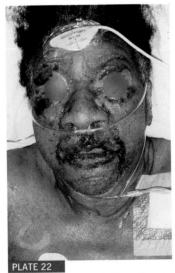

PLATE 22

Toxic epidermal necrolysis. Mucosal erosions involve the mouth, nose, and eyes.

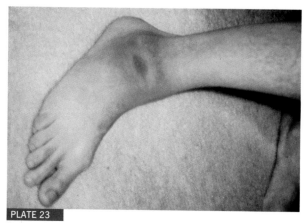

PLATE 23

Brown recluse spider bite. Early changes include a targetoid erythema with mild swelling of the joint.

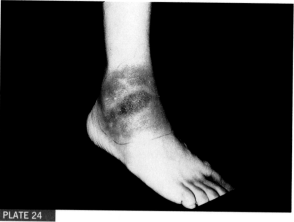

PLATE 24

Brown recluse spider bite. The same patient as in Plate 23, a few days later. The bite site is more purpuric, with more pronounced ankle swelling.

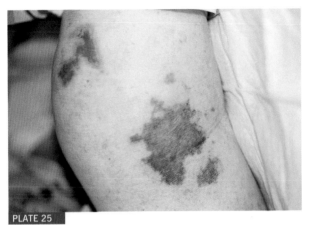

PLATE 25

Antiphospholipid antibody syndrome. This patient had an underlying myeloproliferative disorder.

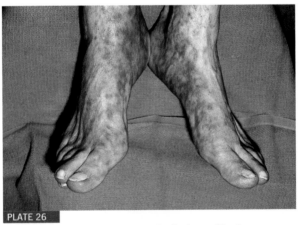

PLATE 26

Cholesterol emboli. Livedo is present on the distal extremities. In some patients these areas progress to necrosis. *(From Johns Hopkins Dermatology Residents Study Set.)*

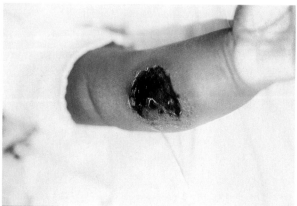

PLATE 27

Mucormycosis in an immunosuppressed infant. The geographical morphology of the eschar is a consequence of the vascular occlusion of the underlying vessel by fungus. This pattern may be seen in any vasoocclusive disorder (e.g., calciphylaxis, cholesterol emboli). *(Courtesy Bernard Cohen, MD/Dermatlas.com.)*

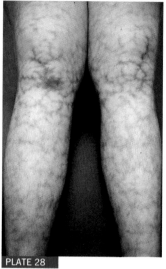

PLATE 28

Livedo reticularis. The classic fishnet pattern is demonstrated.

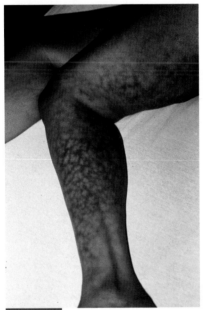

PLATE 29

Erythema ab igne. Although morphologically similar to livedo reticularis, the pattern is caused by the deposition of melanin and hemosiderin and is usually permanent. *(Courtesy Ciro Martins, MD.)*

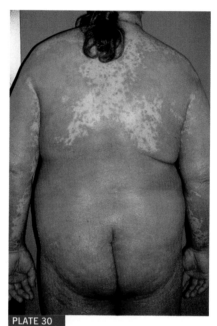

PLATE 30

Erythroderma from psoriasis. Clues in the clinical history (this patient had a history of classic plaque psoriasis) and examination may point to the correct diagnosis, but a biopsy is often necessary to make a definitive diagnosis.

Inpatient Dermatology

Keliegh S. Culpepper, MD, and Susan Laman, MD, MPH

FAST FACTS

- Definitive diagnosis of many cutaneous diseases requires evaluation and biopsy by a dermatologist.
- Many common systemic illnesses may have accompanying cutaneous manifestations (Table 19-1 and Plates 1 to 6).
- Incidence of cutaneous drug reactions is 1% to 3% and for certain drugs approaches 10%.[1]
- Cutaneous metastases occur in 10% of patients with metastatic cancer (Plates 7 and 8).[2]
- Patients with human immunodeficiency virus infection (HIV) have a higher incidence of cutaneous diseases and drug reactions than non-HIV-infected individuals.[3]

19

Infection

CELLULITIS

1. Cellulitis is an infection of the soft tissue of the skin, often of an extremity or operative site.

I. CLINICAL PRESENTATION

1. Cellulitis is usually painful, warm to touch, ill defined, and unilateral. Patients are often unaware of any antecedent trauma. Edema and bullae may form. When on the lower extremity, cellulitis may coexist with underlying venous disease consisting of edema, varicosities, and an ill-defined hyperpigmentation caused by hemosiderin deposition. Fever is present in 26% of patients, and 46% have leukocytosis.[4] Patients with multiple comorbidities may be at risk for necrotizing fasciitis (see later discussion).

II. DIAGNOSTICS

1. Erysipelas is a sharply demarcated, bright red, superficial streptococcal infection that may progress to cellulitis. Antibiotics to cover *Streptococcus* spp. are indicated.
2. Stasis dermatitis is frequently misdiagnosed as cellulitis. Patients have venous disease. Erythema (Plate 9) is present, and pruritus may be severe. There are no systemic manifestations, and pain is not a feature. Stasis dermatitis is often bilateral, in contrast to cellulitis. Risk of venous stasis increases in patients with a history of leg trauma or surgery; therefore stasis dermatitis may be unilateral. Topical steroids and prescription compression stockings are indicated.

TABLE 19-1

COMMON CUTANEOUS MANIFESTATIONS OF INTERNAL DISEASE

Disease	Cutaneous Manifestations
Human immunodeficiency virus infection	Prurigo nodules (Plate 1), ichthyosis (Plate 2), seborrheic dermatitis, psoriasis, herpes simplex virus, condyloma, histoplasmosis, cryptococcosis, Kaposi's sarcoma (Plate 3)
Hepatitis C	Porphyria cutanea tarda, erythema nodosum, leukocytoclastic vasculitis (Plate 4), cryoglobulinemia, polyarteritis nodosa, and possibly lichen planus
Hepatitis B	Polyarteritis nodosa, leukocytoclastic vasculitis (Plate 4), cryoglobulinemia, serum sickness reaction with urticaria
Chronic liver disease	Striae, spider "nevi," gynecomastia (men), acne, localized scleroderma
Renal failure	Pseudoporphyria, calcinosis cutis, calciphylaxis (Plate 5), pruritus, perforating disorders
Endocarditis	Splinter hemorrhages, conjunctival hemorrhages, Osler nodes, Janeway lesions
Diabetes	Acanthosis nigricans, diabetic bullae, necrobiosis lipoidica diabeticorum (Plate 6), eruptive xanthoma

3. Contact or irritant dermatitis is caused by topical products such as antibiotic preparations, steroids, or emollients. Contact dermatitis can mimic cellulitis, usually without associated systemic symptoms. Discontinuation of all topical products and dermatology consultation are indicated. Topical steroids may be helpful but may also contain the contactant.

4. Lymphedema verrucosa nostra is a slowly progressive condition characterized by woody edema, hyperkeratosis, and verrucous nodules (Plate 10). Classic venous stasis is not a feature, since the primary insufficiency is lymphatic, not venous.

III. MANAGEMENT

1. Treatment is generally oral or intravenous (IV) antibiotics to cover *Staphylococcus* spp. or *Streptococcus* spp. (see Chapter 47).

NECROTIZING FASCIITIS

1. Necrotizing fasciitis is a rapidly progressive infection of the subcutaneous and fascial layers. It is commonly caused by group A *Streptococcus* or may be a mixed infection.

I. CLINICAL PRESENTATION

1. Patients may be of any age and often have an underlying condition such as vascular disease, alcoholism, diabetes, injection drug use, or an immunocompromised state. Patients are quite ill with fever, leukocytosis, tachycardia, and anemia.[5] They may have a history of minor antecedent trauma or recent surgery.

2. Although the limbs are a common site, necrotizing fasciitis may occur

on the perineum (Fournier's gangrene), face, or abdomen. The involved area is an ill-defined painful region of woody edema and erythema that may change to a dusky hue over days. Vesicles and bullae may develop. Skin crepitance suggests presence of a gas-forming organism such as *Clostridium*. Anesthesia occurs if cutaneous sensory nerves are damaged. At later stages skin over involved areas may progress to necrosis (Plate 11) and may slough (in contrast to cellulitis).

II. DIAGNOSTICS AND MANAGEMENT

1. *Necrotizing fasciitis requires immediate surgical treatment and cannot be treated with antibiotics alone.* Biopsies performed by dermatologists at the bedside are not deep or large enough to assist with diagnosis. General surgeons can obtain deep specimens at the bedside to send for frozen section analysis or can evaluate for necrosis via a deep incision along the fascial plane ("finger test").[6]
2. Ultrasound, computed tomography, and magnetic resonance imaging have been shown to be helpful with diagnosis,[7] but if immediate imaging is not available, surgical intervention should not be delayed. Treatment with broad-spectrum antibiotics should begin promptly while a surgery consultation is requested.
3. If a toxin-producing organism is suspected, clindamycin may be added to decrease synthesis of toxins. Hemodynamic support and cultures of blood and surgical specimens are also indicated.

HERPES ZOSTER

1. Herpes zoster is reactivation of the varicella-zoster virus in the ganglion. It spreads along the sensory nerve and thus has a dermatomal distribution.

I. CLINICAL PRESENTATION

1. Herpes zoster usually begins with pain or paresthesia and can mimic internal causes of pain such as a myocardial infarction or gastrointestinal pain. After a few days vesicles arise. These are small vesicles in clusters on an erythematous base. They may coalesce into larger vesicles. After several days they may turn into pustules that become crusted over. The hallmark is the dermatomal distribution. The most common sites are the face and the lower thoracic and lumbar regions (Plate 12).

II. DIAGNOSTICS

1. Herpes zoster is a clinical diagnosis, but dermatologists can use a Tzanck preparation to look for giant cells (multinucleated keratinocytes; Plate 13). Alternatively, the clinician may use a no. 15 scalpel blade to reflect the roof of the blister (Plate 14), scrape the base of a vesicle, and gently smear it on a slide. The slide is then submitted to the microbiology laboratory for evaluation. The presence of multinu-

cleated keratinocytes does not establish a diagnosis of herpes zoster. A positive Tzanck preparation is also seen with herpes simplex infections. A culture or direct fluorescent antibody test can differentiate between varicella-zoster and herpes simplex.

2. Culture specimens from intact vesicles should also be obtained by reflecting the blister roof and swirling the culture swab on the base. Special viral culture medium is required. Typically, if patient does not experience discomfort from the swabbing, the specimen may not have enough material and may yield a false-negative culture.

III. MANAGEMENT

1. Treatment should be initiated as soon as possible (Table 19-2). Valacyclovir and famciclovir are given three times a day, which is more convenient than the five times a day dosage of acyclovir. In immunocompetent patients valacyclovir and famciclovir are equivalent in reducing postherpetic neuralgia and zoster-related pain.[8] The benefit of systemic steroids is controversial, and they are currently not recommended.[9]

Infestation

SCABIES

1. Scabies is infestation of the skin with the *Sarcoptes scabiei* mite.

I. CLINICAL PRESENTATION

1. In common scabies, transmission is from human to human and requires close physical contact. Pruritus is present and is often worse at night. Burrows (linear 4-mm red welts with a gray speck at the end, which may be seen with the unassisted eye; Plate 15) and inflammatory papules may be found in the web spaces, lateral hands and feet, volar wrists, elbows, axillae, genitalia, areolae, and umbilicus.

TABLE 19-2
TREATMENT RECOMMENDATIONS FOR HERPES ZOSTER INFECTION

Immunocompetence of Patient	Valacyclovir	Famciclovir	Acyclovir
Immunocompetent	1 g PO tid × 7 days	500 mg PO tid × 7 days	800 mg PO 5 times a day × 7 days
Immunocompromised, dermatomal (excluding V_1 distribution)*		500 mg PO tid × 10 days	800 mg PO 5 times a day × 10 days
Immunocompromised involving V_1 or disseminated			5-10 mg/kg IV q8h

*Data from Tyring S et al: Cancer Invest 2001; 19(1):26.

2. Immunocompetent individuals may have only a few mites, which often makes definitive diagnosis difficult.
3. Norwegian or crusted scabies (Plate 16) occurs in immunocompromised or physically or mentally debilitated patients. It is often misdiagnosed as psoriasis. A sand-colored hyperkeratosis is present on the skin. The hands and feet demonstrate hyperkeratosis and nail deformity. Itch may not be a prominent feature.
4. Transmission occurs easily in this variant because thousands of mites are on the patient and mites are also present in fomites, bedclothes, and the patient's room.

II. DIAGNOSTICS

1. Diagnosis is often difficult in common scabies. Skin scrapings are evaluated in mineral oil under the microscope. The clinician uses a no. 15 blade dipped in mineral oil to scrape burrows vigorously and then smears the scrapings gently on a glass slide for microscopy. Identification of mites, ova, or feces is diagnostic (Plate 17). If mineral oil is not readily available, a clear liquid soap may be substituted.
2. Norwegian or crusted scabies is easy to diagnose because of the large number of mites and distinctive clinical appearance (Table 19-3).

19

INPATIENT DERMATOLOGY

TABLE 19-3

FEATURES OF COMMON SCABIES VERSUS NORWEGIAN SCABIES

	Common Scabies	Norwegian Scabies
Host	Immunocompetent adults, nursing home or mentally debilitated patients	Immunocompromised (human immunodeficiency virus, transplant, or malignancy), mentally or physically debilitated patients
Average number of mites per host	10	Thousands
Most common lesion sites	Burrows or inflammatory papules may occur on palms and soles, wrists, ankles, web spaces, penis, areolae, axillae, and waistline	Sandy hyperkeratosis over entire body; often misdiagnosed as psoriasis
Pruritus	May be mild or severe	Not present, or patients are unable to complain or scratch
Ease of transmission	Close personal contacts	Highly contagious via skin and fomite contact
Treatment	Permethrin, topical steroids, antihistamines	Permethrin; may need multiple treatments; consider ivermectin

III. MANAGEMENT

1. Nursing and support staff and household contacts should be treated. Family members and friends not living in the patient's household may be affected and should be contacted. If the patient lives in a chronic care facility, the institution should be notified that the patient has scabies. Patients with common scabies must be placed on contact precautions until 24 hours after the first treatment.

2. Patients with Norwegian scabies must have contact precautions maintained until 24 hours after the second treatment.[10]

3. Permethrin 5% cream (30 g per person per application) is applied to the entire body from the neck down and left on for 10 hours. This must be applied thoroughly, including axillae, genital area, and under every fingernail and toenail (which may harbor mites from scratching).

4. Patients with Norwegian scabies should have the permethrin applied to the face and scalp as well (avoiding the eyes and mouth). All linens must be changed after the first treatment. A second treatment 1 week later is recommended.

5. After the first treatment with a topical scabicide the patient may be given oral antihistamines (Box 19-1) and a midpotency topical steroid such as triamcinolone 0.1% cream may be applied twice a day to help with pruritus. Oral antibiotics may be necessary to treat any secondary infection from scratching. Pruritus may persist weeks to months after the scabies infection has been appropriately treated. If not all affected contacts are appropriately treated, reinfection with the mite may occur.

6. Patients with Norwegian scabies require multiple serial treatments with various scabicides, ivermectin, and possibly keratolytics. Ivermectin is an antiparasitic medication approved by the U.S. Food and Drug Administration for onchocerciasis. For scabies it is administered as a single dose of 200 to 400 μg/kg. The total number of doses and intervals required remain controversial, but ease of administration and few side effects make ivermectin logistically feasible.[11] For inpatients it may be most useful as adjunctive therapy in patients with Norwegian scabies. A dermatology consultation to assist with the treatment strategy may be helpful.

BOX 19-1

ANTIHISTAMINES COMMONLY USED IN DERMATOLOGY

SEDATING

Diphenhydramine 25-50 mg PO q 4-6h

Hydroxyzine 25-50 mg PO q 4-6h

NONSEDATING

Fexofenadine 60 mg PO bid or 180 mg PO qd

Loratadine 10 mg PO qd

Cetirizine 10 mg PO qd (somnolence affects 14%)

Drug Reactions

Medications cause myriad cutaneous reactions. The most common are discussed here.

MORBILLIFORM DRUG ERUPTION

1. Morbilliform drug eruption is the most common drug-induced eruption. Its resemblance to measles accounts for its name.

I. CLINICAL PRESENTATION

1. Erythematous macules and papules are present on the upper trunk and extremities (Plate 18) and may involve the palms and soles. They blanch with pressure and may become confluent.
2. Pruritus and fever are features, and in contrast to more severe drug reactions (see later discussion), skin pain is not present. The eruption develops within 7 to 14 days of beginning a medication and may persist for up to 2 weeks after the medication is discontinued. It does not progress to a more serious reaction. Antibiotics are typical offenders.

II. DIFFERENTIAL DIAGNOSTICS

1. The differential diagnosis includes measles, viral exanthem, folliculitis, miliaria, disseminated candidiasis, graft versus host disease, and Rocky Mountain spotted fever.

III. MANAGEMENT

1. Class II or III topical steroids and oral antihistamines (Box 19-1) are helpful. The best course of action with respect to the offending drug is to discontinue it.

ERYTHEMA MULTIFORME AND STEVENS-JOHNSON SYNDROME

I. CLINICAL PRESENTATION

1. The mild form (erythema multiforme minor) has localized cutaneous involvement that is usually acral. The patient has erythematous, annular or targetoid macules that may itch. Mucous membrane involvement is limited to one site, often the mouth. The eruption is self-limited. Although this minor form may be drug related, patients who have recurrent episodes usually have a history of recurrent herpes simplex virus (HSV) infections. The HSV outbreak predates or is concurrent with the eruption.[12]
2. Stevens-Johnson syndrome (SJS; also called erythema multiforme major) is the more severe form. Erythematous targetoid macules and patches can form bullae (Plate 19) and may coalesce, leading to widespread cutaneous involvement (Plate 20). Patients may complain of pain or burning. Subsequently the skin sloughs. Gentle pressure on a bulla or erythematous skin may cause sloughing (Nikolsky's sign). In contrast to erythema multiforme minor, SJS

BOX 19-2

SOME CAUSES OF ERYTHEMA MULTIFORME AND STEVENS-JOHNSON
SYNDROME

MEDICATIONS

Sulfonamides

Penicillin

Nonsteroidal antiinflammatory drugs

Phenytoin

Allopurinol

Other antibiotics

INFECTIONS

Herpes simplex virus

Mycoplasmal pneumonia[13]

Hepatitis C[14]

Histoplasmosis[15,16]

Epstein-Barr virus[17]

Adenovirus

---

affects two or more mucous membrane areas (eyes, mouth, or
genitalia).

3. Differentiation between SJS and toxic epidermal necrolysis (TEN)
   is difficult in severe cases. The dermatology literature is fraught
   with controversy regarding the exact classification of TEN and SJS.
   In many instances the two conditions are regarded together to
   simplify the matter, since the approach to management is the same
   for both.

4. Numerous medications or infections, some of which are listed in
   Box 19-2,[13-17] cause SJS.

II. DIAGNOSTICS

1. As the name "multiforme" implies, the clinical presentation varies. If
   the diagnosis is in doubt, a dermatology consultation to evaluate the
   need for biopsy may be valuable.

III. MANAGEMENT

1. Erythema multiforme minor is self-limited. Suppressive treatment of
   HSV infection with antiviral medications may prevent future outbreaks.
   Topical steroids may relieve local symptoms. Viscous lidocaine can
   alleviate discomfort from oral erosions.

2. Treatment of SJS includes identification and treatment of the
   underlying infection or discontinuation of a suspected medication.
   Other interventions are discussed in the treatment section of the
   following discussion of TEN.

TOXIC EPIDERMAL NECROLYSIS

I. CLINICAL PRESENTATION

1. TEN is a rapidly progressive, widespread eruption with erythematous macules that develop vesicles and bullae. These coalesce, and the skin sloughs in large sheets (Plate 21). Patients may complain about burning or pain of skin and mucosal sites before clinical involvement.

2. Mucous membranes of the mouth, eyes, and anogenital area become denuded and have hemorrhagic crusting (Plate 22). Any part of the respiratory tree may be involved. Nikolsky's sign is present.

3. Microscopic examination reveals full-thickness epidermal necrosis.

II. DIAGNOSTICS

1. TEN is usually induced by medication. Common offenders are the same as for SJS, but TEN has also been associated with dozens of other medications.[18] Information about any nonprescription medications and supplements the patient may be taking (e.g., ibuprofen) must be elicited.

III. MANAGEMENT

1. The causative drug should be identified if possible and discontinued. Any unnecessary medications should also be discontinued. Potential underlying infection should be treated. Dermatology, ophthalmology, and nutrition consultation should be sought. Oxygenation and respiratory involvement are monitored, and a low threshold for the decision to transfer the patient to the intensive care unit or burn unit is appropriate. If a large body surface area is involved, transfer to a burn unit should be considered because delay in such a transfer is associated with higher mortality.[19]

2. Prophylactic antibiotic treatment, avoiding the use of high-risk sensitizers (e.g., sulfa-based drugs) should be instituted. Bedside suction to assist with secretions should be available. Sputum, blood, urine, and skin specimens are taken regularly for culture. Serum electrolyte levels and urine output are monitored.

3. Foley catheterization is usually unnecessary, and use of central lines should be avoided if possible. Wounds may be dressed with silver-coated dressings (e.g., Acticoat) or a nonstick wound dressing (e.g., Xeroform gauze). Any skin débridement should be postponed until disease progression has stopped.

Tissue Necrosis

I. CLINICAL PRESENTATION

1. Tissue necrosis is a hemorrhagic infarction of the skin with many possible causes. Large ecchymoses with geographical (angulated) borders develop. Diagnosis is based on clinical appearance, although

19

INPATIENT DERMATOLOGY

the history and other systemic manifestations are helpful in elucidating the etiology.

2. Skin biopsy is helpful, but the results may take many days. Treatment should not be delayed unnecessarily.

II. DIAGNOSTICS

1. Skin necrosis has numerous causes, some of which are discussed in the following sections. Other conditions to consider include disseminated intravascular coagulation, cryoglobulinemia, anticoagulant-induced skin necrosis, spider bite (Plates 23 and 24), and antiphospholipid antibody syndrome (Plate 25).

CALCIPHYLAXIS

1. Calciphylaxis is painful retiform purpura with histological evidence of calcium deposition in small and medium-sized cutaneous vessels, as well as superficial vascular thrombosis.

I. CLINICAL PRESENTATION

1. Tender induration of the skin progresses to ulcers and eschars (Fig. 19-5), which may become very large. The surrounding skin may appear livedoid. Occasionally calcification is seen on plain film x-ray examination.

2. Calciphylaxis usually affects the abdomen or legs. It most often occurs in patients with end-stage renal disease who are receiving dialysis (hemodialysis more commonly than peritoneal) and who in many cases have secondary hyperparathyroidism. Calciphylaxis has also been reported in patients with a decrease in functional protein C,[20] primary hyperparathyroidism in the absence of renal disease,[21] and metastatic breast cancer.[22]

II. DIAGNOSTICS

1. The list of differential diagnoses includes hyperoxaluria,[23] vasculitis, anticoagulant-induced skin necrosis, disseminated intravascular coagulation, antiphospholipid antibody syndrome (Plate 25), cholesterol emboli (Plate 26), and deep fungal infection (Plate 27).

III. MANAGEMENT

1. Patients with calciphylaxis generally have a poor prognosis and commonly die from sepsis. A dermatology consultation is needed to evaluate for biopsy.

2. Calcium and phosphate imbalance should be corrected.[24] Subtotal parathyroidectomy may be beneficial[25] and should be considered. Hyperbaric oxygen treatment has been used for patients without underlying hyperparathyroidism.[26]

3. If the functional protein C level is abnormal, a hematology consultation should be considered.

CHOLESTEROL EMBOLI

1. Unstable atherosclerotic plaques embolize to skin and other organs.

I. CLINICAL PRESENTATION

1. Patients have a history of atherosclerotic disease. Thrombolytic agents and anticoagulants can destabilize plaques, which then embolize. A frequent scenario is the discovery of purpuric lesions on the legs and feet after cardiac catheterization (Plate 26).
2. Livedo reticularis (Plate 28) is the presenting finding in 50% of patients[27] and may be elicited by having the patient stand.[28] Lesions may progress to ulceration and gangrene.

II. MANAGEMENT

1. The patient should be evaluated for manifestations of systemic embolization (neural, renal, gastrointestinal, and ocular). Hypertension and hyperlipidemia should be controlled.
2. The use of anticoagulants is controversial because they are a cause of cholesterol emboli. Oral corticosteroids may be of benefit.[29] Aggressive local wound care is necessary for ulcerations.

DEEP FUNGAL INFECTIONS

I. CLINICAL PRESENTATION

1. Immunocompromised patients may be at risk for fungal infections, most commonly aspergillosis or mucormycosis. The organisms may spread hematogenously and occlude vessels, causing secondary infarction and ulceration with eschar formation (Plate 27). Localized infection may occur at sites of occlusion, such as intravenous catheters,[30] and from penetrating trauma.
2. Mucormycosis also causes ulceronecrotic lesions of the central face among patients with insulin-dependent diabetes, particularly those with ketoacidosis (see Chapter 22). Skin biopsy and culture are necessary for diagnosis.
3. Disseminated candidiasis may lead to skin lesions, as may other fungal infections such as cryptococcosis and histoplasmosis.

VASCULITIS

I. CLINICAL PRESENTATION

1. The cutaneous manifestations of vasculitis vary with the size of the vessel involved. Vessels of various sizes may be involved concurrently, resulting in a mixed presentation. Small vessel vasculitis is characterized by purpura and palpable purpura. Examples include Henoch-Schoenlein purpura (Plate 4) and cryoglobulinemia.
2. Vasculitis of medium-sized vessels may manifest itself as livedo

reticularis (Plate 28), tender inflammatory nodules, ulcers, or digital infarcts. Diagnoses to consider include Wegener's granulomatosis, Churg-Strauss syndrome, polyarteritis nodosa, or a connective tissue disease such as lupus erythematosus or rheumatoid arthritis. Behçet's disease should also be considered, since it may involve vessels of any size.

II. DIAGNOSTICS

1. A thorough history and physical examination are required, with special attention to possible underlying viral hepatitis, connective tissue or rheumatic diseases, and recent bacterial infections. A dermatology consultation should be obtained to evaluate the need for skin biopsy. A rheumatology consultation may be necessary.
2. Laboratory testing should be based on the history and physical examination and may include serological tests for cryoglobulins, rheumatoid factor, antinuclear antibodies, complement, and hepatitis.

Livedo Reticularis

I. CLINICAL PRESENTATION

1. Livedo reticularis (Plate 28) is a clinical finding that has myriad underlying causes (Box 19-3), some of which represent medical urgencies.[31]
2. Erythema ab igne (Plate 29) mimics livedo reticularis. Chronic thermal damage to the skin produces a marbled pigmentation of the skin. Radiators and heating pads are common causes.

Erythroderma

I. CLINICAL PRESENTATION

1. Erythroderma is a cutaneous reaction pattern common to many skin conditions (Box 19-4), although often the underlying cause is not found.[32] Patients have inflammation of more than 90% of their skin.

BOX 19-3

COMMON CAUSES OF LIVEDO RETICULARIS

Cutis marmorata (physiological livedo)
Polyarteritis nodosa
Connective tissue disease–associated vasculitis
Antiphospholipid antibody syndrome
Sneddon's syndrome
Calciphylaxis
Hyperoxaluria
Cholesterol emboli
Disseminated intravascular coagulation

Scaling, weeping, and fissuring may be present. Honey-colored crusting may indicate secondary impetiginization.

2. Erythroderma increases cardiac output, and this may exacerbate underlying cardiac disease. Patients may be hypothermic or have electrolyte abnormalities. Discomfort may limit mobility.

3. Most cases of erythroderma are subacute. Acute onset of erythroderma should prompt consideration of scarlet fever, toxic epidermal necrolysis, scalded skin syndrome (staphylococcus or streptococcus associated), sunburn, graft versus host disease, or drug reaction. Usually a little scale is found on the skin in these conditions because the onset of erythroderma is acute.

II. DIAGNOSTICS

1. The history may reveal a preexisting condition, such as psoriasis (Plate 30), or a causative medication. A dermatology consultation is necessary to evaluate the need for biopsy and treatment.

III. MANAGEMENT

1. Treatment is tailored to the underlying condition. Antibiotic treatment of bacterial superinfection should be administered. Hypothermia and fluid-electrolyte imbalance should be corrected.

2. Patients at risk for cardiac compromise should be evaluated. Midpotency topical steroids may alleviate symptoms, but definitive diagnosis is necessary to target the appropriate treatment.

PEARLS AND PITFALLS

- Herpes zoster.
  - Patients are contagious to those who have not been exposed to the varicella virus. They should be placed on contact precautions. Once the lesions are crusted over, the patients are no longer contagious, although universal precautions should still be observed.
  - Although cultures and a Tzanck preparation to look for multinucleated giant cells are helpful, this approach is generally not required if the clinical appearance is obvious. Treatment may therefore be initiated on the basis of clinical appearance alone.

19

INPATIENT DERMATOLOGY

BOX 19-4

SOME CAUSES OF ERYTHRODERMA

Drug reaction
Cutaneous T cell lymphoma or Sézary syndrome
Atopic dermatitis
Psoriasis
Seborrheic dermatitis
Ichthyosis
Contact dermatitis
Dermatomyositis
Paraneoplastic association with internal malignancy

- Patients who have more than 25 vesicles outside the primary affected dermatome may have disseminated zoster. Patients with disseminated zoster are generally immunocompromised. Investigation for HIV or underlying malignancy is warranted. These patients may also be at risk for visceral involvement and require IV treatment with acyclovir.
- If herpes zoster is on the face, the tip of the nose should be checked for vesicles. If they are found, an ophthalmology consultation is needed because the eye may be involved.
- Toxic epidermal necrolysis.
  - Rapidity of discontinuing the causative medication is related to improved survival.[33]
  - Treatment with steroids is controversial and is not indicated.
  - Prompt treatment with IV immunoglobulin may be of benefit.[34,35] Discuss with a dermatology consultant.
- Useful websites.
  - www.dermatlas.com. An excellent resource for clinical images.
  - www.eMedicine.com/derm. A good resource for further diagnostic and treatment related information. Some photos are included at the end of the topics.
  - www.telemedicine.org/stamfor1.htm. Online dermatology textbook.

REFERENCES

[c] 1. Svensson CK, Cowen EW, Gaspari AA. Cutaneous drug reactions. Pharmacol Rev 2001; 53(3):357.

[b] 2. Lookingbill D, Spangler N, Helm KF. Cutaneous metastases in patients with metastatic carcinoma: a retrospective study of 4020 patients. J Am Acad Dermatol 1993; 29:228.

[b] 3. Coopman SA et al. Cutaneous disease and drug reactions in HIV infection. N Engl J Med 1993; 328:1670.

[b] 4. Hook EW 3rd et al: Microbiologic evaluation of cutaneous cellulitis in adults. Arch Intern Med 1986; 146:295.

[c] 5. Mahan KT. Infectious diseases of the lower extremity. Baltimore: Williams & Wilkins; 1991.

[c] 6. Andreasen TJ, Green SD, Childers BJ. Massive infectious soft-tissue injury: diagnosis and management of necrotizing fasciitis and purpura fulminans. Plast Reconstr Surg 2001; 107(4):1025.

[c] 7. Struk DW et al. Imaging of soft tissue infections. Radiol Clin North Am 2001; 39(2):277.

[a] 8. Tyring SK et al. Antiviral therapy for herpes zoster: randomized, controlled clinical trial of Valacyclovir and famciclovir therapy in immunocompetent patients 50 years and older. Arch Fam Med 2000; 9:863.

[a] 9. Whitley RJ et al. Acyclovir with and without prednisone for the treatment of herpes zoster: a randomized, placebo-controlled trial. The National Institute of Allergy and Infectious Diseases Collaborative Antiviral Study Group. Ann Intern Med 1996; 125:376.

[b] 10. Obasanjo OO et al. An outbreak of scabies in a teaching hospital: lessons learned. Infect Control Hosp Epidemiol 2001; 22(1):13.

[b] 11. Meinking TL et al. The treatment of scabies with ivermectin. N Engl J Med 1995; 333(1):26.

[b] 12. Schofield JK, Tatnall FM, Leigh I M. Recurrent erythema multiforme: clinical features and treatment in a large series of patients. Br J Dermatol 1993; 128:542.

[c] 13. Tay YK et al: *Mycoplasma pneumoniae* infection is associated with Stevens-Johnson syndrome, not erythema multiforme (von Hebra). J Am Acad Dermatol 1996; 35:757.

[b] 14. Dumas V et al. Recurrent erythema multiforme and chronic hepatitis C: efficacy of interferon alpha. Br J Dermatol 2000: 142;1248.

[b] 15. Friedman SJ, Black JL, Duffy J. Histoplasmosis presenting as erythema multiforme and polyarthritis. Cutis 1984; 34:396.

[b] 16. Sellers TF et al: An epidemic of erythema multiforme and erythema nodosum caused by histoplasmosis. Ann Intern Med 1965; 62:1244.

[b] 17. Williamson DM: Erythema multiforme in infectious mononucleosis. Br J Dermatol 1974; 91:345.

[c] 18. Litt JZ. Drug eruption reference manual. New York: Parthenon; 1998.

[b] 19. McGee T, Munster A. Toxic epidermal necrolysis syndrome: mortality rate reduced with early referral to regional burn center. Plast Reconstr Surg 1998; 102(4):1018.

[b] 20. Mehta R et al. Skin necrosis associated with acquired protein C deficiency in patients with renal failure and calciphylaxis. Am J Med 1990; 88(3):252.

[b] 21. Winkelmann RK, Keating FR. Cutaneous vascular calcification, gangrene, and hyperparathyroidism. Br J Dermatol 1970; 83:263.

[b] 22. Mastruserio DN et al. Calciphylaxis associated with metastatic breast carcinoma. J Am Acad Dermatol 1999; 41:295.

[b] 23. Somach SC et al. Fatal cutaneous necrosis mimicking calciphylaxis in a patient with type 1 primary hyperoxaluria. Arch Dermatol 1995; 131(7):821.

[b] 24. Block GA. Prevalence and clinical consequences of elevated Ca x P product in hemodialysis patients. Clin Nephrol 2000; 54(4):318.

[b] 25. Girotto JA et al. Parathyroidectomy promotes wound healing and prolongs survival in patients with calciphylaxis from secondary hyperparathyroidism. Surgery 2001; 130(4):645.

[b] 26. Podymow T, Wherrett C, Burns KD. Hyperbaric oxygen in the treatment of calciphylaxis: a case series. Nephrol Dial Transplant 2001; 16 (11):2176.

[b] 27. Falanga V, Fine MJ, Kapoor WN. The cutaneous manifestations of cholesterol crystal embolization. Arch Dermatol 1986; 122(10):1194.

[b] 28. Sheehan MG, Condemi JJ, Rosenfeld SI. Position dependent livedo reticularis in cholesterol emboli syndrome. J Rheumatol 1993; 20(11):1973.

[b] 29. Mann SJ, Sos TA. Treatment of atheroembolization with corticosteroids. Am J Hypertens 2001; 14(8 Pt 1):831.

[b] 30. Allo MA et al. Primary cutaneous aspergillosis associated with Hickman intravenous catheters. N Engl J Med 1987; 317:1105.

[c] 31. Fleischer AB, Resnick SD. Livedo reticularis. Dermatol Clin 1990; 8:347.

[c] 32. Rothe MJ, Bialy TL, Grant-Kels JM. Erythroderma. Dermatol Clin 2000; 18:405.

[b] 33. Garcia-Duval I et al. Toxic epidermal necrolysis and Stevens-Johnson syndrome: does early withdrawal of causative drugs decrease the risk of death? Arch Dermatol 2000; 136:323.

[b] 34. Viard I et al. Inhibition of toxic epidermal necrolysis by blockade of CD95 with human intravenous immunoglobulin. Science 1998; 282:490.

[b] 35. Stella M et al. Toxic epidermal necrolysis treated with intravenous high-dose immunoglobulins: our experience. Dermatology 2001; 203:45.

19

INPATIENT DERMATOLOGY

Management of Chronic Wounds

Amanda M. Clark, RN, BSN, CWCN

FAST FACTS

- Normal healing should occur within 4 to 6 weeks. Wounds that do not heal in that time are considered chronic wounds and may require intervention of a specialist.
- Chronic wounds often have an underlying cause, such as pressure, vascular disease, infection, autoimmune disease, or diabetes.[1] Management of chronic wounds requires attention to the primary problem or cause of the wound, appropriate medical and surgical management, and local wound care.

20

I. EPIDEMIOLOGY

1. Most chronic wounds are a result of pressure, venous stasis, arterial insufficiency, or diabetic-neuropathic changes.

2. Pressure ulcers are a serious complication of chronic illness and hospitalization. A recent national benchmark survey of pressure ulcers determined that the incidence of pressure ulcers in acute care settings is approximately 7%.[2] Most of these ulcers developed on the sacrum and coccyx within a 5-day length of stay. Critical care patients have even higher occurrences of ulcers, with an incidence of 33% and a prevalence of 41%.

3. In the United States the total cost of pressure ulcer treatment has been estimated at $1.3 to $1.6 billion annually.[3] Incident pressure ulcers are associated with a hospital cost that is 2.7 times greater and a hospitalization that is 2.4 times longer than if no pressure ulcer developed.

4. Nosocomial infections and other complications are more likely to develop in patients with pressure ulcers.[4]

5. Venous stasis ulcers account for 70% to 90% of all lower extremity ulcers. An estimated 1% of the population has venous stasis ulcers.[5] These ulcers can remain for months to years and have a high rate of recurrence. The most difficult aspect of treating these ulcers is the lifestyle changes the patient must make to prevent recurrence.

6. Arterial ulcers comprise approximately 5% of lower extremity ulcers. Many of these patients have diabetes mellitus in addition to other atherogenic risk factors.

7. Of the 7.5 million U.S. residents who have diabetes, 30% have peripheral vascular disease and 15% have lower extremity ulcers.[6] These wounds are virtually impossible to heal unless arterial flow is restored to the affected limb.

8. Management of diabetic, also referred to as neuropathic, ulcers accounts

for nearly 25% of hospital days for the 11 to 16 million diabetic patients in the United States.[7]

9. Foot ulcers develop in 15% of patients with diabetes. Diabetic foot wounds account for 50% of all nontraumatic amputations in the United States.[8]

II. CLINICAL PRESENTATION AND BASIC WOUND ASSESSMENT

A. APPEARANCE

1. These macroscopic indices apply to all wounds, regardless of origin.
2. Color (red/yellow/black system).[9] If more than one color is present, treat for the least healthy color.
a. Red wound base: Characteristic of the healthy wound. Granulation tissue is often described as beefy red and shiny.[10] Goals for wound care are gentle cleansing and dressings to protect the wound and provide a moist wound environment.
b. Yellow wound base: Color may be deep yellow or brown to creamy white. Yellow covering is unhealthy and composed of devitalized tissue, fibrin slough, or purulent exudate. Goals for wound care are aggressive cleansing and débridement of devitalized tissue.
c. Black wound base: Indicative of necrotic wound base. Eschar may be moist or dry. Dry eschar is often indicative of ischemia. The goal for wound care is débridement except in the presence of ischemia.
3. **Exudate:** Note volume, color, odor, and consistency. Some bacteria have a characteristic odor and color. For example, drainage from *Pseudomonas aeruginosa* has a characteristic blue-green color and sweet odor.[11] Extremely foul odor and purulent drainage can be suggestive of anaerobic infection.[9]
4. **Size, depth, and location:** Include the presence and direction of sinus tracts (also called tunnels), which can extend in any direction from the wound, or of undermining (destruction of tissue under wound margins, which creates a shelf).
5. **Surrounding skin:** Evaluate for presence of induration, fluctuance (may signal deeper tissue damage), maceration (may indicate failure of dressing to absorb exudate), or erythema.
6. **Presence of edema:** May be associated with venous insufficiency, inflammation, or infection.

B. HISTORY OF WOUND

1. Onset and duration.
2. Pain.
3. **Comorbidities of patient:** For example, diabetes, known venous or arterial insufficiency, autoimmune disease, malnutrition, incontinence.

C. PARTIAL- VERSUS FULL-THICKNESS ULCERS

1. Refers only to the level of skin injured, not to the type of tissue in the wound bed.
2. **Partial thickness:** Tissue loss is confined to the epidermis and part of the dermis. Healing occurs by epithelialization.

3. **Full thickness:** Tissue loss extends below the dermis and may include subcutaneous tissue, muscle, and bone. Healing occurs through the healing cascade and includes scar formation.[10]

III. COMMON TYPES OF CHRONIC WOUNDS

A. PRESSURE ULCERS

1. **Definition:** "A pressure ulcer is any lesion caused by unrelieved pressure resulting in damage of underlying tissue. Pressure ulcers usually occur over bony prominences and are graded or staged to classify the degree of tissue damage observed."[3]

2. **Pressure ulcer staging:** This system of wound classification refers only to pressure ulcers. It was accepted at a consensus conference of the National Pressure Ulcer Advisory Panel (NPUAP) in 1989 and adopted by the AHCPR in the Pressure Ulcer Guidelines of 1992 and 1994 (Fig. 20-1).[3]

a. A pressure ulcer cannot be staged accurately until the necrotic tissue is removed (Fig. 20-2).

b. Pressure ulcers cannot be "reverse-staged," since the stages are based on layers of tissue damage that can never be regenerated. That is, these wounds fill with granulation tissue, not the original tissue layers present, so a stage IV ulcer will never heal to become a stage III.

3. **Causes of pressure ulcers** (Fig. 20-3).

a. Pressure: Major cause of pressure ulcer formation, although many factors help determine whether pressure will create an ulcer. These include intensity of pressure, duration of pressure, and tissue tolerance. An inverse relationship exists between duration and intensity of pressure in causing ischemia. Tissue tolerance is the condition or integrity of skin and supporting structures that influences ability to redistribute the applied pressure.[13]

b. Shear, friction, and nutritional debilitation: Contributors to ulcer formation. Friction is the force of two surfaces moving across one another and by itself causes only superficial injury. Shear is the interplay of gravity and friction. It is the mechanical force by which bony structures move and accounts for tunnels and sinus tracts that occur on the overlying skin. Moisture is often considered the primary risk factor for pressure ulcer development, especially when secondary to fecal incontinence. Other contributing factors include advanced age, low blood pressure, psychosocial status, smoking, and increased body temperature.[13]

4. **Risk assessment and prevention.**

a. A pressure ulcer prevention program that uses a risk assessment scale should be implemented.[13] Interventions are designed to decrease the amount of pressure, friction, shear, and moisture and maximize nutritional status. This can be accomplished through proper positioning techniques and support surfaces, proper incontinence care and moisture control, and a nutritional program. At-risk patients should be turned every 2 hours while in bed and every hour while in a chair.[3]

20

MANAGEMENT OF CHRONIC WOUNDS

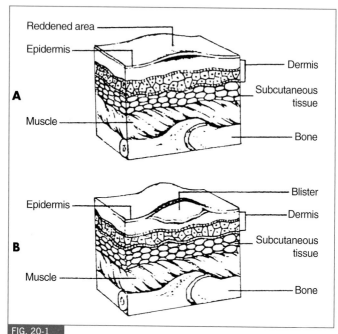

FIG. 20-1

A, Stage I. Observable pressure-related alteration of intact skin whose indicators as compared with the adjacent or opposite area on the body may include changes in one or more of the following: skin temperature (warmth or coolness), tissue consistency (firm or boggy feel), and sensation (pain, itching). The ulcer appears as a defined area of persistent redness in lightly pigmented skin, whereas in darker skin tones, the ulcer may appear with persistent red, blue, or purple hues. **B,** Stage II. Partial thickness skin loss involving epidermis or dermis. The ulcer is superficial and manifested clinically as an abrasion, blister, or shallow crater.

cont'd

b. Several instruments have been designed that use summative rating scales based on contributing factors and that specify critical scores to identify patients at risk.[13] Some examples are the Braden (Fig. 20-4), Norton, and Gosnell Scales.

5. Support surfaces.

a. To *heal* a pressure ulcer, relieve the pressure.

b. The goals of providing support surfaces are to increase the area of support; reduce moisture retention, heat accumulation, shearing, and pressure; promote dynamic (versus static) properties; and keep costs down.[3]

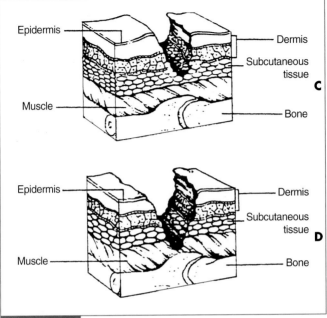

FIG. 20-1—cont'd

C, Stage III. Full-thickness skin loss involving damage or necrosis of subcutaneous tissue, which may extend down to, but not through, underlying fascia. The ulcer is manifested clinically as a deep crater with or without undermining of adjacent tissue. **D,** Stage IV. Full-thickness skin loss with extensive destruction, tissue necrosis, or damage to muscle, bone, or supporting structures (e.g., tendon or joint capsule). Tunneling and sinus tracts may also be associated with stage IV pressure ulcers. *(Drawings from Hess CT. Wound care: nurse's clinical guide. Springhouse, Pa: Springhouse; 1995. Text from National Pressure Ulcer Advisory Panel Consensus Conference 1998: Staging of pressure ulcers.)*

   c. The AHCPR recommends these criteria for selecting support surfaces.
     (1) Pressure-reducing surfaces for all patients at risk.
     (2) Static support if the patient can assume a variety of positions without bearing weight on the ulcer or "bottoming out" (i.e., compressing the mattress fully). Static support surfaces spread the load over a larger area through the use of foam, gel, water, or air.
     (3) Dynamic support if the patient cannot assume a variety of positions without placing weight on the ulcer, if the ulcer "bottoms out" on a static surface, or if the ulcer is not healing. Dynamic support sur-

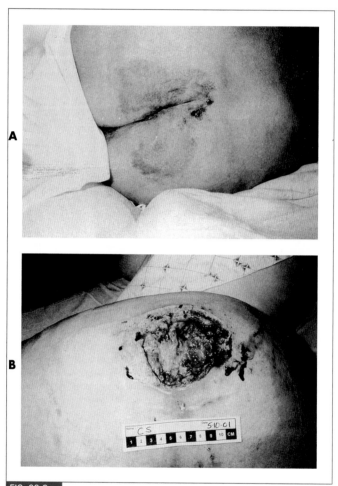

FIG. 20-2

Common types of wounds. **A,** Stage I pressure ulcer, indicative of deep tissue damage. **B,** Necrotic pressure ulcer of left ischium, which could not be staged before débridement.

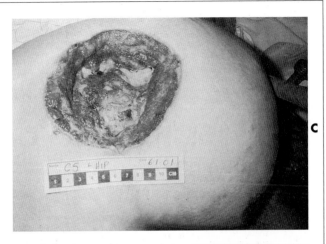

C

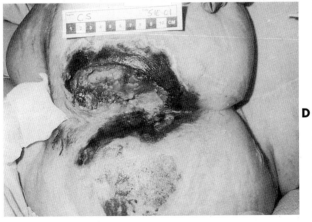

D

FIG. 20-2—cont'd

C, Stage IV pressure ulcer of left ischium after surgical débridement and 2 weeks of daily pulsatile lavage. **D,** Necrotic pressure ulcer of sacrum before surgical débridement. *cont'd*

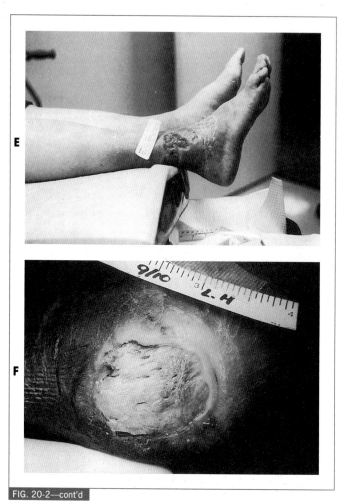

E, Venous stasis ulcer after initiation of compression therapy. F, Stage IV pressure ulcer of heel.

faces minimize static support by inflating and deflating an air-based support surface.

(4) Low air loss or air-fluidized therapy if the patient has large stage III or IV ulcers or multiple surfaces are affected.

d. Surfaces can be overlays (lie on top of standard hospital mattress), replacement mattresses (complete hospital mattresses with more pressure reduction than standard mattresses), or specialty mattresses (entire units used in place of the hospital bed).

e. Outdated methods such as "donuts," which increase intensity of pressure, and sheepskin, which is ineffective on pressure, should be avoided.

B. LOWER EXTREMITY ULCERS

1. These are caused by venous stasis, arterial insufficiency, and diabetic-neuropathic changes. See Table 20-1 for details.

IV. MANAGEMENT OPTIONS

A. GOALS OF TOPICAL THERAPY[14]

1. Remove necrotic tissue and foreign bodies, which prolong the inflammatory process and serve as a medium for bacterial growth.
2. Identify and eliminate infection.
3. Obliterate dead space, which can lead to abscesses and sinus tracts and acts as a fluid medium for bacteria.
4. Absorb excess exudates to protect surrounding skin from maceration.
5. Maintain a moist wound surface.
6. Provide thermal insulation to maintain normal tissue temperature, which improves blood flow to the wound and enhances epidermal migration.
7. Protect the healing wound from trauma and bacterial invasion.

B. MOIST WOUND HEALING

1. Moist wound healing is the mainstay of advanced wound care techniques.[14]
a. Maintains tissue hydration and temperature.
b. Prevents eschar and scab formation.
c. Promotes rapid epithelialization and contraction and decreases pain.
d. Autolysis softens necrotic debris.
e. Provides better vascular supply and maintenance of tissue viability to resist infection.
f. Causes a slightly acidotic pH (better because this is normal for tissue).
g. Permits growth factors to be functional.
h. "A dry wound is a dead wound."

C. TYPES OF DÉBRIDEMENT[14]

1. The wound must be free of necrotic tissue for healing to begin.
2. **Autolytic débridement:** The body's own white blood cells break down necrotic tissue. This can be accomplished with any moisture-retentive dressing and is a function of advanced wound care.
3. **Conservative sharp instrumental débridement:** Removal of loose

Text continued on p. 359

20

MANAGEMENT OF CHRONIC WOUNDS

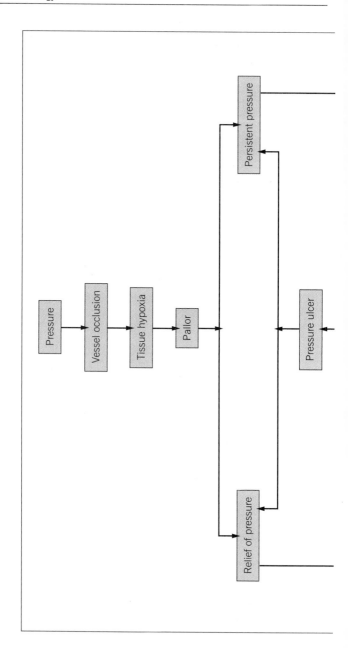

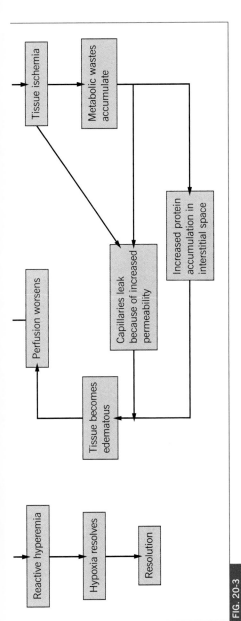

FIG. 20-3

Cellular response to pressure. *(From Bryant RA et al. Pressure ulcers. In Bryant RA. Acute and chronic wounds—nursing management. St Louis: Mosby; 1992.)*

20

MANAGEMENT OF CHRONIC WOUNDS

Braden Pressure Ulcer Risk Assessment[1]

Patient Name _____

Age _____ Address _____

Date _____

(Indicate appropriate numbers below)

NOTE: Bed- and chairbound individuals with impaired ability to reposition themselves should be assessed for risk of developing pressure ulcers.

Patients with established pressure ulcers should be reassessed periodically.

	1	2	3	4	
SENSORY PERCEPTION ability to respond meaningfully to pressure-related discomfort	**1. Completely Limited:** Unresponsive (does not moan, flinch, or grasp) to painful stimuli, due to diminished level of consciousness or sedation. OR limited ability to feel pain over most of body surface.	**2. Very Limited:** Responds only to painful stimuli. Cannot communicate discomfort except by moaning or restlessness. OR has a sensory impairment which limits the ability to feel pain or discomfort over 1/2 of body.	**3. Slightly Limited:** Responds to verbal commands, but cannot always communicate discomfort or need to be turned. OR has some sensory impairment which limits ability to feel pain or discomfort in 1 or 2 extremities.	**4. No Impairment:** Responds to verbal commands, has no sensory deficit which would limit ability to feel or voice pain or discomfort.	
MOISTURE degree to which skin is exposed to moisture	**1. Constantly Moist:** Skin is kept moist almost constantly by perspiration, urine, etc. Dampness is detected every time patient is moved or turned.	**2. Very Moist:** Skin is often, but not always, moist. Linen must be changed at least once a shift.	**3. Occasionally Moist:** Skin is occasionally moist, requiring an extra linen change approximately once a day.	**4. Rarely Moist:** Skin is usually dry, linen only requires changing at routine intervals.	
ACTIVITY degree of physical activity	**1. Bedfast:** Confined to bed.	**2. Chairfast:** Ability to walk severely limited or non-existent. Cannot bear own weight and/or must be assisted into chair or wheelchair.	**3. Walks Occasionally:** Walks occasionally during day, but for very short distances, with or without assistance. Spends majority of each shift in bed or chair.	**4. Walks Frequently:** Walks outside the room at least twice a day and inside room at least once every 2 hours during waking hours.	

	1. Completely Immobile: Does not make even slight changes in body or extremity position without assistance.	2. Very Limited: Makes occasional slight changes in body or extremity position but unable to make frequent or significant changes independently.	3. Slightly Limited: Makes frequent though slight changes in body or extremity position independently.	4. No Limitations: Makes major and frequent changes in position without assistance.	
MOBILITY ability to change and control body position					
NUTRITION usual food intake pattern	**1. Very Poor:** Never eats a complete meal. Rarely eats more than 1/3 of any food offered. Eats 2 servings or less of protein (meat or dairy products) per day. Takes fluids poorly. Does not take a liquid dietary supplement. OR is NPO and/or maintained on clear liquids or IV's for more than 5 days.	**2. Probably Inadequate:** Rarely eats a complete meal and generally eats only about 1/2 of any food offered. Protein intake includes only 3 servings of meat or dairy products per day. Occasionally will take a dietary supplement. OR receives less than optimum amount of liquid diet or tube feeding.	**3. Adequate:** Eats over half of most meals. Eats a total of 4 servings of protein (meat, dairy products) each day. Occasionally will refuse a meal, but will usually take a supplement if offered. OR is on a tube feeding or TPN regimen which probably meets most of nutritional needs.	**4. Excellent:** Eats most of every meal. Never refuses a meal. Usually eats a total of 4 or more servings of meat and dairy products. Occasionally eats between meals. Does not require supplementation.	
FRICTION AND SHEAR	**1. Problem:** Requires moderate to maximum assistance in moving. Complete lifting without sliding against sheets is impossible. Frequently slides down in bed or chair, requiring frequent repositioning with maximum assistance. Spasticity, contractures or agitation lead to almost constant friction.	**2. Potential Problem:** Moves feebly or requires minimum assistance. During a move skin probably slides to some extent against sheets, chair, restraints, or other devices. Maintains relatively good position in chair or bed most of the time but occasionally slides down.	**3. No Apparent Problem:** Moves in bed and in chair independently and has sufficient muscle strength to lift up completely during move. Maintains good position in bed or chair at all times.		

NOTE: Patients with a total score of 16 or less are considered to be at risk of developing pressure ulcers. (15 or 16 = low risk, 13 or 14 = moderate risk, 12 or less = high risk)

© 1988 Barbara Braden and Nancy Bergstrom. Reprinted with permission.
1. Braden BJ, Bergstrom N. Clinical utility of the Braden Scale for Predicting Pressure Sore Risk. *Decubitus.* 1989;2:44-51.

TOTAL SCORE:

FIG. 20-4

Braden pressure ulcer risk assessment. *(From Braden BJ, Bergstrom N. Decubitus 1989; 2:44.)*

MANAGEMENT OF CHRONIC WOUNDS **20**

TABLE 20-1

QUICK ASSESSMENT OF LEG ULCERS

	Venous Insufficiency (Stasis)	Arterial Insufficiency	Diabetic-Neuropathic
History	Previous deep venous thrombosis and varicosities	Diabetes	Diabetes
	Reduced mobility	Anemia	Spinal cord injury
	Obesity	Arthritis	Hansen's disease
	Vascular ulcers	Increased pain with activity or elevation	Relief of pain with ambulation
	Phlebitis	Cerebrovascular accident	Paresthesia of extremities
	Traumatic injury	Smoking	
	Congestive heart failure	Intermittent claudication	
	Orthopedic procedures	Traumatic injury to extremity	
	Pain reduced by elevation	Vascular procedures, surgeries	
		Hypertension	
		Hyperlipidemia	
		Arterial disease	
Location	Medial aspect of lower leg and ankle	Toe tips or web spaces	Plantar aspect of foot
	Superior to medial malleolus	Phalangeal heads around lateral malleolus	Metatarsal heads
		Areas exposed to pressure or repetitive trauma	Heels
			Altered pressure points and sites of painless trauma or repetitive stress

Appearance	Color: base ruddy Surrounding skin: erythema (venous dermatitis) or brown staining (hyperpigmentation) Depth: usually shallow Wound margins: irregular Exudate: moderate to heavy Edema: pitting or nonpitting; possible induration and cellulitis Skin temperature: normal; warm to touch Granulation tissue: frequently present Infection: less common	Color: base of wound, pale or pallid on elevation; dependent rubor Surrounding skin: shiny, taut, thin, dry, hair loss on lower extremities, atrophy of subcutaneous tissue Depth: deep Wound margins: even Exudate: minimal Edema: variable Skin temperature: decreased, cold Granulation tissue: rarely present Infection: frequent (signs may be subtle) Necrosis, eschar, gangrene may be present	Color: normal skin tones; trophic skin changes; fissuring and callus formation Depth: variable Wound margins: well defined Exudate: variable Edema: cellulitis, erythema, and induration common Skin temperature: warm Granulation tissue: frequently present Infection: frequent Necrotic tissue variable, gangrene uncommon Reflexes usually diminished Altered gait; orthopedic deformities common
Perfusion	Pain: minimal unless infected or desiccated Peripheral pulses: present and palpable Capillary refill: normal (<3 seconds)	Pain: intermittent claudication, resting, positional, nocturnal Peripheral pulses: absent or diminished Capillary refill: delayed (>3 seconds); ankle/brachial index <0.8	Pain: diminished sensitivity to touch; reduced response to pinprick (usually painless) Peripheral pulses: present and palpable Capillary refill: normal

Data from Clinical fact sheet: quick assessment of leg ulcers. www.wocn.org. Accessed on Jan. 31, 2003.

cont'd

MANAGEMENT OF CHRONIC WOUNDS 20

TABLE 20-1

QUICK ASSESSMENT OF LEG ULCERS—cont'd

	Venous Insufficiency (Stasis)	Arterial Insufficiency	Diabetic-Neuropathic
Treatment	Measures to improve venous return: surgical obliteration of damaged veins; elevation of legs; compression therapy to provide at least 30 mm Hg compression at ankle (options: short stretch bandages [e.g., Setopress, Surepress, Comprilan], therapeutic support stockings, Unna's boot, Profore four-layer wrap, compression pumps) Topical therapy: goals are to absorb exudate, maintain moist wound surface (e.g., alginate, foam, hydrocolloid dressings)	Measures to improve tissue perfusion: revascularization if possible; medications to improve red blood cell transit through narrowed vessels; lifestyle changes (no tobacco, no caffeine, no constrictive garments, avoidance of cold); hydration; measures to prevent trauma to tissues (appropriate footwear at *all times*) Topical therapy: dry uninfected necrotic wound: keep dry; dry infected wound: immediate referral for surgical débridement and aggressive antibiotic therapy; open wound: moist wound healing, nonocclusive dressings (e.g., solid hydrogels) or *cautious* use of occlusive dressings, aggressive treatment of any infection	Measures to eliminate trauma: pressure relief for heel ulcers; "offloading" for plantar ulcers (bed rest or contact casting or orthopedic shoes); appropriate footwear Tight glucose control Aggressive infection control (débridement of any necrotic tissue, orthopedic consultation for exposed bone, antibiotic coverage) Topical therapy: cautious use of occlusive dressings, dressing to absorb exudate and keep surface moist

Data from Clinical fact sheet: quick assessment of leg ulcers. www.wocn.org. Accessed on Jan. 31, 2003.

necrotic tissue may be done by a physician, nurse, or physical therapist who is properly trained and qualified. It is often adjunctive with hydrotherapy.

4. **Enzymatic débridement:** Use of enzyme ointment requires a prescription or physician's order. Most forms need a moist environment to be active, and saline gauze may be used to provide this. Eschar must be cross-hatched with a scalpel.

5. **Surgical débridement:** This is the most rapid and effective form of débridement. It converts a chronic wound to an acute wound when enough devitalized tissue is débrided to reveal a clean (bleeding) wound base. Disadvantages are greater cost and risks to patient from anesthesia.

6. **Mechanical débridement:** Mechanical débridement is performed with wound irrigation and hydrotherapy. A traditional "wet to dry" dressing also mechanically débrides but is nonselective for necrotic tissue.

7. **Pulsatile lavage:** Irrigation with concurrent suction cleanses wounds and promotes formation of granulation tissue. It is indicated in the presence of necrotic tissue, foreign material, excessive drainage, or chronic wounds that need a "jump start" to heal.

a. Whirlpool: The whirlpool is indicated for large wounds with heavy drainage and without undermining or tunneling. It is often used on extremities. The presence of appliances, such as central lines or ostomies, that would contraindicate soaking must be considered.

b. Stable eschar on extremity: Stable eschar should *not* be débrided if poor vascular supply, as with diabetes or arterial disease, is suspected. The goal of topical therapy is to keep the wound dry and prevent infection. Occlusive dressings are also contraindicated because of their ability to débride by autolysis.

D. **GUIDELINES FOR TOPICAL THERAPY** (Table 20-2)

1. Topical therapy is a continually changing field, and new products are introduced frequently. Table 20-2 gives examples of some commonly used product categories but is not all-inclusive.

2. Advanced wound care products achieve goals of greater patient comfort, cost effectiveness, and fewer nursing hours required. Saline gauze dressing can also be used but must be changed frequently enough to prevent drying of the wound and to absorb drainage.

PEARLS AND PITFALLS

- Management of chronic wounds requires attention to the primary problem or cause of the wound, appropriate medical and surgical management, and local wound care.
- Patients with pressure ulcers are more likely to have nosocomial infections and other complications.[4]
- All chronic wounds are contaminated, although not all are infected. A positive wound culture does not necessarily indicate infection, and a colonized wound can heal.[15]
- Obtaining swab specimens from wounds is a common method of determining the likelihood of infection but poses several limitations if not per-

20

MANAGEMENT OF CHRONIC WOUNDS

TABLE 20-2
GUIDELINES FOR TOPICAL THERAPY

	Red	Yellow	Black
Appearance	Red or pink wound with or without granulation tissue	Soft necrotic tissue, "slough," or thick tenacious exudate from creamy ivory to yellow green; pus, fibrous material, and cellular components may be present	Black, gray, or brown adherent necrotic tissue (eschar); pus, fibrous material and cellular components may be present
Goal	Protection (débridement not necessary)	Elimination of necrotic tissue	Elimination of necrotic tissue Débridement
Wound cleansing	Atraumatic gentle cleansing	Cleansing (débridement appropriate) Aggressive wound cleansing	Débridement depends on location and type of eschar
Shallow wound, stage I or II	**DRY WOUND** For fragile skin: nonadherent, impregnated dressing appropriate for fragile skin (i.e., Xeroform, Adaptic, Vaseline gauze); change bid and prn; may cover with secondary dressing Transparent film or hydrocolloid dressing (change as recommended by manufacturer, usually every 3-4 days and prn); may first apply a thin layer of hydrogel over wound surface for added moisture; not recommended for fragile skin Solid hydrogel sheet: cut to fit wound, apply cover dressing, change qod and prn **MOIST WOUND** Hydrocolloid: change every 3-5 days and prn	**DRY WOUND** Hydrocolloid dressing: change every 3-5 days and prn; may first apply a thin layer of hydrogel over wound surface; not recommended on fragile skin Enzymatic débridement cream: apply to necrotic wound bed and cover with saline gauze; expect increased drainage **MOIST WOUND** Calcium alginate or hydrofiber: change every 1-3 days or when strikethrough to secondary dressing occurs Enzymatic débriding cream: apply to necrotic wound base and cover with gauze; expect increased drainage Hydrocolloid: change every 2-5 days and prn; limited absorptive capacity	**TIPS OF EXTREMITY (FINGERS OR TOES)** Keep dry; open to air; allow to autolyse; monitor for signs of infection **HEELS** Relieve pressure to area and monitor changes If dry, hard, black eschar is present without drainage or erythema, leave dry If open, moist, or draining; hydrocolloid every 2-3 days or hydrogel-impregnated gauze every day **OTHER AREAS** If unsure of depth, sharp débridement as soon as possible to minimize infection risk

Polyurethane foam: apply to wound and secure with wrap bandage, change every 2-5 days and prn

MODERATELY TO HEAVILY EXUDATIVE WOUND

Calcium alginate or hydrofiber: change every 1-3 days and prn for strikethrough to secondary dressing

Foam: secure with wrap and change every 2-5 days and prn

DRY WOUND

Hydrogel-impregnated gauze with secondary dressing qd; may change every 3 days if secondary dressing is thin film or hydrocolloid

MOIST WOUND

Calcium alginate or hydrofiber packing; change every 1-3 days and prn for strikethrough to secondary dressing

Negative-pressure system

Deep wound, stage III or IV

DRY WOUND

Hydrogel with secondary dressing of gauze (change qd) or transparent film or hydrocolloid (change every 3 days)

Enzymatic débriding cream: apply to necrotic wound and cover with gauze packing; expect increased drainage

MOIST WOUND

Calcium alginate or hydrofiber: change every 1-3 days or prn for strikethrough to secondary dressing

Enzymatic débriding cream: apply to necrotic base and cover with gauze; expect increased drainage

Superficial eschar: film or hydrocolloid dressing over area may accelerate autolysis; change every 1-2 days to monitor eschar deterioration

MANAGEMENT OF CHRONIC WOUNDS

20

Modified from Johns Hopkins Hospital. Management of a patient requiring wound care. Appendix B. Guidelines for wound management. 2000.

formed correctly. Caution should be exercised in the interpretation of results from these sources.

- Antibiotics should be used only when clinical wound infection is present and should be administered systemically. Topical antimicrobials are not advocated for chronic wounds.[17]
- Wound must be free of necrotic tissue for healing to begin. Besides surgical débridement, other types include conservative sharp, enzymatic, autolytic, and mechanical débridement.
- Stable eschar on an extremity should *not* be débrided if poor vascular supply is suspected, as in diabetes or arterial disease. The goal of topical therapy is then to keep the wound dry and prevent infection.
- Referrals to consider.
  - Wound care nurse specialist: For recommendations regarding topical therapy and general patient care related to nonhealing wounds.
  - Plastic surgery: For extensive débridement of necrotic wounds or consideration of other surgical interventions, such as a flap or graft.
  - Vascular surgery: For evaluation of vascular flow in an arterial or diabetic ulcer and for bypass grafting to allow healing to occur.
  - Orthopedic surgery: For exposed bone in the wound bed and evaluation for amputation of a severely gangrenous extremity.
  - Podiatry: Can provide evaluation and surgery of foot and ankle as indicated, as well as specialized services for patients whose feet have impaired vascular supply, such as toenail care and diabetic ulcer care.
  - Physical therapy: For pulsatile lavage or whirlpool and conservative sharp débridement. Most physical therapy departments provide advanced wound care, such as compression therapy or electronic stimulation.

REFERENCES

[c] 1. Kane D, Krasner D. Wound healing and wound management. In Krasner D, Kane D. Chronic wound care, 2nd ed. Wayne, Pa: Health Management Publications; 1997.

[b] 2. Whittington K, Patrick M, Roberts J. A national study of pressure ulcer prevalence and incidence in acute care hospitals. J Wound Ostomy Continence Nurs 2000; 27:209.

[d] 3. Agency for Health Care Policy and Research. Treatment of pressure ulcers (Clinical Practice Guideline No. 15). Rockville, Md: AHCPR Public Health Service, US Department of Health and Human Services; 1994, AHCPR Pub. No. 95-0652.

[b] 4. Allman RM et al. Pressure ulcers, hospital complications, and disease severity: impact on hospital costs and length of stay. Adv Wound Care 1999; 12:22.

[c] 5. Baker SR et al. Epidemiology of chronic venous ulcers. Br J Surg 1991; 78:864.

[c] 6. Levin ME. The diabetic foot: pathophysiology, evaluation, treatment. In Levin ME, O'Neal LW. The diabetic foot, 4th ed. St Louis: Mosby; 1988.

[c] 7. Bild DE et al. Lower extremity amputation in people with diabetes: epidemiology and prevention. Diabetes Care 1989; 12:24.

[c] 8. Pecoraro RE, Reiber GE, Burgess EM. Pathways to diabetic limb amputation: basis for prevention. Diabetes Care 1990; 13:513.

[c] 9. Cuzzell J. The new RYB color code. Am J Nurs 1988; 88:1342.

[c] 10. Cooper DM. Wound assessment and evaluation of healing. In Bryant RA. Acute and chronic wounds, nursing management. St Louis: Mosby; 1992.

[c] 11. Mureebe LM, Morris DK. Wound infection: a physician's perspective. Ostomy Wound Manage 1998; 44:56.

[c] 13. Bryant RA et al. Pressure ulcers. In Bryant RA. Acute and chronic wounds—nursing management. St Louis: Mosby; 1992.

[c] 14. Doughty DB. Principles of wound healing and wound management. In Bryant RA. Acute and chronic wounds—nursing management. St Louis: Mosby; 1992.

[c] 15. Gilchrist B. Infection and culturing. In Krasner D, Kane D. Chronic wound care, 2nd ed. Wayne, Pa: Health Management Publications; 1997.

20

MANAGEMENT OF CHRONIC WOUNDS

Adrenal Insufficiency

Assil Saleh, MBBS, and Paul W. Ladenson, MD

Fast Facts

- In 1855 Thomas Addison first reported a syndrome of adrenal cortical destruction that today bears his name.
- Worldwide the most common cause of adrenal insufficiency (AI) is tuberculosis. In the United States the most common causes are auto-immune adrenal destruction in females and adrenoleukodystrophy in males. At least 90% of glandular function must be disrupted before clinical AI becomes evident.
- Up to 40% of critically ill patients in intensive care unit settings have AI.
- Primary AI results from direct destruction of the adrenal glands. Secondary AI is caused by derangement of the hypothalamic-pituitary-adrenal axis.
- Signs and symptoms of AI may be nonspecific and difficult to recognize, yet AI is potentially fatal if unrecognized and untreated. Death usually results from hypotension or cardiac arrhythmia caused by hyperkalemia.
- AI is suspected on the basis of nonspecific symptoms (e.g., weight loss, fatigue, nausea, vomiting, depression) and more specific findings (e.g., hypotension, hypoglycemia, hyponatremia, hyperkalemia, hyperpigmentation, peripheral eosinophilia).
- Glucocorticoid replacement is the mainstay of AI therapy. The goal is to use the smallest dose needed to relieve symptoms yet avoid steroid-related complications (e.g., weight gain, osteoporosis).

21

I. EPIDEMIOLOGY

1. In 1855, Thomas Addison first reported a condition caused by "failure of the suprarenal glands" and characterized by "languor, debility, and remarkable feebleness of the heart," a disorder now recognized as adrenal insufficiency (AI).[1]
2. AI may be primary (in conditions of direct destruction of the adrenal glands, such as Addison's disease) or secondary (caused by derangement of the hypothalamic-pituitary-adrenal axis, as occurs with long-term use of exogenous steroids). The acute presentation of AI is a medical emergency necessitating urgent diagnosis and therapy.
3. Tuberculosis is the leading cause of primary AI worldwide. This is not the case in the United States, where 70% to 90% of cases result from autoimmune destruction of the adrenal glands and only 7% to 20% from tuberculosis.[2,3]

4. Currently Addison's disease has an incidence in Western countries of about 5 to 6 cases per million people per year and a prevalence of 35 to 60 cases per million.[4,5] In adults the mean age at the time of diagnosis is 40.[6]

5. Autoimmune AI may occur alone or in conjunction with other endocrinopathies. Cases of the latter are termed polyglandular failure syndromes and develop in two general ways: type 1, which occurs in childhood and is associated with hypoparathyroidism and mucocutaneous candidiasis, and type 2, which occurs in adulthood and is associated with insulin-dependent diabetes mellitus, autoimmune thyroid disease, alopecia areata, and vitiligo.[7,8] In one series nearly half of patients in whom autoimmune Addison's disease was diagnosed were found to have another autoimmune condition.[2]

6. AI has been described as "the unforgiving master of nonspecificity and disguise" because of its multitude of possible clinical presentations.[9]

II. PATHOPHYSIOLOGY AND ETIOLOGY

1. The hypothalamic-pituitary-adrenal (HPA) axis is integral to a diverse range of body functions and is crucial for maintaining homeostasis, especially in response to unexpected stressors such as infection, injury, and hypotension. The hormonal end products of this axis are produced by the adrenal glands.

2. The adrenal cortex consists of three discrete layers: the outer zona glomerulosa, which secretes mineralocorticoids (principally aldosterone) and the underlying zona fasciculata and zona reticularis, which produce glucocorticoids, chiefly cortisol, as well as adrenal androgens. The inner adrenal medulla produces catecholamines, mainly epinephrine.

3. Destruction of adrenal cortical tissue results in primary AI, which becomes clinically apparent when greater than 90% of glandular function is lost.[10] In autoimmune adrenalitis this destruction is caused by cytotoxic lymphocytes, which generally spare the adrenal medulla.[11]

4. The principal hormone of the HPA axis, cortisol, is produced in a rhythmic and highly regulated fashion. Fig. 21-1 illustrates the circadian rhythm of cortisol secretion. The highest serum concentration occurs between 6 and 8 AM. Fig. 21-2 depicts the regulation of cortisol secretion and lists the major effects of cortisol on the body.

5. Only about 10% of circulating cortisol is free and physiologically active. The remaining 90% is bound to cortisol-binding globulin and thus is affected by factors that raise plasma levels of this globulin, such as estrogen therapy.[12] Inadequate cortisol is a source of significant morbidity and mortality, particularly in critically ill patients, and complete absence of cortisol production is lethal.[10] A diverse range of insults can cause AI. Representative examples are listed in Box 21-1.

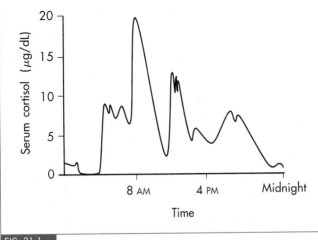

FIG. 21-1

Diurnal rhythm of cortisol secretion. *(Modified from Weitzman ED et al. J Endocrinol Metab 1971; 33:14.)*

III. CLINICAL PRESENTATION AND DIAGNOSTICS

1. AI may manifest itself in varying degrees of severity along a broad clinical continuum, ranging from mild constitutional symptoms elicited only with stress to frank hemodynamic collapse. Major clinical features of AI are listed in Box 21-2.
2. Definitive diagnosis of suspected AI consists of two steps: ascertaining whether cortisol production is adequate and localizing the culprit anatomical lesion. The relevant methods are presented in Figs. 21-3 and 21-4, respectively.

IV. MANAGEMENT[11,14-17]

A. MANAGEMENT OF SYMPTOMATIC CHRONIC ADRENAL INSUFFICIENCY

1. Glucocorticoid replacement is indicated for all patients with AI. The goal is to use the smallest dose needed to relieve symptoms yet avoid steroid-related complications (e.g., weight gain and osteoporosis).
a. Hydrocortisone 15 to 20 mg PO qam and 5 to 10 mg PO qpm (alternative glucocorticoid preparations may be used per the equivalency guide in Table 21-1.)
b. Follow clinical symptoms.
2. Mineralocorticoid replacement should be included for patients with primary AI only.
a. Fludrocortisone (Florinef) 100 μg PO qd (50 to 200 μg).

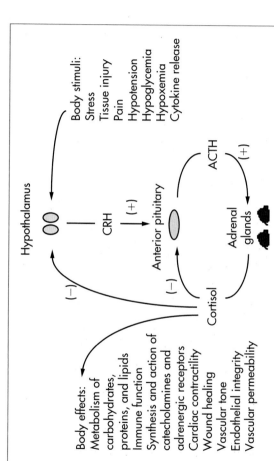

FIG. 21-2

Hypothalamic-pituitary-adrenal axis. Corticotropin-releasing hormone (CRH) and arginine vasopressin are produced by the hypothalamus in response to a variety of stimuli. CRH induces the anterior pituitary to release adrenocorticotropin (ACTH), which triggers cortisol secretion from the adrenal glands. Cortisol exerts a negative-feedback effect on the anterior pituitary and hypothalamus, inhibiting release of CRH and ACTH and thereby regulating its own secretion.

BOX 21-1

CAUSES OF ADRENAL INSUFFICIENCY

PRIMARY ADRENAL INSUFFICIENCY

Autoimmune
  Autoimmune adrenalitis (isolated or as part of type I and type II autoimmune
    polyglandular disease)
Infection
  Tuberculosis
  Fungal infections (e.g., histoplasmosis, cryptococcosis, blastomycosis)
  Human immunodeficiency virus related (e.g., cytomegalovirus, *Mycobacterium
    avium-intracellulare, Cryptococcus, Toxoplasma,* Kaposi's sarcoma)
Adrenal hemorrhage
  Waterhouse-Friderichsen syndrome
  Lupus anticoagulant, antiphospholipid antibodies
  Idiopathic thrombocytopenic purpura, heparin-induced thrombocytopenia
  Iatrogenic (e.g., anticoagulation)
Metastatic disease
  Particularly lung, breast, kidney, lymphoma, malignant melanoma
Infiltrative disease (e.g., hemachromatosis, amyloidosis)
Drugs
  Ketoconazole, etomidate, aminoglutethimide, metyrapone, mitotane (reduce
    steroid synthesis)
  Rifampin, dilantin, phenobarbital (increase steroid catabolism)
Familial
  Familial glucocorticoid deficiency
  Adrenoleukodystrophy and the milder variant adrenomyeloneuropathy (both
    usually inherited as an X-linked recessive trait)

SECONDARY ADRENAL INSUFFICIENCY

Cessation of prior glucocorticoid therapy
Pituitary and hypothalamic disorders
  Infiltrative tumor (adenoma, craniopharyngioma)
  Sarcoidosis, histiocytosis X
  Lymphocytic hypophysitis
  Hemorrhage
  Autoimmune destruction
  Empty-sella syndrome
  Postpartum pituitary necrosis (Sheehan's syndrome)
  Head trauma
Isolated adrenocorticotropic hormone deficiency
Surgery
  After transsphenoidal pituitary surgery
  Removal of functional adrenal adenoma

Data from Oelkers W. N Engl J Med 1996; 335:1206; and Werbel SS, Ober KP. Endocrinol Metab Clin North Am 1993; 22:303.

BOX 21-2
CLINICAL FEATURES OF ADRENAL INSUFFICIENCY

Both Primary and Secondary Adrenal Insufficiency

Fatigue, weakness

Depression, apathy, confusion

Anorexia, weight loss

Dizziness, orthostatic hypotension

Nausea, vomiting, diarrhea

Hypoglycemia, hyponatremia*

Mild normocytic anemia, lymphocytosis, eosinophilia

Primary Adrenal Insufficiency

Hyperpigmentation

Hyperkalemia

Vitiligo

Autoimmune thyroid disease

Central nervous system symptoms in adrenomyeloneuropathy (e.g., spastic paralysis)

Secondary Adrenal Insufficiency

Pallor without significant anemia

Amenorrhea, diminished libido, impotence

Reduced axillary and pubic hair

Small testes

Secondary hypothyroidism

Prepubertal growth deficit, delayed puberty

Headache, visual changes

Diabetes insipidus

Acute Adrenal Crisis

Dehydration, hypotension, shock (out of proportion to severity of current illness)

Abdominal pain (mimicking acute abdomen)

Unexplained hypoglycemia

Unexplained fever

Electrolyte derangements

Hyperpigmentation or vitiligo

Autoimmune endocrine deficiencies (e.g., hypothyroidism, gonadal failure)

Data from Oelkers W. N Engl J Med 1996; 335:1206; and Zaloga GP, Marik P. Crit Care Clin 2001; 17:25.

*Hyponatremia in primary adrenal insufficiency is a consequence of aldosterone deficiency and resultant sodium wasting; in secondary adrenal insufficiency it is a consequence of cortisol deficiency, vasopressin release, and water retention.[11]

b. Encourage salt and fluid intake.

c. Follow blood pressure, serum potassium level, and plasma renin level, with upper-normal range as the target.

3. Androgen replacement in women (may be needed in women to reduce malaise and sexual dysfunction).

a. Dehydroepiandrosterone (DHEA) 25 to 50 mg PO qd.

4. If a minor febrile illness or injury occurs in a patient being treated for AI, the glucocorticoid dosage should be increased by two to three times during the event. If the patient is also being treated with mineralocorticoids or androgens, the dosages of these agents should be maintained and not be increased.

5. Supplementation for surgical procedures (supplement on call to operating room and continue postoperatively with intermittent or continuous IV dose).

a. For most radiographic studies and minor procedures under local anesthesia, no supplementation is necessary.

b. For minor operations such as herniorrhaphy, administer hydrocortisone 25 mg IV with the induction of anesthesia, then resume usual oral doses.

c. For moderate surgeries such as cholecystectomy or joint replacement, hydrocortisone 50 to 75 mg IV qd should be given on call to the operating room and continued for 1 to 2 days postoperatively.

d. For major procedures such as coronary bypass, hydrocortisone 100 to 150 mg IV qd for 2 to 3 days. Taper as stress resolves.

6. Emergency precautions.

a. Supplementary ampules of glucocorticoid for self-injection (e.g., dexamethasone 4 mg IM) in case of vomiting should be given to all patients.

b. All patients should wear a Medic-Alert or similar warning bracelet.

B. EMERGENCY MANAGEMENT OF ACUTE ADRENAL INSUFFICIENCY (ADRENAL CRISIS)

1. Establish large-bore intravenous access.

2. Order and send for immediate assessment a basic metabolic panel plus routine plasma cortisol and adrenocorticotropic hormone (ACTH) levels. Continue therapy while laboratory work is being processed.

3. Infuse 2 to 3 L of 5% dextrose in normal saline as rapidly as can be safely administered.

4. Administer hydrocortisone 100 mg q6h IV. Alternatively, give one dose of dexamethasone 4 mg IV, perform ACTH stimulation test, then switch to hydrocortisone 100 mg q6h IV.

5. Taper steroids as rapidly as conditions permit.

6. Identify and treat triggers.

C. EMPIRICAL STEROID WITHDRAWAL PROTOCOL

1. Significant interpatient variability exists in tolerating withdrawal, and no well-controlled studies are available to establish practice guidelines.

Text continued on p. 376

21

ADRENAL INSUFFICIENCY

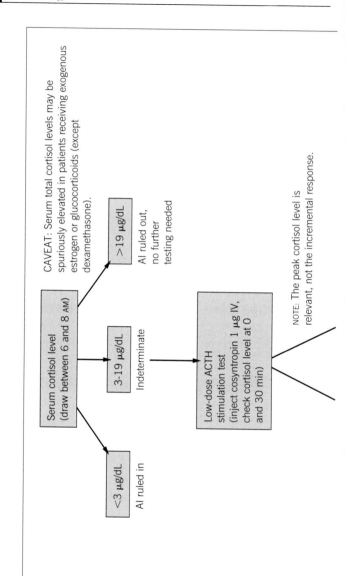

CAVEAT: Serum total cortisol levels may be spuriously elevated in patients receiving exogenous estrogen or glucocorticoids (except dexamethasone).

Serum cortisol level (draw between 6 and 8 AM)

<3 μg/dL
AI ruled in

3-19 μg/dL
Indeterminate

>19 μg/dL
AI ruled out, no further testing needed

Low-dose ACTH stimulation test (inject cosyntropin 1 μg IV, check cortisol level at 0 and 30 min)

NOTE: The peak cortisol level is relevant, not the incremental response.

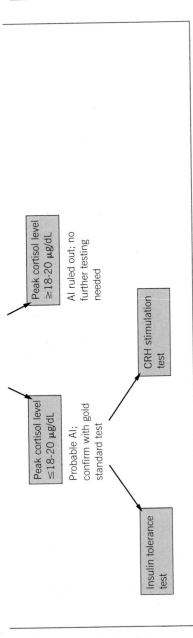

FIG. 21-3

Diagnostic step 1: confirming adrenal insufficiency. *ACTH,* Adrenocorticotropin; *CRH,* corticotropin-releasing hormone. *(Data from Grinspoon SK, Biller BM. J Clin Endocrinol Metab 1994; 79:923; Oelkers W. N Engl J Med 1996; 335:1206; and Werbel SS. Ober KP. Endocrinol Metab Clin North Am 1993; 22:303.)*

21

ADRENAL INSUFFICIENCY

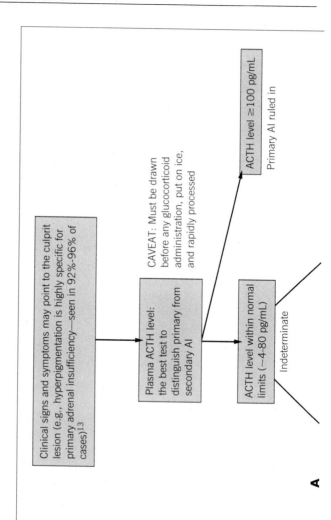

Clinical signs and symptoms may point to the culprit lesion (e.g., hyperpigmentation is highly specific for primary adrenal insufficiency—seen in 92%-96% of cases)[13]

Plasma ACTH level: the best test to distinguish primary from secondary AI

CAVEAT: Must be drawn before any glucocorticoid administration, put on ice, and rapidly processed

ACTH level ≥100 pg/mL

Primary AI ruled in

ACTH level within normal limits (~4-80 pg/mL)

Indeterminate

A

21

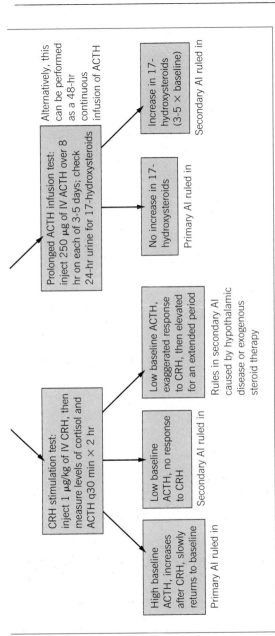

FIG. 21-4

Diagnostic step 2: **A,** localizing anatomical lesion within the hypothalamic-pituitary-adrenal axis. *(Data from Grinspoon SK, Biller BM. J Clin Endocrinol Metab 1994; 79:923; and Werbel SS, Ober KP. Endocrinol Metab Clin North Am 1993; 22:303.)* cont'd

ADRENAL INSUFFICIENCY

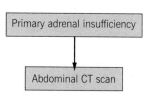

Adrenal glands may be small and atrophied (e.g., autoimmune AI), large or calcified (e.g., tuberculosis, fungal disease), infiltrated (infiltrative or metastatic disease), or hemorrhagic (sepsis, coagulopathy)

B

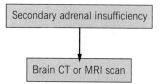

Pituitary or hypothalamic pathological conditions best visualized by MRI; CT may better reveal calcifications associated with craniopharyngioma or pituitary invasion of the sella

FIG. 21-4—cont'd

B, localizing anatomical lesion radiographically. *ACTH,* Adrenocorticotropin; *AI,* adrenal insufficiency; *CRH,* corticotropin-releasing hormone; *CT,* computed tomography; *MRI,* magnetic resonance imaging. *(Data from Grinspoon SK, Biller BM. J Clin Endocrinol Metab 1994; 79:923; and Werbel SS, Ober KP. Endocrinol Metab Clin North Am 1993; 22:303.)*

2. If daily dose is greater than the equivalent of 60 mg prednisone, decrease dose by 10 mg/day every 1 to 2 weeks.
3. If daily dose is 20 to 60 mg prednisone equivalents, decrease dose by 5 mg/day every 1 to 2 weeks.
4. If daily dose is 10 to 20 mg prednisone equivalents, decrease dose by 2.5 mg/day every 1 to 2 weeks.
5. If daily dose is 5 to 9 mg prednisone, decrease dose by 1 mg/day every 1 to 2 weeks.

PEARLS AND PITFALLS

- Human immunodeficiency virus (HIV)-positive patients.
  - AI is considerably more common in HIV-positive patients than in the general population. Prevalence estimates have ranged from 5% to 20%.[19-21] A high index of suspicion for AI is needed for these individuals because glucocorticoid therapy may be lifesaving. This is particularly the case for patients who have disseminated opportunistic in-

TABLE 21-1			
RELATIVE STEROID POTENCIES AND BIOLOGICAL HALF-LIVES			
Steroid	Equivalent Glucocorticoid Dose (mg)	Relative Mineralocorticoid Activity	Biological Half-Life (hr)
SHORT ACTING			
Cortisol	20	1	0.5-1.5
Cortisone	25	2	8-12
Hydrocortisone	20	2	8-12
Prednisone	5	1	18-36
Prednisolone	5	1	18-36
Methylprednisolone	4	0	18-36
INTERMEDIATE ACTING			
Triamcinolone	4	0	18-36
LONG ACTING			
Betamethasone	0.6-0.75	0	36-54
Dexamethasone	0.75	0	36-54

Data from Tarascon. Tarascon pocket pharmacopoeia. Loma Linda, Calif: Tarascon Publishing; 2001; and Werbel SS, Ober KP. Endocrinol Metab Clin North Am 1993; 22:303.

fections, such as *Mycobacterium avium-intracellulare* infection, tuberculosis, histoplasmosis, or cytomegalovirus infection, and appear to be responding inadequately to standard therapies.[22]

- Critically ill (intensive care unit) patients.
  - AI is highly prevalent in the intensive care unit (ICU) setting, where it has been reported to affect up to 40% of critically ill patients.[23,24] Prolonged ICU stays (more than 14 days) and age greater than 55 are associated with a three-fold increased risk of AI.[25] AI in these individuals may be due to suppression of the HPA axis by cytokines (e.g., interleukin-1 [IL-1], IL-6, and tumor necrosis factor alpha) or primary adrenal destruction and hemorrhage (e.g., Waterhouse-Friderichsen syndrome in sepsis).
  - AI should be suspected when a critically ill patient has refractory hypotension, unexplained high fever, hyponatremia, hyperkalemia, hypoglycemia, hyperpigmentation, or eosinophilia. When suspicion is high, treatment should be initiated promptly (even in the absence of definitive diagnosis) with hydrocortisone 100 mg IV q8h for 2 to 3 days, then tapered accordingly.[10]
- Hypoaldosteronism.
  - Adrenal secretion of aldosterone is regulated by the renin-angiotensin system and serum potassium concentration. Deficient secretion may result from hyporeninemia (i.e., owing to destruction of juxtaglomerular cells or use of nonsteroidal antiinflammatory drugs) or disordered aldosterone biosynthesis (e.g., in hypotensive adrenal ischemia, heparin therapy, diabetes, or metastatic cancer). Isolated hypoaldosteronism can clinically mimic the electrolyte and volume abnormalities of pri-

mary AI, yet cortisol secretion is unaffected. It should be considered in refractory hyperkalemia not explained by renal or adrenal insufficiency.[13]

REFERENCES

[b] 1. Addison T. On the constitutional and local effects of diseases of the supra-renal capsules. London: Samuel Highley; 1855.

[b] 2. Zelissen PM, Bast EJ, Croughs RJ. Associated autoimmunity in Addison's disease. J Autoimmun 1995; 8:121.

[a] 3. Kasperlik-Zaluska AA et al. Association of Addison's disease with autoimmune disorders—a long-term observation of 180 patients. Postgrad Med J 1991; 67:984.

[b] 4. Kong MF, Jeffcoate W. Eighty-six cases of Addison's disease. Clin Endocrinol (Oxf) 1994; 41:757.

[b] 5. Willis AC, Vince FP. The prevalence of Addison's disease in Coventry, UK. Postgrad Med J 1997; 73:286.

[c] 6. Oelkers W, Diederich S, Bahr V. [Diagnosis of adrenal cortex insufficiency]. Dtsch Med Wochenschr 1994; 119:555.

[b] 7. Ahonen P et al. Clinical variation of autoimmune polyendocrinopathy–candidiasis–ectodermal dystrophy (APECED) in a series of 68 patients. N Engl J Med 1990; 322:1829.

[b] 8. Betterle C et al. Type 2 polyglandular autoimmune disease (Schmidt's syndrome). J Pediatr Endocrinol Metab 1996; 9(suppl 1):113.

[b] 9. Brosnan CM, Gowing NF. Addison's disease. Br Med J 1996; 312:1085.

[b] 10. Zaloga GP, Marik P. Hypothalamic-pituitary-adrenal insufficiency. Crit Care Clin 2001; 17:25.

[b] 11. Oelkers W. Adrenal insufficiency. N Engl J Med 1996; 335:1206.

[a] 12. Grinspoon SK, Biller BM. Clinical review 62: laboratory assessment of adrenal insufficiency. J Clin Endocrinol Metab 1994; 79:923.

[b] 13. Werbel SS, Ober KP. Acute adrenal insufficiency. Endocrinol Metab Clin North Am 1993; 22:303.

[b] 14. Graham GW, Unger BP, Coursin DB. Perioperative management of selected endocrine disorders. Int Anesthesiol Clin 2000; 38:31.

[b] 15. Oelkers W, Diederich S, Bahr V. Therapeutic strategies in adrenal insufficiency. Ann Endocrinol (Paris) 2001; 62:212.

[b] 16. Salem M et al. Perioperative glucocorticoid coverage: a reassessment 42 years after emergence of a problem. Ann Surg 1994; 219:416.

[b] 17. Arlt W et al. Dehydroepiandrosterone replacement in women with adrenal insufficiency. N Engl J Med 1999; 341:1013.

[c] 18. Tarascon. Tarascon pocket pharmacopoeia. Loma Linda, Calif: Tarascon Publishing; 2001.

[b] 19. Dobs AS et al. Endocrine disorders in men infected with human immunodeficiency virus. Am J Med 1988; 84:611.

[a] 20. Findling JW et al. Longitudinal evaluation of adrenocortical function in patients infected with the human immunodeficiency virus. J Clin Endocrinol Metab 1994; 79:1091.

[a] 21. Raffi F et al. Endocrine function in 98 HIV-infected patients: a prospective study. AIDS 1991; 5:729.

[b] 22. Eledrisi MS, Verghese AC. Adrenal insufficiency in HIV infection: a review and recommendations. Am J Med Sci 2001; 321:137.

[b] 23. Barquist E, Kirton O. Adrenal insufficiency in the surgical intensive care unit patient. J Trauma 1997; 42:27.

[b] 24. Moran JL et al. Hypocortisolaemia and adrenocortical responsiveness at onset of septic shock. Intensive Care Med 1994; 20:489.

[b] 25. Rivers EP et al. Adrenal insufficiency in high-risk surgical ICU patients. Chest 2001; 119:889.

Diabetic Ketoacidosis and Hyperosmolar Hyperglycemic State

Gregory O. Clark, MD, and Christopher D. Saudek, MD

FAST FACTS

- Diabetic ketoacidosis (DKA) is characterized by the triad of hyperglycemia (>250 mg/dL), acidemia (arterial pH <7.3; serum bicarbonate <18 mEq/L), and ketonemia.
- Hyperosmolar hyperglycemic state (HHS) consists of severe hyperglycemia (>600 mg/dL), increased osmolarity (>330 mOsm/kg), and when hyperosmolarity is greater than approximately 350 mOsm/kg, altered mental status.
- Mortality rates are 9% to 14% for DKA and 10% to 50% for HHS.[1]
- Infection is the most common precipitant of DKA and HHS (Boxes 22-1 and 22-2). Nonadherence to insulin therapy is the most common precipitant of DKA and HHS in urban blacks.[2] Severe dehydration also predisposes to HHS.
- Treatment of DKA and HHS includes administration of intravenous (IV) fluid to correct dehydration and hyperosmolarity, administration of insulin to reverse hyperglycemia and ketoacidosis (in DKA), correction of electrolyte abnormalities, identification of precipitants, and frequent patient monitoring.
- Complications of treatment include hypoglycemia, hypokalemia, and, rarely, cerebral edema.
- The diagnosis and treatment of DKA and HHS outlined in this chapter are based on American Diabetes Association recommendations.[3]

I. EPIDEMIOLOGY

1. The incidence of DKA is 4.6 to 8 episodes per 1000 people with diabetes per year, with higher rates in younger age groups. HHS occurs more frequently in those over 65 years old.
2. Mortality rates are approximately 9% to 14% for DKA and 10% to 50% for HHS, with higher mortality rates for those with comorbidities and at extremes of age.[2]

II. CLINICAL PRESENTATION

A. PATHOPHYSIOLOGY

1. DKA usually occurs in patients with type 1 diabetes mellitus but can occur in those with type 2 diabetes. Hyperglycemia is caused by severe insulin deficiency and counterregulatory hormone (i.e., gluca-

---

BOX 22-1

COMMON PRECIPITATING FACTORS OF DIABETIC KETOACIDOSIS

Infection

Inadequate insulin delivery (nonadherence to therapy, insulin pump nondelivery)

New-onset type 1 diabetes

Surgery

Pregnancy

Severe illness (trauma, myocardial infarction, cerebrovascular accident, pancreatitis)

Medications (corticosteroids, sympathomimetic agents, phenytoin, estrogens, thiazides, nicotinic acid, danazol, diazoxide, growth hormone, pentamidine, indomethacin, thyroid hormone, chlorpromazine, salicylates)

BOX 22-2

COMMON PRECIPITATING FACTORS OF HYPEROSMOLAR HYPERGLYCEMIC STATE

Impaired thirst (elderly patients)

Patients prone to dehydration (dialysis, excess diuresis, burns)

Infection

Surgery

Pregnancy

Severe illness (trauma, myocardial infarction, cerebrovascular accident, pancreatitis)

Medications (corticosteroids, sympathomimetic agents, phenytoin, estrogens, thiazides, nicotinic acid, danazol, diazoxide, growth hormone, pentamidine, indomethacin, thyroid hormone, chlorpromazine, salicylates)

---

gon and catecholamine) excess that results in increased glucose production and decreased glucose utilization. Virtually complete insulin deficiency also causes the uncontrolled release of free fatty acids from adipose tissue. Oxidation of free fatty acids leads to ketonemia and acidosis. Glycosuria causes dehydration and loss of electrolytes. Ketoacidosis further exacerbates electrolyte abnormalities, specifically an extracellular shift of potassium. DKA typically develops over 1 to 2 days.

2. HHS usually develops among patients with type 2 diabetes mellitus. It is characterized by extreme hyperglycemia, often to more than 1000 mg/dL, with dehydration causing serum hyperosmolarity. Mental status correlates with serum osmolality. Stupor and coma are typically present with osmolality greater than 340 to 350 mOsm/kg H_2O.[3] The pathophysiological mechanism is insulin activity insufficient to prevent hyperglycemia yet sufficient to prevent severe lipolysis and ketosis. The commonly used term "hyperosmolar nonketotic coma" is misleading, since mild ketosis can exist and coma is unusual.

B. SYMPTOMS

1. **Acute hyperglycemia:** Polyuria, polydipsia, weight loss, dehydration, weakness, fatigue.
2. **Acidosis:** Nausea, vomiting, "air hunger," abdominal pain, fatigue.
3. **Neurological manifestations:** Stupor, coma, seizures (more common in severe HHS).

C. SIGNS

1. **Dehydration:** Poor skin turgor, dry mucous membranes, absence of axillary sweat, tachycardia, orthostatic hypotension.
2. **Signs of ketoacidosis:** Kussmaul's respirations (rapid and deep breathing as respiratory compensation for metabolic acidosis); fruity breath odor (an indication of ketonemia in DKA); emesis and abdominal pain (common in DKA); guaiac-positive stools resulting from hemorrhagic gastritis.
3. **Signs of severe hyperosmolarity:** Altered mental status ranging from mild confusion to coma.
4. **Hypothermia (hyperthermia indicates infection).**
5. **Other evidence of a precipitating factor (e.g., infection) must be sought.**

III. DIAGNOSTICS

A. LABORATORY TESTS

1. **Tests for all patients with suspected DKA or HHS.**
   a. After the history and physical examination.
      (1) Arterial blood gases: To assess acidosis and respiratory compensation.
      (2) Serum and urine ketones: To specify ketosis as cause of acidosis.
      (3) Serum chemistries, including glucose, electrolytes, blood urea nitrogen (BUN), and creatinine: To assess, particularly, extent of hyperglycemia, dehydration, serum potassium, and prerenal azotemia.
         (a) Serum sodium: Levels are normally lowered in the presence of hyperglycemia because the osmolar load of glucose causes an extracellular shift of free water. The "corrected" serum sodium should be calculated by adding 1.6 mEq/L to the measured Na^+ for each 100 mg/dL that the glucose level is elevated above normal. Elevation of the "corrected" serum sodium indicates severity of dehydration.
         (b) Serum potassium: Shifted extracellularly by acidosis, so hyperkalemia may exist even when total body potassium is significantly diminished. Conversely, insulin treatment shifts potassium into cells, causing a real risk of hypokalemia as acidosis is corrected.
      (4) Anion gap and serum osmolality should be calculated to assess acid-base status and whether hyperosmolarity is sufficient to explain

changes in mental status. Calculated osmolality should be compared with measured osmolality to rule out an osmolar gap.

$$\text{Anion gap} = Na^+ - (Cl^- + HCO_3^-) \text{ (mEq/L)}$$

$$\text{Serum osmolality} = 2[Na^+ \text{ (mEq/L)}] + \frac{\text{Glucose (mg/dL)}}{18} + \frac{\text{BUN (mg/dL)}}{2.8}$$

Note: Some individuals do not advocate adding BUN/2.8, since urea is freely permeable across cell walls and may not contribute to effective serum osmolarity.

    (5) Complete blood cell count (CBC) with differential (white blood cell [WBC] count is often elevated even in the absence of infection and is proportional to the degree of ketonemia).

    (6) Urinalysis, particularly to rule out urinary tract infection.

    (7) Cultures of blood, urine, or sputum if infection is suspected.

    (8) Serum amylase and lipase with abdominal pain; amylase and less frequently lipase levels may be elevated from nonpancreatic sources.

b. During therapy.

    (1) Serum glucose should be checked hourly while IV insulin is titrated.

    (2) Electrolytes, BUN, and creatinine should be checked every 2 to 4 hours until stable.

    (3) In DKA, acidosis is monitored by measurement of venous pH every 2 hours.

    (4) Ketone monitoring is unnecessary after diagnosis of DKA, since correction of acidosis shifts redox equilibrium toward acetoacetate, which is measured by many bedside sensors, and may appear to increase as total ketosis decreases.

2. Tests for diagnosis of DKA.

a. Plasma glucose >250 mg/dL.

b. The degree of acidosis (along with mental status) determines the severity of DKA.

c. Mild.

    (1) Arterial pH 7.25 to 7.30.

    (2) Serum bicarbonate 15 to 18 mEq/L.

    (3) Anion gap >10.

d. Moderate.

    (1) Arterial pH 7.00 to 7.24.

    (2) Serum bicarbonate 10 to 14 mEq/L.

    (3) Anion gap >12.

e. Severe.

    (1) Arterial pH <7.00.

    (2) Serum bicarbonate <10 mEq/L.

    (3) Anion gap >12.

f. Urine and serum ketones: Tests on undiluted blood and urine are at least moderately positive. Presence of urine ketones is not diagnostic of DKA, since they may occur in normal fasting.

3. Tests for diagnosis of HHS.

a. Plasma glucose >600 mg/dL.

b. Serum osmolality >330 mOsm/kg H_2O.

c. Arterial pH >7.3 and serum bicarbonate >15 mEq/L.

d. Mild ketonuria or ketonemia may be present.

e. Sometimes DKA and HHS overlap, with ketosis, acidosis, and hyperosmolality.

B. ELECTROCARDIOGRAM

1. An electrocardiogram should be obtained to rule out MI as a precipitating factor and to evaluate electrolyte abnormality.

C. RADIOGRAPHY

1. Chest x-ray examination should be performed if clinically indicated.

D. DIFFERENTIAL DIAGNOSIS

1. Ketosis.

a. Alcoholic ketoacidosis: Ketosis exists and acidosis can be severe, but hyperglycemia is absent.

b. Starvation ketosis: Distinguished from DKA by the absence of both hyperglycemia and significant acidosis.

2. Acidosis.

a. High anion gap (>14).

    (1) Lactic acidosis.

        (a) Tissue hypoxia (shock, respiratory failure).

        (b) Sepsis.

        (c) Neoplasm (leukemia or lymphoma).

        (d) Liver or renal failure.

        (e) Seizure.

        (f) Metformin.

    (2) Ketoacidosis: As for lactic acidosis.

    (3) Uremia: Chronic renal failure.

    (4) Ingestion: Salicylate, methanol, ethylene glycol.

        (a) Salicylate: Combined respiratory alkalosis and metabolic acidosis exist after aspirin ingestion.

        (b) Methanol: Blood methanol level is elevated, and an osmolar gap (measured serum osmolality – calculated total osmolality) is present. Visual disturbance may exist.

        (c) Ethylene glycol: Urine calcium oxalate crystals and an osmolar gap help establish the diagnosis.

b. Nonanion gap: Usually results from the loss of bicarbonate.

    (1) Renal tubular acidosis.

    (2) Diarrhea.

IV. MANAGEMENT

A. FLUID

1. Fluid deficits average 6 L in DKA and 9 L in HHS.[4]

2. Evaluate corrected serum sodium upon admission, after history and physical examination. Even with severe dehydration, give 1 L

22

DKA AND HYPEROSMOLAR HYPERGLYCEMIC STATE

normal saline (0.9% NaCl) over 1 hour (15-20 mL/kg) to restore intravascular volume and renal perfusion. Continue normal saline at this rate until blood pressure and organ perfusion are restored (as evidenced by urine output and physical examination). More conservative rehydration may be necessary in the presence of cardiac or renal compromise.

3. If corrected serum sodium level is normal to high, switch to half normal saline (0.45% NaCl) at a rate of 4 to 14 mL/kg/hr. If corrected serum sodium is low, continue normal saline at a rate of 4 to 14 mL/kg/hr.

4. Change IV fluid to 5% dextrose with 0.45% NaCl when glucose level reaches 250 mg/dL in DKA and 300 mg/dL in HHS. Use of 10% dextrose may be necessary to maintain the glucose level between 150 and 200 mg/dL until DKA has resolved or to maintain the glucose level between 250 and 300 mg/dL until patients with HHS are mentally alert and serum osmolality is less than 315 mOsm/kg.

5. Fluid deficits should be replaced at a slower rate (i.e., over 48 hours) in patients younger than 20 years because of an increased risk of cerebral edema. Osmolality should not decrease more than 3 mOsm/kg H_2O per hour, and mental status should be evaluated frequently.

B. INSULIN

1. Exclude hypokalemia (K^+ <3.3 mEq/L) before administration of insulin.

2. Administer regular insulin 0.15 U/kg as an IV bolus (~10 U on average).

3. Infuse 0.1 U/kg/hr (~7 U/hr).

4. Check glucose hourly.

5. Double the insulin infusion hourly until the glucose level falls by 50 to 70 mg/dL/hr.

6. **DKA:** When the glucose level reaches 250 mg/dL, adjust insulin infusion to maintain the glucose level between 150 and 200 mg/dL until acidosis has resolved (bicarbonate >18 mEq/L, venous pH >7.30, anion gap <12). Add 5% or 10% dextrose to IV fluids if necessary. Once DKA has resolved, administer subcutaneous insulin and continue IV insulin for an additional 1 to 2 hours. IV insulin has a half-life of minutes, and if it is discontinued before subcutaneous administration begins, ketoacidosis may recur.

7. **HHS:** When the glucose level reaches 300 mg/dL, adjust insulin infusion to maintain the glucose level between 250 and 300 mg/dL until serum osmolality is less than 315 mOsm/kg and mental status is normal.

8. If patients remain on a nothing by mouth status (NPO) despite resolution of DKA or HHS, IV administration of insulin should continue. Alternatively, regular insulin can be administered subcutaneously every 4 hours based on blood glucose levels while the patient is NPO.[5]

9. When DKA has resolved and the patient is able to drink, previous subcutaneous insulin regimens may be resumed. Patients with newly diagnosed type 1 diabetes should be treated with a total insulin dose of 0.6 to 0.7 U/kg/day as a multidose regimen of short-acting and longer acting insulin. Doses should be modified based on subsequent glucose levels.

C. ELECTROLYTES

1. **Potassium:** Serum potassium levels can be low, normal, or high, yet total body deficits average 3 to 5 mEq/kg in DKA and 4 to 6 mEq/kg in HHS.[4,6] Hypokalemia may cause cardiac arrhythmias and is a common cause of mortality, especially in DKA. Serum potassium levels fall during treatment with insulin, bicarbonate, or IV fluid.
a. Hold insulin if K^+ level is less than 3.3 mEq/L. Administer 40 mEq K^+ hourly until K^+ level is 3.3 mEq/L or higher.
b. If K^+ is 5.5 mEq/L or higher, withhold potassium. Monitor K^+ every 2 hours.
c. If K^+ is 3.3 to 5.5 mEq/L, administer 20 to 30 mEq K^+ per liter of IV fluid. Goal serum K^+ is 4 to 5 mEq/L.
d. K^+ supplementation may require lower doses in the presence of renal compromise.

2. **Bicarbonate:** Bicarbonate should be considered only for life-threatening acidosis, and its use is controversial even when the pH is 6.9 to 7.1. Studies are also inadequate to prove benefit in patients with a pH below 6.9.[5] The American Diabetes Association recommends treatment with sodium bicarbonate as follows.
a. When pH is less than 6.9, 100 mmol $NaHCO_3$ over 2 hours.
b. When pH is 6.9 to 7.0, 50 mmol $NaHCO_3$ over 1 hour.
c. Repeat every 2 hours until pH is greater than 7.0.
d. Monitor K^+ (bicarbonate therapy lowers serum K^+).
e. In patients younger than 20 years of age, bicarbonate should be given only if pH is less than 7.0 after 1 hour of hydration. Give 1 to 2 mEq/kg in half normal saline over 1 hour.

3. **Phosphate:** DKA depletes total body phosphate. Serum phosphate levels decrease with insulin therapy. Treatment with phosphate may cause hypocalcemia and has been shown not to affect clinical outcome in DKA.[7] For prevention of cardiac and skeletal muscle weakness, however, potassium phosphate at 20 to 30 mEq per liter of replacement fluid can be given when the serum phosphate level is less than 1 mg/dL or when the patient has cardiac dysfunction, anemia, or respiratory depression.

D. OUTPATIENT PREVENTION

1. Improvement of access to medical care, especially during illness.
2. Education of patients and their family members about sick-day management: Specifically, patients should be advised never to discontinue insulin and should be educated about the use of supplemental short-acting insulin based on self-monitoring of blood

22

DKA AND HYPEROSMOLAR HYPERGLYCEMIC STATE

glucose. Avoidance of dehydration and awareness and avoidance of other precipitants of DKA and HHS should be emphasized.

3. **Increased public awareness of the signs and symptoms of diabetes:** May lead to earlier diagnoses and reduce morbidity.

PEARLS AND PITFALLS

- Initiate volume resuscitation with 1 L normal saline over 1 hour.
- Administer a regular insulin bolus of 0.15 U/kg IV followed by 0.1 U/kg/hr IV.
- If the serum K^+ level is 3.3 mEq/L or higher but less than 5.5 mEq/L, give 20 to 30 mEq K^+ per liter of IV fluid to keep K^+ between 4 and 5 mEq/L. Be watchful for hypokalemia.
- Bicarbonate should be repleted only when serum pH is less than 7.0 in DKA.
- Hypoglycemia commonly complicates the overtreatment of DKA and HHS. It can be prevented by adding dextrose to rehydration fluid as plasma glucose improves and adjusting insulin doses to maintain mild hyperglycemia until DKA or HHS has resolved.
- Hyperglycemia and ketoacidosis may recur if intravenous administration of insulin is stopped before subcutaneous administration is started. Give insulin subcutaneously for 1 to 2 hours before stopping IV administration.
- Hypokalemia is a common cause of death, especially in DKA, and results from treatment with fluid, insulin, and especially bicarbonate. Supplementation with K^+ should begin with hydration while serum K^+ levels are still in the normal range.
- Cerebral edema is rare but frequently fatal and occurs in both DKA and HHS, most commonly in pediatric patients. It may be prevented by avoidance of early and excessive use of hypotonic fluid and a gradual reduction of serum hyperosmolarity. Mental status should be monitored frequently because cerebral edema may develop rapidly. Diagnosis can be confirmed by CT scan of the brain.

REFERENCES

[b] 1. Diabetes in America, 2nd ed. Bethesda, Md: National Diabetes Data Group, National Institutes of Health; 1995.
[b] 2. Umpierrez GE et al. Hyperglycemic crises in urban blacks. Arch Intern Med 1997; 157(6):669.
[d] 3. American Diabetes Association: Position statement: hyperglycemic crises in patients with diabetes mellitus. Clin Diabetes 2001; 19(2):82.
[c] 4. Kreisberg PA. Diabetic ketoacidosis: new concepts and trends in pathogenesis and treatment. Ann Intern Med 1978; 88(5):681.
[c] 5. Kitabchi AE et al. Management of hyperglycemic crises in patients with diabetes. Diabetes Care 2001; 24(1):131.
[c] 6. Ennis ED, Stahl EJ, Kreisberg RA. The hyperosmolar hyperglycemic syndrome. Diabetes Rev 1994; 2:115.
[a] 7. Fisher JN, Kitabchi AE. A randomized study of phosphate therapy in the treatment of diabetic ketoacidosis. J Clin Endocrinol Metab 1983; 57(1):177.

Thyroid Disorders

Gail V. Berkenblit, MD, PhD, and W. Tabb Moore, MD

FAST FACTS

- An outpatient screening for thyroid-stimulating hormone (TSH) is recommended for all women over age 60, patients with other autoimmune disorders or strong family history, patients with dementia, and patients with elevated cholesterol levels.
- Diagnosis of thyroid disorders in inpatients is complicated by the effects of nonthyroidal illness and medications.
- In primary thyroid disease, hyperthyroidism is characterized by excessively high thyroxine (T_4) levels and suppressed TSH; conversely, hypothyroidism has a deficiency of T_4 and an elevation of TSH.
- TSH measurement is the most sensitive test of thyroid dysfunction; TSH demonstrates a log-linear relationship with T_4.
- TSH levels do not accurately reflect the thyroid status in patients who are receiving dopamine or steroids, have pituitary or hypothalamic dysfunction, are in an unstable metabolic state such as recovery from nonthyroid illness, or are being treated for hyperthyroidism or hypothyroidism.
- The most common causes of hyperthyroidism are Graves' disease, toxic multinodular goiter, subacute thyroiditis, postpartum thyroiditis, and medication-induced thyrotoxicosis (Table 23-1).
- The most common causes of hypothyroidism are Hashimoto's disease and thyroid ablation (Table 23-2).
- Thyrotoxicosis is treated medically with β-blockers and methimazole, propylthiouracil, or radioactive iodine thyroid ablation. In rare cases surgery is still necessary.
- Hypothyroidism is treated with thyroxine hormone replacement, begun at full dose in patients younger than 50 and without heart disease and at a reduced dose otherwise. Patients with hypothyroidism that is mild or of recent onset can almost always be started on full doses.

23

I. EPIDEMIOLOGY

1. Thyroid disease is more common in women, the elderly, patients with other autoimmune disorders, and those with a family history of thyroid disease.
2. Hyperthyroidism has a prevalence of 2% in women and 0.2% in men. Hypothyroidism is more common and is seen in 5% to 8% of randomly screened populations.
3. Postpartum thyroiditis, a painless form of thyroiditis, occurs in 5% of women, generally 2 to 6 months after delivery.

TABLE 23-1

CAUSES OF THYROTOXICOSIS

Cause	Mechanism	Thyroid Examination
Graves' disease	Stimulatory anti-TSH receptor antibodies	Diffuse goiter
Toxic multinodular goiter	Activating mutations of TSH receptor or Gs-α gene	Nodule(s)
Subacute thyroiditis	Destruction that releases stored hormone	Minimal goiter
DeQuervain's	Postviral	Tender
Painless	Autoimmune	Nontender
CT dye or amiodarone	Iodine surplus (Jod-Basedow) or toxic thyroiditis	Nodular or diffuse goiter or normal
Hydatidiform mole	hCG cross-activation of TSH receptors	Minimal goiter
Pituitary tumor	TSH overproduction	Minimal goiter
Struma ovarii	Ectopic thyroid tissue in ovarian tumor	Normal
Exogenous thyrotoxicosis		Normal
Iatrogenic	Oversupplementation of thyroxine	
Factitious	Surreptitious ingestion of thyroxine	

CT, Computed tomography; *hCG,* human chorionic gonadotropin; *TSH,* thyroid-stimulating hormone.

TABLE 23-2

CAUSES OF HYPOTHYROIDISM

Cause	Mechanism	Thyroid Examination
Hashimoto's disease	Autoimmune destruction	Firm bosselated gland with pyramidal lobe
Ablation or resection	Removal of functioning thyroid tissue	Atrophic or cervical scar
Central hypothyroidism	Pituitary or hypothalamic failure	Atrophic
Iodine deficiency	Low substrate for iodination	Goiter
Lithium	Decreased thyroid hormone synthesis	Goiter
Amiodarone	Wolff-Chaikoff effect; thyroiditis	Goiter or normal
Peripheral resistance	Rare genetic defect in T_3 nuclear receptor	Normal

T_3, Triiodothyronine.

II. CLINICAL PRESENTATION

A. HYPERTHYROIDISM

1. Symptoms of classic hyperthyroidism include fatigue, heat intolerance, weight loss, palpitations, exertional dyspnea, increased bowel motility, hair loss, diaphoresis, oligomenorrhea, anxiety, irritability, and tremulousness. Patients with Graves' ophthalmopathy may also complain of gritty eyes, diplopia, or blurry vision.
2. Classic symptoms generally decrease with advancing age, making diagnosis more difficult. Older patients usually have marked weight

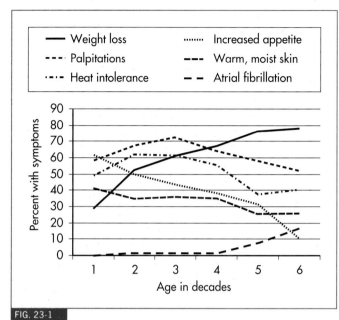

FIG. 23-1

Presentation of hyperthyroidism varies by decade of life. (Modified from Nordyke R, Gilbert F, Harada A. Arch Intern Med 1988; 148:626.)

loss and cardiovascular symptoms, including atrial fibrillation and congestive heart failure, a presentation that has been termed apathetic hyperthyroidism.

3. Nordyke and associates examined prevalence of signs and symptoms by age and found a decrease in all except weight loss and atrial fibrillation (Fig. 23-1).[1] Occasionally a single manifestation of hyperthyroidism predominates, such as headache, cardiovascular or gastrointestinal symptoms, urticaria, orbitopathy, myasthenia, or hypokalemic periodic paralysis.

4. Physical signs of hyperthyroidism include tachycardia, hyperactivity, stare and lid lag, warm moist skin, proximal muscle weakness, tremor, and hyperreflexia. A palpable goiter is present in 95% of patients except in the group with apathetic hyperthyroidism, 50% of whom do not have an enlarged thyroid gland. A bruit over the gland is indicative of increased blood flow and is usually associated with Graves' disease.

5. Patients with Graves' disease may also exhibit exophthalmos, perior-bital edema, gynecomastia, clubbing, and pretibial myxedema. Hyper-

thyroidism is present in 5% of patients with new-onset atrial fibrillation.[2]

6. Associated laboratory findings may include hypercalcemia, increased alkaline phosphatase, anemia, and mild granulocytopenia. Decreased bone density measurements may be found.

7. In rare cases severe hyperthyroidism produces a life-threatening condition characterized by hyperthermia, delirium, tachyarrhythmias, and high-output cardiac failure. This so-called thyroid storm is most commonly seen in patients with poor access to health care. Often thyroid crisis is precipitated by a physiological stress, such as myocardial infarction, infection, or surgery, or by an acute iodine load. Levels of thyroid hormone do not distinguish between patients with thyroid storm and uncomplicated thyrotoxicosis. A clinical diagnostic scoring system for thyroid storm has been proposed (Table 23-3).[3]

B. HYPOTHYROIDISM

1. In contrast to hyperthyroidism, hypothyroidism causes fatigue, weight gain, cold intolerance, hoarseness, constipation, dry skin, arthralgias and myalgias, menometrorrhagia, decreased libido, and mood alterations. Symptoms often occur so insidiously that the condition goes unnoticed.

2. Physical findings include bradycardia, cool dry skin, brittle nails and hair, macroglossia, and delayed relaxation of reflexes. Pericardial effusion, ascites, and congestive failure may be present.

3. Laboratory tests may demonstrate hyponatremia, macrocytic anemia, an elevated creatine phosphokinase level, hyperprolactinemia, and abnormal results of liver function tests. In the Colorado Thyroid Prevalence Study, cholesterol levels were observed to rise in direct proportion to TSH (Fig. 23-2).[4] Such an increase may contribute to an increased risk of coronary artery disease.

4. Severe hypothyroidism may culminate in myxedema coma, which more commonly develops in the winter months. Patients manifest hypothermia, hypotension, bradycardia, and altered mental status. Risk factors for myxedema coma include old age, poor access to health care, and long-standing thyroid disease; acute cases have been reported to occur after thyroid resection. Often sepsis, myocardial infarction, or other stressors precipitate myxedema coma.

5. Schmidt's syndrome is a polyglandular endocrinopathy comprising both thyroid and adrenal failure. This entity should be considered especially in patients with hypothyroidism and weight loss or salt cravings. Measurement of cortisol is crucial before treatment because thyroxine supplementation can increase cortisol metabolism and precipitate adrenal crisis in patients in coma or near coma.

III. DIAGNOSTICS

1. TSH and T_4 levels are the mainstay of diagnosis (Table 23-4). T_4 has a log-linear relationship with TSH, so that twofold changes in T_4 levels

TABLE 23-3

DIAGNOSTIC CRITERIA FOR THYROID STORM

Criterion	Points
THERMOREGULATORY DYSFUNCTION	
Temperature	
99°-99.9° F	5
100°-100.9° F	10
101°-101.9° F	15
102°-102.9° F	20
103°-103.9° F	25
≥104.9° F	30
CENTRAL NERVOUS SYSTEM EFFECTS	
Mild (agitation)	10
Moderate (delirium, psychosis, extreme lethargy)	20
Severe (seizure, coma)	30
GASTROINTESTINAL-HEPATIC DYSFUNCTION	
Moderate (diarrhea, nausea and vomiting, abdominal pain)	10
Severe (unexplained jaundice)	20
CARDIOVASCULAR DYSFUNCTION	
Tachycardia	
99-109 beats/min	5
110-119 beats/min	10
120-129 beats/min	15
130-139 beats/min	20
≥140 beats/min	25
CONGESTIVE HEART FAILURE	
Mild (pedal edema)	5
Moderate (bibasilar rales)	10
Severe (pulmonary edema)	15
Atrial fibrillation	10
PRECIPITANT HISTORY	
Negative	0
Positive	10

Data from Burch HB, Wartofsky L. Endocrinol Metab Clinic North Am 1993; 22:263.
In the setting of low thyroid-stimulating hormone and high thyroxine levels, a composite score of 45 or more is strongly suggestive of the diagnosis, a score of 25 to 44 supports the diagnosis, and a score of less than 24 makes the diagnosis unlikely.

23

THYROID DISORDERS

result in 50-fold changes in TSH levels. Thus TSH is the most sensitive marker of thyroid dysfunction.

2. In the general population, current guidelines recommend screening for TSH elevation of all women over age 60, patients with other autoimmune disorders or strong family history, patients with dementia, and all patients with elevated cholesterol levels.[5,6] Periodic screening of patients taking lithium or amiodarone is also recommended.

3. Although total serum T_4 concentrations are affected by changes in thyroxine-binding globulins and inhibitory proteins, alterations in hormone metabolism, and concurrent medications, free T_4 levels allow more accurate assessment of the physiological state. Total T_4 levels,

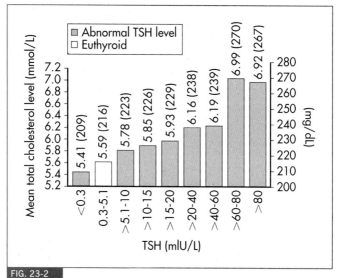

Total cholesterol levels rise with increasing severity of thyroid dysfunction. *TSH,* Thyroid-stimulating hormone. *(From Canaris G et al. Arch Intern Med 2000; 160:526.)*

TABLE 23-4

DIAGNOSTIC TESTS IN THYROID DISEASE

Diagnosis	Thyroid-Stimulating Hormone	Free Thyroxine
Hypothyroidism		
Overt	Increased	Decreased
Subclinical	Increased	Normal
Euthyroid	Normal	Normal
Hyperthyroidism		
Subclinical	Decreased	Normal
Overt	Decreased	Increased

Normal values for thyroid-stimulating hormone are 0.5 to 5 mIU/L. Normal values for free thyroxine are 0.9 to 1.9 ng/dL.

the T_3 resin (thyroid hormone binding ratio) test, and the derived free thyroxine index are no longer being used. They have been replaced by the free T_4 level. This eliminates abnormalities in testing associated with changes in thyroid-binding globulin. It should be noted that 5% to 10% of patients with hyperthyroidism have elevations only of T_3 level. Thus measurement of T_3 is important when the diagnosis of hyperthyroidism is suspected and the free T_4 level is normal.
4. Measurement of radioiodine uptake is usually necessary to

differentiate forms of thyrotoxicosis. The presence of a bruit over the gland may obviate the need to measure uptake. Iodine uptake is high with increased T_4 production, as in Graves' disease, whereas in thyroiditis there is destruction of thyroid tissue with a low uptake. Radioactive iodine uptake is also low in cases of exogenous T_4 supplementation and very rarely because of ectopic T_4 production from struma ovarii. Measurement of thyroglobulin can be useful in distinguishing thyroiditis from factitious hyperthyroidism, since thyroglobulin is released with tissue destruction.

5. The presence of antithyroid antibodies can provide supporting data for the diagnosis of autoimmune thyroid disorders. High levels of antithyroid peroxidase antibodies and antithyroglobulin antibodies are found in Hashimoto's disease and to a lesser extent in Graves' disease. Autoantibodies can also be useful in predicting progression to overt hypothyroidism in patients with subclinical hypothyroidism.

IV. MANAGEMENT

A. HYPERTHYROIDISM

1. Individual forms of thyrotoxicosis require different treatment. Subacute thyroiditis is usually transient and can be treated with β-blockers to control symptoms. Graves' disease and toxic multinodular goiter rarely resolve spontaneously but rather require treatment with medications, radioactive iodine ablation, or surgical resection. Antithyroid medications can restore a euthyroid state in 4 to 12 weeks, but prolonged therapy may be necessary and induction of a permanent remission is less likely than with radioactive iodine treatment. Patients are commonly treated with radioactive iodine ablation because it is safe and usually restores euthyroidism in 3 to 6 months. Because of the morbidity, expense, and availability of alternative modes of treatment, thyroidectomy is less frequently used.

2. Since many of the symptoms of hyperthyroidism are due to increased sympathetic activity from upregulation of β-adrenergic receptors, β-blockers are a mainstay in the management of symptoms. Highly lipid-soluble β-blockers, such as propranolol, also reduce peripheral conversion of T_4 to T_3, although they require more frequent doses than metoprolol and atenolol. β-Blockers are efficacious in management of symptoms, but they do not ameliorate all thyroxine effects and are not used as the sole therapy in Graves' disease.

3. Both propylthiouracil and methimazole inhibit the synthesis of thyroid hormones. Propylthiouracil is also a potent inhibitor of the peripheral conversion of T_4 to T_3. This feature makes it useful in severe thyrotoxicosis, but its dosage requirement (100-200 mg q8h) makes it less preferable for routine therapy than methimazole (10-30 mg qd). Side effects of both propylthiouracil and methimazole include allergic dermatitis, hepatotoxicity, arthritis, vasculitis, and agranulocytosis.

4. In thyroid storm and severe hyperthyroidism, adjunctive therapies may be required (Box 23-1). Iodine, given in the form of Lugol's solution or saturated solution of potassium iodide, blocks release of T_4 and T_3 from the thyroid. Pretreatment with methimazole or propylthiouracil must be given at least 1 hour before administration of iodides to prevent the iodine from fueling new thyroid hormone synthesis. As additional therapy, corticosteroids are commonly given to decrease conversion of T_4 to T_3 and because of the increased turnover of cortisol. Acetaminophen may be used as an antipyretic, but aspirin displaces thyroid hormones from binding proteins and should not be given in thyroid storm.

5. Consideration should be given to treatment of subclinical hyperthyroidism (suppressed TSH with normal T_4). Osteoporosis and atrial fibrillation have been reported as complications of subclinical hyperthyroidism.[7] Assessment of the overall clinical picture will determine whether to treat this condition.

B. HYPOTHYROIDISM

1. Usual daily requirements for thyroxine are 1.7 μg/kg lean body weight for most adults and 1 μg/kg lean body weight for elderly patients because of their decreased clearance. Full-dose therapy from the start is currently recommended for adults younger than 50 years and without heart disease. For patients older than 50 or with heart disease, the dose should start at 25 μg or less and be increased gradually at 4-week intervals. TSH should be measured at 4 weeks to assess therapy. Concurrent medications can affect thyroxine uptake by decreasing absorption (iron, bile acid sequestrants, antacids) and altering metabolism (rifampin, many antiepileptic drugs).

2. In myxedema coma, treatment should begin with intravenous administration of thyroxine (500-μg bolus followed by 1.5-2 μg/kg/day) alone or with triiodothyronine (10 μg IV q8h). Although direct administration of T_3 has a theoretical advantage of faster onset of action, no controlled trials exist comparing the two regimens. As with treatment of severe thyrotoxicosis, supportive measures and treatment of comorbid conditions are crucial. Glucocorticoids should be coadministered because of the possibility of Schmidt's syndrome and also because severe hypothyroidism may itself depress adrenal function.

3. Current guidelines recommend treatment of subclinical

BOX 23-1

ACUTE MEDICAL MANAGEMENT OF THYROID STORM

Propranolol 60-80 mg PO q4h

Methimazole 30 mg q6h or propylthiouracil 250 mg PO q4h

Lugol's iodine solution or saturated solution of potassium iodide 10 gtt PO q8h

Hydrocortisone 100 mg IV q8h

Cooling blanket and other supportive measures

hypothyroidism, especially when patients are symptomatic or have hypercholesterolemia. Supporting the need for treatment is the Rotterdam Study of 1149 women, which found a greater prevalence of aortic atherosclerosis and myocardial infarction in women with subclinical disease.[8] Three randomized, controlled clinical trials demonstrating improvement in overall symptom scores and memory with treatment are reviewed in McDermott and Ridgway.[9]

PEARLS AND PITFALLS

- Diagnosis of thyroid disease in hospitalized patients is fraught with pitfalls. Dopamine, corticosteroids, and octreotide all inhibit pituitary release of TSH and result in low TSH levels, independent of metabolic status. Diagnosis is further complicated by the effects of nonthyroidal illness on the thyroid axis. In the "euthyroid sick" state, first T_3 and then, with more severe illness, T_4 levels decline in patients with nonthyroidal illness. The TSH level is initially normal or occasionally low (15%) and rises during recovery (Fig. 23-3).[10] Although low T_4 levels do correlate

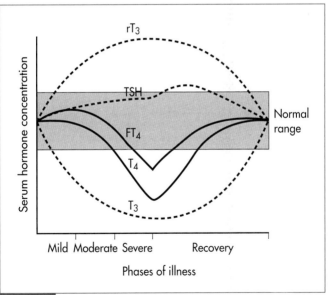

FIG. 23-3

Thyroid hormone levels change with course and severity of nonthyroidal illness. *FT₄*, Free thyroxine; *rT₃*, reverse triiodothyronine; *T₃*, triiodothyronine; *T₄*, thyroxine; *TSH*, thyroid-stimulating hormone. *(From Moore WT, Eastman R. Diagnostic endocrinology, 2nd ed. St Louis: Mosby; 1996.)*

with an adverse prognosis, studies have failed to demonstrate a mortality benefit from thyroxine supplementation.

- One study of 1580 patients in a large urban hospital demonstrated the magnitude of the problem of inpatient thyroid testing (Fig. 23-4).[11],[12] Abnormal TSH levels were observed in 17%. TSH levels less than 0.1 mIU/mL were attributed to nonthyroidal illness in 41%, glucocorticoid therapy in 35%, and actual thyroid disease in only 24%. Conversely, of patients with an elevated TSH of 7 to 20 mIU/mL, fully 72% had nonthyroidal illness, 14% had received glucocorticoid therapy, and only 14% had hypothyroidism. Therefore, if thyroid testing is done on a

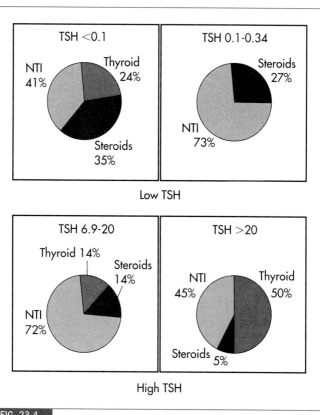

FIG. 23-4

Nonthyroidal illness (NTI) and glucocorticoids in hospitalized patients can result in both suppressed and elevated thyroid-stimulating hormone (TSH) levels. *(Modified from Spencer C et al. Clin Chem 1987; 33:1391.)*

critically ill patient, clinical correlation is important. The presence of a goiter, a history of pituitary disease, or thyroid ablation may help the clinician make the correct diagnosis. For patients who do not meet clinical criteria, retesting 6 to 8 weeks after recovery is recommended. It may be necessary to treat the patient and establish a definitive diagnosis later.

REFERENCES

[b] 1. Nordyke RF et al. Graves disease: influence of age on clinical findings. Arch Intern Med 1988; 148:626.

[b] 2. Kahn AD et al. How useful is thyroid function testing in patients with recent onset atrial fibrillation? The Canadian Registry of Atrial Fibrillation Investigators. Arch Intern Med 1996; 156:2221.

[c] 3. Burch HB, Wartofsky L. Life-threatening thyrotoxicosis: thyroid storm. Endocrinol Metab Clinic North Am 1993; 22:263.

[b] 4. Canaris G et al. The Colorado Thyroid Disease Prevalence Study. Arch Intern Med 2000; 160:526.

[d] 5. Surks M et al. American Thyroid Association guidelines for use of laboratory tests in thyroid disorders. JAMA 1990; 263:1529.

[c] 6. Surks M, Sievert R. Drugs and thyroid function. N Engl J Med 1995; 333:1688.

[b] 7. Sawin C et al. Low serum thyroptropin concentrations as a risk factor for atrial fibrillation in older persons. N Engl J Med 1994; 331:1249.

[b] 8. Hak AE et al. Subclinical hypothyroidism is an independent risk factor for atherosclerosis and myocardial infarction in elderly women: the Rotterdam Study. Ann Intern Med 2000; 132:270.

[c] 9. McDermott M, Ridgway EC. Subclinical hypothyroidism is mild thyroid failure and should be treated. J Clin Endocrinol Metab 2001; 86:4585.

[c] 10. Moore WT, Eastman R. Diagnostic endocrinology, 2nd ed. St Louis: Mosby; 1996.

[b] 11. Spencer C et al. Specificity of sensitive assays of thyrotropin used to screen for thyroid disease in hospitalized patients. Clin Chem 1987; 33:1391.

[d] 12. Singer P et al. Treatment guidelines for patients with hyperthyroidism and hypothyroidism. JAMA 1995; 273:808.

23

THYROID DISORDERS

Approach to Abdominal Pain

Vandana R. Long, MD, Anastasio Saliaris, MD, and Francis Giardiello, MD

FAST FACTS

- Within the first few minutes of evaluation, determine if the abdominal pain is an emergency, urgent, or low-risk chronic issue and act accordingly.
- Maintain a low threshold for ordering imaging of immunosuppressed patients.
- *All* women of childbearing age should have a pregnancy test, and most should have a pelvic examination.
- Always think of nonabdominal causes of abdominal pain such as esophageal spasm or rupture, myocardial ischemia, pericarditis, pneumonia, uremia, diabetic ketoacidosis, hyperparathyroidism, and herpes zoster.

24

I. GENERAL APPROACH TO ABDOMINAL PAIN

A. HISTORY

1. **Description of abdominal pain:** Time and rapidity of onset, character (severity, constancy, quality), site (Box 24-1), radiation (e.g., hepatobiliary diseases often radiate to the right shoulder and scapula; pancreatitis radiates to the back), aggravating and relieving factors (change of position, stress, association with meals or menstrual cycle).
2. **Associated symptoms:** Nausea; vomiting; diarrhea; constipation; hematemesis; melena; hematochezia; dysphagia; odynophagia; changes in appetite; early satiety; weight loss; jaundice; itching; belching; flatulence; dysuria; hematuria; vaginal or penile discharge; fevers and chills; skin, joint, or eye symptoms.
3. **Past medical history:** Prior abdominal surgeries, immunosuppression (steroids, human immunodeficiency virus/acquired immunodeficiency syndrome [HIV/AIDS], posttransplant state, chemotherapy), peripheral vascular disease, diabetes mellitus, history of sexually transmitted diseases, medications such as nonsteroidal antiinflammatory drugs or antibiotics.
4. **Social history:** Alcohol, tobacco, illicit drug use, travel and dietary history.
5. **Family history:** Inflammatory bowel disease, familial Mediterranean fever, vascular disease.

B. PHYSICAL EXAMINATION

1. **General inspection:** Level of distress, position (patient will be immobile in peritonitis, writhing in pain in renal colic, in fetal position in pancreatitis), body habitus, jaundice, spider angiomata, palmar erythema.

BOX 24-1
ABDOMINAL PAIN BY LOCATION*

Right Upper Abdomen	Middle Upper Abdomen	Left Upper Abdomen
Choledocholithiasis	Gastroesophageal reflux disease	Splenic rupture
Acute cholecystitis	Esophagitis	Splenic infarct
Cholangitis	Hiatal hernia	Pancreatitis
Hepatitis	Gastritis	Pneumonia
Hepatic congestion	Pancreatitis	Myocardial infarction
Pneumonia	Peptic ulcer (gastric, duodenal)	Gastric ulcer
Myocardial infarction	Gastric outlet obstruction	Pyelonephritis
Appendicitis	Choledocholithiasis	
Pyelonephritis	Superior mesenteric artery syndrome	
	Myocardial infarction	
	Appendicitis	
	Aortic aneurysm	
	Aortic dissection	
	Middle Abdomen	
	Small bowel obstruction	
	Gastroenteritis	
	Irritable bowel syndrome	
	Malabsorption	
	Bowel perforation	
	Peritonitis	
	Mesenteric ischemia	
Right Lower Abdomen	**Middle Lower Abdomen**	**Left Lower Abdomen**
Appendicitis	Dysmenorrhea	Diverticulitis
Ureteral colic	Pelvic inflammatory disease	Ureteral colic
Pyelonephritis	Ectopic pregnancy	Pyelonephritis
Inflammatory bowel disease	Ovarian cyst rupture	Inflammatory bowel disease
Diverticulitis	Bladder distention	Pelvic inflammatory disease
Pelvic inflammatory disease	Cystitis	Ectopic pregnancy
Ectopic pregnancy	Strangulated hernia	Ovarian cyst rupture
Ovarian cyst rupture		Strangulated hernia
Strangulated hernia		

*This is a general guide to abdominal pain by location. Each box represents a region of the abdomen and common causes of pain in that location. These lists are not all-inclusive, and considerable overlap occurs in the areas where pain is perceived.

2. **Vital signs:** Temperature, blood pressure, pulse rate, respirations, oxygen saturation.
3. **Abdominal examination.**
a. Inspection: Surgical scars, distention, masses, distended veins (caput medusae), visible peristalsis, ecchymosis (Cullen's sign indicates periumbilical ecchymosis; Grey Turner's sign indicates flank discoloration), hernias (inguinal, femoral, obturator, abdominal wall).
b. Palpation: Guarding and rigidity, tenderness, rebound, superficial masses, organomegaly, pulsatile liver, pulsatile mass (aortic aneurysm), bladder distention, costovertebral angle tenderness, McBurney's point (two thirds of the way from umbilicus to iliac crest) tenderness (sign of appendicitis), Murphy's sign (arrest of inspiration with right upper quadrant [RUQ] palpation) in cholecystitis, shifting dullness.
c. Percussion: Liver span, bladder distention.
d. Auscultation: Presence and quality of bowel sounds, bruits.
4. **Rectal examination:** Tenderness, masses, stool color and consistency, occult blood.
5. **Pelvic examination:** Discharge, cervical motion tenderness, ovarian masses and cysts.

C. INITIAL DIAGNOSTIC STUDIES

1. **Laboratory tests:** Complete blood cell count (CBC) with differential, urinalysis and culture, liver and renal function tests in most patients. All women of childbearing age should have a pregnancy test.
2. **Electrocardiogram:** All patients with risk factors for cardiovascular disease.
3. **Chest radiograph and upright abdominal film:** Pneumonia and free air (bowel perforation).
4. **Abdominal plain film:** Bowel dilation, cecal diameter, air-fluid levels, urinary stones, gallbladder stones (rarely radiopaque), pneumatosis intestinalis (air in the bowel wall seen in cases of bowel infarction), thumbprinting (intestinal ischemia).
5. **Ultrasound:** Hepatobiliary and renal disease; pelvic causes of abdominal pain in women.
6. **Computed tomography (CT) scan:** Aortic aneurysm, intestinal ischemia, diverticulitis, inflammatory bowel disease, bowel obstruction, intraabdominal abscess.

II. CLINICAL PRESENTATION, DIAGNOSTICS, AND MANAGEMENT

Within the first few minutes of evaluating a patient's abdominal pain, the physician must decide if the pain is an emergency or is a low-risk or chronic issue.

A. EMERGENCIES

1. **Bowel perforation.**
a. Clinical presentation: The patient may have a history of ulcer disease, inflammatory bowel disease, diverticulitis, recent abdominal surgeries, or endoscopic procedures. The abdominal pain may be localized or

24

APPROACH TO ABDOMINAL PAIN

diffuse, depending on the extent of inflammation. The physical examination suggests peritonitis if the patient is motionless, is febrile, has tenderness to palpation with rebound and guarding, and is without bowel sounds.

b. Diagnostics: Upright or left lateral decubitus film can reveal free air. X-ray examination is only 38%[1] sensitive in diagnosing free air, perhaps because patients are not kept upright for 5 to 10 minutes before the film is taken. If the radiograph does not show free air but bowel perforation is suspected, a CT scan should be ordered.

c. Management: Supportive therapy, intravenous (IV) antibiotics, emergency surgical consultation.

2. **Ruptured ectopic pregnancy.**

a. Clinical presentation: Suggestive features in a woman of reproductive age include abdominal pain, a history of amenorrhea, and acute vaginal bleeding. Many patients are asymptomatic before tubal rupture. After perforation, guarding, rigidity, and hypotension are common. Adnexal tenderness, mass, and uterine enlargement should be sought on pelvic examination.

b. Diagnostics: Serum β human chorionic gonadotropin level is greater than 1500 IU/L, and transvaginal ultrasound does not show *intrauterine* pregnancy.

c. Management: Tubal pregnancy may resolve spontaneously or rupture. Rupture leads to hemorrhage and is associated with high mortality. An emergency gynecological consultation is needed if tubal rupture is suspected.

3. **Ruptured abdominal aortic aneurysm.**

a. Clinical presentation: Patients with a history of vascular disease, tobacco use (fivefold increased risk[2]), and positive family history (fourfold increased risk[3]) are more likely to have an aortic aneurysm. Symptoms are throbbing, pulsatile pain in the epigastric or lumbar region that changes to steady and continuous pain after rupture. On examination, pulsatile mass above the umbilicus and hypotension are common.

b. Diagnostics: Patients should be observed closely if this diagnosis is being seriously entertained. Aneurysms 6 cm or larger in diameter are more likely to rupture. Ultrasound is almost 100% sensitive, except in obese patients or in the presence of overlying bowel gas.[4] A CT scan can be useful if the ultrasound findings are nondiagnostic.

c. Management: Emergency surgical consultation should be obtained. Other interventions include fluid resuscitation with two wide-bore IV lines, normalization of anticoagulation if indicated, and transfusion of packed red blood cells. Much disagreement exists as to whether the use of β-blockers is beneficial for individuals who present without hypotension. Currently there are no clinical data suggesting improved survival in patients who have ruptured abdominal aortic aneurysms and are treated with β-blockers.

4. **Strangulated hernia.**

a. Clinical presentation: The patient is usually male (inguinal hernias are the most common type and are 10 times more common in men). Patients with a history of abdominal straining (lifting, constipation, coughing), pregnancy, obesity, and ascites are at greater risk for hernias. Symptoms of strangulation are severe abdominal pain and nonreducible hernia that is tender, erythematous, and swollen because of obstruction of venous flow.

b. Diagnostics: History and physical examination are adequate in the majority of cases. A CT scan can be obtained in the rare case of an unclear diagnosis.

c. Management: Emergency surgery is critical to save the strangulated bowel before it becomes necrotic.

5. **Toxic megacolon.**

a. Clinical presentation: Patients with inflammatory bowel disease (IBD), infection with *Clostridium difficile* or other infectious colitis, ischemic colitis, diverticulitis, colon cancer, and HIV are at risk. Patients often have at least 1 week of abdominal pain caused by one of the above conditions, then complain of bloody diarrhea, severe pain, and distention. Patients appear ill and often are hypotensive with fever and signs of peritonitis (abdominal tenderness, guarding, rebound).

b. Diagnostics: Colonic dilation of more than 6 cm and three of the following: fever, tachycardia (>120 beats/min), leukocytosis, and anemia, plus one of the following: dehydration, mental status changes, hypotension, and electrolyte disturbances.[5] A stool sample should be sent for Gram's staining, fecal leukocytes, and assays for *C. difficile* toxin.

c. Management: The patient should be given nothing by mouth (NPO), and a nasogastric (NG) tube should be inserted for decompression. Supportive therapy includes IV fluids, electrolyte repletion, and broad-spectrum antibiotics. Antimotility agents and narcotics should not be used because they may further decrease motility and increase the likelihood of perforation and peritonitis. Immediate surgical consultation should be obtained and colectomy performed if the patient exhibits signs of perforation or persistent symptoms after 48 hours of conservative management.

B. URGENT CONDITIONS

1. **Cholecystitis.**

a. Clinical presentation: Symptoms are RUQ pain radiating to the right shoulder and scapula, nausea, anorexia, fever, and vomiting. On physical examination, RUQ tenderness, a positive Murphy's sign, and mild jaundice may be present.

b. Diagnostics: Patients have leukocytosis with a left shift and mildly elevated levels of bilirubin, alkaline phosphatase, transaminases, and amylase. RUQ ultrasound may show a thickened gallbladder wall (>4 mm) (in a patient with a normal albumin level), sonographic Murphy's sign,

24

APPROACH TO ABDOMINAL PAIN

and presence of pericholecystic fluid in acute cholecystitis. If ultrasound does not establish the diagnosis, a technetium dimethyl iminodiacetic acid scan should be obtained. This test involves IV injection of radio-labeled isotope to evaluate biliary excretion and cystic duct patency. In cholecystitis the gallbladder is not visualized because of obstruction of the cystic duct. This test is 95% sensitive and 90% specific for acute calculous cholecystitis.[6] False negative results occur with acalculous cholecystitis, and false positive results occur when patients are receiving total parenteral nutrition.[7]

c. Management: The patient is kept NPO and started on IV fluids. NG suctioning should be applied if the patient is vomiting. Antibiotics and analgesia are administered as needed. Surgical consultation for cholecystectomy should be obtained.

2. Cholangitis (stasis and infection in the biliary tract).

a. Clinical presentation: Fever, RUQ pain, and jaundice (Charcot's triad) occur in 50% to 75% of patients with cholangitis.[8] The presence of Reynolds' pentad (Charcot's triad plus mental status changes and hypotension) is indicative of suppurative cholangitis and is associated with high morbidity and mortality.

b. Diagnostics: Leukocytosis and elevated alkaline phosphatase and direct bilirubin levels are present, and blood cultures are positive. RUQ ultrasound shows common bile duct dilation and stones. Endoscopic retrograde cholangiopancreatography (ERCP) can be performed to confirm the diagnosis.

c. Management: Antibiotics and supportive treatment with IV fluids should be initiated. NPO status is maintained. Vitamin K is given if needed. Urgent biliary duct drainage by stone removal or sphincterotomy can be performed with ERCP or percutaneously. Open surgical drainage is reserved for cases in which these modalities have failed.

3. Pancreatitis (see Chapter 26).

a. Clinical presentation: The patient typically has a history of alcohol abuse or biliary stones. Epigastric pain radiating to the back, nausea, and vomiting are common symptoms. In hemorrhagic pancreatitis, Grey Turner's and Cullen's signs may be present.

b. Diagnostics: Amylase and lipase levels may be elevated. Amylase is not specific for pancreatitis and can be elevated in peptic ulcer disease, intestinal obstruction, bowel ischemia, and other conditions. Amylase and lipase may not be elevated in chronic pancreatitis. Determine Ranson's criteria for risk stratification by ordering a CBC, liver function tests, measurement of calcium, lactic dehydrogenase, and blood urea nitrogen, and arterial blood gas determinations. An abdominal film can show absence of psoas shadows, a sentinel loop adjacent to the pancreas (ileus), and calcification in chronic pancreatitis. A CT scan may show edema, necrosis, a phlegmon, or pseudocysts. Although not urgent for a stable patient, a CT scan can be obtained within 72 hours after admission for evaluation of pancreatic necrosis.[9]

c. Management: There is ongoing debate about whether patients need to be kept NPO.[10] NG suctioning, IV fluid administration, and analgesics are provided. A surgical consultation is needed if the patient's condition is deteriorating or there is concern about a necrotic pancreas or abscess that would require surgical intervention.

4. Hepatitis.

a. Clinical presentation: The patient should be asked about alcohol and acetaminophen use, blood exposures, recent dietary history, autoimmune diseases, and medications. Common symptoms are anorexia, nausea, vomiting, malaise, myalgias, fever, RUQ pain, diarrhea, dark urine, light-colored stools, pruritus, tender hepatomegaly, and jaundice.

b. Diagnostics: Levels of transaminases, bilirubin (direct and indirect), and alkaline phosphatase are elevated. Prothrombin time and albumin and glucose levels should be checked for signs of hepatic dysfunction. Further investigations depend on the history and degree of elevation of alanine aminotransferase and aspartate aminotransferase levels but may include hepatitis serological tests, ethanol and acetaminophen levels, and autoimmune markers (antinuclear antibody, anti–smooth muscle antibody, anti–liver-kidney microsomal antibody). Liver biopsy may be needed to make the diagnosis.

c. Management: Therapy is supportive, including IV hydration. Hypoglycemia is treated with dextrose, and coagulation defects with vitamin K. Specific therapy depends on the type of hepatitis. For example, autoimmune and alcoholic hepatitis are often treated with steroids, whereas acetaminophen toxicity is treated with N-acetylcysteine (see Chapter 25).

5. Bowel obstruction.

a. Clinical presentation: Anorexia, nausea, vomiting (especially with more proximal obstruction), colicky abdominal pain, constipation or diarrhea, and obstipation are common symptoms. On physical examination the abdomen is distended and bowel sounds may be absent or high pitched and "tinkling," as in small bowel obstruction (SBO). If the patient is febrile and has signs of peritonitis, the possibility of bowel perforation, strangulation, or necrosis should be considered.

b. Diagnostics: Abdominal radiograph examination can help differentiate large bowel obstruction (haustra that do not cross the lumen) and SBO (valvulae conniventes that cross the entire lumen). In SBO, plain film x-ray shows central gas shadows and no gas in the large bowel, air-fluid levels, and bowel distention. Cecal diameter greater than 10 to 12 cm raises concern for bowel necrosis and perforation and should prompt consideration of bowel decompression or surgical intervention. If suspicion is high for obstruction, x-ray examination should be followed by an abdominal CT scan. The radiograph is 77% sensitive and 50% specific for bowel obstruction, whereas CT is 93% sensitive and 100% specific. CT can predict the level of obstruction in 93% of cases, whereas the radiography can predict the level only 60% of the time.

24

APPROACH TO ABDOMINAL PAIN

Cause of the obstruction can be determined 87% of the time with CT and only 7% with plain film.[11]

c. Management: Treatment includes NPO status, NG tube decompression, aggressive IV fluid administration, electrolyte repletion, and surgical evaluation. Note: Colonic pseudoobstruction, or Ogilvie's syndrome, is a *functional* bowel obstruction. Neostigmine therapy should be considered in these cases.

6. **Appendicitis.**

a. Clinical presentation: Symptoms include nausea, anorexia, fever, and central abdominal pain and cramping that migrate to the right lower quadrant (RLQ) and later change in character to sharp pain exacerbated by movement. On physical examination the patient has pain and guarding in the RLQ on palpation at McBurney's point, as well as pain in the RLQ on palpation of the left lower quadrant (Rovsing's sign), pain in the RLQ on extension of the right hip (iliopsoas sign), and pain with internal rotation of the hip (obturator sign). There can be tenderness on rectal examination if the inflamed appendix is adjacent to the rectum.

b. Diagnostics: The white blood cell count is often elevated. CT scan may show for a thick-walled appendix (>2 mm), appendicolith, phlegmon, abscess, free fluid, and fat stranding in the RLQ. The CT scan is 96% to 98% sensitive and 83% to 89% specific for appendicitis.[12] Plain films are usually not helpful. The appendix is visualized by ultrasound in only one third of cases. However, if it is visualized and more than 6 mm in diameter, appendicitis is likely.[13]

c. Management: Immediate surgical consultation for appendectomy is needed.

7. **Diverticulitis.**

a. Clinical presentation: Patients report left lower quadrant (LLQ) pain (rarely RLQ pain) and typically have had such symptoms before. They have nausea, vomiting, and changes in bowel habits. On physical examination LLQ tenderness and occasionally a palpable mass are found. If the bowel has perforated, patients may have a toxic appearance and will have localized or diffuse rebound and guarding.

b. Diagnostics: Leukocytosis is present. Free air will be seen on plain film if there is perforation. The CT scan shows focal thickening, fluid collections, fistulae, or obstruction.

c. Management: Treatment is oral antibiotics and a clear liquid diet initially. If no improvement occurs, NPO status and IV administration of antibiotics should be tried. Surgical consultation is indicated for perforation, abscess, obstruction, or fistula.

8. **Mesenteric ischemia.**

a. Clinical presentation: Hypercoagulable states, potential embolic sources (atrial fibrillation or endocarditis), or vascular disease should be sought. Patients have diffuse abdominal pain that is often out of proportion to physical findings. Physical examination findings include abdominal distention, occult blood in the stool, rebound and guarding, and absent bowel sounds if the ischemia is progressing to peritonitis.

b. Diagnostics: Patients may have leukocytosis with a left shift, metabolic acidosis (lactic acid), and elevated levels of amylase, LDH, or CK with continued ischemia. Plain film may show ileus, bowel wall thickening, or pneumatosis intestinalis. CT has a sensitivity of 64% and a specificity of 92% for bowel ischemia.[14] Mesenteric angiography is the gold standard, but magnetic resonance angiography or venography is a new modality that can help make the diagnosis and obviates the need for exposure to IV contrast agents.

c. Management: Therapy is supportive, with correction of metabolic acidosis, antibiotic administration, and insertion of an NG tube for decompression. Anticoagulation should be initiated unless there is bleeding or surgery will be performed immediately. An early surgical consultation should be obtained, given risk of bowel necrosis and perforation. Interventional radiology may offer additional options, including thrombolytic agents, embolectomy, angioplasty, and stent placement.

C. LOW-RISK AND CHRONIC CONDITIONS

1. Peptic ulcer disease and gastritis.

a. Clinical presentation: The patient has epigastric or left upper quadrant pain that may be improved (duodenal ulcers) or worsened (gastric ulcers) with eating. Anorexia, nausea, and vomiting are more common with gastric ulcers. Mild epigastric tenderness is found on physical examination.

b. Diagnostics: If signs of peritonitis are present, an upright x-ray examination is needed immediately to rule out perforation. Otherwise, esophagogastroduodenoscopy and biopsy to look for *Helicobacter pylori* are performed.

c. Management: An H_2 blocker or proton pump inhibitor is administered. If test results show *H. pylori*, treatment for eradication of infection is initiated (see Chapter 31).

2. Nephrolithiasis.

a. Clinical presentation: The patient writhes in bed from excruciating colicky pain that begins in the flank and radiates to the scrotum or labia. Dysuria, hematuria, difficulty urinating if stone is obstructing, nausea, vomiting, and diaphoresis are common symptoms.

b. Diagnostics: Urinalysis shows hematuria. Kidney, ureter, and bladder (KUB) radiography shows 90% of stones (calcified, struvite, and cystine stones are radiopaque). Ultrasound is equivalent to and less expensive than CT[15] and therefore is the most cost-efficient screening tool after KUB. Noncontrast CT is 91% sensitive and 95% specific for renal stones. CT has better sensitivity and specificity than IV pyelography[16] and can show radiolucent stones missed on KUB.

c. Management: Therapy is supportive with IV fluids and pain control if the stone is less than 5 mm. If it is greater than 5 mm, urological evaluation for possible lithotripsy should be obtained. If uric acid stone is present, the urine should be alkalinized.

3. **Pyelonephritis.**

a. Clinical presentation: Symptoms include flank pain, nausea, vomiting, fever, costovertebral angle tenderness, urinary frequency, dysuria, and suprapubic pain.

b. Diagnostics: Laboratory findings include leukocytosis, pyuria and hematuria on urinalysis, and a positive urine culture if obtained before antibiotics are administered. If the patient fails to improve on standard therapy, renal ultrasound should be performed to rule out renal abscess or obstruction.

c. Management: Antibiotics are given for 14 days. Indications for hospitalization include the patient's inability to maintain hydration or take medications, extreme illness, or an unclear diagnosis.

4. **Pelvic inflammatory disease.**

a. Clinical presentation: Patients at high risk include women who are younger than 35 years, use no or nonbarrier contraception, have new, multiple, or symptomatic sexual partners, and have a prior history of pelvic inflammatory disease (PID) or sexually transmitted disease. Patients have bilateral lower abdominal pain associated with menses, coitus, or jarring movements. Fever and chills, vaginal discharge, urethritis, proctitis, and uterine bleeding can be present. On physical examination there is tenderness in the lower quadrants with or without rebound or guarding. Purulent vaginal discharge, cervical motion tenderness, and uterine and adnexal tenderness may be found on pelvic examination. Among patients with PID, 10% have Fitz-Hugh–Curtis syndrome (perihepatitis associated with PID) and will have RUQ pain as well.

b. Diagnostics: The presence of leukocytosis should be sought. Other diagnostic tests include pelvic examination with cultures for gonorrhea and chlamydia, urinalysis, and measurement of urine β-hCG. Transvaginal ultrasound should be performed if pelvic abscess is a concern.

c. Management: Treatment is with antibiotics. Patients should be screened for other sexually transmitted diseases and educated about safe sex practices.

5. **Inflammatory bowel disease (IBD)** (see Chapter 29).

a. Clinical presentation: Patients may have crampy abdominal pain, fever, diarrhea, rectal bleeding and mucus, rectal ulcers and fistulae, constipation, fecal urgency, signs of peritonitis if perforation is present, and associated symptoms such as arthralgias, arthritis, ocular symptoms, and skin disorders (erythema nodosum and pyoderma gangrenosum).

b. Diagnostics: Ulcerative colitis is diagnosed by colonoscopy with biopsy. Findings include confluent erythematous mucosa, pseudopolyps, inflammatory infiltrate, crypt abscesses, and mucosal ulcers. In Crohn's disease, colonoscopy and upper gastrointestinal series with small bowel follow-through show narrowing of the lumen (string sign), cobblestoning, fistulae, and skip lesions. Biopsy shows focal ulcerations, acute and chronic inflammation, and granulomas, which can be found from the mouth to the anus.

c. Management: Treatment may include NPO status, IV fluids, TPN, oral or IV administration of steroids depending on acuity of the illness, topical or systemic administration of 5-aminosalicylic acid agents, and antibiotics if the patient does not respond to initial management. Azathioprine, mercaptopurine, methotrexate, or infliximab is administered for refractory disease.

6. **Biliary colic:** The name "biliary colic" is a misnomer because pain is continuous. Biliary colic is caused by a stone impacted in the gallbladder neck, cystic duct, or common bile duct (CBD).

a. Clinical presentation: Biliary colic is common in obese, multiparous, middle-aged women (the five "Fs": female, fat, forty, fertile, and flatulent). Patients complain of nausea, vomiting, dyspepsia, flatulence, belching, and RUQ or epigastric pain radiating to the back and right shoulder that is aggravated by fatty food intake. Each attack usually lasts 2 to 4 hours. On examination the patient may be writhing in pain, tachycardic, diaphoretic, jaundiced, and tender in the RUQ.

b. Diagnostics: RUQ ultrasound is only 50% sensitive if ductal dilation is absent and is 75% sensitive when dilation is present. The CT scan is 75% sensitive for detecting a CBD stone, regardless of dilation. Despite normal findings on noninvasive radiological testing, ERCP reveals a retained CBD stone with 90% sensitivity.[17] Magnetic resonance cholangiopancreatography uses magnetic resonance to evaluate the biliary and pancreatic ducts. It is an excellent noninvasive alternative to ERCP, with a sensitivity of 92% and specificity of 100%.[18]

c. Management: Therapy is supportive with analgesics, as well as antiemetics if the patient is nauseated. The stone often spontaneously passes back into the gallbladder or forward into the duodenum. If symptoms do not abate spontaneously, ERCP with or without sphincterotomy should be performed and the stone should be removed. Prophylactic cholecystectomy should be considered, especially for diabetic patients.

7. **Gastroenteritis.**

a. Clinical presentation: Patients have a recent history of travel or work at a daycare center or a history of unusual food consumption (e.g., uncooked meats, fish, or unpasteurized dairy products). Abdominal pain, fever, nausea, vomiting, and watery diarrhea (more than six loose stools a day for >48 hours) with or without blood or mucus are common complaints.

b. Diagnostics: Fecal leukocytes and occult blood should be sought. Stool Gram's stain and culture are needed only if symptoms persist or if patients are immunosuppressed or have IBD. Stool for ova and parasite examination should be obtained from international travelers, immunosuppressed patients, and patients with bloody diarrhea. *C. difficile* toxin should be checked in patients who have recently used antibiotics.

c. Management: Aggressive oral rehydration therapy or IV fluids should be given if the patient is unable to tolerate oral intake. Empirical antibiotics should be considered only for immunocompromised patients. If the patient has persistent symptoms or severe illness, stool culture should be obtained and treatment should be based on the results. If *C. difficile* toxin is present, metronidazole should be administered orally. Antimotility agents should be used only if the patient shows no signs of inflammatory diarrhea (fever, bloody stools, or fecal leukocytes) and is negative for *C. difficile* toxin.

8. **Irritable bowel syndrome.**

a. Clinical presentation: Patients may have mood or anxiety disorders. Symptoms are crampy abdominal pain, bloating, feeling of incomplete evacuation, diarrhea or constipation, mucus production, and pain relieved by defecation. Patients may also experience straining or urgency.

b. Diagnostics: Patients must have abdominal pain for at least 12 weeks (not necessarily consecutive) of the year and must have two of three of the following symptoms: pain relieved by defecation, change in stool frequency, and change in stool appearance. This is a diagnosis of exclusion. Structural and metabolic abnormalities should be ruled out before this diagnosis is made.[19]

c. Management: Treatment includes symptom control with dietary modification (i.e., increase in fiber and avoidance of foods that precipitate symptoms or increase flatulence), stress management, and medications (e.g., anticholinergics, antidepressants, antidiarrheals), depending on symptoms.

III. UNUSUAL CAUSES OF ABDOMINAL PAIN

1. **Lead poisoning:** Patients have diffuse and poorly localized pain, with a rigid abdomen. They may also have mental status changes, peripheral neuropathy, and anemia.

2. **Porphyria:** Presenting symptoms include colicky abdominal pain, vomiting and diarrhea or constipation, proximal muscle pain, peripheral neuropathy, mental status changes, and diaphoresis. Patients often have ileus with abdominal distention.

3. **Familial Mediterranean fever:** In this autosomal recessive disorder, recurrent and severe episodes of abdominal pain and fever occur in patients of Mediterranean background.

4. **Angioneurotic edema:** Severe episodic abdominal pain is caused by C1 esterase inhibitor deficiency. The C4 level should be checked.

5. **Oddi's sphincter dysfunction:** The common bile duct pressure is elevated because of Oddi's sphincter spasm or stricture. Patients have symptoms of biliary colic. Liver function tests reveal cholestasis, and RUQ ultrasound shows ductal dilation.

6. **Eosinophilic gastroenteritis:** Eosinophilic infiltrate is present in the small intestine mucosa. Patients have abdominal pain, diarrhea, nausea, fever, malabsorption, and eosinophilia.

7. **Mesenteric adenitis:** Acute diarrhea and fever associated with joint and skin abnormalities (erythema nodosum and multiforme) are caused by infection with *Yersinia* spp. Patients have RLQ tenderness as a result of enlarged mesenteric lymph nodes, and this condition is often misdiagnosed as appendicitis.

8. **Collagenous colitis:** Middle-aged women with crampy abdominal pain and watery diarrhea. Collagenous colitis is often confused with irritable bowel syndrome.

PEARLS AND PITFALLS

- When HIV-positive patients with low CD4 cell counts have abdominal pain, the clinician must have a lower threshold of suspicion and obtain imaging earlier than for nonimmunosuppressed patients. If the CD4 count is less than $100/mm^3$, the possibility of cytomegalovirus, fungi, *Mycobacterium avium* complex, *Cryptosporidium*, microsporidia, *Isospora belli*, and lymphoma should be considered in addition to all the usual pathogens. Also, many of the medications used to treat patients with HIV/AIDS can cause abdominal pain (i.e., producing such conditions as pancreatitis and renal stones).

- Steroids place patients at an increased risk of gastritis, peptic ulcer disease, pancreatitis, and bowel perforation. Steroids mask symptoms of many intraabdominal pathological conditions. Therefore the clinician should obtain a CT scan early in the presentation.

- All patients with ascites and abdominal pain should have a diagnostic paracentesis performed (with specimens sent for cell count and differential, Gram's staining, culture, and albumin evaluation) to rule out spontaneous bacterial peritonitis (see Chapter 27).

- Typhlitis, inflammation of the cecum, should be considered in the differential diagnosis when neutropenic patients have fever, RLQ pain, and tenderness. This condition is frequently misdiagnosed as appendicitis. *Pseudomonas* bacteremia is common. Treatment is antibiotics with or without surgery.

- After bone marrow transplantation, graft-versus-host disease can manifest itself as abdominal pain and diarrhea. Diagnosis is made by endoscopy with biopsy.

REFERENCES

[b] 1. Stapakis JC, Thickman D. Diagnosis of pneumoperitoneum: abdominal CT scan versus upright chest film. J Comput Assist Tomography 1992; 16:713.

[b] 2. Lederle FA et al. Prevalence and associations of abdominal aortic aneurysm detected through screening. Aneurysm Detection and Management (ADAM) Veterans Affairs Cooperative Study Group. Ann Intern Med 1997; 126:441.

[b] 3. Salo JA et al. Familial occurrence of abdominal aortic aneurysm. Ann Intern Med 1999; 130:637.

[c] 4. La Roy LL et al. Imaging of abdominal aortic aneurysms. AJR Am J Roentgenol 1989; 152:785.

[b] 5. Jalan KN et al. An experience with ulcerative colitis: toxic dilatation in 55 cases. Gastroenterology 1969; 57:68.

[b] 6. Swayne LC, Ginsberg HN. Diagnosis of acute cholecystitis by cholescintigraphy: significance of pericholecystic hepatic uptake. AJR Am J Roentgenol 1989; 152:1211.

[c]   7. Ahmed A et al. Management of gallstones and their complications. Am Fam Physician 2000; 61:1673.

[b]   8. Saik RP et al. Spectrum of cholangitis. Am J Surg 1975; 130:143.

[d]   9. Lankisch PG et al. Do we need a computed tomography examination in all patients with acute pancreatitis within 72 h after admission to hospital for the detection of pancreatic necrosis? Scand J Gastroenterol 2001; 36:432.

[c] 10. Lobo DN et al. Evolution of nutritional support in acute pancreatitis. Br J Surg 2000; 87:695.

[b] 11. Suri S et al. Comparative evaluation of plain films, ultrasound and CT in the diagnosis of intestinal obstruction. Acta Radiol 1999; 40:422.

[b] 12. Balthazar EJ et al. Acute appendicitis: CT and ultrasound correlation in one hundred patients. Radiology 1994; 190:31.

[b] 13. Jeffrey RB Jr et al. Acute appendicitis: sonographic criteria based on 250 cases. Radiology 1988; 167:327.

[b] 14. Taourel PG et al. Acute mesenteric ischemia: diagnosis with contrast-enhanced CT. Radiology 1996; 199:632.

[b] 15. Patlas M et al. Ultrasound vs CT for the detection of ureteric stones in patients with renal colic. Br J Radiol 2001; 74:901.

[b] 16. Chen MY, Zagoria RJ. Can noncontrast helical computed tomography replace intravenous urography for evaluation of patients with acute urinary tract colic? J Emerg Med 1999; 17:299.

[c] 17. Goroll AH, Mulley AG. Primary care medicine, 4th ed. Philadelphia: Lippincott, Williams & Wilkins; 2000.

[c] 18. Marks JM, Ponsky JL. Benign surgical disorders of the gallbladder. In DiMarino AJ Jr, Benjamin SB, editors. Gastrointestinal disease: an endoscopic approach, vol 2. Malden, Mass: Blackwell Science; 1997.

[c] 19. Thompson WG et al. Functional bowel disorders. In Drossman DA et al, editors. Rome II: the functional gastrointestinal disorders, 2nd ed. McLean, Va: Degnon Associates; 2000.

Acute Liver Failure and Metabolic Liver Disease

David E. Kaplan, MD, and Thomas Faust, MD

FAST FACTS

- Fulminant hepatic failure (FHF) carries an 80% mortality rate without transplantation.
- Most cases in the United States are due to acute viral hepatitis, drug reaction, or acetaminophen overdose or are idiopathic.
- *N*-Acetylcysteine therapy has proven benefit within 15 hours of acetaminophen ingestion but may also reduce morbidity and mortality if given after the 15-hour window.
- Supportive care should be administered while the need to refer the patient to the intensive care unit (ICU) or a tertiary referral center for transplantation evaluation is assessed.
- Patients with Wilson's disease, idiosyncratic drug reactions, or grade III or IV hepatic encephalopathy on presentation should be immediately referred for transplantation.

25

I. EPIDEMIOLOGY

1. Each year an estimated 10,000 to 20,000 cases of FHF occur in the United States.[1] The most common cause in developed nations is acetaminophen overdose, followed by cryptogenic causes, idiosyncratic drug reactions, acute hepatitis B, and hepatitis A.[2] In developing countries acute viral hepatitis is responsible for the majority of cases.

2. Overall mortality without transplantation in most series approximates 75% to 80% but depends highly on the cause of FHF. Spontaneous recovery occurs in as many as 60% of patients with acetaminophen overdose and 40% of patients with fulminant hepatitis A. In contrast, transplant-free survival occurs in only 12% of cases of idiosyncratic drug reaction and is nearly nonexistent in Wilson's disease. In the largest American series of patients with FHF of all causes, 25% survived spontaneously, 41% underwent orthotopic liver transplantation (OLT) with 76% having 1-year survival, and 34% died without undergoing OLT.[2]

II. CLINICAL PRESENTATION

1. At presentation patients with acute hepatic failure have new-onset jaundice (Box 25-1), frequently associated with systemic symptoms or right upper quadrant (RUQ) abdominal discomfort. In addition to scleral, sublingual, or generalized icterus, physical examination may reveal fetor hepaticus, RUQ tenderness, or asterixis (Box 25-2).

BOX 25-1

DIFFERENTIAL DIAGNOSIS OF JAUNDICE

NONHEPATIC

Hemolysis (any cause)

Ineffective erythropoiesis

Neonatal

EXTRAHEPATIC BILIARY (OBSTRUCTIVE)

Intraluminal Obstruction

Choledocholithiasis

Parasites

Luminal Obstruction

Benign stricture

Cholangiocarcinoma

Primary sclerosing cholangitis

Choledochal cyst

Extraluminal Obstruction

Pancreatic tumor

Pancreatitis

Ampullary carcinoma

Porta hepatis adenopathy or mass

HEPATOCELLULAR

Acute hepatitis

   Alcohol

   Viral

   Toxic

   Ischemic

Cirrhosis (all causes)

2. Stigmata of chronic liver disease, such as spider angiomata, palmar erythema, caput medusae, and testicular atrophy, are characteristically absent. The liver may be shrunken, normal, enlarged, or pulsatile, depending on the cause of failure. Mental status changes, which are required to make the diagnosis of FHF, may be present at admission or may develop within days to weeks.

3. Cases of FHF having certain causes may have specific prodromal symptoms (Box 25-3). For example, patients who have ingested *Amanita* spp. or *Lepiota* spp. mushrooms may have a latent period of 24 hours, followed by abdominal cramps, diarrhea, and emesis, then progress to FHF. Acute viral hepatitis is often manifested as malaise, fatigue, myalgias, arthralgias, and fever, with subsequent jaundice and FHF. Acetaminophen overdose is often a suicide attempt, usually involving ingestion of 20 to 25 g. However, therapeutic ingestions of as little as 4 g may be toxic in patients on long-term anticonvulsant therapy or in alcoholics.[3]

BOX 25-1—cont'd

DIFFERENTIAL DIAGNOSIS OF JAUNDICE

INTRAHEPATIC BILIARY AND CHOLESTATIC DISORDERS

Primary sclerosing cholangitis

Caroli's disease

Medications (not inclusive list)

  Clavulanic acid

  Methlytestosterone

  Total parenteral nutrition

  Chemotherapy

Sepsis and systemic infection

Infiltrative processes

  Tumor metastases

  Amyloid

  Lymphoma

  Sarcoidosis

Metabolic disorders

  Gilbert's disease (unconjugated)

  Inborn errors of metabolism (many)

  Benign recurrent intrahepatic cholestasis (BRIC)

  Paroxysmal familial intrahepatic cholestasis (PFIC)

  Thyroidopathy

  Renal disease

Postoperative jaundice

Cholestasis of pregnancy

Posthepatocellular injury

BOX 25-2

CONN'S GRADING OF PORTOSYSTEMIC ENCEPHALOPATHY

GRADE	CHARACTERISTICS
I	Asterixis, slow thought and affect
II	Drowsiness, inappropriate behavior, confusion
III	Somnolence or semistupor
IV	Coma, but may respond to deep pain

Data from Conn HO. The syndrome of portal-systemic encephalopathy. In Conn HO, Lieberthal MM, editors. The hepatic coma syndromes and lactose. Baltimore: Williams & Wilkins; 1979.

BOX 25-3

ABBREVIATED LIST OF CAUSES OF ACUTE HEPATIC FAILURE

INFECTION

Viral hepatitis: hepatitis A to G, non-A to non-G

Herpesviruses: cytomegalovirus, herpes simplex virus, varicella-zoster virus, Epstein-Barr virus

Adenovirus

Paramyxovirus

Parvovirus B19

Tuberculosis

VASCULAR OR POSTHEPATIC DISEASE

Budd-Chiari syndrome

Venoocclusive disease

Congestive hepatopathy

Shock

NEOPLASIA

Melanoma

Lymphoproliferative disorders

After bone marrow transplantation

DRUG-INDUCED

Analgesic drugs: acetaminophen, nonsteroidal antiinflammatory drugs

Anticonvulsant drugs: valproic acid, carbamazepine, phenytoin, felbamate

Sulfonamides: sulfasalazine

Antitubercular drugs: isoniazid, pyrazinamide

Antifungal drugs: ketoconazole, terbinafine

Antihypertensive drugs: lisinopril, methyldopa

Antiretroviral drugs: didanosine

Miscellaneous drugs: omeprazole, troglitazone, flutamide, disulfiram, methotrexate, nefazodone, halothane, propylthiouracil, tetracycline

EXPOSURES

Mushrooms: *Amanita phalloides, Lepiota* spp.

Herbal: pyrrolizidine alkaloids, chaparral, Jin Bu Huan

Yellow and white phosphorus

Carbon tetrachloride

Copper salts, arsenicals

3,4-Methelenedioxymethamphetamine (MDMA; Ecstasy)

OTHER

Autoimmune hepatitis

Wilson's disease

Reye's syndrome

Extensive hepatectomy

Acute fatty liver of pregnancy

Heatstroke

III. DIAGNOSTICS

1. The diagnosis is confirmed by laboratory studies, which reveal abnormally elevated levels of aspartate aminotransferase and alanine aminotransferase (usually >1000 IU/L) or alkaline phosphatase, as well as evidence of hepatocyte dysfunction, including hyperbilirubinemia, coagulopathy, hyperammonemia, lactic acidosis, and hypoglycemia. Signs of impending complications, such as renal insufficiency and sepsis, are common (Table 25-1).

TABLE 25-1

PATHOGENESIS AND MEDICAL MANAGEMENT OF THE MAJOR COMPLICATIONS OF ACUTE LIVER FAILURE

Major Complications	Pathogenesis	Management
Hypoglycemia	Diminished glucose synthesis	Blood glucose monitoring; intravenous glucose administration
Encephalopathy	Cerebral edema	CT scan (if advanced encephalopathy); ICP monitoring (if patient is in a coma); careful positioning of patient; consideration of osmotherapy (mannitol) or barbiturates
	Other common reversible factors	Standard therapy; avoidance of benzodiazepines and other sedative medications
Sepsis, pneumonia, other organ system infections	Bacterial or fungal infection	Aseptic medical and nursing care; surveillance cultures; antimicrobial agents
Hemorrhage (e.g., gastrointestinal, intracerebral)	Stress ulceration	H_2 receptor antagonists; proton pump inhibitors; nasogastric aspiration
	Coagulopathy	Vitamin K; platelet or fresh-frozen plasma infusions
Hypotension	Hypovolemia	Hemodynamic monitoring of central pressures; volume repletion with blood or colloid
	Decreased vascular resistance	α-Adrenergic agents
Respiratory failure	Acute respiratory distress syndrome	Hemodynamic monitoring of central pressures; mechanical ventilation
Renal failure	Hypovolemia	Hemodynamic monitoring of central pressures; volume repletion with blood or colloid
	Hepatorenal syndrome or acute tubular necrosis	Avoidance of nephrotoxic agents (e.g., aminoglycosides, aspirin, contrast dye); hemofiltration and dialysis

From Feldman M, Friedman LS, Sleisenger MH. Sleisenger & Fordtran's gastrointestinal and liver disease, 7th ed. Philadelphia: WB Saunders; 2003.

ACUTE LIVER FAILURE AND METABOLIC LIVER DISEASE

25

2. The initial workup must focus on identification of the underlying cause and on risk stratification. A thorough history focusing on medication use and exposures may quickly narrow the differential diagnosis. Key clues may include recent travel or camping; medication changes; ill contacts; ingestion of shellfish, mushrooms, or herbal products; intravenous (IV) drug use; receipt of blood products or history of needlestick injury; recent or current pregnancy; depression with suicidal ideation; or underlying malignancy.

3. When acetaminophen overdose is suspected, gastric lavage for pill fragments followed by activated charcoal is indicated. Serum and urine toxicological studies, including serum acetaminophen levels, must be obtained for all patients. In overdose cases acetaminophen levels should be obtained if possible at 4 and 15 hours after ingestion to estimate risk by widely published nomograms (Fig. 25-1).

4. In addition to the routine hematological tests with comprehensive metabolic panels and prothrombin and activated partial thromboplastin times, laboratory evaluation should include arterial blood gases, hepatitis serological tests, antinuclear antibody titers, ceruloplasmin level, serum copper level, blood type and screen, and blood cultures. Obtaining factor V and VIII levels should be considered because they may be helpful for risk assessment.

5. Liver duplex sonography should be performed to assess liver size and vascular patency and to rule out underlying cirrhosis or a space-occupying lesion. Other noninvasive studies may include slit-lamp examination, other viral serological tests, echocardiography, chest x-ray examination, and purified protein derivative of tuberculin testing.

6. Transjugular liver biopsy may be required in cryptogenic cases and may help distinguish autoimmune hepatitis from idiosyncratic drug reactions to identify candidates for corticosteroid treatment. Necrosis of more than 70% of the liver portends poor survival.

IV. MANAGEMENT (Fig. 25-2)

A. INITIAL CONSIDERATIONS

1. Risk stratification should begin in the emergency department and continue on the ward. In acetaminophen overdose, pH greater than 7.3 at admission, grade III encephalopathy, prothrombin time greater than 35 seconds, or creatinine level greater than 300 µmol/L (3.4 mg/dL) predicts poor outcome and should prompt immediate referral for transplantation.[3]

2. The London (also known as King's College) criteria, the most widely accepted schema for nonacetaminophen FHF, are based on age, etiology, duration of delay in onset of hepatic encephalopathy (HE), coagulopathy, and bilirubin concentration (Box 25-4).[3] The presence of high-grade encephalopathy, although often a late finding, portends a poor prognosis and identifies patients who require more immediate transplant referral, as well as immediate ICU referral.

BOX 25-4

MODIFIED LONDON CRITERIA FOR TRANSPLANT REFERRAL (NOT INCLUDING ACETAMINOPHEN OVERDOSE)

I. Prothrombin time >35 sec (INR 7.7)

II. Grade III or IV encephalopathy

III. Or three of the following:

    A. Age <10 years or >40 years

    B. Non-A, non-B hepatitis

    C. Halothane-induced

    D. Idiosyncratic drug reactions

    E. Duration of jaundice before onset of encephalopathy >7 days

    F. Prothrombin time >25 sec (INR 3.85)

    G. Bilirubin level >300 μmol/mL (17.5 mg/dL)

Data from O'Grady JG et al. Gastroenterology 1989; 97:439; Pauwels A et al. J Hepatol 1993; 17:124.

INR, International normalized ratio.

3. Levels of factor V, a vitamin K–independent, hepatically synthesized clotting factor, have been prospectively validated in one study as an alternative criterion for referral for emergency OLT. According to guidelines known as the Clichy criteria,[4] patients with coma or confusion and factor V levels less than 20% of normal if younger than 30 years old or less than 30% of normal if older than 30 years old should be referred for emergency OLT. Factor V levels should be followed serially. Return to 50% normal levels at 48 hours and to normal levels at day 4 predicts recovery.[5]

4. A single retrospective comparison of the London and Clichy criteria in acetaminophen overdose suggested superiority of the London criteria.[6] However, diagnostic accuracy for the Clichy and London criteria appear to be similar in non-acetaminophen-related FHF.[7]

5. The duration of time between onset of jaundice and onset of encephalopathy defines four distinct clinical subclassifications that prognosticate both survival and certain complications: hyperacute liver failure (HALF; <1 week), acute liver failure (ALF; 1-4 weeks), subacute liver failure (SALF; 4-12 weeks), and late-onset failure (>12 weeks).[8] Intracranial hypertension develops in 49% of patients with HALF, compared with 16% of those with SALF, but ascites develops in only 20% of patients with HALF, compared with 79% of those with SALF.[9] Survival also varies by subclass: HALF, 36% to 37%; ALF, 7% to 22%; SALF, 14% to 21%.[8,9] These differences are reflected in the London criteria.

B. TOXIC INGESTIONS

1. Effects of toxin ingestions, including acetaminophen, may be aborted if gastric lavage and activated charcoal administration are performed within several hours of the ingestion.

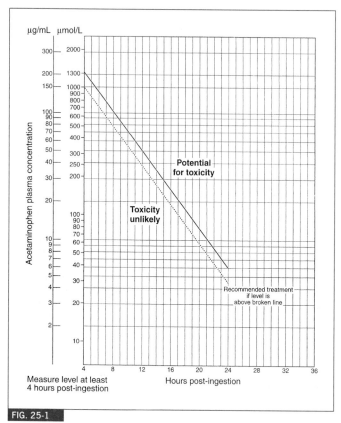

FIG. 25-1

Rumack-Matthew nomogram for acetaminophen poisoning. *(From Rumack BH, Matthew H: Pediatrics 1975; 55:871.)*

2. Patients with toxic acetaminophen overdose must be treated promptly with *N*-acetylcysteine. Toxin levels over 200 mg/L at 4 hours or over 30 mg/L at 15 hours predict toxicity; however, lower limits must be used in patients with chronic alcoholism or taking anticonvulsants.[8]

3. When *N*-acetylcysteine is administered within 15 hours of ingestion, preventive efficacy nears 100%.[10,11] Given after 15 hours, it reduces the risk of grade IV encephalopathy (from 75%-77% to 40%-68%).[12]

Retrospective data also suggest a survival benefit and reduction in need for hemodialysis.[13]

4. N-Acetylcysteine is administered orally with 140 mg/kg as an initial dose, then 70 mg/kg q4h for 17 doses. Activated charcoal reduces bioavailability of N-acetylcysteine and should not be given simultaneously.

5. The role of N-acetylcysteine as a nonspecific antoxidant in the treatment of nonacetaminophen FHF remains under investigation.[14] A multicenter study in the United States is ongoing. Given the benign safety profile of N-acetylcysteine, we recommend consideration of its use in all cases of FHF.

C. ENCEPHALOPATHY

1. Mild encephalopathy may be managed with restriction of dietary protein, lactulose 30 g PO qid, and selective bowel decontamination with neomycin or metronidazole.[15] Neomycin is less preferable because it may contribute to renal insufficiency.

2. Grade II or greater HE should prompt ICU referral.[16,17] Once high-grade HE ensues, management includes frequent neurological checks, avoidance of agitation, and in many centers placement of an intra-cranial pressure (ICP) monitor. If clinical or ICP data suggest intracra-nial hypertension, mannitol 0.3 to 1.0 mg/kg IV is given and re-peated to attain serum osmolarity approaching 320 mOsm/L. If the patient is anuric, mannitol must be coupled with ultrafiltration or he-modialysis. Hyperventilation to $Paco_2$ of 25 to 30 mm Hg should be reserved for patients with evidence of impending herniation.

3. Inotropic support to maintain a cerebral perfusion pressure of 50 mm Hg may be needed, and occult seizure activity should be treated.[11,15] Small studies suggest a possible therapeutic role for induced hypother-mia for uncontrolled intracranial hypertension.[18] Cooling patients to a core temperature near 32° C reduces intracranial pressure, decreases cerebral blood flow, and normalizes cerebral perfusion autoregula-tion.[19] The use of this modality in human subjects is still purely ex-perimental. Cerebral edema is responsible for the majority of deaths from FHF.

D. INFECTIONS

1. Bacterial and fungal infections, particularly aspergillosis, are common in FHF and frequently fatal. The use of prophylactic antibiotics and selective bowel decontamination remains controversial,[20] but authors universally endorse empirical antibiotics when any sign of infection is seen.[11,15] Some authors recommend empirical antifungal therapy for leukocytosis (leukocyte count >20,000/µL).[11] Specimens for surveillance blood, urine, and endotracheal cultures should be ob-tained at least every other day from the critically ill patient with FHF.

E. RENAL FAILURE

1. Acute renal failure (ARF) develops in up to 50% of patients with FHF[21] and 75% of patients with grade III or IV encephalopathy.[8]

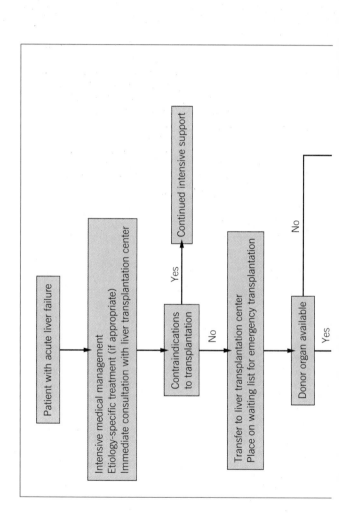

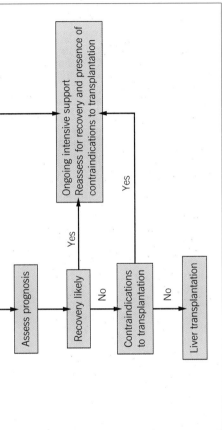

FIG. 25-2

Management of acute liver failure. The initial approach to patient management includes intensive care support and prompt contact with a liver transplantation center. Even if contraindications to liver transplantation are present at the time of admission, urgent patient transfer to a transplantation center may be beneficial in selected circumstances. *(From Feldman M, Friedman LS, Sleisenger MH: Sleisenger & Fordtran's gastrointestinal and liver disease, 7th ed. Philadelphia: WB Saunders; 2003.)*

ACUTE LIVER FAILURE AND METABOLIC LIVER DISEASE **25**

Renal failure portends poor survival (50%), prolonged mechanical ventilation, and longer stay in the ICU and hospital.[21] Preventive measures include treatment of infections, avoidance of nephrotoxins (i.e., aminoglycosides), treatment of hypotension with colloid,[10] and dopamine 2 to 4 μg/kg $\cdot$ min IV.[11,22] When dialysis is necessary, continuous venovenous or arteriovenous hemodialysis should be used to avoid aggravation of intracranial hypertension associated with acute hemodialysis.

F. HYPOTENSION

1. Hypotension may require use of colloid or vasopressors (see Chapter 12). Systemic sepsis must be aggressively treated with empirical antibiotics, potentially including antifungal therapy.

G. GASTROINTESTINAL BLEEDING PROPHYLAXIS

1. Prophylaxis against gastrointestinal hemorrhage with H_2 blockers, sucralfate, or proton pump inhibitors should be initiated on admission (see Chapter 31). An active blood type and screen must be maintained. Fresh frozen plasma should be used only for clinically significant bleeding or invasive procedures. Desmopressin may be beneficial if uremia coexists.

H. MISCELLANEOUS

1. Hypoglycemia may require hypertonic glucose infusion. Supportive therapy may be required for pulmonary edema, pancreatitis, and other metabolic abnormalities. Adult respiratory distress syndrome (ARDS) and multiorgan system failure can complicate the clinical course and contribute to mortality. Care of patients with FHF requires the coordination of multiple consulting services, all of which assist in the management of specific facets of the patient's treatment.

I. LIVER REPLACEMENT THERAPY

1. **Orthotopic liver transplantation:** Criteria for transplantation in FHF, whether or not it is caused by acetaminophen overdose, are discussed in detail above (Box 25-5). Contraindications to transplantation in FHF are equivalent to those for OLT in chronic liver disease. Serious bacterial or fungal infections are the most common reasons that otherwise acceptable candidates are denied OLT. OLT yields 46% to 92% 1-year survival rates in FHF,[2,23-25] which although suboptimal are markedly better than the natural history of severe FHF.

BOX 25-5

LONDON CRITERIA FOR TRANSPLANT REFERRAL (ACETAMINOPHEN OVERDOSE)

I. Prothrombin time >35 sec (INR 7.7)

II. Grade III or IV encephalopathy

III. pH 7.3

IV. Creatinine level >300 μmol (3.4 mg/dL)

INR, International normalized ratio.

2. **Experimental approaches:** Controlled trials of charcoal hemoperfusion have failed to demonstrate any benefit of this modality.[26] Liver replacement therapies with a bioartificial liver (BAL) or extracorporeal liver assist device (ELAD) system consist of cartridges that allow perfusion of the patient's plasma over columns of human hepatoblastoma or porcine hepatocyte cells. Phase I trial data demonstrate that the neurological status stabilizes in most patients, that this modality shows promise as a bridge to transplantation, and that a few patients recover spontaneously when given additional time for hepatocyte regeneration.[27,28] The MARS albumin dialysis system has been studied in acute-on-chronic liver failure.[29] Auxiliary liver transplantation[30] and living donor liver transplantation[31] may prove, after prospective investigation, to have advantages over primary cadaveric OLT.

PEARLS AND PITFALLS

- A thorough initial history is critical because this may be the last opportunity to identify a specific cause.
- The London and Modified London criteria have excellent positive predictive value but poor negative predictive value. Since failure to meet criteria does not predict survival, continued observation is critical.
- A diagnosis of Wilson's disease should be considered in patients of appropriate age, and if Wilson's disease is fulminant, the patient should be referred for transplantation immediately.
- *N*-Acetylcysteine may have benefit in acetaminophen overdose, even after 15 hours, and has no toxicity.
- Anticipation of expected complications and early intervention may reduce morbidity and mortality.
- The use of benzodiazepines and other sedatives should be avoided because they may obscure critical neuropsychiatric signs of decompensation.
- All patients should be referred to the nearest tertiary care or liver transplant center as soon as possible.
- A recent single-center study from Denmark found that a serum phosphate level greater than 1.2 mmol/L (3.7 mg/dL) at 48 to 96 hours after acetaminophen overdose had 89% sensitivity, 100% specificity, 100% positive-predictive value, and 98% accuracy in predicting death without transplantation in acetaminophen overdose. This indicator outperformed the London criteria in the study population.[32] If these data are confirmed at other centers, risk stratification in acetaminophen overdose would be greatly simplified.

REFERENCES

[d] 1. Hoofnagle JH et al. Fulminant hepatic failure: summary of a workshop. Hepatology 1995; 21:240.

[b] 2. Schiodt FV et al. Etiology and outcome for 295 patients with acute liver failure in the United States. Liver Transplant Surg 1999; 5:29.

[b] 3. O'Grady JG et al. Acute liver failure: redefining the syndromes. Lancet 1993; 342:252.

[b] 4. Bernuau J et al. Criteria for emergency liver transplantation in patients with acute viral hepatitis and factor V (FV) below 50% of normal: a prospective study. Hepatology 1991; 14:49.

[b] 5. Pereira LM et al. Coagulation factor V and VIII/V ratio as predictors of outcome in paracetamol induced fulminant hepatic failure: relation to other prognostic indicators. Gut 1992; 33:98.

[b] 6. Izumi S et al. Coagulation factor V levels as a prognostic indicator in fulminant hepatic failure. Hepatology 1996; 23:1507.

[b] 7. Pauwels A et al. Emergency liver transplantation for acute liver failure: evaluation of London and Clichy criteria. J Hepatol 1993; 17:124.

[c] 8. O'Grady J. Acute liver failure. J R Coll Physicians Lond 1997; 31:603.

[b] 9. Dhiman RK et al. Prognostic evaluation of early indicators in fulminant hepatic failure by multivariate analysis. Dig Dis Sci 1998; 43:1311.

[b] 10. Prescott LF et al. Intravenous *N*-acetylcysteine: the treatment of choice for paracetamol poisoning. BMJ 1979; 2:1097.

[b] 11. Smilkstein MJ et al. Efficacy of oral *N*-acetylcysteine in the treatment of acetaminophen overdose: analysis of the national multicenter study (1976 to 1985). N Engl J Med 1988; 319:1557.

[a] 12. Keays R et al. Intravenous acetylcysteine in paracetamol induced fulminant hepatic failure: a prospective controlled trial. BMJ 1991; 303:1026.

[b] 13. Harrison PM et al. Improved outcome of paracetamol-induced fulminant hepatic failure by late administration of acetylcysteine. Lancet 1990; 335:1572.

[b] 14. Ben-Ari Z, Vaknin H, Tur-Kaspa R. *N*-Acetylcysteine in acute hepatic failure (non-paracetamol-induced). Hepatogastroenterology 2000; 47:786.

[c] 15. Mas A, Rodes J. Fulminant hepatic failure. Lancet 1997; 349:1081.

[b] 16. Daas M et al. Acute liver failure: results of a 5-year clinical protocol. Liver Transplant Surg 1995; 1:210.

[b] 17. Makin AJ et al. A 7-year experience of severe acetaminophen-induced hepatotoxicity (1987-1993). Gastroenterology 1995; 109:1907.

[b] 18. Jalan R et al. Treatment of uncontrolled intracranial hypertension in acute liver failure with moderate hypothermia. Lancet 1999; 354:1164.

[b] 19. Jalan R et al. Restoration of cerebral blood flow autoregulation and reactivity to carbon dioxide in acute liver failure by moderate hypothermia. Hepatology 2001; 34:50.

[a] 20. Rolando N et al. Prospective study comparing the efficacy of prophylactic parenteral antimicrobials, with or without enteral decontamination, in patients with acute liver failure. Liver Transplant Surg 1996; 2:8.

[b] 21. Mendoza A et al. Liver transplantation for fulminant hepatic failure: importance of renal failure. Transplant Int 1997; 10:55.

[c] 22. Munoz SJ. Difficult management problems in fulminant hepatic failure. Semin Liver Dis 1993; 13:395.

[b] 23. O'Grady JG et al. Liver transplantation after paracetamol overdose. BMJ 1991; 303:221.

[b] 24. McCashland TM et al. The American experience with transplantation for acute liver failure. Semin Liver Dis 1996; 16:427.

[b] 25. Ascher NL et al. Liver transplantation for fulminant hepatic failure. Arch Surg 1993; 128:677.

[a] 26. O'Grady JG et al. Controlled trials of charcoal hemoperfusion and prognostic factors in fulminant hepatic failure. Gastroenterology 1988; 94:1186.

[b] 27. Watanabe FD et al. Clinical experience with a bioartificial liver in the treatment of severe liver failure: a phase I clinical trial. Ann Surg 1997; 225:484.

[b] 28. Watanabe FD et al. Treatment of acetaminophen-induced fulminant hepatic failure with a bioartificial liver. Transplant Proc 1997; 29:487.

[a] 29. Heemann U et al. Albumin dialysis in cirrhosis with superimposed acute liver injury: a prospective, controlled study. Hepatology 2002; 36:949.

[b] 30. Pereira SP et al. Auxiliary partial orthotopic liver transplantation for acute liver failure. J Hepatol 1997; 26:1010.

[b] 31. Fuchinoue W et al. Living-related liver transplantation for fulminant hepatic failure. Transplant Proc 1997; 29:424.

[a] 32. Schmidt LE, Dalhoff K. Serum phosphate is an early predictor of outcome in severe acetaminophen-induced hepatotoxicity. Hepatology 2002; 36:659.

Acute Pancreatitis

Geoffrey C. Nguyen, MD, and Mary L. Harris, MD

FAST FACTS

- Acute pancreatitis is a potentially fatal disease with a mortality rate of 5% to 10%.
- Gallstones and alcohol account for up to 80% of cases of acute pancreatitis.
- Diagnosis is based on clinical findings and confirmed by amylase or lipase levels three times the upper limit of normal or radiographic findings.
- Assessment of severity by Ranson's score, APACHE-II criteria, or computed tomography (CT) scan is a crucial step in management.
- Prophylactic antibiotics are indicated in acute necrotizing pancreatitis.

I. EPIDEMIOLOGY

1. Acute pancreatitis is defined as inflammation of the pancreas, which may involve peripancreatic tissue or remote organs and may also have local complications, such as pancreatic necrosis.
2. Acute pancreatitis is common, responsible for 108,000 hospitalizations and 2251 deaths in the United States in 1987.[1] The incidence varies from 4.8 to 24.2 per 100,000, with a mortality rate as high as 5% to 10%.[2,3] The vast majority of patients have mild pancreatitis, and most recover within 5 to 7 days.
3. Gallstones and alcohol intake account for more than 80% of acute pancreatitis cases. Most episodes of gallstone pancreatitis are associated with transient impaction of a stone in the pancreatic ampulla.
4. Biliary pancreatitis is more common in women, with a peak incidence between 50 and 60 years of age. Other causes include hypertriglyceridemia, hypercalcemia, drugs, trauma, previous endoscopic retrograde cholangiopancreatography (ERCP), Oddi's sphincter dysfunction, viral infections, and anatomical abnormalities. Box 26-1 outlines the conditions that cause pancreatitis.[4] Drugs that are definitely associated with acute pancreatitis include azathioprine, 6-mercaptopurine, asparaginase, pentamidine, and didanosine.

II. CLINICAL PRESENTATION

1. The hallmark of acute pancreatitis is continuous, boring, epigastric, right upper quadrant (RUQ), or diffuse abdominal pain. Onset of pain is gradual, peaks in 30 to 60 minutes, and then remains steady. In about half of cases a bandlike radiation to the back occurs. Abdominal pain is accompanied by nausea and vomiting in almost 90% of cases. Patients may find relief by bending forward.

427

BOX 26-1

CAUSES OF PANCREATITIS

Bacterial infection (*Mycoplasma,* Legionnaire's disease, *Campylobacter)* infection

Cardiopulmonary bypass

Cholelithiasis, choledocholithiasis

Crohn's disease

Cystic fibrosis

Drugs and toxins (thiazides, azathioprine, ethacrynic acid, furosemide, tetracycline, oral contraceptives, scorpion venom, methyl alcohol, 6-mercaptopurine, asparaginase, pentamidine, and didanosine)

Endoscopic retrograde cholangiopancreatography

End-stage renal failure

Ethanol abuse

Familial pancreatitis

Hypercalcemia

Hyperlipidemia (especially hypertriglyceridemia)

Hyperparathyroidism

Hypothermia

Idiopathic

Intraductal parasites

Major abdominal surgery

Mesenteric ischemia or embolism

Organ transplantation (cytomegalovirus)

Pancreas divisum

Pancreatic tumors

Penetrating gastric or duodenal ulcer

Pregnancy

Shock

Sphincter of Oddi dysfunction

Trauma

Upper gastrointestinal endoscopy

Vasculitis

Viral infection (mumps, Coxsackie virus, human immunodeficiency virus, viral hepatitis)

---

2. Systemic signs include fever, tachycardia, tachypnea, and in severe cases hypotension. The abdominal findings vary from minimal tenderness to distention with peritoneal signs, depending on severity. Intraabdominal hemorrhage manifests itself as periumbilical (Cullen's sign) or flank (Grey Turner's sign) ecchymoses.[2]

3. The differential diagnosis includes acutely perforated ulcer, acute cholecystitis, acute intestinal obstruction, acute mesenteric ischemia, and renal colic. Hyperamylasemia may also be seen in other conditions such as mumps, ectopic pregnancy, and renal failure.

4. Acute pancreatitis is diagnosed on the basis of clinical features and confirmed by either serum biological markers or radiographic findings.

III. DIAGNOSTICS
A. LABORATORY TESTS

1. Serum amylase levels rise within 6 to 12 hours of onset of pain. Levels greater than three times the upper limit of normal are characteristic of pancreatitis and usually do not occur in other conditions, such as salivary injury, viscous perforation, mesenteric ischemia, or renal failure.[5] Amylase levels usually normalize within 5 to 7 days in uncomplicated cases. High triglyceride levels (>1000 mg/dL) may mask high serum amylase levels.

2. Serum lipase levels that exceed three times the upper limit of normal are also a diagnostic indicator of acute pancreatitis and have greater sensitivity and specificity than amylase. The serum lipase level remains elevated for 7 to 14 days. The levels of amylase and lipase *do not* correlate with severity and can actually be normal in severe necrotizing pancreatitis.[6] Furthermore, daily measurement of levels has no clinical value.

3. An alanine aminotransferase level greater than 150 IU/L is highly suggestive of gallstone pancreatitis.[7] A lipase/amylase ratio greater than 2 suggests alcohol as the etiology.[8,9]

B. IMAGING

1. An abdominal radiograph should be obtained to evaluate for other causes of abdominal symptoms. A "sentinel loop" may be suggestive of severe pancreatitis.

2. An RUQ ultrasound is the test of choice for detecting gallstone pancreatitis. It should be obtained within 24 to 48 hours of an initial bout to evaluate for gallstones and dilation of the common bile duct.

3. Contrast-enhanced CT is the radiographic imaging modality of choice for both the diagnosis and assessment of severity of acute pancreatitis. Although it may not detect 15% to 30% of mild cases, abnormal findings are almost always detected in moderate and severe cases. Abdominal CT is indicated for the following patients: (1) those in whom the clinical diagnosis is uncertain; (2) those with hyperamylasemia and severe clinical pancreatitis, abdominal distention, tenderness, high fever (>39° C), and leukocytosis; (3) those with a Ranson's score of greater than 3 or an APACHE-II score of greater than 8; (4) those who do not show improvement after 72 hours of initial conservative therapy; and (5) those demonstrating acute deterioration after initial clinical improvement (Table 26-1 and Box 26-2).[10] Abdominal CT allows for assessment of degree of pancreatic inflammation and presence of peripancreatic fluid. Addition of intravenous (IV) contrast medium can distinguish between pancreatic edema and necrosis, since the latter is not enhanced.

26

ACUTE PANCREATITIS

TABLE 26-1
APACHE-II SEVERITY OF DISEASE CLASSIFICATION SYSTEM

Physiological Variable	SCORE								
	+4	+3	+2	+1	0	+1	+2	+3	+4
1. Rectal temperature (° C)	≥41	39.0-40.9		38.5-38.9	36.0-38.4	34.0-35.9	32.0-33.9	30.0-31.9	≤29.9
2. Mean arterial blood pressure (mm Hg)	≥160	130-159	110-129		70-109		50-69		≤49
3. Heart rate (beats/min)	≥180	140-179	110-139		70-109		55-69	40-54	≤39
4. Respiratory rate (breaths/min)	≥50	35-49		25-34	12-24	10-11	6-9		≤5
5. Oxygenation (mm Hg) (if Fio_2 ≥0.5, record A-aDo_2; if Fio_2 <0.5, record only Pao_2)	A-aDo_2 ≥500	A-aDo_2 350-499	A-aDo_2 200-349		A-aDo_2 <200; Pao_2 >70	Pao_2 61-70		Pao_2 55-60	Pao_2 <55
6. Arterial pH or	≥7.7	7.6-7.69		7.5-7.59	7.33-7.49		7.25-7.32	7.15-7.24	<7.15
Serum HCO_3^- (not preferred, but use in lieu of arterial pH if arterial blood gas measurement is not available)	≥52	41.0-51.9		32.0-40.9	22.0-31.9		18.0-21.9	15.0-17.9	<15
7. Serum sodium (mmol/L)	≥180	160-179	155-159	150-154	130-149		120-129	111-119	<110
8. Serum potassium (mmol/L)	≥7	6.0-6.9		5.5-5.9	3.5-5.4	3.0-3.4	2.5-2.9		<2.5

	+4	+3	+2	+1	0	+1	+2	+3	+4
9. Serum creatinine (mg/dL) (double the point score for acute renal failure)	>3.5	2.0-3.4	1.5-1.9		0.6-1.4		<0.6		
10. Hematocrit (%)	≥60		50.0-59.9	46.0-49.9	30.0-45.9		20.0-29.9		<20
11. White blood count	≥40		20.0-39.9	15.0-19.9	3.0-14.9		1.0-2.9		<20
12. Glasgow Coma Scale (GCS) (score = 15 minus actual GCS)									

A. Total Acute Physiology Score (APS): Sum of the 12 individual variable points

B. Age Points

Assign point to age as follows:

Age (yr)	Points
≤44	0
45-54	2
55-64	3
65-74	5
≥75	6

26

ACUTE PANCREATITIS

cont'd

TABLE 26-1

APACHE-II SEVERITY OF DISEASE CLASSICATION SYSTEM—cont'd

C. Chronic Health Points

If the patient has a history of severe organ system insufficiency or is immunocompromised, assign points as follows:

a. For nonoperative or emergency postoperative patients: 5 points

b. For elective postoperative patients: 2 points

Organ insufficiency or immunocompromised state must have been evident before this hospital admission and conform to the following criteria:

Liver: Biopsy-proven cirrhosis and documented portal hypertension; episodes of past upper gastrointestinal bleeding attributed to portal hypertension; or prior episodes of hepatic failure, encephalopathy, or coma.

Cardiovascular: New York Heart Association class IV.

Respiratory: Chronic restrictive, obstructive, or vascular disease resulting in severe exercise restriction (e.g., unable to climb stairs or perform household duties, or documented chronic hypoxia, hypercapnia, secondary polycythemia, severe pulmonary hypertension, or respirator dependency).

Renal: Recurring chronic dialysis.

Immunocompromised:. The patient has received therapy that suppresses resistance to infection (e.g., immunosuppression, chemotherapy, radiation, long-term or recent high-dose steroids) or has a disease that is sufficiently advanced that the patient is unable to suppress infection (e.g., leukemia, lymphoma, acquired immunodeficiency syndrome).

APACHE-II Score = A + B + C

Severe acute pancreatitis is suggested by score ≥8 on initial presentation; peak score >9.

BOX 26-2

RANSON'S CRITERIA

AT ADMISSION

Age >55 years

White blood cell count >16,000/mm^3

Glucose level >200 mg/dL

Lactate dehydrogenase level >350 IU/L

Aspartate aminotransferase level >250 IU/L

AT 48 HOURS

Hematocrit decrease of >10%

Blood urea nitrogen level increase of >5 mg/dL

Calcium level <8 mg/dL

Pao_2 <60 mm Hg

Base deficit >4 mEq/L

Fluid sequestration >6 L

RISK FACTORS	MORTALITY RATE
0-2	<1%
3-4	≈15%
5-6	≈40%
>6	≈100%

IV. MANAGEMENT

1. The initial step in management of acute pancreatitis is assessment of severity (Fig. 26-1). Most episodes of acute pancreatitis are mild, and patients typically recover within 5 to 7 days with supportive management. Severe necrotizing pancreatitis, however, is associated with significantly higher rates of complications and mortality. According to a 1992 symposium, severe acute pancreatitis is characterized by a Ranson's score of 3 or higher or an APACHE-II score of 8 or higher; organ failure; or local complications, such as necrosis, abscess, or pseudocyst. Organ failure is the most important indicator of severity and is defined by (1) shock with systolic blood pressure less than 90 mm Hg; (2) pulmonary insufficiency with Pao_2 of 60 mm Hg or less; (3) renal failure with creatinine level greater than 2 mg/dL; (4) gastrointestinal bleeding of more than 500 mL/24 hr.[6] Scoring systems, CT imaging, and serum biochemical markers are all used in conjunction with clinical assessment in predicting severity.

2. The APACHE-II scoring system provides instantaneous assessment of severity of pancreatitis and should be implemented on the day of admission. The Ranson's criteria system is much simpler than the APACHE-II but requires 48 hours for completion. Thus the latter has superior sensitivity and specificity in distinguishing mild from severe

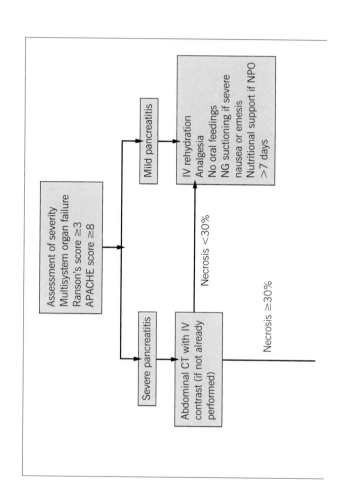

Assessment of severity
Multisystem organ failure
Ranson's score ≥3
APACHE score ≥8

Mild pancreatitis

Severe pancreatitis

Abdominal CT with IV contrast (if not already performed)

Necrosis <30%

Necrosis ≥30%

IV rehydration
Analgesia
No oral feedings
NG suctioning if severe nausea or emesis
Nutritional support if NPO >7 days

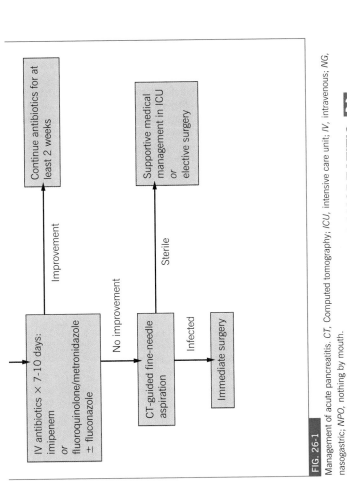

FIG. 26-1
Management of acute pancreatitis. *CT*, Computed tomography; *ICU*, intensive care unit; *IV*, intravenous; *NG*, nasogastric; *NPO*, nothing by mouth.

ACUTE PANCREATITIS

26

pancreatitis during the initial evaluation. At 48 hours either the APACHE-II or Ranson's criteria can be used. The APACHE-II has the advantage that it can be monitored every day. An initial score of 8 or less suggests minimal risk of death. A peak APACHE-II score higher than 9 was the best indicator of severe pancreatitis.[6,10-13]

3. The CT severity index is based on a combination of prognostic indicators, including extent of pancreatic necrosis and degree of peripancreatic inflammation (Box 26-3). The score has strong correlation with risk of both local complications and death.[14] A CT scan should always be obtained within 72 hours for further risk stratification when severe pancreatitis is suspected on the basis of Ranson's score or APACHE-II criteria.

4. The C-reactive protein (CRP) is an acute-phase reactant that is readily measurable and is a sensitive marker for necrotizing pancreatitis. A peak CRP level of 210 mg/L on the second, third, or fourth day or a level higher than 120 mg/L on the seventh day is predictive of severe disease.[15,16] A hematocrit value of 47% or higher at the time of admission is also a risk factor for severe pancreatic necrosis.[17]

BOX 26-3

COMPUTED TOMOGRAPHIC SEVERITY INDEX (CTSI)

CT Grade	CTSI Points
A—Normal pancreas	0
B—Focal or diffuse enlargement of pancreas	1
C—Pancreatic abnormalities accompanied by mild peripancreatic inflammation	3
D—Single fluid collection usually within anterior pararenal space	4
E—Two or more fluid collections near the pancreas or the presence of gas in or adjacent to the pancreas	5

Necrosis	
None	0
<33%	2
33%-50%	4
>50%	6

CTSI = CT Grade (0-4) + Necrosis (0-6)

Total Points	Complications	Mortality
0-3	8%	<3%
4-6	35%	6%
7-10	92%	17%

A. MANAGEMENT OF MILD PANCREATITIS

1. Patients who do not have evidence of organ failure, whose APACHE-II score is 8 or less, and who have no evidence of pancreatic necrosis or high-grade pancreatic inflammation on CT benefit from supportive measures. This involves pain management, often requiring IV narcotics and patient-controlled analgesia. Adequate IV fluid repletion is essential to prevent hypovolemia from third-space losses or emesis. Nasogastric tube placement may be indicated if severe vomiting or ileus is a prominent feature.

2. Patients should be given nothing by mouth until their requirement for IV narcotics is minimal or being tapered off. As long as abdominal pain has subsided, bowel sounds have returned, and the patient is hungry, a clear liquid diet can be started and advanced as tolerated over several days.[6]

B. MANAGEMENT OF SEVERE PANCREATITIS

1. In addition to supportive management, patients with severe necrotizing pancreatitis require nutritional support, systemic antibiotics, and possibly surgery while being carefully monitored in an intensive care setting.

2. Nutrition: Patients who will likely be unable to tolerate oral intake for more than 7 days should receive either enteral nutrition through a nasojejunal tube or total parenteral nutrition. The former is safe even in severe acute pancreatitis and is preferred because it reduces the risk of catheter-related infections, and enteral nutrients are thought to maintain the intestinal barrier.[6,10,18,19]

3. Prophylactic antibiotics: Localized infection develops in approximately one third of patients with severe necrotizing pancreatitis and is a leading cause of morbidity and mortality. Patients with severe pancreatitis, as defined by organ failure or by an APACHE-II score greater than 9 and evidence of necrosis of more than 30% of the pancreas, should be started on meropenem or imipenem for these agents' broad-spectrum coverage and pancreatic tissue penetration.[6,10,20-22] Fluoroquinolones are an alternative but appear to be less effective and should be used in conjunction with metronidazole.[23] IV antibiotics should be continued for at least 14 days. Fluconazole should also be considered because broad-spectrum antibiotics predispose to fungal infection, which has a higher mortality in necrotizing pancreatitis.[24,25]

4. Severe pancreatitis without improvement: Infected necrotic tissue develops in 40% to 70% of cases of necrotizing pancreatitis and is a leading cause of mortality.[26] Patients who do not improve clinically within 7 to 14 days on antibiotics should undergo a CT-guided aspiration of the necrotic pancreas to distinguish between sterile and infected necrosis.[22,27,28] Infected pancreatic necrosis evident by Gram's stain and confirmed later by culture requires immediate surgical débridement. Patients with sterile necrosis can be

26

ACUTE PANCREATITIS

managed with continued medical therapy or elective surgery in several weeks.

C. MANAGEMENT OF GALLSTONE PANCREATITIS

1. Most cases of gallstone pancreatitis do not require ERCP because common bile duct stones usually pass spontaneously into the duodenum. Patients should undergo prompt ERCP only if there is evidence of obstructive jaundice or cholangitis.[29-31] Among patients with persistent common bile duct stones but without cholangitis or progressive jaundice, ERCP may be performed electively.
2. Patients with mild gallstone pancreatitis should undergo elective cholecystectomy within 7 days after recovery. Surgery may be delayed for at least 3 weeks in severe gallstone pancreatitis because of an increased risk of infection.[32]

PEARLS AND PITFALLS

- Idiopathic acute pancreatitis.
  - A patient is allowed one episode of pancreatitis of unclear etiology without an exhaustive workup for underlying causes.
  - ERCP should be performed if a recurrent episode of "idiopathic" pancreatitis takes place.[33]
  - After ERCP, only 10% of cases of acute pancreatitis are truly idiopathic.
- Acute pancreatitis and human immunodeficiency virus (HIV).
  - Acute pancreatitis is 35 to 800 times more common in patients with HIV than in the general population.[34]
  - Drugs such as didanosine and pentamidine are the most common causes of acute pancreatitis in the HIV population.[34]
  - In patients with HIV, opportunistic infections such as cytomegalovirus should be identified as potential causes of acute pancreatitis and treated aggressively.

REFERENCES

[c] 1. Steinberg W, Tenner S. Acute pancreatitis. N Engl J Med 1994; 330:1198.
[d] 2. Mergener K, Baillie J. Acute pancreatitis. BMJ 1998; 316:44.
[d] 3. Neoptolemos JP et al. Acute pancreatitis: the substantial human and financial costs. Gut 1998; 42:886.
[c] 4. Sakorafas GH, Tsiotou AG. Etiology and pathogenesis of acute pancreatitis: current concepts. J Clin Gastroenterol 2000; 30:343.
[d] 5. Vissers RJ et al. Amylase and lipase in the emergency department evaluation of acute pancreatitis. J Emerg Med 1999; 17:1027.
[d] 6. Banks PA. Practice guidelines in acute pancreatitis. Am J Gastroenterol 1997; 92:377.
[b] 7. Tenner S, Dubner H, Steinberg W. Predicting gallstone pancreatitis with laboratory parameters: a meta-analysis. Am J Gastroenterol 1994; 89:1863.
[b] 8. Gumaste VV et al. Lipase/amylase ratio: a new index that distinguishes acute episodes of alcoholic from nonalcoholic acute pancreatitis. Gastroenterology 1991; 101:1361.
[b] 9. Tenner SM, Steinberg W. The admission serum lipase: amylase ratio differentiates alcoholic from nonalcoholic acute pancreatitis. Am J Gastroenterol 1992; 87:1755.
[c] 10. Wyncoll DL. The management of severe acute necrotising pancreatitis: an evidence-based review of the literature. Intensive Care Med 1999; 25:146.

[b] 11. Larvin M, McMahon MJ. APACHE-II score for assessment and monitoring of acute pancreatitis. Lancet 1989; 2:201.

[c] 12. Dervenis C, Bassi C. Evidence-based assessment of severity and management of acute pancreatitis. Br J Surg 2000; 87:257.

[b] 13. Wilson C et al. Prediction of outcome in acute pancreatitis: a comparative study of APACHE II, clinical assessment and multiple factor scoring systems. Br J Surg 1990; 77:1260.

[b] 14. Balthazar EJ et al. Acute pancreatitis: value of CT in establishing prognosis. Radiology 1990; 174:331.

[b] 15. Pezzilli R et al. Serum interleukin-6, interleukin-8, and beta 2-microglobulin in early assessment of severity of acute pancreatitis: comparison with serum C-reactive protein. Dig Dis Sci 1995; 40:2341.

[b] 16. Wilson C et al. C-reactive protein, antiproteases and complement factors as objective markers of severity in acute pancreatitis. Br J Surg 1989; 76:177.

[b] 17. Baillargeon JD et al. Hemoconcentration as an early risk factor for necrotizing pancreatitis. Am J Gastroenterol 1998; 93:2130.

[a] 18. Kalfarentzos F et al. Enteral nutrition is superior to parenteral nutrition in severe acute pancreatitis: results of a randomized prospective trial. Br J Surg 1997; 84:1665.

[d] 19. Guillou PJ. Enteral versus parenteral nutrition in acute pancreatitis. Baillieres Best Pract Res Clin Gastroenterol 1999; 13:345.

[a] 20. Sainio V et al. Early antibiotic treatment in acute necrotising pancreatitis. Lancet 1995; 346:663.

[a] 21. Pederzoli P et al. A randomized multicenter clinical trial of antibiotic prophylaxis of septic complications in acute necrotizing pancreatitis with imipenem. Surg Gynecol Obstet 1993; 176:480.

[c] 22. Ratschko M et al. The role of antibiotic prophylaxis in the treatment of acute pancreatitis. Gastroenterol Clin North Am 1999; 28:641.

[a] 23. Bassi C et al. Controlled clinical trial of pefloxacin versus imipenem in severe acute pancreatitis. Gastroenterology 1998; 115:1513.

[b] 24. Grewe M et al. Fungal infection in acute necrotizing pancreatitis. J Am Coll Surg 1999; 188:408.

[b] 25. Gloor B et al. Pancreatic infection in severe pancreatitis: the role of fungus and multiresistant organisms. Arch Surg 2001; 136:592.

[d] 26. Isenmann R, Beger HG. Natural history of acute pancreatitis and the role of infection. Baillieres Best Pract Res Clin Gastroenterol 1999; 13:291.

[b] 27. Gerzof SG et al. Early diagnosis of pancreatic infection by computed tomography–guided aspiration. Gastroenterology 1987; 93:1315.

[c] 28. Widdison AL, Karanjia ND. Pancreatic infection complicating acute pancreatitis. Br J Surg 1993; 80:148.

[a] 29. Folsch UR et al. Early ERCP and papillotomy compared with conservative treatment for acute biliary pancreatitis. The German Study Group on Acute Biliary Pancreatitis. N Engl J Med 1997; 336:237.

[c] 30. Nitsche R, Folsch UR. Role of ERCP and endoscopic sphincterotomy in acute pancreatitis. Baillieres Best Pract Res Clin Gastroenterol 1999; 13:331.

[a] 31. Neoptolemos JP et al. Controlled trial of urgent endoscopic retrograde cholangiopancreatography and endoscopic sphincterotomy versus conservative treatment for acute pancreatitis due to gallstones. Lancet 1988; 2:979.

[b] 32. Uhl W et al. Acute gallstone pancreatitis: timing of laparoscopic cholecystectomy in mild and severe disease. Surg Endosc 1999; 13:1070.

[d] 33. Somogyi L et al. Recurrent acute pancreatitis: an algorithmic approach to identification and elimination of inciting factors. Gastroenterology 2001; 120:708.

[c] 34. Dassopoulos T, Ehrenpreis ED. Acute pancreatitis in human immunodeficiency virus–infected patients: a review. Am J Med 1999; 107:78.

26

ACUTE PANCREATITIS

Ascites

Michal L. Melamed, MD, Stephen Moff, MD, and F. Fred Poorad, MD

Fast Facts

- Cirrhosis is the major cause of ascites, but other conditions can also cause ascites.
- Among patients with ascites, 80% have cirrhosis.[1]
- The two most common causes for cirrhosis in the United States are hepatitis C and alcohol, which often coexist.
- A cell count with greater than 250 polymorphonuclear cells (PMNs) is consistent with spontaneous bacterial peritonitis (SBP).
- The prevalence of SBP in cirrhotic patients admitted to the hospital ranges between 10% and 30%. Half the cases of SBP are present at the time of admission, and the rest are acquired during hospitalization.[2]

27

I. EPIDEMIOLOGY

1. Ascites is due to portal hypertension in 90% of cases. Of those with ascites, 80% have cirrhosis as an underlying disorder.
2. Ascites has many etiologies (Table 27-1).

II. CLINICAL PRESENTATION

A. HISTORY

1. The term "ascites" comes from the Greek *askos,* meaning bag or sack. The word is used to describe a pathological accumulation of fluid within the peritoneal space. Patients should be asked about risk factors for ascites, both current and often forgotten past ones. These include the following.

a. Alcohol abuse.

b. Intravenous drug use.

c. Sexual orientation.

d. Tattoos.

e. Recent travel and country of origin (foreign endemic exposures).

f. Past blood transfusions: Among cases of idiopathic liver failure, 4% are the result of viral hepatitis from a long-forgotten blood transfusion.

g. History of malignancy: Breast, lung, pancreatic, and colon primaries can cause ascites via peritoneal metastases. Malignancy-based ascites is often painful, whereas cirrhotic ascites is not (unless a superimposed infection, such as SBP, is present). If ascites develops suddenly in a patient with stable cirrhosis, underlying liver cancer may be the cause.

h. A history of congestive heart failure with right heart failure, constrictive pericarditis, or restrictive cardiomyopathy.

i. Renal disease: Nephrogenic ascites can occur in the setting of anasarca.

TABLE 27-1

CAUSES OF ASCITES

Cause of Ascites	Comments
Portal hypertension	
Cirrhosis	Accounts for 80% of ascites in the United States
Fulminant hepatic failure	Rarely causes ascites
Hepatic outflow obstruction	Ascites is a characteristic clinical feature of hepatic outflow obstruction
Congestive heart failure	
Constrictive or restrictive cardiomyopathy	
Budd-Chiari syndrome—hepatic vein or inferior vena cava occlusion	Most commonly associated with an underlying thrombotic disorder
Venoocclusive disease	Important cause of ascites in bone marrow transplant recipients
Portal vein occlusion	Rarely causes ascites
Malignancy	Accounts for 10% of ascites in the United States; peritoneal carcinomatosis causes 50% of malignant ascites
Infection	
Peritoneal tuberculosis	See Tables 27-2 and 27-3
Fitz-Hugh–Curtis syndrome	Perihepatitis associated with fibrous perihepatic exudate usually caused by *Neisseria gonorrhoeae* or *Chlamydia trachomatis*
Infectious peritonitis in patients infected with human immunodeficiency virus	
Renal	
Nephrotic syndrome	Covert cirrhosis should be excluded
Nephrogenous in hemodialysis recipients	Covert cirrhosis should be excluded
Endocrine	
Myxedema	
Meigs' syndrome	
Struma ovarii	
Ovarian stimulation syndrome	
Pancreatic ascites	Associated with pancreatitis, raised ascitic amylase concentration
Biliary leak	Previous surgery, including laparoscopic cholecystectomy, gangrenous gallbladder, trauma, percutaneous liver biopsy
Urine ascites	Urinary leak into the peritoneum
Systemic lupus erythematosus	
Miscellaneous	Idiopathic chronic nonspecific peritonitis in patients infected with human immunodeficiency virus
Mixed causes	See text

From Goldman L, Bennett JC. Cecil textbook of medicine, 21st ed. Philadelphia: WB Saunders; 2000.

TABLE 27-2

CLINICAL CHARACTERISTICS OF PERITONEAL TUBERCULOSIS

Clinical Characteristic	Percent*
Ascites	80-100
Abdominal swelling	65-100
Abdominal pain	36-93
Weight loss	37-87
Fever	56-100
Diarrhea	9-27
Abdominal tenderness	65-87
Anemia	46-68
Positive purified protein derivative test	55-100

From Goldman L, Bennett JC. Cecil textbook of medicine, 21st ed. Philadelphia: WB Saunders; 2000.

*The percentages represent the frequency with which these features have been observed in peritoneal tuberculosis. These data antedate studies of tuberculosis in patients infected with human immunodeficiency virus.

27

ASCITES

TABLE 27-3

DIAGNOSTIC TESTS OF PERITONEAL TUBERCULOSIS

Diagnostic Test	Comments
Paracentesis	
With smear	<3% positive
With culture	<20%-80% positive
With measurement of ascitic adenosine deaminase	≤32.3 U/L; low ascitic protein levels (i.e., cirrhosis) may cause false negative results; not validated in U.S. patients
With lactate dehydrogenase level ≤90 U/L	
Laparoscopy with biopsy	Best test; up to 100% positive
Needle biopsy of the peritoneum	Largely replaced by laparoscopy
Diagnostic laparotomy	Should be considered if laparoscopy not available

From Goldman L, Bennett JC. Cecil textbook of medicine, 21st ed. Philadelphia: WB Saunders; 2000.

j. Clotting disorders: Vascular thrombosis of the inferior vena cava, hepatic veins, or portal veins can cause ascites.

k. Recent or unusual infections: Tuberculosis-associated ascites is rare in the United States (Tables 27-2 and 27-3).

B. PHYSICAL EXAMINATION

1. Physical examination findings for ascites are often unreliable. In fact, accuracy for detection of ascites is less than 60%. The first step in detection is inspection for a full, bulging abdomen. The most telling finding, however, is flank dullness to percussion; if it is absent, the probability of ascites is less than 10%.[3]

2. Dullness requires 1500 mL of fluid. Without flank dullness there is no reason to check for shifting. The test for a fluid wave is not useful.[4]

Gaseous distention and ovarian masses can mimic ascites. On percussion the presence of gas is apparent as diffuse tympani and the presence of ovarian masses as central dullness and tympanitic flanks.

3. It is important to look for signs of advanced liver disease, such as palmar erythema, spider angiomas, large collateral veins in the abdominal wall, mild encephalopathy, and fetor hepaticus (peculiar breath odor in persons with severe liver disease). Visible veins on the patient's back suggest blockage of the inferior vena cava. An immobile mass at the umbilicus (termed a Sister Mary Joseph nodule, after a scrub nurse who assisted the famous surgeon William Mayo) is highly suggestive of peritoneal carcinomatosis. Elevated jugular venous pressures point to concomitant heart failure or constrictive pericarditis. Patients with nephrotic syndrome as the cause of their ascites may have anasarca.

4. SBP, which often has a subtle history, is an important consideration. A high index of suspicion for SBP must be maintained, since it can develop in any patient with ascites. Signs and symptoms of SBP include complaints of abdominal pain, fever, and gastrointestinal complaints, such as nausea, vomiting, and diarrhea. Signs of impaired liver function, such as hepatic encephalopathy or renal failure, may be the sole presenting feature.

III. DIAGNOSTICS

A. ULTRASOUND

1. Ultrasound can detect as little as 100 mL of abdominal fluid.

B. PARACENTESIS

1. Paracentesis is the gold standard for the proper diagnosis and is often important in the treatment of discomfort from intraabdominal pressure from ascites. Sampling of the ascitic fluid should be attempted on patients with the following conditions.

a. New-onset ascites (for diagnosis of cause).

b. Fever in a patient with known ascites to rule out SBP.

c. Symptomatic relief.

d. Decompensated liver failure, including new renal failure or encephalopathy, to evaluate for SBP.

2. Information on how to perform paracentesis can be found in Chapter 2. Ascitic fluid should be sent for a complete blood cell count with differential, albumin levels, and cultures. Studies show that inoculation of 10 to 20 mL of ascitic fluid into two blood culture bottles at the bedside optimizes results.[5]

3. Other tests, depending on the clinical setting, include total protein, glucose, lactate dehydrogenase (LDH), amylase, triglycerides, Gram's stain, acid-fast bacteria smear and culture, and cytological examination. If a concurrent serum albumin level is ordered, the serum-ascites gradient (SAAG) can be calculated.

4. The (SAAG) (subtract the ascites albumin from the serum albumin)

BOX 27-1
CAUSES OF ASCITES BASED ON SERUM-ASCITES ALBUMIN GRADIENT
HIGH GRADIENT (≥1.1 g/dL)
Cirrhosis
Alcoholic hepatitis
Cardiac failure
Massive liver metastases
Fulminant hepatic failure
Budd-Chiari syndrome
Portal vein thrombosis
Venoocclusive disease
Fatty liver of pregnancy
Myxedema
"Mixed" ascites
LOW GRADIENT (<1.1 g/dL)
Peritoneal carcinomatosis
Peritoneal tuberculosis
Pancreatic ascites
Biliary ascites
Nephrotic syndrome
Serositis
Bowel obstruction or infarction

Data from Runyon BA et al. Ann Intern Med 1992; 117(3):215.

27

ASCITES

has been found useful in determining the cause of ascites.[6] If the SAAG is greater than 1.1 g/dL, the patient has portal hypertension with approximately 97% accuracy (Box 27-1).

IV. MANAGEMENT

A. ASCITES AND REFRACTORY ASCITES

1. The treatment of ascites in cirrhosis should proceed in a step-wise fashion from diuretics and sodium restriction to the eventual development of refractory ascites requiring large-volume paracentesis and possibly to transjugular intrahepatic portosystemic shunt (TIPS) and liver transplantation if available. The initial aim is to create a negative sodium and water balance. General treatment recommendations include the following.
   a. Complete abstinence from alcohol.
   b. Sodium-restricted diet (88 mmol/day or 2000 mg/day).
   c. Orally administered spironolactone and furosemide (ideally in a 100:40 ratio; maximum 400:160).
   d. Free water restriction (necessary only if the serum sodium level is <130 mmol/L).
2. Measurement of 24-hour urine sodium excretion can be used to deter-

mine patient compliance with diet restrictions and diuretics (sodium excretion should not be >78 mmol/day if the patient is truly adhering to the 88 mmol/day limit and when a nonurinary sodium excretion of 10 mmol/day in an afebrile patient without diarrhea is taken into account). This strategy is effective in controlling fluid overload in 90% of patients.[7] Bed rest is not recommended.

3. Patients with a low SAAG usually do not have portal hypertension, and they do not respond to the treatment just outlined unless they have the nephrotic syndrome.

4. In the 10% of patients whose ascites is truly resistant to diet restrictions and diuresis, serial therapeutic paracenteses (as frequently as every 2 weeks) are recommended. Support for routine postparacentesis albumin infusion is still controversial, but it is useful in patients with hypotension or renal failure and those undergoing weekly paracentesis.

5. Peritoneovenous shunting to decrease portal pressure is another option for refractory ascites, but it is rarely used now because of the high morbidity associated with shunt malfunction and infection. It should not be considered for patients who are transplant candidates or those with marked encephalopathy. In a randomized study patients who underwent the TIPS procedure had a lower mortality rate than those receiving serial large-volume paracenteses,[8] but the mortality rate is high in patients with Childs class C cirrhosis undergoing TIPS with refractory ascites as the sole indication. Liver transplantation should be considered for all patients with refractory ascites when appropriate.[9]

B. SPONTANEOUS BACTERIAL PERITONITIS

1. Patients with an ascitic fluid PMN count greater than 250/mm^3 are considered to have SBP and should receive empirical treatment with a third-generation cephalosporin, cefotaxime 2 g IV q8h.[10] When culture and sensitivity results return, the antibiotic coverage can be narrowed. The three most common isolates from ascitic fluid are *Escherichia coli, Klebsiella pneumoniae,* and *Streptococcus pneumoniae.* Inability to identify an organism from ascitic fluid cultures does not rule out SBP.

2. After 48 hours of appropriate antimicrobial treatment the ascites neutrophil count should decrease. Patients with a neutrophil count less than 250/mm^3 but with signs and symptoms of systemic illness also need empirical antibiotic treatment until ascites culture results are reported.

3. In patients with cirrhosis and SBP, treatment with intravenous albumin (1.5 g/kg within 6 hours of the diagnostic paracentesis, followed by 1 g/kg on day 3) in addition to an antibiotic reduces the incidence of renal impairment and death in comparison with treatment with an antibiotic alone.[11]

4. Secondary peritonitis differs from SBP in that the ascites neutrophil count in the former is usually much higher (in the thousands). In addition, the culture data often reveal polymicrobial infection, and two or three of the following are usually present in the ascites: total pro-

tein level greater than 1 g/dL, LDH level greater than the upper limit of normal for serum, or glucose level less than 70 mg/dL. These criteria offer 100% sensitivity but only 45% specificity for secondary peritonitis. Presence of these findings should prompt an evaluation for the source of infection, which is often a perforated viscous.

5. SBP prophylaxis is a controversial topic. High-risk patients include those with ascitic total protein measurements less than 1 g/dL, a prior history of SBP, or acute variceal hemorrhage. Treatment for patients with acute variceal hemorrhage is norfloxacin 400 mg PO bid for 7 days, and treatment for patients with an ascitic protein level below 1 g/dL or a prior history of SBP is norfloxacin 400 mg PO qd. Long-term outpatient prophylaxis with quinolones remains controversial, and most authorities recommend reserving this treatment for patients who have survived an episode of SBP.

PEARLS AND PITFALLS

- The history and physical examination can suggest the etiology of ascites, but the gold standard for diagnosis is paracentesis.
- A patient admitted to the hospital with new-onset ascites or ascites with a fever needs a diagnostic paracentesis.
- SBP is a common complication of ascites and must be considered whenever clinical deterioration occurs in a patient with ascites.
- When a patient with ascites has marked hypotension in comparison to an often hypotensive baseline (unresponsive to fluid boluses), a medical intensive care unit consultation should be considered.
- Aminoglycosides should not be used to treat SBP because of the risk of exacerbating underlying renal dysfunction.
- Patients receiving appropriate antibiotic treatment for SBP should show clinical improvement within 48 hours. If a patient does not improve, a sample of the ascites can be obtained to see if the neutrophil count has decreased and to culture the fluid for the possibility of another microbiological etiology.

REFERENCES

[c] 1. Feldman M, Friedman LS, Sleisenger MH. Sleisenger and Fordtran's gastrointestinal and liver disease. Philadelphia: WB Saunders; 2002.

[d] 2. Rimola A et al. Diagnosis, treatment and prophylaxis of spontaneous bacterial peritonitis: a consensus document. International Ascites Club. J Hepatol 2000; 32(1):142.

[b] 3. Williams JW, Simel DL. Does this patient have ascites? How to divine fluid in the abdomen. JAMA 1992; 267:2645.

[a] 4. Cattau EL Jr et al. The accuracy of the physical examination in the diagnosis of suspected ascites. JAMA 1982; 247(8):1164.

[b] 5. Runyon BA, Canawati HN, Akriviadis EA. Optimization of ascitic fluid culture technique. Gastroenterology 1988; 95(5):1351.

[a] 6. Runyon BA et al. The serum-ascites albumin gradient is superior to the exudate-transudate concept in the differential diagnosis of ascites. Ann Intern Med 1992; 117(3):215.

[c] 7. Runyon BA. Management of adult patients with ascites caused by cirrhosis. Hepatology 1998; 27:264.

[a] 8. Rossle M et al. A comparison of paracentesis and transjugular intrahepatic portosystemic shunting in patients with ascites. N Engl J Med 2000; 342:1701.

27

ASCITES

[c] 9. Menon KV, Kamath PS. Managing the complications of cirrhosis. Mayo Clin Proc 2000; 75:501.

[a] 10. Felisart J et al. Cefotaxime is more effective than is ampicillin-tobramycin in cirrhotics with severe infections. Hepatology 1985; 5(3):457.

[a] 11. Sort P et al. Effect of intravenous albumin on renal impairment and mortality in patients with cirrhosis and spontaneous bacterial peritonitis. N Engl J Med 1999; 341:403.

Diarrhea

Gregory B. Ang, MD, Mark Donowitz, MD, and Cynthia L. Sears, MD

FAST FACTS

- Diarrhea is a change in bowel habits with stool weight greater than 200 g per day.
- Diarrhea may be classified as acute (lasting ≤14 days), persistent (lasting 14-28 days), or chronic (lasting >4 weeks).
- Acute diarrheal illnesses are usually due to infections, are self-limited, and often do not require medications for cure,[1] but they nevertheless require oral rehydration solution (ORS) for symptomatic therapy.
- Chronic diarrhea is often classified into three major categories.[2]
  - Watery diarrhea: secretory or osmotic.
  - Inflammatory diarrhea.
  - Fatty diarrhea.
- Chronic secretory diarrhea may be distinguished from nonsecretory diarrhea by the response of the diarrhea to fasting. Secretory diarrhea persists after 48 hours of fasting, whereas nonsecretory diarrhea ceases by 48 to 72 hours of fasting.[3]

28

I. EPIDEMIOLOGY

1. Diarrheal diseases constitute the fourth leading cause of deaths worldwide.[4]
2. The annual rate of acute diarrheal illness in adults in industrialized countries is estimated to be one episode per person per year,[5] with 211,000,000 cases per year in the United States.[6] The prevalence of chronic diarrhea is estimated to be 3,080,000 cases per year in the United States.[6]

II. ACUTE DIARRHEA: CLINICAL PRESENTATION AND DIAGNOSTICS

1. Most cases of acute diarrhea do not require medical attention. Medical evaluation should be undertaken in patients with more severe illness as indicated by any of the following features.
a. Profuse watery diarrhea with volume depletion (as evidenced by orthostatic hypotension).
b. Dysentery (frequent stools with blood and mucus).
c. Fever.
d. Diarrhea with severe abdominal pain.
e. Diarrhea in the elderly.
f. Immunocompromised patients (e.g., acquired immunodeficiency syndrome [AIDS], posttransplant state, chemotherapy, diabetes).
2. Historical, epidemiological, and laboratory features aid in the

BOX 28-1

DIFFERENTIAL DIAGNOSIS OF ACUTE NONINFECTIOUS DIARRHEA

Drugs and toxins (e.g., magnesium, caffeine, theophylline, laxatives, opiates,
  lactulose, colchicines, metformin, digitalis, iron, methyldopa, hydralazine, sorbitol,
  quinidine, fructose, mannitol, arsenic, cadmium, mercury, mushrooms)
Irritable bowel syndrome
Inflammatory bowel disease
Ischemic bowel disease
Food allergies
Lactase deficiency
Onset of chronic diarrhea of any cause (e.g., VIPoma)

      evaluation and management of acute diarrhea (Table 28-1[7,8] and Box 28-1).

3. Laboratory evaluation should be undertaken only for patients who are severely ill and meet any of the criteria outlined above.

a. Check stools for fecal leukocytes, lactoferrin, or occult blood to determine the need for obtaining stool cultures.

b. Obtain stool cultures only for patients with severe diarrhea, fever, or dysentery or for patients with stools positive for fecal leukocytes, lactoferrin, or occult blood.[9]

c. Evaluation of stools for ova and parasites is indicated in the setting of persistent or chronic diarrhea, travel to developing countries or mountainous areas, exposure to children attending day care centers, male homosexual sex or patients with AIDS, community waterborne outbreaks, and bloody diarrhea with few or no fecal leukocytes.

d. Stool should be assayed for *Clostridium difficile* toxin if patients have received antimicrobial therapy within the past 2 months. (The sensitivity in detecting *C. difficile* toxin increases with successive consecutive stool specimens, with estimated sensitivities of 79% on the first stool specimen, 91% on the second specimen, and 100% on the third specimen.[10])

e. Flexible sigmoidoscopy with or without endoscopy should be considered for homosexual men and patients with persistent diarrhea (>14 days) not responding to antimicrobial therapy or without a diagnosis after laboratory evaluation.

III. ACUTE INFECTIOUS DIARRHEA: MANAGEMENT

1. Empirical antimicrobial therapy may be considered in the following patients.

a. Patients with moderate to severe traveler's diarrhea may be treated empirically with a fluoroquinolone (e.g., ciprofloxacin 500 mg PO bid) for 3 to 5 days.

b. Patients with diarrhea lasting more than 10 to 14 days and with suspected giardiasis may be treated empirically with metronidazole 250 to 750 mg PO tid for 7 days.

c. Patients with severe febrile diarrheal illnesses may be treated empirically with a fluoroquinolone if they are in a toxic or unstable condition, preferably once Shiga toxin–producing *Escherichia coli* is ruled out by fecal testing (because of concern for inducing hemolytic-uremic syndrome).[7]

2. All patients with diarrhea who require medical evaluation and are volume depleted (i.e., orthostatic) should receive fluid and electrolyte repletion, preferably via the oral route with solutions containing water, salt, and sugar or amino acids (or both). The rationale is that intestinal sodium-glucose and sodium-amino acid absorption via sodium-glucose and sodium-amino acid transporters remains largely intact in most diarrheal illnesses.

3. The use of antimotility agents for adult patients with febrile dysentery is controversial. Several studies have shown no adverse effects of antimotility agents in adults with dysentery,[11-13] whereas one study suggested that they may prolong disease.[14] In children and the elderly the hemolytic-uremic syndrome may be triggered by antimotility agents with enterohemorrhagic *E. coli* infection[15] and neurological symptoms may be worsened.[16] In adults with nondysenteric diarrhea, antimotility agents such as loperamide (4 mg initially, then 2 mg after each unformed stool not to exceed 16 mg qd) or diphenoxylate with atropine (4 mg qid) may be safely used.

4. Specific antimicrobial therapy is used when a treatable pathogen is identified in stool samples (Table 28-1).

5. A systematic approach to the evaluation and management of acute diarrhea is outlined in Fig. 28-1.[17-19]

IV. CHRONIC DIARRHEA: DIAGNOSTICS AND MANAGEMENT

1. Evaluation of patients with chronic diarrhea is more complex than that of patients with acute diarrhea because of the larger differential diagnosis involved (Box 28-2). Furthermore, any acute cause of diarrhea can result in chronic diarrhea. The first step in evaluating chronic diarrhea is to rule out infectious causes by sending stool samples taken at two separate times for cultures, sending samples taken at two or three times for evaluation for ova and parasites, acid-fast staining (to evaluate for *Cryptosporidium, Cyclospora,* and *Isospora belli*), and *Giardia* antigen testing (enzyme-linked immunosorbent assay). *C. difficile* testing is performed if there is a history of any antibiotic use within the past 2 months.

2. In addition to the history, physical examination, and routine laboratory blood work, a quantitative stool collection and analysis is often necessary to classify the diarrhea and to assist in making specific diagnoses once infectious causes are ruled out (Table 28-2).[20]

Text continued on p. 457

TABLE 28-1

DIFFERENTIAL DIAGNOSIS OF ACUTE INFECTIOUS DIARRHEA

Agent	Clinical Features	Treatment*
VIRUSES		
Norwalk agent	Schools; waterborne; foodborne	None; consider lactose-free diet for 6 weeks, especially if diarrhea persists
Rotavirus	Day care centers; contact with young children	None; consider lactose-free diet for 6 weeks, especially if diarrhea persists
Adenovirus		None
BACTERIA		
Salmonella (non-typhi)	Foodborne (many vehicles, e.g., eggs, raw milk, ice cream)	No therapy for healthy host with mild to moderate symptoms; TMP/SMX 1 DS bid or FQ × 5-7 days if severe illness
Shigella	20% foodborne; primarily person-to-person (e.g., daycare centers)	TMP/SMX 1 DS bid × 3 days (if acquired in U.S.); FQ (if acquired outside U.S.)
Campylobacter jejuni	Foodborne (e.g., undercooked poultry); associated with Guillain-Barré syndrome	Erythromycin 500 mg bid, FQ, or azithromycin × 5 days
Staphylococcus aureus	Food poisoning; emesis more prominent than diarrhea within 6 hr of exposure to ingested toxin	None
Bacillus cereus	Two syndromes: (1) similar to S. aureus, onset of emesis within 6 hr, vehicle often fried rice; (2) similar to C. perfringens, watery diarrhea, longer incubation	None
Clostridium perfringens	Food poisoning; incubation period 8-24 hr	None
Vibrio cholerae O1 or O139	Contaminated shellfish, raw seafood (e.g., sushi)	Doxycycline 300 mg × 1 dose or TMP/SMX 1 DS bid × 3 days
Escherichia coli O157:H7 (EHEC or STEC)	Foodborne dysentery (e.g., undercooked hamburger); associated with HUS	Avoid use of antibiotics because of increased risk of HUS[7]
ETEC, EAEC	Travelers	FQ × 1 dose to 3-5 days or TMP/SMX 1 DS bid × 3-5 days
Clostridium difficile	Recent antimicrobial therapy (within the past 2 months)	Metronidazole 250 mg qid to 500 mg tid × 10 days
Yersinia enterocolitica	Pseudoappendicitis	Usually none

PROTOZOA

Cryptosporidium parvum	HIV; foodborne; waterborne; daycare	Consider paromomycin 500 mg tid × 7 days if severe
Microsporidia	HIV (importance in immunocompetent host is unclear)	Albendazole 400 mg bid × 3 weeks if immunocompromised
Isospora belli	HIV; travel	TMP/SMX 1 DS bid × 7-10 days
Cyclospora	Foodborne; travel; duration >3 weeks	TMP/SMX 1 DS bid × 7 days
Giardia lamblia	Ingestion of stream water; travel to Russia, mountainous areas	Metronidazole 250 mg tid × 5-7 days
Entamoeba histolytica	Travel to endemic areas; male homosexual intercourse; few or no fecal leukocytes	Metronidazole 750 mg tid × 5-10 days, plus paromomycin 500 mg tid × 7 days

Modified from Guerrant RL et al. Clin Infect Dis 2001; 32:331.

DS, Double strength; *EAEC*, enteroadherent *Escherichia coli*; *EHEC*, enterohemorrhagic *E. coli*; *ETEC*, enterotoxigenic *E. coli*; *FQ*, fluoroquinolone, such as ciprofloxacin 500 mg PO bid; *HIV*, human immunodeficiency virus; *HUS*, hemolytic-uremic syndrome; *STEC*, Shiga toxin–producing *E. coli*; *TMP/SMX*, trimethoprim-sulfamethoxazole.

*Treatment in immunocompetent patients. Hydration, preferably oral, is essential in all cases.

28

DIARRHEA

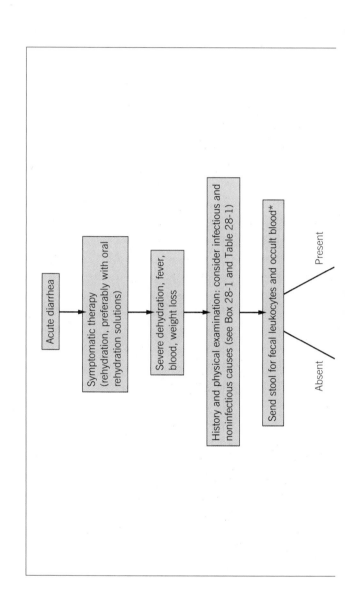

Acute diarrhea

Symptomatic therapy (rehydration, preferably with oral rehydration solutions)

Severe dehydration, fever, blood, weight loss

History and physical examination: consider infectious and noninfectious causes (see Box 28-1 and Table 28-1)

Send stool for fecal leukocytes and occult blood*

Present

Absent

28

DIARRHEA

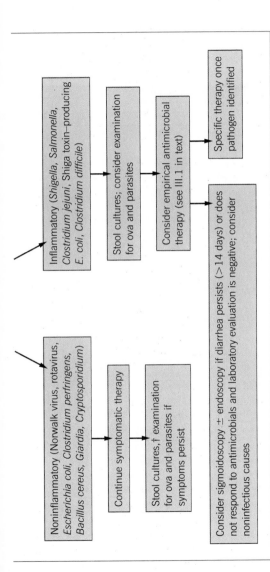

FIG. 28-1

Approach to acute diarrhea. *Send stool for *Clostridium difficile* toxin test if the patient has a history of antibiotic use within the past 2 months. Twenty-five percent of *C. difficile* disease occurs in the outpatient setting. †Of patients with *Shigella, Salmonella,* and *C. difficile* infections, 30% or more do not have fecal leukocytes or occult blood.[18,19] *(Modified from Guerrant RL, Bobak DA. N Engl J Med 1991; 325:327.)*

BOX 28-2

CAUSES OF CHRONIC DIARRHEA

OSMOTIC WATERY DIARRHEA

Osmotic laxatives (magnesium, phosphate, sulfate)

Carbohydrate malabsorption

SECRETORY WATERY DIARRHEA

Congenital syndromes

Bacterial toxins

Inflammatory bowel disease

Vasculitis

Drugs and poisons (see Box 28-1)

Laxative abuse

Disordered motility or regulation

Endocrine diarrhea (hyperthyroidism, hypothyroidism, Addison's disease, gastrinoma, VIPoma, somatostatinoma, carcinoid syndrome, medullary thyroid carcinoma, mastocytosis)

Other tumors (colon carcinoma, lymphoma, villous adenoma)

Idiopathic secretory diarrhea

Epidemic secretory (Brainerd's) diarrhea

INFLAMMATORY DIARRHEA

Inflammatory bowel disease

Infectious diseases

Ischemic colitis

Radiation colitis

FATTY DIARRHEA (50% WATERY)

Malabsorption syndromes (celiac disease, Whipple's disease, short bowel syndrome, small bowel bacterial overgrowth)

Maldigestion (pancreatic exocrine insufficiency, inadequate luminal bile acids)

Modified from Schiller LR. Med Clin North Am 2000; 84:1259.

TABLE 28-2

STOOL STUDIES IN NONINFECTIOUS CHRONIC DIARRHEA

Study	Comments
Stool Na, K	Osmotic gap <50 mOsm/kg suggestive of secretory diarrhea; >50 mOsm/kg suggestive of osmotic diarrhea; fecal osmotic gap = 290 − 2(stool Na + K)*
Stool pH	pH <5.6 suggestive of carbohydrate malabsorption*
Fecal occult blood	Positive test suggests the presence of inflammatory bowel disease, neoplastic diseases, ischemia, radiation
Fecal leukocytes	Presence suggests inflammatory or infectious diarrhea
Sudan stain; 72-hr fecal fat (on 75-100 g fat/day diet)	>14 g fat/day (steatorrhea) indicates malabsorption (normally <7 g fat/day)
Stool alkalinization or thin-layer chromatography	Evaluation for laxative abuse (bisacodyl, phenolphthalein, anthraquinones)
Stool weight	Diarrhea defined by stool weight >200 g/day
Stool osmolality	Osmolality <250 mOsm/kg implies dilution of stool with water or urine
Stool Mg, sulfate, phosphate	Stool Mg >45 mM suggests inadvertent Mg ingestion in mineral supplements or antacids, or surreptitious laxative abuse

K, Potassium; *Mg*, magnesium; *Na*, sodium.
*Data from Eherer AJ, Fordtran JS. Gastroenterology 1992; 103:545.

28

DIARRHEA

3. Additional radiological, urine, blood, endoscopic, or other studies may be considered for further evaluation of chronic diarrhea (Table 28-3).
4. The response to fasting is often used to distinguish secretory from nonsecretory diarrhea. Secretory diarrhea persists after 48 hours of fasting, whereas nonsecretory diarrhea ceases by 48 to 72 hours of fasting.[3]
5. A systematic approach to the evaluation of chronic diarrhea is outlined in Fig. 28-2.
6. As with acute diarrhea, patients with chronic diarrhea must be adequately hydrated, preferably with ORS. Empirical therapy for chronic diarrhea is recommended in three situations.[2]
   a. As a temporizing or initial treatment before diagnostic testing.
   b. After diagnostic testing has failed to confirm a diagnosis.
   c. When no specific treatment is available or specific treatment fails to effect a cure.
7. Options for empirical treatment include the following.
   a. Antimicrobials (e.g., metronidazole, fluoroquinolone, or trimethoprim-sulfamethoxazole) if the prevalence of bacterial or protozoal infection is high.
   b. Bile acid–binding resins (e.g., cholestyramine).
   c. Opiates (e.g., loperamide) for symptomatic control.

TABLE 28-3

ADDITIONAL STUDIES IN THE EVALUATION OF CHRONIC DIARRHEA

Radiological	Urine	Blood	Endoscopic	Other
Abdominal radiographic findings (for pancreatic calcification)	5-HIAA (for carcinoid syndrome)	Gastrin,* calcitonin,* VIP,* somatostatin*	Sigmoidoscopy with biopsy	Test of bile acid or other breath test for bacterial overgrowth
Barium studies of the upper gastrointestinal tract, small bowel, and colon	Thin-layer chromatography (for laxatives)	Erythrocyte sedimentation rate	Colonoscopy and ileoscopy with biopsy (for right-sided colitis, amebiasis, Crohn's disease, and microscopic and collagenous colitis)	Nutritionist-supervised lactose-free diet for 3-5 days
Abdominal computed tomography		Thyroid function tests	Upper endoscopy, including small bowel biopsy	

5-HIAA, 5-Hydroxyindoleacetic acid; *VIP,* vasoactive intestinal peptide.
*Should not be performed unless stool volume is >1 L/day or severe hypokalemia is present.

d. Octreotide reserved as a secondary agent, usually in secretory diarrhea, dumping syndrome, and chemotherapy-induced diarrhea.

PEARLS AND PITFALLS

- Homosexual men with diarrhea who have been the recipients of anal intercourse are at risk for proctitis and colitis resulting from direct rectal inoculation of pathogens. In addition to the more common bacterial enteropathogens, *Neisseria gonorrhoeae*, herpes simplex virus, *Chlamydia trachomatis*, and *Treponema pallidum* should be considered as possible causative agents.
- Antibiotic prophylaxis is not generally recommended for otherwise healthy individuals traveling to high-risk areas, unless the traveler has a significant predisposing illness, such as AIDS, inflammatory bowel disease, hypochlorhydria induced by prior gastric surgery or use of a proton pump inhibitor, diabetes mellitus for which insulin is taken, or malignancy, or the traveler cannot afford to get diarrhea during the trip.[21] Fluoroquinolones are recommended for empirical self-therapy for traveler's diarrhea.
- Symptomatic food handlers and health care workers with infectious diarrhea should be excluded from directly handling food and from caring for patients. Asymptomatic food handlers and health care workers with infectious diarrhea should have two consecutive negative stool samples taken 24 hours apart and at least 48 hours after resolution of symptoms before returning to their jobs.[8]
- In immunocompromised patients, such as transplant recipients, patients undergoing chemotherapy, patients with human immunodeficiency virus infection, and patients with primary immunodeficiencies, the differential diagnosis of diarrhea is altered; a discussion is beyond the scope of this chapter.

28

DIARRHEA

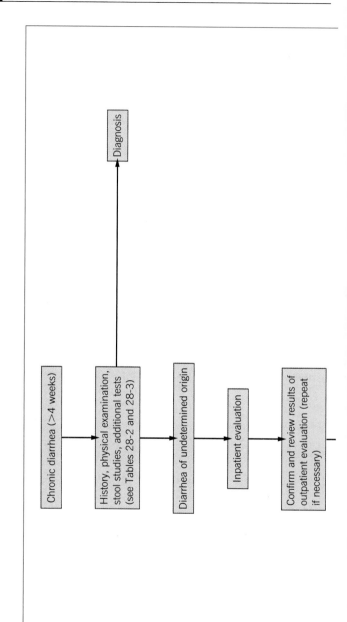

Chronic diarrhea (>4 weeks)

History, physical examination, stool studies, additional tests (see Tables 28-2 and 28-3)

Diagnosis

Diarrhea of undetermined origin

Inpatient evaluation

Confirm and review results of outpatient evaluation (repeat if necessary)

28

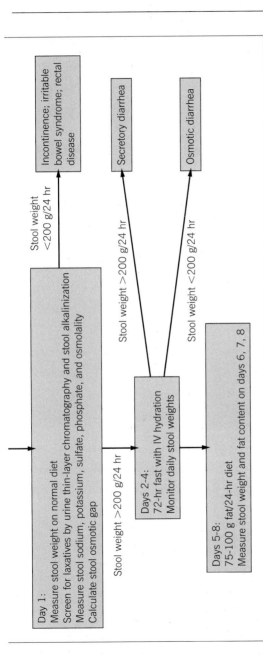

FIG. 28-2

Approach to chronic diarrhea. *(Modified from Donowitz M et al. N Engl J Med 1995; 332:725.)*

REFERENCES

[c] 1. Schiller LR. Diarrhea. Med Clin North Am 2000; 84:1259.

[d] 2. American Gastroenterological Association Medical Position Statement: guidelines for the evaluation and management of chronic diarrhea. Gastroenterology 1999; 116:1461.

[c] 3. Donowitz M et al. Evaluation of patients with chronic diarrhea. N Engl J Med 1995; 332:725.

[b] 4. Murray CJL, Lopez AD. Mortality by cause for eight regions of the world. Global Burden of Disease Study. Lancet 1997; 349:1269.

[b] 5. Feldman R, Banatvala N. The frequency of culturing stools from adults with diarrhoea in Great Britain. Epidemiol Infect 1994; 113:41.

[d] 6. The burden of gastrointestinal diseases. Bethesda, Md: American Gastroenterological Association; 2001.

[b] 7. Wong CS et al. The risk of the hemolytic-uremic syndrome after antibiotic treatment of *Escherichia coli* O157:H7 infections. N Engl J Med 2000; 342:1930.

[d] 8. Guerrant RL et al. Practice guidelines for the management of infectious diarrhea. Clin Infect Dis 2001; 32:331.

[d] 9. DuPont HL. Guidelines on acute infectious diarrhea in adults. Am J Gastroenterol 1997; 92:1962.

[b] 10. Manabe YC et al. *Clostridium difficile* colitis: an efficient clinical approach to diagnosis. Ann Intern Med 1995; 123:835.

[a] 11. Taylor DN et al. Treatment of traveler's diarrhea: ciprofloxacin plus loperamide compared with ciprofloxacin alone; a placebo-controlled, randomized trial. Ann Intern Med 1991; 114:731.

[a] 12. Petruccelli BP et al. Treatment of traveler's diarrhea with ciprofloxacin and loperamide. J Infect Dis 1992; 165:557.

[a] 13. Murphy GS et al. Ciprofloxacin and loperamide in the treatment of bacillary dysentery. Ann Intern Med 1993; 118:582.

[a] 14. DuPont H, Hornick R. Adverse effect of Lomotil therapy in shigellosis. JAMA 1973; 226:1525.

[b] 15. Cimolai N et al. Risk factors for the progression of *Escherichia coli* O157:H7 enteritis to hemolytic-uremic syndrome. J Pediatr 1990; 116:589.

[b] 16. Cimolai N et al. Risk factors for the central nervous system manifestations of gastroenteritis-associated hemolytic-uremic syndrome. Pediatrics 1992; 90:616.

[c] 17. Guerrant RL, Bobak DA. Bacterial and protozoal gastroenteritis. N Engl J Med 1991; 325:327.

[b] 18. Slutsker L et al. *Escherichia coli* O157:H7 diarrhea in the United States: clinical and epidemiologic features. Ann Intern Med 1997; 126:505.

[b] 19. Talan DA et al. Etiology of bloody diarrhea among patients presenting to United States emergency departments: prevalence of *Escherichia coli* O157:H7 and other enteropathogens. Clin Infect Dis 2001; 32:573.

[a] 20. Eherer AJ, Fordtran JS. Fecal osmotic gap and pH in experimental diarrhea of various causes. Gastroenterology 1992; 103:545.

[c] 21. DuPont H, Ericsson C. Prevention and treatment of traveler's diarrhea. N Engl J Med 1993; 328:1821.

Inflammatory Bowel Disease

Geoffrey C. Nguyen, MD, Rachel Y. Chong, MD, and Mary L. Harris, MD

Fast Facts

- Inflammatory bowel disease (IBD) refers to ulcerative colitis and Crohn's disease, idiopathic diseases affecting the gastrointestinal tract that are distinguished from each other by clinical, histological, and endoscopic characteristics (Table 29-1).
- Although the clinical course of IBD is chronic and frequently relapsing and remitting, mortality is generally not greater than in the general population.
- Ulcerative colitis is confined to the mucosa and submucosa of the colon and invariably involves the rectum.
- Crohn's disease may affect any component of the gastrointestinal tract in a discontinuous pattern of "skip lesions."
- Ulcerative colitis and Crohn's disease have clinical and therapeutic similarities, and approximately 10% of patients have indeterminate IBD in which the clinical picture does not allow distinction between the two entities.

I. EPIDEMIOLOGY

1. The incidence and prevalence of ulcerative colitis in the United States are 7.3 and 116 per 100,000, respectively. The incidence of Crohn's disease is 7.0/100,000 and the prevalence is 104/100,000.[1]
2. The peak age at onset for both diseases is between 15 and 25 years with a smaller second peak between the ages of 50 and 80. Males and females are affected equally.
3. The incidence of ulcerative colitis and Crohn's disease is higher among persons of Ashkenazi Jewish and Scandinavian descent and lower among Hispanics and African-Americans. Urban regions tend to have a higher incidence of IBD than rural areas.
4. Interestingly, there is an increased association between Crohn's disease and cigarette smoking but a decreased association between ulcerative colitis and tobacco use.

II. CLINICAL PRESENTATION

A. ULCERATIVE COLITIS

1. The typical presentation of ulcerative colitis is bloody diarrhea characterized by frequent small loose stools and often associated with tenesmus. However, symptoms depend on severity and location of disease. Severity of disease is assessed by clinical, physical, and laboratory criteria as shown in Table 29-2.
2. Ulcerative colitis invariably involves the rectum and is termed

ulcerative proctitis when it is limited to this area. Proctosigmoiditis extends into the mid–sigmoid colon, and left-sided ulcerative colitis involves the regions up to the splenic flexure. Pancolitis refers to inflammation that affects colonic mucosa beyond the splenic flexure.

3. More than half of patients initially have a mild and indolent disease

TABLE 29-1

COMPARISON OF ULCERATIVE COLITIS AND CROHN'S DISEASE

	Ulcerative Colitis	Crohn's Disease
CLINICAL FEATURES		
Diarrhea	Frequently bloody	Usually occult blood
Constitutional symptoms	In severe disease	Frequent
Abdominal pain	In severe disease	Frequently prominent
Perianal disease	None	Common
Fistulae	None	Common
Small bowel involvement	Never with exception of backwash ileitis	Frequent
Surgery	Curative	Recurs after surgery
Increased cancer risk	Yes	Yes
ENDOSCOPIC FEATURES		
Rectal involvement	Always	Rectal sparing common
Lesions	Continuous and circumferential	Skip lesions
Aphthous ulcers	Infrequent	Common
Cobblestoning	No	Yes
PATHOLOGICAL FEATURES		
Inflammation	Mucosal and submucosal	Transmural
Granuloma	No	Diagnostic when present

TABLE 29-2

CRITERIA FOR EVALUATING THE SEVERITY OF ULCERATIVE COLITIS

Criteria	Mild Disease	Severe Disease	Fulminant Disease
Stool frequency (per day)	≤4	5-10	>10
Hematochezia	Intermittent	Frequent	Continuous
Temperature (° C)	Normal	>37.5	>37.5
Heart rate (beats/min)	Normal	>90	>90
Hematocrit value	Normal	<75% of normal	Transfusion required
Erythrocyte sedimentation rate	Normal	Elevated	Elevated
Colonic features on radiography	—	Air, edematous wall, thumbprinting	Dilation
Clinical signs	—	Abdominal tenderness	Abdominal distention and tenderness

Modified from Hanauer SB. N Engl J Med 1996; 334:841.

that involves the rectum and sigmoid. These patients may have self-limited episodes of rectal bleeding and tenesmus, although nonbloody diarrhea is not uncommon. At presentation approximately one third have moderately severe disease that is manifest as more frequent bloody stools (up to 10 per day), a mild anemia, low-grade fever, and some abdominal tenderness. Severe or fulminant ulcerative colitis is characterized by more than 10 bloody stools per day, severe abdominal cramping, severe anemia, high-grade fever, hypo-albuminemia, and weight loss.

4. The rectal examination may reveal bright red blood, but the physical examination is usually normal in mild ulcerative colitis. Patients with moderate disease may have low-grade fever and abdominal tenderness. In severe cases, however, presenting features of ulcerative colitis may include fever, tachycardia, orthostatic hypotension, severe abdominal tenderness with rebound over the colon, and decreased bowel sounds.

5. A deadly complication of ulcerative colitis is toxic megacolon resulting from transmural inflammation. The inflammation paralyzes smooth muscle layers, resulting in colonic dilation associated with systemic symptoms. Bloody diarrhea with abdominal distention and tenderness is typical, and patients appear acutely toxic. Diagnosis is based on radiographic evidence of colonic dilation and the clinical criteria outlined in Box 29-1.

6. The differential diagnosis of ulcerative colitis depends on the presentation. If the patient has proctitis, the physician should consider other causes of rectal blood, including internal hemorrhoids, diverticulosis, arteriovenous malformations, colorectal cancer, infectious proctitis, and radiation proctitis in those with history of exposure. For patients with bloody diarrhea, infectious colitis (e.g., *Shigella, Campylo-*

BOX 29-1

CRITERIA FOR TOXIC MEGACOLON

1. Chronic dilation

    and

2. Three of the following:

    Fever >38° C

    Tachycardia >120 beats/min

    Leukocytosis >10,500/mm^3

    Anemia

    and

3. One of the following:

    Dehydration

    Altered mental status

    Hypotension

    Electrolyte disturbances

bacter, Yersinia) and ischemic colitis should be included in the differential diagnosis. See Chapter 30 for discussion of other causes of lower gastrointestinal bleeds.

B. CROHN'S DISEASE

1. The clinical presentation of Crohn's disease is more variable than that of ulcerative colitis. The predominant symptoms are diarrhea, abdominal pain, and weight loss, often associated with low-grade fever and malaise.

2. Crohn's disease most frequently affects the ileum and colon (40%) but may be confined to the distal ileum (30%) or limited to the colon (25%).[2] The clinical course can follow three patterns: (1) inflammatory, (2) perforating and fistulizing, and (3) stenosing or stricturing. The inflammatory type involves diarrhea caused by multiple factors, including increased secretion and impaired fluid reabsorption resulting from inflammation of the ileum or colon. Bile malabsorption and steatorrhea may also result from ileal disease or resection. Patients with inflammatory Crohn's disease also frequently have colicky abdominal pain, often in the right lower quadrant. Perforating disease may occur when transmural inflammation leads to serosal penetration and subsequent localized peritonitis with fever and abdominal pain with rebound or guarding. Penetration of the bowel wall may also result in fistulization.

3. Although enteroenteric fistulae may be asymptomatic, enterovesicular fistulae may lead to recurrent polymicrobial urinary tract infections and pneumaturia. Psoas and retroperitoneal abscesses may arise from fistulae in the retroperitoneum. Perianal disease—perianal abscesses, fissures, ulcers, strictures, and stenoses—may occur in one third of patients and is characterized by pain and drainage.

4. The differential diagnosis of Crohn's disease includes infections, caused by such organisms as *Yersinia, Shigella, Campylobacter,* and *Giardia*, and ileocecal tuberculosis. Other diseases that may mimic Crohn's disease include intestinal lymphoma, amyloidosis, lymphocytic and collagenous colitis, and diverticulitis. Behçet's disease, in particular, can be manifested as inflammation of the terminal ileum and aphthous ulcers, as well as having such extraintestinal manifestations as uveitis, arthritis, erythema nodosum, and iridocyclitis.

C. EXTRAINTESTINAL MANIFESTATIONS

1. IBD is commonly associated with extraintestinal manifestations.[3] The sacroiliac joints are frequently affected, resulting in a seronegative spondyloarthropathy. Patients may also have peripheral oligoarthritis in larger joints such as the knees, hips, elbows, and wrists.

2. Common skin manifestations include erythema nodosum and pyoderma gangrenosum. Inflammation may also involve the eyes, resulting in anterior uveitis or episcleritis.

3. Sclerosing cholangitis is a serious hepatic complication more

commonly seen in ulcerative colitis than in Crohn's disease. Patients initially have an elevated alkaline phosphatase level. Nephrolithiasis is commonly seen in Crohn's disease and results from calcium malabsorption and increased absorption of oxalate. The incidence of thromboembolism is also increased in IBD.[4]

III. DIAGNOSTICS

A. LABORATORY TESTS

1. Stool studies, including fecal leukocytes, culture, ova and parasites, and *C. difficile* toxin screen, should be obtained for patients with suspected IBD to rule out an infectious etiology. Nonspecific markers of inflammation, such as the erythrocyte sedimentation rate and the C-reactive protein level, may be elevated during acute flare-ups. In addition, patients with suspected IBD should have a complete blood cell count to evaluate for leukocytosis and severe anemia. Hypoalbuminemia may reflect poor nutritional status, and electrolyte abnormalities may indicate severe diarrhea.

2. The serological markers perinuclear antineutrophilic cytoplasmic antibody (P-ANCA) and anti–*Sacchromyces cerevisiae* antibody (ASCA) may help distinguish between ulcerative colitis and Crohn's disease, especially in indeterminate cases. In several studies patients with positive tests for P-ANCA and negative tests for ASCA were more likely to have ulcerative colitis, whereas those who were P-ANCA negative and ASCA positive were more likely to have Crohn's disease.[5] Although these tests have a specificity greater than 90%, they have a low sensitivity (40%-60%) and should be used only as an adjunct to endoscopy and radiography in diagnosis.

B. ENDOSCOPY

1. Colonoscopy with ileoscopy and biopsy is the primary tool for the diagnosis of IBD and determination of the extent of disease. In most cases endoscopy can be used to differentiate between ulcerative colitis and Crohn's disease. Endoscopic features that may be observed in both diseases include pseudopolyps, fibrotic strictures, loss of haustral folds, and linear superficial scars.

2. Findings that may be more specific to Crohn's disease include aphthous ulcers, which may involve the entire wall of the colon; cobblestoning; and the presence of discontinuous lesions.[6] Sparing of the rectum is also more suggestive of Crohn's disease, since ulcerative colitis invariably involves the rectum. However, patients with ulcerative colitis who have been treated with 5-aminosalicylic acid (ASA)/steroid suppositories may also demonstrate rectal sparing. Isolated involvement of the terminal ileum is also suggestive of Crohn's disease. In ulcerative colitis, inflammation of the terminal ileum usually occurs only in the presence of pancolitis. Normal mucosal vasculature adjacent to affected regions is also more typical of Crohn's disease.

3. Typical endoscopic findings in ulcerative colitis include erythema, mucosal edema, friability, loss of fine vascular pattern, and mucosal granularity. These features typically begin at the anal verge and extend proximally in a continuous and circumferential manner. In addition to its utility in the diagnosis, colonoscopy during an ulcerative colitis flare may predict clinical severity and need for surgery.[7] Biopsy may also detect superimposed cytomegalovirus colitis. In severe cases of suspected ulcerative colitis, sigmoidoscopy is preferable to colonoscopy because of the reduced risk of perforation. Colonoscopy is contraindicated in suspected cases of toxic megacolon.

C. **IMAGING**

1. Fluoroscopic studies play an important role in the diagnosis of Crohn's disease. The dedicated small bowel series and upper gastrointestinal series are particularly important in detecting Crohn's disease proximal to the terminal ileum and not accessible by ileoscopy. Findings may include multiple aphthous ulcers, a cobblestone appearance, fistulae, and a "string sign" caused by luminal narrowing.

2. Radiographic imaging is a powerful adjunct in diagnosing many of the complications of IBD. Plain films are helpful in the assessment of suspected toxic megacolon or small bowel obstruction. Single contrast studies are particularly valuable in defining strictures, fistulae, and tumors. Abdominal computed tomography with contrast medium may be used to identify abscesses, microperforations, fluid collections, or colonic thickening. Findings consistent with ulcerative colitis on double-contrast radiographic studies include pseudopolyps, mucosal granularity, fibrosis, and loss of haustral folds.

IV. MANAGEMENT

1. IBD is managed predominantly in the outpatient setting. Hospitalized patients with IBD tend to have more severe manifestations of the disease. Some patients are admitted for severe exacerbations of known disease, whereas in other hospitalized patients the disease is diagnosed for the first time.

2. The goal of treatment is to achieve remission and then to maintain this state with a variety of agents. In general, the first line of treatment for both Crohn's disease and ulcerative colitis is the use of 5-ASA acid derivatives. Steroids are often used for acute flare-ups, and immunomodulators are used to maintain remission of severe refractory disease.

A. **MANAGEMENT OF ULCERATIVE COLITIS** (Fig. 29-1)

1. Mild to moderate cases of ulcerative colitis may be encountered in the inpatient setting when patients are initially admitted for lower gastrointestinal bleeding. The 5-ASA (mesalamine) drugs are the first-line agents in both induction and remission therapy for mild to moderate ulcerative colitis.[8,9] The parent compound, sulfasalazine, is a less expensive alternative but has more frequent side effects. In

Condition	Treatment		
Proctitis	5-ASA enemas or 5-ASA suppositories or oral 5-ASA drugs or corticosteroid enemas	*Continued activity* → Prednisone or immunomodulators	*Continued activity* → Proctectomy
Mild to moderate pancolitis	Oral 5-ASA drugs	*Continued activity* → Prednisone	*Continued activity or* → Immunomodulators *Steroid dependence* or colectomy
Severe or fulminant pancolitis	Parenteral steroids	*Continued activity* → Cyclosporine or colectomy	
Disease in remission	Maintenance with oral 5-ASA drugs		

FIG. 29-1

Treatment of ulcerative colitis. ASA, Aminosalicylic acid. *(From Goldman L, Bennett JC. Cecil textbook of medicine, 21st ed. Philadelphia: WB Saunders; 2000.)*

29

INFLAMMATORY BOWEL DISEASE

patients with ulcerative proctitis, topical 5-ASA drugs such as FIV-ASA suppositories or topical corticosteroids (Cortifoam) applied twice daily are effective in achieving remission.[10] Rowasa enemas (5-ASA) may be implemented at 4 g daily for disease extending to the proctosigmoid and distal colon.[11] In patients with moderate to severe ulcerative colitis, prednisone may be initiated at a dose of 40 to 60 mg PO daily and then slowly tapered after remission is achieved.

2. Patients with fulminant ulcerative colitis requiring hospitalization are at increased risk for severe gastrointestinal bleeding, toxic megacolon, and perforation. The mainstays of treatment for these patients are parenteral steroids, strict bowel rest, and nutritional support. Those with severe gastrointestinal bleeding require immediate assessment of their hemodynamic status and management of the bleeding. Parenteral steroids (methylprednisolone 20 mg IV q8h or prednisolone 30 mg IV q12h) can be administered. For patients who do not improve within 7 to 10 days, cyclosporine 4 mg/kg given as a continuous IV infusion over 24 hours may be used in conjunction with steroids. This therapy may yield an initial response in 50% to 80% of patients.[12] The serum total cholesterol level should be checked before initiation of therapy, since levels less than 120 mg/dL may predispose to seizures.

3. Once hospitalized, patients with fulminant ulcerative colitis should be monitored for signs and symptoms of toxic megacolon and perforation as discussed previously. Vital signs should be measured as often as every 4 to 6 hours, and abdominal examinations should be performed frequently.

4. In cases where the diagnosis of toxic megacolon is established, nasogastric suction should be initiated for decompression. In unstable patients broad-spectrum antibiotics should be started. Daily abdominal plain film radiographs are needed for these patients. The surgical service should be promptly consulted, and colectomy should be considered if the patient does not respond to medical therapy within 72 hours.

5. Once remission is achieved, patients should be started on a maintenance regimen. Since steroids are ineffective as maintenance agents, orally administered prednisone should be initiated and gradually tapered and a 5-ASA agent should be started. Patients who initially respond to cyclosporine should be switched to orally administered cyclosporine for several months and simultaneously be started on a regimen of 6-mercaptopurine or its prodrug azathioprine for maintenance.

6. Surgical intervention should be considered for patients whose fulminant ulcerative colitis is refractory to medical therapy. Other indications for surgery include toxic megacolon, severe bleeding, impending perforation, strictures, high-grade dysplasia, and severe extraintestinal manifestations. It should be noted that the progressive course of primary sclerosing cholangitis is unchanged

by surgery. Among the more common surgical options are the proctocolectomy with permanent ileostomy and the colectomy with mucosal proctectomy and subsequent ileal pouch–anal anastomosis. In emergency situations the latter may be performed in multiple stages with an initial abdominal colectomy and formation of a Hartmann's pouch. Surgery is curative for ulcerative colitis.

B. MANAGEMENT OF CROHN'S DISEASE (Fig. 29-2)

1. The management of Crohn's disease depends on the clinical presentation. In patients with mild inflammatory symptoms of abdominal pain and diarrhea, the 5-ASA agents are the first line of therapy and the choice of formulation depends on the target region.[13] Pentasa is a sustained-released granular formulation that targets the upper gastrointestinal tract, as well as the ileum and colon. Asacol is pH sensitive and targets the ileum and colon, whereas sulfasalazine is active only in the colon.

2. Patients who do not respond to mesalamine at maximum doses of 4.8 g/day after 3 to 4 weeks should be started on metronidazole at 10 mg/kg in divided doses alone or in combination with ciprofloxacin 500 mg bid.[14] For patients who do not respond to antibiotics or who have moderately severe symptoms, prednisone 40 mg/day PO should be started. A slow-release form of budesonide (Entocort EC), at a dose of 9 mg/day, is also effective in achieving remission in patients with disease affecting the ileum to the ascending colon. This corticosteroid is associated with fewer systemic side effects because more than 90% is metabolized by the liver via first-pass effect.[15]

3. Patients whose disease is refractory to the preceding measures or who are chronically dependent on steroids should be started on immuno-modulators, including azathioprine or its metabolite 6-mercaptopurine at 50 mg/day. Myelosuppression is a common adverse effect, and patients need monthly monitoring of blood cell counts. Methotrexate, at an initial weekly dose of 25 mg IM, is an alternative for patients who cannot tolerate azathioprine.[16]

4. The tumor necrosis factor–α antagonist infliximab is the next line of therapy for moderate to severe Crohn's disease that is refractory to the above measures. Infliximab is administered as 5 mg/kg at 0, 2, and 6 weeks and then subsequently given every 8 weeks. For those who continue to have active disease despite immunomodulator therapy, long-term low-dose steroid therapy or complete bowel rest with total parenteral nutrition may be needed.

5. Once remission has been achieved, maintenance therapy should be initiated with mesalamine. Patients who achieve remission with azathioprine or 6-mercaptopurine (6-MP) should be maintained on these regimens.[17] Similarly, patients with refractory disease who required infliximab to achieve remission should continue to receive infusions at 6- to 8-week intervals.[18]

6. Perineal abscesses and draining fistulae that are not amenable to

Condition	Treatment
Colitis or ileocolitis	Oral 5-ASA drug or metronidazole → *Continued activity* Prednisone → *Continued activity or Steroid dependence* Immunomodulator → *Continued activity* Surgery
Ileitis	Prednisone → *Continued activity* Immunomodulator → *Continued activity* Surgery
Fistula	TPN or immunomodulator → *Failure to close* Surgery
Abscess	Antibiotics, drainage, and resection
Obstruction caused by inflammation	IV fluids, nasogastric suction, parenteral steroids → *Failure to respond* Surgery

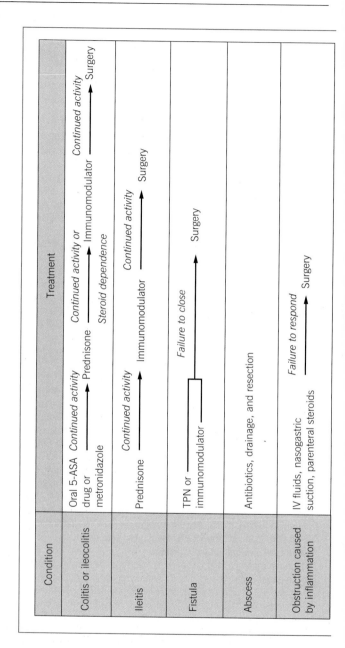

Obstruction caused by scarring	IV fluids, nasogastric suction
Perianal disease	Antibiotics and surgical drainage
Disease in remission	Maintenance with oral 5-ASA drugs or immunomodulators

Failure to respond ⟶ Surgery

FIG. 29-2

Treatment of Crohn's disease. *ASA,* Aminosalicylic acid; *TPN,* total parenteral nutrition. *(From Goldman L, Bennett JC. Cecil textbook of medicine, 21st ed. Philadelphia: WB Saunders; 2000.)*

29

INFLAMMATORY BOWEL DISEASE

surgery are initially managed with metronidazole, ciprofloxacin, or both. Relapse after discontinuation of antibiotics is common, however, and long-term therapy may be required. If perineal disease remains refractory, 6-MP, infliximab, or surgery may be indicated. Other fistulization in Crohn's disease should be treated with azathioprine or 6-MP, since fistulae are generally not successfully closed with steroids or sulfasalazine. If this therapy is unsuccessful, infliximab should be initiated.[19] Patients with enterovesical fistulae and resultant urinary tract infections need antibiotics and often surgery.

7. Patients with Crohn's disease commonly require hospitalization for microperforation, obstructive symptoms, or severe bleeding. Those with evidence of localized abscesses or microperforation should be treated with bowel rest and broad-spectrum antibiotics and may require surgery. Whether steroids should be used in this situation is controversial. Initially, pelvic and abdominal abscesses should be managed conservatively. Although surgical resection of affected bowel segments yields a lower rate of recurrence, medical therapy and percutaneous drainage have been found to avert subsequent surgery in the majority of patients and may be an alternative to surgery.[20] Unless small bowel obstruction occurs in the setting of previous adhesions, it is usually partial and is managed initially with intravenous fluids, parenteral nutrition, and nasogastric suction. Failure to improve or development of complete obstruction is an indication for surgery. Ulceration in Crohn's disease may also lead to severe bleeding and requires supportive management, parenterally administered steroids, and possibly surgery.

8. The most common indications for surgery in Crohn's disease are high-grade small bowel obstruction, perforation, massive hemorrhage, and refractoriness to medical therapy. High-grade dysplasia on surveillance biopsy also requires surgical intervention. Surgical options depend on the regions involved. Perforation or stricture of the small bowel may be managed by segmental resection and anastomosis. Stricturoplasty may relieve intestinal obstruction while averting short gut syndrome. Treatment of colorectal involvement ranges from segmental colectomy to total proctocolectomy, depending on extent of the disease. Unlike ulcerative colitis, Crohn's disease commonly recurs after surgery; endoscopically discovered relapse occurs at a rate of 70% per year and clinically apparent recurrence at 15% per year. Postoperative prophylaxis with mesalamine or metronidazole may reduce this recurrence rate.[21,22]

C. SURVEILLANCE FOR COLORECTAL CANCER

1. Both ulcerative colitis and Crohn's colitis predispose patients to colorectal cancer. The cancer risk for ulcerative colitis is 0.5% to 1% per year after 10 years.[23] Patients who have had ulcerative colitis and Crohn's disease involving the colon for more than 8 years should

undergo annual examination with colonoscopy. Multiple contiguous surveillance biopsy specimens should be obtained.

PEARLS AND PITFALLS

- Colonoscopy with ileoscopy is the primary diagnostic tool in IBD.
- Patients taking steroids on a long-term basis should also take calcium and vitamin D supplements and undergo dual-energy x-ray absorptiometry during the first 3 to 6 months of steroid therapy because maximal bone loss occurs in this period.
- Patients with Crohn's disease of the small bowel have a predisposition to iron, folate, and vitamin B_{12} malabsorption and should be screened for these deficiencies.
- Bile salt malabsorption is a common cause of diarrhea in patients who have undergone ileal resections of less than 100 cm. This diarrhea may respond to cholestyramine.
- Steroids, sulfasalazine, or mesalamine is the therapy of choice for IBD during pregnancy.
- Surgery is curative for ulcerative colitis but not for Crohn's disease, which has a clinical recurrence as high as 20% 1 year after surgery.
- Prophylaxis against deep venous thrombosis is an important aspect of management, since patients with IBD have an increased risk of thromboembolic events.
- The risk of colorectal cancer is increased in both ulcerative colitis and Crohn's colitis, and patients who have had disease longer than 8 years should have annual colonoscopies.
- Irritable bowel syndrome occurs in 15% to 20% of the general population and is a common comorbid condition in IBD.[24]
- If patients have symptoms of irritable bowel syndrome, this does not exclude the diagnosis of IBD or vice-versa.
- Irritable bowel syndrome occurring concomitantly with IBD may not respond to antiinflammatory agents, but supportive care with antidiarrheal or antispasmodic medications may alleviate symptoms.
- Endoscopy may be useful in distinguishing irritable bowel symptoms from active IBD.

29

INFLAMMATORY BOWEL DISEASE

REFERENCES

[c] 1. Farrokhyar R, Swarbrick ET, Irvine EJ. A critical review of epidemiological studies in inflammatory bowel disease. Scand J Gastroenterol 2001; 36:2.

[b] 2. Farmer RG, Hawk WA, Turnbull RBJ. Clinical patterns in Crohn's disease: a statistical study of 615 cases. Gastroenterology 1975; 68:627.

[b] 3. Bernstein CN et al. The prevalence of extraintestinal diseases in inflammatory bowel disease: a population-based study. Am J Gastroenterol 2001; 96:1116.

[c] 4. Koutroubakis IE. Role of thrombotic vascular risk factors in inflammatory bowel disease. Dig Dis 2000; 18:161.

[b] 5. Peeters M et al. Diagnostic value of anti–*Saccharomyces cerevisiae* and antineutrophil cytoplasmic autoantibodies in inflammatory bowel disease. Am J Gastroenterol 2001; 96:730.

[b] 6. Pera A et al. Colonoscopy in inflammatory bowel disease: diagnostic accuracy and proposal of an endoscopic score. Gastroenterology 1987; 92:181.

[b] 7. Carbonnel F et al. Colonoscopy of acute colitis: a safe and reliable tool for assessment of severity. Dig Dis Sci 1994; 39:1550.

[a] 8. Schroeder KW, Tremaine WJ, Ilstrup DM. Coated oral 5-aminosalicylic acid therapy for mildly to moderately active ulcerative colitis: a randomized study. N Engl J Med 1987; 317:1625.

[c] 9. Hanauer SB, Dassopoulos T. Evolving treatment strategies for inflammatory bowel disease. Annu Rev Med 2001; 52:299.

[a] 10. Campieri M et al. Mesalazine (5-aminosalicylic acid) suppositories in the treatment of ulcerative proctitis or distal proctosigmoiditis: a randomized controlled trial. Scand J Gastroenterol 1990; 25:663.

[a] 11. Sutherland LR et al. 5-Aminosalicylic acid enema in the treatment of distal ulcerative colitis, proctosigmoiditis, and proctitis. Gastroenterology 1987; 92:1894.

[a] 12. Lichtiger S et al. Cyclosporine in severe ulcerative colitis refractory to steroid therapy. N Engl J Med 1994; 330:1841.

[a] 13. Prantera C et al. Mesalamine in the treatment of mild to moderate active Crohn's ileitis: results of a randomized, multicenter trial. Gastroenterology 1999; 116:521.

[a] 14. Sutherland L et al. Double blind, placebo controlled trial of metronidazole in Crohn's disease. Gut 1991; 32:1071.

[a] 15. Thomsen OO et al. A comparison of budesonide and mesalamine for active Crohn's disease. N Engl J Med 1998, 339:370.

[a] 16. Feagan BG et al. Methotrexate for the treatment of Crohn's disease. North American Crohn's Study Group Investigators. N Engl J Med 1995; 332:292.

[a] 17. Candy S et al. A controlled double blind study of azathioprine in the management of Crohn's disease. Gut 1995; 37:674.

[a] 18. Rutgeerts P et al. Efficacy and safety of retreatment with anti–tumor necrosis factor antibody (infliximab) to maintain remission in Crohn's disease. Gastroenterology 1999; 117:761.

[a] 19. Present DH et al. Infliximab for the treatment of fistulas in patients with Crohn's disease. N Engl J Med 1999; 340:1398.

[b] 20. Garcia JC et al. Abscesses in Crohn's disease: outcome of medical versus surgical treatment. J Clin Gastroenterol 2001; 32:409.

[a] 21. McLeod RS et al. Prophylactic mesalamine treatment decreases postoperative recurrence of Crohn's disease. Gastroenterology 1995; 109:404.

[a] 22. Rutgeerts P et al. Controlled trial of metronidazole treatment for prevention of Crohn's recurrence after ileal resection. Gastroenterology 1995; 108:1617.

[d] 23. Kornbluth A, Sachar DB. Ulcerative colitis practice guidelines in adults. American College of Gastroenterology, Practice Parameters Committee. Am J Gastroenterol 1997; 92:204.

[c] 24. Bayless TM, Harris ML. Inflammatory bowel disease and irritable bowel syndrome. Med Clin North Am 1990; 74:21.

Lower Gastrointestinal Bleed

Kerri L. Cavanaugh, MD, Vandana R. Long, MD, and Mary L. Harris, MD

FAST FACTS

- The first step in managing a lower gastrointestinal bleed (LGIB) is to assess the stability of the patient and resuscitate if needed.
- Early colonoscopy may offer both diagnostic and therapeutic options.
- In severe bleeding, tagged red blood cell scan or angiography should be used to locate the source, especially if the patient may undergo surgery.
- Overall, mortality rates are usually lower (<5% of patients) for LGIB than for upper gastrointestinal bleeds (UGIBs).[1]
- Bleeding ceases spontaneously in approximately 75% to 85% of LGIB cases.[2]

I. EPIDEMIOLOGY

1. Information regarding the epidemiology of LGIB is difficult to interpret because criteria for the verification of the location of bleeding are neither standardized nor often reported.
2. The annual incidence of LGIB is 21 to 27 cases per 100,000 adults.[3]
3. LGIB accounts for approximately 24% to 33% of all hospital admissions for gastrointestinal (GI) bleeding.[4]
4. LGIB occurs more often in men, and the incidence increases with age. A 200-fold increase in incidence occurs between ages 30 and 90 years.[3]

II. CLINICAL PRESENTATION

A. DEFINITIONS

1. LGIB is bleeding below the ligament of Treitz (suspensory ligament between third and fourth parts of the duodenum).
2. Hematochezia is the presence of bright red blood from the rectum. It is usually caused by a LGIB, but an estimated 10% are the result of a brisk UGIB.
3. Melena is the occurrence of black tarry stools, which results from metabolism of blood in the GI tract by hydrochloride to produce hematin. At least 50 mL of blood is necessary to produce melena. Melena usually indicates that the bleeding source is proximal to the cecum.[5]

B. DIFFERENTIAL DIAGNOSIS

1. Conditions causing LGIB are summarized in Box 30-1.[6]
2. Because the location of bleeding is difficult to verify, many diagnoses are "presumptive" rather than "definitive."

BOX 30-1

CONDITIONS THAT CAUSE LOWER GASTROINTESTINAL BLEEDING

COMMON CAUSES

Diverticulosis	42%-55% (60% of bleeding diverticula are in the right side of the colon)
Angiodysplasia	3%-12% (>50% occur in the right side of the colon)
Cancer, polyp	8%-26%
Inflammatory bowel disease (ulcerative colitis more often than Crohn's disease)	2%-8%
Anorectal disease	3%-9%
Small bowel disease	3%-5%
Infectious colitis (e.g., typhoid, *Escherichia coli* O157:H7, CMV)	1%-5%
Radiation colitis	1%-5%
Vasculitis (e.g., polyarteritis nodosa, Wegener's granulomatosis, rheumatoid arthritis)	1%-3%

RARE CAUSES

Postpolypectomy bleeding
Aortocolonic fistula
Trauma
Colonic ischemia

PATIENTS WITH HUMAN IMMUNODEFICIENCY VIRUS OR ADULT IMMUNODEFICIENCY SYNDROME*

CMV colitis	39%
Idiopathic colonic ulcers	28%
Anorectal disease	23%
Colonic histoplasmosis	
Kaposi's sarcoma	
Colitis, bacterial	

CMV, Cytomegalovirus.
*Data from Chalasani N, Wilcox CM. Am J Gastroenterol 1998; 93(2):175.

C. INITIAL EVALUATION

1. **Stability of the patient:** As with UGIB, assessment of vital signs is the critical first step. Further evaluation should be delayed until the patient is stable. Presenting signs of LGIB are listed in Box 30-2.[7-9]
2. **Evaluation once the patient is stable.**
a. History.
   (1) Characteristics of bleeding, including onset, duration, and color. One study found that patients and physicians used 23 different terms; even with a color card (5 colors) there was little agreement. Only the brightest red was predictive of a coloanorectal source.[5]

BOX 30-2

SIGNS OF LOWER GASTROINTESTINAL BLEEDING AT PRESENTATION

Decrease in hemoglobin *and* hemodynamic abnormality	50%
Orthostatic changes	30%
Syncope	10%
Shock	9%

The initial blood pressure correlates with mortality rates (systolic blood pressure >100 mm Hg in 8%; 80-99 mm Hg in 17%; <80 mm Hg in >30%).

Orthostatic measurements may help determine whether volume loss is significant.

Tachycardia is an important risk factor for morbidity and mortality.

Data from Bramley PN et al. Scand J Gastroenterol 1996; 31(8):764; Richter JM et al. Gastrointest Endosc 1995; 41(2):93; and Schiller KFR, Truelove SC, Williams DG. Br Med J 1970; 2(700):7.

    (2) Nonsteroidal antiinflammatory drugs, acetylsalicylic acid, and steroids are risk factors, especially for diverticular bleeding.[10]

    (3) History of radiation therapy: Bleeding usually follows within months but can occur up to 3 years later.

    (4) Vascular surgery: Does the patient have an aortic graft? (Bleeding often occurs as a "sentinel bleed.")

    (5) Colonoscopy history; recent polypectomy.

    (6) Comorbid conditions, such as alcoholism, liver disease, bleeding disorders, trauma, cardiac disease, or renal disease.

b. Physical and rectal examination, including anoscopy.

    (1) Anoscopy should be a routine procedure and often is performed in the initial evaluation.

    (2) In a prospective study among patients with LGIB, 2% had palpable rectal cancers.[11]

    (3) In one series of 17,941 patients, 11% had anorectal disease such as hemorrhoids or fissures.[12]

c. Exclusion of upper GI source.

    (1) Nasogastric tube aspiration: An aspirate is considered positive with the presence of any red blood, dark coffee grounds material, or pink flecks. A negative aspirate is clear or bilious.

    (2) If aspirate is positive: 93% upper GI source, 7% source undetermined; none with a lower GI source.[13]

    (3) If aspirate is negative: 60% lower GI source, 40% source undetermined; 1% upper GI source.[13]

III. DIAGNOSTICS

A. LABORATORY TESTS

1. Hemoglobin and hematocrit.

a. These may not accurately reflect blood loss (Fig. 30-1). It may be several hours before a drop in a patient's hematocrit is evident.

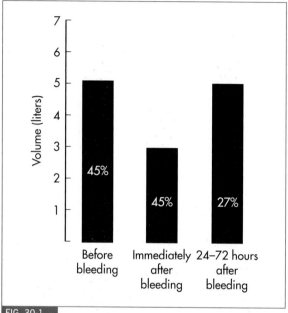

FIG. 30-1
Plasma volumes *(solid bars)*, red blood cell volumes *(stippled bars)*, and hematocrits before bleeding and after 2-L blood loss. A baseline hematocrit of 45% is assumed. *(From Feldman M, Scharschmidt BF, Sleisenger MH: Sleisenger & Fordtran's gastrointestinal and liver disease, 7th ed. Philadelphia: WB Saunders; 2001.)*

b. Hemoglobin level below 10 g/dL may be associated with increased mortality (especially for UGIB).[14]
c. Hematocrit should be followed closely (i.e., measured every 6 hours).
d. Transfusion raises the hematocrit value approximately 2% to 3% per unit transfused. A check of coagulation times and ionized calcium levels should be considered for patients who receive multiple units of blood (typically ≥5 units).

2. **Platelet count:** If it is less than 50,000/mm^3, transfusion should be considered, usually beginning with 6 units for the average person. No randomized controlled trials have been presented to support this recommendation.

3. **Prothrombin time and activated partial thromboplastin time:** If these are abnormal, administration of fresh frozen plasma should be considered (the quantity is often based on weight).

4. **Blood urea nitrogen/creatinine ratio:** A ratio greater than 36 suggests UGIB (when renal disease is absent). However, this measurement has

a large degree of overlap in its association with UGIB and LGIB and should not be relied on to make the diagnosis.[15]

B. SIGMOIDOSCOPY

1. Use of sigmoidoscopy is often recommended in a less urgent setting.
2. Sigmoidoscopy is not usually performed on patients admitted to the hospital.

C. COLONOSCOPY

1. Colonoscopy was introduced in the 1970s but was not used initially because of concern about the risks of colon preparation.
2. More recently, evidence has shown that an oral GI preparation is indeed safe. Several studies have looked at colonoscopy as the primary diagnostic evaluation. A review compiled 13 studies; of 1561 colonoscopy examinations, 68% documented a source or a presumed source (range 48%-90%).[16] Complications (overall 1.3%) included heart failure, bowel perforation, exacerbation of bleeding, and septicemia.

D. TAGGED RED BLOOD CELL SCAN

1. The technetium label remains in the bloodstream for 48 hours and is not taken up by the liver or spleen.
2. This method can detect rates of bleeding as low as 0.1 mL/min, but usually needs higher rates of bleeding for accurate detection and localization.
3. A review of 16 studies looked at 1418 scans, 45% of which were positive. Whether this identifies a higher morbidity and mortality risk is unclear.[16] The test is most accurate when a positive result is obtained within 2 hours of injection.
4. Reliability: Pooled studies showed an accuracy of approximately 78%[16]; thus additional studies to localize the bleeding source are recommended before surgical management.
5. No studies comparing colonoscopy with tagged red blood cell scans are available.

E. ANGIOGRAPHY

1. Angiography is performed to determine location of bleeding, especially if surgical management is needed.
2. It detects rates as low as 0.5 mL/min.
3. Results are more likely to be positive if patient also has a positive tagged red cell scan.
4. A review of 14 studies showed mean positivity to be 47% (range 27%-77%).[16]
5. Complications (overall 9.3%) included hematoma, femoral artery thrombosis, contrast reaction, renal failure, and transient ischemic attack.[17]

F. BARIUM ENEMA

1. Barium enema has a very low diagnostic yield, and results are often misleading.

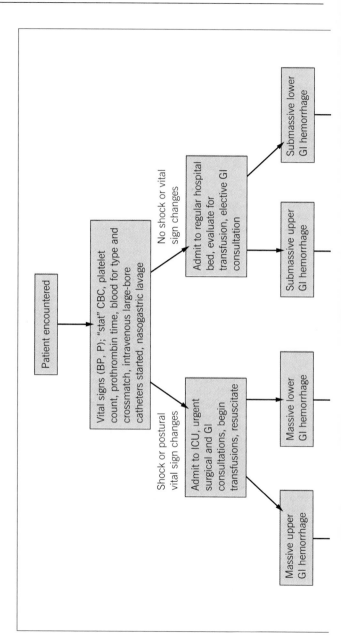

Patient encountered

→

Vital signs (BP, P); "stat" CBC, platelet count, prothrombin time, blood for type and crossmatch, intravenous large-bore catheters started, nasogastric lavage

Shock or postural vital sign changes

Admit to ICU, urgent surgical and GI consultations, begin transfusions, resuscitate

Massive upper GI hemorrhage

Massive lower GI hemorrhage

No shock or vital sign changes

Admit to regular hospital bed, evaluate for transfusion, elective GI consultation

Submassive upper GI hemorrhage

Submassive lower GI hemorrhage

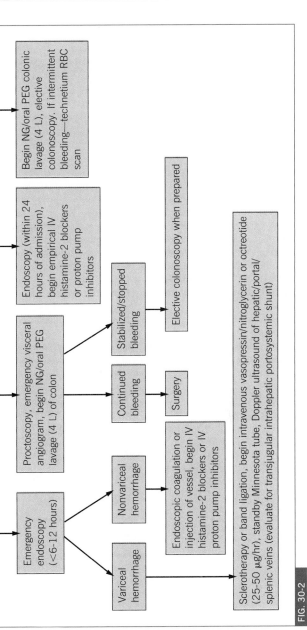

FIG. 30-2

Approach to the patient with gastrointestinal hemorrhage. *BP,* Blood pressure; *CBC,* complete blood cell count; *GI,* gastrointestinal; *ICU,* intensive care unit; *NG,* nasogastric; *P,* pulse; *PEG,* polyethylene glycol; *RBC,* red blood cell. *(From Goldman L, Bennett JC. Cecil textbook of medicine, 21st ed. Philadelphia: WB Saunders; 1999.)*

2. It interferes with colonoscopy and angiography and thus should be avoided for initial diagnosis.

IV. MANAGEMENT (Fig. 30-2)

A. CONSULTATION

1. The intensive care unit team should be consulted if there is any concern about hemodynamic instability.

B. VOLUME RESUSCITATION

1. Two large-bore peripheral intravenous catheters, preferably 16-gauge, should be inserted.
2. Volume resuscitation versus blood transfusion.
   a. In the acute setting, fluid resuscitation with normal saline is performed, but blood typing and crossmatch for 2 to 6 units of blood should be ordered.
   b. Transfusions are necessary for 36% of patients with LGIB.[4]
   c. Patients should generally receive transfusions to a goal hematocrit between 25% and 30%, depending on existing comorbidities.
3. Vasopressors are often not recommended initially because hypotension is a result of volume loss. Replacement of volume is the priority.

C. CORRECTION OF COAGULOPATHY

1. Reversal of coagulopathy with platelets or fresh frozen plasma may be necessary.
2. No studies have established the optimal coagulation parameters or platelet count.
3. Patients who have normal platelet counts and coagulation parameters at presentation and receive several units of packed red blood cells (>5 units) may require fresh frozen plasma or platelet transfusions because of a dilution effect.

D. COLONOSCOPY

1. Signs of recent hemorrhage such as active bleeding, visible vessels, and adherent clots should be sought.[18]
2. Therapeutic options include thermal contact probe, laser, monopolar electrocautery, and injection sclerotherapy.
3. One recent study of therapeutic colonoscopy showed that in diverticular disease, colonoscopy performed within 6 to 12 hours resulted in a significant decrease in rebleeding.[19]

E. ANGIOGRAPHY

1. This modality provides both diagnostic and therapeutic options and is recommended in settings of rapid bleeding.
2. **Vasoconstrictors:** Initial control of bleeding is obtained in 62% to 100%, and rebleeding occurs in 16% to 50%.[6] Complications include fluid retention, hyponatremia, transient hypertension, sinus bradycardia, arrhythmia, pulmonary edema, and myocardial ischemia.
3. **Embolization:** Agents include gelatin-sponge pledgets, microcoils, and polyvinyl alcohol particles. Complications include abdominal pain, fever, and ischemic infarction.

F. SURGERY

1. A surgical consultation is needed for continued severe bleeding with high transfusion requirements.
2. Surgical options include directed segmental resection (if the bleeding location is known), blind segmental resection, or a total abdominal colectomy with ileorectal anastomosis in emergency cases.
3. Localization of the bleeding source by scanning or angiography is helpful because rebleeding rates are higher after blind surgery than after directed surgery (42% versus 14%).[16]

PEARLS AND PITFALLS

- Although a number of studies of the findings in LGIB have been performed, no gold standard for diagnosis and verification of the bleeding source has been established.
- Colonoscopy offers promising therapeutic options, even in urgent and possibly emergency situations. Development of practice guidelines is still needed.
- In patients receiving multiple units of packed red blood cells, hypocalcemia may develop because of chelation with citrate (additive in blood units). In addition, coagulation times may be prolonged because of a dilution effect.

REFERENCES

[d] 1. Zuccaro G Jr. Management of the adult patient with acute lower gastrointestinal bleeding. Am J Gastroenterol 1998; 93(8):1202.

[c] 2. Jensen DM, Machicado GA. Colonoscopy for diagnosis and treatment of severe lower gastrointestinal bleeding: routine outcomes and cost analysis. Gastrointest Endosc Clin North Am 1997; 7(3):477.

[b] 3. Longstreth GF. Epidemiology and outcome of patients hospitalized with acute lower gastrointestinal hemorrhage: a population-based study. Am J Gastroenterol 1997; 92(3):206.

[c] 4. Peura DA et al: The American College of Gastroenterology Bleeding Registry: preliminary findings. Am J Gastroenterol 1997; 92(6):924.

[a] 5. Zuckerman GR et al. An objective measure of stool color for differentiating upper from lower gastrointestinal bleeding. Dig Dis Sci 1995; 40(8):1614.

[c] 6. Zuckerman GR, Prakash C. Acute lower intestinal bleeding. II. Etiology, therapy, and outcomes. Gastrointest Endosc 1999; 49(2):228.

[b] 7. Bramley PN et al. The role of an open access bleeding unit in the management of colonic haemorrhage: a 2-year prospective study. Scand J Gastroenterol 1996; 31(8):764.

[b] 8. Richter JM et al. Effectiveness of current technology in the diagnosis and management of lower gastrointestinal hemorrhage. Gastrointest Endosc 1995; 41(2):93.

[b] 9. Schiller KFR, Truelove SC, Williams DG. Hematemesis and melena with special reference to factors influencing the outcome. Br Med J 1970; 2(700):7.

[b] 10. Foutch PG. Diverticular bleeding: are nonsteroidal anti-inflammatory drugs risk factors for hemorrhage and can colonoscopy predict outcome for patients? Am J Gastroenterol 1995; 90(10):1779.

[a] 11. Cheung PS et al. Frank rectal bleeding: a prospective study of causes in patients over the age of 40. Postgrad Med J 1988; 64(751):364.

[c] 12. Vernava AM et al. Lower gastrointestinal bleeding. Dis Colon Rectum 1997; 40(7):846.

[b] 13. Luk GD, Bynum TE, Hendrix TR. Gastric aspiration in localization of gastrointestinal hemorrhage. JAMA 1979; 241(6):576.

30

LOWER GASTROINTESTINAL BLEED

[b] 14. Rockall TA et al. Risk assessment after acute upper gastrointestinal haemorrhage. Gut 1996; 38(3):316.

[b] 15. Chalasani N, Clark WS, Wilcox CM. Blood urea nitrogen to creatinine concentration in gastrointestinal bleeding: a reappraisal. Am J Gastroenterol 1997; 92(10):1796.

[c] 16. Zuckerman GR, Prakash C. Acute lower intestinal bleeding. I. Clinical presentation and diagnosis. Gastrointest Endosc 1998; 48(6):606.

[b] 17. Egglin TKP et al. Complications of peripheral arteriography: a new system to identify patients at increased risk. J Vasc Surg 1995; 22(6):787.

[d] 18. Gostout CJ. The role of endoscopy in managing acute lower gastrointestinal bleeding. N Engl J Med 2000; 342(2):125.

[b] 19. Jensen DM. Urgent colonoscopy for the diagnosis and treatment of severe diverticular hemorrhage. N Engl J Med 2000; 342(2):78.

Upper Gastrointestinal Bleed

Jean S. Wang, MD, and David M. Cromwell, MD

FAST FACTS

- Upper gastrointestinal (GI) hemorrhage is defined by bleeding proximal to the ligament of Treitz.
- Clinical presentation usually involves hematemesis and melena.
- The most common causes are peptic ulcers, gastric erosions, and varices.
- With most forms of upper GI hemorrhage, bleeding stops spontaneously in 80% to 90% of cases.
- Overall, upper GI bleeding from all causes leads to death in 6% to 10% of patients. However, an acute variceal bleeding episode is associated with a 30% to 50% mortality rate.[1,2]

I. EPIDEMIOLOGY

1. Upper GI bleeding results in approximately 300,000 hospital admissions or 150 cases per 100,000 population annually in the United States.[3] Mortality from upper GI bleeding is 6% to 10%.[4-6] Table 31-1 lists the most common causes of acute upper GI hemorrhage.[4,5,7,8]

II. CLINICAL PRESENTATION

1. The presence of acute upper GI hemorrhage is suggested by hematemesis (vomiting of bloody or coffee grounds material), which is seen in 56% of patients.[4]
2. Distinguishing between upper and lower GI bleeding based on stool color can be difficult.
   a. Melena (black, tarry stools): As little as 50 to 100 mL of blood deposited into the gastric lumen for at least 14 hours can cause melena,[9] which occurs in 70% of patients with upper GI bleeding but may also be seen with proximal lower GI bleeding.
   b. Hematochezia (bright red blood per rectum): Hematochezia can be seen with massive upper GI bleeding if 1000 mL or more of blood is deposited into the gastric lumen.[10] This more commonly signifies a lower GI source of bleeding, particularly in severe upper GI bleeding episodes.
3. Syncope (14%) or presyncope (43%) may be part of the history, particularly in severe upper GI bleeding episodes.[4]

III. DIAGNOSTICS

1. Nasogastric aspirate and lavage.
   a. When upper GI bleeding is strongly suspected, a nasogastric tube

TABLE 31-1	
CAUSES OF ACUTE UPPER GASTROINTESTINAL HEMORRHAGE[4,5,7,8]	
Diagnosis	Incidence (%)
MOST COMMON CAUSES	
Peptic ulcer disease (stomach or duodenum)	47-79
Gastric erosions	6-30
Esophageal varices	8-16
No diagnosis determined	8-22
OTHER CAUSES	
Esophagitis	
Erosive duodenitis	
Mallory-Weiss tear	
Neoplasm	
Esophageal ulcer	
Stomal ulcer	
Osler-Weber-Rendu telangiectasia	

should be placed and lavage should be performed with 500 mL tap water. Nasogastric lavage that reveals bright red blood confirms the diagnosis of active upper GI bleeding.[11] If nasogastric lavage produces only coffee grounds material, this probably represents old blood from recent upper GI bleeding (which may no longer be actively bleeding).

b. If nasogastric lavage reveals large amounts of fresh blood, gastric lavage with tap water should be continued in an attempt to clear the stomach contents before upper endoscopy. Endotracheal intubation should be considered for airway protection during endoscopy.

c. A negative lavage finding does not exclude the diagnosis of upper GI bleeding, since the bleeding may have stopped or may be occurring at a site beyond the gastric pylorus.[5] Nasogastric lavage that is clear and has a bilious appearance is more reassuring for the exclusion of upper GI bleeding because the presence of bilious fluid implies that the lavage includes evaluation for bleeding beyond the pylorus.

2. **Laboratory studies.**

a. Hemoglobin level and hematocrit: Initially the hemoglobin level and hematocrit may not accurately reflect blood loss because the body requires 24 to 72 hours to equilibrate intravascular volume (see Fig. 30-1).[12]

b. Coagulation studies (prothrombin time, partial thromboplastin time).

c. Platelet count.

d. Blood urea nitrogen (BUN) and creatinine levels: Elevated BUN with a normal creatinine level, especially with a ratio greater than 35 in patients without renal failure, suggests upper GI bleeding. This finding is caused by volume depletion and absorbed blood proteins.[13,14]

e. Blood typing and screening in preparation for transfusion.

3. **Diagnostic studies.**

a. Endoscopy: Patients should be given nothing by mouth (NPO), and once they are hemodynamically stable, upper endoscopy (esophagogastroduodenoscopy) should be performed to localize the site of bleeding and allow possible therapeutic intervention.

b. Tagged red blood cell scan: This alternative test may be helpful in localizing the site of bleeding in patients with brisk bleeding (>0.1 mL/min) if endoscopy is not available, although its utility and accuracy are controversial.[15,16]

c. Selective mesenteric arteriography: This is another alternative to endoscopy. It is reported to be approximately 75% sensitive but again is helpful only in the setting of brisk bleeding (arterial blood loss of 0.5-0.6 mL/min).

d. Chest x-ray examination: This should be performed in patients with significant hematemesis or altered mental status to rule out aspiration.

e. Barium contrast studies: These should not be performed because they may interfere with subsequent endoscopy, angiography, or surgery.

IV. MANAGMENT

1. **Hemodynamic stabilization.**

a. All patients with GI bleeding should have two large-bore (18-gauge or larger) peripheral IV lines or a central venous line at all times for immediate IV access in case of sudden GI hemorrhage.

b. Hemodynamic status should be assessed, and resuscitation with blood products or intravenous fluids should be the first priority.

c. Elective endotracheal intubation should be considered to reduce the risk of aspiration in patients with massive bleeding, altered mental status, or severe agitation.

2. **Supportive transfusions.**

a. Transfusion with packed red blood cells is performed to keep the hematocrit greater than 25% (>30% if the patient has a history of coronary artery disease or advanced renal disease).

b. If coagulopathy is present, transfusion with fresh frozen plasma and administration of vitamin K to keep the international normalized ratio below 1.5.

c. If thrombocytopenia is present, transfusion with platelets is performed to keep the platelet count above $50,000/mm^3$.

d. Calcium levels should be monitored after multiple transfusions because calcium-citrate chelation may cause hypocalcemia.

3. **Management of specific conditions.**

a. Ulcers.

   (1) Endoscopic appearance of ulcers has been correlated with the risk of rebleeding and mortality (Table 31-2).

   (2) Clean-based ulcers: These carry little risk for recurrent bleeding, so the patient may resume eating and be discharged from the hospital once he or she is adequately resuscitated.[17]

   (3) Flat spots or adherent clots: Observation in the hospital on a general medical floor for 2 to 3 days is needed to ensure that rebleeding does not occur.

TABLE 31-2

ASSOCIATION BETWEEN ENDOSCOPIC APPEARANCE OF ULCERS AND RISK OF REBLEEDING AND MORTALITY

Endoscopic Characteristic	Prevalence (%)	Further Bleeding (%)	Underwent Surgery (%)	Mortality (%)
Clean base	42	5	0.5	2
Flat spot	20	10	6	3
Adherent clot	17	22	10	7
Nonbleeding visible vessel	17	43	34	11
Active bleeding	18	55	35	11

Data from Laine L, Peterson WL. N Engl J Med 1994; 331:717.

(4) Visible vessels or actively bleeding ulcers: These are associated with the highest risk for rebleeding and should be monitored in the intensive care unit for at least the first day. After 3 days of stability, discharge can be considered, since most episodes of rebleeding occur within 3 days of the initial episode. Although feeding does not influence the rate of rebleeding, patients should be kept NPO or given only clear liquids for the first 2 days in case they require urgent endoscopy for recurrent bleeding.[18]

(5) Follow-up endoscopy on an outpatient basis should be performed in patients found to have a gastric ulcer to ensure healing and exclude an underlying malignancy. Repeat endoscopy is unnecessary in patients with only duodenal ulcers.

b. Prevention of recurrent bleeding.

(1) Control of gastric acidity can promote healing and prevent recurrent bleeding in high-risk patients.

(2) Oral H_2 receptor antagonists such as ranitidine[19] and proton pump inhibitors such as omeprazole[20] have been found to be equally effective.[21]

(3) For patients with severe bleeding an intravenous proton pump inhibitor may be considered. Omeprazole, given as an IV bolus of 80 mg followed by a continuous infusion of 8 mg/hr for 72 hours, has been shown to reduce recurrent bleeding after endoscopic management of bleeding ulcers.[22] Pantoprazole is another proton pump inhibitor available in intravenous formulation.

(4) The two primary risk factors for ulcers are *Helicobacter pylori* infection and use of nonsteroidal antiinflammatory drugs (NSAIDs). Therefore, when endoscopic biopsy reveals *H. pylori,* the patient should be treated for eradication of the organism. All NSAIDs (including aspirin) should be avoided.[23]

c. Management of recurrent bleeding from ulcers.

(1) Patients with recurrent bleeding after initial endoscopic control should undergo a second attempt at endoscopic retreatment.[24]

(2) Surgery should be performed if bleeding persists after two

therapeutic endoscopies or if the patient remains hemodynamically unstable despite aggressive resuscitation.

(3) If surgery is not an option because of other serious comorbidities, angiographic therapy such as arterial embolization can be considered if interventional radiologists experienced in the technique are available.[25]

7. Esophageal varices.

a. In a patient with known cirrhosis and portal hypertension, the most likely source of bleeding is esophagogastric varices. Intravenous octreotide (a long-acting analog of somatostatin) should be started once the patient is hemodynamically stable. It is generally administered as an initial 50-μg bolus followed by 50 μg/hr continuous infusion for 5 days. A combination of octreotide and endoscopic therapy appears to be more effective than either modality alone.[26,27] Esophagogastroduodenoscopy can offer therapeutic interventions such as sclerotherapy and band ligation. If these techniques do not stop bleeding, balloon tamponade (e.g., with a Sengstaken-Blakemore or Minnesota tube) should be instituted and transjugular intrahepatic portosystemic shunt (TIPS) should be attempted to decrease portal pressure,[28] since this procedure has significantly lower mortality rates than does surgery.[29]

b. Once the patient has stopped actively bleeding, combination medical treatment with a nonselective β-blocker (e.g., nadolol or propranolol) plus isosorbide mononitrate has been found to be more effective than recurrent endoscopic therapy as prophylaxis against rebleeding.[30] The β-blocker should be started first and titrated to a goal heart rate of 55 to 60 beats/min. The isosorbide mononitrate can then be added and titrated upward as tolerated on the basis of blood pressure to achieve a goal systolic blood pressure of 95 to 105 mm Hg. Patients with recurrent variceal bleeding should consider TIPS, which has been found to be more effective than recurrent endoscopic therapy in prophylaxis against rebleeding, although no difference in overall mortality between the two therapies has been found.[31,32]

c. Bleeding from varices stops spontaneously in about 50% of patients, but without intervention the rebleeding rate is 60% to 70%. If variceal bleeding is continuous, the mortality rate is high (70%-80%). The incidence of rebleeding is highest in the first 3 days after the initial episode and decreases thereafter.

PEARLS AND PITFALLS

- In patients with a history of coronary artery disease, special care should be taken to assess the patient for myocardial ischemia in the setting of upper GI bleeding. However, recent history of myocardial infarction does not preclude endoscopy unless the patient is hypotensive or very ill (APACHE-II score ≥16; see Table 26-1).[33]
- Indications for intensive care unit monitoring.
  - Hemodynamic instability.
    - Orthostasis (definition varies): In general, when the patient changes

position from supine to standing, if after 2 minutes the pulse rate increases by more than 20 beats/min, the systolic blood pressure drops more than 20 mm Hg, and diastolic blood pressure drops more than 10 mm Hg, orthostasis is present. This indicates at least a 20% loss of intravascular volume and is associated with an increased mortality rate of 13% compared to 9% when no orthostasis is present.[4]

- Shock: If supine blood pressure is less than 100 mm Hg and pulse is greater than 100 beats/min, shock is probably present. This indicates at least a 40% loss of intravascular volume and is associated with mortality rates up to 30%.[4]
- Active bleeding.
  - Ongoing hematemesis or hematochezia.
  - Nasogastric lavage with bright red blood that does not clear after a 500-ml lavage.
- Predictors of adverse outcome (defined as death, the need for any operation, recurrent hematemesis, recurrent melena after initial clearing, or a falling hematocrit value despite transfusion) at initial evaluation include the following.[34]
  - Initial hematocrit less than 30%.
  - Initial systolic blood pressure less than 100 mm Hg.
  - Red blood in the nasogastric lavage.
  - Evidence of portal hypertension (e.g., history of cirrhosis or ascites on examination).
  - Hematemesis.
- Predictors of mortality.[4]
  - Age greater than 60 years: Mortality rate 12% to 25% (compared with <10% for age <60 years).
  - Serious comorbidities (cardiac, central nervous system, GI, hepatic, neoplastic, pulmonary, renal, physiological stress): As the number of comorbidities increased from none to six, mortality rates increased dramatically from 3% to 7%, 10%, 15%, 27%, 44%, and 67%, respectively.
- Theoretical concern has been raised regarding the safety of inserting a nasogastric tube in patients with known esophageal varices. Our experience indicates that this is safe but should be avoided in patients with varices that were recently banded.

REFERENCES

[b] 1. Graham DY, Smith JL. The course of patients after variceal hemorrhage. Gastroenterology 1981; 80:800.

[b] 2. Thomsen BL, Moller S, Sorensen TIA. Copenhagen Esophageal Varices Sclerotherapy Project: optimized analysis of recurrent bleeding and death in patients with cirrhosis and esophageal varices. J Hepatol 1994; 21:367.

[b] 3. Cutler JA, Mendeloff AI. Upper gastrointestinal bleeding: nature and magnitude of the problem in the U.S. Dig Dis Sci 1981; 26(suppl):90S.

[b] 4. Silverstein FE et al. The national ASGE survey on upper gastrointestinal bleeding. II. Clinical prognostic factors. Gastrointest Endosc 1981; 27:80.

[b] 5. Gilbert DA et al. The national ASGE survey on upper gastrointestinal bleeding. III. Endoscopy in upper gastrointestinal bleeding. Gastrointest Endosc 1981; 27:94.

[b] 6. Yavorski RT et al. Analysis of 3,294 cases of upper gastrointestinal bleeding in military medical facilities. Am J Gastroenterol 1995; 90:568.

[b] 7. Vreeburg EM et al. Acute upper gastrointestinal bleeding in the Amsterdam area: incidence, diagnosis, and clinical outcome. Am J Gastroenterol 1997; 92:236.

[b] 8. Longstreth GF, Feitelberg SP. Hospital care of acute nonvariceal upper gastrointestinal bleeding: 1991 and 1981. J Clin Gastroenterol 1994; 19:189.

[b] 9. Daniel WA Jr, Egan S. The quantity of blood required to produce a tarry stool. JAMA 1939; 113:2232.

[b] 10. Schiff L et al. Observations on the oral administration of citrated blood in man. II. The effect on the stools. Am J Med Sci 1942; 203:409.

[b] 11. Luk GD, Bynum TE, Hendrix TR. Gastric aspiration in localization of gastrointestinal hemorrhage. JAMA 1979; 241:576.

[b] 12. Ebert RV, Stead EA, Gibson JG. Response of normal subjects to acute blood loss. Arch Intern Med 1941; 68:687.

[b] 13. Richards RJ, Donica MB, Grayer D. Can the blood urea nitrogen/creatinine ratio distinguish upper from lower gastrointestinal bleeding? J Clin Gastroenterol 1990; 12:500.

[b] 14. Chalasani N, Clark WS, Wilcox CM. Blood urea nitrogen-to-creatinine concentration in gastrointestinal bleeding: a reappraisal. Am J Gastroenterol 1997; 92:1796.

[b] 15. Emslie JT et al. Technetium-99m-labeled red blood cell scans in the investigation of gastrointestinal bleeding. Dis Colon Rectum 1996; 39:750.

[b] 16. Garofalo TE, Abdu RA. Accuracy and efficacy of nuclear scintigraphy for the detection of gastrointestinal bleeding. Arch Surg 1997; 132:196.

[c] 17. Laine L, Peterson WL. Medical progress: bleeding peptic ulcer. N Engl J Med 1994; 331:717.

[a] 18. Laine L et al. Prospective evaluation of immediate versus delayed refeeding and prognostic value of endoscopy in patients with upper gastrointestinal hemorrhage. Gastroenterology 1992; 102:314.

[a] 19. Jensen DM et al. A controlled study of ranitidine for the prevention of recurrent hemorrhage from duodenal ulcer. N Engl J Med 1994; 330:382.

[a] 20. Khuroo MS et al. A comparison of omeprazole and placebo for bleeding peptic ulcer. N Engl J Med 1997; 336:1054.

[a] 21. Villanueva C et al. Omeprazole versus ranitidine as adjunct therapy to endoscopic injection in actively bleeding ulcers: a prospective and randomized study. Endoscopy 1995; 27:308.

[a] 22. Lau JY et al. Effect of intravenous omeprazole on recurrent bleeding after endoscopic treatment of bleeding peptic ulcers. N Engl J Med 2000; 343:310.

[b] 23. Somerville K, Faulkner G, Langman M. Non-steroidal anti-inflammatory drugs and bleeding peptic ulcer. Lancet 1986; 1:462.

[a] 24. Lau JYW et al. Endoscopic retreatment compared with surgery in patients with recurrent bleeding after initial endoscopic control of bleeding ulcers. N Engl J Med 1999; 340:751.

[b] 25. Lieberman DA et al. Arterial embolization for massive upper gastrointestinal tract bleeding in poor surgical candidates. Gastroenterology 1984; 86(5 Pt 1):876.

[a] 26. Besson I et al. Sclerotherapy with or without octreotide for acute variceal bleeding. N Engl J Med 1995; 333:555.

[a] 27. Avgerinos A et al. Early administration of somatostatin and efficacy of sclerotherapy in active oesophageal variceal bleeds: the European Acute Bleeding Oesophageal Variceal Episodes (ABOVE) randomised trial. Lancet 1997; 350:1495.

[b] 28. Rossle M et al. The transjugular intrahepatic portosystemic stent-shunt procedure for variceal bleeding. N Engl J Med 1994; 330:165.

[b] 29. Jalan R et al. A comparative study of emergency TIPSS and esophageal transection in the management of uncontrolled variceal hemorrhage. Am J Gastroenterol 1995; 90:1932.

[a] 30. Villanueva C et al. Nadolol plus isosorbide mononitrate compared with sclerotherapy for the prevention of variceal rebleeding. N Engl J Med 1996; 334:1624.

31

UPPER GASTROINTESTINAL BLEED

[a] 31. Cabrera J et al. Transjugular intrahepatic portosystemic shunt versus sclerotherapy in the elective treatment of variceal hemorrhage. Gastroenterology 1996; 110:832.

[a] 32. Rossle M et al. Randomised trial of transjugular-intrahepatic-portosystemic shunt versus endoscopy plus propranolol for prevention of variceal rebleeding. Lancet 1997; 349:1043.

[b] 33. Cappell MS, Iacovone FM Jr. Safety and efficacy of esophagogastroduodenoscopy after myocardial infarction. Am J Med 1999; 106:29.

[b] 34. Corley DA et al. Early indicators of prognosis in upper gastrointestinal hemorrhage. Am J Gastroenterol 1998; 93:336.

Anemia

Hetty Carraway, MD, and Michael Streiff, MD

FAST FACTS

- The most common cause of anemia in women in the United States is iron deficiency anemia.
- Criteria for anemia are a hematocrit value below 37% in women and below 40% in men or a hemoglobin level below 12 g/dL in women and below 14 g/dL in men.
- Blood transfusion is associated with a lower short-term mortality rate among elderly patients with acute myocardial infarction if the hematocrit value on admission is 30% or lower. The goal for any patient with coronary artery disease is to keep the hematocrit value above 30%.[1]
- Patients with sickle cell anemia have a "usual baseline." They do not need transfusions to raise the hematocrit to "normal" values.
- Analysis of the peripheral blood smear will help with the diagnosis of thalassemia, hemoglobinopathy, and sideroblastic anemia.
- Classic patterns (Fig. 32-1).
  - Iron deficiency: Low serum iron level, high total iron binding capacity (TIBC), low transferrin percent saturation, low ferritin level, low reticulocyte count.
  - Anemia of chronic disease (ACD): Low-normal serum iron level, low-normal TIBC, low-normal transferrin percent saturation, normal to high ferritin level, low reticulocyte count.
  - Sideroblastic anemia: High total body iron level, high transferrin saturation, high ferritin level, increased serum iron level.

I. EPIDEMIOLOGY

1. Iron deficiency anemia is the most common anemia in the United States. Iron deficiency anemia affects 10% of premenopausal women, 25% of pregnant women, 5% of children, and 2.5% to 5% of men and menopausal women. Children, pregnant women, and the elderly are the most commonly affected by anemia.
2. All patients with anemia deserve to have an evaluation, and data show that after evaluation, 40% of elderly patients with anemia will have a change in therapy. African-Americans, immigrants, and the socioeconomically deprived are also at risk.

II. CLINICAL PRESENTATION

1. History and physical examination.
a. Patients often have presenting symptoms of fatigue or low energy. An adequate history is vital, and this should include evaluation of energy level, cold intolerance, history of substance abuse (including alcohol

ingestion, type of diet, medications, and vitamins), pica, neurological complaints (which may occur with vitamin B_{12} or iron deficiency), family history of anemia or hemoglobinopathies, gastrointestinal bleeding, menorrhagia, or kidney problems. Allergies or medications can precipitate hemolysis, especially in patients with glucose-6-phosphate dehydrogenase (G6PD) deficiency or hemolytic anemia.

b. Physical examination should include assessment of pallor, skin creases, nails (spoon nails are consistent with iron deficiency), angular stomatitis (iron deficiency), glossitis (iron deficiency and megaloblastic anemia), orthostatic hypotension (acute bleeding), jaundice (hemolytic anemia, liver disease), bruising (leukemia, myelodysplastic syndrome), telangiectasias, and splenomegaly.

III. DIAGNOSTICS (Fig. 32-1)

1. The American Task Force Guidelines recommend that all infants and pregnant women be screened for anemia. Routine screening of other persons is not recommended unless they are symptomatic. Hemoglobin analysis should be performed at the first prenatal visit in all pregnant African-American women.

2. All patients with anemia should have a complete blood cell count with differential, basic metabolic panel (to evaluate renal function), reticulocyte count, peripheral blood smear, and screening stool for occult blood. After results of these tests are available, the anemia can be classified as belonging to one of four categories (hemolytic, macrocytic, normocytic, or microcytic) and can be approached with additional specific tests.

3. A peripheral blood smear is useful as long as the patient has not received a blood transfusion recently. The peripheral blood smear is a thin smear processed with Wright's stain. It is helpful in distinguishing the type of anemia based on the size, shape, and color of the red blood cells. For example, patients with iron deficiency have abnormally shaped red blood cells (poikilocytosis), small red blood cells (microcytosis), increased red blood cell distribution width (RDW) (anisocytosis), and lack of pigmentation (hypochromia). In megaloblastic anemia, macroovalocytes, hypersegmented neutrophils, and Howell-Jolly bodies are seen. A peripheral blood smear from a patient with anemia of chronic disease would be expected to have normal or microcytic red blood cells. In patients with liver disease, thin macrocytes, target cells, and acanthocytes (spur cells) may be present.

4. The red blood cell shape is frequently the most helpful clue in the differential diagnosis of hemolytic disorders. Diagnostic findings include fragmentation of red blood cells from traumatic hemolysis on artificial heart valves, spherocytosis as a marker of hereditary spherocytosis, sickle cells and oakleaf cells of sickle cell disease, target cells in thalassemia, and blister forms in G6PD deficiency.

Examination of the peripheral blood smear is a simple and inexpensive undertaking that often provides critical clues to the etiology of anemia. This tool should not be ignored.

5. The mean corpuscular volume (MCV) is a direct measure of the average size of the red blood cell. Normal value of MCV ranges from 80 to 100 fL. The characterization of anemia according to the size of the erythrocytes is an efficient and organized approach to diagnosing causative factors in anemia. Microcytic anemia (MCV <80 fL), macrocytic anemia (MCV >100 fL), and normocytic anemia (MCV 80-100 fL) are discussed in detail below.

6. A reduced mean corpuscular hemoglobin concentration (MCHC) often points to a diagnosis of iron deficiency, thalassemia, or sideroblastic anemia.

7. The RDW reveals the variation of red cell volumes. A high RDW suggests possible iron, vitamin B_{12}, or folate deficiency.

8. The reticulocyte count is determined after a blood film is stained for reticulin (the remains of the cellular RNA). Early reticulocytes are bigger than mature red cells, so a high reticulocyte count elevates the MCV. Reticulocyte count is usually expressed as a percentage of cells examined in an individual patient. This number must be corrected for the presence of anemia because the initial count, expressed as a percentage of RBCs present, is spuriously elevated when it is related to a reduced anemic RBC pool. The corrected reticulocyte count, or reticulocyte index, is equal to the patient's hematocrit (Hct) divided by 45 and multiplied by the percentage of reticulocytes.

$$\text{Reticulocyte index} = \% \text{ Reticulocytes} \times \frac{\text{Patient's Hct}}{45}$$

A reticulocyte index of less than 1 is consistent with inadequate RBC production in the setting of anemia. A reticulocyte index of greater than 2 is consistent with adequate RBC production and points to ongoing RBC loss from either bleeding or hemolysis. A reticloctye index between 1 and 2 is indeterminate.

9. Ferritin is the major iron storage protein. The ferritin assay is the most sensitive and specific laboratory test for the assessment of iron stores. A low ferritin level (<12 ng/mL in females and <30 ng/mL in males) is evidence of iron deficiency. Ferritin is also an acute-phase reactant. Elevated levels of ferritin can be seen in acute illness, inflammation, and infection, even in the presence of iron deficiency. However, high ferritin levels make iron deficiency unlikely.

10. The measurement of serum iron is affected by many variables, including free hemoglobin, inflammation, infection, and iron ingestion. Often a low serum iron level is helpful in the diagnosis of anemia of chronic disease. Logically, low levels of serum iron are also seen in iron deficiency anemia.

11. TIBC is a laboratory measurement of the ability of serum iron to bind.

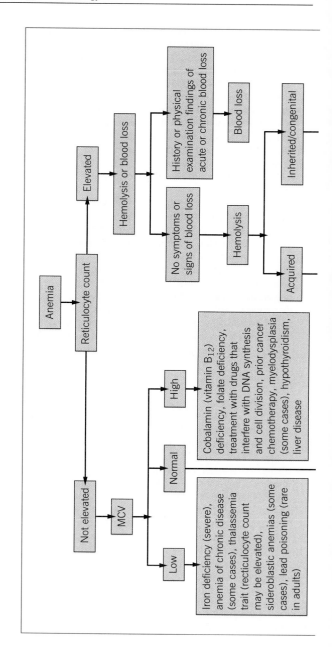

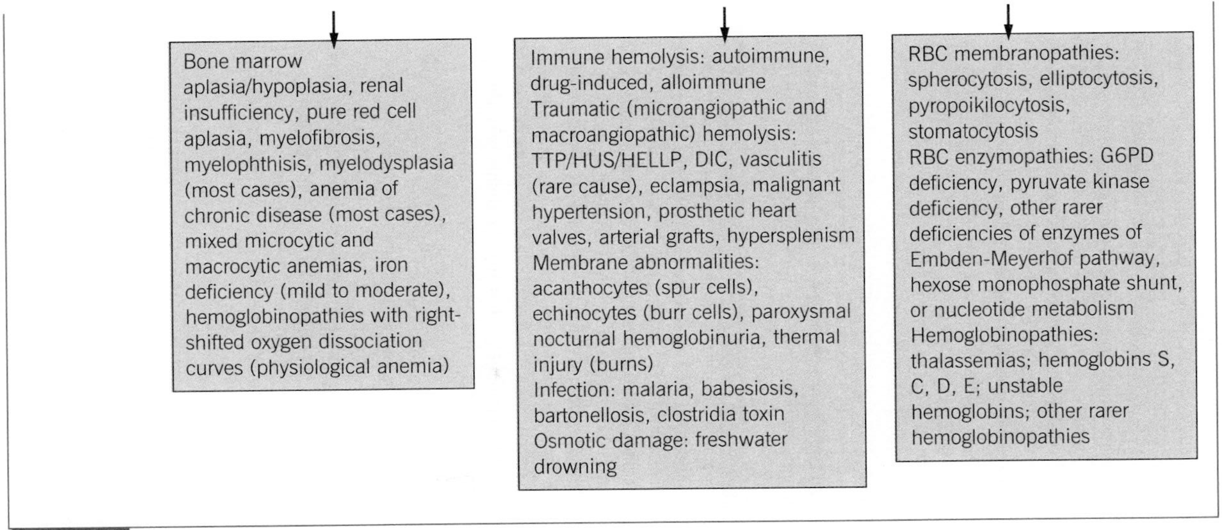

32

ANEMIA

FIG. 32-1

Diagnosis of anemias. *DIC,* Disseminated intravascular coagulation; *HELLP,* hepatomegaly, elevated liver (function tests), low platelets; *HUS,* hemolytic-uremic syndrome; *TTP,* thrombotic thrombocytopenic purpura. *(Data from Goldman L, Bennett JC. Cecil textbook of medicine, 21st ed. Philadelphia: WB Saunders; 2000.)*

Bone marrow aplasia/hypoplasia, renal insufficiency, pure red cell aplasia, myelofibrosis, myelophthisis, myelodysplasia (most cases), anemia of chronic disease (most cases), mixed microcytic and macrocytic anemias, iron deficiency (mild to moderate), hemoglobinopathies with right-shifted oxygen dissociation curves (physiological anemia)

Immune hemolysis: autoimmune, drug-induced, alloimmune Traumatic (microangiopathic and macroangiopathic) hemolysis: TTP/HUS/HELLP, DIC, vasculitis (rare cause), eclampsia, malignant hypertension, prosthetic heart valves, arterial grafts, hypersplenism Membrane abnormalities: acanthocytes (spur cells), echinocytes (burr cells), paroxysmal nocturnal hemoglobinuria, thermal injury (burns) Infection: malaria, babesiosis, bartonellosis, clostridia toxin Osmotic damage: freshwater drowning

RBC membranopathies: spherocytosis, elliptocytosis, pyropoikilocytosis, stomatocytosis RBC enzymopathies: G6PD deficiency, pyruvate kinase deficiency, other rarer deficiencies of enzymes of Embden-Meyerhof pathway, hexose monophosphate shunt, or nucleotide metabolism Hemoglobinopathies: thalassemias; hemoglobins S, C, D, E; unstable hemoglobins; other rarer hemoglobinopathies

TIBC is affected largely by transferrin, a β-globulin that regulates absorption and transport of iron. TIBC is typically low in anemia of chronic disease and elevated in iron deficiency anemia.

12. Transferrin saturation is equal to the serum iron divided by the TIBC. A transferrin saturation of less than 10% suggests iron deficiency. This is not specific, however, since up to 30% of patients with a low saturation are not iron deficient. Transferrin is also an acute-phase reactant like ferritin, so illness, medication, and nutritional status affect TIBC. A falsely elevated TIBC falsely lowers the transferrin saturation. In addition, a low TIBC and a low serum iron level (both seen in anemia of chronic disease) result in a normal transferrin saturation. As might be expected, normal transferrin saturation is frequently seen in anemia of chronic disease.

13. A bone marrow aspirate stained for hemosiderin is the gold standard test for diagnosis of iron deficiency anemia, but this test is not always performed because it is painful and expensive and because sampling errors are associated with the procedure.

IV. MANAGEMENT[2]

1. The role of transfusion in anemia is somewhat unclear. Transfusions are often used in the acute setting of blood loss and are also used to improve the clinical condition of patients who have been admitted to the hospital, especially if they are critically ill. The evidence to support such therapy is not strong, but the perceived potential loss if treatment is withheld is often what drives therapy. A randomized controlled clinical trial was performed to evaluate the benefits of blood transfusion for critically ill patients. This study concluded that transfusions provided no benefit to critically ill patients with the possible exception of patients with unstable angina and acute myocardial infarction.[3]

2. In the United States, erythropoietin therapy has been approved by the Food and Drug Administration for patients with select medical conditions,[4] including those with chronic renal failure (1989-1990), those with HIV infection receiving zidovudine therapy (1990), patients with cancer (1993), and patients undergoing surgery (1996). In one study erythropoietin was most beneficial for surgical patients whose initial hematocrit value was 33% to 39% and whose anticipated blood losses were 1 to 3 L.

3. Iron deficiency anemia.[5-7]

a. Diagnosis of iron deficiency anemia is made when a patient has a low hematocrit value along with microcytic anemia (MCV <80 fL) and a low ferritin level (<12 ng/mL in women and <30 ng/mL in men). Iron saturation is less than 15%. A bone marrow examination is almost never indicated, since a trial of iron therapy usually establishes the diagnosis with less discomfort and expense to the patient. Iron deficiency anemia results from any condition in which the dietary iron intake does not meet the body's demands.

b. The average adult has 2 to 5 g of iron (1 g in storage form). Blood loss is the only way to excrete iron. The total iron cost in pregnancy is 1 g, including the estimated blood loss at delivery. Pregnant women are placed on a folate and iron regimen. The average loss of blood with each menstrual cycle in women is 22 mg. Menstruating young women with microcytic anemia can be treated presumptively with iron if they will be available for follow-up to determine their response. A careful family history should be obtained to identify cases of thalassemia. Most patients with iron deficiency anemia, however, should be assumed to have a gastrointestinal blood loss. Testing these patients for fecal occult blood is essential.

c. Iron is absorbed in the duodenum. Treatment for iron deficiency anemia is ferrous sulfate 325 mg (60 mg elemental iron) PO tid with meals for 6 to 12 months. This equates to an elemental iron treatment dose of 180 to 200 mg/day. Scratching the tablet or having patients take it with an acidic beverage is thought to increase gastrointestinal absorption. Leading causes of treatment failure are poor compliance (because of nausea and constipation from iron) and poor absorption (caused by concomitant antacid use). The reticulocyte count increases in 1 week and peaks at 10 days after iron therapy has begun. Hemoglobin levels should normalize in about 2 months. If iron therapy fails, gastrointestinal malabsorption (e.g., sprue) should be considered as a possible etiology of anemia. If oral iron therapy is unsuccessful, IV or IM iron replacement can be considered.

4. **Anemia of chronic disease.**[8,9]

a. Diagnosis of anemia of chronic disease is made when a patient has a low hematocrit value along with microcytic or normocytic anemia and a normal or high ferritin level. Transferrin and iron saturation are normal with a low TIBC. Bone marrow biopsy is not usually indicated, but if one is performed, the results are normal. Anemia of chronic disease is a diagnosis of exclusion; drug toxicity and chronic blood loss should be excluded before a final diagnosis of anemia of chronic disease is established.

b. Anemia of chronic disease has a slow onset with minimal symptoms. The pathophysiology is not well understood, but this condition probably evolved as a cytokine-mediated defense against microbial pathogens. The result is that iron is withheld from microbes as well as from erythroid precursors. Ultimately, RBC survival is shortened and marrow compensatory response is impaired because of disturbed iron metabolism and impaired erythropoietin production.

c. Anemia of chronic disease improves only when the underlying disorder has been identified and treated and the hematocrit value has increased.

5. **Megaloblastic anemia.**[10,11]

32

ANEMIA

a. Macrocytic anemia (MCV >100 fL) can be divided into two major groups, the megaloblastic anemias and nonmegaloblastic anemias. The presence of hypersegmented neutrophils and large platelets on peripheral blood smear leads to the diagnosis of megaloblastic anemia. Megaloblastic anemia affects all three cell lines, and pancytopenia may be found at presentation. Normal neutrophils and platelets in the presence of an elevated MCV signify that the patient has a nonmegaloblastic anemia.

b. Nonmegaloblastic anemias usually reflect membrane cholesterol defects related to systemic abnormalities such as liver or hypothyroid disease, and patients with this disease may benefit from evaluation with liver function tests and thyroid function tests.

c. Further evaluation of megaloblastic anemia includes assays for serum vitamin B_{12} and red blood cell folate levels. Deficiency of vitamin B_{12} (usually because of impaired absorption) or folate (because of poor nutrition or increased demand) is the most common cause of this anemia. Intestinal malabsorption or defective secretion of intrinsic factor may cause vitamin B_{12} deficiency. Defective secretion of intrinsic factor can be caused by autoimmune destruction of stomach parietal cells (pernicious anemia) or by surgical removal of the parietal cells when part of the stomach is removed (gastrectomy). Patients who have small bowel disease, blind loop syndrome, or intestinal parasites may have vitamin B_{12} deficiency because of lack of absorption in the ileum. The Schilling test can distinguish these conditions: if vitamin B_{12} absorption does not become normal after administration of intrinsic factor, intestinal disease is the culprit. In vitamin B_{12} deficiency, patients may have symptoms of neurological compromise that predates the onset of anemia or macrocytosis. The daily vitamin B_{12} requirement is 2 to 5 μg. Liver stores house 2 to 5 mg, so clinical manifestations of vitamin B_{12} deficiency may take years to develop.

d. Folate deficiency may be caused by poor nutrition (alcoholism), malabsorption (jejunal disease), or increased requirements (pregnancy, dialysis, hemolytic anemia). Anticonvulsant drugs and oral contraceptives have been associated with megaloblastic anemia caused by folate deficiency.

e. Within 48 hours of parenteral vitamin B_{12} or folate administration, marrow abnormalities begin to normalize. Complete normalization occurs within 2 to 3 days. Reticulocyte count peaks in 4 to 10 days. If response is blunted, an underlying iron deficiency anemia should be suspected. Folate treatment of vitamin B_{12}–deficient patients may partially correct the anemia and marrow abnormalities but may accelerate the development of neurological abnormalities. The vitamin B_{12} dosage is 1000 μg/day for 1 to 2 weeks, then 1000 μg/week for 4 weeks, then maintenance dosage of 100 or 1000 μg/month subcutaneously for life. Folate replacement is 1 mg/day PO.

PEARLS AND PITFALLS

- For patients with chronic renal failure, anemia workup should be performed when the hematocrit value has fallen to 80% of the mean value for a healthy person (<33% in premenopausal females and prepubertal patients, <37% in adult males and postmenopausal women.) In a patient with renal disease, evaluation of anemia should include a complete blood cell count, reticulocyte count, iron parameters (serum iron level, TIBC, percent saturation, ferritin level), and testing for fecal occult blood. This evaluation should take place before initiation of erythropoietin therapy to exclude any component of anemia not caused by renal insufficiency. In addition, it is important to recognize that patients receiving erythropoietin therapy need adequate iron stores to support erythropoiesis. As renal failure worsens, likelihood of erythropoietin deficiency increases. If no cause for anemia is found other than chronic renal failure and the creatinine level is greater than 2 mg/dL, the anemia is most likely the result of renal failure and erythropoietin therapy is indicated. In patients with chronic renal failure and normochromic, normocytic anemia, the erythropoietin level is rarely elevated. Thus a determination of the serum erythropoietin level is not needed before initiation of therapy.
- HIV-infected patients.
  - Incidence of anemia is as high as 70% in patients with acquired immunodeficiency syndrome (AIDS). Often the incidence of various cytopenias correlates directly with the degree of immunosuppression. In a review of more than 32,000 patients infected with HIV, the annual incidence of anemia increased with disease progression; anemia developed in 3% of all patients with asymptomatic HIV infection, 12% of asymptomatic patients with CD4 count less than 200 cells/mm^3, and 37% of patients with AIDS-related illnesses.[12] The presence of anemia was associated with an increased morbidity and mortality in patients with HIV infection. Anemia was associated with increased risk of death when patients were stratified by CD4 counts. In addition, when anemia was treated, mortality rates decreased to the same levels as in patients who were not anemic (regardless of CD4 count).
  - Anemia in HIV-infected patients is usually a multifactorial process. Possible causes of the anemia include infections (*Mycobacterium avium, Mycobacterium tuberculosis, Histoplasma capsulatum,* cytomegalovirus, Epstein-Barr virus, parvovirus B19), malignancy (non-Hodgkin's lymphoma, Hodgkin's lymphoma, or plasma cell dyscrasias), and nutritional effects (anorexia, wasting, malabsorption, deficiency of vitamin B$_{12}$ or folate). Other causes include abnormal iron metabolism, hemolysis (antibody mediated, drug induced, or in patients with G6PD deficiency receiving inciting drugs such as Bactrim, dapsone, or primaquine), and medications (by direct marrow-toxic effects). Patients receiving zidovudine (AZT) often have bone marrow suppression or

macrocytosis.[13] Bone marrow evaluation may be helpful in determining the cause of anemia and may provide useful histological information, especially in cases of malignancy. Some evidence has indicated that bone marrow evaluation may lead to earlier diagnosis in patients with febrile illness.

- Recombinant human erythropoietin can increase the hematocrit and reduce transfusion requirements in HIV-infected patients. The findings of four prospective, randomized, double-blind, placebo-controlled clinical trials support the use of erythropoietin in the HIV population when symptomatic anemic patients have baseline serum erythropoietin levels less than 500 IU/L. In these studies 70% of patients had significant increases over baseline hematocrit and a reduction in transfusion requirements as a result of erythropoietin therapy. Erythropoietin should be given as 100 IU/kg subcutaneously three times a week.[14-16]

REFERENCES

[b] 1. Wu W-C et al. Blood transfusion in elderly patients with acute myocardial infarction. N Engl J Med 2001; 345:1230.

[c] 2. Beutler E. The common anemias. JAMA 1988; 259:2433.

[a] 3. Hebert PC et al. A multicenter, randomized, controlled clinical trial of transfusion requirements in critical care. N Engl J Med 1999; 340:409.

[b] 4. Goodnough L et al. Erythropoietin therapy. N Engl J Med 1997; 336:933.

[b] 5. Guyatt GH. Diagnosis of iron-deficiency anemia in the elderly. Am J Med 1990; 88:205.

[b] 6. Lipshitz DA et al. A clinical evaluation of serum ferritin as an index of iron stores. N Engl J Med 1974; 290:1213.

[c] 7. Brown RG. Determining the cause of anemia: general approach, with emphasis on microcytic hypochromic anemias. Postgrad Med 1991; 89:161.

[b] 8. Cash JM et al. The anemia of chronic disease: spectrum of associated diseases in a series of unselected hospitalized patients. Am J Med 1989; 87:638.

[c] 9. Andrews N. Disorders of iron metabolism. N Engl J Med 1999; 341:1986.

[b] 10. Carmel R. Pernicious anemia: the expected findings of very low serum cobalamin levels, anemia, and macrocytosis are often lacking. Arch Intern Med 1988; 148:1712.

[b] 11. Ledrele FA. Oral cobalamin for pernicious anemia: medicine's best kept secret? JAMA 1991; 265:94.

[c] 12. Zon LI, Arkin C, Groopman JE. Haematologic manifestations of the human immunodeficiency virus. Br J Haematol 1987; 66:251.

[c] 13. Sullivan PS, Hanson DL, Chu SY. Epidemiology of anemia in HIV infected persons: results from the Multistate Adult and Adolescent Spectrum of HIV Disease Surveillance Project. Blood 1998; 91:301.

[b] 14. Henry DH. Experience with epoetin alfa and acquired immunodeficiency syndrome anemia. Semin Oncol 1998; 25:64.

[b] 15. Henry DH et al. Recombinant human erythropoietin in the treatment of anemia associated with HIV infection and zidovudine therapy: overview of four clinical trials. Ann Intern Med 1992; 117:739.

[b] 16. Fischl M et al. Recombinant human erythropoietin for patients with AIDS treated with zidovudine. N Engl J Med 1990; 323:1069.

Sickle Cell Anemia

Rosalyn Juergens, MD, and Sophie Lanzkron, MD

FAST FACTS

- Vasoocclusion is the most common reason for hospital admission and is treated with aggressive hydration, parenteral pain control, and oxygen if the patient is hypoxic as well as treatment of the precipitating cause.
- Indications for transfusion and exchange transfusion include chest crisis, strokes and transient ischemic attacks (TIAs), priapism, splenic sequestration crisis, and fulminant liver vasoocclusion.
- Chronic sickling can affect every organ system.

33

I. EPIDEMIOLOGY[1]

1. One in every 400 African-Americans in the United States has sickle cell disease (SCD). Current mean survival for individuals with sickle cell anemia is 48 years for women and 42 years for men.
2. SCD is defined as hemoglobin SS disease (sickle cell anemia), hemoglobin SC disease, or sickle cell–β-thalassemia.
3. Eight percent of African-Americans are heterozygous carriers of the sickle cell trait.
4. Hemoglobin S results from a substitution of a valine for glutamic acid as the sixth amino acid of the β-globin chain.
5. Two of these abnormal β-globin chains when part of a tetramer with two α-globin chains form a polymer that is poorly soluble when deoxygenated and distorts the erythrocyte into a sickled form (Fig. 33-1).

II. CLINICAL PRESENTATION, DIAGNOSTICS, AND MANAGEMENT OF ACUTE CRISES

A. VASOOCCLUSIVE CRISIS

1. Vasoocclusive crisis is the most common reason for patients with SCD to seek medical care.
2. The frequency of attacks varies from patient to patient, but in one large study 33% of patients with SCD rarely had pain, 33% had two to six pain crises requiring hospitalization per year, and 33% had more than six pain-related crises per year.[2]
3. Increased mortality is associated with higher numbers of annual pain crises.[3]
4. Acute pain is a result of tissue ischemia caused by occlusion of capillaries by sickled erythrocytes.[1]
5. Chronic pain is the residua of destroyed bones, joints, and visceral organs from previous pain crises.
6. Acute pain crisis episodes typically last 5 to 7 days.

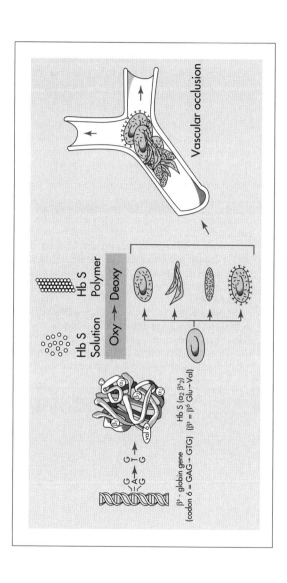

FIG. 33-1

Schematic view of the pathophysiological characteristics of sickle cell disease. The double-stranded DNA molecule on the left represents a β-globin gene in which a GAG→GTG substitution in the sixth codon has created the sickle cell gene. The product of this gene is the β^s-globin variant, in which valine is substituted for glutamic acid as the sixth amino acid. The mutant hemoglobin tetramer $\alpha_2\beta^s_2$ is HbS, which loses solubility and polymerizes when deprived of oxygen. Upon deoxygenation, most sickle cells accumulate polymer and lose deformability; some cells sickle; a fraction of cells become dehydrated, irreversibly sickled, and poorly deformable; and a few cells accrue cytoadherence molecules on their surface. Dehydrated and highly adherent cells also may be generated by polymerization-independent processes. Vasoocclusion, shown on the right, is initiated by adherent cells sticking to the vascular endothelium, thereby creating a nidus that traps rigid cells and facilitates polymerization. *(From Goldman L, Bennett JC. Cecil textbook of medicine, 21st ed. Philadelphia: WB Saunders; 1999.)*

SICKLE CELL ANEMIA

33

7. Factors that can precipitate acute pain crises include dehydration, infections, low oxygen tension, acidosis, pregnancy, alcohol, stress, and cold weather.
8. Treatment of acute crises.[4]
   a. Treatment is mainly supportive and includes aggressive hydration and adequate pain management (Table 33-1).[5,6]
   b. Patient-controlled analgesia is a way to meet the dual goals of prompt delivery of pain medication and prevention of oversedation.[5]
   c. Supplemental oxygen has been shown to have benefit only when hypoxia is present; it can cause rebound sickling if the Po_2 decreases precipitously.[7]
   d. Transfusion has not been shown to shorten the duration of acute pain crises.[5]
9. Hydroxyurea increases the production of hemoglobin F and can be used as a means of decreasing the number and severity of acute pain crises in the chronic setting (Table 33-2). The dosage is started at 500 mg PO each day and can be increased either by 500 mg every 2 weeks until the patient's white blood cell count falls to 3000/mm^3 or to a maximum of 2000 mg per day.[8] A hematology consultation should be considered when this medication is used.

B. CHEST CRISIS[9,10]
1. Chest crisis is diagnosed when patients have all of three criteria.
   a. Pulmonary infiltrates on chest radiograph.
   b. Chest pain.
   c. Fever.
2. Causes in adults include bacterial and viral infection, pulmonary fat embolism, pulmonary edema, and microvascular/macrovascular lung infarction.
3. The mainstay of treatment on presentation is analgesia (with care taken to avoid respiratory depression), cautious administration of intravenous (IV) fluids, oxygen supplementation, and empirical antibiotics while culture results are awaited.
4. If the patient has multilobar involvement in the setting of anemia, thrombocytopenia, or both; rapidly progressive disease; underlying cardiac disease; or respiratory failure, transfusion is indicated.
5. Standard transfusions can be used for patients who at presentation are more anemic than baseline measurements.
6. Exchange transfusions can be used for patients who are not significantly more anemic than baseline but who need to have their concentration of hemoglobin SS reduced (<30%).
7. Unless there is a proven diagnosis of venous thromboembolism, anticoagulation is not indicated.

C. APLASTIC CRISIS[11]
1. Aplastic crisis is caused by a transient arrest in erythropoiesis with a secondarily abrupt fall in hemoglobin concentrations.
2. Most cases are associated with parvovirus B19, but aplastic crisis has

TABLE 33-1

RECOMMENDED DOSE AND INTERVAL OF ANALGESICS NECESSARY TO OBTAIN
ADEQUATE PAIN CONTROL IN SICKLE CELL DISEASE

Analgesic	Dose or Rate	Comments
SEVERE OR MODERATE PAIN		
Morphine	Parenteral: 0.1-0.15 mg/kg q3-4h; recommended maximum single dose 10 mg PO: 0.3-0.6 mg/kg q4h	Drug of choice for pain; lower doses in the elderly and in patients with liver failure or impaired ventilation
Meperidine	Parenteral: 0-75-1.5 mg/kg q2-4h; recommended maximum dose 100 mg PO: 1.5 mg/kg q4h	Increased incidence of seizures; avoid use in patients with renal or neurological disease or those who receive monoamine oxidase inhibitors
Hydromorphone	Parenteral: 0.01-0.02 mg/kg q3-4h	
Oxycodone	PO: 0.04-0.06 mg/kg q4h PO: 0.15 mg/kg/dose q4h	
Ketorolac	Intramuscular: adults: 30 or 60 mg initial dose, followed by 15-30 mg; children: 1 mg/kg load, followed by 0.5 mg/kg q6h	Equal efficacy to 6 mg morphine sulfate; helps narcotic-sparing effect; not to exceed 5 days; maximum 150 mg first day, 120 mg subsequent days; may cause gastric irritation
Butorphanol	Parenteral: adults: 2 mg q3-4h	Agonist-antagonist; can precipitate withdrawal if given to patients who are being treated with agonists
MILD PAIN		
Codeine	PO: 0.5-1 mg/kg q4h; maximum dose 60 mg	Mild to moderate pain not relieved by aspirin or acetaminophen; can cause nausea and vomiting
Aspirin	PO: adults: 0.3-6 mg q4-6h; children: 10 mg/kg q4h	Often given with a narcotic to enhance analgesia; can cause gastric irritation; avoid use in febrile children
Acetaminophen	PO: adults: 0.3-0.6 mg q4h; children: 10 mg/kg	Often given with a narcotic to enhance analgesia
Ibuprofen	PO: adults: 300-400 mg q4h; children: 5-10 mg/kg q6-8h	Can cause gastric irritation
Naproxen	PO: adults: 500 mg/dose initially, then 250 mg q8-12h; children: 10 mg/kg/ day (5 mg/kg q12h)	Long duration of action; can cause gastric irritation
Indomethacin	PO: adults: 25 mg q8h; children: 1-3 mg/kg/day given 3 or 4 times	Contraindicated in psychiatric, neurological, and renal diseases; high incidence of gastric irritation; useful in gout

Data from Charache S et al. Medicine (Baltimore) 1996; 75:300. In Hoffman R et al: Hematology: basic principles and practice, 3rd ed. New York: Churchill Livingstone; 2000.

33

SICKLE CELL ANEMIA

TABLE 33-2

CLINICAL EFFECTS OF HYDROXYUREA THERAPY

Variable	Hydroxyurea	Placebo	p Value
Acute pain crisis rate	2.5/yr	4.5/yr	<.0001
Hospitalization rate for acute pain crisis	1.0/yr	2.4/yr	<.0001
Interval to first pain crisis	3.0 mo	1.5 mo	<.0001
Interval to second pain crisis	8.8 mo	4.6 mo	<.0001
Acute chest syndrome	25.0	51.0	<.0001
Subjects receiving transfusions	48.0	73.0	=.0001
Blood units transfused	336.0	586.0	=.0004

Data from Charache S et al. Medicine (Baltimore) 1996; 75:3 00. In Hoffman R et al: Hematology: basic principles and practice, 3rd ed. New York: Churchill Livingstone; 2000.

also been reported with *Streptococcus pneumoniae, Salmonella,* and Epstein-Barr virus.

3. Treatment is with transfusions, which can be intermittently necessary for several weeks.
4. If the patient has a refractory parvovirus B19 infection, IV immune globulin can be administered.

D. SPLENIC SEQUESTRATION CRISIS[12]

1. Vasoocclusion in the spleen causes a marked decrease in hemoglobin concentration. This occurs primarily in those who have not undergone autoinfarction (more common in Hb SC or sickle-cell thalassemia).
2. The crisis is treated with exchange transfusion.
3. This type of crisis is recurrent, and splenectomy is usually recommended after an acute episode.

III. ORGAN SYSTEM INVOLVEMENT

A. CENTRAL NERVOUS SYSTEM

1. Ischemic strokes.
   a. Strokes affect 6% to 12% of patients with SCD and are one of the leading causes of death in both children and adults with SCD.[13]
   b. Most of the data is on SCD and strokes in children and includes information regarding primary prevention and secondary prevention of strokes with transfusions.
   c. Prophylactic transfusion for strokes has not been studied in adults and is generally not recommended.[14]
   d. Use of exchange transfusion to keep the HbS concentration below 30% during an acute stroke is beneficial.[15]
   e. The following major risk factors for ischemic stroke were identified on multivariate analysis in the Cooperative Study of Sickle Cell Disease.[16]
      (1) Previous TIA: relative risk (RR) 56.
      (2) Low steady state hemoglobin: RR 1.9 per 1 g/dL decrease.
      (3) Rate of acute chest syndrome: RR 2.4 per event per year.
      (4) An episode of acute chest syndrome within the previous 2 weeks: RR 7.0.

(5) Elevated systolic blood pressure: RR 1.3 per 10 mm Hg increase.

f. The efficacy of aspirin or warfarin therapy in prevention of recurrent stroke has not been established.

g. Evaluation of stroke in the SCD population is the same as in the general population and includes non-contrast-enhanced computed tomography (CT) acutely to evaluate for hemorrhage followed by magnetic resonance imaging (MRI).[5] A transcranial Doppler flow study to detect subclinical neurological disease should be considered.

2. **Intracranial hemorrhage (ICH).**

a. ICH accounts for one third of strokes in patients with SCD and has a very high immediate mortality.

b. The peak incidence of ICH is between the ages of 20 and 29 years, whereas ischemic infarction is much more common in children.

c. In the Cooperative Study of Sickle Cell Disease two major risk factors for hemorrhagic stroke were identified on multivariate analysis.[16]

   (1) Low steady state hemoglobin: RR 1.6 per 1 g/dL decrease.

   (2) Increased steady state leukocyte count: RR 1.9 per 5000/μL increase.

d. Immediate exchange transfusion is recommended for patients with ICH.

e. Presentation includes headache, increased intracranial pressure, altered level of consciousness, and focal neurological deficits.

f. Evaluation is with CT scan and follow-up MRI or magnetic resonance angiography.[5]

B. EYES

1. **Proliferative sickle retinopathy.**

a. This is the most common ocular sequela of SCD (increased frequency in Hb SC disease).[17]

b. Treatment is with laser photocoagulation.

c. Vitreous hemorrhage and retinal detachment may result from this condition.

C. LUNGS

1. **Acute chest syndrome:** see acute crises section.

2. **Chronic restrictive lung disease.**[18]

a. This is a sequela of recurrent chest crises.

b. It is one of the major complications of SCD in older patients.

c. Prognosis is poor: 50% 2-year mortality.

d. Pulmonary hypertension and cor pulmonale develop in these patients.

D. CARDIOVASCULAR SYSTEM

1. **Hypertension.**

a. Hypertension is common in SCD and may reflect underlying renal disease.

b. Treatment differs in that diuretics are to be used with caution so that dehydration and sickling are not precipitated.

c. β-Blockers and calcium channel blockers are the mainstays of therapy.

d. Angiotensin-converting enzyme inhibitors can be useful if the patient has proteinuria.

33

SICKLE CELL ANEMIA

2. **Cardiac disease.**
a. Exercise capacity is generally reduced from multifactorial causes in SCD.
b. Atherosclerotic coronary disease is less common in this population, but myocardial infarctions with clean coronary arteries still occur.[19]
c. If a stress test is indicated, radionuclide or echocardiographic studies are more helpful than electrocardiography-based tests because of the high rate of false-positive results.[5]

E. **HEPATOBILIARY SYSTEM**

1. **Gallstones.**[20]
a. Increased bilirubin production from chronic hemolysis puts SCD patients at increased risk of gallstones.
b. Incidence is 75% by age 30.
c. Presentation is the same as in patients without SCD.
d. For surgical recommendations see the section on surgery below.

2. **Acute liver disease.**
a. The liver can be the site of vasoocclusion, causing an acute rise in levels of transaminases, bilirubin, and alkaline phosphatase.
b. Other causes of acute liver disease (e.g., cholecystitis, viral hepatitis) must be excluded before this diagnosis can be made.
c. Acute liver disease is usually self-limited but on rare occasion can progress to fulminant liver failure (see Chapter 25) and necessitate exchange transfusion.[21]
d. Treatment otherwise is the same as in any vasoocclusive crisis.

F. **RENAL SYSTEM**

1. **Hyposthenuria.**[22]
a. Hyposthenuria is the inability to maximally concentrate urine.
b. It generally manifests itself by age 3 and is characterized by increased obligatory daily urine output of more than 2 L per day.
c. It may predispose patients to dehydration and more frequent sickling.

2. **Renal tubular acidosis.**[22]
a. Renal tubular acidosis is the most common cause of metabolic acidosis in SCD.
b. It should be corrected by sodium bicarbonate therapy if acidemia is present.
c. It is also associated with hyperkalemia that is generally unresponsive to loop diuretics.

3. **Gross hematuria.**[23]
a. Painless hematuria is commonly seen in SCD. In 80% of cases bleeding is unilateral in the left kidney.
b. Hematuria can also develop in sickle cell trait carriers.
c. Evaluation includes renal ultrasound, cystoscopy, and culture.
d. Treatment includes aggressive hydration to keep urine flow high, alkalinization of the urine, and bed rest.
e. If the bleeding is refractory, aminocaproic acid can be used but is associated with an increased risk of clot formation in the urinary tract.

4. **Proteinuria.**[24]
a. Proteinuria is present in 25% of adults with SCD.

b. It can progress to nephrotic syndrome from membranoproliferative glomerulonephritis.

5. **Renal papillary necrosis.**

a. Renal papillary necrosis is a common and usually asymptomatic cause of hematuria and proteinuria in SCD.

b. It is associated with interstitial nephritis from nonsteroidal antiinflammatory drug (NSAID) use.

6. **Chronic renal failure.**[25]

a. SCD is not a contraindication for hemodialysis or renal transplant.

b. Prevalence is greater in SCD than in the African-American population.

G. MUSCULOSKELETAL SYSTEM

1. **Leg ulcers.**[26]

a. Leg ulcers are found in 10% to 20% of patients with SCD and are more prevalent in men.

b. The mainstay of treatment is aggressive wound care (see Chapter 20).

c. Transfusions may be used when ulcers are refractory to therapy for longer than 6 months.

2. **Avascular necrosis of the femoral and humeral heads.**[27]

a. Peak incidence is between ages 25 and 35.

b. Evaluation is by MRI.

c. Total joint replacement may be necessary both to treat pain and to improve function.

3. **Joint effusions.**

a. Joint effusions may be caused by synovial infarction, but gout, septic arthritis, osteoarthritis, or rheumatic causes should be considered (see Chapter 70).

b. Treatment is NSAIDs and local heat.

H. GENITOURINARY SYSTEM[25]

1. **Acute priapism.**

a. The most common form is acute recurrent priapism that subsides spontaneously.

b. It occurs most commonly in children with SCD.

c. Between 30% and 50% of male patients with SCD report at least one episode in their lifetime.

d. Failure of an erection to subside after several hours is a urological emergency.

e. Management includes aggressive IV hydration, IV narcotics for pain relief, and if necessary exchange transfusion.

f. If these measures do not work, penile aspiration may be required.

2. **Impotence.**

a. Partial or complete impotence may result from recurrent or prolonged priapism.

b. Management of impotence can include penile prostheses.

I. BLOOD SYSTEM[28]

1. Anemia in SCD is a chronic hemolytic anemia with an appropriate reticulocyte response.

2. Mean hemoglobin concentrations are approximately 8 g/dL.

3. Folate deficiency is common and 20% of patients with SCD are iron deficient, so supplementation is required.

4. White blood cell counts are higher than normal (12,000 to 15,000/mm^3) even in the absence of infection.

5. Thrombocytosis may be present.

6. Bone marrow transplantation is potentially curative for SCD, but the short- and long-term complications remain as barriers to widespread use.[29]

J. INFECTIOUS DISEASE

1. Fevers can occur as a result of vasoocclusion, but a persistent fever higher than 38.3° C should prompt an evaluation for infection.

2. Infections tend to occur in already damaged areas such as lungs, kidneys, and bones.

3. These patients should be considered functionally asplenic because in general their spleens have undergone autoinfarction by early childhood.

4. Common infections.

a. Pneumonia (see Chapter 43): Common organisms include many atypical bacteria such as *Mycoplasma, Chlamydia,* and *Legionella.* Because of immunizations, *Streptococcus pneumoniae* and *Haemophilus influenzae* are becoming less common pathogens.[9]

b. Urinary tract infections can be recurrent and can lead to urosepsis. Follow-up urine cultures 2 weeks after treatment are recommended (see Chapter 48).

c. Osteomyelitis (see Chapter 47) and septic arthritis (see Chapter 72) must be differentiated from vasoocclusive bony pain. The organisms that cause osteomyelitis in SCD are different in that *Salmonella* species are the most common causative organisms whereas *Staphylococcus aureus* is the infectious agent in approximately 25% of cases. Chronic *Salmonella* osteomyelitis requires prolonged antibiotic therapy with 1 month of recommended IV treatment followed by months of oral therapy.[30]

PEARLS AND PITFALLS

- Chronic pain management.[31]
  - Chronic pain can be a component in SCD and must be adequately treated.
  - Medications that can be helpful in treating chronic pain in outpatients include long-acting narcotics such as morphine sulfate sustained release bid or methadone on a bid or tid schedule.
  - Short-acting analgesics (see the pain management scheme) should be used for breakthrough pain.
- Surgery.[32]
  - Patients with SCD have been shown to have a higher rate of surgical complications compared with the general population (30% rate of serious complications).
  - Studies have compared transfusion to a hemoglobin level greater than

10 g/dL with exchange transfusion (goal Hb SS <30%) and have found no significant change in operative morbidity after either of these modalities is received.

- Preoperative transfusion (either exchange or standard) is recommended.
- Postoperative acute chest syndrome develops in 10% of patients who undergo surgery.
- The main complication of transfusion is the increased incidence of new alloantibody formation.
- Health maintenance.
  - All adults should be immunized against *S. pneumoniae,* hepatitis B virus, and influenza.
  - Folic acid should be given daily (1 mg PO each day).
  - Annual retinal examinations are needed to detect early proliferative retinopathy.
  - No additional risk of oral contraceptive use is associated with SCD.
  - Genetic counseling should be offered to all patients with SCD.

REFERENCES

[c] 1. Bunn HF. Pathogenesis and treatment of sickle cell disease. N Engl J Med 1997; 337:762.

[c] 2. Powars DR. Natural history of sickle cell disease—the first ten years. Semin Hematol 1975; 12:267.

[c] 3. Platt OS et al. Pain in sickle cell disease: rates and risk factors. N Engl J Med 1991; 325:11.

[c] 4. Steinberg M. Management of sickle cell disease. N Engl J Med 1999; 340:1021.

[d] 5. Reid CD et al. Management and therapy of sickle cell disease. 3rd Ed. NIH Pub No 96-2117. Rockville, Md: National Institutes of Health, National Heart, Lung and Blood Institute, Public Health Service, Dept of Health and Human Services; rev 1995.

[c] 6. Yale SH et al. Approach to the vaso-occlusive crisis in adults with sickle cell disease. Am Fam Physician 2000; 61:1349.

[b] 7. Embury SH et al. Effects of oxygen inhalation on endogenous erythropoiesis, and properties of blood cells in sickle-cell anemia. N Engl J Med 1984; 311:291.

[a] 8. Charache S et al. Effect of hydroxyurea on the frequency of painful crises in sickle cell anemia. N Engl J Med 1995; 332:1317.

[a] 9. Vichinsky EP et al. Causes and outcomes of the acute chest syndrome in sickle cell crisis. N Engl J Med 2000; 342:1855.

[c] 10. Stuart MJ et al. Acute chest syndrome of sickle cell disease: new light on an old problem. Curr Opin Hematol 2001; 8:111.

[b] 11. Serjeant GR et al. Human parvovirus infection in homozygous sickle cell disease. Lancet 1993; 41:1237.

[c] 12. Emond AM et al. Acute splenic sequestration in homozygous sickle cell disease: natural history and management. J Pediatr 1985; 107:201.

[c] 13. Powars DR et al. The natural history of stroke in sickle cell disease. Am J Med 1978; 65:461.

[c] 14. Adams RJ. Stroke prevention in sickle cell disease. Curr Opin Hematol 2000; 7:101.

[c] 15. Cohen AR et al. A modified transfusion program for prevention of stroke in sickle cell disease. Blood 1992; 79:1657.

[c] 16. Ohene-Frempong F et al. Cerebrovascular accidents in sickle cell disease: rates and risk factors. Blood 1998;91:288.

[c] 17. Hayes RJ et al. Haematological factors associated with proliferative retinopathy in homozygous sickle cell disease. Br J Ophthalmol 1981; 65:712.

33

SICKLE CELL ANEMIA

[c] 18. Minter KR et al. Pulmonary complications of sickle cell anemia. Am J Respir Crit Care Med 2001; 164:2016.

[c] 19. O'Neill B et al. Myocardial infarction in sickle cell anemia. Am J Hematol 1984; 16:139.

[b] 20. Haberkern CM et al. Perioperative outcome of 364 cases from the National Preoperative Transfusion Study. Blood 1997; 89:1533

[c] 21. Sheehy TW et al. Exchange transfusion for sickle cell intrahepatic cholestasis. Arch Intern Med 1980; 140:1364.

[c] 22. Allon M. Renal abnormalities in sickle cell disease. Arch Intern Med 1990; 150:501.

[c] 23. Pham PT et al. Renal abnormalities in sickle cell disease. Kidney Int 2000; 57:1.

[c] 24. Falk RH et al. Sickle cell nephropathy. Adv Nephrol 1994; 23:133.

[c] 25. Bruno D et al. Genitourinary complications of sickle cell disease. J Urol 2001; 166:803.

[c] 26. Koshy M et al. Leg ulcers in patients with sickle cell disease. Blood 1989; 74:1403.

[b] 27. Milner PF et al. Sickle cell disease as a cause of osteonecrosis of the femoral head. N Engl J Med 1991; 325:1476.

[b] 28. West MS et al. Laboratory profile of sickle cell disease: a cross-sectional analysis. The Cooperative Study of Sickle Cell Disease. J Clin Epidemiol 1992; 45:893

[c] 29. Hoppe CC et al. Bone marrow transplantation in sickle cell disease. Curr Opin Oncol 2001; 13:85.

[c] 30. Anand AJ, Glatt AE. *Salmonella* osteomyelitis and arthritis in sickle cell disease. Semin Arthritis Rheum 1994; 24:211.

[c] 31. Brookoff D et al. Treating sickle cell pain like cancer pain. Ann Intern Med 1992; 116:364.

[b] 32. Vichinsky EP et al. A comparison of conservative and aggressive transfusion regimens in the perioperative management of sickle cell disease. N Engl J Med 1995; 333:206.

Thrombocytopenia

Susan Lee Limb, MD, Luis A. Diaz, Jr., MD, and Lawrence Gardner, MD

FAST FACTS

- Keep platelet counts above 20,000/µL in patients with systemic illness (i.e., infection).
- To minimize bleeding risk, platelet counts should be above 50,000/µL for any procedure.
- In heparin-naïve patients, type 2 heparin-induced thrombocytopenia should take at least 5 days to develop.
- Mucosal and cutaneous bleeding are the most common physical findings of thrombocytopenia.
- Platelets survive approximately 8 to 10 days in circulation.
- Central nervous system bleeding is the most common cause of death in thrombocytopenia.
- Posttransfusion purpura affects women 26 times more frequently than men.
- Spontaneous bleeding usually does not occur until platelet counts are below 10,000/µL.

34

I. DEFINITIONS

1. Thrombocytopenia is defined as a platelet count less than 150,000/µL of whole blood, with normal values ranging from 150,000 to 450,000/µL.
2. Variations in the platelet count may be physiological or pathological.
   a. Platelet numbers fluctuate with the different stages of the menstrual cycle or in certain nutritional deficiencies.
   b. As acute-phase reactants, platelets increase in the setting of systemic inflammation.
3. Thrombocytopenia may occur with anemia, leukopenia, or both, or may be isolated.
4. Likely causes of pancytopenia include hypersplenism, a systemic illness, a bone marrow toxin, bone marrow replacement (e.g., leukemia, metastatic tumor), or a bone marrow failure state (e.g., myelodysplasia, aplastic anemia).
5. Thrombocytopenia accompanied by anemia may indicate Evans' syndrome (hemolytic anemia and immune thrombocytopenia) or a microangiopathic hemolytic anemia.

II. CLINICAL PRESENTATION

1. For the most part thrombocytopenia is an incidental discovery on laboratory testing. Most patients are asymptomatic.

2. Generally, increased bleeding from minimal trauma is not observed until counts decrease below 50,000/µL.[1] Spontaneous bleeding usually occurs when counts are less than 10,000/µL.

3. Intracranial bleeding is the main cause of death from thrombocytopenia, but fortunately, it is exceedingly rare.

4. Self-limited, small vessel bleeding in the gastrointestinal and genitourinary tract is the usual manifestation of thrombocytopenia. Common examples are gingival bleeding, epistaxis, and menorrhagia.

5. Gross hematuria or gastrointestinal bleeding in the absence of trauma is uncommon.

6. Petechiae and ecchymoses may also be present.

a. Petechiae.
   (1) Petechiae are nonpalpable red lesions 1 to 3 mm in diameter. They are caused by the extravasation of red blood cells into the skin.
   (2) They do not blanch under pressure.
   (3) They arise in dependent areas such as the lower extremities or over the sacral area in the bedridden.

b. Ecchymoses.
   (1) Ecchymoses are larger areas of subcutaneous bleeding, greater than 3 mm in diameter.
   (2) These areas do not blanch under pressure.

c. Palpable purpura.
   (1) Purpura is the presence of raised, tender lesions that originate from inflamed blood vessels with subsequent hemorrhage into the surrounding skin.
   (2) Purpura is not typical of isolated thrombocytopenia and should raise the suspicion of vasculitis or other systemic inflammation.

7. Patients with thrombocytopenia and functional platelet disorders rarely exhibit the deep bleeding into muscles and joints and severe postoperative bleeding seen in patients with coagulation disorders such as hemophilia.

8. Patients with a consumptive process (e.g., idiopathic thrombocytopenic purpura [ITP], hypersplenism) have a lower risk of bleeding than patients with poor platelet production.

9. Bleeding from thrombocytopenia is more likely if an additional coagulopathic condition, such as anemia, uremia, or hemophilia, is present.

III. DIAGNOSTICS (Fig. 34-1)

A. PLATELET LIFE CYCLE

1. Platelets arise from megakaryocytes in the bone marrow.

2. Approximately 40,000 platelets per microliter of whole blood are generated each day in healthy individuals. Approximately 30% to 40% of the released platelets are sequestered in the spleen.[2]

3. The remaining platelets circulate for 7 to 10 days, although the half-

life of transfused platelets is considerably less (even for human leukocyte antigen matched).

4. Only a small fraction of circulating platelets is consumed by thrombosis.

5. Most platelets are cleared by macrophage-mediated phagocytosis.

B. TYPES OF THROMBOCYTOPENIA BY PATHOGENESIS

1. Pseudothrombocytopenia.

a. Pseudothrombocytopenia should be considered a potential explanation for reduced platelet counts before the physician embarks on an extensive workup.

b. It is usually due to platelet clumping in the blood sample, leading to an underestimation of platelets by automated cell counters.

   (1) Clumping may arise from inadequate anticoagulation of the sample or immunoglobulin-mediated agglutination.

   (2) Certain otherwise healthy individuals express an autoantibody to a concealed epitope on the IIb/IIIa glycoprotein found on platelet membranes. In the presence of EDTA the epitope is exposed and the autoantibodies mediate platelet agglutination.

c. Pseudothrombocytopenia is confirmed by collection of a blood sample in a tube containing heparin or sodium citrate as the anticoagulant or by a check of a peripheral blood smear taken directly from a fingerstick.[3,4]

d. Much more rare is the May-Hegglin syndrome, a condition of leukocyte and immune deficiencies. It is associated with large platelets that are often miscounted with automated analyzers, resulting in an artifactual thrombocytopenia.

2. **Dilution of the platelet population caused by transfusion or splenomegaly.**

a. Transfusion-related thrombocytopenia is the result of large transfusions of packed red blood cells or plasma because stored blood contains few viable platelets. This is readily corrected by platelet transfusions, although transfusion is not always necessary in the absence of active bleeding.

b. Splenomegaly caused by liver disease, portal vein thrombosis, or any other cause (including splenic lymphoma or Gaucher's disease) results in a mild thrombocytopenia accompanied by a mild anemia and leukopenia.

3. **Decreased production (Box 34-1).**

a. Decreased production is usually the result of congenital or acquired bone marrow suppression.

b. In the general medicine inpatient population the bone marrow suppression is most likely caused by infection, toxic agents, or poor nutritional status.

c. Evaluation of new thrombocytopenia should include consideration of recent infections, chemotherapy and radiation, alcohol intake, and underlying vitamin B_{12} or folate deficiency.

Text continued on p. 524

34

THROMBOCYTOPENIA

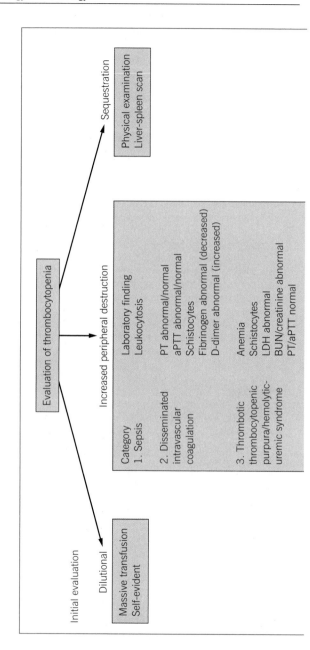

Initial evaluation

Evaluation of thrombocytopenia

Dilutional

Increased peripheral destruction

Sequestration

Massive transfusion
Self-evident

Category	Laboratory finding
1. Sepsis	Leukocytosis
2. Disseminated intravascular coagulation	PT abnormal/normal aPTT abnormal/normal Schistocytes Fibrinogen abnormal (decreased) D-dimer abnormal (increased)
3. Thrombotic thrombocytopenic purpura/hemolytic-uremic syndrome	Anemia Schistocytes LDH abnormal BUN/creatinine abnormal PT/aPTT normal

Physical examination
Liver-spleen scan

4. Cardiac: post cardiac bypass, prosthetic heart valve

Anemia
Schistocytes
LDH abnormal

5. Platelet antibodies: drug-induced, posttransfusion purpura, collagen-vascular disease, idiopathic thrombocytopenic purpura

Normal screening studies

FIG. 34-1

Evaluation of thrombocytopenia. *aPTT*, Activated partial thromboplastin time; *BUN*, blood urea nitrogen; *LDH*, lactate dehydrogenase; *PT*, prothrombin time. (*Data from Goldman L, Bennett JC. Cecil textbook of medicine, 21st ed. Philadelphia: WB Saunders; 1999.*)

34

THROMBOCYTOPENIA

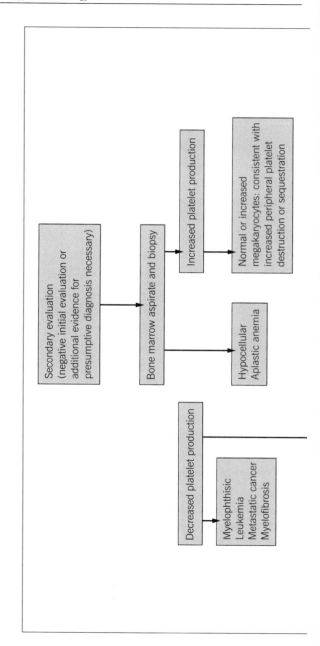

34

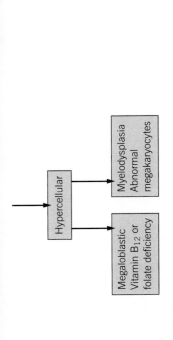

FIG. 34-1—cont'd

Evaluation of thrombocytopenia. *(Data from Goldman L, Bennett JC. Cecil textbook of medicine, 21st ed. Philadelphia: WB Saunders; 1999.)*

BOX 34-1

CAUSES OF DECREASED PLATELET PRODUCTION

CONGENITAL

Increased platelet size

    Bernard-Soulier syndrome (loss of glycoprotein 1b)

    Alport's syndrome

    May-Hegglin anomaly

Normal platelet size

    Thrombocytopenia with absent radius

    Wiskott-Aldrich syndrome (immunodeficiency, eczema, and thrombocytopenia)

ACQUIRED

Bone marrow infiltration

    Metastatic cancer

    Hematological malignancy (e.g., leukemia)

    Myelofibrosis

    Gaucher's disease

    Granulomatous process

Aplastic anemia

Amegakaryocytic thrombocytopenia

    Viral (e.g., parvovirus)

    Drug-induced (e.g., chemotherapy)

Ineffective thrombopoiesis

    Folate and vitamin B_{12} deficiency

    Paroxysmal nocturnal hemoglobinuria

    Myelodysplastic syndrome

    Iron deficiency (late and rare)

---

d. Patients with chronic illnesses such as lupus (see Chapter 73) and human immunodeficiency virus (HIV) infection also frequently have decreased megakaryopoiesis.

e. One study showed that thrombocytopenia in patients admitted to the intensive care unit was often associated with histiocyte engulfment of megakaryocytes (hemophagocytic syndromes).[5]

f. In amegakaryocytic thrombocytopenia, autoantibodies are directed against megakaryocytes and lead to decreased megakaryopoiesis and platelet production. Some degree of this is also seen in classic ITP, but peripheral destruction is much more important (see below).

g. Primary problems with megakaryopoiesis, such as thrombocytopenia with absent radius (TAR) syndrome, are rare. The TAR syndrome arises from faulty production of early megakaryocyte precursors.

4. Increased destruction (Box 34-2).

a. Increased destruction is generally an immune-mediated process, resulting in premature clearance of platelets from circulation.

b. In the inpatient population, drugs are common culprits because they

---

BOX 34-2

CAUSES OF PLATELET DESTRUCTION

IMMUNE MECHANISMS

Idiopathic

Autoimmune

  Chronic lymphocytic leukemia

  Systemic lupus erythematosus

  Thyroid disease

  Hypogammaglobulinemia

  Antiphospholipid syndrome

  Allogeneic bone marrow transplant

Human immunodeficiency virus

Drug-dependent immune

Posttransfusion purpura

Sepsis

Neonatal alloimmune thrombocytopenia

NONIMMUNE MECHANISMS

Disseminated intravascular coagulation

Cardiopulmonary bypass surgery

Thrombotic thrombocytopenic purpura

Hemolytic-uremic syndrome

Preeclampsia

Acute or hyperacute graft rejection

Syndrome of hemolysis, elevated liver enzymes, and low platelet count

Cavernous hemangioma (Kasabach-Merritt) syndrome

---

    activate complement and lead to peripheral platelet destruction (Box 34-3).

c. Autoimmune conditions such as ITP and antiphospholipid syndrome can increase platelet clearance as well.

d. A rare cause of increased destruction of platelets is type IIB von Willebrand disease, in which an autosomally transmitted thrombocytopenia is accompanied by a bleeding history out of proportion to the thrombocytopenia present.

e. Destructive, immune-mediated thrombocytopenia can also be seen after certain infections and is common in HIV infection.

f. In microangiopathic hemolytic anemias caused by thrombotic thrombocytopenia purpura (TTP), vasculitis, disseminated intravascular coagulopathy (DIC), or malignant hypertension, thrombocytopenia is accompanied by fragmented red blood cells and a reticulocytosis.

g. Physical destruction (nonimmune) from shear stress may occur during cardiopulmonary bypass or from prosthetic heart valves. During cardiovascular surgery, bypass pumps can activate platelets and augment their destruction.

BOX 34-3

DRUGS THAT MAY ALTER HEMOSTASIS

DRUGS REPORTED TO CAUSE THROMBOCYTOPENIA

Immune Mechanism Proposed*

Quinine and quinidine
Sulfa compounds
Ampicillin
Penicillin
Thiazide diuretics
Furosemide
Chlorthalidone
Phenytoin
α-Methyldopa
Heparin
Digitalis derivatives
Aspirin
Valproic acid
Ranitidine
Cimetidine
Danazol
Procainamide
Carbamazepine
Acetaminophen
Phenylbutazone
p-Aminosalicylate
Rifampin
Acetazolamide
Anazolene
Arsenicals

Nonimmune Mechanisms (hemolytic-uremic syndrome, thrombotic thrombocytopenic purpura)

Ticlopidine
Mitomycin
Cisplatin
Cyclosporine

Mechanism Undefined

Gold compounds
Indomethacin

From Goldman L, Bennett JC. Cecil textbook of medicine, 21st ed. Philadelphia: WB Saunders; 1999.

*The list is limited to drugs for which there are multiple reports and in vitro or in vivo evidence of antiplatelet antibodies.

BOX 34-3—cont'd

DRUGS THAT MAY ALTER HEMOSTASIS

DRUGS THAT ALTER PLATELET FUNCTION

Primary Antiplatelet Agents

Aspirin

Dextran

Dipyridamole

Sulfinpyrazone

Ticlopidine

Drugs in Which Inhibition of Platelet Function Is Associated with Prolongation of the Bleeding Time

Nonsteroidal antiinflammatory agents

β-Lactam antibiotics

ε-Aminocaproic acid (>24 g/day)

Heparin

Plasminogen activators (streptokinase, urokinase, tissue plasminogen activator)

DRUGS THAT AFFECT COAGULATION FACTORS

Induction of Antibodies Inhibiting Function

Lupus anticoagulant††‡

  Phenothiazines

  Procainamide

Factor VIII antibodies

  Penicillin

Factor V antibodies

  Aminoglycosides

Factor XIII antibodies

Isoniazid

Inhibitors of Synthesis of Vitamin K–Dependent Clotting Factors (Factors II, VII, IX, X; Proteins C and S)

Coumarin compounds

Moxalactam

Inhibitor of Fibrinogen Synthesis

L-Asparaginase‡

From Goldman L, Bennett JC. Cecil textbook of medicine, 21st ed. Philadelphia: WB Saunders; 2000.
†Does not cause bleeding.
‡May cause thrombosis.

h. In cases of increased platelet destruction the bone marrow should reveal normal or increased megakaryocytes.

IV. MANAGEMENT OF COMMON CAUSES OF THROMBOCYTOPENIA

A. DRUGS AND TOXINS

1. **Immune-mediated destruction.**

a. Immune-mediated destruction is the most common mechanism for drug-induced thrombocytopenia.

b. Antibody-drug complexes on the surface of platelets trigger complement activation and subsequent removal from the circulation.

c. Drug-induced thrombocytopenia typically develops 2 to 3 weeks after initial exposure to the drug.[6,7]

d. One exception to this is the antithrombotic glycoprotein IIb/IIIa receptor inhibitors. In the EPIC trial[8] the study investigators reported thrombocytopenia occurring within 30 minutes to 24 hours of abciximab administration. The rapidity of this thrombocytopenia is attributed to preformed antibodies that exist against glycoprotein neoepitopes exposed during normal platelet reactions.[9]

2. **Several drugs and toxins can suppress platelet production (Box 34-3).**

a. The list of potential offending drugs is continually expanding with varying amounts of clinical evidence to support each one.

b. Almost every drug has been associated with some degree of thrombocytopenia.

c. The medications that are best established as common causes of thrombocytopenia are heparin, quinine and quinidine, cimetidine, rifampin, and anticonvulsants such as valproic acid.[6]

d. Chemotherapeutic agents cause varying degrees of bone marrow suppression.

e. Large quantities of ethanol can cause a generalized suppression of marrow function and induce a transient drop in platelet generation.

f. Thiazide diuretics can impair megakaryocyte production, leading to a mild thrombocytopenia that may persist for several months after the drug is discontinued.

g. Generally, thrombocytopenia caused by drug antibodies resolves within 7 to 10 days after discontinuation of the medication[10] but can persist longer. Patients with more severe cases may benefit from a course of prednisone, starting at 1 mg/kg PO qd and tapering over several weeks. In critical situations treatment may include platelet transfusions, intravenous immune globulin therapy, and parenteral corticosteroids, similar to the management of severe ITP.

h. Various antiplatelet antibody tests are available, although their role in clinical decision making has yet to be established. These tests are expensive, and the results may not be obtained in a timely manner. More important, the presence of drug antibodies is not proof of a drug-induced thrombocytopenia, especially in sick patients who have multiple reasons to have thrombocytopenia. In hospitalized patients the elimination of useful drugs from the arsenal because of a questionable allergy can limit and adversely affect clinical management. If these tests are ordered, their results should be used to confirm rather than diagnose drug-related thrombocytopenia.

i. An increase in platelet counts after discontinuation of the drug is still the key to diagnosis.

B. HEPARIN-INDUCED THROMBOCYTOPENIA (Table 34-1)

1. Heparin, in particular, requires close surveillance.

2. Type 1 heparin-induced thrombocytopenia (HIT).

a. Mild thrombocytopenia occurs in the first 3 days of heparin administration.

b. This is a nonimmune disease.

c. It is caused by direct effects of heparin on platelet activation.[11]

d. It is relatively common, occurring in up to 30% of patients receiving low molecular weight or unfractionated heparin.

e. Type 1 HIT resolves spontaneously without thrombosis or other sequela, even with continued heparin exposure.

3. Type 2 HIT.

a. Type 2 HIT can be severe.

b. The incidence of true type 2 varies according to study, ranging from 0.3% to 3%.[12]

c. It is an immune-mediated process.

   (1) Antibodies form against a complex of heparin and platelet factor 4.[13]
   (2) Antibodies then bind to the Fc receptors on platelets, causing platelet release of prothrombic microparticles.

d. Even in small doses, such as the amount used in IV flushes, heparin can produce severe thrombocytopenia and thrombosis.

e. When type 2 HIT occurs in heparin-naïve patients, a decrease in platelet count does not occur before day 5 of heparin administration, although thrombosis can occur before the onset of true (platelet count <150,000/μL) thrombocytopenia.[12]

TABLE 34-1		
HEPARIN-INDUCED THROMBOCYTOPENIA		
Variable	HIT Type 1	HIT Type 2
Frequency	~25%	~3%
Mechanism	Nonimmunogenic	Fc portion of antibody binding to platelets
Positive for HIT antibodies	No (~30% false positives)	Yes (~75%)
Platelet nadir	~90,000	~70,000
Day of onset	<Day 5	>Day 5
Treatment	None; continue heparin	Alternative anticoagulation
Thrombosis	No	~30%

HIT, Heparin-induced thrombocytopenia.

f. A more rapid decline (10.5 hours) in platelet count may be seen in patients exposed to heparin within 100 days of presentation.[14]

g. Diagnostics.

(1) Several laboratory tests are available for the diagnosis of type 2 HIT.

(2) The gold standard is the ^{14}C-serotonin release assay.[12] Radio-labeled, normal platelets are combined with patient serum and therapeutic heparin concentrations. Induction of ^{14}C-serotonin release from platelets constitutes a positive test result.[15] The high cost of radiolabeled products hampers their widespread use.

(3) Another commercially available test is an enzyme-linked immunosorbent assay (ELISA) kit to document the presence of these antibodies. Although both these tests are approximately 75% sensitive, neither is very specific. A positive test result may not be accompanied by clinical HIT or even by thrombocytopenia. One study showed that after cardiac surgery approximately 50% of patients had an ELISA positive for HIT, whereas only 1% met the clinical criteria for type 2 HIT 2, giving a positive predictive value of 2%.[16]

h. Management.

(1) Although cessation of all forms of heparin is the first step in management, it is not sufficient.

(2) The presence of type 2 HIT is the most potent hypercoagulable risk factor known.

(3) Thrombosis, either arterial or venous, develops in up to 50% of patients with type 2 HIT and has a fatality rate of up to 20%. Thus anticoagulation is necessary until the platelet count increases and plateaus (or longer, if thrombosis has occurred).

(4) Unfortunately, up to 90% of patients with HIT display cross-reactivity with low molecular weight heparin as well,[17] necessitating the use of alternative anticoagulants such as the direct thrombin inhibitors hirudin or argatroban (Table 34-2).

(5) Warfarin should be started only after the patient has achieved therapeutic levels of these other agents because of the transient hypercoagulable state caused by the initial warfarin-mediated decline in protein C and an association of gangrene with early warfarin use in patients with HIT.[18]

TABLE 34-2

ALTERNATIVE ANTICOAGULANTS USED IN HEPARIN-INDUCED THROMBOCYTOPENIA

Variable	Hirudin (Leuperidin)	Argatroban
Mechanism	Thrombin inhibitor	Thrombin inhibitor
Monitoring	aPTT	aPTT
Dose reductions	Renal dysfunction	Hepatic dysfunction
Caveats		Elevates PT

aPTT, Activated partial thromboplastin time; *PT,* prothrombin time.

C. IDIOPATHIC THROMBOCYTOPENIC PURPURA

1. Primary autoimmune thrombocytopenia is referred to as idiopathic thrombocytopenic purpura (ITP).
2. Drugs can cause secondary autoimmune thrombocytopenia.
3. Primary ITP may be associated with lupus, autoimmune thyroid disorders, indolent or aggressive lymphomas, hepatitis C, HIV, or large granular lymphocytosis. ITP can be divided into acute and chronic disease.
4. Acute ITP.
   a. Acute ITP is more common in the pediatric population.
   b. It is characterized by an abrupt reduction in platelet counts after recovery from an upper respiratory infection or viral exanthem.
   c. Two main processes are responsible for acute ITP.
      (1) Antibodies generated against the infectious agent cross-react with platelet antigens.
      (2) Immune complexes are formed from viral antigens binding Fc-receptors located on platelet surfaces.[19]
   d. Over 90% of patients with acute ITP make a full recovery within 2 to 8 weeks.[20]
5. Chronic ITP.
   a. Chronic ITP is a more indolent disease.
   b. It accounts for over 90% of cases of ITP in adults.
   c. An incidence of 66 million cases per year has been estimated based on extrapolation of pediatric data, but the true incidence is difficult to document because many cases are asymptomatic and no gold standard for diagnosis exists.[21]
   d. Pathophysiology.
      (1) Autoantibodies bind to glycoprotein IIb/IIIa or glycoprotein Ib to IX complexes on platelets.
      (2) This binding promotes phagocytic clearance of platelets and in some individuals may directly impair platelet function by blocking critical portions of the glycoproteins.
   e. Like other autoimmune diseases, chronic ITP is more common in women (70% of reported cases) and the majority of these patients are under 40 years of age.[21]
   f. To an extent the diagnosis of chronic ITP is a diagnosis of exclusion.
   g. Laboratory tests measuring antiplatelet antibodies have not been proved to have predictive value and are not recommended for diagnosis by the American Society of Hematology.[22]
   h. Basic evaluation should include careful history, physical examination, complete blood cell count, and peripheral blood smear to look for other causes of isolated thrombocytopenia.
   i. Bone marrow aspiration is generally reserved for patients over 50 years of age to rule out myelodysplasia.[23,24] It should be performed when thrombocytopenia is accompanied by an otherwise unexplained anemia

or leukopenia or when abnormalities are seen in the peripheral blood smear.

6. **Management.**

a. Treatment depends on the severity of the illness.

b. In HIV-associated thrombocytopenia, treatment with antiretroviral agents can be effective in resolving the ITP. Mild, asymptomatic cases of ITP with platelet counts ranging from 30,000 to 50,000/μL generally do not require intervention.[25]

c. Steroids: The mainstay of symptomatic therapy is glucocorticoids. A 4- to 6-week course of prednisone 1 mg/kg qd that is then tapered slowly is adequate for most cases of increased bleeding. About half of patients respond to steroids and achieve full or partial remission. The goal should be to maintain a safe platelet count with the minimal amount of steroid use.

d. Aminocaproic acid: Bleeding patients should be given the antifibrinolytic agent ε-aminocaproic acid (Amicar).

e. Platelet transfusions are usually ineffective but may be attempted in actively bleeding patients.

f. IV immune globulin: Other treatment in urgent situations should include 1 g/kg intravenous immune globulin (IVIG) for 2 to 5 days; Rh-positive patients should be given 50 to 75 μg/kg anti-Rh(D), a component of IVIG. Both of these treatments are thought to block phagocytosis and downregulate Fc receptors.[22] Approximately 70% of patients respond transiently to IVIG or anti-D, but neither agent achieves a long-term remission.[26,27]

g. Unfortunately, the majority of patients have relapses after the withdrawal of steroids. A repeat trial of steroids may be attempted, including high-dose Decadron (40 mg PO every day for 4 days), but no standard regimen exists and usage varies widely among practitioners.[22]

h. Splenectomy: In steroid-dependent patients elective splenectomy may be a viable option. Roughly two thirds of patients achieve normal platelet counts within a week of surgery,[22] but recurrent thrombocytopenia develops in some of these patients. Persistent or recurrent thrombocytopenia after splenectomy may be due to accessory spleens or growth of splenic tissue left behind from the initial operation. Splenic remnants can be detected by radionuclide scanning.

i. Many other immunosuppressive agents have been attempted for patients not responding to treatment, but no large trials proving efficacy exist. Small series or case reports have described the use of vincristine, low-dose (100 mg PO every day) or high-dose cyclophosphamide, cyclosporine, and Rituxamab (an anti-CD20 antibody).

D. **MICROANGIOPATHIC HEMOLYTIC ANEMIAS**

1. Microangiopathic hemolytic anemias occur in thrombotic thrombocytopenic purpura (TTP), hemolytic-uremic syndrome, vasculitis, malignant hypertension with renal disease, and disseminated intravascular coagulation (DIC).

2. The cause of a microangiopathic hemolytic anemia is usually easily determined on the basis of clinical history, examination, and laboratory data.

3. TTP.

a. Diagnosis (the pentad).

   (1) Fever.
   (2) Change in mental status.
   (3) Renal abnormalities.
   (4) Thrombocytopenia.
   (5) Hemolytic anemia.

b. The hemolytic-uremic syndrome (HUS) is clinically similar, although renal failure is more usually more pronounced. HUS usually occurs in younger patients, and it is more often associated with infection (including *Escherichia coli* H7:O157).

c. Recently, TTP has been found to be closely associated with a deficiency in a protease activity directed against von Willebrand factor.[27,28]

d. TTP is fatal unless prompt treatment is initiated. The combination of steroids with plasmapheresis and plasma exchange has been found to be very effective.[29] Platelet transfusions are considered contraindicated, although much of the evidence is anecdotal.

4. DIC.

a. DIC is the systemic activation of coagulation, as well as the depletion of platelets and coagulation proteins as a result of ongoing coagulation.

b. DIC is an acquired disorder.

c. DIC has two difficult-to-manage sequelae.

   (1) Intravascular formation of fibrin, thrombotic occlusion of small and medium-sized vessels, and subsequent organ ischemia.
   (2) Bleeding.

d. The depletion of platelets is problematic, and typically platelet numbers are less than 100,000 cells/μL at the time of diagnosis.

e. DIC is associated with multiple disease states and conditions, most commonly infection, cancer, and pregnancy (Box 34-4).

f. Treatment is supportive, and prophylactic transfusions with platelets are not recommended.[30] However, patients with fewer than 20,000 platelets/μL or with bleeding complications should be given platelet transfusions (goal >100,000/μL).

E. POSTTRANSFUSION PURPURA

1. Posttransfusion purpura (PTP) is an uncommon transfusion reaction that results in severe thrombocytopenia.

2. PTP lasts days to weeks.

3. PTP develops approximately 7 days after transfusion of platelets or red blood cells (which may also contain platelets).

4. It is an immune-mediated process that mimics drug-induced thrombocytopenia and ITP, especially because the peripheral blood smears and bone marrow aspirates are the same.

BOX 34-4

MAJOR CAUSES OF DISSEMINATED INTRAVASCULAR COAGULATION

Infections
  Gram-negative bacterial sepsis
  Other bacteria, fungi, viruses, Rocky Mountain spotted fever, malaria
Obstetrical complications
  Amniotic fluid embolism
  Retained dead fetus
  Abruptio placentae
  Toxemia
  Septic abortion
Malignancies
  Pancreatic carcinoma
  Adenocarcinomas
  Acute promyelocytic leukemia
  Other neoplasms
Liver failure
Acute pancreatitis
Envenomation
Transfusion reactions
Respiratory distress syndrome
Trauma, shock
  Brain injury
  Crush injury
  Burns
  Hypothermia, hyperthermia
  Fat embolism
  Hypoxia, ischemia
  Surgery
Vascular disorders
  Giant hemangioma (Kasabach-Merritt syndrome)
  Vascular tumors

From Goldman L, Bennett JC. Cecil textbook of medicine, 21st ed. Philadelphia: WB Saunders; 1999.

5. Patients with PTP are sensitized to foreign antigens during pregnancy or by previous transfusion.
6. PTP affects women (white) more often than men.[31]
7. First-line treatment is IVIG in high doses. A response is seen in 4 to 5 days.
8. Corticosteroids and exchange transfusion are also effective but take 1 to 2 weeks for a response.[32]
9. Patients with PTP should receive only washed cells in the future.

PEARLS AND PITFALLS

- Before low platelet counts are evaluated, causes of pseudothrombocytopenia should be ruled out.
- Heparin-induced thrombocytopenia can develop at very low doses of heparin, such as the amount used in intravenous line flushes.
- Isolated thrombocytopenia usually suggests immune thrombocytopenia or pseudothrombocytopenia.
- HIV-associated thrombocytopenia may be due to decreased production as well as increased destruction.
- DIC treatment is primarily supportive, and interventions should be aimed at treating the underlying disorders.

34

THROMBOCYTOPENIA

REFERENCES

[c] 1. Lacey JV, Penner JA. Management of idiopathic thrombocytopenic purpura in the adult. Semin Thromb Haemost 1977; 3(3):160.

[c] 2. Bell WR. Bleeding disorders. In Stobo JD et al, editors. The principles and practice of medicine, 23rd ed. Stamford, Conn: Appleton & Lange; 1996.

[e] 3. Payne BA, Pierre RV. Pseudothrombocytopenia: a laboratory artifact with potentially serious consequences. Mayo Clinic Proc 1984; 59(2):123.

[e] 4. Casonato A et al. EDTA dependent pseudothrombocytopenia caused by antibodies against the cytoadhesive receptor GPIIb-IIIa. J Clin Pathol 1994; 47(7):625.

[b] 5. Francois B et al. Thrombocytopenia in the sepsis syndrome: role of hemophagocytosis and macrophage colony–stimulating factor. Am J Med 1997; 103(2):114.

[d] 6. George JN et al. Idiopathic thrombocytopenic purpura: a practice guideline developed by explicit methods for the American Society of Hematology. Blood 1996; 88(1):3.

[c] 7. Rivzi MA, Kojouri K, George JN. Drug-induced thrombocytopenia: an updated systematic review. Ann Intern Med 2001; 134(4):346.

[a] 8. Berkowitz SD et al. Occurrence and clinical significance of thrombocytopenia in a population undergoing high-risk percutaneous coronary revascularization: evaluation of c7E3 for the Prevention of Ischemic Complications (EPIC) Study Group. J Am Coll Cardiol 1998; 32(2):311.

[e] 9. Curtis BR et al. Thrombocytopenia after second exposure to abciximab is caused by antibodies that recognize abciximab-coated platelets. Blood 2002; 99(6):2054.

[b] 10. Pedersen-Bjergaard U, Andersen M, Hansen PB. Drug-induced thrombocytopenia: clinical data on 309 cases and the effect of corticosteroid therapy. Eur J Clin Pharmacol 1997; 52:183.

[e] 11. Greinacher A et al. Laboratory diagnosis of heparin-associated thrombocytopenia and comparison of platelet aggregation test, heparin-induced platelet activation test, and platelet factor 4/heparin enzyme-linked immunosorbent assay. Transfusion 1994; 71(5):641.

[a] 12. Warkentin TE et al. Heparin-induced thrombocytopenia in patients treated with low-molecular-weight heparin or unfractionated heparin. N Engl J Med 1995; 332(20):1330.

[e] 13. Amiral J et al. Platelet factor 4 complexed to heparin is the target for antibodies generated in heparin-induced thrombocytopenia. Thromb Haemost 1992; 68(1):95.

[b] 14. Warkentin TE, Kelton JG. Temporal aspects of heparin-induced thrombocytopenia. N Engl J Med 2001; 344:1286.

[e] 15. Sheridan D, Carter C, Kelton JG. A diagnostic test for heparin-induced thrombocytopenia. Blood 1986; 67(1):27.

[b] 16. Warkentin TE et al. Impact of the patient population on the risk for heparin-induced thrombocytopenia. Blood 2000; 96(5):1703.

[c] 17. Warkentin TE. Clinical presentation of heparin-induced thrombocytopenia. Semin Hematol 1998; 4 (suppl 5):9.

[b] 18. Warkentin TE et al. The pathogenesis of venous limb gangrene associated with heparin-induced thrombocytopenia. Ann Intern Med 1997; 127(9):804.

[e] 19. Wright JF, Blanchette VS, Wang H. Characterization of platelet-reactive antibodies in children with varicella-associated acute idiopathic thrombocytopenic purpura (ITP). Br J Haematol 1996; 95(1):145.

[c] 20. George JN, El-Harake MA, Aster RH. Thrombocytopenia due to enhanced platelet destruction by immunologic mechanisms. In Beutler E et al, editors. Williams hematology, 5th ed. New York: McGraw-Hill; 1995.

[c] 21. George JN et al. Drug-induced thrombocytopenia: a systematic review of published case reports. Ann Intern Med 1998; 129(11):886.

[a] 22. Godeau B et al. Intravenous immunoglobulin for adults with autoimmune thrombocytopenic purpura: results of a randomized trial comparing 0.5 and 1 g/kg body weight. Br J Haematol 1999; 107(4):716.

[b] 23. Najean Y, Lecompte T. Chronic pure thrombocytopenia in elderly patients: an aspect of myelodysplastic syndrome. Cancer 1989 ;64(12):2506.

[b] 24. Menke DM et al. Refractory thrombocytopenia: a myelodysplastic syndrome that may mimic immune thrombocytopenic purpura. Am J Clin Pathol 1992; 98(5):502.

[b] 25. Stasi R et al. Long-term observation of 208 adults with chronic idiopathic thrombocytopenic purpura. Am J Med 1995; 98(5):436.

[e] 26. Scaradavou A et al. Intravenous anti-D treatment of idiopathic thrombocytopenic purpura: experience in 272 patients. Blood 1997; 89(8):2689.

[b] 27. Furlan M et al. Von Willebrand factor–cleaving protease in thrombotic thrombocytopenic purpura and the hemolytic-uremic syndrome. N Engl J Med 1998; 339(22):1578.

[e] 28. Tsai HM, Lian EC. Antibodies to von Willebrand factor–cleaving protease in acute thrombotic thrombocytopenic purpura. N Engl J Med 1998 ;339(22):1585.

[b] 29. Bell WR et al. Improved survival in thrombotic thrombocytopenic purpura–hemolytic uremic syndrome: clinical experience in 108 patients. N Engl J Med 1991; 325(6):398.

[c] 30. Levi M, ten Cate H. Disseminated intravascular coagulation. N Engl J Med 1999; 341:586.

[c] 31. McCrae KR, Herman JH. Post-transfusion purpura: two unusual cases and a literature review. Am J Hematol 1996; 52(3):205.

[e] 32. Becker T et al. High-dose intravenous immunoglobulin for post-transfusion purpura. Br J Haematol 1985; 61(1):149.

Neutropenic Fever

Tatiana M. Prowell, MD, and B. Douglas Smith, MD

FAST FACTS

- Neutropenic fever is defined as one temperature of 38.3° C or higher, or 1 hour of temperatures of 38° C or higher, in the setting of an absolute neutrophil count (ANC) less than 500/mm³.
- The prognosis of neutropenic fever is determined primarily by the severity and duration of neutropenia. An ANC below 100/mm³ and neutropenia of greater than 7 days' duration are associated with the poorest outcomes.[1]
- Patients with neutropenic fever often have infection without any localizing signs or symptoms because of their inability to mount an inflammatory response.
- Risk factors for infection in neutropenic patients include advanced age, medical comorbidities, leukemia induction or bone marrow transplant, inpatient status, indwelling catheter, malnutrition, loss of mucosal integrity, neurological impairment, and atelectasis or aspiration.[2]

35

I. EPIDEMIOLOGY

1. Neutropenic fever is the most common indication for nonelective admission of oncology patients, both during and after chemotherapy.[3]
2. Patients with neutropenia of more than 2 weeks' duration have nearly a 100% incidence of documented bacterial or fungal infection.[4,5]
3. The pathogens infecting neutropenic patients have changed in the past few decades.
   a. Historically, gram-negative organisms such as *Escherichia coli, Klebsiella,* and *Pseudomonas aeruginosa* have been the bacterial organisms most often isolated in patients with neutropenic fever, but over the past decade *Streptococcus viridans* and *Staphylococcus epidermidis* have become the most common isolates. This is thought to be due to increased use of indwelling catheters and antimicrobial prophylaxis against gram-negative organisms.[3]
   b. Among patients with leukemia, a threefold to eightfold increase in the incidence of fungal infections has occurred in recent decades, with approximately 80% of fungal infections caused by *Candida* species.[6]

II. CLINICAL PRESENTATION

1. Neutropenia is defined as an ANC less than 500/mm³. In a patient with neutropenia a fever is defined as one temperature of 38.3° C or higher, or an hour of persistent temperatures of 38° C or higher.[7]
2. Fever is frequently an incidental finding during a routine assessment of

vital signs at home or by a health care provider. Because patients lack the ability to mount an inflammatory response, localized signs and symptoms of infection may be absent. For example, the absence of an infiltrate on radiography does not rule out pneumonia.

3. The most commonly identified sites of infection in a neutropenic host are the oropharynx, sinuses, lungs, urinary tract, perirectal area, and skin, especially around the site of an indwelling catheter. Thus the physical examination and initial diagnostic studies should focus on these areas, although the majority of infections in neutropenic fever are manifested solely as bacteremia.[6]

III. DIAGNOSTICS

1. The diagnosis of neutropenic fever is easily defined, but determination of its source can be challenging. Current guidelines from the Infectious Disease Society of America recommend that in addition to a thorough history and physical examination, the initial workup include cultures of blood (peripheral and from all catheter ports), urine, any lesions noted, and stools (if diarrhea is present) before initiation of antimicrobial agents, as well as a complete blood cell (CBC) count, chemistries (to assess electrolytes and renal and hepatic function), and a chest radiograph. Additional testing should be guided by the results of the history and physical examination.[1] Current guidelines can be found online at www.idsociety.org.

2. Recent studies suggest that low serum protein concentrations at the initial evaluation for neutropenic fever are associated with an increased risk for septic shock, even before the development of clinical signs or symptoms. Although not yet widely used, protein C levels may become an important tool in early identification of patients requiring more aggressive therapy.[8]

IV. MANAGEMENT

1. Withholding empirical antibiotics from febrile patients with neutropenia is associated with a mortality rate greater than 80% to 90%.[3,9,10] With the use of empirical antibiotics, however, the mortality rate associated with neutropenic fever has fallen to less than 10%.[5]

2. The optimal treatment regimen and duration of therapy have not been established by randomized trials, but most experts recommend continuation of broad-spectrum antimicrobial agents until the patient becomes afebrile and neutropenia resolves (ANC >500/mm^3) or until clinically indicated, whichever is longer (Fig. 35-1).[5]

a. Conventional therapy for neutropenic fever has been an antipseudomo-nal β-lactam combined with an aminoglycoside,[11] such as piperacillin-tazobactam 3.375 g IV q4h and tobramycin 2 mg/kg IV load followed by 1.7 mg/kg IV q8h (goal peak level 4-10 μg/mL and goal trough level 1-2 μg/mL).

b. As a consequence of the nephrotoxicity associated with aminoglycosides and the increasing prevalence of gram-positive culture isolates, alternative parenteral regimens have been studied.[12] Those shown in clinical trials to have equivalent or superior efficacy with less toxicity include monotherapy with imipenem-cilastatin 500 mg IV q6h[13] or ceftazidime 2 g IV q8h.[14,15]

3. **No evidence has been presented to support routine use of vancomycin as part of the initial empirical regimen for neutropenic fever.**

a. Even patients whose cultures subsequently grew gram-positive bacteria resistant to the therapy they had received had no difference in survival with empirical inclusion of vancomycin at the start of therapy.[16]

b. Vancomycin should be considered in the initial regimen for patients who have severe mucositis, hypotension, or obvious catheter-associated infection, are receiving current fluoroquinolone prophylaxis, or are being treated in a center with a high prevalence of methicillin-resistant *Staphylococcus* or cephalosporin-resistant *Streptococcus.*[1]

4. **In patients with persistent fever despite 72 hours or more of broad-spectrum antibiotics, empirical antifungal coverage should be added because the risk for disseminated fungal infections increases both with increasing duration of neutropenia and with the use of broad-spectrum antibiotics.**

a. Treatment should begin with amphotericin B at a dose of 1 mg/kg/day and be increased to a maximum dose of 1.5 mg/kg/day for persistent fever after 24 hours at a given dose.[17,18]

b. Liposomal amphotericin B at 3 mg/kg/day is as effective as conventional amphotericin B in terms of treatment success and survival with less nephrotoxicity, fewer infusion-associated side effects, and fewer breakthrough fungal infections.[19]

c. Voriconazole was also compared to amphotericin B in a randomized multicenter trial and found to have improved efficacy, as well as an absolute mortality benefit of 13% in the treatment of suspected invasive aspergillosis. It has the benefit of being available in an oral form. As management of neutropenic fever increasingly shifts to the outpatient setting, voriconazole may eventually replace amphotericin as the drug of choice for empirical therapy for suspected fungal pathogens.[20]

5. **Many attempts have been made to devise a prediction rule to identify febrile neutropenic patients at low risk of complications.**

a. The best known of these is the Talcott prediction rule, which classified patients into four groups. The "low-risk" group (patients with a malignancy responding to therapy and no medical comorbidities) had a mortality rate of zero and a complication rate below 3%, as compared with the higher risk groups who had approximately a 15% mortality rate and a greater than 30% complication rate.[21]

b. A more comprehensive prediction model was designed and validated in an international prospective study by the Multinational Association of Supportive Care in Cancer (MASCC) (Table 35-1).[22]

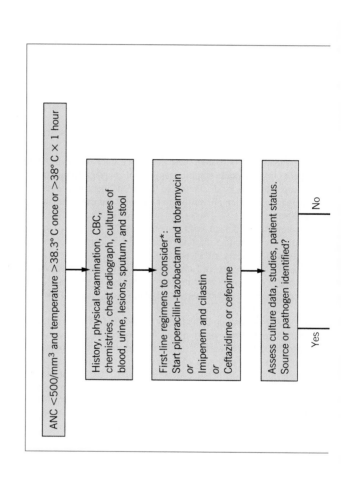

ANC <500/mm³ and temperature >38.3° C once or >38° C × 1 hour

History, physical examination, CBC, chemistries, chest radiograph, cultures of blood, urine, lesions, sputum, and stool

First-line regimens to consider*:
Start piperacillin-tazobactam and tobramycin
or
Imipenem and cilastin
or
Ceftazidime or cefepime

Assess culture data, studies, patient status. Source or pathogen identified?

Yes   No

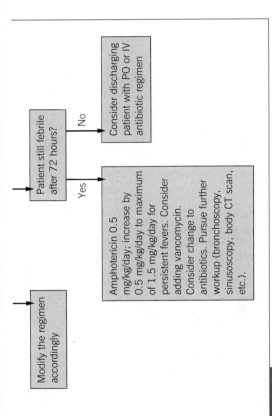

FIG. 35-1

Treatment of neutropenic fever. *Specific antibiotic choices will vary based on hospital formulary and local trends in pathogens and antibiotic resistance.

NEUTROPENIC FEVER 35

TABLE 35-1

FACTORS ASSOCIATED WITH LOW RISK OF COMPLICATIONS FROM
NEUTROPENIC FEVER AND THEIR PREDICTIVE VALUE

Factor	Odds Ratio	95% Confidence Interval	Weight
Minimal or no symptoms from cancer	8.21	4.15-16.38	5
No hypotension	7.62	2.91-19.89	5
No chronic obstructive pulmonary disease	5.35	1.86-15.46	4
Solid tumor, or if a heme tumor, no history of fungal infection	5.07	1.97-12.95	4
No dehydration	3.81	1.89-7.73	3
Moderate symptoms from cancer	3.70	2.18-6.29	3
Outpatient	3.51	2.02-6.04	2
Age <60 years	2.45	1.51-4.01	2

Data from Klatersky J et al for Multinational Association of Supportive Care in Cancer. J Clin Oncol 2000; 18:3038.

The total score is the sum of the weights, with a higher score indicating lower risk. Any score of 21 or higher is considered "low-risk." Using a MASCC risk index score of 21 or greater, the positive predictive value was 91%, sensitivity 71%, and specificity 68% in identifying patients alive and without serious complications at 5 days. The prediction rule outperforms the Talcott prediction rule in all parameters except specificity (90%).

6. Some low-risk patients[23] can safely be treated with oral antibiotics on an inpatient basis or even as outpatient therapy.

a. Several trials have shown that for low-risk patients hospitalized with fever and neutropenia expected to resolve within 10 days, oral therapy (ciprofloxacin 750 mg PO bid or tid, combined with amoxicillin-clavulanate 500-625 mg PO tid) is equivalent to conventional IV antibiotics in terms of treatment success, duration of fever and therapy, and survival.[24,25]

b. If low-risk patients are in a stable social situation, an outpatient antibiotic regimen, preceded by a brief observation period in an ambulatory care setting, is safe, effective, and associated with considerable financial savings and improved patient satisfaction.[1,26]

7. Trials evaluating the routine use of hematopoietic growth factors such as granulocyte colony–stimulating factor or granulocyte-macrophage colony–stimulating factor in febrile neutropenic patients have failed to show any significant improvement in clinical outcomes or survival, although one showed a reduction in duration of neutropenia by 1 day.[27-29] Use of growth factors in the subset of high-risk patients, defined as those expected to have neutropenia of 10 or more days' duration with fevers higher than 40° C or documented infection, does appear to have some value.[30]

PEARLS AND PITFALLS

- Routine pharmacological prophylaxis against bacterial infections, although of variable efficacy in preventing bacteremia, has not been shown to decrease infection-related mortality and selects for antimicrobial resistance both in the community and in the individual patient.[7,31] Outside of the bone marrow transplantation setting, it is not recommended. Some experts are in favor of using prophylactic antibiotics in the subset of patients undergoing cyclic chemotherapy who have had multiple prior episodes of neutropenic fever, although no evidence is available to support this practice.

- Prophylaxis against fungal infections by use of amphotericin B nasal spray, low-dose IV amphotericin B, or fluconazole has no effect on the rate of invasive mycoses.[6,32,33] Although fluconazole clearly decreases the risk of colonization and superficial infection with *Candida* species, it is generally not regarded as cost effective.[34,35]
- In neutropenic patients with positive serological tests for herpes simplex virus (HSV), acyclovir 1000 mg PO daily in divided doses has been found to prevent HSV outbreaks and reduce the severity of mucositis.[36]
- Neutropenic patients are routinely advised to wash raw fruits and vegetables thoroughly before eating them, although no data have been presented to support this practice.
- Patients should be counseled to maintain an active lifestyle, since data show that improved performance status is associated with better tolerance of chemotherapy and its complications.

REFERENCES

[c] 1. Bodey G et al. Quantitative relationships between circulating leukocytes and infections in patients with acute leukemia. Ann Intern Med 1996; 64:328.

[c] 2. Tice A. Outpatient parenteral antibiotic therapy for fever and neutropenia. Infect Dis Clin North Am 1998; 12:963.

[c] 3. Pizzo P. Drug therapy: management of fever in patients with cancer and treatment-induced neutropenia. N Engl J Med 1993; 328:1323.

[c] 4. Rubin R et al. Understanding and diagnosing infectious complications in the immunocompromised host: current issues and trends. Hematol Oncol Clin North Am 1993; 7:795.

[c] 5. Chanock S et al. Fever in the neutropenic host. Infect Dis Clin North Am 1996; 10:777.

[c] 6. Emmanouilides C et al. Opportunistic infections in oncologic patients. Hematol Oncol Clin North Am 1996; 10:841.

[d] 7. Hughes W et al. 1997 Guidelines for the use of antimicrobial agents in neutropenic patients with unexplained fever. Clin Infect Dis 1997; 25:551.

[b] 8. Mesters R et al. Prognostic value of protein C concentrations in neutropenic patients at high risk of severe septic complications. Crit Care Med 2000; 28:2209.

[a] 9. Schimpff S et al. Empiric therapy with carbenicillin and gentamicin for febrile patients with cancer and granulocytopenia. N Engl J Med 1971; 284:1061.

[d] 10. Hughes W et al. Guideline for the use of antimicrobial agents in neutropenic patients with unexplained fevers. J Infect Dis 1990; 161:381.

[a] 11. Bodey G et al. Beta-lactam regimens for the febrile neutropenic patient. Cancer 1990; 65:9.

[a] 12. EROTC International Antimicrobial Therapy Cooperative Group E: Ceftazidime combined with a short or long course of amikacin for empiric therapy of gram-negative bacteremia in cancer patients with granulocytopenia. N Engl J Med 1987; 317:1692.

[a] 13. Winston D et al. Beta-lactam antibiotic therapy in febrile neutropenic patients: a randomized trial comparing cefoperazone plus piperacillin, ceftazidime plus piperacillin, and imipenem alone.

[b] 14. Sanders J et al. Ceftazidime monotherapy for empiric treatment of febrile, neutropenic patients: a meta-analysis. J Infect Dis 1992; 164:907.

[a] 15. DePauw B et al. Ceftazidime compared with piperacillin and tobramycin for the empiric treatment of fever in neutropenic patients with cancer. Am J Med 1994; 120:834.

[a] 16. EROTC International Antimicrobial Therapy Cooperative Group and the National Cancer Institute of Canada: Vancomycin added to empirical combination antibiotic therapy for fever in granulocytopenic cancer patients. J Infect Dis 1991; 163:951.

[c] 17. Walsh T et al. Empiric therapy with amphotericin B in febrile granulocytopenic patients. Rev Infect Dis 1991; 13:496.

[a] 18. Pizzo P et al. Empiric antibiotic and antifungal therapy for cancer patients with prolonged fever and granulocytopenia. Am J Med 1982; 72:101.

[a] 19. Walsh T et al. Liposomal amphotericin B for empirical therapy in patients with persistent fever and neutropenia. N Engl J Med 1999; 340:764.

[b] 20. Herbrecht R et al. Voriconazole versus amphotericin B for primary therapy of invasive aspergillosis. N Engl J Med 2002; 347:408.

[b] 21. Talcott J et al. Risk assessment in cancer patients with fever and neutropenia: a prospective, two-center validation of a prediction rule. J Clin Oncol 1992; 10:316.

[b] 22. Klatersky J et al for Multinational Association of Supportive Care in Cancer. The Multi-national Association of Supportive Care in Cancer risk index: a multinational scoring system for identifying low-risk febrile neutropenic cancer patients. J Clin Oncol 2000; 18:3038.

[c] 23. Rolston K et al. Early empiric antibiotic therapy for febrile neutropenia patients at low risk. Infect Dis Clin North Am 1996; 10:223.

[a] 24. Freifeld A et al. A double-blind comparison of empirical oral and intravenous antibiotic therapy for low-risk febrile patients with neutropenia during cancer chemotherapy. N Engl J Med 1999; 341:305.

[a] 25. Kern W et al. Oral versus intravenous empirical antimicrobial therapy for fever in patients with granulocytopenia who are receiving cancer chemotherapy. N Engl J Med 1999; 341:312.

[c] 26. Rubenstein E et al. Outpatient treatment of febrile episodes in low-risk neutropenic patients with cancer. Cancer 1993; 71:3640.

[b] 27. Gruson D et al. Impact of colony-stimulating factor therapy on clinical outcome and frequency rate of nosocomial infections in intensive care unit neutropenic patients. Crit Care Med 2000; 28:3155.

[a] 28. Anaissie E et al. Randomized comparison between antibiotics alone and antibiotics plus granulocyte-macrophage colony–stimulating factor in cancer patients with fever and neutropenia. Am J Med 1996; 100:17.

[a] 29. Maher D et al. Filgrastim in patients with chemotherapy-induced febrile neutropenia: a double-blind, placebo-controlled trial. Ann Intern Med 1994; 121:492.

[d] 30. American Society of Clinical Oncology: American Society of Clinical Oncology recommendations for the use of hematopoietic colony-stimulating factors: evidence-based clinical practice guidelines. J Clin Oncol 1994; 12:2471.

[c] 31. Cruciani M et al. Prophylaxis with fluoroquinolones for bacterial infections in neutropenic patients: a metaanalysis. Clin Infect Dis 1996; 23:795.

[a] 32. Perfect J et al. Prophylactic intravenous amphotericin-B in neutropenic autologous bone marrow transplant recipients. J Infect Dis 1992; 165:891.

[b] 33. Rousey S et al. Low-dose amphotericin-B prophylaxis against invasive *Aspergillus* infections in allogeneic marrow transplantation. Am J Med 1991; 91:484.

[a] 34. Schaffner A et al. Effect of prophylactic fluconazole on the frequency of fungal infections, amphotericin-B use, and health care costs in patients undergoing intensive chemotherapy for hematologic neoplasias. J Infect Dis 1995; 172:1035.

[a] 35. Winston D et al. Fluconazole prophylaxis in patients with acute leukemia: results of a randomized, placebo-controlled, double-blind, multicenter trial. Ann Intern Med 1993; 118:495.

[c] 36. Meyers J. Chemoprophylaxis of viral infections in immunocompromised patients. Eur J Cancer 1989; 25:1369.

Oncological Emergencies

David Wang, MD, Phil Nivatpumin, MD,
Josh Lauring, MD, PhD, and Carole Miller, MD

FAST FACTS

- Tumor lysis syndrome.
  - Tumor lysis syndrome, sometimes seen in malignant disease, is a group of metabolic abnormalities that includes hyperkalemia, hyperuricemia, hyperphosphatemia, and hypocalcemia.
  - The syndrome is usually associated with hematological malignancies but can be seen with some solid tumors, especially after therapy.
  - In highly metabolically active diseases, tumor lysis syndrome can occur with steroid treatment alone.
  - Acute, oliguric renal failure may develop from uric acid crystallization in the distal tubules and collecting system or calcium phosphate deposition in the tubules and interstitium. This causes an obstructive uropathy.
  - Patients at risk for tumor lysis syndrome should be treated with aggressive hydration and allopurinol.
  - The syndrome is potentially fatal but is treatable and often reversible.
- Hyperviscosity syndrome (HVS).
  - Viscosity is the resistance that a fluid exhibits to the flow of one layer over another.
  - HVS results from excessive paraproteinemia.
  - Symptoms are directly related to sludging within and decreased perfusion of the microcirculation, especially of the central nervous system (CNS), visual system, and cardiopulmonary system.
  - Relative plasma viscosity over 4.0 is often an indication for plasmapheresis.
  - Clinical symptoms of HVS in a susceptible patient, regardless of the plasma viscosity, should make the physician consider treatment.
- Epidural spinal cord compression (ESCC).
  - ESCC is defined as compression of the thecal sac by tumor in the epidural space at the level of the spinal cord or the cauda equina.
  - This complication occurs in 5% of patients with cancer.[1]
  - Corticosteroids and radiation therapy are the mainstays of treatment.
  - In the majority of cases the compression occurs in the thoracic spine, followed by the lumbosacral and cervical spine.

36

cont'd

FAST FACTS—CONT'D

- *Awareness of the possibility is essential.* The median delay from the onset of back pain to the diagnosis of ESCC is 2 months. The median delay from the onset of symptoms of actual spinal cord compression to the diagnosis of ESCC is 10 days.[2]
- Superior vena cava (SVC) syndrome.
  - Cancer is the most common cause of SVC syndrome.
  - Lung cancer and lymphoma account for over 90% of cases of SVC syndrome caused by malignancy.
  - SVC syndrome is not a true emergency unless evidence of airway obstruction or cerebral edema is present.
  - In the absence of airway obstruction or cerebral edema, the most important consideration is to make an accurate tissue diagnosis of cancer, since 60% of patients with SVC syndrome do not have a previously known diagnosis of cancer.
- Hypercalcemia.
  - Hypercalcemia is the most common metabolic complication of malignancy.
  - The most common pathophysiological mechanism is secretion of parathyroid hormone–related protein (PTHrP) by tumor cells.
  - Common presenting symptoms are lethargy, dehydration, constipation, and altered mental status. Acute renal failure is common.
  - Treatment involves volume resuscitation, initiation of diuresis with saline, and administration of bisphosphonates with or without calcitonin.
- Hemorrhagic cystitis.
  - Hemorrhagic cystitis is an acute or insidious diffuse bladder inflammation with hemorrhage.[3]
  - It can be caused by chemotherapy, radiation, malignancy, infiltrative processes (such as amyloid), or infections.
  - Radiation and chemotherapeutic agents account for the majority of severe bladder hemorrhages. Hemorrhage can occur immediately after or years after therapy.[4]
  - Cyclophosphamide commonly causes hemorrhagic cystitis.
  - Patients have urinary symptoms such as dysuria, urinary frequency, and urinary urgency along with hematuria. Development of urinary retention from clots may cause suprapubic or flank pain.
- Neoplastic meningitis.
  - Patients typically have signs and symptoms involving multiple levels of the CNS.
  - Lumbar puncture is the most important diagnostic test. Cytological tests on cerebrospinal fluid (CSF) are positive in up to 90% of cases after three lumbar punctures.

Fast Facts—cont'd

- Treatment generally involves focal craniospinal radiation and intrathecal chemotherapy.
- The prognosis is poor, but prompt recognition and treatment can improve the quality of life.
- Intracranial metastases.
  - Malignancies that commonly metastasize to the brain include melanoma, sarcoma, and cancers of the lung (40%), breast (40%), kidney, and colon.
  - Intracranial metastases are a common complication, affecting 18% to 22% of patients with cancer.[5]

Tumor Lysis Syndrome

I. EPIDEMIOLOGY AND CLINICAL PRESENTATION

1. Tumor lysis syndrome occurs in patients with acute leukemia and high-grade lymphoma (i.e., Burkitt's) because of the heavy tumor burden and rapid cell turnover rate. It has also been reported in patients with small cell lung carcinoma, breast carcinoma, sarcoma, ovarian malignancies, germ cell tumors, and medulloblastoma.

2. Tumor lysis syndrome occurs either spontaneously or after therapy (including preparative regimens for bone marrow transplantation). The incidence of hyperphosphatemia is lower in the spontaneous form, presumably because new malignant cells can utilize the excess phosphate. The incidence of spontaneously occurring tumor lysis syndrome is unknown. In one case series the syndrome developed in 8 of 33 patients with lymphoblastic lymphoma or "undifferentiated" lymphoma before treatment and 2 required hemodialysis.[6] Another case series of patients with Burkitt's lymphoma reported the development of spontaneous tumor lysis syndrome in 33% of patients.[7]

3. Risk factors for the syndrome include young age (<25 years), male sex, advanced disease with abdominal involvement, high lactate dehydrogenase (LDH) level, prior volume depletion (from anorexia, fever, tachypnea, or "nothing by mouth" status for staging workup), and concentrated acidic urine.[8]

4. Metabolic derangements arise from rapid tumor cell death and release of intracellular potassium, phosphate, and purines. The kidneys normally excrete these products, but the excretory process becomes overwhelmed.

a. Hyperuricemia: Uric acid is the end product of purine metabolism (Fig. 36-1). It has been reported that patients with lymphoid malignancies have increased urinary excretion of uric acid even at lower serum levels than control subjects.[9,10] Urine uric acid concentrations are more accurate than plasma uric acid levels in predicting the risk of develop-

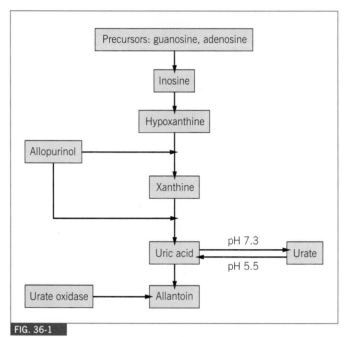

FIG. 36-1

Metabolic pathway for uric acid. *(Modified from Jones DP et al. Pediatr Nephrol 1995; 9:206.)*

ing uric acid nephropathy. Patients with uric acid nephropathy may have a urine uric acid/creatinine ratio above 1.0, whereas patients with acute renal failure from other causes have ratios less than 1.0.[10] Hyperuricosuria leads to crystallization of uric acid in renal tubules and collecting ducts, which is promoted by the acidic environment of the renal medulla. Crystallization leads to intraluminal tubular obstruction and damage to renal tubular epithelial cells, which phagocytose the crystals. Allopurinol inhibits xanthine oxidase, which decreases the production of uric acid.

b. Calcium phosphate deposition: This was discovered after renal failure developed in patients who were pretreated with allopurinol.[11] Calcium phosphate complexes form in the interstitium and in the renal tubules.

c. Acute renal failure worsens the hyperkalemia, hyperphosphatemia, and hypocalcemia.

d. Severity of the metabolic derangements depends on the timing and intensity of chemotherapy, intracellular electrolyte and solute levels, prophylactic measures, acid-base status, and glomerular filtration rate.[12]

BOX 36-1

CAUSES OF RENAL FAILURE IN PATIENTS WITH CANCER

Urinary obstruction

Severe volume depletion

Parenchymal disease

  Glomerulonephritis (e.g., cryoglobulinemia)

  Vasculitis

  Hypercalcemic nephropathy

  Tumor replacement

  Tumor lysis syndrome

    Acute uric acid nephropathy

    Calcium and phosphate nephropathy

  Myeloma kidney (cast nephropathy)

  Drug nephrotoxicity

    Methotrexate

    Cis-platinum

    Mitomycin C

    Interferon-alfa

    Interleukin-2

    Antibiotics

Modified from Arrambide K, Toto RD. Semin Nephrol 1993; 13(3):273.

II. DIAGNOSTICS

1. Tumor lysis syndrome should be suspected in a patient who has a tumor known to cause the syndrome and at presentation has a high LDH level, hyperuricemia (usually >15 mg/dL), hyperphosphatemia (usually >8 mg/dL), hyperkalemia, hypocalcemia, and renal failure.
2. Other causes of renal failure in patients with cancer must be ruled out (Box 36-1).

III. MANAGEMENT

1. Management of tumor lysis syndrome is divided into prevention and conservative therapy versus hemodialysis.[8]
2. Prevention includes an initial dose of allopurinol 600 to 900 mg PO followed by doses of 300 to 600 mg PO every day and aggressive hydration with intravenous fluids containing bicarbonate 50 to 100 mEq/L administered at a rate of 200 to 300 mL/hr. The goal urine pH should be 7.0 to 7.5. Daily urine output should exceed 2500 mL. If possible, allopurinol should be started at least 48 hours before initiation of cytoreductive therapy.[13] Often, however, chemotherapy cannot be delayed. Overzealous alkalinization should be avoided because this can precipitate further calcium phosphate deposition and worsen hypocalcemia by shifting calcium to its nonionized form.
3. Acetazolamide 5 mg/kg/day to maintain the solubility of uric acid can be considered. Because acetazolamide alkalinizes urine, it can also

paradoxically cause calcium phosphate deposition and shift calcium to its nonionized form.

4. Hyperkalemia should be aggressively treated with potassium restriction, Kayexalate, and loop diuretics. Maneuvers to shift potassium intracellularly should be used only as a temporizing measure.

5. For hyperphosphatemia, phosphate binders such as Amphojel should be used.

6. Only symptomatic hypocalcemia should be treated because exogenous calcium in the setting of hyperphosphatemia may produce metastatic calcification.

7. Indications for hemodialysis include metabolic acidosis, electrolyte imbalances, fluid overload, and uremia. At present, hemodialysis is preferred over peritoneal dialysis because of the higher uric acid and phosphorus clearance rates. Peritoneal dialysis can also be contraindicated in patients with abdominal disease. The role of continuous venovenous hemodialysis is being evaluated. Dialysis should be performed early because the duration of oliguria before initiation of dialysis correlates with the duration of oliguria after dialysis is initiated. Dialysis, once initiated, may be needed daily.

8. Fluid intake and output should be strictly monitored, and electrolyte levels (potassium, phosphate, uric acid, calcium) and patient weight should be checked twice daily.

Hyperviscosity Syndrome

I. EPIDEMIOLOGY

1. Elevated paraproteinemia is the most common cause of HVS. Of the paraproteinemias, Waldenström's macroglobulinemia/ lymphoplasmacytic lymphoma (immunoglobulin M [IgM] gammopathy associated with low-grade B-cell lymphoma) accounts for the majority of cases.[14]

2. The incidence of HVS in Waldenström's macroglobulinemia is nearly 20%.[15]

3. The second most common paraproteinemia related to HVS is multiple myeloma. The incidence of HVS is 4.2% in patients with IgG myeloma and up to 25% in those with IgA myeloma.[16]

II. CLINICAL PRESENTATION

1. The classic triad of symptoms includes visual disturbances, bleeding, and neurological manifestations.

2. Visual disturbances with occasional visual loss can be due to retinopathy characterized by "sausage-link" or "boxcar" venous engorgement of the retinal veins that leads to bleeding, exudates, microaneurysms, and rarely papilledema.

3. Bleeding from mucosal surfaces, including the gastrointestinal tract, is thought to be related to impaired platelet function.

4. Neurological manifestations include headache, dizziness, vertigo, hearing impairment, somnolence, seizures, stroke, and coma.
5. Cardiopulmonary findings may include pulmonary edema, myocardial infarction, and valvular abnormalities.

III. DIAGNOSTICS

1. Laboratory evaluation should include complete blood cell count, serum chemistries, plasma viscosity, whole blood viscosity, and coagulation profiles. Serum and urine protein electrophoresis should be requested if the patient is being evaluated for paraproteinemia.
2. Although values for absolute viscosity are measurable, plasma (or serum) viscosity or whole blood viscosity is measured clinically and reported as a value relative to that of water (in the case of serum) or blood at a certain hematocrit (in the case of whole blood).
3. Measurement of relative plasma viscosity involves placing a sample of the patient's serum in a capillary tube and a sample of water in another capillary tube. The time the serum and the water take to leave their respective tubes is measured. Relative plasma viscosity is the time for the serum divided by the time for the water.
4. Normal relative plasma viscosity is between 1.4 and 1.8. Values from 2.0 to 4.0 are abnormal but rarely symptomatic. Values above 4.0 are frequently symptomatic and are an indication for emergency treatment.[17]
5. Relative whole blood viscosity is measured in the same way as plasma viscosity except that rather than water in a standard tube, blood with a known hematocrit is used. The relative whole blood viscosity is calculated by a comparison of the time the sample takes to flow through the capillary tube with a standard curve of various blood samples with varying hematocrits. Therefore whole blood viscosity is reported as being comparable to a sample with a certain hematocrit (e.g., a patient's whole blood has a viscosity comparable to that of a patient with a hematocrit of 65%).
6. Relative whole blood viscosity of 55% or greater increases the risk of HVS.

IV. MANAGEMENT

1. Plasmapheresis is the gold standard of treatment.
2. Large-bore access is required for exchange. A dialysis catheter is adequate in the emergency setting. More permanent catheters (e.g., Quinton) are often placed by surgeons or interventional radiologists.
3. A larger percentage of IgG and IgA is extravascular (smaller molecules than IgM), and therefore paraproteinemia from IgG or IgA may require larger plasmapheresis volumes and repeated procedures to adequately reduce viscosity.[18] IgM is predominantly intravascular and can often be cleared in one or two treatments.
4. Packed red blood cell transfusions increase blood viscosity and ex-

acerbate symptoms. They should be withheld until the viscosity is measured and appropriately lowered.

5. Diuretics and volume depletion increase viscosity, and their use should be avoided.

Epidural Spinal Cord Compression

I. EPIDEMIOLOGY

1. Metastatic prostate cancer, breast cancer, and lung cancer each account for approximately 15% to 20% of cases.[19]
2. Renal cell cancer, non-Hodgkin's lymphoma, and multiple myeloma each account for approximately 5% to 10% of cases.
3. In an estimated 20% of cases of ESCC, the compression is the initial presentation of malignancy.[20]
4. Arterial seeding of bone is the most common route of entry into the vertebrae. In approximately 10% of cases, cells from paraspinal masses can enter directly via the neural foramen.
5. Tumors ultimately encircle the thecal sac, obstructing the epidural venous plexus and causing vasogenic edema and subsequent necrosis of white and gray matter.[21]
6. Corticosteroids may reduce vasogenic edema.

II. CLINICAL PRESENTATION

1. Pain is by far the most common complaint, occurring in up to 95% of patients with ESCC.[1]
2. Features of pain that suggest malignancy include worsening with recumbency (whereas pain from a herniated disk or degenerative disk disease usually improves with lying down).
3. Acute worsening of the pain may imply pathological vertebral fracture.
4. Unfortunately, the majority of patients with ESCC already have weakness at the time of diagnosis, with a high proportion no longer ambulatory.[22]
5. Weakness is usually symmetrical, and hemicord syndromes are rare (as opposed to intramedullary metastases).
6. Radicular symptoms occur more commonly in the lumbosacral spine than in the thoracic spine.
7. Commonly reported sensory symptoms include ascending numbness and paresthesias. Lhermitte's sign (sudden electric-like shocks extending down the spine with neck flexion) is rarely present. Saddle sensory findings are common in cauda equina syndrome.
8. Hyperreflexia below the level of the lesion is common.
9. Bladder and bowel dysfunction is a late symptom.

III. DIAGNOSTICS

1. Plain radiographs, computed tomography (CT), and bone scans are not sensitive in the detection of ESCC. The false negative rates are high.

If imaging shows obvious vertebral collapse or pedicle fracture, it is useful. However, a negative result should not deter further evaluation.
2. Magnetic resonance imaging (MRI) with gadolinium is the definitive study in evaluation for ESCC. It is widely available and easily tolerated. Evidence of physical compression of the spinal cord or the cauda equina in a symptomatic patient should prompt therapy.
3. CT myelography is useful when MRI is contraindicated.

IV. MANAGEMENT

1. Analgesics, including opiates, are often necessary for pain.
2. Aggressive bowel regimens are essential, given that autonomic dysfunction and limited mobility may increase the occurrence of constipation, ileus, and even abdominal viscus perforation.
3. Prophylaxis against deep venous thrombosis is strongly indicated for all paraparetic patients.
4. Bed rest is often unnecessary because patients know what maneuvers will exacerbate their pain.
5. Corticosteroids are frequently given. Debate exists as to the optimal dose. Only one randomized clinical trial has addressed the use of steroids in ESCC, and it demonstrated a significant benefit in ambulation at both 3 and 6 months.[23]
6. A typical steroid regimen consists of a 10-mg bolus of dexamethasone, followed by 16 to 40 mg daily in divided doses with a taper in the dose every 3 to 4 days.
7. Radiation is the therapy of choice for ESCC. Prompt consultation with the radiation oncology department is advised whenever ESCC is suspected.
8. Vertebrectomy should be considered for patients with spinal instability, local recurrence after spinal radiation therapy, a known radiation-resistant tumor (e.g., renal cell carcinoma), or deterioration during radiation therapy.

Superior Vena Cava Syndrome

I. EPIDEMIOLOGY

1. Malignant tumors account for approximately 80% of cases of the SVC syndrome. The remainder are caused by thrombosis or infection and its sequelae, such as fibrosing mediastinitis.
2. Among malignancies, lung cancer and lymphoma cause 94% of cases.[24]
3. Small cell lung cancer is more likely than non–small cell lung cancer to cause SVC syndrome because the former tends to develop centrally and the latter peripherally. SVC syndrome develops in up to 20% of patients with small cell lung cancer.
4. Among lymphomas, Hodgkin's disease rarely causes SVC obstruction, whereas diffuse large cell and lymphoblastic lymphomas are the usual

culprits. The remainder of malignant tumors that cause SVC syndrome include other mediastinal tumors such as thymomas, germ cell tumors, and metastases.

II. CLINICAL PRESENTATION

1. Dyspnea is the most common presenting symptom, followed by edema of the face, trunk, or extremities.
2. The most common signs are facial and upper extremity edema, jugular venous distention, distention of thoracic veins, and dyspnea. Less common is facial plethora.[25-27]

III. DIAGNOSTICS

1. Radiographic studies are necessary to demonstrate SVC compression or obstruction, to assess collateral blood flow, and to determine the location of the tumor or lymph nodes causing the obstruction. Chest radiographs are abnormal in approximately 80% of cases. The most common findings are superior mediastinal and right hilar masses, mediastinal widening, and pleural effusion. Contrast-enhanced CT gives the greatest information about the extent of tumor, the exact location of compression, and collateral vessels. MRI is an alternative if the patient cannot receive contrast dye. Radionuclide venography provides information about the vascular structures and flow but does not define the tumor.
2. A tissue diagnosis can be obtained in two thirds of cases by sputum cytology, pleural fluid cytology, or biopsy of enlarged peripheral lymph nodes. Bone marrow biopsy may be used to diagnose non-Hodgkin's lymphoma or small cell lung cancer, as well as provide staging information. Bronchoscopy, mediastinoscopy, thoracotomy, or CT-guided biopsy can facilitate the diagnosis in almost all other cases.[28] These procedures may also be indicated to provide staging information. Invasive diagnostic procedures may be performed with little risk of serious complications.

IV. MANAGEMENT

1. If there is no evidence of central airway obstruction or cerebral edema, therapy can safely be deferred until diagnostic tissue samples have been obtained.[29,30] Radiation therapy may prevent the determination of a tissue diagnosis in over 40% of cases.[31]
2. If stridor is present, prompt otolaryngology consultation should be obtained for possible tracheostomy. Administration of steroids to decrease laryngeal edema should be considered. Positive-pressure ventilation, with 20% oxygen/80% helium, and frequent suctioning as necessary to control secretions are other measures that may be helpful in the interim.
3. Supportive measures, such as diuretics and elevation of the head of the bed, may provide symptomatic relief. Nonemergency therapy

depends on the tissue diagnosis. Tumors that most commonly cause SVC syndrome are sensitive to chemotherapy, and chemotherapy is superior to radiation alone. Combination therapy decreases local recurrence rates of non-Hodgkin's lymphomas and improves survival in limited-stage small cell lung cancer. Radiation relieves symptoms in 70% of patients within 2 weeks. Non–small cell lung cancers respond poorly to therapy, and the development of SVC syndrome is a poor prognostic factor. With treatment most patients with SVC syndrome die as a result of progression of their underlying disease rather than from complications of SVC syndrome.

4. Endovascular stent placement may be considered for patients who cannot tolerate radiation or chemotherapy or for whom such treatments are unlikely to be successful. Studies have reported success rates of 68% to 100%, with most patients remaining symptom free until death.[32]

Hypercalcemia

I. EPIDEMIOLOGY

1. Hypercalcemia occurs in 10% to 20% of patients with cancer.
2. The most common associated tumors are breast and lung cancer and multiple myeloma.
3. Malignant tumors can increase serum calcium levels through several mechanisms.
a. Bone metastases produce local osteolysis mediated by cytokines and locally produced PTHrP. Multiple myeloma and lymphomas may secrete other osteoclast-activating factors.
b. Nonmetastatic solid tumors and non-Hodgkin's lymphomas may secrete PTHrP, which mimics many of the actions of PTH to increase serum calcium levels.
c. Hodgkin's lymphoma and some non-Hodgkin's lymphomas produce calcitriol, leading to increased calcium absorption from the intestine.
d. Use of estrogen or tamoxifen to treat patients with breast cancer and extensive bony metastases can lead to hypercalcemia.
4. PTHrP inhibits the tubular reabsorption of calcium, which potentiates osmotic diuresis and results in sodium and water loss. With worsening dehydration, often compounded by anorexia, vomiting, and immobility, renal function worsens and calcium excretion is further impaired.

II. CLINICAL PRESENTATION

1. Symptoms and signs develop when the serum calcium level increases to greater than 12 mg/dL. Clinical manifestations involve the gastrointestinal, renal, cardiovascular, and nervous systems. Anorexia, nausea and vomiting, constipation, and acute pancreatitis may develop. Polyuria leading to dehydration is common, and nephrolithiasis may

result. Hypertension may occur, although patients frequently have intravascular volume depletion. The QT interval on the electrocardiogram is shortened. Neurological manifestations include weakness, lethargy, fatigue, confusion, stupor, psychosis, and coma.

III. DIAGNOSTICS

1. Most patients already have a diagnosis of cancer because hypercalcemia is frequently a late complication. If cancer has not been diagnosed, rapid development of hypercalcemia with a low serum PTH level suggests malignancy.
2. The serum calcium and albumin levels should be obtained. The serum calcium concentration should be adjusted by 0.8 mg/dL for each 1 g/dL by which the albumin level differs from 4 g/dL.
3. Measurement of serum PTH or PTHrP has little clinical utility unless the cause of the hypercalcemia is in doubt.

IV. MANAGEMENT

1. **Saline:** Initial treatment involves restoration of intravascular volume with 0.9% saline. This lowers the calcium concentration by dilution and increases renal calcium excretion by restoring the glomerular filtration rate. Administration of 3 to 4 L/day should lead to euvolemia and maintain a brisk diuresis. Fluid intake and output should be closely monitored. Serum electrolyte, calcium, magnesium, and phosphorus levels should be checked two or three times a day.
2. **Diuretics:** Use of thiazide diuretics should be avoided because they worsen hypercalcemia. Loop diuretics, such as furosemide 80 to 100 mg q1-2h, have been shown to lower calcium levels.[33] Intense diuresis should be used cautiously because it may lead to persistent hypovolemia, as well as life-threatening hypokalemia and hypomagnesemia.
3. **Bisphosphonates:** These drugs inhibit bone resorption, thereby acting directly on the source of the hypercalcemia. Several agents have been shown to reduce serum calcium levels in the setting of malignancy. Pamidronate is the most effective bisphosphonate commonly used. A single dose of pamidronate is more effective than 3 days of etidronate and has a longer duration of action.[34] Zolendronate, which was recently approved for use, was shown to have better efficacy and duration of effect than pamidronate in pooled data from two phase III trials.[35] Zoledronic acid also has a shorter infusion time of 15 minutes. A dose of 90 mg of pamidronate normalized calcium concentrations in 100% of patients with malignancy who had a serum calcium level greater than 12 mg/dL after normal saline hydration.[36] Pamidronate is equally effective if given as a 4-hour or 24-hour infusion in normal saline. It may cause fever, hypomagnesemia, and hypophosphatemia. The maximum effect on calcium levels occurs in 2 to 4 days. Pamidronate 30 mg is sufficient for calcium levels less than 12 mg/dL. For levels between

12 and 13.5 mg/dL, 60 mg of pamidronate should be given, and for levels greater than 13.5 mg, 90 mg should be given.

4. **Calcitonin:** Salmon calcitonin works more rapidly than pamidronate and should be used for severe hypercalcemia. It inhibits bone resorption and increases urinary calcium excretion. Doses of 4 to 8 IU/kg IM or SC q6-12h lower the calcium concentration by 1 to 2 mg/dL within 4 to 6 hours. Calcitonin's usefulness is limited by tachyphylaxis, which develops in most patients. Calcitonin has a prolonged effect when a bisphosphonate is administered concomitantly.[37] Calcitonin also has potent analgesic effects on bone pain caused by skeletal metastases. Side effects include flushing, nausea, and abdominal cramping. Allergic reactions have been reported.

5. **Plicamycin:** This drug inhibits osteoclast function. A dose of 25 µg/kg infused over 4 to 6 hours and repeated every 24 to 48 hours will begin to lower calcium levels within 12 hours. Maximum effect occurs in 48 to 72 hours and lasts for days to weeks. Plicamycin has several important side effects, including hepatotoxicity, nephrotoxicity, and thrombocytopenia. Pamidronate was shown to be more effective and less toxic than plicamycin in a randomized crossover trial.[38] For these reasons it is used less frequently than pamidronate.

6. **Glucocorticoids:** For hypercalcemia associated with multiple myeloma and lymphoma, prednisone 20 to 40 mg/day reduces calcium concentration within 2 to 5 days.

7. **Dialysis:** For patients with calcium concentrations of 18 to 20 mg/dL, hemodialysis or peritoneal dialysis with a calcium-free dialysate bath can be effective. Dialysis may also play a role in patients with renal insufficiency or congestive heart failure who cannot tolerate saline diuresis.

8. **Other agents:** Gallium nitrate inhibits bone resorption. It must be administered as a continuous infusion over 5 days and has a slow onset of action and the potential to cause nephrotoxicity. Orally administered phosphate may modestly decrease serum calcium levels by decreasing intestinal calcium absorption. Its use is limited by dose-related diarrhea, and it should not be used if the serum phosphorus level is greater than 3 mg/dL or in the setting of renal insufficiency. Phosphate should not be administered intravenously because of the risk of metastatic soft tissue calcification, except in cases of life-threatening hypercalcemia when other treatments have failed.

Hemorrhagic Cystitis

I. EPIDEMIOLOGY

1. Hemorrhagic cystitis can occur in up to 20% of patients receiving cyclophosphamide or busulfan. Another chemotherapeutic agent that commonly causes hemorrhagic cystitis is ifosfamide.

2. Approximately 20% of patients who receive pelvic irradiation will develop a urological complication. Hematuria develops in 3%.[39]

3. Viruses that may be implicated in hemorrhagic cystitis include adenovirus, influenza, cytomegalovirus, herpes simplex virus, and BK virus. This should be considered in bone marrow transplant recipients.

4. Cyclophosphamide can cause hemorrhage, bladder fibrosis, and secondary bladder tumors. The effect is caused by acrolein, a degradation product of cyclophosphamide. Hemorrhagic cystitis developed in up to 40% of patients receiving the medication in early years.[40] In a Mayo Clinic review of 100 serial patients in whom hemorrhagic cystitis developed after cyclophosphamide administration, 20% required transfusion support and hemorrhage began on average after a cumulative oral dose of 90 g or intravenous dose of 18 g.[41] Cyclophosphamide-induced mucosal edema is followed by mucosal hyperplasia, papillary proliferation, and smooth muscle fiber contraction. Sloughing of the mucosa leads to hematuria.

5. Radiation therapy initially causes diffuse mucosal edema, which is followed by formation of vascular telangiectasias, submucosal hemorrhage, interstitial fibrosis, smooth muscle fibrosis, and obliterative endarteritis. Rupture of one of these ectatic vessels can lead to massive hemorrhage.

II. DIAGNOSTICS

1. Workup includes urinalysis, urine culture, coagulation parameters, plain radiographs, ultrasonography, and cystoscopy.

III. MANAGEMENT

1. Prophylaxis of cyclophosphamide-induced hemorrhagic cystitis includes IV hydration with forced diuresis or bladder irrigation. IV hydration should begin 12 to 24 hours before administration of cyclophosphamide and continue for 24 to 48 hours after completion of the dose. Loop diuretics should be used to maintain a urine output greater than $100 \text{ mL/m}^2/\text{hr}$.

2. In addition to IV hydration, diuresis, and bladder irrigation, mesna (2-mercaptoethane sulfonate) is administered. Mesna binds the metabolized product of cyclophosphamide, acrolein, which is toxic to the bladder. Mesna is first oxidized to an inactive disulfide, which becomes activated once it is excreted into urine. A dose of mesna 20% of the total cyclophosphamide dose (i.e., 200 mg mesna for 1000 mg of cyclophosphamide) is given at the time of cyclophosphamide administration, and then two or three additional 20% doses are given at intervals of 4 hours. Side effects include mild nausea and occasional vomiting. Mesna has decreased the incidence of hematuria and hemorrhagic cystitis after use of cyclophosphamide. In a randomized trial comparing IV hydration with mesna and with continuous bladder irrigation (CBI), mesna had a lower rate of mild to

moderate hematuria and there was no significant difference in the rate of severe hemorrhagic cystitis. Patients with CBI had a higher rate of urinary tract infections (27% versus 14%), bladder spasm, restriction of mobility, and severe discomfort (84% and 2%).[42]

3. In patients undergoing BMT, bladder irrigation and mesna equally decrease the incidence of severe bladder hemorrhage.

4. In general, when drug-induced hemorrhagic cystitis is suspected, management includes discontinuation of the offending agent, optimization of coagulation parameters, repletion of platelets, and symptomatic treatment (use of antispasmodics or narcotic analgesics). Packed red blood cells should be transfused as needed.

5. Hematuria may be classified as mild, moderate, or severe depending on response to therapeutic maneuvers and transfusion requirements.

6. For mild hematuria (defined as a stable hematocrit), bladder irrigation with water, saline, silver nitrate, or alum is performed. Silver nitrate may be instilled as a 0.5% to 1.0% solution made in sterile water for 10 to 20 minutes followed by saline irrigation. Alum is delivered by continuous bladder irrigation (300-1000 mL/hr) for 24 hours with a 1% solution of the ammonium or potassium salt made up in sterile water. Alum causes protein precipitation, vasoconstriction, and decreased capillary permeability but may take up to 7 days to cause cessation of hematuria.[3] Adverse effects of alum include suprapubic pain, fever, bladder spasm, urinary retention, and aluminum toxicity.

7. For moderate hematuria (defined as a decrease in hematocrit over days and requiring less than 6 units of packed red blood cells), any clots are evacuated and further clot formation is prevented by means of continuous bladder irrigation with water or saline. Aminocaproic acid or bladder instillation with alum or silver nitrate should be considered.

8. For severe hematuria (defined as hemorrhage refractory to simple irrigations, instillations, or aminocaproic acid and requiring more than 6 units of packed red blood cells), formalin instillation should be performed. Formalin works by fixing the bladder mucosa in vivo but can cause extreme pain. Instillation should be done by a urologist in the operating room with the patient under general anesthesia. Formalin concentrations of 1% or 10% are used. Complications of formalin therapy such as renal papillary necrosis, renal failure, ureteral stenosis, bladder contracture, and bladder rupture are decreased when formalin concentrations less than 4% are used. If formalin fails, selective embolization of the anterior branches of the hypogastric artery can be considered. Surgical options include cystotomy with bladder packing or urinary diversion and partial cystectomy.

9. Clots can be evacuated at the bedside with irrigation if bleeding has not been prolonged. If bleeding has continued for several days, cystoscopy may be necessary to determine the location of clots and cauterize bleeders.

36

ONCOLOGICAL EMERGENCIES

10. Aminocaproic acid (Amicar) inhibits fibrinolysis by inhibiting plasminogen activator substances. The loading dose is 5 g PO followed by 1 to 1.5 g hourly to a maximum of 30 g in a 24-hour period. Upper urinary tract bleeding must be ruled out because aminocaproic acid may cause clots to become more dense and difficult to pass.

11. Treatment of hemorrhagic cystitis is summarized in Fig. 36-2 and Table 36-1.

Neoplastic Meningitis

I. EPIDEMIOLOGY

1. As systemic treatment of cancer has improved with the use of chemotherapeutic agents that often do not penetrate the CSF, the incidence of neoplastic meningitis has risen dramatically. This has been particularly evident in the case of childhood leukemias, where 75% of those treated experienced relapse in the CNS before the introduction of routine CNS prophylaxis.

2. Almost any tumor can invade the meninges, but the most common are breast cancer, small cell lung cancer, melanoma, lymphoma, and leukemias.

II. CLINICAL PRESENTATION

1. The characteristic feature of neoplastic meningitis is the presence of neurological signs and symptoms at multiple levels of the neuraxis.[43,44]

2. Common presenting symptoms include headache, mental status changes, weakness, diplopia, paresthesias, radicular pain, and bowel or bladder dysfunction.

3. Common presenting signs include altered mental status, cranial nerve palsies (most commonly causing extraocular and facial muscle paresis), asymmetrical reflexes, and weakness. Neurological signs are typically more numerous and extensive than patient symptoms.

4. Signs and symptoms of raised intracranial pressure and seizures may also be present, but nuchal rigidity and signs of meningeal irritation are relatively uncommon (15%).

III. DIAGNOSTICS

1. Approximately 95% of patients with neoplastic meningitis already carry a diagnosis of cancer, and most have other metastases. A high index of suspicion is required to make the diagnosis in the other 5%. Early diagnosis of meningeal involvement is important for those with known cancer because progressive, irreversible neurological dysfunction and death occur within 4 to 6 weeks without treatment. The history and physical examination elucidate the symptoms and signs of neurological dysfunction and suggest the areas of nervous system involvement at multiple levels of the neuraxis.[43,44]

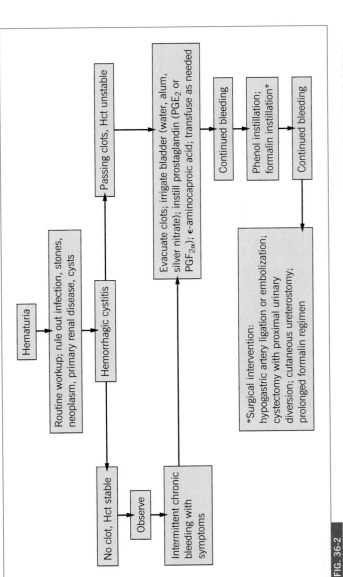

FIG. 36-2

Hematuria. *Hct,* Hematocrit; *PGE,* prostaglandin E; *PGF,* prostaglandin F. *(Modified from DeVries CR, Freiha FS. J Urol 1990; 143:1.)*

TABLE 36-1

TREATMENT OF HEMORRHAGIC CYSTITIS

Therapy	Administration	Duration	Advantages	Disadvantages
Normal saline	Continuous bladder irrigation	Until urine is clear	No adverse effects	Not effective as monotherapy in severe hemorrhagic cystitis
Alum	Continuous bladder irrigation with 1% solution	Until urine is clear	Mild adverse effects; no anesthesia required	Recurrence common; aluminum toxicity rare
Prostaglandins	Prostaglandin E₁ 375-750 μg; carboprost tromethamine 0.1-0.8 mg/dL instilled into bladder daily with dwell time of 1-4 hours	4-7 days	Very few adverse effects; no anesthesia required	Expensive; close monitoring required; uncertain efficacy
Silver nitrate	0.5%-1.0% solution instilled into bladder with dwell time of 10-20 minutes	Single application; repeat if no response	Patients may respond after other therapies fail	Short duration of response; anesthesia required; limited data in literature
Estrogens	5 mg/day PO, with or without 1 mg/kg IV bid for first 2 days of therapy	Until bleeding ceases; 7-10 days	Easily administered	Increased risk of cardiovascular complications; limited data in literature
Formalin	1%-10% solution instilled into bladder with dwell time of 5-30 minutes	Single application; repeat if no response	Successful response common	Anesthesia required; painful; risk of vesicoureteral reflux
Phenol	Bladder instillation of 100% solution	Single application	Used in refractory hemorrhagic cystitis	Limited data in literature
Vasopressin	Continuous IV infusion at 0.4 U/min	Until bleeding ceases	Used in refractory hemorrhagic cystitis	Limited data in literature; systemic adverse effects; limited duration of response
Aminocaproic acid	5 g IV q6h, then 300 mg/kg/day PO or continuous bladder irrigation (12 g/L) at 50 mL/hr	Until bleeding ceases	Used in refractory hemorrhagic cystitis	Limited data in literature; systemic adverse effects; limited duration of response

Modified from West NJ. Pharmacotherapy 1997; 17(4):696.

2. The most important diagnostic test is the lumbar puncture. The CSF is abnormal in more than 95% of cases, as defined by high opening pressure, elevated cell count or protein level, low glucose level, or positive cytological findings. Most patients have more than one abnormal value. Cytological study results are positive in more than 50% of initial CSF samples, and the yield increases to approximately 90% after three lumbar punctures.[43] Cytological study results may be falsely positive when reactive lymphocytes in the setting of infectious or inflammatory meningitis are mistaken for malignant lymphocytes. In these cases specimens should be sent for flow cytometry.

3. A variety of CSF biochemical markers, such as β-glucuronidase and lactate dehydrogenase, have been evaluated, but they are not sensitive or specific enough to be clinically useful.[45] An elevated CSF carcino-embryonic antigen level is specific for carcinomatous meningitis if it exceeds the serum level.[46]

4. Imaging studies are less sensitive and specific than lumbar puncture. Approximately one half of patients have abnormalities on CT, MRI, or myelography. The most common findings are hydrocephalus and contrast enhancement of the basilar cisterns or cortical convexities. Meningeal enhancement may be seen for several weeks after lumbar puncture, so imaging should be performed before lumbar puncture to avoid this potential confounder.[47] MRI of the brain and relevant portions of the spinal cord should be performed in patients with suspected neoplastic meningitis to determine the presence of brain metastases and the risk of herniation before lumbar puncture.

5. A positive CSF cytological result or appropriate neurological signs and symptoms with associated CSF or radiographic abnormalities establish the diagnosis.

IV. MANAGEMENT

1. Prognosis is generally poor. Without treatment, median survival is 4 to 6 weeks. Standard therapy extends survival to 3 to 6 months. In one series median 1-year survival was only 21%. Some patients with more indolent tumors, such as breast cancer and certain lymphomas, survive much longer. As with spinal cord compression from epidural metastases, neurological deficits become irreversible in a short time, necessitating prompt treatment to reduce the associated morbidity, even if the survival benefit is not great. As with all cancer therapy, evaluation of the patient's performance status, extent of systemic disease, and overall prognosis must be a prerequisite to the decision to pursue aggressive treatment or palliation.

2. Craniospinal radiation has become a cornerstone of therapy for leukemia and lymphoma with CNS involvement. However, solid tumors are more radiation resistant than hematological neoplasms and myelosuppression limits the dose. Instead radiation is focused on areas of bulky disease or symptomatic involvement.

36

ONCOLOGICAL EMERGENCIES

3. Intrathecal (IT) administration of chemotherapy through a subcutaneous (Ommaya) reservoir and intraventricular catheter has become standard because most chemotherapeutic agents do not achieve high or reliable levels in CSF when administered systemically. In clinical trials patients with leukemic meningitis have had better responses when IT chemotherapy was administered by Ommaya reservoir than when it was given by lumbar injection. Methotrexate, cytosine arabinoside (Ara-C), and thiotepa are the agents commonly used. Ara-C is effective mainly against leukemias and lymphomas. Methotrexate and thiotepa appear to be equivalent in efficacy and toxicity.[48] One open-label randomized trial showed a doubling of the time to neurological progression when IT depot Ara-C was used rather than IT methotrexate.[49]

4. Because tumor can obstruct CSF flow and therefore limit delivery of IT chemotherapy to all affected areas of the neuraxis, a radionuclide CSF flow scan is recommended. If results are abnormal, IT therapy can be delayed until radiation treatments are administered to sites of obstruction.

5. CSF is analyzed monthly until cytological studies become negative, and every 2 months thereafter.

6. Although the use of IT chemotherapy has become the standard of care for carcinomatous meningitis, no randomized, controlled studies have been published to support its use. One early series from Memorial Sloan-Kettering used historical control subjects to argue for improved survival with IT chemotherapy.[43] A retrospective analysis comparing two groups of patients with solid tumors and leptomeningeal metastases found no difference in response rate or survival between groups treated with and without IT chemotherapy. Both groups received radiation and systemic chemotherapy. The incidence of leukoencephalopathy, a complication of IT chemotherapy combined with radiation, was higher in the IT chemotherapy group.[50] One recent study compared patients with lymphomatous and carcinomatous meningitis treated with IT methotrexate against those treated with high-dose systemic methotrexate and found median survival improved in the IT methotrexate group. Randomized, prospective studies are needed to validate this finding.

Intracranial Metastases

I. CLINICAL PRESENTATION AND DIAGNOSTICS

1. Patients may complain of headache, focal weakness or sensory loss, or gait instability.

2. Findings on clinical neurological examination may be obvious or subtle.

3. Brain CT with contrast medium or MRI should be performed.

4. Signs of increasing intracranial pressure include decreased conscious-

ness, papilledema, pupillary abnormalities, ophthalmoplegia, posturing, nausea and vomiting, meningismus, and the Cushing reflex.[51]

II. MANAGEMENT

1. The physician should determine whether the mass is a new metastasis in a patient with known malignancy, a simultaneous presentation of a primary tumor and a brain metastasis, or a brain metastasis from an unknown primary tumor.

2. **Known malignancy:** The patient may have a single metastasis or multiple metastases. For a single brain metastasis, randomized trials suggest that if the primary tumor does not progress for 3 months, resection of the intracranial mass followed by radiation is the treatment of choice. One study compared surgery plus radiation versus radiation alone in 86 patients with non–small cell lung carcinoma.[52] Median survival with the combined treatment modality was 40 weeks, versus 15 weeks with radiation alone. A second study looked at patients with a variety of primary tumors and compared surgical resection plus radiation to radiation alone.[53] Median survival with the combined modality was 10 months, versus 6 months for radiation alone. Radiation surgery (proton beam, gamma knife, or linear accelerator) is another option. For multiple brain metastases, radiation therapy is the standard treatment and the median survival is 2 to 6 months.

3. **Simultaneous presentation:** When this occurs, the primary malignancy is often in the lung. With a single brain metastasis, both primary and metastatic lesions should be excised. Five-year survival in this population is 45%.[54] Craniotomy should precede thoracotomy.

4. **Unknown primary tumor:** A priority should be obtaining a tissue diagnosis from the intracranial lesion. An alternative is a workup for an unknown primary tumor, including basic laboratory tests, chest radiography, and thoracic and abdominal CT scans.

5. Cranial irradiation is usually given as 3000 cGy in divided fractions over a 2-week period.

6. Steroids should be used when the patient has significant brain edema. Brain edema results from increased permeability of the blood-brain barrier. Steroids are thought to stabilize the endothelial cells lining the blood-brain barrier, minimizing permeability. The standard dexamethasone dosage is 16 mg/day divided bid or qid.[55] Therapeutic effects should be seen within 48 hours. Proton pump inhibitors should be considered when high-dose steroids are being used.

7. Surgery is limited to patients with a solitary brain metastasis and those undergoing emergency craniotomy for increased intracranial pressure.

PEARLS AND PITFALLS

- Tumor lysis syndrome.
  - Allopurinol may cause rash (including Stevens-Johnson syndrome) or interstitial nephritis, lead to xanthine stone formation, or cause pneu-

mopathy. The IV form of allopurinol is available for patients unable to tolerate oral medications.

- Uricase 50 to 100 units/kg IV or IM is being used experimentally. Uricase converts uric acid to the water-soluble metabolite allantoin. One potential complication of uricase is anaphylaxis. Pegylated uricase can be given IM, which has a longer half-life and may allow the use of lower doses.[56]

- The role of prophylactic dialysis should be investigated. In pediatric populations continuous arteriovenous or venovenous hemodialysis has been used prophylactically. In one case series continuous venovenous hemodialysis (CVVHD) was initiated before chemotherapy for five children with either Burkitt's or acute lymphoblastic leukemia. Four maintained normal uric acid, potassium, blood urea nitrogen, and creatinine levels. Azotemia developed in the fifth child, who had an occluded CVVHD filter.[57]

- SVC syndrome.
  - SVC syndrome develops in some patients with malignancy because of clot extension from central venous catheters. Such patients can be treated with thrombolytic therapy with or without percutaneous transluminal angioplasty, followed by anticoagulant therapy.

- Hemorrhagic cystitis.
  - The role of prostaglandins in treatment of cyclophosphamide-induced cystitis continues to be investigated. PGE_2 (0.75 mg in 200 mL normal saline) has been instilled into the bladder and left for 4 hours.[58] This was repeated daily until bleeding stopped. Another case series reports use of PGF_2.[59] Carboplast is a synthetic derivative of PGF_2 that is administered as a solution of 0.1 to 0.8 mg/dL.[60] It is instilled into the bladder and left for several hours. Proposed mechanisms of prostaglandin infusions include protection of the microvasculature and epithelium and inhibition of the development of tissue edema.[3]
  - Investigational therapies for treatment of radiation-induced hemorrhagic cystitis include sodium pentosulfanpolysulfate, which mimics the bladder's normal glycosaminoglycan lining,[61] conjugated estrogen at 5 mg/day,[62] and hyperbaric oxygen at 2 to 2.5 atm.[63]

- Neoplastic meningitis.
  - Patients with hydrocephalus require placement of ventricular shunts. Shunts can be equipped with valves that allow the shunts to be turned off during IT chemotherapy sessions.
  - A leukoencephalopathy syndrome can develop after IT methotrexate therapy and brain irradiation.

- Intracranial metastases.
  - Cerebellar metastases may cause more severe symptoms than supratentorial metastases and be more difficult to identify because there are fewer localizing symptoms. Symptoms may include nausea and vomiting, headache, and gait disturbance.

- Intracranial hemorrhage occurs in 14% of patients with intracerebral metastases.[64]
- Seizures occur in 15% to 25% of patients with intracerebral metastases.[5] Phenytoin does not seem to alter the incidence.[65] Phenytoin interacts with dexamethasone, producing lower effective concentrations,[66] and can cause erythema multiforme in patients receiving cranial irradiation.[67] Because of this, phenytoin should not be used prophylactically but only after the initial seizure.
- Emergency treatment of increased intracranial pressure includes hyperventilation to a P_{CO_2} between 25 and 30 mm Hg, osmotic diuresis with mannitol (20%-25% solution given as 0.5-2.0 g/kg IV over 20-30 minutes), and dexamethasone at a dose of 40 to 100 mg.[3]

- Hyperviscosity syndrome: hyperleukocytosis.
  - The large number of myeloid or lymphoid cells in leukemia can result in leukostasis and compromise oxygen delivery to tissues. The packed cell volume of white blood cells (WBCs), or leukocrit, depends on both the number and size of cells. Large cells (e.g., monoblasts) increase the leukocrit more than small cells (e.g., lymphocytes). Therefore symptoms are most common in acute myeloid leukemia, followed by acute lymphocytic leukemia (AML), the blastic phase of chronic myelogenous leukemia, and chronic lymphocytic leukemia. There is no absolute WBC count cutoff for clinical symptoms, although symptoms are usually seen at counts greater than 100,000/mm³.[68]
  - Symptoms are similar to those of HVS. Clinical symptoms are usually related to CNS and pulmonary involvement. Oxygen delivery may be further hampered by the high metabolic activity of dividing blast cells. Hyperleukocytosis, particularly in AML, is a risk factor for intracerebral or pulmonary hemorrhage.[69] Patients with acute promyelocytic leukemia are particularly prone to disseminated intravascular coagulopathy. The initial mortality rate for patients with AML and symptomatic hyperleukocytosis is high.[70]

36

ONCOLOGICAL EMERGENCIES

REFERENCES

[c] 1. Schiff D, Batchelor T, Wen PY. Neurologic emergencies in cancer patients. Neurol Clin North Am 1998; 16(2):449.

[b] 2. Husband DJ. Malignant spinal cord compression: prospective study of delays in referral and treatment. Br Med J 1998; 317:18.

[c] 3. Russo P. Urologic emergencies in the cancer patient. Semin Oncol 2000; 27:284.

[c] 4. DeVries CR, Freiha FS. Hemorrhagic cystitis: a review. J Urol 1990; 143:1.

[b] 5. Zimm S et al. Intracerebral metastases in solid-tumor patients: natural history and results of treatment. Cancer 1981; 48:384.

[b] 6. Tsokos GC et al. Renal and metabolic complications of undifferentiated and lymphoblastic lymphomas. Medicine (Baltimore) 1981; 60:218.

[b] 7. Cohen LF et al. Acute tumor lysis syndrome: a review of 37 patients with Burkitt's lymphoma. Am J Med 1980; 68:486.

[c] 8. Arrambide K, Toto RD. Tumor lysis syndrome. Semin Nephrol 1993; 13(3):273.

[b] 9. Mir MA. Renal excretion of uric acid and its relation to relapse and remission in acute myeloid leukemia. Nephron 1977; 19:69.

[b] 10. Kelton J, Kelley WN, Holmes EW. A rapid method for the detection of acute uric acid nephropathy. Arch Intern Med 1978; 138:612.

[b] 11. Kanfer A et al. Extreme hyperphosphatemia causing acute anuric nephrocalcinosis in lymphosarcoma. BMJ 1979; 1:1320.

[c] 12. Jones DP, Mahmoud H, Chesney RW. Tumor lysis syndrome: pathogenesis and management. Pediatr Nephrol 1995; 9:206.

[b] 13. Razis E et al. Incidence and treatment of tumor lysis syndrome in patients with acute leukemia. Acta Haematol 1994; 91:171.

[c] 14. Pimentel L. Medical complications of oncologic disease. Emerg Med Clin North Am 1993; 11:407.

[b] 15. Preston FE et al. Myelomatoses and the hyperviscosity syndrome. Br J Haematol 1978; 38:517.

[b] 16. Whittaker JA, Puddenham EGD, Bradley J. Hyperviscosity syndrome in IgA multiple myeloma. Lancet 1973; 2:572.

[c] 17. Bloch KJ, Maki DG. Hyperviscosity syndromes associated with immunoglobulin abnormalities. Semin Hematol 1973; 10:113.

[c] 18. Kaplan AA. Towards a rational prescription of plasma exchange: the kinetics of immunoglobulin removal. Semin Dial 1992; 5:227.

[c] 19. Posner JB. Neurologic complications of cancer. Philadelphia: FA Davis; 1995.

[b] 20. Schiff D, O'Neill BP, Suman VJ. Spinal epidural metastasis as the initial manifestation of malignancy: clinical features and diagnostic approach. Neurology 1997; 49:452.

[c] 21. Siegal T. Spinal cord compression: from laboratory to clinic. Eur J Cancer 1995; 31A:1748.

[b] 22. Gilbert RW, Kim JH, Posner JB. Epidural spinal cord compression from metastatic tumor: diagnosis and treatment. Ann Neurol 1978; 3:40.

[a] 23. Sorensen S et al. Effect of high-dose dexamethasone in carcinomatous metastatic spinal cord compression treated with radiotherapy: a randomized trial. Eur J Cancer 1994; 30A:22.

[c] 24. Abner A. Approach to the patient who presents with superior vena cava obstruction. Chest 1993; 103:394S.

[b] 25. Armstrong BA et al. Role of irradiation in the management of superior vena cava syndrome. Int J Radiat Oncol Biol Phys 1987; 13:531.

[b] 26. Chen JC, Bongard F, Klein SR. A contemporary perspective on superior vena cava syndrome. Am J Surg 1990; 160:207.

[b] 27. Fincher RE. Superior vena cava syndrome: experience in a teaching hospital. South Med J 1987; 80:1243.

[b] 28. Porte H et al. Superior vena cava syndrome of malignant origin: which surgical procedure for which diagnosis? Eur J Cardiothorac Surg 2000; 17(4):384.

[b] 29. Schraufnagel DE et al. Superior vena caval obstruction: is it a medical emergency? Am J Med 1981; 70:1169.

[c] 30. Ahmann FR. A reassessment of the clinical implications of the superior vena caval syndrome. J Clin Oncol 1984 ;2:961.

[b] 31. Loeffler JS et al. Emergency prebiopsy radiation for mediastinal masses: impact on subsequent pathologic diagnosis and outcome. J Clin Oncol 1986; 4:716.

[c] 32. Yim CD, Sane SS, Bjarnason H. Superior vena cava stenting. Radiol Clin North Am 2000; 38:409.

[b] 33. Suki WN et al. Acute treatment of hypercalcemia with furosemide. N Engl J Med 1970; 283:836.

[a] 34. Gucalp R et al. Comparative study of pamidronate disodium and etidronate disodium in the treatment of cancer-related hypercalcemia. J Clin Oncol 1992; 10:134.

[a] 35. Major P et al. Zoledronic acid is superior to pamidronate in the treatment of hypercalcemia of malignancy: a pooled analysis of two randomized, controlled clinical trials. J Clin Oncol 2001; 19:558.

[a] 36. Nussbaum SR et al. Single-dose intravenous therapy with pamidronate for the treatment of hypercalcemia of malignancy: comparison of 30-, 60-, and 90-mg dosages. Am J Med 1993; 95:297.

[c] 37. Bilezikian JP. Management of hypercalcemia. J Clin Endocrinol Metab 1993; 77:1445.

[a] 38. Thurlimann B et al. Plicamycin and pamidronate in symptomatic tumor-related hypercalcemia: a prospective randomized crossover trial. Ann Oncol 1992; 3:619.

[b] 39. Dean RJ, Lytton B. Urologic complications of pelvic irradiation. J Urol 1978; 119:64.

[b] 40. Watson NA, Notley RG. Urologic complications of cyclophosphamide. Br Urol 1973; 45:606.

[b] 41. Stillwell TJ, Benson RC. Cyclophosphamide induced hemorrhagic cystitis: a review of 100 patients. Cancer 1988; 61:451.

[a] 42. Vose JM et al. Mesna compared with continuous bladder irrigation as uroprotection during high-dose chemotherapy and transplantation: a randomized trial. J Clin Oncol 1993; 11:1306.

[b] 43. Wasserstrom WR, Glass JP, Posner JB. Diagnosis and treatment of leptomeningeal metastases from solid tumors: experience with 90 patients. Cancer 1982; 49:759.

[b] 44. Olson ME, Chernik NL, Posner JB. Infiltration of the leptomeninges by systemic cancer: a clinical and pathologic study. Arch Neurol 1974; 30:122.

[c] 45. Grossman SA, Krabak MJ. Leptomeningeal carcinomatosis. Cancer Treat Rev 1999; 25:103.

[b] 46. Jacobi C, Reiber H, Felgenhauer K. The clinical relevance of locally produced carcinoembryonic antigen in cerebrospinal fluid. J Neurol 1986; 233:358.

[c] 47. DeAngelis LM. Current diagnosis and treatment of leptomeningeal metastasis. J Neurol Oncol 1998; 38:245.

[a] 48. Grossman SA et al. Randomized prospective comparison of intraventricular methotrexate and thiotepa in patents with previously untreated neoplastic meningitis. J Clin Oncol 1993; 11:561.

[a] 49. Glantz MJ et al. A randomized controlled trial comparing intrathecal sustained-release cytarabine (DepoCyt) to intrathecal methotrexate in patients with neoplastic meningitis from solid tumors. Clin Cancer Res 1999; 5:3394.

[b] 50. Bokstein F, Lossos A, Siegal T. Leptomeningeal metastases from solid tumors: a comparison of two prospective series treated with and without intra-cerebrospinal fluid chemotherapy. Cancer 1998; 82:1756.

[c] 51. Quinn JA, DeAngelis LM. Neurologic emergencies in the cancer patient. Semin Oncol 2000; 27(3):311.

[a] 52. Patchell RA et al. A randomized trial of surgery in the treatment of single metastases to the brain. N Engl J Med 1990; 322:494.

[a] 53. Vecht CJ et al. Treatment of single brain metastasis: radiotherapy alone or combined with neurosurgery? Ann Neurol 1993; 33:583.

[b] 54. Hankins JR et al. Surgical management of lung cancer with solitary cerebral metastasis. Ann Thorac Surg 1988; 46:24.

[c] 55. Vecht CJ. Clinical management of brain metastasis. J Neurol 1998; 245:127.

[b] 56. Chua CC et al. Use of polyethylene glycol–modified uricase (PEG-uricase) to treat hyperuricemia in a patient with non-Hodgkin lymphoma. Ann Intern Med 1988; 109:114.

[b] 57. Saccente SL, Kohaut EC, Berkow RL. Prevention of tumor lysis syndrome using continuous veno-venous hemofiltration. Pediatr Nephrol 1995; 9:569.

[b] 58. Mohiuddin J et al. Treatment of cyclophosphamide-induced cystitis with prostaglandin E_2. Ann Intern Med 1984; 101:142.

[b] 59. Shurafa M, Shumaker E, Cronin S. Prostaglandin F_2-alpha bladder irrigation for control of intractable cyclophosphamide-induced hemorrhagic cystitis. J Urol 1987; 137:1230.

[c] 60. West NJ. Prevention and treatment of hemorrhagic cystitis. Pharmacotherapy 1997; 17(4):696.

[b] 61. Parsons CL. Successful management of radiation cystitis with sodium pentosanpolysufate. J Urol 1986; 136:813.

[b] 62. Liu YK et al. Treatment of radiation or cyclophosphamide induced cystitis using conjugated estrogen. J Urol 1990; 144:41.

[b] 63. Mathews R et al. Hyperbaric oxygen therapy for radiation induced hemorrhagic cystitis. J Urol 1999; 161:435.

[b] 64. Mandybur TI. Intracranial hemorrhage caused by metastatic tumors. Neurology 1977; 27:650.

[b] 65. Cohen N et al. Should prophylactic anticonvulsants be administered to patients with newly diagnosed cerebral metastases: a retrospective analysis. J Clin Oncol 1988; 6:1621.

36

ONCOLOGICAL EMERGENCIES

[b] 66. Chalk JB et al. Phenytoin impairs the bioavailability of dexamethasone in neurological and neurosurgical patients. J Neurol Neurosurg Psychiatry 1984; 47:1087.

[b] 67. Delattre JY, Safai B, Posner JB. Erythema multiforme and Stevens-Johnson syndrome in patients receiving cranial irradiation and phenytoin. Neurology 1988; 38:194.

[b] 68. Cuttner J et al. Association of monocytic leukemia in patients with extreme leukocytosis. Am J Med 1980; 69:555.

[b] 69. Bunin NJ, Pui C-H. Differing complications of hyperleukocytosis in children with acute lymphoblastic or acute nonlymphoblastic leukemia. J Clin Oncol 1985; 3:1590.

[b] 70. Vaughan WP et al. Factors affecting survival of patients with acute myelocytic leukemia presenting with high WBC counts. Cancer Treat Rep 1981; 65:1007.

Primary Human Immunodeficiency Virus Infection

Amy C. Weintrob, MD, and Charles B. Hicks, MD

FAST FACTS

- Primary (or acute) human immunodeficiency virus (HIV) infection is the period after acquisition of HIV that is characterized by high levels of HIV replication, an expansive immunological response, and in the majority of patients a symptomatic illness.
- Between 50% and 90% of persons with primary HIV infection are symptomatic.[1,2]
- The most common presenting symptoms are fever, lymphadenopathy, pharyngitis, fatigue, rash, myalgia, arthralgia, and headaches.[1,3]
- Common laboratory abnormalities during primary HIV infection include lymphopenia, thrombocytopenia, atypical lymphocytes, and elevated levels of liver enzymes (alanine aminotransferase [ALT] and aspartate aminotransferase [AST]).[1,3]
- Routine screening assays for HIV (enzyme-linked immunosorbent assay [ELISA]) are often negative during primary HIV infection, and confirmatory tests (Western blot) may be negative or indeterminate.[4-6]
- Diagnosis of primary HIV infection requires the detection of p24 antigen in serum or high levels of HIV RNA or DNA in blood with either a negative HIV ELISA or a positive ELISA with a negative or indeterminate confirmatory Western blot.
- Current consensus panels advise that antiretroviral therapy be initiated during primary HIV infection. Referral to an HIV specialist is warranted.[7]

I. EPIDEMIOLOGY

1. Sexual intercourse is the most common way HIV is transmitted. Other modes of transmission include intravenous drug use, oral-genital contact, transfusion of contaminated blood or blood products, and vertical transmission.[8]

2. To minimize the risk of transfusion-related HIV infection, U.S. blood banks screen donated blood with both an antibody assay and a nucleic acid antigen assay that detects HIV RNA. The risk of transfusion-related infection is estimated to be 1:493,000 (personal communication, American Red Cross National Testing Laboratory).[9]

3. Signs, symptoms, and laboratory manifestations of primary HIV infection are similar for all routes of transmission.[10]

II. CLINICAL PRESENTATION

A. PATHOPHYSIOLOGY

1. HIV virions bind to specific combinations of receptors present on host cells. CD4[+] T lymphocytes and macrophages are the primary cellular targets for HIV because they possess high-affinity cellular receptors. The HIV surface envelope protein gp120 binds directly to CD4; however, a coreceptor is required for viral fusion and entry. Two G-protein–coupled chemokine coreceptors, CXCR4 and CCR5, determine viral tropism for certain cell types. HIV strains that display tropism for T cells (termed X4 viruses) generally use the CXCR4 coreceptor, and strains that display tropism for macrophages (termed R5 viruses) use the CCR5 coreceptor. R5 viruses are preferentially transmitted and are present in the early stages of infection.[11-13]

2. Virus is transported to regional lymph nodes within 48 hours of acquisition. Systemic dissemination follows soon thereafter.[11]

3. After dissemination of HIV, seeding of lymphoid tissues occurs. The virus is shed into genital and oropharyngeal fluids early during primary infection, and levels of HIV RNA are higher in these compartments during primary HIV infection than in chronic HIV infection.[14]

4. Levels of HIV RNA in the plasma begin to increase about 1 week after infection with HIV. Clinical symptoms of primary HIV infection (see below) usually appear 2 to 4 weeks after infection as the viral load continues to increase.[15]

5. Approximately 3 to 4 weeks after infection the viral load begins to decline rapidly. This is followed by a slower decline in viral load that occurs from approximately 5 weeks to 2 months after infection. During this time, HIV RNA levels approach a steady state between viral production and clearance. The steady-state HIV RNA level, called the viral set point, is established by 3 to 6 months after infection.[15]

6. The initial decline in viral load is at least partly due to virus-specific immune responses that limit viral replication. The number of HIV-specific cytotoxic T lymphocytes increases sharply as the host cellular immune system attempts to contain viral replication.[16]

7. Animal studies suggest that lowering the peak viral load during primary HIV infection results in a lower viral set point, which is associated with slower rates of CD4[+] cell loss and progression to acquired immunodeficiency syndrome (AIDS).[17]

B. SYMPTOMS

1. Between 50% and 90% of individuals with primary HIV infection are symptomatic.[1,2]

2. Clinical illness usually appears approximately 2 weeks after HIV acquisition, although it may appear as early as 1 week or as late as 6 weeks after acquisition.[1]

3. The duration of the illness is usually 1 to 2 weeks, although it has been reported to last for 10 weeks or more.[1]

4. The most common clinical feature of primary HIV infection is fever, which is present in 80% to 90% or more of infected persons.[1]
5. Other common symptoms include fatigue, pharyngitis, weight loss, myalgias, headache, nausea, night sweats, diarrhea, vomiting, and rash (Table 37-1).[1,3,18]
6. Most symptoms are self-limited, although fatigue may be persistent.
7. Symptom onset is typically abrupt rather than gradual.
8. The classic rash associated with primary HIV infection is maculopapular and symmetrical. It affects primarily the face or trunk but can affect the extremities. The rash may last only a few days.
9. An illness lasting longer than 14 days portends a worse prognosis.[2]

C. SIGNS

1. Findings on physical examination include lymphadenopathy, oral ulcers, oral candidiasis, genital ulcers, and splenomegaly (Table 37-2).[3]

D. LABORATORY FINDINGS

1. Laboratory studies during primary HIV infection may show lymphopenia, thrombocytopenia, increase in atypical lymphocytes, elevated AST or ALT levels, and elevated amylase or lipase levels (Table 37-2).
2. The CD4$^+$ cell count usually decreases during primary HIV infection but may remain within the normal range. The ratio of CD4$^+$ cells to CD8$^+$ cells is almost always inverted (less than 1) during primary HIV infection.
3. Cerebrospinal fluid examination may be consistent with an aseptic meningitis.[3]

TABLE 37-1

FREQUENCY OF SYMPTOMS ASSOCIATED WITH PRIMARY HUMAN IMMUNODEFICIENCY VIRUS INFECTION

Symptom	Percent of Patients
Fever	>80-90
Fatigue	90
Pharyngitis	50-70
Weight loss	24-70
Rash	40-60
Myalgias	50-60
Headache	50-60
Nausea	30-60
Night sweats	20-50
Diarrhea	20-50
Vomiting	10-40
Abdominal pain	20
Depression	5-10

37

PRIMARY HUMAN IMMUNODEFICIENCY VIRUS INFECTION

TABLE 37-2

FREQUENCY OF SIGNS ASSOCIATED WITH PRIMARY HUMAN IMMUNODEFICIENCY VIRUS INFECTION

Sign	Percent of Patients
Lymphadenopathy	40-50
Thrombocytopenia	40-50
Leukopenia	40-50
Aseptic meningitis	20-30
Elevated liver enzyme levels	20-30
Oral ulcers	10-30
Oral candidiasis	10-20
Genital ulcers	5-10
Splenomegaly	<5

III. DIAGNOSIS

A. DIFFERENTIAL DIAGNOSIS

1. Epstein-Barr virus mononucleosis.
2. Cytomegalovirus mononucleosis.
3. Toxoplasmosis.
4. Rubella.
5. Viral hepatitis.
6. Secondary syphilis.
7. Disseminated gonococcal infection.
8. Primary herpes simplex virus infection.
9. Influenza.
10. Other viral infections.
11. Drug reaction.

B. DIAGNOSTICS (Fig. 37-1)

1. Primary HIV infection remains difficult to diagnose because the signs and symptoms associated with the illness are nonspecific. *A high index of suspicion is crucial.*
2. The HIV ELISA, the most commonly used diagnostic test, detects antibodies generated against HIV. These antibodies do not appear until 20 to 30 days after HIV acquisition. Because primary HIV infection typically occurs 14 days after HIV acquisition, the ELISA test result is negative early in primary HIV infection.[4]
3. If the HIV ELISA result is positive, a confirmatory Western blot is performed. The Western blot detects antibodies to specific HIV antigens such as core (p17, p24, p55), polymerase (p31, p51, p66), and envelope (p41, gp120, gp160) proteins. In acute HIV infection, no or only a few bands may be present and the test may be interpreted as negative or indeterminate.[19]
4. HIV p24 antigen can be detected before seroconversion and can therefore be used to diagnose primary HIV infection. The p24 antigen is detectable in serum as early as the first day of symptomatic primary HIV infection. Levels decrease after the second week of

symptoms as antibodies appear and immune complexes are formed. Thus the p24 antigen assay is most useful for detecting early primary HIV infection.[4]

5. Plasma levels of HIV RNA (measured by polymerase chain reaction [PCR]) are extremely high during primary HIV infection and decrease over the following 2 months concurrent with the resolution of symptoms and the appearance of a specific immune response against HIV. The presence of high levels of HIV RNA or DNA in the blood in conjunction with either a negative HIV ELISA result or a positive ELISA result with a negative or indeterminate Western blot establishes the diagnosis of primary HIV infection.[20]

6. Plasma levels of HIV RNA measured by PCR are often greater than 10^6 copies/mL in primary HIV infection. Low levels of HIV RNA (<5000 copies/mL) are sometimes seen in individuals with repeatedly negative HIV ELISA and Western blot results and most likely represent false positive results.

7. HIV RNA PCR is considerably more sensitive than the p24 antigen assay, may be positive 3 to 5 days earlier, and remains positive throughout the entire illness. However, it is more expensive.[4,20]

8. To diagnose primary HIV infection, the physician must first consider the possibility. A history of potential exposure to HIV within the previous 8 weeks increases the possibility of the diagnosis. If primary HIV infection is suspected, HIV-specific antibody assay (ELISA confirmed, if positive, by Western blot) and HIV RNA PCR should be ordered. If HIV RNA PCR is unavailable, a p24 antigen assay may be ordered with the understanding that test results are positive only in early primary HIV infection.

9. If the HIV ELISA or Western blot result is negative or inconclusive and the diagnosis is still suspected, the test should be repeated in 2 to 4 weeks to assess for seroconversion.

IV. MANAGEMENT

A. LABORATORY EVALUATION

1. Individuals with primary HIV infection should have baseline HIV genotyping performed to evaluate for resistance to antiretroviral therapy. Recent reports suggest that the incidence of resistance in HIV isolates from persons with acute HIV infection may be increasing.[21,22]

2. Other laboratory evaluations routinely performed in persons with chronic HIV infection should also be performed in those with primary HIV infection, including serological tests for viral hepatitis and syphilis and a tuberculin (purified protein derivative) test.

B. ANTIRETROVIRAL THERAPY

1. Current consensus guidelines recommend that highly active antiretroviral therapy (HAART) be initiated during primary HIV infection.[7] Support for this recommendation stems from several lines of research. First, virus isolated from individuals with primary HIV infection has

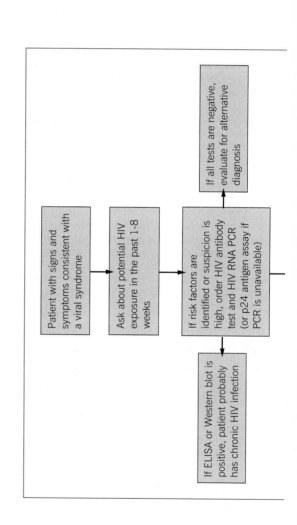

Patient with signs and symptoms consistent with a viral syndrome

Ask about potential HIV exposure in the past 1-8 weeks

If risk factors are identified or suspicion is high, order HIV antibody test and HIV RNA PCR (or p24 antigen assay if PCR is unavailable)

If all tests are negative, evaluate for alternative diagnosis

If ELISA or Western blot is positive, patient probably has chronic HIV infection

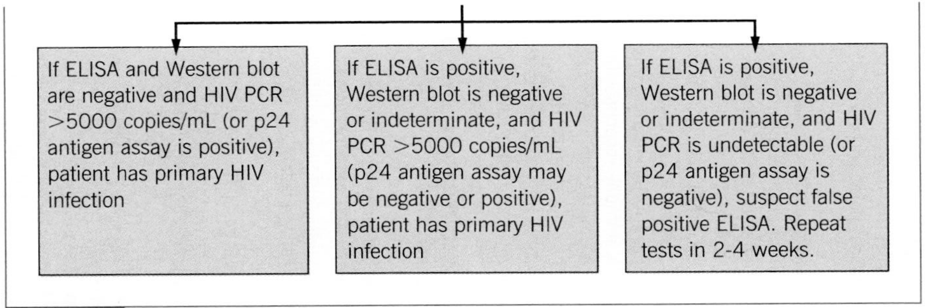

FIG. 37-1.

Diagnosis of primary human immunodeficiency virus infection. *ELISA,* Enzyme-linked immunosorbent assay; *HIV,* human immunodeficiency virus; *PCR,* polymerase chain reaction.

37

PRIMARY HUMAN IMMUNODEFICIENCY VIRUS INFECTION

been shown to be relatively homogeneous compared with that isolated from individuals with chronic HIV infection.[23] This homogeneity may allow a more effective response to combination antiretroviral therapy. Second, early treatment may limit damage to the immune system and may allow the production and maintenance of virus-specific cellular immune responses that help suppress viremia.[24] Third, higher viral set points are associated with more rapid progression to AIDS and death.[25] Some research suggests that lowering the viral load during primary HIV infection results in a lower viral set point and perhaps a slower progression of disease.[17]

2. When combination therapy with either two nucleoside reverse transcriptase inhibitors plus a protease inhibitor or three agents targeted against reverse transcriptase was initiated during primary HIV infection, viral loads were reduced to undetectable levels and $CD4^+$ cell counts increased significantly. The control of viremia was associated with HIV-specific $CD4^+$ T helper cell responses to p24 antigen.[24,26] These data suggest that initiating HAART during primary HIV infection may preserve or restore specific immune responses that help to control viremia and may slow disease progression.

3. The main disadvantage of beginning therapy during primary HIV infection is that it may increase the time patients receive antiretroviral therapy because some patients would otherwise not require therapy for years. Increasing the duration of therapy increases the cost of the medicine, may increase side and adverse effects of the medicine, and requires strict adherence to prevent resistance.

4. Besides receiving antiretroviral therapy, patients need education about HIV, including the means and prevention of transmission. They require close follow-up to ensure adherence to therapy and monitor for adverse effects of the medicines. Referral to centers performing clinical trials should be considered if they are reasonably available.

PEARLS AND PITFALLS

- Between 50% and 90% of persons with primary HIV infection are symptomatic.[1,2]
- The risk of sexual transmission from an individual with chronic HIV infection is estimated to be 0.1% per contact. The risk of sexual transmission from an individual with primary HIV infection may be as high as 5% to 30% per contact.[27]
- Symptoms usually begin approximately 2 weeks after exposure to HIV.[15]
- The signs and symptoms of primary HIV infection resemble those of many other viral infections and include fever, fatigue, myalgias, rash, headache, pharyngitis, lymphadenopathy, nausea, abdominal pain, elevated hepatic enzyme levels, leukopenia, thrombocytopenia, and presence of atypical lymphocytes.
- A patient whose signs or symptoms suggest mononucleosis should also be considered to possibly have primary HIV infection. A retrospective study of individuals who had signs or symptoms consistent with

mononucleosis but had a negative Monospot test result showed that 1.2% of the individuals probably had primary HIV infection.[28] False positive Epstein-Barr virus heterophil tests (Monospot tests) in patients with primary HIV infection have also been reported.[29]

- Atypical lymphocytes may be seen in both Epstein-Barr virus mononucleosis and primary HIV infection. In primary HIV infection, the percentage of atypical lymphocytes is usually less than 10%, whereas in cases of mononucleosis the percentage is often much higher.

- Routine HIV (HIV ELISA) test results are often negative during primary HIV infection. The diagnosis of primary HIV infection should include an HIV ELISA (to evaluate for chronic infection), as well as an HIV RNA PCR (or p24 antigen assay if PCR is unavailable) (Fig. 37-1). The p24 antigen is found early in primary HIV infection but becomes undetectable later in primary infection as antibody complexes are formed.

- HIV RNA levels in plasma peak approximately 2 to 3 weeks after acquisition of HIV. Levels then decrease over the next month concomitant with the formation of immune responses to the virus and the resolution of symptoms of primary HIV infection.[15]

- Genital ulcer disease, urethritis, and cervicitis increase the risk of transmitting and acquiring HIV; therefore consideration of other sexually transmitted diseases is appropriate when primary HIV infection is diagnosed.[30]

- HIV can be transmitted by oral sex with an HIV-infected person.[31,32]

- Individuals with primary HIV infection should be advised about the possible advantages and disadvantages of antiretroviral therapy. Close follow-up is needed to ensure adherence with medicines, to monitor for adverse effects of the medicines, and to provide continued psychosocial counseling.

REFERENCES

[b] 1. Schacker T et al. Clinical and epidemiologic features of primary HIV infection. Ann Intern Med 1996; 125:257.

[b] 2. Pedersen C et al. Clinical course of primary HIV infection: consequences for subsequent course of infection. BMJ 1989; 299:154.

[b] 3. Vanhems P et al. Acute HIV-1 disease as a mononucleosis-like illness: is the diagnosis too restrictive? Clin Infect Dis 1997; 24:965.

[b] 4. Von Sydow M et al. Antigen detection in primary HIV infection. Br Med J 1988; 296:238.

[b] 5. Henrard DR et al. Detection of HIV-1 p24 antigen and plasma RNA: relevance to indeterminate serologic tests. Transfusion 1994; 34:376.

[b] 6. Busch MP et al. Time course of detection of viral and serologic markers preceding human immunodeficiency virus type 1 seroconversion: implications for screening of blood and tissue donors. Transfusion 1995; 35:91.

[d] 7. Department of Health and Human Services. Available at www.hivatis.org/guidelines/adult/pdf/Atajani.pdf.

[c] 8. Royce RA et al. Sexual transmission of HIV. N Engl J Med 1997; 336:1072.

[b] 9. Schreiber GB et al. The risk of transfusion-transmitted viral infections: the retrovirus epidemiology donor study. N Engl J Med 1996; 334:1685.

[b] 10. Routy P et al. Comparison of clinical features of acute HIV-1 infection in patients infected sexually or through injection drug use. J Acquir Immune Def Syndr 2000; 24:425.

[b] 11. Spira AI et al. Cellular targets of infection and route of viral dissemination after an intravaginal inoculation of simian immunodeficiency virus into rhesus macaques. J Exp Med 1996; 183:215.

[b] 12. Frankel SS et al. Replication of HIV-1 in dendritic cell derived syncytia at the mucosal surface of the adenoid. Science 1996; 272:115.

[b] 13. Zaitseva M et al. Expression and function of CCR5 and CXCR4 on human Langerhans cells and macrophages: implications for HIV primary infection. Nat Med 1997; 3:1369.

[b] 14. Pilcher CD et al. HIV in body fluids during primary HIV infection: implications for pathogenesis, treatment, and public health. AIDS 2001; 15:837.

[b] 15. Lindback S et al. Viral dynamics in primary HIV-1 infection. AIDS 2000; 14:2283.

[b] 16. Koup RA et al. Temporal association of cellular immune responses with the initial control of viremia in primary human immunodeficiency virus type 1 syndrome. J Virol 1994; 68:46505.

[b] 17. Haigwood NL et al. Passive immune globulin therapy in the SIV/macaque model: early intervention can alter disease profile. Immunol Lett 1996; 51:107.

[b] 18. Clark SJ et al. High titers of cytopathic virus in plasma of patients with symptomatic primary HIV-1 infection. N Engl J Med 1991; 324:954.

[b] 19. Celum CL et al. Indeterminate human immunodeficiency Western blots: seroconversion risk, specificity of supplemental tests, and an algorithm for evaluation. J Infect Dis 1991; 164:656.

[b] 20. Bollinger RC et al. Risk factors and clinical presentation of acute primary HIV infection in India. JAMA 1997; 278:2085.

[b] 21. Boden D et al. HIV-1 drug resistance in newly infected individuals. JAMA 1999; 282:1135.

[b] 22. Little S et al. Reduced antiretroviral drug susceptibility among patients with primary HIV infection. JAMA 1999; 282:1142.

[b] 23. Zhu T et al. Genotypic and phenotypic characterization of HIV-1 patients with primary infection. Science 1993; 261:1179.

[b] 24. Rosenberg ES et al. Vigorous HIV-1 specific CD4+ T cell responses associated with control of viremia. Science 1997; 278:1447.

[b] 25. Mellors JW et al. Prognosis in HIV-1 infection predicted by the quantity of virus in plasma. Science 1996; 272:1167.

[b] 26. Lafeuillade A et al. Effects of a combination of zidovudine, didanosine, and lamivudine on primary human immunodeficiency virus type 1 infection. J Infect Dis 1997; 175:1051.

[c] 27. Jacquez JA et al. Role of the primary infection in epidemics of HIV infection in gay cohorts. J Acquir Immune Def Syndr 2000; 7:1169.

[b] 28. Rosenberg ES, Caliendo AM, Walker BD. Acute HIV infection among patients tested for mononucleosis. N Engl J Med 1999; 340:969.

[b] 29. Walensky RP et al. Investigation of primary HIV infection in patients who test positive for heterophile antibody. Clin Infect Dis 2001; 33:570.

[b] 30. Mehendale SM et al. Incidence and predictors of HIV type 1 seroconversion in patients attending sexually transmitted disease clinics in India. J Infect Dis 1995; 172:1486.

[b] 31. Berrey MM, Shea T. Oral sex and HIV transmission. J Acquir Immune Def Syndr 1997; 14:475.

[b] 32. Lifson AR et al. HIV seroconversion in two homosexual men after oral intercourse with ejaculation: implications for counseling concerning safe sexual practices. Am J Public Health 1990; 80:1509.

Central Nervous System Involvement in Human Immunodeficiency Virus Infection

Nimalie D. Stone, MD, and Justin McArthur, MBBS, MPH

FAST FACTS

- As many as two thirds of patients with human immunodeficiency virus (HIV) infection may have clinically relevant neurological disease, and patients frequently have multiple or concurrent neurological disorders.[1]
- Cerebrospinal fluid (CSF) findings are abnormal in approximately 90% of HIV-positive patients, especially during the clinically asymptomatic phase of infection.[2]
- Given the overlap in the clinical presentation of many of the central nervous system (CNS) processes occurring in HIV, a cranial imaging study is recommended as the first step in diagnostic evaluation.[3]
- *Cryptococcus neoformans* is the most common opportunistic organism infecting the CNS in HIV-infected patients.
- Toxoplasmosis is the most common cause of intracranial mass lesions in HIV-infected patients.[4]

I. EPIDEMIOLOGY

1. Neurological processes considered acquired immunodeficiency virus (AIDS)-defining illnesses include the following (Table 38-1).[5]
   a. HIV-associated dementia.
   b. Extrapulmonary cryptococcal infection (most often cryptococcal meningitis).
   c. Cytomegalovirus (CMV) infection (including encephalitis, retinitis, and polyradiculitis).
   d. Primary CNS lymphoma (PCNSL).
   e. CNS toxoplasmosis.
   f. Progressive multifocal leukoencephalopathy (PML).
2. Some of these CNS processes, such as PML, CNS toxoplasmosis, and CMV encephalitis, are considered reactivation of latent infectious processes as a result of declining cell-mediated immunity, whereas others, such as cryptococcal meningitis, are new opportunistic infections.
3. Despite its association with Epstein-Barr virus (EBV) and possibly human herpes virus 8, primary CNS lymphoma has not been defined as an opportunistic infection. EBV proteins may trigger malignant transformation in host cells.[6]

TABLE 38-1

REPORTS OF CENTRAL NERVOUS SYSTEM PROCESSES AS ACQUIRED IMMUNODEFICIENCY DISEASE–DEFINING ILLNESSES AND ESTIMATED CD4$^+$ NADIR

CNS Process	Prevalence[5] (%)	CD4$^+$ Count at Presentation (Cells/μL)
Cryptococcal meningitis	5	<100
CNS toxoplasmosis	4	<200
Primary CNS lymphoma	1	<50
Progressive multifocal leukoencephalopathy	1	<200
Cytomegalovirus encephalitis	2*	<100
Human immunodeficiency virus–associated dementia	5*	<500

CNS, Central nervous system.
*Probably estimated.

4. CNS infection by the HIV virus is believed to cause HIV-associated dementia; however, host response producing indirect mechanisms, such as macrophage activation causing cytokine release within the brain, may also play an important role.[7]
5. Usually the occurrence of neurological disease in HIV is related to the degree of host immunocompromise; in some cases, however, neurological disease is the presenting illness or even develops after immune reconstitution. The CD4$^+$ nadir may be more important than the current CD4$^+$ count in predicting the patient's risk of CNS opportunistic infections.
6. Most CNS opportunistic infections develop only when CD4$^+$ counts fall below 200 cells/μL, and some diseases, such as PCSNL and CMV encephalitis, do not occur until CD4$^+$ counts are less than 100 cells/μL.
7. The possibility of acute bacterial meningitis (including that caused by *Listeria monocytogenes*) and viral meningoencephalitis should be considered in immunocompromised patients.
8. Differential diagnosis of acute meningitis is covered in Chapter 44. *Listeria monocytogenes* and *Mycobacterium tuberculosis* should be in the differential diagnosis of acute meningitis in patients with HIV.
9. Differential diagnosis of encephalitis includes toxic and metabolic processes, viruses (herpes simplex virus [HSV], CMV, arbovirus, enterovirus), toxoplasmosis, and *Listeria* rhombencephalitis (rare). In the appropriate clinical setting, CSF polymerase chain reaction (PCR) testing can help establish a diagnosis. Available PCR tests include those for EBV, CMV, arbovirus, and HSV.

II. CLINICAL PRESENTATION

1. In general the common CNS diseases that may be occurring in an HIV-infected patient are difficult to differentiate by history and physical examination alone (Table 38-2).[8-11]

TABLE 38-2

CLINICAL FINDINGS AND TIME OF DISEASE PROGRESSION

CNS Process	Common Clinical Signs and Symptoms	Progression of Disease
Cryptococcal meningitis[8]	Headache (75%), fever (>65%), nausea, altered mentation, meningismus	Days to weeks
CNS toxoplasmosis[9]	Headache (55%), seizures (30%), confusion, fever, focal neurological deficits; patients are usually not taking trimethoprim-sulfamethoxazole prophylaxis	Days to weeks
Primary CNS lymphoma[10]	Mental status changes (60%), focal neurological deficits, headache	Weeks
Progressive multifocal leukoencephalopathy	Slowly progressive focal neurological deficits (i.e., ataxia, aphasia, or hemiparesis)	Weeks to months
Cytomegalovirus encephalitis	Acute or subacute confusion, memory and attention deficits, headache	Days
Human immunodeficiency virus–associated dementia[11]	Slowly progressive cognitive, motor, and behavioral changes (poor concentration, forgetfulness, loss of balance, apathy); often occurs with HIV-associated myelopathy and sensory neuropathy	Months

CNS, Central nervous system.

CNS INVOLVEMENT IN HIV INFECTION

38

2. Fig. 38-1 provides an algorithm for the approach to an HIV-infected patient with a headache.

III. DIAGNOSTICS

1. As shown in Fig. 38-1, both neuroimaging and CSF studies provide diagnostic information about the etiology of CNS infections in HIV. Table 38-3 summarizes CSF, radiological, and other study findings.[10,12,13]

2. Common CSF abnormalities seen in HIV, which are not specific to any particular secondary process, include evidence of intrathecal synthesis of anti-HIV antibody (90%), detection of viral RNA (~75%), pleocytosis (50%-65%), and elevated CSF protein level (35%).[2]

3. Empirical treatment of toxoplasmosis should be initiated when ring-enhancing CNS lesions are seen on neuroimaging studies unless the lesion is solitary and the patient was previously known to be seronegative for *Toxoplasma* immunoglobulin G (IgG). In this situation a stereotactic brain biopsy is indicated.[3]

4. If available, thallium-201 single-photon emission computed tomography (SPECT) imaging may provide another noninvasive method to differentiate CNS lymphoma from CNS toxoplasmosis. A positive uptake represents ongoing cell activity as would be expected in a growing tumor, whereas a negative SPECT scan would be more consistent with an abscess. Sensitivity and specificity are both ~90%.[14]

5. The presumptive diagnosis of CNS toxoplasmosis is made if a clinical response to induction therapy is demonstrated on follow-up imaging after 2 weeks of treatment.[4,15]

6. The diagnosis of HIV-associated dementia is based on clinical presentation and the exclusion of all other opportunistic processes. The dementia can be further characterized by neuropsychological tests and a typical magnetic resonance imaging appearance. The CSF HIV RNA level is typically elevated.[16]

7. Measurement of the CSF HIV RNA may be useful in assessing the response to highly active antiviral therapy (HAART) in HIV-associated dementia.

IV. MANAGEMENT

Table 38-4 outlines recommended and alternative therapies.[4,15,17-21]

PEARLS AND PITFALLS

- Neurosyphilis and tuberculous meningitis are other potential CNS processes that must be considered in the differential diagnosis of a patient with HIV who has mental status changes, especially with normal CD4+ cell counts. If there is clinical evidence of syphilis, neurosyphilis is suspected, or serological tests of peripheral blood show increasing titers, a Venereal Disease Research Laboratory (VDRL) test of CSF is needed to evaluate for neurosyphilis. Evidence of pulmonary tuberculosis infection

Text continued on p. 589

TABLE 38-3
IMPORTANT DIAGNOSTIC TESTS

CNS Process	CSF Findings[10]	Radiological Findings[12]	Other Studies
Cryptococcal meningitis	Culture positive for *Cryptococcus* (95%); reactive CSF *Cryptococcus* antigen; India ink positive (60%-80%)	Punctate lesions in basal ganglia; no enhancement	Reactive serum *Cryptococcus* antigen
CNS toxoplasmosis	Possible *Toxoplasma* antigen for CSF detection (PCR) is being studied	Many 1- to 2-cm "simple" ring lesions; moderate enhancement	Response to empirical therapy within first 2 weeks (by MRI); known positive for *Toxoplasma* IgG; brain biopsy is definitive
Primary CNS lymphoma	PCR positive for EBV (still experimental, negative result does not rule out PCNSL); CSF cytological tests positive (<5%)	Solitary to several large heterogeneous mass lesions in periventricular white matter; strong enhancement	Failure to respond to empirical therapy for toxoplasmosis, especially if patient is known to be IgG seronegative; T-201 SPECT scan; brain biopsy is definitive
Progressive multifocal leukoencephalopathy	PCR positive for JC virus (60%)	Changes in subcortical white matter; no mass effect; no enhancement	Characteristic findings on imaging; brain biopsy is definitive but unnecessary
CMV encephalitis	Increased protein level; decreased glucose level; PCR positive for CMV (95%)	Several confluent lesions in periventricular white matter; moderate enhancement; scans may be normal in 30%-50%[13]	Positive for CMV viremia (60%); retinitis, radiculitis, or other organ infection with CMV in >70%
Human immunodeficiency virus–associated dementia	Elevated protein level; pleocytosis; CSF may be normal	Diffuse, ill-defined lesions in deep white matter; no enhancement	Diagnosis of exclusion; neuropsychological testing showing subcortical dementia

CMV, Cytomegalovirus; *CNS*, central nervous system; *CSF*, cerebrospinal fluid; *EBV*, Epstein-Barr virus; *IgG*, immunoglobulin G; *MRI*, magnetic resonance imaging; *PCNSL*, primary central nervous system lymphoma; *PCR*, polymerase chain reaction; *T-201 SPECT*, thallium-201 single-photon emission computed tomography.

38

CNS INVOLVEMENT IN HIV INFECTION

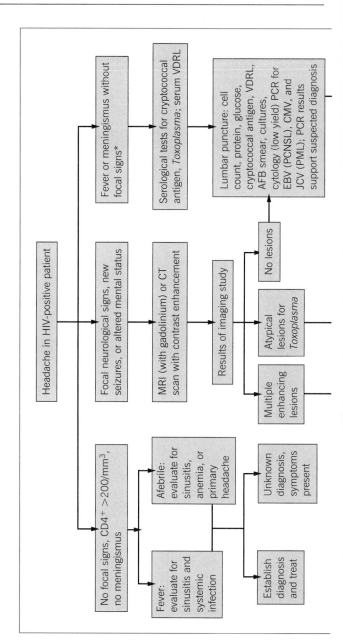

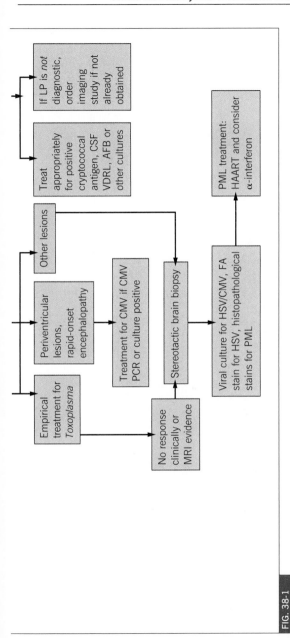

FIG. 38-1

Diagnosis of primary human immunodeficiency virus infection. *AFB*, Acid-fast bacillus; *CMV*, cytomegalovirus; *CSF*, cerebrospinal fluid; *CT*, computed tomography; *FA*, fluorescent antibody; *PCR*, polymerase chain reaction; *EBV*, Epstein-Barr virus; *HAART*, highly active antiviral therapy; *HSV*, herpes simplex virus; *JCV*, JC virus; *LP*, lumbar puncture; *MRI*, magnetic resonance imaging; *PCNSL*, primary central nervous system lymphoma; *PML*, progressive multifocal leukoencephalopathy; *VDRL*, Venereal Disease Research Laboratory.

38

CNS INVOLVEMENT IN HIV INFECTION

TABLE 38-4

MANAGEMENT OF CNS PROCESSES IN HIV

CNS Process	Recommended Therapy	Alternative Therapy	Suppression
Cryptococcal meningitis[17]	Amphotericin B 0.7-1.0 mg/kg/day IV, plus flucytosine 100 mg/kg/day PO in 4 doses for 2 weeks' induction, followed by fluconazole 400 mg/day PO for 10-week course	Fluconazole 400-800 mg/day plus flucytosine 100 mg/kg/day for 6-week course (for mild cryptococcal meningitis); liposomal amphotericin B may be used for renal compromise	Fluconazole 200 mg/day PO lifelong
CNS toxoplasmosis[4]	Pyrimethamine 100-200 mg/day PO load for 2 days, then 75-100 mg/day, plus sulfadiazine 1.5-2 g PO qid, plus folinic acid 10 mg/day PO for 6-week course	For sulfa-allergic patients, may substitute clindamycin 600-900 mg PO qid for sulfadiazine[15]	Pyrimethamine 25-50 mg/day PO, plus sulfadiazine 1 g PO qid (or clindamycin 300-450 mg PO tid-qid), plus folinic acid 5 mg/day PO lifelong
Primary CNS lymphoma	Irradiation is standard therapy; a recent trial demonstrated possible improvement of lesions with combined HAART (including AZT), ganciclovir, and interleukin-2[18]	Other trials are exploring combined radiation therapy and chemotherapy	Not applicable
PML	No proven treatment exists, although antiretroviral therapy has been shown to improve survival	Interferon-α has been suggested to provide additional benefit[19]	Not applicable
CMV encephalitis	Ganciclovir 5 mg/kg IV bid for 3-6 weeks with or without foscarnet 60 mg/kg IV q8h or 90 mg/kg IV q12h for 3-6 weeks	If treatment with one drug fails, may try in combination (especially if patient has had prior treatment for CMV)	Ganciclovir 5 mg/kg/day with or without foscarnet 90 mg/kg/day
HIV-associated dementia[20]	HAART, especially agents with increased CNS penetration such as AZT, stavudine (D4T), abacavir, nevirapine, and efavirenz	For treatment failure, may recheck CSF HIV RNA level; adjunctive therapy with selegiline 5 mg twice a week[21]	Some patients need supervised HAART administration

AZT, Zidovudine; *CMV,* cytomegalovirus; *CNS,* central nervous system; *CSF,* cerebrospinal fluid; *HAART,* highly active antiretroviral therapy; *HIV,* human immunodeficiency virus; *PML,* progressive multifocal leukoencephalopathy.

increases the risk for tuberculous meningitis. CSF monocytosis also increases the likelihood of tuberculous meningitis.

- In patients who have $CD4^+$ counts below 100 cells/μL and are positive for *Toxoplasma* IgG, primary prophylaxis with trimethoprim-sulfamethoxazole (Bactrim, Septra) double strength, one tab PO qd, is recommended.

- Cryptococcal meningitis causes a communicating hydrocephalus because of blockage of the arachnoid granulations by the polysaccharide capsule of *Cryptococcus neoformans*. An opening pressure greater than 190 mm H_2O is considered abnormal. Both initial opening pressure and change in opening pressure with therapy are considered predictive of poor outcome. In a subgroup analysis of patients in a study comparing amphotericin B to amphotericin B plus 5-fluorocytosine for treatment of cryptococcal meningitis, those who did not have a decrease of 10 mm H_2O from an initially elevated opening pressure after 2 weeks of therapy had greater clinical failure of therapy and those with an initial opening pressure greater than 350 mm H_2O had higher death rates at 12 months.[22] Patients with cryptococcal meningitis and intracranial pressure (opening pressure) greater than 250 mm H_2O during lumbar puncture should undergo serial lumbar punctures until opening pressure remains stable in normal range. Occasionally, ventricular drainage is required. Increased intracranial pressure in cryptococcal meningitis is potentially fatal and is associated with more frequent papilledema, cranial nerve deficits, higher CSF cryptococcal antigen titers, and positive results on India ink staining.[17,22]

- The most important predictor of good outcome in cryptococcal meningitis is normal mental status at presentation.[23,24] The studies referred to here were performed before the HAART era.

- Serum cryptococcal antigen testing with a kit that pretreats with pronase has a 97% sensitivity and 100% specificity for detecting cryptococcal disease. CSF testing has similar sensitivity and specificity.[25]

- PCR testing for tuberculosis, CSF adenosine deaminase level, and culture for tuberculosis can be helpful in identifying tuberculous meningitis.

- Although this chapter focuses on CNS processes in HIV, the multiple effects of HIV on the peripheral nervous system should not be overlooked. The most common peripheral nervous system process in HIV is distal symmetrical polyneuropathy. Progressive polyradiculopathy, a rapidly progressive process often caused by CMV, can lead to an acute cauda equina syndrome. Other peripheral nervous system processes include HIV-associated myopathy, toxic neuropathies and myopathies related to antiretroviral medication effects, and mononeuritis multiplex, which may be caused either by HIV directly or by opportunistic CMV.[26]

- As advances continue in HAART and the management of HIV infection, the incidence of nervous system processes in HIV infection is likely to continue to decrease.

- See reference 27 for a suggested review article.

38

CNS INVOLVEMENT IN HIV INFECTION

REFERENCES

[c] 1. Berger JR et al. Neurologic disease as the presenting manifestation of acquired immunodeficiency syndrome. South Med J 1987; 80:683.

[c] 2. Fauci AS, Lane HC. Human immunodeficiency virus (HIV) disease: AIDS and related disorders. In Fauci AS et al, editors. Harrison's principles of internal medicine, 15th ed. New York: McGraw-Hill; 2001.

[d] 3. American Academy of Neurology, Quality Standards Subcommittee. Evaluation and management of intracranial mass lesions in AIDS. Neurology 1998; 50(1):21.

[c] 4. Luft BJ, Remington JS. Toxoplasmic encephalitis in AIDS (AIDS commentary). Clin Infect Dis 1992; 15:211.

[b] 5. Centers for Disease Control and Prevention. HIV/AIDS surveillance report. 1997; 9(2):1.

[b] 6. Camilleri-Broet S et al. High expression of latent membrane protein 1 of Epstein-Barr virus and BCL-2 oncoprotein in acquired immunodeficiency syndrome–related primary brain lymphomas. Blood 1995; 86:432.

[b] 7. Adamson DC et al. Immunologic nitric oxide synthase: elevation in severe AIDS dementia and induction by HIV-1 coat protein, gp41. Science 1996; 274:1917.

[c] 8. Chuck SL, Sande MA. Infections with *Cryptococcus neoformans* in the acquired immunodeficiency syndrome. N Engl J Med 1989; 321:784.

[c] 9. Porter SB, Sande MA. Toxoplasmosis of the central nervous system in the acquired immunodeficiency syndrome. N Engl J Med 1992; 327:1643.

[c] 10. Bartlett J, Gallant JE. 2000-2001 Medical management of HIV infection. Baltimore: Port City Press; 2000.

[c] 11. Navia BA et al. The AIDS dementia complex. I. Clinical features. Ann Neurol 1986; 19:517.

[d] 12. Price RW. American Academy of Neurology Annual Course 347, Infections of the Nervous System; May 5, 1995.

[c] 13. Holland NR et al. Cytomegalovirus encephalitis in acquired immunodeficiency syndrome (AIDS). Neurology 1994; 44:507.

[b] 14. Ruiz A et al. Use of thallium-201 brain SPECT to differentiate cerebral lymphoma from toxoplasma encephalitis in AIDS patients. Am J Neuroradiol 1994; 15:1885.

[c] 15. Luft BJ et al. Toxoplasmic encephalitis in patients with acquired immunodeficiency syndrome. N Engl J Med 1993; 329:995.

[b] 16. McArthur JC et al. Relationship between HIV-associated dementia and CSF viral load. Ann Neurol 1997; 42:689.

[d] 17. Saag MS et al. Practice guidelines for the management of cryptococcal disease. Clin Infect Dis 2000; 30:710.

[b] 18. Raez L et al. Treatment of AIDS-related primary central nervous system lymphoma with zidovudine, ganciclovir, and interleukin-2. AIDS Res Hum Retrovirus 1999; 15(8):713.

[b] 19. Huang SS et al. Survival prolongation in HIV-associated progressive multifocal leukoencephalopathy treated with alpha interferon: an observational study. J Neurovirol 1998; 4:324.

[d] 20. McArthur JC. Differential diagnosis and clinical management strategies for common central nervous system infections. Insights HIV Dis Manage 1998; 6(2):23.

[a] 21. Sacktor N et al. Transdermal selegiline in HIV-associated cognitive impairment: pilot placebo-controlled study. Neurology 2000; 54:233.

[d] 22. Graybill JR et al. Diagnosis and management of increased intracranial pressure in patients with AIDS and cryptococcal meningitis. Clin Infect Dis 2000; 30:47.

[a] 23. Dismukes WE, Cloud G, Gallis HA. Treatment of cryptococcal meningitis with combination of amphotericin B and flucytosine for four as compared with six weeks. N Engl J Med 1987; 317:334.

[a] 24. Saag MS et al. Comparison of amphotericin B with fluconazole for the treatment of acute AIDS-associated cryptococcal meningitis. N Engl J Med 1992; 326:83.

[b] 25. Tanner DC et al. Comparison of commercial kits for the detection of cryptococcal antigen. J Clin Microbiol 1994:1680.

[c] 26. Simpson DM, Berger JR. Management of the HIV-infected patient. I. Neurologic manifestations of HIV infection. Med Clin North Am 1996; 80(6):1363.

[c] 27. Skiest DJ. Focal neurological disease in patients with acquired immunodeficiency syndrome. Clin Infect Dis 2002; 34:103.

Pneumocystis carinii (jiroveci) Pneumonia

Josh Lauring, MD, PhD, and Stuart C. Ray, MD

Fast Facts

- *Pneumocystis carinii* has been renamed *Pneumocystis jiroveci* because genetic sequencing has found the human pathogen to differ from the rat pathogen in several DNA sequences. The term "PcP" may be used to refer to *Pneumocystis* pneumonia.[1]
- *Pneumocystis carinii* pneumonia (PCP) remains the most common acquired immunodeficiency syndrome (AIDS)-defining infection in patients infected with human immunodeficiency virus (HIV), despite the reduction in incidence brought about by prophylaxis and highly active antiretroviral therapy (HAART).
- Ninety-five percent of PCP cases occur in HIV-infected patients with $CD4^+$ counts below $200/mm^3$.
- Bronchoalveolar lavage (BAL) is the most sensitive diagnostic technique and confers little risk if transbronchial biopsy is not performed. It should be used for high-risk patients if an induced sputum examination result is negative.
- Empirical therapy will inappropriately treat up to 50% of patients and miss other important lung pathogens in 20%.
- Prophylaxis should be instituted when the $CD4^+$ count falls below $200/mm^3$. Trimethoprim-sulfamethoxazole is the most effective agent. Side effects are common. Acceptable alternative regimens include dapsone, trimethoprim-dapsone, aerosolized pentamidine, and atovaquone.
- Standard treatment for PCP is trimethoprim-sulfamethoxazole. Intravenous pentamidine, trimethoprim-dapsone, trimetrexate-leucovorin, clindamycin-primaquine, and atovaquone are alternatives. Standard treatment duration is 21 days.
- Adjunctive corticosteroids reduce the incidence of respiratory failure and mortality in moderate to severe PCP (Pao_2 <70 mm Hg or PAo_2-Pao_2 gradient >35 mm Hg).
- Respiratory failure carries a poor prognosis, with mortality in the range of 60%.
- Primary and secondary prophylaxis may safely be discontinued in patients who are receiving HAART and whose $CD4^+$ count has increased to greater than $200/mm^3$ for 3 months.

cont'd

Fast Facts—cont'd

- Non-HIV-infected patients with immunosuppression caused by malignancy, chemotherapy, solid organ transplantation, or prolonged high-dose corticosteroid treatment are at high risk for PCP and should receive prophylaxis. Compared with HIV-infected patients, these patients have a more fulminant presentation, higher incidence of respiratory failure, and greater mortality.

I. EPIDEMIOLOGY

1. PCP is the most common AIDS-defining illness.
2. Before the introduction of effective prophylaxis and HAART, PCP developed in 80% of patients with AIDS at some point in their course. With a $CD4^+$ count below $250/mm^3$, the 2-year probability that PCP would develop was 40%.[2]
3. Chemoprophylaxis reduces the risk of PCP by two thirds.[3]
4. The addition of HAART has reduced the incidence of PCP by over 60%.
5. Despite the impact of prophylaxis and HAART, PCP remains a leading cause of mortality related to HIV and other forms of immunosuppression.
6. The majority of cases of PCP occur in patients who are not receiving medical care or who are not receiving prophylaxis.[4]
7. Short-term mortality is 10% to 20%. Since the advent in 1990 of adjunctive corticosteroid therapy for moderate to severe PCP, the rate of respiratory failure and the case-fatality rate have declined. Respiratory failure still carries a grave prognosis, with approximately 60% mortality.[5]
8. Microbiological information regarding PCP is presented in Box 39-1.[6,7]

BOX 39-1

PNEUMOCYSTIS CARINII: MICROBIOLOGICAL INFORMATION

Pneumocystis carinii was originally classified as a protozoan because of its three morphological forms: cysts, sporozoites, and trophozoites.

Analysis of ribosomal RNA and mitochondrial DNA suggests a closer relationship to fungi.

Pneumonia is thought to result from reactivation of latent organisms; most individuals are infected in childhood.

Although case clustering has been reported and studies have demonstrated animal-to-animal transmission, the contribution of communicable infection is thought to be small.[5]

There are currently no recommendations for isolation or contact precautions for PCP.

Histopathological study shows an intraalveolar acellular exudate filling the alveoli in PCP.[6]

II. CLINICAL PRESENTATION

1. The classic symptoms of PCP are fever (79%-100%), progressive dyspnea on exertion (95%), and cough (95%); however, this triad is observed in only 50% to 60% of patients.[8] The cough may be productive in 30% of cases.

2. PCP is characterized by an insidious onset and slow progression, in contrast to the more acute presentation of bacterial pneumonia.

3. The most common physical findings are fever (84% >38.1° C) and tachypnea (62%). Crackles and rhonchi may be heard, but the lungs are clear on auscultation in 50% of cases.

4. Pneumothorax with associated chest pain may occur in 2% to 6%. The presence of pneumothorax in a patient with HIV represents PCP in over 80% of cases.[9]

5. Extrapulmonary pneumocystosis occurs rarely and is more common in patients receiving prophylaxis with aerosolized pentamidine. The heart, skin, spleen, bone marrow, thyroid, eyes, and adrenal glands may be involved. Among patients with PCP, 95% have $CD4^+$ counts below $200/mm^3$ within 2 months of presentation, and patients often have other signs of advanced HIV disease, such as wasting and oral candidiasis.[10]

6. Box 39-2 presents criteria for assessing the severity of PCP.

III. DIAGNOSTICS

1. Several studies have attempted to simplify the diagnosis of PCP through the use of noninvasive assessments. The most informative noninvasive assessments are the presence of classic symptoms (fever, cough, and exertional dyspnea), oral thrush or hairy leukoplakia, lack of prophylaxis for PCP, serum lactate dehydrogenase (LDH) level, arterial oxygen desaturation after exercise, and chest radiography.[11,12]

2. The chest radiograph is abnormal in over 80% of cases. The classic appearance of diffuse bilateral interstitial or perihilar infiltrates is seen in 58% to 68% of cases but is only 84% to 97% specific for PCP. Such infiltrates may be seen in 40% to 60% of cases of bacterial pneumonia, tuberculosis, and pulmonary Kaposi's sarcoma.[11-13] The combination of normal chest radiograph and normal diffusing capacity for carbon monoxide (DLCO) was found to be helpful in ruling out PCP.[14] High-resolution computed tomography (CT) is highly sensitive for PCP; in one study CT had a sensitivity of 100% and a specificity of 89% when the presence of patchy or nodular ground-glass opacities was used to indicate possible PCP.[15]

39

PNEUMOCYSTIS CARINII (JIROVECI) PNEUMONIA

BOX 39-2

SEVERITY OF *PNEUMOCYSTIS CARINII* PNEUMONIA

Mild: Pao_2 >70 mm Hg, PAo_2-Pao_2 <35 mm Hg

Moderate to severe: Pao_2 <70 mm Hg or PAo_2-Pao_2 >35 mm Hg

3. The LDH level exceeds the normal range in 90% to 100% of patients. A normal LDH level may help to rule out the diagnosis if the pretest probability of PCP is low to intermediate, but an elevated LDH level is not specific for PCP, since bacterial pneumonia and tuberculosis may also cause an elevated LDH.[16]

4. Arterial oxygen desaturation after exercise on a defined treadmill protocol has a sensitivity approaching 100% for PCP when appropriate cut-off values are used.[12,17] However, the specificity of such tests is low. Less standardized measurements such as oxygen saturation before and after ambulation in a hospital ward have not been well studied, and a lack of desaturation should not be used to rule out PCP.

5. In summary, noninvasive assessments, particularly in combination, may be used to adjust the pretest probability of PCP. Such assessments are often used to guide the decision to pursue definitive diagnostic testing with induced sputum or BAL. For instance, a patient who does not have diffuse interstitial infiltrates and has a normal LDH level has a less than 5% probability of PCP. Notably, among patients who had had a previous episode of PCP, the previously mentioned noninvasive assessments were as likely to be positive in non-PCP presentations as in recurrent PCP.[12]

6. Although some authors advocate empirical therapy for PCP when the pretest probability is high,[18] there are several reasons to pursue a definitive diagnosis. Even with typical symptoms and infiltrates on chest radiograph, less than half of the patients in one large series had PCP on BAL and 20% had another organism in addition to or instead of *P. (carinii) jiroveci*. Empirical therapy would expose many patients to unnecessary toxicity and would be ineffective or incomplete in many others.[13]

7. Definitive diagnosis is commonly based on examination of induced sputum or BAL. Both methods are 99% to 100% specific for PCP. Induced sputum has reported sensitivities of 55% to 94%, varying with the expertise of the staff at any given institution.[19] The sensitivity of induced sputum testing can be enhanced by the use of immunofluorescent staining and the polymerase chain reaction. Immunofluorescence is generally accepted as the most validated gold standard test.[20] Expectorated sputum was demonstrated to have equivalent sensitivity to induced sputum (52% versus 56%) in a series from one institution.[21] However, the majority of patients have nonproductive cough at presentation.

8. Induced and expectorated sputum examination has been shown to have an acceptable yield, provided that the expectorated sample is a deep specimen. The saline used to facilitate sputum induction does not inhibit the diagnosis of pathogens other than *Pneumocystis*.[22]

9. If sputum induction cannot be performed or is nondiagnostic, BAL should be performed. BAL is 89% to 98% sensitive for PCP. The yield

is increased by lavage of multiple areas of lung and by guiding lavage to the most involved area on chest radiography. If transbronchial biopsy is not performed, the morbidity of BAL is low.[20] In intubated patients endotracheal aspiration or BAL can establish the diagnosis.

10. Although empirical therapy is not recommended, anti-*Pneumocystis* treatment while diagnostic testing is being carried out is certainly advisable for a sick patient who may have PCP. Early initiation of therapy will not compromise the sensitivity of induced sputum examination or BAL. In fact, *P. carinii* cysts were detected in 76% of patients after 3 weeks of appropriate therapy and in 24% 6 weeks after diagnosis. Persistence of cysts was not associated with an increased risk of relapse.[23]

11. Box 39-3 describes the differential diagnosis of pulmonary disease in HIV-positive patients,[24-29] and Box 39-4 outlines the differential diagnosis of pulmonary complications of HIV according to chest radiography.[24] Box 39-5 lists relevant points in the patient history and laboratory tests.[30]

BOX 39-3

DIFFERENTIAL DIAGNOSIS OF PULMONARY DISEASE IN HUMAN IMMUNODEFICIENCY VIRUS–POSITIVE PATIENTS

COMMUNITY-ACQUIRED PNEUMONIA

Causative organisms include *Streptococcus pneumoniae, Haemophilus influenzae, Klebsiella pneumoniae, Chlamydia pneumoniae,* and *Mycoplasma pneumoniae*. The rate of community-acquired pneumonia in human immunodeficiency virus (HIV)-positive persons in the era before highly active antiviral therapy was 5.5 per 100-person years in one study, and the disease was most common in those with CD4+ count below 200/mm^3.[23] See Chapter 43 for further information.

VIRAL PNEUMONITIS

Respiratory viral pathogens include influenza A and B, parainfluenza 1, 2, and 3, respiratory syncytial virus, and adenovirus. Rarely, cytomegalovirus (CMV) causes pneumonia in patients with acquired immunodeficiency syndrome, although CMV can be found frequently in bronchoalveolar lavage fluid; therefore either extra-pulmonary or invasive pulmonary disease should be demonstrated before this diagnosis is made.[24] Respiratory viral pathogens can be detected through naso-pharyngeal wash specimens inoculated into viral media at the bedside.

CAVITARY LUNG DISEASE

Tuberculosis typically cavitates in patients with higher CD4+ counts. Other more common causes of cavitary lung disease (although rare causes of pulmonary infection in general) include *Mycobacterium kansasii, Pseudomonas aeruginosa, Aspergillus, Nocardia asteroides,* and *Rhodococcus equi.* Although cavitary disease is an uncommon presentation of *Pneumocystis* pneumonia, it should always be considered in a susceptible host.[25]

cont'd

BOX 39-3

DIFFERENTIAL DIAGNOSIS OF PULMONARY DISEASE IN HUMAN IMMUNODEFICIENCY VIRUS–POSITIVE PATIENTS—cont'd

MYCOBACTERIAL DISEASE

Tuberculosis can manifest itself as focal infiltrates, reticulonodular infiltrates, cavitary disease, hilar adenopathy, or effusion. In early HIV, tuberculosis occurs as upper lobe cavitary disease; in later stages pneumonitis or a miliary pattern can be seen. *Mycobacterium avium* complex (MAC) may colonize airways without causing disease, a marker for the development of disseminated MAC. *M. kansasii* causes cavitary or nodular disease in patients with CD4+ counts below 50/mm^3.[26]

FUNGAL DISEASE

Aspergillus pneumonia occurs in up to 4% of patients with acquired immunodeficiency syndrome. Focal or cavitary infiltrates, often pleural based, are seen. *Coccidioides immitis* is found in endemic areas; diffuse nodular infiltrates, focal infiltrates, cavities, and hilar adenopathy may be seen.[27] *Candida* rarely causes disease; histopathological evidence of invasive disease is necessary to diagnose *Candida* pneumonia. *Cryptococcus neoformans* can cause infiltrate or nodular disease; lumbar puncture should be performed if *C. neoformans* pneumonia is diagnosed. *Histoplasma capsulatum* can cause pulmonary or disseminated disease.[28]

NONINFECTIOUS DISEASE

Kaposi's sarcoma, lymphoma, and lymphocytic interstitial pneumonitis can cause pulmonary disease.

BOX 39-4

DIFFERENTIAL DIAGNOSIS OF PULMONARY COMPLICATIONS OF HUMAN IMMUNODEFICIENCY VIRUS BASED ON RADIOGRAPHIC FINDINGS

DIFFUSE RETICULONODULAR INFILTRATES

Pneumocystis carinii
Miliary tuberculosis
Histoplasmosis
Coccidioidomycosis
Kaposi's sarcoma
Lymphocytic interstitial pneumonitis
Leishmania donovani
Toxoplasma gondii
Cytomegalovirus

NODULES

Mycobacterium tuberculosis
Cryptococcosis
Kaposi's sarcoma
Nocardia

cont'd

BOX 39-4

DIFFERENTIAL DIAGNOSIS OF PULMONARY COMPLICATIONS OF HUMAN IMMUNODEFICIENCY VIRUS BASED ON RADIOGRAPHIC FINDINGS—cont'd

HILAR ADENOPATHY

M. tuberculosis
Cryptococcosis
Mycobacterium avium complex
Histoplasmosis
Coccidioidomycosis
Kaposi's sarcoma
Lymphoma

NORMAL

P. carinii
M. tuberculosis
Cryptococcosis
M. avium complex

CONSOLIDATION

Common
Pyogenic bacteria
Cryptococcosis
Kaposi's sarcoma
Rare
Nocardia
M. tuberculosis
Mycobacterium kansasii
Bordetella bronchiseptica[23]

PLEURAL EFFUSION

Common
Pyogenic bacteria (*Staphylococcus aureus* > *Streptococcus pneumoniae* > *Pseudomonas aeruginosa*)
M. tuberculosis
Cryptococcosis
Kaposi's sarcoma
P. carinii
Hypoalbuminemia
Septic emboli
Heart failure
Aspergillosis
Rare
Rhodococcus equi
Histoplasmosis
Coccidioidomycosis

Modified from Bartlett JG, Gallant JE. *2000-2001 Medical management of HIV infection*. Baltimore: Port City Press; 2000.

cont'd

BOX 39-4

DIFFERENTIAL DIAGNOSIS OF PULMONARY COMPLICATIONS OF HUMAN IMMUNODEFICIENCY VIRUS BASED ON RADIOGRAPHIC FINDINGS—cont'd

PLEURAL EFFUSION—cont'd

L. donovani

T. gondii

M. avium complex

Lymphoma

Nocardia

Modified from Bartlett JG, Gallant JE. *2000-2001 Medical management of HIV infection*. Baltimore: Port City Press; 2000.

BOX 39-5

DIAGNOSTIC TESTING FOR *PNEUMOCYSTIS CARINII* PNEUMONIA

HISTORY

Is the patient an appropriate host?

Human immunodeficiency virus (HIV) positive with CD4+ count <200/mm³ or <13% total CD4+ cells

Taking appropriate prophylaxis?

For non-HIV-infected hosts, see risk factors in Pearls and Pitfalls section

Is the time course of disease appropriate?

Generally subacute onset of shortness of breath

PHYSICAL EXAMINATION

Evaluate for respiratory distress and pneumothorax

Check oxygen saturation

LABORATORY TESTS

Arterial blood gases

Lactate dehydrogenase level (normal helps to rule out *Pneumocystis carinii* pneumonia in a low- or moderate-probability case)

RADIOGRAPHY

Chest radiograph divided into four quadrants; abnormalities in more quadrants increase the likelihood of *P. carinii* pneumonia[29]

Look for pneumothoraces

High-resolution chest computed tomography if the diagnosis is in question

---

MICROBIOLOGY

Expectorated or induced sputum for immunofluorescence testing

Bronchoalveolar lavage if sputum findings are negative

IV. MANAGEMENT (Table 39-1)

1. **Prophylaxis.**

a. Prophylaxis is highly effective at preventing both primary and secondary PCP cases in high-risk populations. Prophylaxis is recommended for HIV-infected patients with CD4$^+$ counts below 200/mm^3, unexplained fever (temperature >37.8° C) for more than 2 weeks, oropharyngeal candidiasis, or a history of PCP. HAART suppresses HIV replication and causes a concomitant rise in the CD4$^+$ count. Discontinuation of both primary and secondary prophylaxis is safe when the CD4$^+$ count has been over 200/mm^3 for more than 3 months.[31-35]

b. Trimethoprim-sulfamethoxazole is the preferred agent for prophylaxis. Two metaanalyses concluded that this drug combination was more effective than dapsone-containing regimens or aerosolized pentamidine.[3,36] Adverse reactions, which are generally not allergic in nature, are common. Symptomatic treatment with antihistamines, dose reduction, desensitization, and drug holidays may be beneficial. One single-strength (SS) tablet daily is as effective as one double-strength (DS) tablet daily.[3] Although the regimen is less well studied, one SS tablet three times weekly appears to be as effective as one SS tablet daily.[37] The lower dose regimens are better tolerated, although they do not provide adequate prophylaxis against toxoplasmosis for patients with CD4$^+$ counts below 100/mm^3 and positive anti-*Toxoplasma* immunoglobulin G (IgG) antibody. Full-dose trimethoprim-sulfamethoxazole has the additional advantages of providing anti-*Toxoplasma* prophylaxis and preventing many bacterial infections.

c. Dapsone plus pyrimethamine and atovaquone is also effective for toxoplasmosis prophylaxis, although dapsone is less effective than trimethoprim-sulfamethoxazole for PCP prevention. Atovaquone was as effective as dapsone and aerosolized pentamidine in head-to-head comparisons in patients who could not tolerate trimethoprim-sulfamethoxazole.[38,39]

d. Aerosolized pentamidine is less effective but much better tolerated than systemic prophylaxis, which increases compliance. Pentamidine prophylaxis increases the risk of extrapulmonary pneumocystosis (which remains extremely rare) and pneumothorax and decreases the diagnostic sensitivity of BAL. It offers no protection against toxoplasmosis. Patients should be screened for active tuberculosis to prevent transmission to health care workers. Bronchospasm is common and may be prevented by the preadministration of bronchodilators.

2. **Treatment.**

a. For moderate to severe PCP, trimethoprim-sulfamethoxazole is the agent of choice. Intravenous, not aerosolized, pentamidine is an alternative for severe PCP in patients who cannot tolerate or have not responded to trimethoprim-sulfamethoxazole. Both drugs are associated with a high frequency of major adverse effects, approaching 50%. Trimetrexate-leucovorin is inferior to trimethoprim-sulfamethoxazole but is an option

TABLE 39-1

DRUG THERAPY FOR *PNEUMOCYSTIS CARINII* PNEUMONIA

Indication	Drug	Dosage and Route	Adverse Effects
Prophylaxis	Trimethoprim-sulfamethoxazole	1 DS PO qd or 1 SS PO qd or 1 SS PO 3 times per week	Rash, fever, bone marrow suppression, hepatitis, nausea, vomiting, hyperkalemia
	Dapsone	100 mg po qd	Nausea, vomiting, fever, rash, bone marrow suppression, hepatitis, hemolysis, methemoglobinemia
	Dapsone-pyrimethamine-leucovorin	Dapsone 50 mg qd plus pyrimethamine 50 mg/week plus leucovorin 25 mg/week or dapsone 200 mg/week plus pyrimethamine 75 mg/week plus leucovorin 25 mg/week	As for dapsone
	Atovaquone	1500 mg PO qd	Nausea, vomiting, rash, diarrhea
	Pentamidine	300 mg once a month aerosolized via Respirgard II nebulizer	Cough, bronchospasm
Treatment	Trimethoprim-sulfamethoxazole	Trimethoprim 15 mg/kg/day plus sulfamethoxazole 75 mg/kg/day PO or IV, divided tid or qid; usual oral dose is 2 DS tid	As above for prophylaxis
	Pentamidine	4 mg/kg/day IV	Hypoglycemia, hyperglycemia, QT interval prolongation, arrhythmias, pancreatitis, leukopenia, bone marrow suppression, hepatitis, fever, hyperkalemia
	Trimethoprim-dapsone	Trimethoprim 15 mg/kg/day PO plus dapsone 100 mg PO qd	As for dapsone
	Clindamycin-primaquine	Clindamycin 600 mg IV q8h or 300-450 mg PO q6h plus primaquine base 30 mg/day PO	Rash, anemia, neutropenia, hemolysis, methemoglobinemia
	Atovaquone	750 mg suspension PO tid with meals	As above for prophylaxis
	Trimetrexate-leucovorin	Trimetrexate 45 mg/m²/day plus leucovorin 20 mg/m² PO or IV q6h. Continue leucovorin for 72 hours after last trimetrexate dose	Neutropenia, thrombocytopenia

DS, Double strength; *SS*, single strength.

for intravenous therapy in patients with moderate to severe PCP who cannot tolerate first-line agents.[40]

b. For mild to moderate PCP, trimethoprim-sulfamethoxazole, trimethoprim-dapsone, and clindamycin-primaquine are equally effective (failure rate 7%-12%) and have similar rates of dose-limiting toxicity (24%-33%), although the specific side effects differ among the three regimens and may allow tailoring of therapy toward the individual patient.[41] Atovaquone is less effective, but better tolerated, than trimethoprim-sulfamethoxazole for mild to moderate PCP.[42]

c. Drug toxicity limits the effectiveness of PCP therapy. Common adverse effects may be managed with antihistamines, antipyretics, and antiemetics. Patients should be carefully monitored for treatment-limiting toxicities and switched to an alternative regimen if necessary.

d. Corticosteroids decrease the incidence of respiratory failure and mortality in moderate to severe PCP (Pao_2 <70 mm Hg or PAo_2-Pao_2 >35 mm Hg) if they are started within 24 to 72 hours of the initiation of anti-*Pneumocystis* therapy.[43-46] The beneficial effect of corticosteroids is postulated to derive from their ability to blunt the increased inflammatory response that follows the initiation of antimicrobial therapy. Corticosteroid treatment increases the risk of *Candida* esophagitis but does not significantly increase the incidence of other opportunistic infections or malignancies.[47] The standard regimen is prednisone 40 mg bid on days 1 to 5, 40 mg qd on days 6 to 10, and 20 mg qd on days 11 to 21.

e. Clinical deterioration with worsening oxygenation is common in the first few days of therapy, reaching its nadir at 72 hours.[44] If clinical improvement has not occurred after 7 days of therapy, BAL should be considered to assess for coexisting pathogens or refractory PCP. Data on salvage therapy are limited, but a metaanalysis suggests that clindamycin-primaquine is approximately 90% effective in patients who have failed to respond to trimethoprim-sulfamethoxazole, pentamidine, or both.[48] Mutations in the *P. carinii* dihydropteroate synthase gene have been identified, but there are conflicting data as to whether such mutations confer clinically significant resistance to trimethoprim-sulfamethoxazole.[49,50]

PEARLS AND PITFALLS

- The incidence of PCP in non-HIV-infected patients has increased in the past two decades with increased use of chemotherapy and immunosuppressive agents for organ transplantation and treatment of chronic inflammatory conditions. Indeed, before the AIDS epidemic, PCP was a well-recognized complication after intensive chemotherapy for childhood acute lymphocytic leukemia. The most common predisposing conditions to PCP in non-HIV-infected patients are hematological malignancies, solid tumors, organ or bone marrow transplantation, and autoimmune or inflammatory conditions. More than 90% of patients had been treated with corticosteroids, and many others had been treated with cytotoxic agents or immunosuppressants such as cyclosporine.[5,51,52]

39

PNEUMOCYSTIS CARINII (JIROVECI) PNEUMONIA

- Compared with HIV-infected patients, non-HIV-infected patients have a more fulminant presentation. They have a lower burden of organisms but more severe lung inflammation and hypoxemia. They are more likely to require BAL for diagnosis because of the lower number of organisms.[53,54] The incidence of respiratory failure and death is significantly higher than in HIV-infected patients. In one series respiratory failure occurred in 43% and was associated with a mortality of 66%; overall mortality in these patients is 35% to 40%.[51]

- The mainstay of treatment is trimethoprim-sulfamethoxazole at standard doses. Alternative regimens are acceptable, but in general they have not been studied extensively in this population. Treatment duration is 2, rather than 3, weeks. The use of corticosteroids is controversial. As noted, most of these patients are taking fairly high doses of steroids at the time of presentation. Two small retrospective studies have attempted to examine outcomes in patients who were maintained at their baseline dose or who had their dose tapered versus those who had their dose increased. One study found no benefit for high-dose steroids.[55] The other showed no difference in rates of intubation, intensive care unit (ICU) admission, or mortality, but the increased-dose group had a shorter duration of mechanical ventilation and ICU stay.[56] Data are insufficient to support the use of adjunctive corticosteroids in non-HIV PCP. However, no data have been presented suggesting that a short-term increase in steroids increases risk, and many physicians would elect to maintain patients at their previous steroid doses.

- Prophylaxis is highly effective in non-HIV-infected patients, and the same regimens used for HIV-infected patients apply. Patients with acute leukemia, Hodgkin's disease, or aggressive non-Hodgkin's lymphoma, solid organ transplant recipients, and patients with brain tumors taking high-dose corticosteroids are at high risk and should receive prophylaxis. Although prolonged courses of high-dose corticosteroids for autoimmune or inflammatory diseases are a clear risk factor for PCP, the overall attack rate is low and there are no clear indications from the literature about how much steroid for how long places a patient at a high enough risk to merit prophylaxis. In one series patients had received a median of 30 mg of prednisone for a median of 12 weeks before PCP developed, but 25% were receiving less than 16 mg and 25% had been treated for less than 8 weeks.[51] One prospective study found that 91% of non-HIV PCP cases were associated with a CD4+ count below 300/mm^3. CD4+ counts below 300/mm^3 were also seen in 80% of chemotherapy recipients who did not have PCP and 64% of organ transplant recipients (within 12 months of transplant). Of patients receiving long-term corticosteroids for inflammatory conditions, 39% had CD4+ counts below 300/mm^3.[57] Further study is necessary to decide whether baseline CD4+ counts in non-HIV-infected patients can be used to determine who needs prophylaxis. At present prophylaxis should be offered to individuals receiving the equivalent of 20 mg or more of prednisone for more than 1 month.

REFERENCES

[d] 1. Stringer JR et al. A new name (*Pneumocystis jiroveci*) for *Pneumocystis* from humans. Emerg Infect Dis 2002; 8:891.

[c] 2. Gallant J, Moore R, Chaisson R. Prophylaxis for opportunistic infections in patients with HIV infection. Ann Intern Med 1994; 120:932.

[c] 3. Ioannidis J et al. A meta-analysis of the relative efficacy and toxicity of *Pneumocystis carinii* prophylactic regimens. Arch Intern Med 1996; 156:177.

[c] 4. Kaplan J et al. Epidemiology of human immunodeficiency virus–associated opportunistic infections in the United States in the era of highly active antiretroviral therapy. Clin Infect Dis 2000; 30:S5.

[a] 5. Mansharamani N et al. Management and outcome patterns for adult *Pneumocystis carinii* pneumonia, 1985-1995: comparison of HIV-associated cases to other immunocompromised states. Chest 2000; 118:704.

[b] 6. Helweg-Larsen J et al. Clusters of *Pneumocystis carinii* pneumonia: analysis of person-to-person transmission by genotyping. Q J Med 1998; 91:813.

[c] 7. Kovacs JA et al. New insights into transmission, diagnosis, and drug treatment of *Pneumocystis carinii* pneumonia. JAMA 2001; 286:2450.

[c] 8. Wilkin A, Feinberg J. *Pneumocystis carinii* pneumonia: a clinical review. Am Fam Physician 1999; 60:1699.

[b] 9. Metersky M et al. AIDS-related spontaneous pneumothorax: risk factors and treatment. Chest 1995; 108:946.

[b] 10. Masur H et al. CD4 counts as predictors of opportunistic pneumonias in human immunodeficiency virus (HIV) infection. Ann Intern Med 1989; 111:223.

[b] 11. Katz M, Baron R, Grady D. Risk stratification of ambulatory patients suspected of *Pneumocystis carinii* pneumonia. Arch Intern Med 1991; 151:105.

[b] 12. Smith D et al. Diagnosis of *Pneumocystis carinii* pneumonia in HIV antibody positive patients by simple outpatient assessments. Thorax 1992; 47:1005.

[b] 13. Baughman R, Dohn M, Frame P. The continuing utility of bronchoalveolar lavage to diagnose opportunistic infection in AIDS patients. Am J Med 1994; 97:515.

[b] 14. Huang L et al. Performance of an algorithm to detect *Pneumocystis carinii* pneumonia in symptomatic HIV-infected persons. Chest 1999; 115:1025.

[b] 15. Gruden J et al. High-resolution CT in the evaluation of clinically suspected *Pneumocystis carinii* pneumonia in AIDS patients with normal, equivocal, or nonspecific radiographic findings. AJR 1997; 169:967.

[b] 16. Quist J, Hill A. Serum lactate dehydrogenase (LDH) in *Pneumocystis carinii* pneumonia, tuberculosis, and bacterial pneumonia. Chest 1995; 108:415.

[b] 17. Stover D, Greeno R, Gagliardi A. The use of a simple exercise test for the diagnosis of *Pneumocystis carinii* pneumonia in patients with AIDS. Am Rev Respir Dis 1989; 139:1343.

[c] 18. Tu J, Biem H, Detsky A. Bronchoscopy versus empirical therapy in HIV-infected patients with presumptive *Pneumocystis carinii* pneumonia: a decision analysis. Am Rev Respir Dis 1993; 148:370.

[b] 19. Huang L et al. Suspected *Pneumocystis carinii* pneumonia with a negative induced sputum examination: is early bronchoscopy useful? Am J Respir Crit Care Med 1995; 151:1866.

[b] 20. Arasteh KN et al. Sensitivity and specificity of indirect immunofluorescence and Grocott-technique in comparison with immunocytology (alkaline phosphatase anti alkaline phosphatase = APAAP) for the diagnosis of *Pneumocystis carinii* pneumonia in bronchoalveolar lavage. Eur J Med Res 1998; 3:559.

[b] 21. Metersky M, Aslenzadeh J, Stelmach P. A comparison of induced and expectorated sputum for the diagnosis of *Pneumocystis carinii* pneumonia. Chest 1998; 113:1555.

[b] 22. Fishman JA, Roth RS, Zanzot E. Use of induced sputum specimens for microbiologic diagnosis of infection due to organisms other than *Pneumocystis carinii*. J Clin Microbiol 1994; 32:131.

[b] 23. Gallant J, Chaisson R, Moore R. The effect of adjunctive corticosteroids for the treatment of *Pneumocystis carinii* pneumonia on mortality and subsequent complications. Chest 1998; 114:1258.

39

[b] 24. Hirschtick RE et al. Bacterial pneumonia in persons infected with the human immunodeficiency virus. Pulmonary Complications of HIV Infection Study Group. N Engl J Med 1995; 333:845.

[b] 25. Rodriguez-Barradas MC. Diagnosing and treating cytomegalovirus pneumonia in patients with AIDS. Clin Infect Dis 1996; 23:76.

[c] 26. Gallant JE, Ko AH. Cavitary pulmonary lesions in patients infected with human immunodeficiency virus. Clin Infect Dis 1996; 22:671.

[c] 27. Bartlett JG, Gallant JE. 2000-2001 Medical management of HIV infection. Baltimore: Port City Press; 2000.

[b] 28. Singh VR et al. Coccidioidomycosis in patients infected with human immunodeficiency virus: review of 91 cases at a single institution. Clin Infect Dis 1996; 23:563.

[c] 29. Wheat LJ et al. Disseminated histoplasmosis in the acquired immune deficiency syndrome: clinical findings, diagnosis and treatment, and review of the literature. Medicine 1990; 69:361.

[b] 30. Boldt MJ, Bai TR. Utility of lactate dehydrogenase vs radiographic severity in the differential diagnosis of *Pneumocystis carinii* pneumonia. Chest 1997; 111:1187.

[a] 31. Bernaldo de Quiros J et al. A randomized trial of the discontinuation of primary and secondary prophylaxis against *Pneumocystis carinii* pneumonia after highly active antiretroviral therapy in patients with HIV infection. N Engl J Med 2001; 344:159.

[a] 32. Ledergerber B et al. Discontinuation of secondary prophylaxis against *Pneumocystis carinii* pneumonia in patients with HIV infection who have a response to antiretroviral therapy. N Engl J Med 2001; 344:168.

[a] 33. Furrer H et al. Discontinuation of primary prophylaxis against *Pneumocystis carinii* pneumonia in HIV-1 infected adults treated with combination antiretroviral therapy. N Engl J Med 1999; 340:1301.

[a] 34. Weverling G et al. Discontinuation of *Pneumocystis carinii* prophylaxis after start of highly active antiretroviral therapy in HIV-1 infection. Lancet 1999; 353:1293.

[b] 35. Yangco B et al. Discontinuation of chemoprophylaxis against *Pneumocystis carinii* pneumonia in patients with HIV infection. Ann Intern Med 2000; 132:201.

[c] 36. Bucher H et al. Meta-analysis of prophylactic treatments against *Pneumocystis carinii* pneumonia and *Toxoplasma* encephalitis in HIV-infected patients. J Acquir Immune Defic Syndr Hum Retrovirol 1997; 15:104.

[a] 37. El-Sadr W et al. A randomized trial of daily and thrice weekly trimethoprim-sulfamethoxazole for the prevention of *Pneumocystis carinii* pneumonia in HIV-infected individuals. Clin Infect Dis 1999; 29:775.

[a] 38. El-Sadr W et al. Atovaquone compared with dapsone for the prevention of *Pneumocystis carinii* pneumonia in patients with HIV infection who cannot tolerate trimethoprim, sulfonamides, or both. N Engl J Med 1998; 339:1889.

[a] 39. Chan C et al. Atovaquone suspension compared with aerosolized pentamidine for prevention of *Pneumocystis carinii* pneumonia in human immunodeficiency virus–infected subjects intolerant of trimethoprim or sulfonamides. J Infect Dis 1999; 180:369.

[a] 40. Sattler F et al. Trimetrexate with leucovorin versus trimethoprim-sulfamethoxazole for moderate to severe episodes of *Pneumocystis carinii* pneumonia in patients with AIDS: a prospective, controlled multicenter investigation of the AIDS Clinical Trials Group Protocol 029/031. J Infect Dis 1994; 170:165.

[a] 41. Safrin S et al. Comparison of three regimens for treatment of mild to moderate *Pneumocystis carinii* pneumonia in patients with AIDS: a double blind randomized trial of oral trimethoprim-sulfamethoxazole, dapsone-trimethoprim, and clindamycin-primaquine. Ann Intern Med 1996; 124:792.

[a] 42. Hughes W et al. Comparison of atovaquone (566C80) with trimethoprim-sulfamethoxazole to treat *Pneumocystis carinii* pneumonia in patients with AIDS. N Engl J Med 1993; 328:1521.

[a] 43. Gagnon S et al. Corticosteroids as adjunctive therapy for severe *Pneumocystis carinii* pneumonia in the acquired immunodeficiency syndrome. N Engl J Med 1990; 323:1444.

[a] 44. Bozette S et al. A controlled trial of early adjunctive treatment with corticosteroids for *Pneumocystis carinii* pneumonia in the acquired immunodeficiency syndrome. N Engl J Med 1990; 323:1451.

[a] 45. Montaner J et al. Corticosteroids prevent early deterioration in patients with moderately severe *Pneumocystis carinii* pneumonia and the acquired immunodeficiency syndrome (AIDS). Ann Intern Med 1990; 113:14.

[d] 46. National Institutes of Health–University of California Expert Panel for Corticosteroids as Adjunctive Therapy for *Pneumocystis* Pneumonia. Consensus statement on the use of corticosteroids as adjunctive therapy for *Pneumocystis* pneumonia in the acquired immunodeficiency syndrome. N Engl J Med 1990; 323:1500.

[b] 47. O'Donnell W et al. Clearance of *Pneumocystis carinii* cysts in acute *P. carinii* pneumonia: assessment by serial sputum induction. Chest 1998; 114:1264.

[c] 48. Smego R, Nagar S, Popara M. A meta-analysis of salvage therapy for *Pneumocystis carinii* pneumonia. Arch Intern Med 2001; 161:1529.

[b] 49. Helweg-Larsen J et al. Effects of mutations in *Pneumocystis carinii* dihydropteroate synthase gene on outcome of AIDS-associated *P. carinii* pneumonia. Lancet 1999; 354:1347.

[b] 50. Navin T et al. Effect of mutations in *Pneumocystis carinii* dihydropteroate synthase gene on outcome of *P. carinii* pneumonia in patients with HIV-1: a prospective study. Lancet 2001; 358:545.

[b] 51. Yale S, Limper A. *Pneumocystis carinii* pneumonia in patients without acquired immunodeficiency syndrome: associated illnesses and prior corticosteroid therapy. Mayo Clin Proc 1996; 71:5.

[b] 52. Arend S, Kroon F, van't Wout J. *Pneumocystis carinii* pneumonia in patients without AIDS, 1980 through 1993: an analysis of 78 cases. Arch Intern Med 1995; 155:2336.

[b] 53. Kovacs J et al. *Pneumocystis carinii* pneumonia: a comparison between patients with the acquired immunodeficiency syndrome and patients with other immunodeficiencies. Ann Intern Med 1984; 100:663.

[b] 54. Limper A et al. *Pneumocystis carinii* pneumonia: differences in lung parasite number and inflammation in patients with and without AIDS. Am Rev Respir Dis 1989; 140:1204.

[b] 55. Delclaux C et al. Corticosteroids as adjunctive therapy for severe *Pneumocystis carinii* pneumonia in non–human immunodeficiency virus–infected patients: a retrospective study of 31 patients. Clin Infect Dis 1999; 29:670.

[b] 56. Pareja J, Garland R, Koziel H. Use of adjunctive corticosteroids in severe adult non-HIV *Pneumocystis carinii* pneumonia. Chest 1998; 113:1215.

[b] 57. Mansharamani N et al. Peripheral blood CD4+ T-lymphocyte counts during *Pneumocystis carinii* pneumonia in immunocompromised patients without HIV infection. Chest 2000; 118:712.

39

PNEUMOCYSTIS CARINII (JIROVECI) PNEUMONIA

Central Venous Line Infections

Aimee Zaas, MD, and Stuart C. Ray, MD

FAST FACTS

- Ninety percent of intravascular device–related infections are due to central venous catheters (CVCs).[1]
- The skin insertion site is the most common source of infection for CVCs left in place for less than 10 days.[2]
- Hub contamination is the primary source of catheter colonization and infection for CVCs left in place for more than 10 days.[2]
- Coagulase-negative staphylococci are the most common cause of catheter-related bloodstream infections (CR-BSIs).
- Blood cultures from specimens drawn through CVCs have 90% sensitivity and 92% specificity for diagnosing CR-BSI.[3]
- Mortality rate of catheter-related *Staphylococcus aureus* bloodstream infections is 8.2%, significantly higher than for any other organism.[4]

I. DEFINITIONS

1. **Catheter-related bloodstream infection (CR-BSI):** Isolation of the same organism from a semiquantitative or quantitative culture of a catheter segment and from the blood of a patient with clinical symptoms of a BSI and no apparent other source of infection. One of the following should be present.
   a. Positive semiquantitative (≥15 colony-forming units [CFUs] per segment) or quantitative (≥10^2 CFUs per segment) blood culture growing the same organism as the peripheral blood culture.
   b. Simultaneous quantitative blood cultures with a CVC/peripheral blood ratio greater than or equal to 5:1.
   c. Differential time to positivity (i.e., CVC culture becomes positive at least 2 hours earlier than the peripheral culture).[5]
2. **Colonized catheter:** Growth of at least 15 CFUs (semiquantitative culture) or more than 1000 CFUs (quantitative culture) from a proximal or distal catheter segment in the absence of accompanying clinical symptoms.
3. **Exit site infection:** Erythema, tenderness, purulence, or induration within 2 cm of the catheter exit site.

II. EPIDEMIOLOGY

1. Intravascular catheters are the source of most primary bloodstream infections.[1] The skin insertion site is the most common source of colonization and infection for CVCs left in place less than 10 days, whereas hub contamination becomes a predominant factor in CVC

colonization and BSI when catheters are left in place longer than 10 days.

2. Microbial epidemiology of CR-BSI is outlined in Fig. 40-1.

3. Coagulase-negative staphylococci are the leading pathogens of indwelling catheter and prosthetic device infection, probably because of these organisms' ubiquity as human commensals and their propensity to adhere to polymers and form biofilm (bacteria and extracellular glycoprotein matrix). Biofilm enhances bacterial adherence and provides protection from antibiotic and white blood cell action.

III. CLINICAL PRESENTATION

1. Central venous line infections should be suspected when a patient with a central venous line has unexplained fever, leukocytosis, or hypotension.

2. Catheter exit site infections are generally manifested clinically as purulence, erythema, or induration at the site.

IV. DIAGNOSIS

1. The Centers for Disease Control and Prevention advises culturing of catheters only when clinically indicated (presence of fever, hypotension) because surveillance cultures in asymptomatic patients have not been shown to have clinical benefit.

2. In the setting of fever, guidewire exchange with semiquantitative culture of the catheter tip is another acceptable method for diagnosing CR-BSI. If the catheter culture indicates colonization or infection, the new catheter should be removed and a catheter inserted at a new site.[1]

3. Semiquantitative culture ("roll plate") is used at most institutions to diagnose catheter colonization. Semiquantitative culture involves rolling the tip (distal 4 cm) of the catheter across an agar plate and counting the colonies that form after an overnight incubation. Significant catheter colonization is defined as growth of 15 or more colonies.

a. Semiquantitative culture is the preferred method for diagnosing CR-BSI because of the ease of performing the study. Drawbacks of this technique include the need to remove the catheter, the necessity for overnight incubation to obtain results, and the detection of extraluminal but not intraluminal organisms.

b. Using blood cultures and the semiquantitative roll plate technique, Collignon and associates found a sensitivity of 85%, specificity of 83%, and negative predictive value of 99.7% for the cutoff value of at least 15 colonies to diagnose catheter-related bacteremia in patients in the intensive care unit (ICU).[6]

4. CR-BSI can be diagnosed without removal of the CVC by the simultaneous collection of peripheral blood and blood drawn through the central venous line for culture. In 200 ICU patients with indwelling CVCs, Wormser and associates found a 96% sensitivity (95% confi-

40

CENTRAL VENOUS LINE INFECTIONS

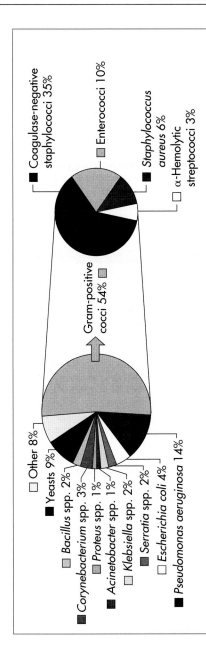

FIG. 40-1

Microbial epidemiology of catheter-related bloodstream infection. *(Modified from Pearson ML. Am J Infect Control 1996; 24:262.)*

dence interval [CI] 89%-100%) and 98% specificity (95% CI 96%-100%) when the peripheral blood culture result was used as the true positive or true negative.[3] In oncology patients with indwelling catheters (most often Hickman or Broviac catheters), the negative predictive value of blood cultures drawn from these catheters was 99%; however, the positive predictive value of such cultures was not as favorable (63%).[7] When CR-BSI is a suspected cause of infection, paired peripheral and catheter blood should be drawn for culture. Results of these cultures should be interpreted in light of the clinical scenario.

5. Differential time to positivity (central venous line blood culture turning positive before a paired peripheral culture) was shown to have a specificity of 100% and sensitivity of 96.4% when a cutoff time of +120 minutes was used in a retrospective analysis of 64 paired cultures.[8] This result remains to be validated in prospective studies.

V. MANAGEMENT

1. The practice of routinely changing central lines (new site or guidewire exchange) to prevent infection has not been found to be useful, regardless of whether catheters were changed every 3 days[9] or every 7 days.[10] Guidewire exchange to replace a malfunctioning catheter or convert to a different catheter type should be performed only if the exit site does not appear to be infected (absence of erythema, tenderness, or purulence).[1]

2. Treatment of CR-BSI depends on the organism cultured.

a. Coagulase-negative staphylococci: Vancomycin is the drug of choice, since isolates are generally methicillin resistant. Alternative antimicrobial agents active against methicillin-resistant coagulase-negative staphylococci include linezolid and quinupristin-dalfopristin. No studies regarding optimal length of treatment have been published. Experts recommend treatment for 7 days if the patient is responding after 48 to 72 hours. Length of treatment is less standardized if the patient is not responding within 48 to 72 hours. No studies have looked at the role of echocardiography in persistent coagulase-negative staphylococcal BSI, but an evaluation for endocarditis is reasonable if the patient does not improve within 48 to 72 hours of therapy with vancomycin. Coagulase-negative staphylococcal CR-BSIs are the only CR-BSIs that can be treated safely without removal of the catheter. This recommendation is based on a retrospective case-controlled study of 70 oncology patients in which equal mortality (11%) was observed in the group whose catheters remained in place and the group whose catheters were removed. Treatment without catheter removal is recommended only if the CVC will remain in place for a short time because recurrences of bacteremia were more common in the group who retained their catheters, particularly after 3 weeks.[11]

b. *S. aureus:* Treatment is with an antistaphylococcal penicillin or vancomycin, depending on sensitivities of the isolate. Vancomycin is inferior to antistaphylococcal penicillins for methicillin-susceptible isolates. Alternative antimicrobial agents active against methicillin-resistant staphylococci include linezolid and quinupristin-dalfopristin. *S. aureus* is never considered a contaminant, and metastatic foci are of particular concern (endocarditis, osteomyelitis, septic emboli, abscesses).[2] Retention of the catheter in *S. aureus* CR-BSI can lead to increased mortality, relapse, and persistence of bacteremia.[12] Treatment should continue for at least 10 days because a shorter duration is associated with increased mortality.[13,14] If the patient does not respond clinically after catheter removal and 3 days of antibiotics, a 4-week course of treatment is appropriate. *S. aureus* endocarditis, bacteremia complicated by septic thrombosis, or *S. aureus* bacteremia in patients with underlying cardiac lesions is generally treated with 4 weeks of intravenous (IV) antibiotics. Transesophageal echocardiography may be a cost-effective method for determining length of therapy in patients with clinically uncomplicated catheter-associated *S. aureus* bacteremia (normal native heart valves, nonintravenous drug user, immunocompetent, no known metastatic infection).[15] Synergistic gentamicin 1 mg/kg q8h for 5 days is often used for complicated *S. aureus* bacteremia.

c. Gram-negative bacilli: Gram-negative bacilli are infrequent causes of CR-BSI. An analysis of 149 episodes of CR-BSI caused by *Stenotrophomonas maltophilia* and non-*aeruginosa Pseudomonas* species showed that failure to remove the catheter was associated with increased rates of recurrent bacteremia and treatment failure.[16] Catheter removal and a 7-day course of intravenous antibiotics are recommended for CR-BSI caused by gram-negative bacilli.[2] Specific antibiotic recommendations are listed in Table 40-1.

d. *Candida* species: Removal of the intravascular catheter and treatment with parenteral antifungal therapy are recommended based on results of several studies showing increased persistence of fungemia and increased mortality.[17,18] A nonneutropenic host can be treated with either fluconazole 400 mg/day for 14 days or amphotericin 0.5 mg/kg IV for 14 days. In candidal infections in nonneutropenic hosts, fluconazole was shown to be as effective as amphotericin and to have fewer adverse effects.[19] Newer fungicidal antifungal agents such as the echinocandin caspofungin are an option, particularly for patients with azole-resistant candidal infections and a contraindication to amphotericin B. Caspofungin has been shown to be noninferior to amphotericin B for the treatment of candidemia.[20] Controversy exists regarding implanted catheter removal in oncology patients.[21]

PEARLS AND PITFALLS

- Always make sure you cut the distal 4 to 6 cm of catheter to send for culture.

40

CENTRAL VENOUS LINE INFECTIONS

TABLE 40-1
TREATMENT OF CATHETER-RELATED BLOODSTREAM INFECTION BASED ON PATHOGEN

Organism	Antimicrobial	Rapid Response	Slow Response	Remove Catheter?
*Staphylococcus aureus** (MSSA)	Oxacillin, nafcillin, cefazolin	10-14 days	4 weeks	Yes
*S. aureus** (MRSA)	Vancomycin	10-14 days	4 weeks	Yes
Staphylococcus epidermidis	Vancomycin	7 days	10-14 days	No†
Gram-negative bacilli	According to sensitivity of isolate	10-14 days	Unknown‡	Yes
Escherichia coli and *Klebsiella*	Third-generation cephalosporin or advanced quinolone§			
Enterobacter and *Serratia*	Carbapenem or cefepime or advanced quinolone			
Acinetobacter	Ampicillin-sulbactam or carbapenem			
Streptococcus maltophilia	TMP-SMX or ticarcillin-clavulanate			
Pseudomonas aeruginosa	Third- or fourth-generation cephalosporin or antipseudomonal penicillin plus aminoglycoside			
Candida albicans	Fluconazole or amphotericin B product (includes lipid formulations) or caspofungin	14 days	?? days¶‖	Yes
Non-albicans *Candida* ‖	Amphotericin B product, caspofungin, possibly advanced-generation azole**	14 days	?? days¶	Yes††

Data from Clin Infect Dis 2001; 32:1249.

MRSA, Methicillin-resistant *Staphylococcus aureus*; *MSSA*, methicillin-susceptible *S. aureus*; *TMP-SMX*, trimethoprim-sulfamethoxazole.
*Infections complicated by endocarditis or septic emboli or in patients with underlying cardiac valvular abnormalities are treated for 4 to 6 weeks.
†Unless the patient is not responding to treatment or is critically ill.
‡Continue until clinical response; consider echocardiography and evaluation for metastatic sites of infection.
§Ciprofloxacin or levofloxacin.
‖ *C. glabrata, C. tropicalis,* and *C. parapsilosis* have varied fluconazole susceptibilities. Check your hospital antibiogram. *C. krusei* is always azole resistant. *C. lusitaniae* is amphotericin resistant.
¶Continue until clinical response; evaluate for metastatic sites of infection, including ophthalmological examination.
**Voriconazole, posaconazole, and ravuconazole are advanced-generation azoles; not approved by the U.S. Food and Drug Administration for this indication at the time of publication.
††Catheter removal in oncology patients is a matter of controversy because the gastrointestinal tract is the presumed source. Consultation with an infectious disease specialist is recommended.[21]

- The algorithm in Fig. 40-2 is adapted in part from "Guidelines for the Management of Intravascular Catheter Related Infections," compiled by an expert panel of the Infectious Diseases Society of America.[5]
- If blood culture results are negative and the CVC has not been cultured, remove and culture the CVC if fever persists and no other source is found.
- If blood and CVC culture results are negative, look for another infectious source.
- If blood culture results are negative and the catheter tip has 15 or more CFUs, monitor closely and repeat blood cultures accordingly. High-risk patients in this situation have valvular heart disease, neutropenia, *Candida,* or an *S. aureus*–positive catheter tip.
- If blood cultures results are positive and the catheter tip has 15 or more CFUs, see the following section.
- For known CR-BSI.
  - Complicated CR-BSI (septic thrombosis, endocarditis, osteomyelitis): Remove the CVC and treat the patient with systemic antibiotics for 4 to 6 weeks, or for 6 to 8 weeks in cases of osteomyelitis.
  - Uncomplicated CR-BSI.
    - Coagulase-negative staphylococci: Remove the CVC and treat with systemic antibiotics for 5 to 7 days *or* retain the CVC and treat for 10 to 14 days.
    - *S. aureus*: Remove the CVC and treat with systemic antibiotics for 14 days; if transesophageal echocardiographic findings are positive, treat for 4 to 6 weeks.
    - Gram-negative bacilli: Remove the CVC and treat the patient with systemic antibiotics for 10 to 14 days.
    - *Candida* species: Remove the CVC and treat the patient with systemic antifungal medication for 14 days after the last positive blood culture result.
- Avoidance of error: prevention of central venous line infections.
  - Subclavian central venous lines are less likely than internal jugular lines to become infected. In one study, colonization rates in ICU patients with central venous catheters were 47% for femoral lines, 22% for internal jugular catheters, and 10% for subclavian catheters.[22] A jugular insertion site, as compared with subclavian, was found to have an odds ratio of 2.7 in a multivariate analysis of infection risk in 503 central venous catheters.[23] Contamination with oropharyngeal and tracheostomy secretions and increased movement of the catheter are reasons that the risk of infection is higher with internal jugular catheters than with subclavian catheters.
  - Chlorhexidine is superior to povidone-iodine as a cutaneous antiseptic for skin cleansing at the time of insertion, yielding an 84% decreased rate of subsequent catheter colonization.[24]
  - Povidone-iodine must dry to have an antimicrobial effect, whereas chlorhexidine works immediately.
  - Prophylactic antimicrobial use during catheter insertion does not reduce the risk of infection.[25]

40

CENTRAL VENOUS LINE INFECTIONS

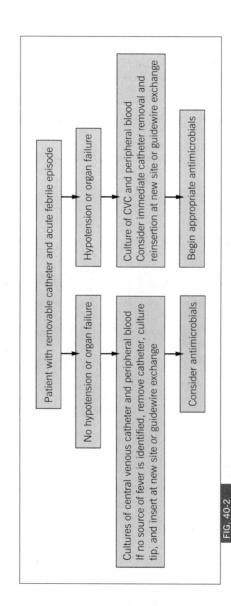

FIG. 40-2

Management of the patient with a removable catheter and acute febrile episode. *CVC,* Central venous catheter.

- The best method for prevention of CR-BSI is use of maximal sterile barriers (MSBs) during catheter insertion. Such barriers include covering the patient with a sterile drape and wearing a mask, cap, sterile gown, and gloves. A landmark randomized, prospective study by Raad and associates[26] compared MSB precautions against standard precautions for nontunneled, noncuffed subclavian and percutaneous indwelling central venous catheter insertion in oncology patients. Colonization occurred in 12 of 167 (7.2%) of the control and 4 of 176 (2.3%) of the MSB group ($p <.04$). Incidence of catheter-related sepsis was six times greater in the control group than in the MSB group, and 83% of the infections or colonizations in the control group were related to skin flora. In the MSB group, 75% of the infections or colonizations were with enteric gram-negative rods and all occurred more than 6 weeks after catheter insertion, which indicates that contamination at the time of insertion was unlikely.
- Special populations.
  - Tunneled catheter management is covered extensively in reference 5.
  - There is no standard for using antibiotic-impregnated catheters for roll plate catheter tip cultures.

REFERENCES

[d] 1. Pearson ML and the Hospital Infection Control Practices Advisory Committee. Guideline for prevention of intravascular device–related infections. Am J Infect Control 1996; 24:262.

[c] 2. Raad II. Intravascular-catheter related infections. Lancet 1998; 351:893.

[a] 3. Wormser GP et al. Sensitivity and specificity of blood cultures obtained through intravascular catheters. Crit Care Med 1990; 18:152.

[a] 4. Byers K et al. Case fatality rate for catheter-related bloodstream infections (CRBSI): a meta-analysis [Abstract 43]. In Proceedings of the fifth annual meeting of the Society for Hospital Epidemiology of America, 1995.

[d] 5. Mermel LA et al. Guidelines for the management of intravascular catheter–related infections. Clin Infect Dis 2001; 32:1249.

[d] 6. Collignon PJ et al. Is semiquantitative culture of central vein catheter tips useful in the diagnosis of catheter associated bacteremia? J Clin Microbiol 1996; 24:532.

[a] 7. DesJardin JA et al. Clinical utility of blood cultures drawn from indwelling central venous catheters in hospitalized patients with cancer. Ann Intern Med 1999; 131:641.

[a] 8. Blot F et al. Earlier positivity of central-venous- versus peripheral-blood cultures is highly predictive of catheter-related sepsis. J Clin Microbiol 1998; 36:105.

[a] 9. Cobb DK et al. A controlled trial of scheduled replacement of central venous and pulmonary artery catheters. N Engl J Med 1992; 327:1062.

[a] 10. Eyer S et al. Catheter related sepsis: prospective, randomized study of three methods of long-term catheter maintenance. Crit Care Med 1990; 18:1073.

[b] 11. Raad II et al. Catheter removal affects recurrence of coagulase negative staphylococcal bacteremia. Infect Control Hosp Epidemiol 1992; 13:215.

[c] 12. Dugdale DC, Ramsey PG. *Staphylococcus aureus* bacteremia in patients with Hickman catheters. Am J Med 1990; 89:137.

[c] 13. Raad II, Sabbagh MF. Optimal duration of therapy for catheter-related *Staphylococcus aureus* bacteremia: a study of 55 cases and review. Rev Infect Dis 1992; 14:75.

[b] 14. Malanoski GJ et al. *Staphylococcus aureus* catheter-associated bacteremia: minimal effective therapy and unusual infectious complications associated with arterial sheath catheters. Arch Intern Med 1995; 155:1161.

[a] 15. Rosen AB et al. Cost-effectiveness of transesophageal echocardiography to determine the duration of therapy for intravascular catheter–associated *Staphylococcus aureus* bacteremia. Ann Intern Med 1999; 130:810.

[b] 16. Elting LS, Bodey GB. Septicemia due to *Xanthomonas* species and non-*aeruginosa* *Pseudomonas* species: increasing incidence of catheter-related infections. Medicine (Baltimore) 1990; 60:196.

[c] 17. Rose HD. Venous catheter–associated candidemia. Am J Med Sci 1978; 275:265.

[b] 18. Nguyen MH et al. Therapeutic approaches in patients with candidemia: evaluation in a multicenter, prospective, observational study. Arch Intern Med 1995; 155:2429.

[a] 19. Rex JH et al. A randomized trial comparing fluconazole with amphotericin B for the treatment of candidemia in patients without neutropenia. Candidemia Study Group and the National Institute. N Engl J Med 1994; 331:1325.

[a] 20. Mora-Duarte J et al. Comparison of caspofungin and amphotericin B for invasive candidiasis. N Engl J Med 2002; 347(25):2020.

[d] 21. Nucci M, Anaissie E. Should vascular catheters be removed from all patients with candidemia? An evidenced-based review. Clin Infect Dis 2002; 34:591.

[a] 22. Gil RT et al. Triple vs single lumen central venous catheters: a prospective study in a critically ill population. Arch Intern Med 1989; 149:1139.

[a] 23. Richet H et al. Prospective multicenter study of vascular-catheter-related complications and risk factors for positive central-catheter cultures in intensive care units. J Clin Microbiol 1990; 28:2520.

[a] 24. Maki DG, Ringer M, Alvarado CJ. Prospective randomised trial of povidone-iodine, alcohol, and chlorhexidine for prevention of infection associated with central venous and arterial catheters. Lancet 1991; 338:339.

[a] 25. Ranson MR et al. Double-blind placebo controlled study of vancomycin prophylaxis for central venous catheter insertion in cancer patients. J Hosp Infect 1990; 15:95.

[a] 26. Raad II et al. Prevention of central venous catheter–related infections by using maximal sterile barrier precautions during insertion. Infect Control Hosp Epidemiol 1994; 15:231.

Infective Endocarditis

David A. Zidar, MD, and Stuart C. Ray, MD

FAST FACTS

- Definition: Infective endocarditis (IE) is an infection of the endothelial surface of the heart. A vegetation of platelet, fibrin, and microorganisms usually forms on the heart valves. Acute bacterial endocarditis (ABE) progresses over days to weeks and is most commonly associated with *Staphylococcus aureus*. The symptoms of subacute bacterial endocarditis (SBE) progress over weeks to months. It is typically caused by less virulent organisms such as viridans streptococci, coagulase-negative staphylococci, enterococci, and gram-negative rods. Because the distinction between ABE and SBE is not reliable enough to be applied in the clinical setting, it is largely of historical interest. In addition, the cause is not always bacterial. Hence the inclusive term "infective endocarditis" (proposed in 1930 by Dr. William S. Thayer) is preferred. In contrast to IE, marantic endocarditis results in a sterile vegetation and is commonly associated with malignancy.
- Complications: The major complications of IE can be divided into three categories: cardiac, complications of septic emboli, and immunological complications (Box 41-1).
- Differential diagnosis: Because of the variability of clinical manifestations, IE can resemble a number of infections, as well as noninfectious processes (Box 41-2).
- Roundsmanship: The so-called HACEK organisms are *Haemophilus* species, *Actinobacillus actinomycetemcomitans*, *Cardiobacterium hominis*, *Eikenella* species, and *Kingella kingae*. This is a popular question on rounds because these organisms are an uncommon cause of IE, but important because they are oxacillin-resistant gram-negative bacilli (GNB). Recent culture techniques have improved the recovery of these organisms, but the microbiology laboratory should be alerted if one of them is suspected.

41

I. EPIDEMIOLOGY

A. INCIDENCE

1. The incidence of infective endocarditis has been estimated to be 4 to 12 cases per 100,000 patients.[1-4] The exact figure, however, depends on the age of a given population[5] and the prevalence of associated risk factors. Men are more frequently affected than women by a ratio between 1.6 and 2.5.
2. Prosthetic valve endocarditis (PVE) occurs in 7% to 25% of total cases of IE.[3,4] The risk for PVE is greatest within the first 6 weeks.

BOX 41-1

COMPLICATIONS OF INFECTIVE ENDOCARDITIS

CARDIAC

Valvular destruction with or without congestive heart failure

Conduction system disruption from myocardial abscess

Purulent pericarditis from extension of myocardial abscess

EMBOLIC

Septic pulmonary emboli resulting from tricuspid or pulmonic valve ("right-sided") endocarditis

Cerebral, renal, splenic, hepatic emboli with concomitant abscess resulting from mitral or aortic valve ("left-sided") endocarditis

---

IMMUNOLOGICAL

Glomerulonephritis

Arthritis

Constitutional symptoms

The cumulative incidence is 1.4% to 3.1% at 12 months and 3.2% to 5.7% after 5 years.[6-11]

3. IE associated with intravenous drug use (IDU) occurs at a rate of 2% to 5% per patient year.[12] In urban populations half the total cases of IE may be related to IDU.[1]

B. RISK FACTORS

1. The majority of patients (55%-75%) have a predisposing condition (Box 41-3).[3,13]

C. LOCATION

1. Important variability exists with regard to which valves are affected. In one study of a non-IDU population in a community hospital, the mitral valve (29%) and aortic valves (22%) or both (7%) were the most commonly affected sites in native valve endocarditis (NVE).[4] In 30% the site of infection was not identified.

2. IDU increases the likelihood of right-sided involvement. In the study just mentioned the tricuspid valve alone (54.5%) was the most common site of infection among IV drug users, followed by both tricuspid and mitral valves (18%). Aortic valves (6%), mitral valves (6%), and both left-sided valves (6%) were much less commonly affected in this population. Other studies, however, have suggested that the incidence of left-sided involvement in this population is higher (57%) than was previously appreciated.[5]

D. MICROBIOLOGY

1. The microbiological features of PVE- and IDU-associated IE differ in several predictable but important ways.

2. PVE within 1 year of valve surgery is most commonly due to

BOX 41-2

"ZEBRAS"* IN THE DIFFERENTIAL DIAGNOSIS OF INFECTIVE ENDOCARDITIS

NONINFECTIVE DISEASE

Atrial myxoma

Acute rheumatic fever

Marantic endocarditis associated with malignancy or collagen-vascular diseases
  (e.g., systemic lupus erythematosus)

Antiphospholipid syndrome

Carcinoid

Thrombotic thrombocytopenic purpura

Renal cell carcinoma

"CULTURE-NEGATIVE" INFECTIVE ENDOCARDITIS

Recent antimicrobial exposure

Fungal endocarditis

Brucella species

Legionella

Bartonella species

Coxiella burnetii (Q fever)

Chlamydia species

Tropheryma whippeli

*From the adage, "If you hear hoofbeats, think horses, not zebras."

41

INFECTIVE ENDOCARDITIS

BOX 41-3

PREDISPOSING CONDITIONS FOR NATIVE VALVE INFECTIVE ENDOCARDITIS

Rheumatic heart disease

Congenital heart disease

Mitral valve prolapse

Degenerative heart disease

Injection drug use

Indwelling catheters and other hardware

coagulase-negative staphylococci (33%), and a large percentage is
methicillin resistant (80%).[14,15]

3. Fungal agents (usually *Candida* species) are also much more common
   in IDU (up to 9%) (Box 41-4).

4. Endocarditis associated with IDU is usually a result of *S. aureus*
   (57%).[14,16-19] Polymicrobial, fungal, or pseudomonal IE also occurs
   more frequently and can be a significant cause of morbidity and
   mortality in this population.

5. Antibiotic use before presentation may complicate interpretation of
   blood culture results.

BOX 41-4	
AGENTS OF NATIVE VALVE ENDOCARDITIS AND THEIR FREQUENCY	
Streptococci	30%-65%
Staphylococcus aureus	25%-30%
Enterococci	15%
Coagulase-negative staphylococci	5%-8%
Gram-negative bacilli	5%
Culture-negative agents	5%
Fungi and polymicrobial infections	Rare

Data from Karchmer AW. Infective endocarditis. In Braunwald E: Heart disease: a textbook of cardiovascular medicine, 6th ed. Philadelphia: WB Saunders; 2001.

II. CLINICAL PRESENTATION

A. SYMPTOMS

1. Most patients have only nonspecific or constitutional symptoms before diagnosis. The most common symptoms are fever (80%-90%), chills (42%-75%), and sweats. Fever may be absent in the elderly or chronically ill.

2. Anorexia, weight loss, and malaise are commonly present (25%-55%). Headaches, confusion, stroke, myalgias, arthralgias, back pain, abdominal pain, nausea, vomiting, chest pain, dyspnea, and cough are also relatively common.[20] Patients with IE generally appear quite ill.

B. SIGNS

1. The most important physical sign is the presence of a heart murmur (80%-90%), but only if it is a new or changing murmur indicative of regurgitation. The absence of a murmur should not preclude consideration of the diagnosis.

2. Surprisingly, a murmur may be absent initially in 55% to 70% of IE cases caused by *S. aureus*.[21,22]

3. Tricuspid valve involvement is often unaccompanied by an audible murmur. In addition, a large proportion of IV drug users have a tricuspid murmur in the absence of IE. As a result, studies of febrile IDU have not demonstrated that cardiac murmurs at the time of initial presentation have significant diagnostic value.[23,24] Nevertheless, careful documentation of the initial cardiac examination is a critical reference point for subsequent care.

4. Other physical examination clues relate to embolic or inflammatory phenomena. These include splenomegaly (15%-50%), petechiae (10%-40%), splinter hemorrhages (5%-15%), Osler nodes (7%-10%), and Roth spots (4%-10%).

5. Focal neurological deficits, ischemic digits, and abdominal tenderness resulting from systemic embolism may also be present.

6. Septic pulmonary embolism, renal embolism, and renal insufficiency

from acute glomerulonephritis are usually unrecognized during physical examination but are also important components of the clinical picture.

III. DIAGNOSTICS

1. The physician should at least consider the diagnosis of IE when encountering any evidence of systemic inflammation or embolization. Usually the diagnosis is pursued when bacteremia is present without an obvious source of infection. However, it is important to recognize that in patients with IE, fever or heart murmur may be absent, blood culture results may be negative, or the clinical picture may be subacute.

2. IE can also mimic rheumatological illness, and corticosteroid use may delay subsequent diagnosis. Therefore a high index of suspicion should be maintained for IE in a variety of settings.

3. The workup should start with a thorough history and physical examination. Blood cultures should be obtained to evaluate for persistent bacteremia, which would be expected in endocarditis, whereas transient bacteremia is seen in focal tissue infections.

4. Persistent bacteremia is defined as either (1) two or more blood culture results positive for the same organism, separated by at least 12 hours, or (2) all of three or the majority of four or more blood culture results positive for the same organism with at least 1 hour between the first and the last culture.[25]

5. If the suspicion is sufficient, echocardiography should be performed. Transthoracic echocardiography (TTE) is noninvasive and highly specific if a vegetation is detected. Therefore it is often the initial test of choice. However, TTE is less than 65% sensitive in NVE and is 16% to 36% sensitive in PVE.

6. In contrast, transesophageal echocardiography (TEE) is 90% to 100% sensitive in NVE and 82% to 96% sensitive in PVE.[26-30] TEE is also the modality of choice for detecting abscess formation (28% versus 87% sensitivity).[30] The utility of these tests and their appropriate use in the clinical setting remain controversial issues.

7. In the absence of pathological data the diagnosis of IE has historically been difficult to make with certainty. Several clinical schemes have been proposed to deal with this issue.

8. The Duke criteria (Box 41-5) are now the most widely accepted.[25] Echocardiographic findings are also used to aid in the diagnosis. On the basis of these criteria, IE can be diagnosed "definitively," even in the absence of histological findings, if two major, one major and three minor, or five minor criteria are present (Box 41-6).

9. The Duke criteria have been validated for use in diagnosis of prosthetic valve endocarditis as well as NVE.[32]

41

INFECTIVE ENDOCARDITIS

BOX 41-5

DUKE CRITERIA

MAJOR CRITERIA

1. Positive blood culture for infective endocarditis
   a. Typical microorganism for infective endocarditis from two separate blood cultures: viridans streptococci, *Streptococcus bovis*, HACEK group, community-acquired *Staphylococcus aureus,* or enterococci in the absence of a primary focus
   b. Persistently positive blood culture, defined as recovery of a microorganism consistent with infective endocarditis from blood cultures drawn more than 12 hours apart, *or* all of three or a majority of four or more separate blood cultures, with first and last being drawn at least 1 hour apart
   c. Culture positive for *Coxiella burnetii* (Q fever) or antiphase I IgG titer >1:800
2. Evidence of endocardial involvement
   a. Positive echocardiogram for infective endocarditis
      i. Oscillating intracardiac mass, on valve or supporting structures, or in the path of regurgitant jets, or on implanted material, in the absence of an alternative anatomical explanation, *or*
      ii. Abscess, *or*
      iii. New partial dehiscence of prosthetic valve, *or*
   b. New valvular regurgitation (increase or change in preexisting murmur not sufficient)

MINOR CRITERIA

1. Predisposition: predisposing heart condition or intravenous drug use
2. Fever: ≥38° C
3. Vascular phenomena: major arterial emboli, septic pulmonary infarcts, mycotic aneurysm, intracranial hemorrhage, conjunctival hemorrhages, Janeway lesions
4. Immunological phenomena: glomerulonephritis, Osler's nodes, Roth spots, rheumatoid factor
5. Microbiological evidence: positive blood cultures but not meeting major criteria (excluding single positive culture for coagulase-negative staphylococci and organisms not known to cause infective endocarditis) as noted previously or serological evidence of active infection with organism consistent with infective endocarditis

Data from Durak DT, Lukes AS, Bright DK. Am J Med 1994; 96:200; and Li J et al. Clin Infect Dis 2000; 30:633.

BOX 41-6

DUKE CRITERIA AND DIAGNOSIS OF INFECTIVE ENDOCARDITIS

DEFINITE INFECTIVE ENDOCARDITIS (PRESENCE OF EITHER NO. 1 OR NO. 2 BELOW)

1. Pathological criteria
   a. Microorganisms: demonstrated by culture or histology in a vegetation, or in a vegetation that has embolized, or in an intracardiac abscess, *or*
   b. Pathological lesions: vegetation or intracardiac abscess present, confirmed by histological tests showing active endocarditis
2. Clinical criteria
   a. Two major criteria, *or*
   b. One major and three minor criteria, *or*
   c. Five minor criteria

POSSIBLE INFECTIVE ENDOCARDITIS

1. Clinical criteria
   a. One major plus one minor, *or*
   b. Three minor criteria

REJECTED INFECTIVE ENDOCARDITIS

1. Firm alternative diagnosis for manifestations of endocarditis, *or*
2. Resolution of manifestations of endocarditis, with antibiotic therapy for 4 days or less, *or*
3. Does not meet criteria for possible infective endocarditis
4. No pathological evidence of infective endocarditis at surgery or autopsy, after antibiotic therapy for 4 days or less

Data from Durak DT, Lukes AS, Bright DK. Am J Med 1994; 96:200; and Li J et al. Clin Infect Dis 2000; 30:633.

IV. MANAGEMENT

A. MEDICAL THERAPY

1. Treatment of IE should be directed at the causative agent, and in most cases blood culture data are available to guide treatment.
2. However, patients with acute IE may require empirical administration of antibiotics after adequate culture specimens are obtained. This may be guided by a patient's risk factors, including prosthetic valves, IDU, or indwelling catheters.
3. At a minimum any empirical therapy should include excellent coverage for *S. aureus,* given its likelihood of causing a rapidly progressive presentation. Oxacillin (2 g IV q4h) plus an aminoglycoside at a dosage for synergy (gentamicin 1 mg/kg q8h) is the regimen of choice for IDU-associated IE at Johns Hopkins. Nafcillin is an acceptable alternative to oxacillin.[33]
4. The likelihood of methicillin-resistant *S. aureus* (or the history of penicillin allergy) should also be determined, and vancomycin can be added or substituted depending on the circumstances.

5. Patients in whom IE is strongly suspected and who have recent (within the preceding year) prosthetic valve implantation or an indwelling vascular catheter may be at high risk for coagulase-negative staphylococcal endocarditis, and empirical therapy with vancomycin (30 mg/kg q24h, in two equally divided doses) should be carefully considered.

6. Cefazolin 2 g IV q8h may be substituted for oxacillin-nafcillin in penicillin-allergic patients who do not have a history of anaphylactic response to penicillin.[33]

7. Ultimately the choice and duration of antibiotics will depend on the microbiological features, allergy history, left- versus right-sided heart involvement, and presence of prosthetic valves or vascular prostheses.

8. Although a complete discussion of the possible treatment regimens for each organism is beyond the scope of this text, several excellent sources are available for more detailed coverage of this issue.[20,34]

9. In general, treatment of gram-positive IE includes a penicillin (or vancomycin) for 4 weeks.[33,34] In cases of uncomplicated right-sided IE caused by staphylococci, however, a 2-week course of penicillin and gentamicin may be as effective as a 4-week regimen.[35] Studies examining short-course therapy always used echocardiography to exclude left-sided involvement.[36]

10. The synergistic affect of aminoglycosides with a penicillin is important for the optimal treatment of enterococcal IE[37,38] and appears to reduce the time until blood culture negativity in cases involving other gram-positive organisms.[39,40]

11. The same is true of endocarditis caused by viridans streptococci with reduced susceptibility to penicillin. The value of aminoglycosides in other forms of endocarditis is less clear, so their use should be avoided for patients at highest risk of toxicity, including those over 65, those with renal dysfunction, and those with preexisting eighth nerve dysfunction.

12. A recent retrospective study of enterococcal endocarditis questions the need for aminoglycosides for the entire duration of enterococcal endocarditis treatment, but shorter courses of aminoglycosides in enterococcal endocarditis have not been studied prospectively.[41]

13. Patients who are receiving appropriate antibiotics for IE may continue to have fever and appear toxic for several days.

14. The rate of thromboembolism declines substantially with initiation of treatment, although the risk continues throughout.[42]

15. Surveillance electrocardiography should be performed daily while the patient is febrile, then periodically during treatment. Particular attention should given to the identification of PR prolongation, which may signify the development of a valve ring abscess.

16. The development of IE-related complications, especially during

appropriate medical therapy, may indicate the need for surgical intervention (Box 41-7).

PEARLS AND PITFALLS

- Key questions to consider in prophylaxis are listed in Box 41-8.
- Fungal endocarditis is a special situation to consider (Box 41-9).
- Avoidance of error: Although this seems obvious, obtaining blood cultures *before* starting antibiotics is critical when infective endocarditis is suspected.
- Special situations: HACEK organisms, penicillin-susceptible viridans streptococci (MIC ≤0.1 µg/mL), and *Streptococcus bovis* are typically treated with ceftriaxone 2 g IV q24h.[33]
- The Austrian syndrome refers to the simultaneous occurrence of pneumonia, meningitis, and endocarditis (specifically aortic valve rupture) caused by *S. pneumoniae*.[43] Mortality from pneumococcal endocarditis in the antibiotic era ranges from 28% to 81%.[44]
- Comorbidities: The association between *S. bovis* endocarditis and colonic pathology has long been recognized. Therefore discovery of *S. bovis* endocarditis should prompt an evaluation for gastrointestinal pathological conditions, particularly malignancies.[45,46]

41

INFECTIVE ENDOCARDITIS

BOX 41-7

SURGICAL INDICATIONS IN INFECTIVE ENDOCARDITIS

Moderate-to-severe congestive heart failure caused by valve dysfunction

Unstable prosthesis

Uncontrolled infection despite optimal antimicrobial therapy

Unavailability of effective antimicrobial therapy: endocarditis caused by fungi, *Brucella*, *Pseudomonas aeruginosa* (aortic or mitral valves)

PVE caused by *Staphylococcus aureus* with an intracardiac complication

Relapse of PVE after optimal therapy

RELATIVE SURGICAL INDICATIONS

Perivalvular extension of infection, or intracardiac fistula

Poorly responsive NVE caused by *S. aureus* (aortic or mitral valves)

Relapse of NVE after optimal antimicrobial therapy

Culture-negative NVE or PVE with persistent fever (≥10 days)

Large (>10 mm diameter) hypermobile vegetation (with or without prior arterial embolus)

Endocarditis caused by highly antibiotic-resistant enterococci

---

Data from Karchmer AW. Infective endocarditis. In Braunwald E, ed. Heart disease: a textbook of cardiovascular medicine, 6th ed. Philadelphia: WB Saunders; 2001.
NVE, Native valve endocarditis; *PVE*, prosthetic valve endocarditis.

BOX 41-8

PROPHYLAXIS FOR INFECTIVE ENDOCARDITIS

WHO?

High-Risk Patients

Prosthetic heart valves

Previous infective endocarditis

Cyanotic congenital heart disease

Patent ductus arteriosus

Aortic regurgitation or stenosis

Mitral regurgitation or stenosis

Ventricular septal defect

Coarctation of the aorta

Previous intracardiac surgery with residual device, hemodynamic abnormality, or systemic-pulmonary shunt

Intermediate-Risk Patients

Mitral valve prolapse with regurgitation or thickened valve leaflets

Pure mitral stenosis

Tricuspid valve disease

Pulmonary stenosis

Asymmetrical septal hypertrophy

Bicuspid aortic valve or calcific aortic sclerosis with minimal hemodynamic abnormality

Degenerative valvular disease in elderly patients

Surgically repaired intracardiac lesions with minimal or no hemodynamic abnormality, <6 months after operation

WHEN?

Dental procedures known to induce gingival or mucosal bleeding, including professional cleaning and scaling

Tonsillectomy or adenoidectomy

Surgery involving gastrointestinal or upper respiratory mucosa

Rigid bronchoscopy

Sclerotherapy for esophageal varices

Esophageal dilation

Endoscopic retrograde cholangiopancreatography

Gallbladder surgery

Cytoscopy, urethral dilation

Urethral catheterization if urinary tract infection is present

Urinary tract or prostate surgery

Incision and drainage of infected tissue

BOX 41-8—cont'd

PROPHYLAXIS FOR INFECTIVE ENDOCARDITIS

WITH WHAT?

Before Dental, Oral, Respiratory Tract, or Esophageal Procedures

Amoxicillin PO (or ampicillin IV): 2 g, 1 hr before procedure (If patient is allergic to penicillin, use clindamycin 600 mg PO, cephalexin 2 g, or azithromycin 500 mg)

Before Genitourinary and Gastrointestinal (Except Esophageal) Procedures in High-Risk Patients

Ampicillin 2 g IM or IV *plus*

Gentamicin 1.5 mg/kg up to 120 mg within 30 minutes of starting procedure, *then* 6 hours later, ampicillin 1 g IM or IV or amoxicillin 1 g PO (If patient is allergic to penicillin, use vancomycin 1 g plus gentamicin 1.5 mg/kg up to 150 mg)

Before Genitourinary and Gastrointestinal (Except Esophageal) Procedures in Moderate-Risk Patients

Amoxicillin 2 g PO 1 hour before procedure or ampicillin 2 g IV or IM within 30 minutes of procedure (If patient is allergic to penicillin, use vancomycin 1 g)

Data from Durack DT. N Engl J Med 1995; 332:38; and Dajani AS et al. JAMA 1997; 277:1794.

41

INFECTIVE ENDOCARDITIS

BOX 41-9

SPECIAL SITUATIONS: FUNGAL ENDOCARDITIS

Fungal endocarditis comprises <10% of all infective endocarditis cases

Risk factors include intravascular catheters, immunocompromise (organ transplant, human immunodeficiency virus, steroid use, malignancy), noncardiac surgery, and intravenous drug use

The aortic valve is the most commonly involved

Clinical presentation includes fever, murmur, emboli (45% of cases in largest series), neurological changes, and heart failure

Microbiological picture includes *Candida albicans* (24%), non-*albicans Candida* (often *C. parapsilosis*) (24%), *Aspergillus* (24%), non-*Aspergillus* fungi (20%), *Histoplasma* (6%)

Treatment of choice is lipid-based amphotericin product and surgery; newer antifungals have not been studied (echinocandins)

Survival rate at 3 years is 41%

Late relapses are possible; some authors recommend suppressive antifungal therapy after initial treatment

Data from Ellis ME et al. Clin Infect Dis 2001; 32:50.

REFERENCES

[b] 1. Berlin JA et al. Incidence of infective endocarditis in the Delaware Valley, 1988-1990. Am J Cardiol 1995; 76:933.

[b] 2. Van der Meer JTM et al. Epidemiology of bacterial endocarditis in the Netherlands. I. Patient characteristics. Arch Intern Med 1992; 152:1863.

[b] 3. Hogevik H et al. Epidemiologic aspects of infective endocarditis in an urban population: a 5-year prospective study. Medicine 1995; 74:324.

[b] 4. Watanakunakorn C, Burkert T. Infective endocarditis at a large community teaching hospital, 1980-1990: a review of 210 episodes. Medicine 1993; 72:90.

[b] 5. Graves MK, Soto L. Left-sided endocarditis in parental drug abusers: recent experience at a large community hospital. South Med J 1992; 85:378.

[b] 6. Rutledge R, Kim J, Applebaum RE. Actuarial analysis of the risk of prosthetic valve endocarditis in 1,598 patients with mechanical and bioprosthetic valves. Arch Surg 1985; 120:469.

[c] 7. Ivert TSA et al. Prosthetic valve endocarditis. Circulation 1984; 69:223.

[b] 8. Arvay A, Lengyel M. Incidence and risk factors of prosthetic valve endocarditis. Eur J Cardiothorac Surg 1988; 2:340.

[b] 9. Calderwood SB et al. Risk factors for the development of prosthetic valve endocarditis. Circulation 1985; 72:31.

[c] 10. Agnihotri AK et al. Surgery for acquired heart disease. J Thorac Cardiovasc Surg 1995; 110:1708.

[b] 11. Horskotte D et al. Late prosthetic valve endocarditis. Eur Heart J 1995; 16(suppl B):39.

[c] 12. Sande MA et al. Endocarditis in intravenous drug users. In Kaye D, ed. Infective endocarditis, 2nd ed. New York: Raven Press; 1992.

[b] 13. Kazanjian P. Infective endocarditis: review of 60 cases treated in community hospitals. Infect Dis Clin Pract 1993; 2:41.

[b] 14. Sandre RM, Shafran SD. Infective endocarditis: review of 135 cases over 9 years. Clin Infect Dis 1996; 22:276.

[c] 15. Karchmer AW. Infections of prosthetic valves and intravascular devices. In Mandell GL, Bennett JE, Dolin R, eds. Principles and practice of infectious diseases. New York: Churchill Livingstone; 2000.

[c] 16. Sande MA et al. Endocarditis in intravenous drug users. In Kaye D, ed. Infective endocarditis, 2nd ed. New York: Raven Press; 1992.

[b] 17. Levine DP, Crane LR, Zervos MJ. Bacteremia in narcotic addicts at the Detroit Medical Center. II. Infectious endocarditis: a prospective comparative study. Rev Infect Dis 1986; 8:374.

[b] 18. Mathew J et al. Clinical features, site of involvement, bacteriologic findings, and outcome of infective endocarditis in intravenous drug users. Arch Intern Med 1995; 155:1641.

[b] 19. Hecht SR, Berger M. Right-sided endocarditis in intravenous drug users: prognostic features in 102 episodes. Ann Intern Med 1992; 17:560.

[c] 20. Karchmer AW. Infective endocarditis. In Braunwald E: Heart disease: a textbook of cardio-vascular medicine, 6th ed. Philadelphia: WB Saunders; 2001.

[b] 21. Roder BL et al. Clinical features of *Staphylococcus aureus* endocarditis: a 10-year experience in Denmark. Arch Intern Med 1999; 159:462.

[b] 22. Fowler VG Jr et al. Infective endocarditis due to *Staphylococcus aureus:* 59 prospectively identified cases with follow-up. Clin Infect Dis 1999; 28:106.

[b] 23. Marantz PR et al. Inability to predict diagnosis in febrile intravenous drug abusers. Ann Intern Med 1987; 106:823.

[b] 24. Weisse AB et al. The febrile parenteral drug user: a prospective study in 121 patients. Am J Med 1993; 94:274.

[b] 25. Durak DT, Lukes AS, Bright DK. New criteria for diagnosis of infective endocarditis: utilization of specific echocardiographic findings. Am J Med 1994; 96:200.

[b] 26. Sochowski RA, Chan KL. Implication of negative results on a monoplane transesophageal echocardiographic study in patients with suspected infective endocarditis. J Am Coll Cardiol 1993; 21:216.

[c] 27. Daniel WG, Mugge A. Transesophageal echocardiography. N Engl J Med 1995; 332:1268.

[b] 28. Vered Z et al. Echocardiographic assessment of prosthetic valve endocarditis. Eur Heart J 1995; 16(suppl B):63.

[a] 29. Morguet AJ et al. Diagnostic value of transesophageal compared with transthoracic echocardiography in suspected prosthetic valve endocarditis. Herz 1995; 20:390.

[a] 30. Daniel WG et al. Comparison of transthoracic and transesophageal echocardiography for detection of abnormalities of prosthetic and bioprosthetic valves in the mitral and aortic positions. Am J Cardiol 1993; 71:210.

[b] 31. Karalis DG et al. Transesophageal echocardiographic recognition of subaortic complications in aortic valve endocarditis: clinical and surgical implications. Circulation 1992; 86:353.

[b] 32. Nettles RE et al. An evaluation of the Duke criteria in 25 pathologically confirmed cases of prosthetic valve endocarditis. Clin Infect Dis 1997; 25:1401.

[d] 33. Wilson WR et al. Antibiotic treatment of adults with infective endocarditis due to streptococci, enterococci, staphylococci and HACEK microorganisms. JAMA 1995; 274:1706.

[c] 34. Scheld WM, Sande MA. Endocarditis and intravascular infections. In Mandell GL, Bennett JE, Dolin R, eds. Mandel, Douglas and Bennett's principles and practice of infectious diseases. 4th ed. New York: Churchill Livingstone; 1995.

[a] 35. Chambers HF, Miller RT, Newman MD. Right-sided *Staphylococcus aureus* endocarditis in intravenous drug abusers: two week combination therapy. Ann Intern Med 1988; 109:619.

[a] 36. Heldman AW et al. Oral antibiotic treatment of right sided staphylococcal endocarditis in injection drug users: prospective randomized comparison with parenteral therapy. Am J Med 1996; 101(1):68.

[c] 37. Eliopoulos GM. Enterococcal endocarditis. In Kaye D, ed. Infective endocarditis, 2nd ed. New York: Raven Press; 1992.

[c] 38. Eliopoulos GM. Aminoglycoside resistant enterococcal endocarditis. Med Clin North Am 1993; 17:117.

[b] 39. Fantin B, Carbon C. In vivo antibiotic synergism: contribution of animal models. Antimicrob Agents Chemother 1992; 36:907.

[b] 40. Korzeniowski O, Sande MA. Combination antimicrobial therapy for *Staphylococcus aureus* endocarditis in patients addicted to parenteral drugs and in nonaddicts: a prospective study. National Collaborative Endocarditis Study Group. Ann Intern Med 1982; 97:496.

[b] 41. Olaison L, Schadewitz K. Enterococcal endocarditis in Sweden 1995-1999: can shorter therapy with aminoglycosides be used? Swedish Society of Infectious Diseases Quality Assurance Study Group for Endocarditis. Clin Infect Dis 2002; 34:159.

[b] 42. Steckelberg JM et al. Emboli in infective endocarditis: the prognostic value of echocardiography. Ann Intern Med 1991; 114:635.

[c] 43. Austrian R. Pneumococcal endocarditis, meningitis and rupture of the aortic valve. Arch Intern Med 1957; 99:539.

[c] 44. Aronin SI et al. Review of pneumococcal endocarditis in adults in the penicillin era. Clin Infect Dis 1998; 26:165.

[c] 45. Murray HW, Roberts RB. *Streptococcus bovis* bacteremia and underlying gastrointestinal disease. Arch Intern Med 1978; 138:1097.

[c] 46. Watanakunakorn C. *Streptococcus bovis* endocarditis. Am J Med 1974; 56:256.

41

INFECTIVE ENDOCARDITIS

Fever of Unknown Origin

Rachel Damico, MD, PhD, and John Mann, MD

FAST FACTS

- In 1961, Petersdorf and Beeson used the following criteria to define a fever of unknown origin (FUO).[1]
  - Body temperature greater than 38.3° C.
  - Fever documented on three separate occasions over a period of at least 3 weeks.
  - No evident diagnosis despite 1 week of inpatient hospital evaluations.
- FUO is frequently an atypical manifestation of a common disease rather than a typical manifestation of unusual disease.
- Neoplasms, collagen-vascular diseases, and infections account for the majority of cases of FUO in immunocompetent patients.[2]
- In human immunodeficiency virus (HIV)-positive patients, mycobacterial infections (tuberculosis and atypical) are the most common causes of FUO.[3]
- In patients older than 65 years temporal arteritis is a significant and treatable cause of FUO, and screening should be performed early in the evaluation.[4]
- Patients with FUO that remains undiagnosed after extensive study tend to have favorable outcomes. For example, in a cohort of 61 patients with FUO who were discharged without diagnosis, the mortality rate at 5 years was only 3.2%.[5]

I. EPIDEMIOLOGY

1. Although the etiological possibilities in FUO remain vast (Box 42-1), the majority of identifiable causes can be grouped into three specific disease categories that have changed little over the past half century.[2]
2. Infections, neoplasms, and noninflammatory diseases, which include collagen-vascular diseases, vasculitides, and granulomatous diseases, account for the majority of cases of diagnosed FUO (Fig. 42-1).[1,6]
3. In contrast, the spectrum of specific diseases that cause FUO is determined by geographical and demographic factors (Fig. 42-2) but also appears to have changed with time. In addition, the proportion of patients for whom no diagnosis can be established is increasing in contemporary series.[6]
4. The foundation of such changes is probably multifactorial and includes the development of improved culture technologies, serological markers, and access to highly sensitive imaging modalities such as computed tomography (CT) and magnetic resonance imaging (MRI).

BOX 42-1

CAUSES OF FEVER OF UNKNOWN ORIGIN

INFECTION

Localized
Appendicitis
Cat-scratch disease
Cholangitis
Cholecystitis
Dental abscess
Diverticulitis
Liver abscess
Osteomyelitis
Pelvic inflammatory disease
Perinephric abscess
Prostatic abscess
Thrombophlebitis
Tuboovarian abscess
Intravascular
Catheter infection
Endocarditis

ORGANISMS

Bacterial
Bartonella
Brucella
Campylobacter
Gonococcus
Legionella
Leptospirosis
Meningococcus
Nocardia
Salmonella
Syphilis
Typhoid
Vibrio
Yersinia
Mycobacterial
Mycobacterium avium-intracellulare infection
Extrapulmonary tuberculosis
Miliary tuberculosis

ORGANISMS—CONT'D

Rickettsial
Ehrlichia
Q fever
Rocky Mountain spotted fever
Viral
Coxsackie virus
Cytomegalovirus
Epstein-Barr virus
Hepatitis viruses
Human immunodeficiency virus
Lymphocytic choriomeningitis virus
Parvovirus
Fungal
Aspergillus
Blastomycoses
Candida
Coccidioidomycoses
Cryptococcus
Histoplasma
Zygomycoses
Sporotrichosis
Pneumocystis
Parasitic
Amebae
Malaria
Trypanosomes
Toxoplasma gondii

TUMOR

Benign
Atrial myxoma
Renal angiomyolipoma
Malignant
Colon
Hepatoma
Leukemia
Lymphoma
Pancreatic
Sarcoma

Modified from Gelfand JA, Dinarello CA, Wolff SM. Fever, including fever of unknown origin. In Isselbacher KJ et al, eds. Harrison's principles of internal medicine, 13th ed. New York: McGraw-Hill; 1994.

BOX 42-1—cont'd

CAUSES OF FEVER OF UNKNOWN ORIGIN

COLLAGEN-VASCULAR

Erythema nodosum
Giant cell arteritis
Polyarteritis nodosa
Rheumatic fever
Rheumatoid arthritis
Still's disease
Systemic lupus erythematosus
Takayasu's disease
Wegener's granulomatosis

MISCELLANEOUS

Aortic dissection
Crohn's disease
Drug fever
Factitious fever
Familial Mediterranean fever
Gout
Hematoma
Pulmonary embolus
Subacute thyroiditis

42

FEVER OF UNKNOWN ORIGIN

Thus advanced diagnostic technologies probably have a prospective influence on the diseases that meet the criteria for FUO.[6]

5. Diseases such as subacute bacterial endocarditis, systemic lupus erythematosus, or occult abscesses that previously manifested themselves as FUO can now be identified before they meet Petersdorf's definition.

6. Other epidemiological factors that have influenced the relative frequency of specific disease entities as causes of FUO include the emergence and recognition of new pathogens such as HIV, HIV-associated opportunistic infections, and Lyme disease. Furthermore, once common diseases such as rheumatic fever have decreased in incidence and diseases unknown in the mid-20th century are now recognized causes of FUO, including drug fever, Kikuchi's disease, and hyperimmunoglobulin D syndrome.[7]

II. CLINICAL PRESENTATION

1. In light of the expense of hospital admissions and the ability to perform much of the diagnostic workup in the outpatient setting, more modern definitions of FUO have eliminated the requirement for hospi-

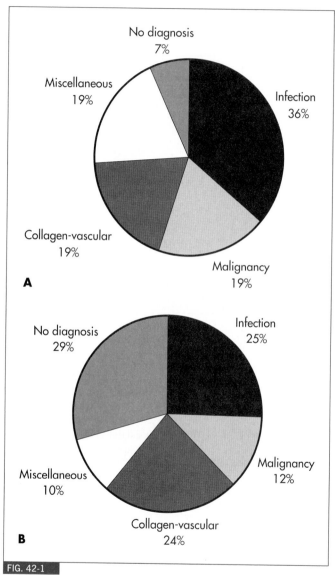

FIG. 42-1

Categories of fever of unknown origin. **A,** In 1961. **B,** In 1997. *(Data from Petersdorf RG, Beeson BP. Medicine 1961; 40:1; and de Kleijn EM, Vandenbroucke JP, van der Meer JW. Medicine 1997; 76:410.)*

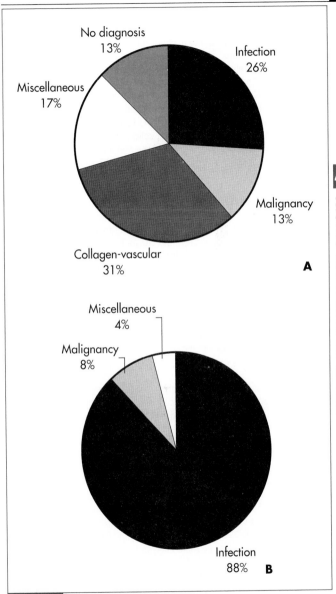

FIG. 42-2

A, Categories of fever of unknown origin in the elderly. **B,** Causes of human immunodeficiency virus–associated fever of unknown origin. *(Data from Knockaert DC, Vanneste LJ, Bobbaers HJ. J Am Geriatr Soc 1993; 41:1187; and Armstrong WS, Katz JT, Kazanjian PH. Clin Infect Dis 1999; 28:341.)*

talization as part of the diagnostic criteria.[8] Some have advocated a new classification of FUO to account for the varied diseases seen in different populations. The four categories in this classification are (1) classically defined FUO, (2) HIV-associated FUO, (3) neutropenic FUO, and (4) nosocomial FUO (Table 42-1).[9]

2. Although FUO has a vast number of causes, mycobacterial infection is among the most common.[1,6] Other common infectious causes are abscesses and endocarditis. Lymphoma is a classic malignant cause of FUO, although in multiple series, solid tumors have been as likely to be identified as lymphoma.[1,10] Of the noninfectious inflammatory diseases, giant cell arteritis, rheumatoid arthritis, and lupus are the most frequently identified causes of FUO.[10]

A. INFECTIONS

1. *Mycobacterium tuberculosis.*

a. Mycobacterial infections are the single most frequent infectious cause of FUO in some series,[1,3,10] and disseminated or miliary tuberculosis may be the most treatable fatal cause of FUO. In patients with miliary tuberculosis manifesting as FUO, the purified protein derivative skin test is positive in less than 50% of cases and sputum is positive in only 25%.[2] Bronchoalveolar lavage samples are commonly culture positive. These cultures can take upward of 4 to 6 weeks to bring results, however, so tissue is necessary for expedient diagnosis. Transbronchial, liver, and bone marrow biopsies often demonstrate granulomas and, less frequently, stain positive for acid-fast organisms. The yield from bone marrow biopsy increases in the setting of ongoing anemia, leukopenia, and monocytosis.[2]

2. **Abscess.**

a. Occult abscesses can form throughout the abdomen and pelvis. The liver is the organ most susceptible to the development of an abscess. Liver abscess forms as the consequence either of hematological spread or of local spread from contiguous infection within the peritoneal cavity or biliary tree. Amebic abscesses are not uncommon, and serological tests can be used to distinguish amebic from pyogenic abscesses. Candidal liver abscesses are seen in patients with chemotherapy-induced neutropenia. Fevers that persist after a patient recovers from a prolonged neutropenia warrant a search for hepatosplenic candidiasis. Although half of patients with liver abscess have symptoms of right upper quadrant tenderness, jaundice, and hepatomegaly, in an equal number FUO is the presenting symptom. This is especially true of the elderly, who are more likely to have a subacute course.[11]

b. Splenic abscesses are far less common than liver abscesses, but if untreated they have a high mortality. Hematogenous spread is the most common means of development and is typically seen in the setting of bacterial endocarditis. Splenic abscesses are manifested as fever and

TABLE 42-1
CLASSIFICATION OF FEVER OF UNKNOWN ORIGIN

Category of Fever of Unknown Origin	Patient Population	Minimal Duration of Investigation	Typical Causes
HIV associated	Confirmed HIV positive	3 days of inpatient investigation or 4 weeks of outpatient studies	Mycobacterial infection (*Mycobacterium avium-intracellulare* and *Mycobacterium tuberculosis*), non-Hodgkin's disease, drug fever
Neutropenic	Absolute neutrophil count ≤500/mm³ or in decline	3 days	Bacterial infections, aspergillosis, candidemia
Nosocomial	Hospitalized in an acute care setting (*not* admitted with infection)	3 days	Pulmonary embolus, sinusitis, *Clostridium difficile* colitis, drug fever
Classic	All others with fever ≥3 weeks	3 days of inpatient investigation or three outpatient visits	Infection, neoplasm, noninfectious inflammatory diseases

Modified from Durack DT, Street AC. Fever of unknown origin—reexamined and redefined. In Remington JS, Swartz MN, eds. Current clinical topics in infectious diseases. Cambridge, Mass: Blackwell; 1991.

FEVER OF UNKNOWN ORIGIN

42

leukocytosis. Only half of patients with liver abscess have left-sided pain and splenomegaly.

c. The majority of perinephric abscesses develop as a consequence of an ascending urinary tract infection. Risk factors for development of perinephric abscess include renal stones, diabetes, previous urological surgery, anatomically abnormal urinary tract, and trauma. Persistent fever and sterile pyuria suggest a perinephric abscess.

B. BACTERIAL ENDOCARDITIS

1. Bacterial endocarditis represents a microbial infection of the endocardial surface of the heart, with platelets, fibrin, inflammatory cells, and microorganisms forming a vegetation, or lesion, on the heart valve. Risk factors for bacterial endocarditis include diabetes mellitus, poor dentition, long-term dialysis, injection drug use, and preexisting valvular heart disease.[12] The valves involved in the infection, as well as the virulence of the organism, determine manifestations of endocarditis.

2. Left-sided vegetations having the capacity to embolize via the systemic circulation lead to mycotic aneurysms and septic abscesses elsewhere. Classic peripheral manifestations of left-sided subacute bacterial endocarditis include splinter hemorrhages under the nail beds, conjunctival petechiae, Osler's nodes (tender nodules on the pulp of the digits), and Janeway's lesion (nontender hemorrhagic lesions on the palms and soles). Isolated right-sided valvular involvement does not result in systemic emboli or peripheral stigmata but may be manifested as pulmonary septic emboli.

3. Even in the absence of previous antibiotic therapy, 5% to 7% of patients who meet strict diagnostic criteria for endocarditis have sterile blood cultures.[13] Administration of antibiotics before blood culture samples are obtained can significantly diminish subsequent yield, and this suppression appears to persist after the antibiotic is no longer present in the blood.[14]

4. If infectious endocarditis is suspected and cultures remain negative for growth after 48 to 72 hours, the pursuit of fastidious and culture-negative organisms may be indicated. This includes prolonged incubation of blood cultures (up to 14 days or even longer), blind subculture onto enriched media, and possibly serological studies for *Coxiella burnetii, Bartonella,* and *Brucella* (Table 42-2). Transesophageal echocardiography (TEE), although invasive, has greater sensitivity than transthoracic echocardiography for vegetations, and the negative predictive value for a negative TEE is greater than 92%.[12] See Chapter 41 for more discussion of endocarditis.

C. MALIGNANCY

1. Lymphoma.

a. Malignancies of reticuloendothelial origin (lymphomas and leukemias) are the cancers most commonly manifested as FUO. Fever is more common in older patients and those with advanced lymphoma. At presen-

---

TABLE 42-2

LABORATORY STUDIES FOR ORGANISMS CAUSING ENDOCARDITIS

Organism	Approach
Abiotrophia species	Grow on supplemented media
Bartonella	Serological assays
Coxiella burnetii (Q fever)	Serological assays
HACEK organisms (*Haemophilus, Actinobacillus, Cardiobacterium, Eikenella, Kingella*)	Prolonged incubation of blood cultures
Chlamydia (*C. psittaci*)	Serological assays
Tropheryma whippelii	
Legionella	Subculture and serological assays
Brucella	Serological assays
Fungi	
Candida	Bacterial or fungal blood cultures
Histoplasma	Urine or serum *Histoplasma* antigen
Aspergillus	Serological tests not approved; rare

Modified from Mylonakis E, Calderwood SB. N Engl J Med 2001; 345:1318.

42

FEVER OF UNKNOWN ORIGIN

tation one fourth to one third of patients with Hodgkin's lymphoma have constitutional symptoms, including low-grade fevers, night sweats, and weight loss (B symptoms). The diagnosis of lymphoma is based on histological evaluation of tissue, typically an excision biopsy of an abnormal lymph node, and not on needle aspiration or needle biopsy because they do not maintain the integrity of the tissue architecture.

2. **Renal cell carcinoma and hypernephroma.**

a. Classic evidence of a renal cell carcinoma includes the triad of flank pain, gross hematuria, and a palpable abdominal mass. These three findings are present in only 10% of the cases, whereas microscopic hematuria is seen in more than half. In the absence of infection, fever may be a presenting manifestation in up to 15% of cases.[2]

D. NONINFECTIOUS INFLAMMATORY DISEASES

1. **Temporal arteritis and giant cell arteritis.**

a. Classic manifestations of giant cell arteritis include headache, fever, anemia, and elevated erythrocyte sedimentation rate. Patients can describe abrupt changes in vision, known as amaurosis fugax, and have systemic symptoms of polymyalgia rheumatica such as proximal muscle stiffness and pain. In some series giant cell arteritis is responsible for FUO in 15% of patients 65 and older.[4]

2. **Still's disease and juvenile rheumatoid arthritis.**

a. Still's disease is a diagnosis of exclusion and is suggested by the triad of arthritis or arthralgias, high fevers (double-quotidian pattern), and an evanescent rash. Fevers may temporally precede the manifestations of arthritis. The patient may have sore throat, lymphadenopathy, splenomegaly, and pleurisy. There are no definitive serological markers, but serum ferritin levels are markedly elevated during flare-ups.

III. DIAGNOSTICS

1. As is true of most of medical diagnoses, the history can provide the most useful diagnostic information.[14] History taking should review past medical illnesses and procedures, medication and alcohol use, family history, occupational exposure history, evidence of immunosuppression and degree, travel history, pets, and any localizing symptoms. Physical examination can also contribute to the diagnosis, and a careful search should be made for evidence of cardiac murmurs, skin lesions, lymphadenopathy, temporal artery thickening or tenderness, and organomegaly.

2. Diagnostic clues may appear over time or become evident with reevaluation, which emphasizes the importance of repeated histories and physical examinations in directing the diagnostic workup.[2,15]

A. FEVER PATTERNS

1. Fever patterns may be helpful in the diagnosis of community-acquired illnesses without localizing features but are not typically useful in nosocomial processes.[16]

2. **Sustained fever:** Sustained fevers are persistently elevated with minimal variation (less than 1° F per day).

3. **Intermittent fever:** Intermittent fevers are an exaggeration of normal circadian rhythms with return to normal body temperature once during most days. Intermittent fevers with extreme variations in temperature are referred to as septic or hectic fevers and are typical of deep-seated or systemic infections, malignancy, or drug reactions.

4. Daily hectic fevers are referred to as quotidian. Double-quotidian fevers (i.e., two extreme variations per day) may be associated with visceral leishmaniasis (kala-azar), Still's disease, and gonococcal endocarditis.[16]

5. **Relapsing fever** (Box 42-2): Relapsing fevers are fevers that recur over intervals of days or weeks.

6. Tertian fevers are fever paroxysms on cycles of day 1 and 3 and are typically seen with *Plasmodium vivax* late in the disease course.[7,16]

7. Quartan fevers are paroxysms occurring in cycles of day 1 and 4 and are seen with *Plasmodium malariae*.[7]

8. Pel-Ebstein fevers are fevers lasting 3 to 10 days with episodes separated by an afebrile period of similar duration and are classically described in Hodgkin's and other lymphomas.[16]

9. A relapsing fever with a periodicity of 21 days is classic for cyclic neutropenia.[16]

10. Pulse-temperature relationship.

a. The absence of an increased pulse rate in the face of fever is referred to as relative bradycardia. This evokes a broad differential diagnosis that includes Legionnaire's disease, drug fever, factitious fever, neoplasms, typhoid, psittacosis, leptospirosis, and brucellosis.

b. Relative bradycardia may be a manifestation of disease directly affecting the cardiac conduction system. For example, relative brady-

BOX 42-2	
RELAPSING FEVER	
INFECTIOUS CAUSES	NONINFECTIOUS CAUSES
Babesiosis	Drug fever
Blastomycosis	Behçet's disease
Borrelia recurrentis	Crohn's disease
Brucellosis	Familial Mediterranean fever
Coccidioidomycosis	Hyperimmunoglobulin D syndrome
Colorado tick fever	Still's disease
Cytomegalovirus	Systemic lupus erythematosus
Dengue fever	
Epstein-Barr virus	
Histoplasmosis	
Lymphocytic choriomeningitis	
Leptospirosis	
Lyme disease	
Malaria	
Q fever (*Coxiella burnetii*)	
Rat-bite fever	
Trench fever	
Tuberculosis	
Typhoid	
Syphilis	
Visceral leishmaniasis	

Modified from Cunha B. Infect Dis Clin North Am 1996; 10:33.

42

FEVER OF UNKNOWN ORIGIN

cardia may be seen in endocarditis complicated by a ring abscess or Lyme disease with associated myocarditis.

B. NONINVASIVE LABORATORY TESTING

1. The definition of FUO does not enumerate the studies that constitute the appropriate initial diagnostic evaluation. Box 42-3 represents a suggested preliminary evaluation.

2. Further testing should be guided by historical, physical, and laboratory clues. Because the etiologies of FUO remain vast and the prevalence of these diseases varies in different populations being evaluated, a diagnostic algorithm remains a clinical challenge.[2]

3. A prospective, multicenter study has attempted to address the utility of different modes of investigation in determining the causes of FUO in an immunocompetent patient population.[6] These data suggest that the primary utility of blood chemistry studies is to direct further investigation and to eliminate diseases from the differential diagnosis.

4. Immunological serological tests appear to have a low yield in establishing the diagnosis of FUO in the absence of diagnostic clues for immunological disorders.

5. Similarly, in the absence of historical, physical, and laboratory clues

---

BOX 42-3

**PRELIMINARY LABORATORY TESTS AND IMAGING IN FEVER
OF UNKNOWN ORIGIN**

Complete blood cell count with differential

Blood chemistries

Liver enzymes with bilirubin

Lactate dehydrogenase

Creatine phosphokinase

Erythrocyte sedimentation rate

Antinuclear antibodies

Rheumatoid factor

Human immunodeficiency virus antibody and polymerase chain reaction

Serological tests for cytomegalovirus and Epstein-Barr virus

Blood cultures from samples taken on three occasions while patient is not receiving
antibiotics

Urinalysis

Purified protein derivative test

Ferritin

Chest radiography

Abdominal and pelvic imaging (computed tomography or ultrasound)

---

pointing to infection, microbiological serological tests tend to have a
low yield in an immunocompetent population. For example, serological
tests for cytomegalovirus were useful only when the presence of
atypical lymphocytes had previously been identified.

C. IMAGING TECHNIQUES

1. Imaging of the chest and abdomen is generally accepted as part of the
   initial screening workup of FUO. Chest radiography is standard and
   can be informative even in the absence of symptoms or abnormal
   examination findings.[17]

2. Abdominal ultrasound is less sensitive than abdominal computed
   tomography (CT)[17] but may be a cost-effective initial screening tool to
   evaluate the hepatobiliary system and gallbladder.

3. CT is more sensitive in detecting small abscesses within the liver and
   spleen, and some authors advocate an abdominal CT in the initial
   screening evaluation. False negative results may rarely occur because
   of failure of oral or intravenous contrast media, deviation from normal
   anatomy, or small size of abscesses. In one study of FUO, abdominal
   CT was generally very sensitive (100%) but had lower specificity than
   ultrasound (80% versus 92%).[17] Because of the widespread and
   repeated use of ultrasound and CT in the workup of FUO, however,
   the yield per imaging test was only 10%.[10]

4. The role of nuclear medicine imaging in the diagnosis of FUO is an
   active area of investigation. Labeled autologous leukocyte scanning

and the newer labeled immune globulin scanning are highly sensitive, image the entire body, and can direct more conventional imaging analysis and invasive investigations.[17] These tests appear to have a relatively high false positive rate.

5. In one study of FUO in the elderly (>65 years of age), nuclear medicine imaging contributed to the diagnosis in 17 of 47 patients while in 11 others the results were considered to be false positives.[4] These authors recommend that nuclear medicine scanning be included in the initial screening evaluation of FUO in the elderly.

6. In another study a positive scan predicted a high likelihood of identifying the etiology of the FUO and a negative scan ruled out an inflammatory disorder with a high degree of certainty.[17]

7. The primary role of imaging modalities is to direct further invasive testing, including biopsy and laparotomy. The contribution of noninvasive laboratory tests in the diagnosis of FUO varies among series.[3,4,18] Typically, one fourth to one half of the diagnoses will be derived from noninvasive means, including serological tests, cultures, radiographic studies, and clinical response to therapy.[2,19]

D. HISTOLOGICAL TECHNIQUES

1. In immunocompetent patients tissue sampling is rarely fruitful as a screening study but may have higher yield when directed by diagnostic clues and noninvasive studies. An exception may be temporal artery biopsy as a screen for giant cell arteritis in elderly patients with FUO and elevated erythrocyte sedimentation rates.[4]

2. Tissue sampling of the lymph nodes, liver, and bone marrow appears to have a higher diagnostic yield in HIV-associated FUO than in classic FUO.[3,20,21] The yield of CT-guided and intraoperative biopsies is higher than that of blind sampling at the bedside (with the exception of temporal artery biopsy).[8] Few tissues and organs have not been sampled at some point in search of the cause of an FUO.

3. Bone marrow biopsy (BmBx): Bone marrow biopsy may be useful in evaluation of miliary tuberculosis, fungal infections, and malignancies. Bone marrow can be evaluated histologically and cultured for bacteria, fungus, and mycobacteria. In immunocompetent patients bone marrow biopsy and culture have low yield and are probably not cost effective as an initial screen.[21] If analysis of blood cultures and more easily obtainable tissues does not reveal a diagnosis, BmBx for culture is an appropriate next intervention. BmBx has a much higher diagnostic yield when performed at this later stage of the workup of classic FUO.[17] In a Spanish case series of patients with HIV-associated FUO, bone marrow examination led to a diagnosis in 30% of the cases and was the only informative diagnostic modality in 20%.[20] In this population bone marrow evaluation is a reasonable screening procedure. Furthermore, in HIV-associated FUO, the presence of thrombocytopenia (<75,000 cells/mm^3) and an aspartate aminotransaminase level higher than 100 U/L

42

FEVER OF UNKNOWN ORIGIN

predicted a high probability of obtaining a diagnosis through bone marrow evaluation.

4. **Skin and muscle biopsy:** Suspicious skin lesions should be sampled and evaluated histologically and by culture. If electromyelography reveals abnormalities, a skin and muscle biopsy is also reasonable. Muscle biopsy has been useful in the diagnosis of polyarteritis nodosa manifest as FUO.

5. **Temporal artery biopsy:** Even in the absence of localizing symptoms, temporal arteritis has been found to be the most common cause of fever in the elderly with FUO and was identified in 15% of the cases in one series.[4] This observation prompted the investigators to advocate temporal artery biopsy as a primary screen in the evaluation of patients age 65 and older. Other series have not found such a high frequency in their older patients,[6] but biopsy is clearly justified before empirical administration of corticosteroids.

6. **Lymph node biopsy:** In the absence of abnormal findings on chest and abdominal imaging, sampling of anterior cervical and inguinal lymph nodes appears to have low diagnostic yield in immunocompetent patients with FUO.[8,15] The presence of generalized adenopathy, even when not detectable on physical examination, significantly increased the yield of lymph node investigations. When generalized adenopathy was present, microbiological and histological evaluation of enlarged lymph nodes had a high diagnostic yield and provided diagnoses in 11 of 14 patients in this prospective series of classic FUO.

7. **Liver biopsy:** Nonspecific liver chemical abnormalities are identified frequently in patients with FUO (50%), whereas specific liver diseases are far less often responsible for the fever (4%).[15] Liver biopsy can help in the diagnosis of granulomatous diseases such as granulomatous hepatitis and sarcoidosis and disseminated infections such as miliary tuberculosis. If the diagnosis of miliary tuberculosis is being entertained, a liver biopsy may be informative. In such cases granulomas, although a nonspecific finding, are identified in 80% to 90% of liver biopsies.[2]

IV. MANAGEMENT

1. Recommending a treatment plan for an FUO is difficult, since this disease by definition represents the absence of a clear diagnosis.

2. A rational approach may include observation of the stable patient after the initial negative diagnostic evaluation (Fig. 42-3). During such a period of observation the clinician should reevaluate for evidence of disease progression or specific organ involvement to narrow the differential diagnosis and direct further, possibly invasive, diagnostic studies such as angiography or exploratory surgery.

3. A therapeutic trial can be cautiously considered if the clinical scenario is consistent with endocarditis, tuberculosis, vasculitis, or Still's disease.

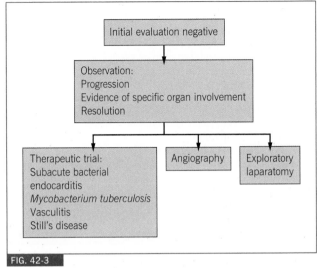

FIG. 42-3

Diagnostic evaluation of patients with fever of unknown origin.

V. OUTCOMES

1. Not surprisingly, the outcomes for patients with FUO depend on the underlying diseases responsible for fever. Patients with FUO whose cause remains undiagnosed after extensive study tend to have favorable outcomes. For example, in a cohort of 61 patients with FUO who were discharged without diagnosis, the mortality rate at 5 years was only 3.2%.[5]

PEARLS AND PITFALLS

- Although it may be tempting to treat FUO empirically with antibiotics, they should not be given to stable patients. The empirical use of antibiotics contributes to the difficulty in identifying the cause of FUO. Antibiotics have the ability to suppress infection and decrease culture yields. Furthermore, they may precipitate drug fever, another cause of FUO. In addition, they may suppress fever without adequately treating the true cause. For example, the fever of miliary tuberculosis may be suppressed by aminoglycosides or fluoroquinolones.
- Eliminate as many medications as possible. For the simple reason that any drug can cause an unexpected reaction, including fever, elimination of all unnecessary medications is prudent.
- Empirical use of corticosteroids should be avoided unless biopsy has shown vasculitis to be present. Corticosteroids have many detrimental side effects, including immunosuppression. Steroids should be used with

extreme caution to treat FUO. High-dose empirical steroids are not encouraged. In the appropriate clinical setting a diagnostic trial of 40 mg of prednisone may be reasonable if temporal arteritis is suspected as the cause of FUO, but a biopsy is still recommended.

- Fever develops with established or occult infection in more than 50% of neutropenic patients.[22] These infections can be rapidly fatal if untreated, so empirical broad-spectrum antibiotics are indicated in febrile neutropenia. Current guidelines for initial antibiotic therapy include one of the following regimens.
  - Vancomycin (if indicated) and ceftazidime.
  - Ceftazidime *or* imipenem.
  - Aminoglycoside *and* antipseudomonal β-lactam.
- Indications for empirical use of vancomycin in febrile neutropenia include severe mucositis, hypotension, quinolone prophylaxis, obvious catheter infection, and documented colonization with MRSA.
- See Chapter 35 for further information on febrile neutropenia.

REFERENCES

[b] 1. Petersdorf RG, Beeson BP. Fever of unexplained origin: report on 100 cases. Medicine 1961; 40:1.
[c] 2. Arnow P, Flaherty JP. Fever of unknown origin. Lancet 1997; 350:575.
[b] 3. Armstrong WS, Katz JT, Kazanjian PH. Human immunodeficiency virus–associated fever of unknown origin: a study of 70 patients in the United States and review. Clin Infect Dis 1999; 28:341.
[b] 4. Knockaert DC, Vanneste LJ, Bobbaers HJ. Fever of unknown origin in elder patients. J Am Geriatr Soc 1993; 41:1187.
[b] 5. Knockaert DC, Dujardin KS, Bobbaers HJ. Long-term follow-up of patients with undiagnosed fever of unknown origin. Arch Intern Med 1996; 156:618.
[b] 6. de Kleijn EM, Vandenbroucke JP, van der Meer JW. Fever of unknown origin. I. A prospective multicenter study of 167 patients with FUO, using fixed epidemiologic entry criteria. Medicine 1997; 76:392.
[c] 7. Cunha B. Fever of unknown origin. Infect Dis Clin North Am 1996; 10:111.
[b] 8. Kanzanjian P. Fever of unknown origin: review of 86 patients treated in community hospitals. Clin Infect Dis 1992; 15:968.
[c] 9. Durack DT, Street AC. Fever of unknown origin—reexamined and redefined. In JS Remington, MN Swartz, eds. Current clinical topics in infectious diseases. Cambridge, Mass: Blackwell; 1991.
[c] 10. Knockaert DC et al. Fever of unknown origin in the 1980s: an update on the diagnostic spectrum. Arch Intern Med 1992; 152:51.
[c] 11. Gelfand JA, Dinarello CA, Wolff SM. Fever, including fever of unknown origin. In Isselbacher KJ et al, eds. Harrison's principles of internal medicine, 13th ed. New York: McGraw-Hill; 1994.
[c] 12. Mylonakis E, Calderwood SB. Infective endocarditis in adults. N Engl J Med 2001; 345:1318.
[b] 13. Hoen B et al. Infective endocarditis in patients with negative blood cultures: analysis of 88 cases from a one-year nationwide survey in France. Clin Infect Dis 1995; 20(3):501.
[c] 14. Jacoby GA, Swartz MN. Fever of undetermined origin. N Engl J Med 1973; 289(26):1407.
[c] 15. de Kleijn EM, van der Meer JW. Inquiry into the diagnostic workup of patients with fever of unknown. Neth J Med 1997; 50:69.
[c] 16. Cunha B. The clinical significance of fever patterns. Infect Dis Clin North Am 1996; 10:33.
[b] 17. de Kleijn EM, Vandenbroucke JP, van der Meer JW. Fever of unknown origin. II. Diagnostic procedures in a prospective multicenter study of 167 patients. Medicine 1997; 76:410.

[b] 18. Bissuel F et al. Fever of unknown origin in HIV-infected patients: a critical analysis of a retrospective series of 57 cases. J Intern Med 1994; 236:529.
[b] 19. Barbado FJ et al. Fever of unknown origin: a survey of 133 patients. J Med 1984; 15:185.
[b] 20. Fernandez-Aviles F et al. The usefulness of the bone marrow examination in the etiological diagnosis of prolonged fever in patients with HIV infection. Med Clin 1999; 112:641.
[b] 21. Volk EE et al. The diagnostic usefulness of bone marrow cultures in patients with fever of unknown origin. Am J Clin Pathol 1998; 110:150.
[d] 22. Huges W et al. 1997 Guidelines for the use of antimicrobial agents in neutropenic patients with unexplained fever. Clin Infect Dis 1997; 25:551.

Community-Acquired Pneumonia

Aimee Zaas, MD, Alan Cheng, MD, and John Bartlett, MD

FAST FACTS

- Treatment for community-acquired pneumonia (CAP) should begin within 4 hours of presentation.
- The diagnosis is based on clinical judgment, supplemented by microbiological and radiologic data.
- The average mortality for hospitalized patients with CAP is 14%.[1]
- The most common etiological agents include *Streptococcus pneumoniae*, *Haemophilus influenzae*, and possibly *Chlamydia pneumoniae*.
- The most common etiological agents in lethal pneumonia are *S. pneumoniae* and *Legionella*.
- Factors indicating a poor prognosis include advanced age, multilobar involvement, bacteremia, and severe associated disease.
- Failure to respond to antibiotics is usually due to delay in initiation of treatment or host factors, not error in antibiotic selection.
- Inpatients should continue to receive intravenous antibiotics until clinically stable and able to take oral medications.

43

I. EPIDEMIOLOGY

1. CAP is defined as an acute infection of the pulmonary parenchyma that is associated with at least some symptoms of acute infection, accompanied by an acute infiltrate on chest radiograph or auscultatory findings consistent with pneumonia in a person who was not hospitalized or residing in a long-term care facility for the 14 days before presentation.[3]
2. Given the emergence of antibiotic resistance and the potential hazards of antibiotic treatment failures, establishment of a definitive diagnosis is desirable. Despite attempts to do so, 40% to 60% of CAP cases have no identified etiological agent.[4] (See "Diagnostics" for further discussion of this point.) Table 43-1 lists the most common etiological agents.[4]
   a. Less common etiological agents of CAP in immunocompetent hosts include fungi, spirochetes, and the causative agents of psittacosis and tularemia.
   b. Seasonal and geographical differences in the etiological agent of CAP also exist. Although *C. pneumoniae* occurs year round, *S. pneumoniae* and *H. influenzae* are more common in the winter months.

TABLE 43-1
MICROBIOLOGICAL PATHOGENS IN COMMUNITY-ACQUIRED PNEUMONIA

Microbiological Agent or Cause	Prevalence (%)
Typical agents	
Streptococcus pneumoniae	20-60
Haemophilus influenzae	3-10
Staphylococcus aureus	3-5
Gram-negative bacilli	3-10
Miscellaneous (*Moraxella catarrhalis,* group A *Streptococcus,* *Neisseria meningitidis*)	3-5
Atypical agents	10-20
Legionella	2-8
Mycoplasma pneumoniae	1-6
Chlamydia pneumoniae	4-6
Viruses (influenza, parainfluenza, respiratory syncytial virus)	2-15
Aspiration	6-10

Data from Bartlett JG, Mundy L. N Engl J Med 1995; 333:1618.
Based on 15 published reports from North America. None of these studies used techniques adequate to detect anaerobes in respiratory secretions; these organisms account for 20% to 30% of cases in some reports. *Pneumocystis carinii* is excluded but may account for up to 15% in recent reports from urban centers.

BOX 43-1

SYMPTOMS OF COMMUNITY-ACQUIRED PNEUMONIA

Fever or hypothermia

Rigors, sweats

New cough with or without sputum production

Hemoptysis

Change in character of respiratory secretions in a patient with chronic cough

Chest discomfort

Dyspnea

Anorexia, fatigue, or myalgias

From Bartlett JG et al. Clin Infect Dis 2000; 31:347.

II. CLINICAL PRESENTATION

1. CAP is a clinical diagnosis based on the patient's history, physical examination, and chest radiography. There is no gold standard method of diagnosis.

2. Data from the Pneumonia Patient Outcomes Research Team (PORT) study show that respiratory symptoms found on presentation of patients with CAP include cough (86%), dyspnea (72%), sputum production (64%), and hemoptysis (16%). Nonpulmonary symptoms included fatigue (91%), fever (74%), sweats (72%), and headaches (58%) (Box 43-1).[5]

3. Thus far no convincing association between a patient's signs and symptoms and a specific etiological agent has been established.[6]

However, a patient's presentation can *suggest* a possible organism. Sudden onset of chills and fever, productive cough, pleuritic chest pain, physical signs of pulmonary consolidation, and focal infiltrates on chest radiograph suggest pneumococcal pneumonia. The symptoms associated with an atypical pneumonia are more insidious and are more likely to include dry cough, sometimes with extrapulmonary symptoms (headaches, myalgias, arthralgias, sore throat, nausea, vomiting, or diarrhea).

4. A chest radiograph is essential for the diagnosis of CAP. Guidelines from the Infectious Disease Society of America (IDSA)[3] require a demonstrable infiltrate on chest radiograph; the only important exception is *Pneumocystis carinii* pneumonia, which may be associated with a false negative chest radiograph in 10% to 30% of cases. However, *Pneumocystis* pneumonia generally has a more subacute presentation (see Chapter 39). The presence or absence of individual findings in a patient's history (cough, dyspnea, sputum production, fever, chills, night sweats, myalgias, sore throat, rhinorrhea, asthma, immunosuppression, or dementia) did not have significant positive or negative predictive value for CAP in an analysis of four major CAP studies.[7]

5. Other laboratory studies that are recommended before treatment include a basic metabolic panel, complete blood cell count, two peripheral blood cultures, sputum Gram's stain and culture, pulse oximetry or arterial blood gas analysis, and serological tests for human immunodeficiency virus (HIV) in patients 15 to 54 years old.

6. Bronchoscopy or transtracheal or transthoracic needle aspiration should be performed only in highly unusual situations.

7. It is recommended that sputum samples be delivered to the laboratory within 2 hours to maximize yield.[8]

III. DIAGNOSTICS

1. A differential diagnosis of CAP includes acute or chronic sinusitis, acute or chronic bronchitis, pulmonary edema, gastroesophageal reflux disease, reactive airway disease, atelectasis, tuberculosis, bronchiolitis obliterans organizing pneumonia, vasculitis, pulmonary embolism, malignancy, or lung abscess (Fig. 43-1).

2. Indicated diagnostic studies for the diagnosis of CAP are based on recommendations from IDSA's practice guidelines and are shown in Box 43-2.

3. The sputum sample should be deep-cough expectorated sputum obtained before antibiotic therapy. Trained personnel should interpret Gram's stain, and culture should be performed only if the specimen is adequate by cytological criteria. For maximum yield, it is important to get the sputum sample to the laboratory within 2 hours of collection.

4. Cytological screening should be done under low-power magnification (×100) to determine the cellular composition. Acceptable specimens have fewer than 10 epithelial cells and more than 25 polymor-

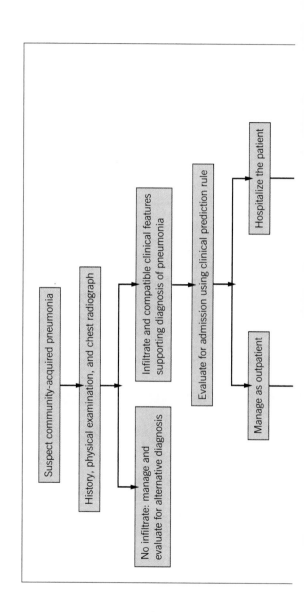

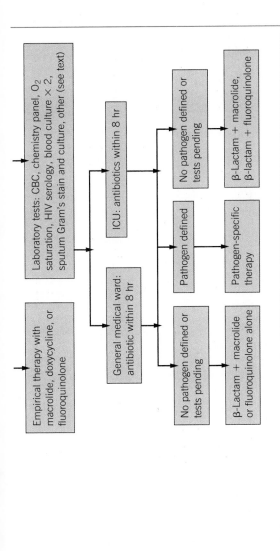

FIG. 43-1

Treatment of patients with community-acquired pneumonia. *CNS*, Central nervous system; *CSF*, cerebrospinal fluid; *CT*, computed tomography; *LP*, lumbar puncture.

43

COMMUNITY-ACQUIRED PNEUMONIA

BOX 43-2

DIAGNOSTIC STUDIES FOR EVALUATION OF COMMUNITY-ACQUIRED PNEUMONIA

BASELINE ASSESSMENT

All patients thought to have pneumonia should have chest radiography to substantiate the diagnosis of pneumonia, detect associated lung diseases, assess response against the known baseline, suggest a pathogen, and assess severity

TESTS FOR ALL HOSPITALIZED PATIENTS (IN ADDITION TO CHEST RADIOGRAPHY)

Complete blood cell count with differential

Chemistry panel, including glucose, serum sodium, liver function tests, and renal function tests

Serological tests for human immunodeficiency virus (HIV) for persons 15 to 54 years of age in hospitals with more than one newly diagnosed case of HIV infection per 1000 discharged patients

Arterial blood gas analysis

Pretreatment blood cultures (two sets)

Gram's stain and culture of sputum

Test for *Mycobacterium tuberculosis* with acid-fast stain and culture for selected patients, especially those with cough for more than 1 month and less than 1 year, other common symptoms, or suggestive radiographs

Test for Legionnaire's disease in selected patients, including any seriously ill patient without another diagnosis, especially if the patient is over 40 years of age, immunocompromised, or nonresponsive to β-lactam antibiotics, if the patient has clinical features suggesting the diagnosis, and in outbreak settings; preferred tests are urine antigen against *Legionella,* direct fluorescent antibody staining of sputum, and culture with selective media

Thoracentesis with Gram's stain, culture, pH determination, and leukocyte count with differential in patient with pleural effusion

Modified from Bartlett JG et al. Clin Infect Dis 2000; 31:347.

phonuclear cells (PMNs) per low-power field. Cytological assessment is not necessary in screening specimens for detection of *Legionella* or mycobacteria. A sputum Gram's stain with many PMNs and no organisms is suggestive of an atypical organism.

5. *S. pneumoniae* is seriously underrepresented by current microbiological testing, as are anaerobes. In patients who are subsequently found to have pneumococcal bacteremia, sputum samples have been falsely negative in 50%.[9] The British Thoracic Society concluded that 148 patients with no identified pathogen had probable *S. pneumoniae.*[10] Similarly, transtracheal aspirate reveals anaerobes in 20% to 33% of cases of CAP.[11] Thus blood cultures are extremely important in the diagnosis of CAP. Blood culture data reveal that 11% of patients hospitalized with CAP have positive blood cultures, with *S. pneumoniae* accounting for 67% of the positive cultures.[4]

6. Pneumococcal urine antigen is a new diagnostic test for CAP. This immunochromatographic assay is a rapid (performed in 15 minutes) noninvasive test for the diagnosis of *S. pneumoniae* infection. Specificity has been reported at 97.2% and sensitivity at 80.4% for detecting antigen in cases of pneumococcal pneumonia.[12]

7. Investigators from the PORT study created a model that can identify patients who should or should not be admitted to the hospital based on data that correlate with mortality.[13] A risk stratification model was derived from data from 14,199 adult inpatients with CAP and validated with 38,039 patients. Patients were over 18 years of age and were excluded if HIV positive. Nursing home patients were included in the analysis. In this two-step model, step 1 (risk class I) was designed to identify very low-risk patients on the basis of history and physical examination and step 2 was designed to assess illness severity on the basis of history, physical examination, and basic laboratory values (Box 43-3). Common sense dictates that certain patients fit "low-risk" classifications but should be treated as inpatients because of unstable social situations.

8. The CAPITAL study validated the PORT prediction rule as a measure to improve the efficiency of medical care for CAP without compromising outcome.[14] In a randomized study the PORT prediction rule was compared with standard care for patients who had CAP and were seen in the emergency department. Investigators found similar mortality, admission to the intensive care unit, and subsequent hospitalization for patients treated in the outpatient setting based on the PORT prediction rule compared with similar patients who were admitted to the hospital. Both the IDSA and the American Thoracic Society endorse the PORT prediction rule.[3,15]

IV. MANAGEMENT

1. Guidelines for antibiotic selection in CAP are provided by the IDSA.[3] When the cause of pneumonia has been determined, antibiotic selections are based on in vitro susceptibility testing or data from clinical trials. If no etiological agent has been detected, the IDSA guidelines offer multiple options from which to choose. *This is done because no clinical trial data clearly demonstrate the superiority of any given regimen.* In addition, allowing choice ensures that a broad range of antibiotics will be used, thus minimizing emergence of resistant pathogens (Table 43-2).

2. Rapid initiation of treatment is imperative. Treatment should begin as soon as possible after the sputum sample is obtained and ideally within 4 hours of presentation. One study of over 14,000 patients found that mortality increased when patients received the first dose of antibiotics more than 8 hours after admission.[16]

3. Preferred antimicrobials for most patients, in no special order (Box 43-4).[3,17-20]

43

COMMUNITY-ACQUIRED PNEUMONIA

BOX 43-3

ASSIGNMENT OF RISK CLASS IN THE PNEUMONIA PATIENT OUTCOMES RESEARCH TEAM (PORT) COHORT

ASSIGNMENT OF PATIENTS WITH CAP TO RISK CLASS I

Is the patient more than 50 years of age? → Yes → Assign to class II-V (see below)

Does the patient have any of the following coexisting conditions: neoplastic disease, congestive heart failure, cerebrovascular disease, renal disease, hepatic disease? → Yes → Assign to class II-V (see below)

Does the patient have any of the following abnormalities on examination: altered mental status, pulse >125 beats/min, respiratory rate >30 breaths/min, systolic blood pressure <90 mm Hg, temperature <35° C or >40° C? → Yes → Assign to class II-V (see below)

If none of the above abnormalities are present, assign patient to class I

ASSIGNMENT TO RISK CLASSES II, III, IV, OR V

Characteristic	Points Assigned
Demographic factor	
Age	
Men	Age (yr)
Women	Age (yr) − 10
Nursing home resident	+10
Coexisting illness	
Neoplastic disease	+30
Liver disease	+20
Congestive heart failure	+10
Cerebrovascular disease	+10
Renal disease	+10
Physical examination findings	
Altered mental status	+20
Respiratory rate >30 breaths/min	+20
Systolic blood pressure <90 mm Hg	+20
Temp <35° C or >40° C	+15
Pulse >125 beats/min	+10
Laboratory and radiographic findings	
Arterial pH <7.35	+30
Blood urea nitrogen level >30 mg/dL (11 mmol/L)	+20
Sodium level <130 mmol/L	+20
Glucose level >250 mg/dL (14 mmol/L)	+10
Hematocrit <30%	+10
Pao$_2$ <60 mm Hg	+10
Pleural effusion	+10

cont'd

BOX 43-3

ASSIGNMENT OF RISK CLASS IN THE PNEUMONIA PATIENT OUTCOMES RESEARCH TEAM (PORT) COHORT—cont'd

ASSIGNMENT TO RISK CLASSES II, III, IV, OR V—CONT'D

Neoplastic disease is defined as any cancer except basal or squamous cell cancer of the skin that was active at the time of presentation or diagnosed within 1 year of presentation. Liver disease is defined as a clinical or histological diagnosis of cirrhosis or another form of chronic liver disease, such as chronic active hepatitis. Congestive heart failure is defined as systolic or diastolic ventricular dysfunction documented by history, physical examination, and chest radiograph, echocardiogram, multiple gated acquisition scan, or left ventriculogram. Cerebrovascular disease is defined as a clinical diagnosis of stroke or transient ischemic attack or stroke documented by computed tomography or magnetic resonance imaging. Renal disease is defined as a history of chronic renal disease or abnormal blood urea nitrogen and creatinine concentrations documented in the medical record. Altered mental status is defined as disorientation to person, place, or time not known to be chronic.

STRATIFICATION OF RISK SCORE

Risk	Risk Class	Points (See Above)	Suggested Treatment Location	Mortality (%)
	I	See above	Outpatient	0.4
Low	II	≤70	Outpatient	0.7
	III	71-90	Inpatient	2.8
Moderate	IV	91-130	Inpatient	8.5
High	V	>130	Inpatient	31.1

Modified from Fine MJ et al. N Engl J Med 1997; 336:243.

a. General medical ward (preferred agents).
   (1) Extended-spectrum cephalosporin combined with a macrolide, *or*
   (2) A β-lactam and β-lactamase inhibitor combined with a macrolide, *or*
   (3) A fluoroquinolone alone.
b. Intensive care unit (preferred agents).
   (1) Extended-spectrum cephalosporin, *or*
   (2) A β-lactam and β-lactamase inhibitor, *plus*
   (3) Either a macrolide or a fluoroquinolone.
c. Modifying factors.
   (1) Structural disease of the lung (bronchiectasis): antipseudomonal agents (piperacillin, piperacillin-tazobactam, carbapenem, or cefepime), *plus* a fluoroquinolone (including high-dose ciprofloxacin).
   (2) β-Lactam allergy: fluoroquinolone with or without clindamycin.
   (3) Suspected aspiration: fluoroquinolone *plus* clindamycin, metronidazole, *or* a β-lactam and β-lactamase inhibitor.
     (a) Extended-spectrum cephalosporin: cefotaxime or ceftriaxone.

TABLE 43-2

PATHOGEN-DIRECTED ANTIMICROBIAL THERAPY FOR COMMUNITY-ACQUIRED PNEUMONIA

Organism	Preferred Antimicrobial	Alternative
Streptococcus pneumoniae		
Penicillin susceptible (MIC <2 µg/mL)	Penicillin G, amoxicillin	Cephalosporins, imipenem, macrolide, clindamycin, doxycycline, or fluoroquinolone
Penicillin resistant (MIC ≥2 µg/mL)	Agents based on in vitro susceptibility tests, including cefotaxime, ceftriaxone, fluoroquinolone, and vancomycin	
Haemophilus influenzae	Cephalosporin (second or third generation), TMP-SMX, doxycycline, β-lactam/β-lactamase inhibitor, macrolide	Fluoroquinolone, clarithromycin
Moraxella catarrhalis	Cephalosporin (second or third generation), TMP-SMX, β-lactam/β-lactamase inhibitor, macrolide	Fluoroquinolone
Anaerobe	β-Lactam/β-lactamase inhibitor, clindamycin	Imipenem
Staphylococcus aureus		
Methicillin-susceptible	Nafcillin/oxacillin ± rifampin or gentamicin	Cefazolin, cefuroxime, vancomycin, clindamycin, TMP-SMX
Methicillin-resistant	Vancomycin ± rifampin or gentamicin	Linezolid
Escherichia coli, Klebsiella, Proteus, or *Enterobacter*	Third-generation cephalosporin ± aminoglycoside, carbapenem	Aztreonam, β-lactam/β-lactamase inhibitor, fluoroquinolone
Pseudomonas aeruginosa	Aminoglycoside ± antipseudomonal β-lactam: ticarcillin, piperacillin, mezlocillin, ceftazidime, cefepime, aztreonam, or carbapenem	Aminoglycoside + ciprofloxacin; ciprofloxacin + antipseudomonal β-lactam
Legionella	Macrolide ± rifampin; fluoroquinolone (including ciprofloxacin)	Doxycycline ± rifampin

Data from Bartlett JG et al. Clin Infect Dis 2000; 31:347.

MIC, Minimum inhibitory concentration; *TMP-SMX,* trimethoprim-sulfamethoxazole.

BOX 43-4

FACTS TO REMEMBER ABOUT ANTIBIOTIC CHOICES

β-Lactams are inactive against *Mycoplasma pneumoniae*, *Chlamydia pneumoniae*, and *Legionella*

Between 10% and 15% of *Streptococcus pneumoniae* is resistant to macrolides[17]

Clindamycin is considered to be the drug of choice for anaerobic pneumonias and lung abscesses[18-20]

(b) Macrolide: azithromycin, clarithromycin, erythromycin.

(c) Fluoroquinolone: levofloxacin, gatifloxacin or moxifloxacin, or another fluoroquinolone with enhanced activity against *S. pneumoniae*.

(d) β-Lactam and β-lactamase inhibitor: ampicillin-sulbactam, or piperacillin-tazobactam.

(e) β-Lactam and β-lactamase inhibitor for structural diseases of the lung: piperacillin-tazobactam.

4. Length of treatment has not been standardized by randomized controlled trials. The generally accepted treatment duration is 5 to 10 days for common bacterial pneumonia, 10 to 14 days for *Mycoplasma* or *Chlamydia*, and 14 to 21 days for *Legionella*. Therapy can change from intravenous to oral when the patient is improving and able to take oral medications.[17]

5. Response to treatment is based on the patient's respiratory symptoms, fever, partial pressure of oxygen, and white blood cell count. Follow-up chest x-ray examination is recommended only for smokers or for selected patients who do not respond to treatment.

6. Box 43-5 outlines poor prognostic factors.

a. Prognostic factors in CAP were determined based on both the PORT cohort and the MedisGroups Comparative Hospital Database of 14,199 patients in 78 U.S. hospitals.

b. Lack of response necessitates a reassessment of the diagnosis and a determination of whether the problem is related to the host (treatment delay, empyema), the medications (inappropriate dosage regimen), or the pathogen (microbiological resistance or misdiagnosis).[3]

PEARLS AND PITFALLS

- Clinical significance of penicillin-resistant *S. pneumoniae*.[21]
  - Penicillin- and cephalosporin-resistant strains of *S. pneumoniae* are an increasing concern. The clinical significance of resistance is less clear.
  - Resistance for "nonmeningitis" isolates of *S. pneumoniae* has been defined by the National Committee of Clinical Laboratory Standards, in part based on outcome studies of pneumococcal pneumonia. Minimum inhibitory concentration (MIC) breakpoints are based on concentrations of penicillin and ceftriaxone required to treat nonmeningitis infections. Penicillin-susceptible isolates have an MIC less than 0.06 μg/mL, intermediate-susceptibility isolates have an MIC of 0.1 to 1 μg/mL, and

---

BOX 43-5

POOR PROGNOSTIC FACTORS IN PATIENTS WITH COMMUNITY-ACQUIRED PNEUMONIA

AGE

Greater than 65 years

COEXISTING DISEASE

Diabetes
Renal failure
Heart failure
Chronic lung disease
Chronic alcoholism
Hospitalization within the previous year
Immunosuppression
Neoplastic disease

CLINICAL FINDINGS

Respiratory rate greater than 30 breaths/min
Systolic blood pressure less than 90 mm Hg or diastolic blood pressure less than 60 mm Hg
Temperature greater than 38.3° C
Altered mental status
Extrapulmonary site of infection (meningitis, septic arthritis)
Laboratory tests
White blood cell count less than 4000/mm^3 or greater than 30,000/mm^3
Pao$_2$ less than 60 mm Hg on room air
Renal failure
Multilobar involvement on chest radiograph
Pleural effusion
Hematocrit value less than 30%
Microbial pathogens: *Streptococcus pneumoniae*, *Staphylococcus aureus*, *Legionella*

Modified from Bartlett JG et al. N Engl J Med 1995; 333:331.

---

penicillin-resistant isolates have an MIC ≥2 μg/mL. Susceptibility to ceftriaxone and cefotaxime is defined as an MIC less than or equal to 1 μg/mL, intermediate as an MIC of 2 μg/mL, and resistant as an MIC ≥ 4 μg/mL. High doses of intravenous penicillin (at least 2 million units q4h in adults with normal renal function) or ampicillin (2 g q6h) are effective in treating pneumococcal pneumonia caused by strains in the intermediate category. The new criteria for resistance in non-meningeal isolates of *S. pneumoniae* (MIC ≥2 μg/mL) apply to 5% to 15% of *S. pneumoniae* in the United States.

- See Chapter 44 for a discussion of pneumococcal meningitis.
- Preferred drugs for penicillin-sensitive strains are β-lactams: amoxicillin, cefotaxime, cefprozil, cefpodoxime, and cefuroxime. Empirical treatment for penicillin-resistant strains should be with a fluoroquinolone, vancomycin, or an agent selected based on in vitro tests.
- Elderly patients may have fewer symptoms of CAP. In a prospective study of 1812 patients with clinical and x-ray evidence of pneumonia at presentation in inpatient and outpatient facilities, advanced age (≥75 years) was associated with significantly fewer symptoms (mean 7.0 as compared with mean 10.3 symptoms) than in patients aged 18 to 44.[22]
- Aspiration pneumonia.
  - The diagnosis should be suspected among patients with depressed levels of consciousness or dysphagia and radiographic evidence of an infiltrate in a dependent pulmonary segment (posterior segment of an upper lobe or superior segment of a lower lobe).
  - Anaerobic infections predominate in out-of-hospital aspiration pneumonia.
  - The drug of choice is clindamycin.[19,20]
  - Metronidazole is associated with treatment failure in aspiration pneumonia caused by aerobic and microaerophilic streptococci.
  - Acceptable alternative regimens include metronidazole plus penicillin or amoxicillin-clavulanate.
  - Patients hospitalized longer than 3 days have "hospital-acquired" oral flora. True aspiration pneumonia in this setting should be treated with a β-lactam and β-lactamase inhibitor or other broad-spectrum antibiotic.
- *Legionella.*
  - *Legionella* is implicated in 2% to 6% of cases in hospital-based series of CAP.
  - Risk is related to exposure, increasing age, smoking, and compromised cell-mediated immunity.
  - All patients admitted to the medical intensive care unit with pneumonia, negative Gram's stain, and immunocompromise should be tested.
  - Clinical factors common in *Legionella* infection include temperature greater than 40° C, hyponatremia, and lactate dehydrogenase level greater than 700 units/mL.[23]
  - Preferred tests are culture on selective media (which often gives false negative results), and *Legionella* urinary antigen testing, which rapidly detects 70% of cases.
  - Doxycycline, azithromycin, ofloxacin, ciprofloxacin, or levofloxacin is the preferred treatment.
  - Treatment duration is 10 to 21 days.
- A review of how to use the PORT prediction rule effectively can be found in reference 24.

43

COMMUNITY-ACQUIRED PNEUMONIA

- The presence of bilateral pleural effusions was an independent marker of 30-day mortality in a subgroup analysis of 1906 patients from the PORT study (RR 2.8; 95% CI 1.4-5.8). Number of involved lobes, bilateral infiltrates, "bronchopneumonia" (patchy consolidation in the distribution of a bronchial lung segment), and air bronchograms were not associated with increased short-term mortality.[25]

REFERENCES

[a] 1. Fine MJ et al. Prognosis and outcomes of patients with community-acquired pneumonia: a meta-analysis. JAMA 1996; 275:134.

[b] 2. Centers for Disease Control and Prevention. Premature deaths, monthly mortality and monthly physician contacts—United States. MMWR Morb Mortal Wkly Rep 1997; 46:556.

[d] 3. Bartlett JG et al. Practice guidelines for the management of community-acquired pneumonia in adults. Clin Infect Dis 2000; 31:347.

[c] 4. Bartlett JG, Mundy L. Community-acquired pneumonia. N Engl J Med 1995; 333:1618.

[a] 5. Fine MJ et al. Processes and outcomes of care for patients with community-acquired pneumonia: results from the pneumonia Patient Outcomes Research Team (PORT) cohort study. Arch Intern Med 1999; 159:970.

[a] 6. Fang GD et al. New and emerging etiologies for community-acquired pneumonia with implications for therapy: a prospective multicenter study of 359 cases. Medicine 1990; 69:307.

[d] 7. Metlay JP, Kapoor WN, Fine MJ. Does this patient have community-acquired pneumonia? Diagnosing pneumonia by history and physical examination. JAMA 1997; 278:1440.

[b] 8. Jefferson H et al. Transportation delay and the microbiological quality of clinical specimens. Am J Clin Pathol 1975; 64:689.

[d] 9. Bartlett JG et al. Community-acquired pneumonia in adults: guidelines for management. Infectious Diseases Society of America. Clin Infect Dis 1998; 28:820.

[d] 10. British Thoracic Society. Guidelines for the management of community-acquired pneumonia in adults admitted to hospital. Br J Hosp Med 1993; 49:346.

[d] 11. Diehr P et al. Prediction of pneumonia in outpatients with acute cough—a statistical approach. J Chronic Dis 1984; 37:215.

[b] 12. Dominguez J et al. Detection of *Streptococcus pneumoniae* antigen by a rapid immunochromatographic assay in urine samples. Chest 2001; 119:243.

[a] 13. Fine MJ et al. A prediction rule to identify low-risk patients with community-acquired pneumonia. N Engl J Med 1997; 336:243.

[a] 14. Marrie TJ et al. A controlled trial of a critical pathway for treatment of CAP: Community Acquired Pneumonia Intervention Trial Assessing Levofloxacin. CAPITAL Study Investigators. JAMA 2000; 283:749.

[d] 15. Niederman MS et al. Guidelines for the management of adults with CAP: diagnosis, assessment of severity, antimicrobial therapy and prevention. AJRCCM 2001; 163:1730.

[b] 16. Meehan TP et al. Quality of care, process and outcomes in elderly patients with pneumonia. JAMA 1997; 278:2020.

[b] 17. Hofmann J et al. The prevalence of drug-resistant *Streptococcus pneumoniae* in Atlanta. N Engl J Med 1995; 333:481.

[c] 18. Bartlett JG. Anaerobic bacterial infections of the lung and pleural space. Clin Infect Dis 1993; 16(suppl 4):3.

[c] 19. Levison ME et al. Clindamycin compared with penicillin for the treatment of anaerobic lung abscesses. Ann Intern Med 1983; 98:466.

[a] 20. Gudiol F et al. Clindamycin vs. penicillin for anaerobic lung infections: high rate of penicillin failures associated with penicillin-resistant *Bacteroides melaninogenicus*. Arch Intern Med 1990; 150:2525.

[b] 21. Butler JC et al. The continued emergence of drug-resistant *Streptococcus pneumoniae* in the United States: an update from the Centers for Disease Control and Prevention's Pneumococcal Sentinel Surveillance System. J Infect Dis 1996; 174:986.

[b] 22. Metlay JP et al. Influence of age on symptoms at presentation in patients with community acquired pneumonia. Arch Intern Med 1997; 157:1453.

[b] 23. Keller DW et al: Clinical diagnosis of Legionnaire's disease using a multivariate model [abstract K55]. In Program and abstracts of the 35th Interscience Conference on Antimicrobial Agents and Chemotherapy (San Francisco). Washington, DC: American Society for Microbiology; 1995.

[a] 24. Fine MJ. Solutions for difficult diagnostic cases of community-acquired pneumonia. Chemotherapy 2001; 47(suppl 4):3.

[b] 25. Hasley PB et al. Do pulmonary radiographic findings at presentation predict mortality in patients with CAP? Arch Intern Med 1996; 156:2206.

43

COMMUNITY-ACQUIRED PNEUMONIA

Meningitis

Alan Cheng, MD, Aimee Zaas, MD, and Paul Auwaerter, MD

FAST FACTS

- Acute bacterial meningitis (ABM) is a medical emergency. Instituting appropriate antibiotic treatment as soon as possible is essential for good outcome.
- The most common etiological agents of community-acquired bacterial meningitis are *Streptococcus pneumoniae, Haemophilus influenzae,* and *Neisseria meningitidis.* The case-fatality rate for ABM is 6% for *H. influenzae,* 3% for *N. meningitidis,* and 21% for *S. pneumoniae.*[1]
- The most common causes of acute viral meningitis are enteroviruses (echovirus or Coxsackie virus).
- Kernig's and Brudzinski's signs are found in about 50% of ABM cases.
- Confusion is a major presenting symptom in the elderly.[2]
- Predictors of acute bacterial (versus viral) meningitis with 99% sensitivity are cerebrospinal fluid (CSF) glucose level below 34 mg/dL, CSF/blood glucose ratio less than 0.23, CSF protein level greater than 220 mg/dL, CSF leukocyte count greater than 2000/mm^3, or CSF polymorphonuclear neutrophil (PMN) count greater than 1180/mm^3.[3]
- Computed tomography of the head is needed before a lumbar puncture is performed in patients older than 60 years and those who are immunocompromised, have a history of central nervous system disease, have had a seizure within 1 week of presentation, are in a coma, have papilledema or focal neurological findings, or have a suspected mass lesion.[4,5]

I. EPIDEMIOLOGY

1. Acute aseptic meningitis typically has a viral cause.[6] Although the enteroviruses (echovirus, Coxsackie virus) are the most common, other viral causes of meningitis include acute human immunodeficiency virus (HIV) infection, Epstein-Barr virus, herpes simplex virus types 1 and 2, mumps virus, lymphocytic choriomeningitis virus, and cytomegalovirus.

2. ABM can be separated into community-acquired and nosocomial causes. Typical pathogens in ABM depend heavily on the age of the host, as well as the presence of comorbid conditions. Community-acquired ABM is most commonly caused by the following organisms (in decreasing order of incidence): *S. pneumoniae, N. meningitidis, Listeria monocytogenes,* and *H. influenzae.*[6] *S. pneumoniae* and *N. meningitidis* are the predominant causes of ABM in patients

1 month of age or older.[7] Gram-negative bacilli and *Staphylococcus aureus* are usually the cause of nosocomial cases (Table 44-1).

3. Subacute and chronic causes of infectious meningitis include *Mycobacterium tuberculosis,* fungi (*Cryptococcus neoformans),* and spirochetes (*Treponema pallidum, Leptospira* species, and *Borrelia burgdorferi).* Noninfectious causes include drugs, carcinoma, and occasionally, rheumatological disorders such as Behçet's disease, systemic lupus erythematosus, and vasculitis.

4. Risk factors for community-acquired ABM include a concurrent or recent history of infection, such as otitis media, sinusitis, pneumonia, endocarditis, and cellulitis. Other risk factors include intravenous drug use, diabetes mellitus, CSF leak, and history of head trauma. The most common cause of meningitis in patients with CSF leak is infection with *S. pneumoniae.* Nosocomial risk factors include recent neurosurgery, indwelling neurosurgical devices, immunocompromised states, CSF leak, and history of head trauma.[6] Comorbid diseases that

TABLE 44-1

COMMON BACTERIAL PATHOGENS BASED ON PREDISPOSING FACTOR IN PATIENTS WITH MENINGITIS

Predisposing Factor	Pathogens
Age	
0-4 weeks	Group B *Streptococcus, Escherichia coli, Listeria monocytogenes, Klebsiella pneumoniae, Enterococcus* spp., *Salmonella* spp.
4-12 weeks	*Streptococcus agalactiae, E. coli, L. mono- cytogenes, Haemophilus influenzae,* * *Streptococcus pneumoniae, Neisseria meningitidis*
3 months–18 years	*S. pneumoniae, N. meningitidis, H. influenzae**
18-50 years	*S. pneumoniae, N. meningitidis*
>50 years	*S. pneumoniae, N. meningitidis, L. mono- cytogenes,* aerobic gram-negative bacilli
Immunocompromised state (non–human immunodeficiency virus)	*S. pneumoniae, N. meningitidis, L. mono- cytogenes,* aerobic gram-negative bacilli (including *Pseudomonas aeruginosa*)
Basilar skull fracture or chronic otitis or sinusitis	*S. pneumoniae, H. influenzae,* group A β-hemolytic streptococci
Head trauma, postneurosurgery	*Staphylococcus aureus, Staphylococcus epidermidis,* aerobic gram-negative bacilli (including *P. aeruginosa*)
Cerebrospinal fluid shunt	*S. epidermidis, S. aureus,* aerobic gram- negative bacilli (including *P. aeruginosa*), diphtheroids, *Propionibacterium acnes*

Data from Tunkel AR, Scheld WM. Acute meningitis. In Mandell GL, Bennett JE, Dolin R. eds. Principles and practice of infectious diseases, 5th ed. Philadelphia: Churchill Livingstone; 2000.
H. influenzae only if patient has not received vaccine.

impair cellular immunity (HIV, steroid use, organ transplantation, cytotoxic chemotherapy) increase the risk of acquiring *L. monocytogenes*. Splenectomy, hypogammaglobulinemia, and multiple myeloma increase the risk of *S. pneumoniae* meningitis.[8]

5. Meningitis was once considered a childhood disease, but the epidemiology has shifted and the median age for bacterial meningitis is now 25 years.[7] The use of conjugated *H. influenzae* type b (Hib) vaccine has virtually abolished this once common infection of infants and children. Nosocomial cases have increased in parallel with the increase in neurosurgical procedures.

6. Patients with a history of alcoholism, intravenous drug use, or other immunocompromised states have an increased risk of less common causes of meningitis, such as *L. monocytogenes*. Eating unpasteurized milk products ("queso fresco") is also associated with *Listeria* infection.

7. A differential diagnosis of acute meningitis includes noninfectious causes of headache, mental status changes, and photophobia. Such causes include intracranial tumors and cysts, lupus cerebritis, seizures, multiple sclerosis, lead or mercury poisoning, drug-induced aseptic meningitis (from intravenous immune globulin, nonsteroidal antiinflammatory drugs), Mollaret's meningitis, post–lumbar puncture headache, subarachnoid bleed, and migraine headache (Box 44-1).

44

MENINGITIS

BOX 44-1

DIFFERENTIAL DIAGNOSIS OF ACUTE MENINGITIS

MAJOR INFECTIOUS ETIOLOGIES

Viruses

Nonpolio enteroviruses*

Mumps virus

Arboviruses†

Herpesviruses‡

Lymphocytic choriomeningitis virus

Human immunodeficiency virus

Adenovirus

Parainfluenza virus types 2 and 3

Influenza virus

Measles virus

Rickettsiae

Rickettsia rickettsii (Rocky Mountain spotted fever)

Rickettsia conorii

Rickettsia prowazekii (epidemic or louse-borne virus)

Rickettsia typhi (endemic or murine typhus)

Rickettsia tsutsugamushi (scrub typhus)

Ehrlichia spp.

cont'd

BOX 44-1

DIFFERENTIAL DIAGNOSIS OF ACUTE MENINGITIS—cont'd

MAJOR INFECTIOUS ETIOLOGIES—cont'd

Bacteria

Haemophilus influenzae

Neisseria meningitidis

Streptococcus pneumoniae

Listeria monocytogenes

Streptococcus agalactiae

Propionibacterium acnes

Staphylococcus epidermidis

Enterococcus faecalis

Escherichia coli

Klebsiella pneumoniae

Pseudomonas aeruginosa

Salmonella spp.

Nocardia spp.

Mycobacterium tuberculosis

Spirochetes

Treponema pallidum (syphilis)

Borrelia burgdorferi (Lyme disease)

Leptospira spp.

Protozoa and Helminths

Naegleria fowleri

Angiostrongylus cantonensis

Strongyloides stercoralis (hyperinfection syndrome)

Other Infectious Syndromes

Parameningeal foci of infection§

Infective endocarditis

Viral postinfectious syndromes

Postvaccination¶

NONINFECTIOUS CAUSES AND DISEASES OF UNKNOWN ETIOLOGY

Intracranial Tumors and Cysts

Craniopharyngioma

Dermoid and epidermoid cysts

Teratoma

Medications

Antimicrobial agents ‖

Nonsteroidal antiinflammatory agents**

Muromonab-CD3 (OKT3)

Azathioprine

Cytosine arabinoside (high dose)

Carbamazepine††

Immune globulin

Ranitidine

Phenazopyridine

BOX 44-1
DIFFERENTIAL DIAGNOSIS OF ACUTE MENINGITIS—cont'd
NONINFECTIOUS CAUSES AND DISEASES OF UNKNOWN ETIOLOGY—cont'd

Systemic Illnesses

Systemic lupus erythematosus

Vogt-Koyanagi-Harada syndrome

Procedure Related

Postneurosurgery

Spinal anesthesia

Intrathecal injections‡‡

Chymopapain infection

Miscellaneous

Seizures

Migraine or migrainelike syndromes

Mollaret's meningitis

From Mandell GL, Bennett JE, Dolin R. Principles and practice of infectious diseases, 5th ed. New York: Churchill Livingstone; 2000.

*Primarily echoviruses and Coxsackie virus.

†In the United States the major etiological agents are the mosquito-borne California, St. Louis, Eastern equine, Western equine, and Venezuelan equine encephalitis viruses and tick-borne Colorado tick fever.

‡Primarily herpes simplex virus type 2, but also herpes simplex virus type 1, varicella-zoster virus, cytomegalovirus, Epstein-Barr virus, and human herpesvirus 6.

§Brain abscess, sinusitis, otitis, mastoiditis, subdural abscess, epidural abscess, venous sinus thrombophlebitis, pituitary abscess, cranial osteomyelitis.

¶Mumps, measles, polio, pertussis, rabies, vaccinia.

‖ Trimethoprim, sulfamethoxazole, trimethoprim-sulfamethoxazole, ciprofloxacin, penicillin, isoniazid.

**Ibuprofen, sulindac, naproxen, tolmetin.

††In patients with connective tissue diseases.

‡‡Air, isotopes, antimicrobial agents, antineoplastic agents, steroids, radiographic contrast media.

II. CLINICAL PRESENTATION

1. Meningitis is considered a medical emergency. Although clinical suspicion may guide management, meningitis is a laboratory diagnosis that is based on CSF analysis (cell count with differential, protein, glucose, Gram's stain, latex agglutination studies, and culture). Data from prospective clinical trials show that clinical history is notoriously nonspecific for the diagnosis of acute meningitis; the history has a reported specificity of 15% for nonpulsatile headache, 50% for generalized headache, and 60% for nausea and vomiting.[9,10] Symptoms include headache, neck stiffness, and lethargy. Signs include meningismus, fever, delirium, obtundation, seizures, and cranial nerve palsies, in addition to Kernig's sign (pain elicited when patient's knee is straightened from a position of flexion at the hip and knee) and Brudzinski's sign (patient flexes hips, knees, or both when

the neck is passively flexed). Several studies have shown that fever, neck stiffness, and change in mental status are highly sensitive findings for acute meningitis; therefore a diagnosis of acute meningitis can be excluded in a patient without any of these symptoms.[9,10] Papilledema is present in less than 1% of cases of ABM, and its presence should suggest an alternative diagnosis.[10]

2. A study of 176 patients with microbiologically proven ABM found three variables to be predictive of poor outcome: hypotension, seizures, and altered mental status. Death or altered neurological status occurred in 5% of patients who had none of these features, in 37% of patients who had one of these features, and in 63% of those who had two of these features (*p* = .001).[11] Thus patients can be classified as low risk (have no hypotension, seizures, or altered mental status), intermediate risk (have one of three high-risk features), or high risk (have at least two high-risk features) (Box 44-2).

3. In addition to the preceding clinical features, individuals with aseptic meningitis may have less common signs, such as chest or abdominal pain (Coxsackie B virus), upper respiratory symptoms, or a rash (Coxsackie A virus type 9 or echovirus type 9). Aseptic meningitis often has a biphasic fever curve and is also associated with constitutional symptoms, myalgias, photophobia, and pharyngitis.[10]

4. *N. meningitidis* is present in 73% of patients with ABM who have a rash (often petechial) at presentation.[6]

5. Subacute meningitis develops over a period of weeks, with mental status changes, headache and neck pain, and fever (Table 44-2). Tuberculous meningitis should be suspected in immigrants from countries in which the infection is endemic, in alcoholics, and in those who are HIV positive. Cryptococcal meningitis occurs in immunosuppressed patients, most commonly patients with acquired immunodeficiency syndrome. Typically occurring when $CD4^+$ counts are below 200 cells/μL, this form of meningitis tends to have a more subtle presentation. See Chapter 38 on central nervous system (CNS) involvement in HIV for a more detailed discussion of cryptococcal meningitis.

6. Fig. 44-1 provides an algorithm for the evaluation of the patient with suspected bacterial meningitis.

TABLE 44-2

PRESENTING SYMPTOMS AND SIGNS IN PATIENTS WITH
BACTERIAL MENINGITIS

Symptom or Sign	Relative Frequency (%)
Headache	>90
Fever	>90
Meningismus	>85
Altered sensorium	>80
Kernig's sign	>50
Brudzinski's sign	>50
Vomiting	35
Seizures	30
Focal neurological findings	10-20
Papilledema	<1

Data from Tunkel AR, Scheld WM. Acute meningitis. In Mandell GL et al, eds. Principles and practice of infectious diseases, 5th ed. New York: Churchill Livingstone; 2000.

44

MENINGITIS

III. DIAGNOSTICS

1. Lumbar puncture (LP) should be performed immediately in a patient who does not have a bleeding diathesis or focal neurological signs. Performing head computed tomography (CT) before LP is controversial, and several authors have attempted to define a population of patients who should undergo the procedures in this order. The most recent investigation of this issue was a prospective cohort study of 301 adults with suspected bacterial meningitis. Of these, 235 underwent CT of the head before LP. Clinical features associated with an abnormal head CT were age greater than 60 years, immunocompromise, history of CNS disease, history of seizure within 1 week of presentation, abnormal level of consciousness, inability to answer two consecutive questions correctly or to follow two consecutive commands, gaze or facial palsy, abnormal visual fields, arm or leg drift, and aphasia. The negative predictive value of these findings was 97%.[5] A study of 111 patients believed to need emergency LP for any reason found that the likelihood ratio for the discovery of a new intracranial mass lesion was significant for the following factors: the presence of mental status changes, papilledema, or focal neurological deficit; a clinician's impression of the patient; or one or more of the features listed in Table 44-3.[4] A third study identified age greater than 60 years, immunocompromised state, recent seizure, a history of CNS disease, and focal neurological deficit as predictors of abnormal head CT results.[8] If head CT is deemed necessary, antibiotics should be administered before the procedure to prevent delay.

2. An antibiotic given before LP does not decrease the likelihood of identifying the causative pathogen. A retrospective review of 177 cases of culture-proven ABM found 39 cases in which antibiotics had been administered before LP. In these patients the combination of

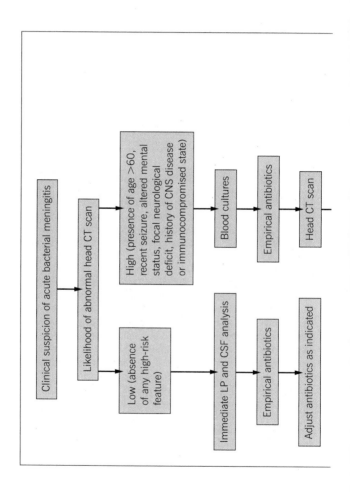

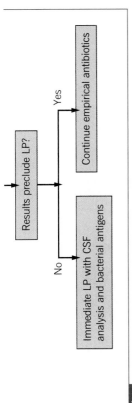

FIG. 44-1

Evaluation of patients with suspected bacterial meningitis. *(Data from Aronin SI, Quagliarello VJ. Hosp Pract 2001; 36(2):43.)*

44

MENINGITIS

TABLE 44-3

PERFORMANCE CHARACTERISTICS OF TEST QUESTIONS, EXAMINATION
FINDINGS, AND PHYSICIAN PREDICTION OF RESULTS OF COMPUTED
TOMOGRAPHY OF THE HEAD

Variable	LR (95% CI)*	Sensitivity (%)	Specificity (%)
HIV risk factors	1.8 (0.9-3.5)	41	77
HIV positivity	1.2 (0.45-3.0)	24	80
Immunosuppression	1.57 (0.88-2.9)	47	70
Malignant neoplasm	0 (0-3.5)	0	93
Head trauma within past 72 hours	0.7 (0.09-5.2)	6	91
Prior central nervous system mass	3.7 (0.67-20.4)	12	97
Seizures within past 72 hours	1.4 (0.4-4.4)	76	65
Altered mentation	2.2 (1.5-3.2)	12	99
Papilledema	11.1 (1.1-115)	18	87
Focal neurodeficit	4.3 (1.9-10.0)	41	90
One or more abnormal findings	1.6 (1.2-1.9)	100	37
New lesion predicted	9.1 (2.4-34)	40	96
Physician believes lumbar puncture is contraindicated	18.8 (4.8-43)	100	95

Data from Gopal AK et al. Arch Intern Med 1999; 159:2681.
CI, Confidence interval; *HIV,* human immunodeficiency virus; *LR,* likelihood ratio.
*Likelihood ratios express odds that the history or physical examination findings would occur in a
patient with, as opposed to without, abnormalities on cranial computed tomography.

blood cultures and Gram's stain of CSF, or latex agglutination alone or
in addition to the preceding, identified the causative pathogen in 92%,
a yield similar to that in the CSF analyses of the untreated group.[12]

3. When LP is performed, CSF should be divided into aliquots in five
sterile tubes. Tube 1—1 mL should be sent for cell count with
differential; tube 2—2 mL should be sent for glucose and protein
determinations; tube 3—5 mL should be sent for Gram's stain and
culture; tube 4—1 mL should be sent for cell count and differential.
An additional tube containing CSF should be sent for the following if
the clinical picture dictates: viral polymerase chain reaction for herpes
simplex virus, enteroviruses, and varicella-zoster virus; Venereal
Disease Research Laboratory (VDRL) testing; acid-fast bacillus smear
and culture (5 mL required); cryptococcal antigen and fungal culture.
Blood, urine, and sputum (if appropriate) cultures should be obtained
before antibiotics are administered. Typical CSF values are given in
Table 44-4; the sensitivities of latex agglutination assays for bacterial
antigens in CSF are summarized in Table 44-5. A complete blood cell
count, serum glucose, and protein level should be determined as well.
If opening pressure is a concern, the physician should make sure that
the patient straightens out his or her legs before measuring. An
opening pressure cannot be accurately obtained if the patient is seated
for LP.

TABLE 44-4

TYPICAL CEREBROSPINAL FLUID VALUES

Determination	Value or Result
NORMAL CEREBROSPINAL FLUID	
Opening pressure	–15 mm Hg or 65-195 mm H_2O
Leukocyte count	<10 mononuclear cells/mm³ (5-10 suspect); ≤1 PMN/mm³
BLOODY TAP	
If peripheral counts normal	WBC/RBC ratio 1:700
If peripheral counts abnormal	True CSF WBC = CSF WBC – blood WBC × CSF RBC/blood RBC
Protein	15-45 mg/dL (higher in elderly); protein level should be less than patient's age if age >35 years
Bloody tap	1 mg protein/1000 RBCs
Glucose	CSF/blood glucose ratio <0.6 (with high serum glucose level, ratio is 0.3)
VIRAL MENINGITIS	
WBC	10-1000/mm³; lymphocytic predominance
Protein	Normal to mildly elevated
Glucose	Normal
BACTERIAL MENINGITIS	
Opening pressure	>180 mm H_2O
WBC	1000-5000/mm³; ≥80% PMNs
Protein	100-500 mg/dL
Glucose	≤40 mg/dL
Lactate	≥35 mg/dL
Gram's stain	Positive in 60%-90%
Culture	Positive in 70%-85%
Bacterial antigen testing	Positive in 50%-100% (depending on pathogen)

Data from Bartlett JG. Pocket book of infectious disease therapy, 10th ed. Baltimore: Williams & Wilkins; 1999.

PMN, Polymorphonuclear cell; *RBC,* Red blood cell count; *WBC,* white blood cell count.

44

MENINGITIS

TABLE 44-5

SENSITIVITY OF LATEX AGGLUTINATION ASSAYS FOR BACTERIAL ANTIGENS IN CEREBROSPINAL FLUID

Organism	Sensitivity (%)
Haemophilus influenzae	78-100
Neisseria meningitidis	50-93
Streptococcus pneumoniae	67-100
Streptococcus agalactiae	69-100

Data from Tunkel AR, Scheld WM. Acute meningitis. In Mandell GL et al, eds. Principles and practice of infectious diseases, 5th ed. New York: Churchill Livingstone; 2000.

4. Up to 30% of cases of listerial meningitis have a lymphocytic predominance in the CSF.[10] Partially treated ABM can have a CSF profile with lymphocytic predominance, similar to acute viral meningitis.

5. WBCs begin to disintegrate in CSF after 90 minutes.

6. The sensitivity of Gram's staining correlates with the bacterial load in the CSF: 25% of patients with fewer than 10^3 colony-forming units (CFUs)/mL have positive Gram's stains, whereas 97% of those with more than 10^5 CFUs/mL have positive Gram's stains.[13] Gram's staining is also pathogen dependent. In two studies Gram's stains were positive in 90% of ABM cases caused by *S. pneumoniae,* 86% of those caused by *H. influenzae,* 75% of those caused by *N. meningitidis,* 50% of those caused by gram-negative bacilli, and less than 50% of those caused by *L. monocytogenes.*[14,15]

7. The following findings predict ABM with 99% certainty: CSF glucose level below 1.9 mmol/L; CSF/serum glucose ratio below 0.23; CSF protein level greater than 2.20 g/dL; CSF leukocyte count greater than 2000×10^6/L; CSF PMN count greater than $1180/mm^3$.[3] This model was verified by another group of investigators and was found to have a receiver operating curve (ROC) of .977.[17] The model remains to be prospectively validated.

IV. MANAGEMENT

1. Prompt initiation of antibiotics is the standard of care for ABM (Table 44-6). When the results of rapid diagnostic tests such as Gram's staining are positive, pathogen-specific therapy should be initiated (Table 44-7). Gram's staining is reliable if the results are positive. If these tests are nondiagnostic, initial therapy should target the most likely organisms demographically.

2. Outcome analysis of 269 patients with ABM found that patients whose prognostic stage did not advance (no development of hypotension, seizures, or altered mental status) from the time of arrival in the emergency department to the time of antibiotic administration did not have a worse outcome if antibiotics were delayed longer than 4 hours. Conversely, if the clinical stage did advance during that time, adverse outcome was directly correlated with delay of antibiotic administration. Thus poor outcome is related to stage of disease at the time of antibiotic administration.[11]

3. Once a specific pathogen is identified, the antibiotic regimen should be tailored to help prevent the emergence of resistant strains. Pathogen-specific therapy should be guided by the local geographical resistance profiles of bacteria.

4. *S. pneumoniae:* Penicillin- and cephalosporin-resistant strains of *S. pneumoniae* are increasingly predominant throughout the world. For example, 25% of *S. pneumoniae* cases in Atlanta in 1994 were intermediately to highly resistant to penicillin (minimum inhibitory concentration [MIC] >2 µg/mL) and 9% were resistant to cefotaxime. In

TABLE 44-6

EMPIRICAL THERAPY IN PATIENTS WITH SUSPECTED ACUTE BACTERIAL
MENINGITIS AND A NONDIAGNOSTIC GRAM'S STAIN

Patient Group	Likely Pathogen	Antibiotic
Immunocompetent		
Age <3 months	Group B *Streptococcus*, *Listeria monocytogenes*, *Escherichia coli*	Ampicillin 100 mg/kg IV q8h + broad-spectrum cephalosporin*
3 months–18 years	*Streptococcus pneumoniae*, *Neisseria meningitidis*, *Haemophilus influenzae*	Broad-spectrum cephalosporin* + vancomycin
18-50 years	*S. pneumoniae*, *N. meningitidis*	Broad-spectrum cephalosporin† + vancomycin
>50 years	*S. pneumoniae*, *L. monocytogenes*, or gram-negative bacilli	Ampicillin‡ + broad-spectrum cephalosporin†
Impaired cellular immunity	*L. monocytogenes* or gram-negative bacilli	Ampicillin + ceftazidime
Head trauma, neurosurgery, cerebrospinal fluid shunt, or nosocomial infection	Staphylococci, gram-negative bacilli, or *S. pneumoniae*	Vancomycin + ceftazidime

Data from Quagliarello VJ, Scheld WM. N Engl J Med 1997; 336:708.
*Cefotaxime 50 mg/kg q6h or ceftriaxone 50-100 mg/kg q12h.
†Cefotaxime 2 g IV q6h or ceftriaxone 2 g IV q12h.
‡Ampicillin 2 g IV q4h.

44

MENINGITIS

Denver, 33% of *S. pneumoniae* isolates were intermediately to highly resistant to penicillin.[18] Given the seriousness of ABM and the increasing prevalence of resistant strains, current recommendations are to start ceftriaxone and vancomycin for suspected pneumococcal meningitis and to discontinue vancomycin if the strain is found to be sensitive to cephalosporins (MIC <0.5 μg/mL) or penicillin (MIC <0.1 μg/mL).[7] Because penetration of vancomycin into CSF is decreased when adjunctive dexamethasone is used,[19] some experts recommend the use of ceftriaxone plus rifampin.[7] Others have found adequate penetration of vancomycin into the CSF of dexamethasone-treated patients.[20] If the *S. pneumoniae* is found to be penicillin or cephalosporin resistant, a repeat LP should be performed 24 to 48 hours after the start of antibiotic therapy to document clearing.[7,21]

5. ***N. meningitidis:*** Penicillin is the drug of choice for *N. meningitidis* meningitis. Resistance is emerging, but the clinical significance of this is unknown. If the patient's response is poor, he or she should be tested for resistance and should instead be given ceftriaxone or cefotaxime if the MIC is 0.1 μg/mL or higher.[7] Strict respiratory isolation should be practiced for those with suspected meningococcal meningitis. Prophy-

laxis with ciprofloxacin or rifampin should be considered for people in close contact.

6. *H. influenzae:* Cefotaxime and ceftriaxone are the drugs of choice because they are superior in sterilizing the CSF when compared with other cephalosporins.[7,22]

7. *L. monocytogenes:* Patients should be given ampicillin plus gentamicin.[7] Patients who are allergic to penicillin should be treated with trimethoprim-sulfamethoxazole 5 mg/kg IV q6h.

8. Gram-negative bacilli: Ceftazidime plus aminoglycoside is preferred because of these agents' high efficacy against *P. aeruginosa.*[7]

9. No specific studies exist on the optimum length of treatment in adults with ABM. A general guideline for duration of IV antibiotics is 7 days for *H. influenzae* and *N. meningitidis* infection, 10 to 14 days for *S. pneumoniae* infection, 14 to 21 days for *L. monocytogenes* or group B streptococcal infection, and 21 days for infection with gram-negative bacilli.[7]

TABLE 44-7

RECOMMENDATIONS FOR ANTIBIOTIC THERAPY IN PATIENTS WITH POSITIVE GRAM'S STAIN OR CULTURE

Type of Bacteria	Antibiotic*
GRAM'S STAIN	
Cocci	
Gram positive	Vancomycin + broad-spectrum cephalosporin
Gram negative	Penicillin G 300,000 U/kg/day IV, up to 24 million units
Bacilli	
Gram positive	Ampicillin + aminoglycoside†
Gram negative	Broad-spectrum cephalosporin + aminoglycoside
CULTURE	
Streptococcus pneumoniae	
Penicillin MIC <0.1 µg/mL	Penicillin G 24 million U q4h
Penicillin MIC 0.1-1.0 µg/mL	Ceftriaxone
Penicillin MIC >2.0 µg/mL	Vancomycin + ceftriaxone
Haemophilus influenzae	
β-Lactamase negative	Ampicillin
β-Lactamase positive	Ceftriaxone
Neisseria meningitidis	Penicillin G
Listeria monocytogenes	Ampicillin + gentamicin
Streptococcus agalactiae	Penicillin G + gentamicin in neonates
Enterobacteriaceae	Broad-spectrum cephalosporin + aminoglycoside‡
Pseudomonas aeruginosa, *Acinetobacter* spp.	Ceftazidime + aminoglycoside

Data from Quagliarello VJ, Scheld WM. N Engl J Med 1997; 336:708.
MIC, Minimum inhibitory concentration.
*Doses are as listed above unless otherwise specified.
†Gentamicin 1.5 mg/kg loading dose, then 1-2 mg/kg q8h; adjust for renal function.
‡If clinical or microbiological response to IV gentamicin is poor, consider intrathecal gentamicin 5-10 mg/day in adults, 1-2 mg/day in neonates.

10. Good evidence has been presented that the use of adjunctive corticosteroids in children older than 2 months of age who are thought to be infected with *H. influenzae* reduces neurological sequelae.[23] The data for adults are less convincing, although administration of corticosteroids before antimicrobials in a group of adults with pneumococcal meningitis did reduce serious sequelae.[24] Expert opinion in an editorial following this article recommends initiation of dexamethasone 10 mg IV q6h for 4 days in adult patients with suspected pneumococcal meningitis and discontinuation of therapy if other types of meningitis are diagnosed. In addition, if the *S. pneumoniae* isolate is penicillin resistant or the physician has a high suspicion of penicillin resistance, dexamethasone should not be used.[25]

PEARLS AND PITFALLS

- Noninfective causes of abnormal CSF to consider are summarized in Box 44-3.
- Response to antibiotics should occur within 24 to 36 hours, with clinical improvement noted.
- Opening pressure is accurate only if the patient's legs are straight and the patient is lying down when this parameter is measured.
- Between 10% and 20% of HIV-infected patients with cryptococcal meningitis have increased intracranial pressure that requires treatment

44

MENINGITIS

BOX 44-3

ABNORMAL CEREBROSPINAL FLUID WITH NONINFECTIOUS CAUSES

Traumatic tap: increased protein and RBCs; WBCs and differential proportionate to RBCs in peripheral blood; clear or colorless supernatant of centrifuged fluid

Chemical meningitis (injection of anesthetics, chemotherapeutic agents, air, radiographic dyes): increased protein, lymphocytes (occasionally neutrophils)

Cerebral contusion, subarachnoid hemorrhage, intracerebral bleed: RBCs, increased protein (1 mg/1000 RBCs); disproportionate increase in neutrophils (peak at 72-96 hours); decreased glucose level in 15%-20%

Vasculitis: increased protein (50-100 mg/dL); increased WBCs (mononuclear cells); normal glucose level

Postictal (repeated generalized seizures): RBCs (0-500/mm^3); WBCs (10-100/mm^3 with variable percentage of polymorphonuclear cells); protein level normal or slightly increased

Tumors (especially glioblastomas, leukemia, lymphoma, breast cancer, pancreatic cancer): low glucose level; increased protein level; moderate neutrophil count

Neurosurgery: blood; increased protein; WBCs (disproportionate to RBCs with predominance of mononuclear cells) up to 2 weeks after operation

Sarcoidosis: increased protein; WBCs (up to 100/mm^3, predominantly mononuclear cells); low glucose level in 10%

Data from Bartlett JG. Pocket book of infectious disease therapy, 10th ed. Baltimore: Williams & Wilkins; 1999.

RBC, Red blood cell; *WBC,* white blood cell.

consisting of serial large-volume LPs or ventriculoperitoneal shunting. If hydrocephalus or focal abscesses are not present, large-volume CSF removal by LP is effective in most patients. It is recommended that CSF pressure be decreased by 50% and maintained at less than 300 cm H_2O.[26-28]

- Treatment of cryptococcal meningitis consists of amphotericin B 0.7 to 1 mg/kg IV daily, plus 5-flucytosine 25 mg/kg PO q6h for 2 weeks. Then the treatment should switch to fluconazole 400 mg/day PO for 10 weeks total, then fluconazole 200 mg/day PO for an indefinite period (suppressive treatment).[28] See Chapter 38 for a more detailed discussion of cryptococcal meningitis.

- College freshmen, splenectomized patients, travelers to endemic areas, those deficient in terminal complement components, and patients with Hodgkin's disease should receive meningococcal vaccination.[29]

- The use of tumor necrosis factor-α inhibitors (e.g., infliximab) has been associated with increased risk of reactivation of *M. tuberculosis*, and tubercular meningitis should be suspected in patients who have received tumor necrosis factor-α inhibitors and show mental status changes at presentation.[30] The CSF tuberculosis polymerase chain reaction and culture are means of diagnosing tubercular meningitis.

- Recent research has been evaluating the role of CSF calcitonin levels in predicting the likelihood of ABM. This test has not been validated and thus is not available for clinical purposes at this time.

- See Chapter 43 for a discussion of the use of pneumococcal urine antigen testing for the diagnosis of invasive pneumococcal disease.

REFERENCES

[d] 1. Schuchat A et al. Bacterial meningitis in the United States in 1995. Active Surveillance Team. N Engl J Med 1997; 337:970.

[d] 2. Behrman RE et al. Central nervous system infections in the elderly. Arch Intern Med 1989; 149:1596.

[a] 3. Spanos A, Harrell FE, Durack DT. Differential diagnosis of acute meningitis: an analysis of the predictive value of initial observations. JAMA 1989; 262:2700.

[a] 4. Gopal AK et al. Cranial computed tomography before lumbar puncture: a prospective clinical evaluation. Arch Intern Med 1999; 159:2681.

[a] 5. Hasbun R et al. Computed tomography of the head before lumbar puncture in adults with suspected meningitis. N Engl J Med 2001; 345:1727.

[c] 6. Durand ML et al. Acute bacterial meningitis in adults: a review of 493 episodes. N Engl J Med 1993; 328:21.

[d] 7. Quagliarello VJ, Scheld WM. Treatment of bacterial meningitis. N Engl J Med 1997; 336:708.

[c] 8. Aronin SI, Quagliarello VJ. New perspectives on pneumococcal meningitis. Hosp Pract 2001; 36:43.

[d] 9. Attia J et al. Does this adult patient have acute meningitis? JAMA 1999; 282:175.

[c] 10. Tunkel AR, Scheld WM. Acute meningitis. In Mandell GL et al, eds. Principles and practice of infectious diseases, 5th ed. Philadelphia: Churchill Livingstone; 2000.

[a] 11. Aronin SI, Peduzzi P, Quagliarello V. Community-acquired bacterial meningitis: risk stratification for adverse clinical outcome and effect of antibiotic timing. Ann Intern Med 1998; 129:862.

[b] 12. Coant PN et al. Blood culture results as determinants in the organism identification of bacterial meningitis. Pediatr Emerg Care 1992; 8:200.

[b] 13. La Scolea LJ, Dryja D. Quantitation of bacteria in cerebrospinal fluid and blood of children with meningitis and its diagnostic significance. J Clin Microbiol 1984; 19:187.

[c] 14. Gray LD, Fedorko DP. Laboratory diagnosis of bacterial meningitis. Clin Microbiol Rev 1992; 5:130.

[c] 15. Greenlee JE. Approach to diagnosis of meningitis: cerebrospinal fluid evaluation. Infect Dis Clin North Am 1990; 4:583.

[c] 16. Bartlett JG. Pocket book of infectious disease therapy, 10th ed. Baltimore: Williams & Wilkins; 1999.

[b] 17. McKinney WP et al. Validation of a clinical prediction rule for the differential diagnosis of acute meningitis. J Gen Intern Med 1994; 9:8.

[c] 18. Redondo E. Drug-resistant *Streptococcus pneumoniae*. N Engl J Med 1996; 334:53.

[b] 19. Paris MM et al. Effect of dexamethasone on therapy of experimental penicillin- and cephalosporin-resistant pneumococcal meningitis. Antimicrob Agents Chemother 1994; 38:1320.

[b] 20. Klugman KP, Friedland IR, Bradley JS. Bactericidal activity against cephalosporin-resistant *Streptococcus pneumoniae* in cerebrospinal fluid of children with acute bacterial meningitis. Antimicrob Agents Chemother 1995; 39:1988.

[c] 21. Paris MM, Ramilo O, McCracken GH. Management of meningitis caused by penicillin-resistant *Streptococcus pneumoniae*. Antimicrob Agents Chemother 1995; 39:2171.

[c] 22. Hervas JA et al. Neonatal sepsis and meningitis due to *Streptococcus equisimilis*. Pediatr Infect Dis 1985; 4:694.

[a] 23. Wald ER et al. Dexamethasone therapy for children with bacterial meningitis. Meningitis Study Group. Pediatrics 1995; 95:21.

[a] 24. de Gans J, van de Beek D. Dexamethasone in adults with bacterial meningitis. European Dexamethasone in Adulthood Bacterial Meningitis Study Investigators. N Engl J Med 2002; 347:1549.

[d] 25. Tunkel AR, Scheld WM. Corticosteroids for everyone with meningitis? N Engl J Med 2002; 347:1613.

[b] 26. Antinori S et al. The role of lumbar puncture in the management of elevated intracranial pressure in patients with AIDS-associated cryptococcal meningitis. Clin Infect Dis 2000; 31:1309.

[d] 27. Graybill JR et al. Diagnosis and management of increased intracranial pressure in patients with AIDS and cryptococcal meningitis. NIAID Mycoses Study Group and AIDS Cooperative Treatment Groups. Clin Infect Dis 2000; 30:47.

[d] 28. Saag MS et al. Practice guidelines for the management of cryptococcal disease. Infectious Diseases Society of America. Clin Infect Dis 2000; 30:710.

[d] 29. Meningococcal disease and college students: recommendations of the Advisory Committee on Immunization Practices (ACIP). MMWR Morb Mortal Wkly Rep 2000; 49:13.

[b] 30. Keane J et al. Tuberculosis associated with infliximab, a TNF-α neutralizing agent. N Engl J Med 2001; 345:1098.

44

MENINGITIS

Sepsis

Sarah B. Noonberg, MD, PhD, and Trish M. Perl, MD, MHS

Fast Facts

- Sepsis is a clinical syndrome arising from an overwhelming systemic inflammatory and procoagulant response to infection that causes widespread tissue injury remote from the site of infection.
- The clinical continuum of disease is as follows: systemic inflammatory response syndrome → sepsis → severe sepsis → septic shock → multisystem organ failure → death.
- An estimated 750,000 cases of sepsis occur in the United States each year, and the average mortality rate is 20% to 40%.[1]
- Despite advances in intensive care, development of broad-spectrum antibiotics, and improved understanding of the pathophysiology of sepsis, mortality and morbidity have been relatively stable over the past several decades.
- The first sepsis-specific therapy to demonstrate significant mortality benefit, activated protein C, has been approved for use in severe sepsis by the U.S. Food and Drug Administration.

45

I. EPIDEMIOLOGY

1. Years of confusing and vague terminology describing clinical syndromes of systemic inflammation and infection have hampered the standardization of research protocols and the analysis of clinical trial data.
2. In 1992 the American College of Chest Physicians and the Society of Critical Care Medicine (ACCP/SCCM) developed a consensus statement on the definition of sepsis and its sequelae.[2] The proposed terminology is presented in Table 45-1.
3. The ACCP/SCCM definitions help to classify patients according to their clinical characteristics and allow comparison of patients from different trials at different centers. Although these terms have been widely adopted, they have also been criticized for their substantial overlap, lack of correlation with pathophysiology, and oversensitivity. In fact, the ACCP/SCCM has recently decided to withdraw their consensus statement.[3] Until a validated case definition of sepsis is developed, however, the current terms remain in use.
4. Despite the importance of sepsis, no population-based prospective cohort studies provide accurate data on incidence, risk factors, and outcome. In 1990, the Centers for Disease Control and Prevention conducted a retrospective review of 1% of U.S. hospital discharges and estimated that the incidence of sepsis had increased from 73.6/ 100,000 patients in 1979 to 175.9/100,000 patients in 1987.[4] The

TABLE 45-1

DEFINITIONS PROPOSED BY THE AMERICAN COLLEGE OF CHEST PHYSICIANS
AND THE SOCIETY OF CRITICAL CARE MEDICINE

Term	Definition
Bacteremia	Presence of viable bacteria in the blood
Systemic inflammatory response syndrome	Severe inflammatory response characterized by two or more of the following: temperature >38° C or <36° C, heart rate >90 beats/min, respiratory rate >20 breaths/min or $Paco_2$ <32 mm Hg, white blood cell count >12,000/mm^3 or <4000/mm^3 or >10% bands
Sepsis	Presence of systemic inflammatory response syndrome with definitive evidence of infection
Severe sepsis	Sepsis associated with organ dysfunction, hypoperfusion, or hypotension (systolic blood pressure <90 mm Hg or >40 mm Hg decrease from baseline systolic blood pressure)
Septic shock	Sepsis with hypotension despite adequate fluid resuscitation and perfusion abnormalities that may include oliguria, altered mental status, or lactic acidosis
Multiple organ dysfunction syndrome	Presence of altered organ function in an acutely ill patient such that homeostasis cannot be maintained without intervention

Data from Bone RC et al. Chest 1992; 101:1644.

reasons for this increase are unclear, but it may be partly due to the large number of immunocompromised patients emerging from the acquired immunodeficiency syndrome epidemic and to enhanced chemotherapeutic regimens.

5. On the basis of more recent data collected from eight United States academic medical centers, a hospital-wide incidence of sepsis was calculated as two cases per 100 admissions,[5] but this is unlikely to reflect the situation in community and general hospitals.

6. Current estimates suggest that 750,000 cases of sepsis occur annually in the United States; 225,000 of these are fatal—similar to the number of deaths after acute myocardial infarction. The annual cost of caring for these patients is estimated at $15 billion.[1]

7. The natural history of sepsis was studied in a population of 3708 patients admitted to a single tertiary care center. On admission, 68% of patients met ACCP/SCCM criteria for systemic inflammatory response syndrome (SIRS). Among these patients, sepsis developed in 26%, severe sepsis in 18%, and septic shock in 4%.

8. The prognostic value of these definitions is reflected in the stepwise progression in mortality, with 7% of patients dying of SIRS, 16% dying of sepsis, 20% dying of severe sepsis, and 46% dying of septic shock.[6]

9. Despite technical advances in intensive care, antimicrobial agents, and diagnostic modalities, overall mortality from sepsis has not changed

TABLE 45-2

MORTALITY AMONG PATIENTS PRESENTING WITH SYSTEMIC INFLAMMATORY RESPONSE SYNDROME

Severity of Disease Progression	Mortality (%)
Systemic inflammatory response syndrome	7
Sepsis	16
Septic shock	20
Severe sepsis	46

Data from Rangel-Frausto MS et al. JAMA 1995; 273:117.

BOX 45-1

RISK FACTORS FOR POOR OUTCOME IN SEPSIS: HOST FACTORS

Hypothermia (temperature <35.5° C)

Leukopenia (white blood cell count <4000/mm^3)

Arterial blood pH <7.33

Shock

Multiorgan dysfunction (renal failure, respiratory failure, cardiac failure)

Age >40 years

Medical comorbidities

CONTROVERSIAL RISK FACTORS

Serum cortisol level

RISK FACTORS UNDER STUDY

Genetic polymorphisms

Data from Kreger BE et al. Am J Med 1980; 68:344; Brun-Buisson C et al. JAMA 1995; 274:968; and Annane D et al. JAMA 2000; 283:1038.

45

SEPSIS

significantly over the past 30 years. However, approximately half of all patients with sepsis have existing fatal comorbid conditions, which hinders the ability to lower mortality rates (Table 45-2).

10. Many studies have identified risk factors for adverse outcomes from sepsis (Box 45-1).[7,8] These can be broadly grouped into host, microbial, and environmental factors.

11. The term "host factors" refers to the degree of physiological derangement induced by infection, and these are highlighted in Box 45-1.[9] Levels of inflammatory mediators, such as interleukin-6 (IL-6) and tumor necrosis factor (TNF), are not useful as prognostic markers, but they may have value in predicting response to upcoming therapies.

12. There is growing interest in the identification of genetic polymorphisms that increase the risk of death from sepsis, including data on the presence of the TNF2 polymorphism in the promoter region of TNF-α.[10] However, the utility of such tests in providing information independent of clinical variables is questionable.

13. Convincing data have shown that the type and source of infection have bearing on the outcome of sepsis. Documented infection with coagulase-negative *Staphylococcus* confers the lowest attributable mortality of 15% to 20%, whereas infection with *Candida,* Enterococcus, and *Pseudomonas* species confers the highest attributable mortality of 30% to 40%.[11]

14. Urosepsis is associated with lower mortality rates than intraabdominal, pulmonary, or unidentified sites of infection.[12] Prognosis was unaffected by whether blood cultures were positive or negative.[13] In patients with positive cultures, however, nosocomial pathogens were associated with a worse outcome than community-acquired pathogens.

15. As yet the only modifiable risk factors are environmental and pertain largely to the timing and the appropriateness of antibiotics. Early recognition and prompt treatment of infection with adequate antibiotics have been shown to positively affect outcome.[14] One study involving 2124 patients with gram-negative bloodstream infections revealed that the mortality rate nearly doubled (18% versus 34%) when antibiotics that did not cover the identified pathogens were used.[15]

16. Even during an international sepsis trial of an anti-TNF monoclonal antibody, inadequate antibiotic coverage was documented in 6% of cases.[16] In one small study the onset of septic shock while patients were in a general ward rather than an intensive care unit was associated with delays in care and adverse outcomes but did not retain significance when the investigators controlled for bloodstream pathogens.[17]

II. CLINICAL PRESENTATION AND PATHOPHYSIOLOGY

1. Patients with sepsis are often first identified because of changes in vital signs that suggest systemic inflammation. Subsequent clinical manifestations result from the loss of autoregulatory capacity and uncontrolled release of plasma immunoregulatory factors. Ultimately, organ dysfunction results from tissue hypoperfusion and lack of adequate tissue oxygenation.

2. The model of a host response to infection is becoming increasingly complex as new inflammatory mediators are being discovered and as new functions for known factors are being elucidated.

3. The primary inciting event in the development of sepsis is the release of a toxic stimulant, such as endotoxin, by an invading microorganism. Once in the circulation, this trigger activates monocytes to produce the major proinflammatory cytokines IL-1 and TNF. These cytokines, among others, cause monocyte and macrophage self-stimulation and activate neutrophils and endothelial cells to produce a wide array of proinflammatory (IL-1, TNF, IL-8, IL-12, prostaglandins, leukotrienes, interferon-γ) and antiinflammatory (IL-4, IL-6, IL-10, transforming growth factor-β) secondary mediators.

4. Endothelial cells express adhesion molecules that facilitate neutrophil attachment and diapedesis. On migration, neutrophils secrete additional factors, including platelet-activating factor and toxic oxygen metabolites, that lead to microvascular permeability and edema formation. Endothelial production of prostacyclins and nitric oxide leads to vasodilatation, hypotension, impaired tissue oxygenation, and ultimately organ dysfunction.[18,19]

5. The mechanism of cell death in sepsis is not fully understood, but it is most likely the result of ischemia from inadequate perfusion and oxygen delivery in the microcirculation.[20]

6. Abnormal oxygen extraction and utilization caused by cytotoxic damage of the mitochondrial electron transport system by endotoxin or TNF have been proposed as an alternative hypothesis, but this finding has been confirmed only in animal studies.[21]

7. Altered cellular apoptosis is another possible hypothesis because exposure to cytokines can cause accelerated apoptosis of endothelial and parenchymal cells while simultaneously causing delayed apoptosis in macrophages and neutrophils.[22]

8. Every organ system is susceptible to the deleterious effects of systemic inflammation and sepsis, and the number of impaired organ systems correlates directly with mortality. Table 45-3 describes organ-specific effects of sepsis.

45

SEPSIS

III. DIAGNOSTICS

1. The clinical manifestations of sepsis arise primarily from the host's response to infection rather than the infection itself. Thus the diagnosis of sepsis should be considered in any patient exhibiting the cardinal signs of systemic inflammation. Unfortunately, because sepsis is a "syndrome" rather than a specific disease entity, no single marker or gold standard for the diagnosis exists.

2. Many patients who appear septic do not have documented infection, and many disease states, such as pancreatitis, can mimic the appearance of sepsis.

3. The diagnosis of SIRS can be made readily on the basis of vital signs and blood counts. Recognition of SIRS should always raise concern for impending sepsis. Its rapid progression and poor prognosis mandate early suspicion of sepsis and prompt evaluation and therapy (Box 45-2).

4. Because sepsis results from infection, a thorough search for a source is the first step in diagnosis (Box 45-3).

5. A history and physical examination may be useful, but they should be focused and expedited. Blood from peripheral sites and through all central lines should be collected in a sterile fashion for aerobic and anaerobic culture.

6. The urinary tract, especially in elderly and immunocompromised patients, is a common and often asymptomatic source of infection.

TABLE 45-3

EFFECTS OF SEPSIS ON INDIVIDUAL ORGAN SYSTEMS

System	Effects
Pulmonary	Increased microvascular permeability leads to deposition of protein-rich edema within the lungs and ventilation-perfusion mismatches; decreased lung compliance leads to development of acute respiratory distress syndrome and hypoxia
Cardiovascular	Hyperdynamic state leads to increased myocardial oxygen demand; loss of vasomotor regulation leads to inability to direct blood to core organs; hypotension leads to tissue hypoperfusion and hypoxia
Neurological	Inadequate oxygen delivery leads to agitation and delirium; decreased responsiveness leads to inability to protect the airway; sedative and analgesic use leads to prolonged altered mental status
Gastrointestinal	Compromised barrier function of the gut leads to bacterial translocation and release of additional systemic endotoxin; liver is unable to clear blood of enteric bacterial by-products and perpetuates systemic inflammation; inability to eat leads to nutritional deficiencies
Hematological	Bone marrow suppression and thrombocytopenia are common; severe sepsis and shock can lead to disseminated intravascular coagulation; altered red blood cell deformability leads to capillary occlusion and thrombosis
Renal	Hypoperfusion and ischemic tubular necrosis lead to oliguria and acute renal failure; use of intravenous contrast dye and aminoglycoside antibiotics also contributes to renal failure

BOX 45-2

DIFFERENTIAL DIAGNOSIS OF SEPSIS

Blood loss
Pancreatitis
Hypothermia
Drug toxicity
Azathioprine hypersensitivity
Cardiogenic shock
Cardiac tamponade
Fulminant hepatic failure

7. The utility of sputum Gram's stain and culture is controversial, but they may be valuable for patients who are able to produce an adequate sample. Suctioning of sputum from patients receiving mechanical ventilation may provide clues to diagnosis, but results must be interpreted with caution because of the frequent colonization of the respiratory tract in intubated patients.

8. Sinus infections are common, especially in patients with nasogastric

BOX 45-3

DIAGNOSTIC STUDIES USEFUL IN DETERMINING CAUSE OF SEPSIS

History and physical examination

Blood cultures (central line, peripheral)

Sputum Gram's stain, cultures (see text)

Paracentesis if appropriate

Lumbar puncture if appropriate

Radiographic studies: chest radiograph, computed tomography of chest, abdomen, pelvis

Evaluation for foreign bodies (hemodialysis, fistula, prosthetic joints)

Skin examination: evaluation for decubiti, perirectal abscess, rash

tubes. Imaging with ultrasound or computed tomography may reveal pleural or peritoneal fluid collections that should be sampled.

9. A full skin examination, especially on the sacrum, may reveal unexpected decubitus ulcers.

10. Knowledge of the patient's past medical history may reveal the presence of prostheses or grafts, which can be a hidden source of infection.

11. Despite thorough evaluation, no source of infection is documented in approximately 20% to 30% of patients who appear septic clinically,[19] which illustrates the difficulty with current definitions.

12. Adequacy of perfusion can best be assessed by clinical parameters, such as mentation, urine output, and capillary refill, and can be supplemented by blood pressure readings.

13. Blood pressure values must be interpreted in the context of baseline values, and electronic determinations should be verified manually with an appropriate-sized cuff.

14. If inadequate perfusion is a concern and blood pressure cannot be readily obtained, an arterial line should be placed for direct intravascular measurements.

15. Occasionally, pulmonary artery (Swan-Ganz) catheters can help to distinguish septic shock from cardiogenic shock when the diagnosis is in doubt, but their routine use in the diagnosis and management of sepsis is controversial (see "Pearls and Pitfalls").

16. Adequacy of tissue oxygenation is harder to assess through clinical parameters. Global measurements of oxygenation delivery and consumption may not adequately reflect ischemia within discrete tissues.

17. New techniques to measure organ-specific hypoxia, such as gastric mucosal pH monitoring (gastric tonometry) to assess splanchnic perfusion, are in use in specialized centers, but they are not widely available and few data support their use.

18. Blood pH and lactate determinations remain the standard means of assessing regional or global tissue hypoxia and the presence of

anaerobic metabolism. Numerous new laboratory markers, such as procalcitonin, phosphate, and IL-6 levels, have been studied as early indicators of sepsis.[23,24]

19. The utility of such markers and of rapid polymerase chain reaction detection of bacteremia has yet to be defined.

IV. MANAGEMENT

1. Infection control and supportive care are the cornerstones of sepsis treatment after the assessment of airway, breathing, and circulation.

2. Empirical broad-spectrum antibiotic coverage should be initiated early, with the choice of agents being determined by the suspected site or source of infection and local resistance patterns.

3. Patients with hospital-acquired sepsis should receive adequate coverage for pseudomonal and methicillin-resistant *Staphylococcus aureus* infections.

4. Once the etiological organism is known, antibiotic coverage should be narrowed to reduce the growing problem of multidrug-resistant pathogens.

5. Lack of clinical response should prompt a search for a persistent source of infection, second site of infection, or resistant organism.

6. Patients with sepsis need close hemodynamic monitoring for the development of septic shock, and transfer to an intensive care unit should be considered early (Box 45-4).

7. Large-bore peripheral or central access is imperative because rapid intravenous infusions may become necessary.

8. At the first sign of hemodynamic compromise, boluses of 250 to 500 mL of normal saline should be given over 5 to 10 minutes each, with clinical evaluation before and after each fluid challenge.

9. Most patients require fluid resuscitation to maintain preload because

---

BOX 45-4

HEMODYNAMIC STABILIZATION AND TOOLS RECOMMENDED FOR HEMODYNAMIC MONITORING IN SEPSIS

TOOLS

Stable, adequate intravenous access—most likely central venous catheter

Arterial line for blood pressure and arterial blood gas monitoring

Urinary catheter to monitor urine output

Swan-Ganz catheter (controversial; see text)

STABILIZATION

Normal saline boluses 250-500 mL infused over 5-10 minutes, with reassessment of hemodynamics after each bolus

Vasopressors as needed, with goal of maintaining systemic vascular resistance; see text, but appropriate initial choice for patients with adequate fluid resuscitation is norepinephrine or dopamine

of the increased vascular permeability, increased venous capacitance, and substantial insensible losses associated with sepsis.

10. Clinical parameters, such as blood pressure, urine output, and lung crackles, can be used to gauge response to therapy. Although colloid solutions may increase intravascular oncotic pressure, they have not been shown to lower mortality more than crystalloid solutions.[25]

11. Patients who remain hypotensive despite adequate fluid resuscitation are in septic shock and require vasopressor therapy. Intensive care monitoring is essential, and all patients should have central venous access and indwelling arterial catheters to allow the administration and titration of vasopressors.

12. There is ongoing debate about the optimal first pressor to use in sepsis,[26] and few randomized controlled trials compare one with another. Vasopressors have varying degrees of effect on α-adrenergic receptors, β-adrenergic receptors, and dopaminergic receptors, and predominant receptor stimulation is often dose dependent.

13. For sepsis the primary goal is increased systemic vascular resistance rather than increased cardiac output, making norepinephrine or dopamine the logical first choice.

14. Dobutamine has no role in sepsis because it is primarily an inotrope and can increase hypotension. When hypoperfusion persists, the general practice is to maximize a first pressor before adding a second agent.

15. All organ systems are at risk of failure in cases of severe sepsis and septic shock, and supportive care should be tailored to each patient's needs.

16. In many patients acute respiratory failure develops, often a result of increased minute ventilatory demand, increased edema, respiratory muscle fatigue, and acute respiratory distress syndrome.

17. Noninvasive ventilation strategies may be tried if patients can cooperate, but altered mental status and persistent hypoxia often necessitate intubation and mechanical ventilation.

18. Efforts to improve tissue hypoxia have led to studies on the use of red blood cell transfusions to increase oxygen delivery, but as yet, no study has demonstrated reduction in mortality or duration of mechanical ventilation.[27,28]

19. Oliguria and acute renal failure frequently accompany sepsis, although less than 5% require dialysis.[29] Most surviving patients ultimately recover renal function.

20. Controversy surrounds the use of "renal dose dopamine" as a means of enhancing renal perfusion. Despite a recent randomized controlled clinical trial demonstrating no benefit of dopamine in preventing renal failure in critically ill patients,[30] some clinicians still use it in specific circumstances.

21. Recent data suggest that the first sepsis-specific therapy may soon be available. After many failed attempts at using adjunctive anti-

45

SEPSIS

inflammatory agents to decrease mortality from sepsis, a large multicenter international trial demonstrated a 6.1% absolute reduction in 28-day mortality with recombinant activated protein C.[31] Recognition of the role of coagulation in the pathogenesis of sepsis led to the development of this antiinflammatory, antithrombotic, and profibrinolytic agent. A clear trend toward increased risk of bleeding was demonstrated in the treated patients, but this did not reach statistical significance. Given the high cost of the medication, its use will probably be controversial, and patients will need to meet strict clinical criteria before it is administered. Trials with inhibitors of platelet-activating factor are under way.

PEARLS AND PITFALLS

- Cytokine therapy in sepsis.
  - Cytokines have been implicated in the pathogenesis of sepsis, leading to the development of cytokine inhibitors as a means of modulating the systemic inflammatory response. The main focus of these efforts has been on strategies to neutralize the effects of TNF-α, a cytokine with a central role in the initiation of sepsis and its progression to multiple organ failure. Initial optimism arose from animal models in which TNF-α neutralization through passive immunization or monoclonal antibodies was shown to lead to improved survival.[32,33] Unfortunately, the efficacy of anti-TNF strategies shown in rheumatoid arthritis and inflammatory bowel disease has not been found in more than 11 clinical trials of sepsis.[34] Analysis of smaller subgroups, such as patients with higher levels of IL-6 or severe sepsis, has shown small but nonsignificant benefits in survival.
  - Recently, Remick and associates[35] showed that a combination of IL-1 receptor antagonist and TNF-soluble receptor decreased lethality in a mouse model of sepsis. These authors hypothesized that patients who have an "excessive uncontrolled hyperinflammatory state" may benefit from this combination antiinflammatory therapy, whereas septic patients who do not mount a significant inflammatory response may need an "immunomodulatory" form of treatment. Whether the combination therapy is beneficial in human subjects awaits clinical trial data.
- Role of low-dose vasopressin in sepsis.
  - Vasopressin, also known as antidiuretic hormone, has recently been studied for the treatment of shock. Vasopressin is a peptide hormone that is released from the posterior pituitary gland in response to increased plasma osmolality, as well as pain, hypovolemia, and various endogenous and exogenous stimuli. Binding of vasopressin to V2 receptor in the renal collecting tubules promotes water resorption, whereas stimulation of V1 receptor on vascular smooth muscle cells causes vasoconstriction.
  - The rationale behind the use of vasopressin in septic shock arose from research demonstrating that plasma levels are inappropriately low in vasodilatory shock, unlike the expected elevation seen in cardiogenic

and hemorrhagic shock. In addition, patients with septic shock are far more sensitive to the vasoconstrictive effects of vasopressin than patients with other forms of shock. These findings led to a recent clinical trial showing that low-level vasopressin infusion (0.04 units/min) resulted in a significant and sustained increase in blood pressure in 14 of 16 patients with septic shock refractory to catecholamines.[36] In the remaining two patients, additional volume repletion was required before a response occurred. The authors did not find any clinical evidence of myocardial, intestinal, or skin ischemia with vasopressin therapy. The small number of patients studied thus far precludes the general use of vasopressin among patients with septic shock until further trials confirm these results.

- Steroid therapy in septic shock.
  - The use of corticosteroids in the treatment of sepsis was proposed as early as 1940 and has remained controversial ever since. Accumulating evidence of the inflammatory pathogenesis of sepsis and demonstration of adrenal insufficiency in significant numbers of patients with sepsis provided a solid scientific basis for steroid therapy. Early animal experiments demonstrated positive effects of corticosteroids and were confirmed by a randomized controlled clinical trial in 1976.[37] In this trial of 172 patients with sepsis who were randomly assigned to intravenous corticosteroids or placebo, mortality was significantly lower in the corticosteroid group (10% versus 38%). Subsequently, in 1987, two large, randomized, multicenter trials[38,39] failed to show any mortality benefit with high-dose corticosteroid therapy and suggested possible deleterious effects. Although routine use of high-dose corticosteroids was largely abandoned, interest remained in the therapeutic potential of low-dose corticosteroids. Over the past 4 years, several small, placebo-controlled trials of prolonged administration of low-dose corticosteroids demonstrated improvement in hemodynamics and reduced pressor requirement but did not show significant mortality benefit.[40,41] In summary, corticosteroids have yet to convincingly prove survival benefit in patients with sepsis. However, as has previously been shown for *Pneumocystis carinii* pneumonia,[42] continued research may identify subgroups of patients that benefit from adjunctive corticosteroid therapy.
  - Most recently, in a large trial, 300 patients with refractory septic shock were assigned at random to receive hydrocortisone 50 mg IV q6h and fludrocortisone 50 μg PO qd for 7 days.[43] Patients were given adrenocorticotropic hormone (ACTH) stimulation testing (250 μg ACTH) and stratified as "responders" if the cortisol level rose 9 μg/dL or more and "nonresponders" if the level rose less than 9 μg/dL. In the nonresponder subgroup (i.e., what authors termed "relative adrenal insufficiency"), at day 28 there were 73 deaths (63%) in the placebo group and 60 deaths (53%) in the corticosteroid group. The median time to death was 12 days in the placebo group and 24 days in the cortico-

steroid group. The HR estimated using a Cox model was 0.67 (95% CI, 0.47-0.95; $p = .02$). The number of patients needed to be treated to save 1 additional life at day 28 was 7 (95% CI, 4-49). However, this study has sparked controversy because the appropriate levels of serum cortisol in critically ill patients have not been defined and because the findings of the study contrast with most prior literature, as summarized in a metaanalysis.[44]

- A recent review of sepsis summarized the controversy by stating, "In summary, clinicians should not use high-dose corticosteroids in patients with sepsis. Low-dose hydrocortisone was effective in one study in patients with septic shock, but that finding has not been confirmed by other groups."[45]
- Insulin therapy and sepsis.
  - Intensive insulin therapy to maintain euglycemic clamp at 80 to 110 mg/dL (as compared with 180-200 mg/dL) has been shown to reduce morbidity, mortality, and episodes of bacterial infection in critically ill patients, regardless of underlying diabetic status.[46] Care should be taken to avoid hypoglycemia.
- Bacterial sepsis in patients with acquired immunodeficiency syndrome.
  - Despite recent advances in the treatment of patients with HIV and acquired immunodeficiency syndrome, pyogenic infections and sepsis in HIV-infected patients remain common. Reasons for this association are unclear but may be a result of several factors. Patients with HIV are often neutropenic because of primary HIV infection of the bone marrow, as well as antiretroviral therapy. Even when neutrophil counts are normal, their function may be suboptimal because of decreased chemotaxis and lower levels of cytokine production. Anticapsular antibodies may also be low in these patients, and the use of long-term antibiotic prophylaxis may lead to colonization with multidrug-resistant organisms. Consequently, HIV-infected patients are more likely to have progression to sepsis from routine infections, and they have a higher mortality rate than HIV-negative patients.[47] Contrary to prior reports, one study suggested that bacterial pathogens are now more common than opportunistic pathogens in HIV-infected patients who are in intensive care. Mortality was not associated with CD4+ count, but it was associated with neutropenia and severity of sepsis.[48]
- Pulmonary artery catheterization in sepsis.
  - Pulmonary artery catheters (PACs) were introduced in 1970 as a means of diagnosing disease and monitoring critically ill patients. About 1.5 million PACs are sold in the United States each year, but only 15% are used in intensive care units.[49] PACs allow the measurement of cardiac output, pulmonary capillary wedge pressure, pulmonary artery pressure, and mixed venous blood gases, providing important information on cardiopulmonary function. However, complications are associated with PAC use, including lung injury, hemorrhage, arrhythmias, infection, and thromboembolism, leading to a mortality rate of

0.02% to 1.5%.[50] Furthermore, management of patients can be adversely affected when data are unreliable or misinterpreted. Several surveys have demonstrated that significant deficits in the understanding of catheter methods and interpretation of the data exist among both physicians and nurses.

- A prospective cohort study[51] and observational studies have suggested that the use of PACs may be associated with higher morbidity and mortality. As a result of continued controversy, the National Heart, Lung, and Blood Institute and the Food and Drug Association conducted the Pulmonary Artery Catheterization and Clinical Outcomes workshop.[48] The workshop called for randomized clinical trials of the use of PACs in patients with decompensated congestive heart failure, acute respiratory distress syndrome, cardiac surgery, and severe sepsis. Such trials are in progress for decompensated heart failure and acute respiratory distress syndrome, but as yet, no trials of PAC use in patients with severe sepsis have been published. Until such studies are performed, the use of the PAC will remain controversial.

45

SEPSIS

REFERENCES

[c] 1. Angus DC et al. Epidemiology of severe sepsis in the United States: analysis of incidence, outcome, and associated costs of care. Crit Care Med 2001; 29:1303.

[d] 2. Bone RC et al. Definitions for sepsis and organ failure and guidelines for the use of innovative therapies in sepsis. ACCP/SCCM Consensus Conference Committee. Chest 1992; 101:1644.

[d] 3. www.chestnet.org/health.science.policy. (Accessed January 2001).

[b] 4. Centers for Disease Control and Prevention. Increase in hospital discharge survey rates for septicemia—United States, 1979-1987. MMWR Morb Mortal Wkly Rep 1990; 39:31.

[b] 5. Sands KE et al. Epidemiology of sepsis syndrome in 8 academic medical centers. JAMA 1997; 278:234.

[b] 6. Rangel-Frausto MS et al. The natural history of the systemic inflammatory response syndrome (SIRS): a prospective study. JAMA 1995; 273:117.

[b] 7. Kreger BE et al. Gram-negative bacteremia. IV. Re-evaluation of clinical features and treatment in 612 patients. Am J Med 1980; 68:344.

[a] 8. Brun-Buisson C et al. Incidence, risk factors, and outcome of severe sepsis and septic shock in adults: a multicenter prospective study in intensive care units. JAMA 1995; 274:968.

[b] 9. Annane D et al. A 3-level prognostic classification in septic shock based on cortisol levels and cortisol response to corticotropin. JAMA 2000; 283:1038.

[b] 10. Mira JP et al. Association of TNF2, a TNF-alpha promoter polymorphism, with septic shock susceptibility and mortality: a multicenter study. JAMA 1999; 282:561.

[c] 11. Rangel-Frausto MS. The epidemiology of bacterial sepsis. Infect Dis Clin North Am 1999; 13:299.

[c] 12. Krieger JN et al. Urinary tract etiology of bloodstream infections in hospitalized patients. J Infect Dis 1983; 148:57.

[c] 13. Bone RC et al. Sepsis syndrome, a valid clinical entity. Crit Care Med 1989; 17:389.

[c] 14. Pittet D. Nosocomial bloodstream infections. In Wenzel RP et al. Prevention and control of nosocomial infections. Baltimore: Williams & Wilkins; 1993.

[a] 15. Leibovici L et al. Monotherapy versus beta-lactam aminoglycoside combination treatment for gram-negative bacteremia: a prospective, observational study. Antimicrob Agents Chemother 1997; 41:1127.

[a] 16. Sprung CL et al. International sepsis trial (Intersept): role and impact of a clinical evaluation committee. Crit Care Med 1996; 24:1441.

[b] 17. Lundberg JS et al. Septic shock: an analysis of outcomes for patients with onset on hospital wards versus intensive care units. Crit Care Med 1998; 26:1020.

[c] 18. Sepsis, SIRS, and septic shock. In Bone RC, ed. Pulmonary and critical care medicine. St Louis: Mosby; 1998.

[c] 19. Wheeler AP, Bernard GR. Treating patients with severe sepsis. N Engl J Med 1999; 340:207.

[a] 20. Katori M et al. Evidence for the involvement of a plasma kallikrein-kinin system in the immediate hypotension produced by endotoxin in anaesthetized rats. Br J Pharmacol 1989; 98:1383.

[c] 21. Sair M et al. Tissue oxygenation and perfusion in severe sepsis. Am J Physiol 1996; 271:1620.

[c] 22. Marshall JC, Watson RW. Apoptosis in the resolution of systemic inflammation. In Vincent JL, ed. Yearbook of intensive care and emergency medicine. New York: Springer-Verlag; 1997.

[c] 23. Von Landenberg P, Shoenfeld Y. New approaches in the diagnosis of sepsis. Isr Med Assoc J 2001; 3:439.

[b] 24. Selberg O et al. Discrimination of sepsis and systemic inflammatory response syndrome by determination of circulating plasma concentrations of procalcitonin, protein complement 3a, and interleukin-6. Crit Care Med 2000; 28:2793.

[c] 25. Choi PT et al. Crystalloids vs. colloids in fluid resuscitation: a systematic review. Crit Care Med 1999; 27:200.

[d] 26. Practice Parameters for Hemodynamic Support of Sepsis in Adult Patients. Task Force of the American College of Critical Care Medicine, Society of Critical Care Medicine. Crit Care Med 1999; 27:639.

[a] 27. Hebert PC et al. A multicenter randomized controlled clinical trial of transfusion requirements in critical care. N Engl J Med 1999; 340:409.

[a] 28. Hebert PC et al. Do blood transfusions improve outcomes related to mechanical ventilation? Chest 2001; 119:1850.

[c] 29. Wheeler A et al. Renal function abnormalities in sepsis. Am J Respir Crit Care Med 1995; 151:A317.

[a] 30. Bellamo R et al. Low dose dopamine in patients with early renal dysfunction: a placebo-controlled randomised trial. Lancet 2000; 356:2139.

[a] 31. Bernard GR et al. Efficacy and safety of recombinant human activated protein C for severe sepsis. N Engl J Med 2001; 344:699.

[a] 32. Beutler B et al. Passive immunization against cachectin/tumor necrosis factor protects mice from lethal effects of endotoxin. Science 1985; 229:869.

[a] 33. Tracey KJ et al. Anti-cachectin/tumor necrosis factor monoclonal antibodies prevent septic shock during lethal bacteremia. Nature 1987; 330:662.

[c] 34. Reinhart K, Karzai W. Anti-tumor necrosis factor therapy in sepsis: update on clinical trials and lessons learned. Crit Care Med 2001; 29:S121.

[c] 35. Remick DG et al. Combination immunotherapy with soluble tumor necrosis factor receptors plus interleukin 1 receptor antagonist decreases sepsis mortality. Crit Care Med 2001; 29:473.

[a] 36. Tsuneyoshi I et al. Hemodynamic and metabolic effects of low dose vasopressin infusions in vasodilatory septic shock. Crit Care Med 2001; 29:487.

[a] 37. Schumer W. Steroids in treatment of clinical septic shock. Ann Surg 1976; 184:333.

[a] 38. Bone RC et al. A controlled trial of high-dose methylprednisolone in the treatment of severe sepsis and septic shock. N Eng J Med 1987; 317:653.

[a] 39. Veterans Administration Systemic Sepsis Cooperative Study Group. Effect of high-dose glucocorticoid therapy on mortality in patients with clinical signs of systemic sepsis. N Engl J Med 1987; 317:659.

[a] 40. Briegel J et al. Stress doses of hydrocortisone reverse hyperdynamic septic shock: a prospective randomized double-blind single center study. Crit Care Med 1999; 27:723.

[a] 41. Bollaert PE et al. Reversal of late septic shock with supraphysiologic doses of hydrocortisone. Crit Care Med 1998; 26:645.

[a] 42. Gagnon S et al. Corticosteroids as adjunctive therapy for severe *Pneumocystis carinii* pneumonia in the acquired immunodeficiency syndrome: a double blind placebo controlled trial. N Engl J Med 1990; 323:1440.

[a] 43. Annane D et al. Effect of treatment with low doses of hydrocortisone and fludrocortisone on mortality in patients with septic shock. JAMA 2002; 288:862.

[d] 44. Cronin L et al. Corticosteroid treatment for sepsis: a critical appraisal and meta-analysis of the literature. Crit Care Med 1995; 23:1430.

[c] 45. Hotchkiss RS, Karl IE. Pathophysiology and treatment of sepsis. N Engl J Med 2003; 348:138.

[a] 46. van den Berghe G et al. Intensive insulin therapy in critically ill patients. N Engl J Med 2001; 345:1359.

[b] 47. Proctor RA. Bacterial sepsis in patients with acquired immunodeficiency syndrome. Crit Care Med 2001; 29:683.

[c] 48. Rosenberg AL et al. The importance of bacterial sepsis in intensive care unit patients with acquired immunodeficiency syndrome: implications for future care in the age of increasing antiretroviral resistance. Crit Care Med 2001; 29:548.

[d] 49. National Heart, Lung, and Blood Institute and Food and Drug Administration workshop report: pulmonary artery catheterization and clinical outcomes. JAMA 2000; 283:2568.

[d] 50. American Society of Anesthesiologists Task Force on Pulmonary Artery Catheters. Anesthesiology 1993; 78:380.

[b] 51. Conners AF et al. The effectiveness of right heart catheterization in the initial care of critically ill patients. SUPPORT Investigators. JAMA 1996; 276:889.

45

SEPSIS

Sexually Transmitted Diseases

Katherine Chang, MD, and Anne Rompalo, MD, ScM

FAST FACTS

- Herpes is the most common cause of genital ulcers in the United States.
- Herpes and chancroid are manifested as painful ulcers, whereas syphilitic ulcers are usually painless.
- Human immunodeficiency virus (HIV) coinfection may alter the presentation and the response to treatment of many sexually transmitted diseases (STDs).
- Newer diagnostic modalities for *Neisseria gonorrhoeae* and chlamydia infections, such as nucleic acid amplification tests, are enabling easier and less invasive testing of symptomatic or asymptomatic infection to be performed.
- Asymptomatic gonorrhea and chlamydia infections are common in women and can result in significant morbidity when pelvic inflammatory disease (PID) ensues. Yearly screening is recommended for sexually active women 25 years or age or less.
- Urethritis is the most common STD syndrome in males, and most cases in the United States are nongonococcal.
- PID develops in 1 million American women each year.[1] Untreated PID results in infertility (20%), ectopic pregnancy (9%), and chronic pain (18%).[2]

46

1. STDs are a diverse group of infections that share common clinical manifestations and epidemiologies. This chapter reviews the most common syndromes that are primarily contracted through sexual contact alone. Not only are STDs important from a public health perspective, but also many may facilitate the transmission of HIV, which places added importance on their identification and control. Complicating the picture is that many infections may be asymptomatic or unidentified by health care providers, resulting in undue morbidity.

Diseases Characterized By Genital Ulcers

HERPES SIMPLEX VIRUS

I. EPIDEMIOLOGY

1. Herpes simplex virus (HSV) is the most common cause of genital ulcers in the United States. An estimated 1 million new cases of genital herpes simplex virus (HSV) infections occur annually, and 40 to 60 million persons are latently infected.

2. HSV-2 accounts for most genital infections; the incidence of those caused by HSV-1 is 10% to 50%.
3. Infection is more common in women. The risk that a woman will contract HSV from an actively infected male after a single contact may be as high as 80%.[3]
4. Most sexual transmission occurs while the contact source is asymptomatic.
5. Ulcerative disease increases the risk of contracting HIV; with herpes infection the relative risk is 1.5 to 2.0.[3]

II. CLINICAL PRESENTATION

1. Primary genital infection can begin as macules and papules and progresses to painful vesicles, pustules, and ulcers. Atypical presentations include urethritis, cervicitis, cystitis, and aseptic meningitis.
2. The incubation period is 2 to 12 days, and the lesions last about 2 to 3 weeks. Viral shedding can persist throughout this period.
3. Other symptoms include fever, dysuria, inguinal adenopathy, and malaise. Women tend to have more severe symptoms and more complications. Lesions in women involve the vulva, perineum, buttocks, cervix, and vagina. As many as 25% of women have aseptic meningitis, and 10% to 15% have a urinary retention syndrome during primary infection.[3] Men classically have vesicular lesions superimposed on an erythematous base on the glans penis or the penile shaft.
4. Complications after a primary episode for both sexes may include meningoencephalitis, neuralgias, and sacral radiculomyelitis.
5. Recurrent infections caused by reactivation of the virus are less severe and resolve more quickly than primary infections. They are preceded by a prodrome and involve a limited number of vesicles (three to five) on the penile shaft in males or vulvar irritation in females. Viral shedding is limited to 2 to 5 days, and the recurrence lasts 8 to 10 days. Complications are uncommon in recurrent disease.
6. After the primary infection approximately one third of patients have more than eight or nine recurrences per year, one third have four to seven recurrences per year, and one third have two to three recurrences per year.
7. HSV-2 infection is much more likely than HSV-1 infection to recur in the genital region.

III. DIAGNOSIS

1. Definitive diagnosis is made by viral culture of vesicle scrapings in patients with genital ulcers or other mucocutaneous lesions. Culture is highly sensitive and specific.
2. HSV polymerase chain reaction (PCR) is the test of choice for detecting HSV in the cerebrospinal fluid (CSF). PCR is more sensitive than culture.

3. Methods that use cytological detection of herpes viral infection, such as the Tzanck smear and cervical Papanicolaou smears, are insensitive and nonspecific.
4. Type-specific g-G1 and g-G2 based serological tests are now available and can confirm a clinical diagnosis of genital herpes when cultures are negative.
5. Antigen detection tests (direct fluorescent antigen or enzyme immunoassay) are rapid and have a greater than 85% sensitivity in symptomatic viral shedders.

IV. MANAGEMENT
A. INITIAL EPISODES
1. Acyclovir, 200 mg PO 5 times per day for 7 to 10 days or 400 mg tid for 7 to 10 days. Symptoms are usually reduced within 48 hours of initiation of acyclovir; however, the natural history of the disease is not affected, nor is the frequency of recurrences.
2. For more severe cases and for those with systemic complications, acyclovir (5 mg/kg IV q8h for 5 days) can be used.
3. Valacyclovir, an ester of acyclovir that increases its bioavailability, appears to be as effective as acyclovir at a dosage of 1 g PO bid for 7 to 10 days.[4]
4. Famciclovir (250 mg PO tid for 7 to 10 days) appears to have efficacy and tolerability that are comparable to those of acyclovir.[5,6]

B. RECURRENT HERPES INFECTION
1. To be effective, treatment should be initiated within 1 day of lesion onset or during the prodrome.
2. Both valacyclovir (500 mg PO bid for 3 to 5 days *or* 1 g PO qd for 5 days) and famciclovir (125 mg PO bid for 5 days) result in faster healing of lesions and shorter duration of symptoms and viral shedding.[5,6]
3. Acyclovir (200 mg PO 5 times/day for 5 days *or* 400 mg PO tid for 5 days) can also be used.

C. SUPPRESSIVE THERAPY
1. For patients with frequent recurrences (six or more per year), suppressive therapy may decrease recurrences by 70% to 80%.[7] Acyclovir, valacyclovir, and famciclovir are effective in suppressing recurrences.[6]
a. Acyclovir 400 mg PO bid.
b. Valacyclovir 500 mg PO qd in those with nine or fewer recurrences per year and 1000 mg PO qd in those with 10 or more recurrences per year.
c. Famciclovir 250 mg PO bid.

D. COUNSELING
1. Counseling of patients is paramount in preventing sexual and perinatal transmission.
2. Natural history, viral shedding, and the possibility of recurrent episodes should be reviewed.

46

SEXUALLY TRANSMITTED DISEASES

3. Patients should be advised to abstain from sexual activity when lesions are present and during prodromes.

E. SPECIAL CONSIDERATIONS

1. HIV-positive patients with genital herpes have a modest increase in frequency and duration of recurrent episodes and a significant increase in the rate of viral shedding.[8]
2. Most HIV-positive patients respond to acyclovir, but the response may be slower.[6]
3. Long-term suppressive therapy in HIV-positive patients may be beneficial. Dosages are higher than those for immunocompetent patients: famciclovir 500 mg PO bid; valacyclovir 500 mg PO bid; and acyclovir 400 to 800 mg PO bid.
4. The incidence of acyclovir resistance is low in HIV-positive patients, and routine acyclovir susceptibility testing is not recommended.
5. The preferred agent in acyclovir-resistant infection is foscarnet. Use is limited by systemic toxicity (renal insufficiency and metabolic disturbances).

SYPHILIS

I. EPIDEMIOLOGY

1. Syphilis, both primary and secondary, is at its lowest rate in the United States since 1941, although it remains a problem in the South and in some metropolitan areas.
2. Outbreaks have been reported in several states, especially in situations involving prostitution or in men who have sex with men.
3. Infection occurs more commonly in men (2.1 times greater incidence) and African-Americans (16 times greater incidence).[9]

II. CLINICAL PRESENTATION

A. PRIMARY SYPHILIS

1. About 21 days after exposure (range 10 to 90 days), a painless papule appears that evolves into the syphilitic chancre, a painless ulcer with an indurated edge. This can occur at any site of inoculation, including the throat, but it usually appears on the penis, labia, or cervix.
2. Firm, rubbery, nontender inguinal adenopathy may accompany the chancre.
3. Within 2 to 6 weeks after exposure the chancre heals without a scar.

B. SECONDARY SYPHILIS

1. Secondary syphilis begins between 6 weeks and 6 months after exposure and lasts 1 to 3 months. Overlap may occur between the first and second stages in 25% of cases.[10]
2. This stage is characterized by a symmetrical maculopapular rash, including the palms and soles, and is associated with fever, malaise, weight loss, and generalized nontender lymphadenopathy. Condylomata lata (flat, wartlike lesions) may be seen in the perianal region

and intertriginous areas. Mucous patches, superficial gray erosions of the mucous membranes, are found in one third of cases.[10] These patches, along with condylomata lata, are particularly infectious, and examiners should avoid contact with them.

3. Abnormal CSF findings of increased protein and cells may occur (15% to 30%), although clinical meningitis involving fever, headache, meningismus, and photophobia is rare.

4. Rarely, hepatitis, arthritis, uveitis, proctitis, periostitis, or immune complex nephropathy is present.

5. After this stage patients enter the latent stage, divided into early (<1 year) and late (>1 year) latent syphilis, in which patients may have relapses of secondary syphilis. These relapses most often occur during early latent disease and are generally milder episodes.

C. TERTIARY SYPHILIS

1. Rarely, patients remain untreated and progress to tertiary syphilis, which includes cardiovascular syphilis, neurosyphilis, and gummas.

2. Cardiovascular syphilis may cause aortitis in 30% to 50% of untreated persons or may cause endarteritis obliterans, which leads to aneurysmal dilatation of the ascending aorta.

D. OTHER CLINICAL MANIFESTATIONS

1. Neurosyphilis can occur at any stage of syphilis. It may be asymptomatic or may present as delirium, seizures, headache, and focal deficits, as in meningovascular syphilis. Tabes dorsalis involves the posterior spinal cord, leading to areflexia, ataxia, lightninglike pain in the extremities, sensory deficits resulting in Charcot joints, and urinary incontinence or retention. General paresis manifests as a dementia syndrome. The Argyll Robertson pupil is a small, irregular pupil that accommodates but does not react to light; this is seen in general paresis and tabes dorsalis. Gummas are nonspecific granulomas that can involve any organ but are more commonly seen in the skin, bones, cartilage, liver, and upper respiratory tract.

III. DIAGNOSIS

1. The diagnosis is made directly via identification of spirochetes in lesions of primary, secondary, or congenital syphilis or indirectly by the detection of antibodies in the serum. Direct examination includes darkfield microscopy and direct fluorescent antibody staining. Indirect testing includes both treponemal (fluorescent treponemal antibody absorption [FTA-ABS], microhemagglutination assay for *Treponema pallidum* [MHA-TP]) and nontreponemal (Venereal Disease Research Laboratory [VDRL]) antibody detection.

2. Darkfield microscopy and direct fluorescent antibody tests are highly sensitive and specific in detecting primary syphilis when samples from active lesions can be obtained.

3. VDRL and its simplified variations (rapid plasma reagin card test, automated reagin test, and unheated serum reagin test) detect

antibodies to purified cardiolipin-lecithin-cholesterol antigen. They are reported as a titer representing the greatest serum dilution that produces a fully reactive test; unlike treponemal titers, nontreponemal titers correlate with disease activity and should be used to assess treatment response. Whichever variation is used, the same variation should be followed throughout a patient's course. VDRL has a sensitivity of 62% to 76% in primary syphilis.[11]

4. False positive results of the nontreponemal serological tests can be caused by advanced age, chronic liver disease, intravenous drug use, Lyme disease, bacterial infections (e.g., endocarditis, tuberculosis, *Mycoplasma),* malignancies, pregnancy, and viral infections (e.g., HIV, varicella, mononucleosis). Titers are usually low (1:1 to 1:4) and occur in 1% to 2% of the population.[12] For this reason, positive results on nontreponemal tests should be confirmed with a treponemal test.

5. FTA-ABS is more sensitive than nontreponemal tests for detecting syphilis. The sensitivity of FTA-ABS is 81% to 100% in primary syphilis and 100% in symptomatic late disease. Once reactive, FTA-ABS usually remains reactive for life, regardless of treatment.[11] However, 24% of patients treated appropriately for primary or secondary syphilis will later have negative FTA-ABS tests.[13]

6. Lumbar puncture and CSF examination should be performed on any patient with syphilis and abnormal CNS signs or symptoms, regardless of stage. CSF abnormalities (including elevated protein level and white blood cell count and reactive serological tests) have not been shown to predict neurological progression or treatment failure in patients with early-stage syphilis and no abnormal CNS signs or symptoms.[14] Thus they are not routinely performed in this population. For latent-stage syphilis, lumbar puncture should precede treatment if patients have neurological, ophthalmic, or psychiatric symptoms; treatment failure (judged by serological or clinical criteria); and HIV seropositivity.

7. CSF VDRL, the standard serological test for detecting neurological involvement, is highly specific (100%) but insensitive (22% to 69%) for active neurosyphilis, which emphasizes the role of clinical judgment in these cases.[15] CSF FTA-ABS is less specific but is believed to be highly sensitive. Several recent studies have suggested that at least 10% of latently infected HIV-positive patients have a reactive CSF-VDRL.[16]

IV. MANAGEMENT (Box 46-1)

1. For early stages (primary, secondary, and early latent) the goal is the resolution of infectious lesions and the prevention of progression. Limited evidence supports the use of alternative therapies for early disease. Both ceftriaxone (for at least 5 to 7 days) and azithromycin have shown promise in preliminary studies, but more data are

BOX 46-1

TREATMENT OF SYPHILIS

PRIMARY, SECONDARY, AND EARLY LATENT SYPHILIS

2.4 MU benzathine penicillin G IM*

LATE LATENT SYPHILIS OR LATENT DISEASE OF UNKNOWN DURATION

2.4 MU benzathine penicillin G IM weekly for 3 weeks*

NEUROSYPHILIS

18-24 MU aqueous penicillin G IV qd for 10-14 days

or

2.4 MU procaine penicillin G IM qd *plus* 500 mg PO probenecid qid for
  10-14 days

followed by

2.4 MU benzathine penicillin G IM weekly for 3 weeks

*Considered adequate for both human immunodeficiency virus–infected and noninfected patients.

46

SEXUALLY TRANSMITTED DISEASES

needed.[17] The goal in more advanced disease (late latent or latent
disease of unknown duration) is to prevent end-organ damage.
2. Treatment failure may be judged on either clinical (recurrence,
persistence, or progression of symptoms) or serological grounds.
A fourfold decline in titer, or a difference of two dilutions, has been
the traditional marker of treatment response. The decline is typically
seen over 6 months to 1 year after treatment.
3. Treatment of partners.
a. Persons exposed within 90 days of the diagnosis of a partner with
primary, secondary, or early latent syphilis should be treated, regardless
of syphilis serostatus.
b. Persons exposed more than 90 days before a partner's diagnosis should
be treated if follow-up is uncertain and test results are not readily
available.
c. Partners of patients with latent syphilis should be evaluated clinically
and serologically.
A. SPECIAL CONSIDERATIONS
1. HIV-seropositive patients with syphilis are less likely to demonstrate
serological improvement, especially with a VDRL titer of 1:32 or less.
This population has a slower response to treatment, a longer interval
between treatments, and a fourfold reduction in VDRL titer compared
with HIV-seronegative individuals.[18]
2. HIV-seropositive patients with genital ulcer disease are more likely
to have multiple lesions at presentation, and those lesions are more
likely to be due to syphilis in HIV-seropositive patients than in HIV-
seronegative patients.[19]
3. Patients with neurosyphilis and a penicillin allergy may be treated with

ceftriaxone 2 g/day either IM or IV for 10 to 14 days, although cross-reaction may occur. If this is a concern, patients should be desensitized and treated with parenteral penicillin.[9]

4. Some experts recommend that HIV-infected patients with late latent syphilis or syphilis of unknown duration undergo lumbar puncture before treatment to rule out neurosyphilis.

CHANCROID

I. EPIDEMIOLOGY

1. Although chancroid is endemic in some areas of the United States (Eastern cities and the South), it usually occurs in discrete outbreaks.
2. Chancroid occurred at epidemic rates in the middle to late 1980s, but rates have steadily declined since 1987. In 2001, only 38 cases of chancroid were reported in the United States; however, it is much more prevalent in other parts of the world, especially Africa, Asia, and Latin America.
3. Uncircumcised men are at increased risk.

II. CLINICAL PRESENTATION (Table 46-1[20])

1. Chancroid is manifested as a small painful papule that ulcerates within 1 to 3 days. In women, ulcers cluster around the cervix.
2. Ulcers have a ragged, undermined border and may have a yellow to gray, foul-smelling exudate covering the base.
3. Unilateral, fluctuant inguinal adenopathy is the presenting feature in 20% to 40% of cases.[21] In 25% of patients the lesion is a suppurative bubo that may spontaneously rupture, leaving thick pus discharge.

III. DIAGNOSIS

1. Definitive diagnosis is based on growth of *Haemophilus ducreyi* (sensitivity ≤80%) on special culture media that are not widely available.
2. A clinical diagnosis can be assumed if examination shows typical clinical findings, including one or more painful ulcers, and tests for syphilis and HSV are negative.[7]
3. Painful ulceration with tender adenopathy is suggestive of chancroid, whereas suppurative adenopathy is almost pathognomonic for the disease.

IV. MANAGEMENT

1. Azithromycin, 1 g PO as a single dose *or*
2. Ceftriaxone, 250 mg IM as a single dose *or*
3. Ciprofloxacin, 500 mg PO bid for 3 days *or*
4. Erythromycin base, 500 mg PO tid for 7 days.

A. SPECIAL CONSIDERATIONS

1. Patients who are uncircumcised or HIV positive do not respond as well to treatment and may require longer treatment courses.
2. Ceftriaxone and azithromycin regimens are not as well studied in HIV-positive patients and should be used only if proper follow-up is ensured in this population.[7]

Diseases Characterized by Urethritis and Cervicitis

GONORRHEA

I. EPIDEMIOLOGY

1. Gonorrhea, along with chlamydia, is a major cause of PID in the United States and may facilitate the transmission of HIV.
2. From 1975 to 1997 a 72% decline occurred in the reported rate of gonorrhea; as of 1999, however, the rate had increased for the second year in a row and had reached 360,000 cases per year.
3. Most cases are seen in adolescents and young adults.[9]

II. CLINICAL PRESENTATION

A. LOCALIZED INFECTION

1. The incubation period is usually 3 to 10 days.
2. Men.
a. Most infected men are overtly symptomatic.
b. Urethritis occurs 2 to 5 days after sexual contact and is characterized by dysuria, frequent urination, meatal irritation, and penile discharge, which initially is thin and mucoid and later becomes purulent.
c. Complications of untreated or undertreated gonococcal urethritis include epididymitis, prostatitis, urethral strictures, penile edema and lymphangitis, and rarely, disseminated disease.
d. Proctitis may lead to pruritus, tenesmus, rectal bleeding, and mucopurulent discharge, but it is asymptomatic in 20% to 50%.[10]
e. Presenting symptoms of pharyngitis may include sore throat, pharyngeal erythema with or without exudates, and cervical adenopathy, although most patients are asymptomatic.
3. Women.
a. Women may be asymptomatic or manifest only minimal symptoms.
b. Urethritis produces symptoms of dysuria and urinary frequency, and cervicitis results in dyspareunia, pelvic pain or discomfort, abnormal menstrual flow, and purulent cervical-vaginal discharge. Cervicitis may be asymptomatic in 50% of infected women.
c. Proctitis may also occur as a result of rectal-vaginal contamination or anal intercourse.
d. PID is a complication in 10% to 40% of infected women.[22] Because

46

SEXUALLY TRANSMITTED DISEASES

TABLE 46-1

CHARACTERISTICS OF GENITAL ULCERS*

	Primary HSV	Recurrent HSV	Primary Syphilis	Chancroid	LGV
Primary lesion	Vesicles, papules, ulcers with an erythematous "punched out" border; superficial with a red, smooth base; not indurated	Grouped vesicles, papules, ulcers with erythematous, "punched out" border; superficial lesions with a red, smooth base; no induration	Ulcer, papule with sharply demarcated border; red, clean base, superficial and indurated	Ulcer, papule with violaceous, ragged, undermined border; yellow to gray exudate-covered base, rare induration, usually soft	Papule, pustule, ulcer; variable border and base; superficial, no induration
Number of lesions	Multiple	Multiple clustered lesions	Usually one	Usually one to three	Usually one
Distribution	Women: bilateral labia, cervix, urethra, perianal; men: penis, urethra, rectum	Unilateral: labia, penis, scrotum, buttocks, perianal	Vulva, penis, anal, perianal, oral	Penis, vulva, cervix	Urethra, cervix, rectum
Local symptoms	Pain, itching, serous discharge	Pain, less severe than primary lesions, itching, serous discharge	Usually painless, serous discharge	Tender, rare itching, purulent to hemorrhagic discharge	Usually painless
Lymph nodes	Tender, firm, bilateral inguinal adenopathy	Unilateral lymphadenopathy (uncommon)	Firm, rubbery, nontender, enlarged	Tender, enlarged, usually unilateral; may suppurate	Tender inguinal and femoral adenopathy, "groove sign," may suppurate with sinus tracts; large painful fluctuant "bubo"

Incubation period	2-7 days		10-90 days	3-7 days	10-14 days
Time course	21 days	7-10 days	2-3 weeks	2-3 weeks	1-2 weeks
Diagnosis	Viral culture	Viral culture	Darkfield microscopy, RPR, VDRL, FTA-ABS, DFA-TP (see text)	Culture of *Haemophilus ducreyi*; Gram's stain of pus from lymph node aspiration	Culture of *Chlamydia trachomatis* L1-3; clinical findings and serology (LGV-CF >1:16)
Treatment	Acyclovir PO or IV, famciclovir PO, valacyclovir PO (see text for dosages)	Acyclovir PO, famciclovir PO, valacyclovir PO (see text for dosages)	Penicillin G (see text for dosages)	Ceftriaxone, ciprofloxacin, azithromycin, erythromycin (see text for dosages)	Doxycycline, 100 mg bid for 21 days or erythromycin base, 500 mg qid for 21 days

Modified from DiCarlo RP, Martin DH. Clin Infect Dis 1997; 25:292.

DFA-TP, direct fluorescent antibody; *FTA-ABS,* fluorescent treponemal antibody absorption; *HSV,* herpes simplex virus; *LGV,* lymphogranuloma venereum; *LGV-CF,* lymphogranuloma venereum complement fixation; *RPR,* rapid plasma reagin; *VDRL,* Venereal Disease Research Laboratory.

*The clinical diagnosis of genital ulcer disease is difficult to make because considerable overlap exists among the major causes of ulceration. Although the classic symptoms and signs of syphilis, chancroid, and herpes simplex are insensitive findings, they are highly specific.[20]

46

SEXUALLY TRANSMITTED DISEASES

gonococcal infections in women are often asymptomatic, those at high
risk for STDs should be routinely screened.

B. DISSEMINATED INFECTION

1. Disseminated infection occurs in less than 1% of gonococcal
   infections.
2. It is characterized by fever, polyarthralgias, and rash consisting of
   petechial, papular, hemorrhagic, or necrotic lesions on the distal
   extremities. Monoarthritis develops in one third of patients; it is a
   common cause of infectious arthritis in young adults. Two thirds have
   tenosynovitis of the wrists, ankles, and knees.
3. Defects in the terminal components of the complement cascade result
   in recurrent episodes of disseminated infection.

III. DIAGNOSIS

1. Culture is performed on selective media. Because cotton tips and
   wooden shafts may be toxic to the organism, the swab should have a
   calcium alginate or synthetic fiber tip and a wire shaft.[23] Cultures
   have good specificity (94%-100%) and sensitivity (95% for
   endocervical specimens). Urethra cultures have better sensitivity in
   symptomatic patients (95%-100%) than in asymptomatic patients
   (50%-70%).[24]
2. Gram's stain reveals gram-negative intracellular diplococci. Sensitivity
   and specificity are similar to those for culture.
3. Nucleic acid amplification tests have sensitivity and specificity that
   are superior to those of culture. Polymerase chain reaction is 95%
   sensitive and 99% to 100% specific.[25] Ligase chain reaction (LCR)
   assays can be performed on urine or vaginal-urethral swabs; the
   sensitivity is 96% to 99%, and the specificity, 98% to 99%.[12]
   Although expensive, LCR allows convenient, noninvasive testing of
   urine specimens. Strand displacement amplification is 89% sensitive
   and 100% specific.[25]
4. DNA probes are widely used, their cost is comparable to that of
   culture, and the sensitivity and specificity are high (>92% sensitivity
   and 100% specificity for endocervical samples).
5. Nonamplified tests, including enzyme immunoassay (EIA), DNA probe,
   and direct fluorescent antibody test, are less sensitive (85%-90%)
   than amplified tests, and their specificity is 95%. Susceptibility testing
   cannot be performed on these tests.

IV. MANAGEMENT (Box 46-2)

1. Routine dual therapy that is effective against gonorrhea and chlamydia
   is recommended because accompanying chlamydial infection is common (10%-30%) and the cost of treatment is less than the cost of
   testing.
2. Quinolone-resistant gonococcal strains are rare in the continental

United States (<0.04% highly resistant, 0.5% with decreased susceptibility). They are now common in Hawaii, and they are far more common in Asia and the Pacific.[9]

3. Hospitalization is recommended during initial therapy for disseminated infection, and patients should be examined clinically for meningitis and endocarditis. Gonococcal meningitis is treated with ceftriaxone 1 to 2 g IV q12h for 10 to 14 days; endocarditis treatment should last at least 4 weeks.

4. Sex partners should be referred for evaluation and treatment.

A. SPECIAL CONSIDERATIONS

1. Patients coinfected with HIV do not require different treatment regimens.

2. Infected patients should also be screened for syphilis.

CHLAMYDIA

I. EPIDEMIOLOGY

1. An estimated 3 to 4 million new chlamydial infections occur each year in the United States, making chlamydia the most common STD in this country.[26]

2. Rates for women are four times those for men, partly because of reporting bias. Infections are most frequently reported in adolescents and young adults. In sexually active adolescent women the prevalence of chlamydia infection is greater than 10%.[26] In asymptomatic men the prevalence is 4% to 10%, whereas in STD clinics it can be as high as 25%.[27,28]

3. Because asymptomatic infection is common and the consequences of untreated infection are significant (PID and resulting infertility, ectopic pregnancy, and chronic pelvic pain), sexually active adolescents and young adults with risk factors for STDs should be screened yearly.

II. CLINICAL PRESENTATION

1. Up to 70% to 80% of women and 50% of men do not have symptoms.[29,30]

2. Clinical manifestations of infection in women include cervicitis, urethritis, endometritis, PID, and Bartholin's gland abscess. Usually the cervix is the initial site of infection, although the urethra and rectum may be infected as well. Presenting symptoms include vaginal discharge, dysuria, postcoital bleeding, and pelvic, uterine, or adnexal pain if PID develops. Signs include mucopurulent cervicitis, easily induced cervical bleeding, culture-negative pyuria, and more than 10 polymorphonuclear neutrophils per oil-immersion field on Gram's stain of a cervical smear.[29,31]

3. PID develops in 10% to 40% of women with untreated chlamydial infection.[22]

46

SEXUALLY TRANSMITTED DISEASES

BOX 46-2

TREATMENT OF GONOCOCCAL INFECTIONS

UNCOMPLICATED GONOCOCCAL INFECTIONS OF THE CERVIX, URETHRA, AND RECTUM

Cefixime 400 mg PO as a single dose

   or

Ceftriaxone 125 mg IM as a single dose

   or

Ciprofloxacin 500 mg PO as a single dose

   or

Ofloxacin 400 mg PO as a single dose

   or

Levofloxacin 250 mg PO as a single dose

Plus, for chlamydial infection, azithromycin 1 g PO as a single dose

   or

Doxycycline 100 mg PO bid for 7 days

If unable to tolerate cephalosporins or quinolones: spectinomycin 2 g IM as a single dose

---

UNCOMPLICATED INFECTIONS OF THE PHARYNX

Ceftriaxone 125 mg PO as a single dose

   or

Ciprofloxacin 500 mg PO as a single dose

   Plus

Azithromycin 1 g PO as a single dose

   or

Doxycycline 100 mg PO bid for 7 days

---

4. In men, infections are usually urethral and symptoms are indistinguishable from those of gonococcal urethritis. Epididymitis, manifested as unilateral scrotal pain with swelling, fever, and tenderness, may occur in young, sexually active men. Rectal discharge and pain during defecation may be signs of rectal infection in participants of receptive anal intercourse.[32] Proctitis may have a similar presentation, along with tenesmus, diarrhea, and rectal bleeding.

III. DIAGNOSIS

1. Historically, culture was the gold standard for diagnosis (sensitivity 50%-90%; specificity near 100%),[33] but it has largely been supplanted by newer, nonculture tests that have greater sensitivity. The Centers for Disease Control and Prevention, however, still recommends that culture be used for urethral specimens for women

---

BOX 46-2—cont'd

TREATMENT OF GONOCOCCAL INFECTIONS

DISSEMINATED GONOCOCCAL INFECTION

Ceftriaxone 1 g IM or IV q24h continued for 24-48 hours after improvement of
  symptoms, then switch to

Cefixime 400 mg PO bid
  or

Ciprofloxacin 500 mg PO bid
  or

Ofloxacin 400 mg PO bid
  or

Levofloxacin 500 mg PO qd

to complete 7 days of therapy

Alternative initial regimens:

Cefotaxime 1 g IV q8h
  or

Ceftizoxime 1 g IV q8h
  or

Ciprofloxacin 500 mg IV q12h
  or

Ofloxacin 400 mg IV q12h
  or

Levofloxacin 250 mg IV qd
  or

Spectinomycin 2 g IM q12h

46

and asymptomatic men, for rectal specimens, and for any cases of
suspected sexual abuse or assault.[26]

2. Nonculture techniques.

a. The direct fluorescent antibody test (sensitivity 50%-70%; specificity
   99.5%) employs direct visualization of the organism by fluorescein-
   labeled antibody staining. Because of the high labor and skill needed to
   perform the test, its use is limited to low volumes of specimens. The
   test is often used as a confirmatory test for other nonculture tests.[33]

b. EIA and rapid tests use antibodies against genus-specific lipopolysac-
   charide. Most EIAs are less sensitive than culture (40%-60%, depending on the test and the site of the specimen), but their specificity is
   99.5%. Positive results should be confirmed with a blocking test or a direct fluorescent antibody test.[36] EIAs can be performed on urine specimens; the best results are achieved with specimens from symptomatic males. Rapid tests use EIA technology but are qualitative and can
   be performed in the office in about 30 minutes. They are less sensitive (52%-85%) and specific (>95%) than laboratory-performed EIAs.[33]

c. DNA probes are 40% to 65% sensitive and 99% specific and have the advantage of being able to test concurrently for *Neisseria gonorrhoeae* with the same specimen.[33] They are less sensitive than DNA amplification tests, and positive results should be confirmed in low-prevalence populations.[26]

d. Nucleic acid amplification tests are extremely sensitive. The sensitivity and specificity of polymerase chain reaction are 90% to 98% and 99% to 100%, respectively. LCR has an overall sensitivity of 90% to 94% and a specificity of 99% to 100%. LCR is highly sensitive and specific for the detection of infection in the urine of both males and females and is a convenient, noninvasive method of detecting asymptomatic infection.[33] Strand displacement amplification has a sensitivity of 94% and a specificity of 100%.[25]

e. Strand displacement amplification is the only amplification test with 100% specificity for the detection of both gonorrhea and chlamydia.[25]

IV. MANAGEMENT

1. Treatment is azithromycin 1 g PO as a single dose *or* doxycycline 100 mg PO bid for 7 days.

2. Alternatives are erythromycin base 500 mg PO qid for 7 days *or* erythromycin ethylsuccinate 800 mg PO qid for 7 days *or* ofloxacin 300 mg PO bid for 7 days *or* levofloxacin 500 mg PO for 7 days. Erythromycin is less efficacious than either azithromycin or doxycycline.

3. Sex *partners* with contact during the 60 days preceding patient symptoms should be referred for evaluation, and the most recent partner should be treated, regardless of time to last contact. Patients should abstain from sex until they are cured (7 days after single-dose treatment or after a 7-day treatment regimen).

4. Test of a cure is not needed if the patient is treated with azithromycin or doxycycline, but it may be considered 3 weeks after erythromycin therapy is completed.

A. SPECIAL CONSIDERATIONS

1. Because doxycycline and ofloxacin are contraindicated in pregnancy, erythromycin base 500 mg qid for 7 days or amoxicillin 500 mg PO tid for 7 days is recommended for pregnant patients.

2. Patients coinfected with HIV do not require different treatment regimens.

NONGONOCOCCAL URETHRITIS

I. EPIDEMIOLOGY

1. Urethritis is the most common STD in men. Incidence is increased during the summer months.

2. In the United States and in much of the developed world, non-

gonococcal urethritis (NGU) is more common than gonococcal urethritis.

3. The ratio of NGU to gonococcal urethritis in the United States is greater in higher socioeconomic status groups. Among college students NGU is more prevalent, whereas in urban STD clinics gonococcal urethritis is more commonly seen.[34]

4. Main causes of NGU are chlamydia (15%-40%), *Ureaplasma urealyticum* (10%-40%), *Mycoplasma genitalium*, and less commonly, *Trichomonas* (13%). Other indeterminate or unidentified pathogens account for an increasing proportion (20%-30%).[35,36]

II. CLINICAL PRESENTATION

1. Dysuria, mucoid or purulent discharge, and urinary frequency may be present.

2. Symptoms may be most marked during the passage of the first morning urine or after ingestion of irritants, such as alcohol.

3. Discomfort between micturitions may manifest itself as itching, pain, frequency, urgency, or a feeling of heaviness of the genitals.

4. Hematuria, deep pelvic pain, pain only during ejaculation, and pain radiating to the back are uncommon in uncomplicated urethritis and should prompt further workup of other parts of the urogenital tract.[34]

III. DIAGNOSIS

See Fig. 46-1.[37]

IV. MANAGEMENT

1. Treatment is azithromycin 1 g PO as a single dose *or* doxycycline 100 mg PO bid for 7 days; these agents have comparable cure rates.[38]

2. Patients with NGU caused by chlamydia have high cure rates with appropriate therapy; in nonchlamydial NGU, however, relapse rates can be as high as 50% at 2 months.[37]

3. For urethritis that does not respond to therapy, wet mount and culture to look for *Trichomonas vaginalis* should be considered or empirical treatment for *Trichomonas* should be initiated. Alternatively, patients may have been reexposed by an untreated sexual partner or may not have complied with treatment.

PELVIC INFLAMMATORY DISEASE

I. EPIDEMIOLOGY

1. An estimated 1 million U.S. women have PID each year.[1]

2. Epidemics of PID directly follow epidemics of gonorrhea or chlamydia.[39]

3. Prevalence rates are highest in adolescents and young adults.

4. PID is most commonly caused by chlamydia and gonorrhea infection.

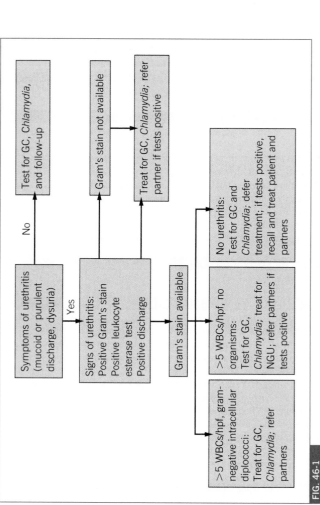

FIG. 46-1

Approach to nongonococcal urethritis. *GC,* Gonococcus; *hpf,* high-power field; *NGU,* nongonococcal urethritis; *WBCs,* white blood cells. *(Modified from Burstein GR, Zenilman JM. Clin Infect Dis 1999; 28(suppl 1):S66.)*

Genital mycoplasmas, endogenous vaginal flora, aerobic streptococci, and *Mycobacterium tuberculosis* are other etiological agents.[40]

II. CLINICAL PRESENTATION

1. The most common presenting symptoms are bilateral lower abdominal pain with or without fever, constitutional symptoms, abnormal vaginal discharge, abnormal uterine bleeding, dyspareunia, dysuria, and nausea and vomiting. Compared with other causes of PID, gonococcal disease has a more dramatic presentation, with peritoneal irritation and fever.[1]

2. Patients may have vague symptoms; 85% of patients delay seeking treatment because of the nonspecific nature of their symptoms. Delaying treatment for 3 days increases by three times the risk that infertility will develop.[41]

3. Factors associated with PID include prior episode of PID, use of an intrauterine device, cigarette smoking, douching, young age, and aspects of sexual behavior that are associated with contracting STDs.[38] Oral contraceptives and barrier methods of contraception protect against upper genital tract infection.[42]

4. Patients should be hospitalized for the following reasons: pregnancy; possible surgical emergency, such as ectopic pregnancy and appendicitis; inability to tolerate an outpatient regimen; lack of response to an outpatient regimen; severe illness with high fever, nausea, and vomiting; adolescence; suspected tuboovarian abscess; and HIV positivity.

5. The sequelae of untreated PID are infertility (20%), ectopic pregnancy (9%), and chronic pelvic pain (18%).[2]

III. DIAGNOSIS

1. The minimal criteria for clinical diagnosis (patient must have all three) are lower abdominal tenderness, adnexal tenderness, and cervical motion tenderness. In patients at high risk for PID the diagnosis of PID should be considered if pelvic tenderness and signs of lower genital tract inflammation are present.

2. Other supporting criteria are oral temperature above 38.3° C, abnormal cervical or vaginal mucopurulent discharge, elevated erythrocyte sedimentation rate, elevated C-reactive protein level, and documented gonococcal or chlamydial infection.

3. The most specific criteria are histological evidence of endometritis, evidence on magnetic resonance imaging or ultrasound, or laparoscopic abnormalities. Direct visual diagnosis is the gold standard, although this is not often practical.[1]

4. Endocervical specimens should be tested for *N. gonorrhoeae* and *Chlamydia trachomatis;* the patient should also be tested for pregnancy.

46

SEXUALLY TRANSMITTED DISEASES

TABLE 46-2

VAGINITIS

	Bacterial Vaginosis	Candidiasis	Trichomoniasis
Etiological agent	Replacement of normal lactobacillus with anaerobic bacteria (e.g., *Prevotella* spp., *Gardnerella vaginalis*, *Mycoplasma hominis*)	*Candida albicans* (80%-92%); other candidal species (e.g., *C. glabrata*) and other yeasts account for the remainder	*Trichomonas vaginalis*
Scope	Most prevalent cause of vaginal discharge or malodor	About 75% of all women have at least one episode; 40%-45% have two or more; <5% have recurrent vulvovaginal candidiasis (see special considerations)	At least 2-3 million symptomatic infections annually among sexually active women in the United States[43]; up to 56% of cases in sexually transmitted disease clinics[44]
Risk factors	Multiple sexual partners, douching, lack of vaginal lactobacilli	Antibiotic use	Multiple sexual partners
Vaginal discharge	Off-white, thin, homogeneous, may be frothy; unpleasant fishy odor, most noticeable after intercourse	White, curdy, adherent to vaginal walls	Malodorous, yellow-green purulent discharge, frothy, "strawberry" cervix
Other symptoms or signs	May be asymptomatic	Pruritus, vulvar erythema and edema, soreness, dyspareunia	Vulvovaginal erythema, dyspareunia
pH	>4.5	4.0-4.5 (normal)	5-6.0
Diagnosis	Clinical criteria (three of the following): (1) homogenous, white, noninflammatory discharge; (2) clue cells on microscopy; (3) pH >4.5; (4) positive whiff test (fishy odor of vaginal discharge before or after addition of 10% KOH) Gram's stain: altered flora typical for bacterial vaginosis	Pseudohyphae on 10% KOH (70%) or saline microscopy (40%); positive cultures in asymptomatic women should not be treated because 10%-20% are colonized	Trichomonads on microscopy (60%-70% sensitivity); culture is the most sensitive commercially available method

46

Treatment	Metronidazole 500 mg PO bid for 7 days	Topical antifungals cure >80%.	Metronidazole 2 g PO as a single dose
	or	Examples:	*Alternatively,* Metronidazole 500 mg PO
	Metronidazole gel 0.75% 5 g	Butoconazole, 2% cream, 5 g	bid for 7 days
	intravaginally qd for 5 days	intravaginally for 3 days	
	or	*or*	Cure rates increased when sexual
	Clindamycin cream 2%, 5 g	Clotrimazole, 1% cream 5 g	partners also treated
	intravaginally qhs for 7 days	intravaginally for 7-14 days	
		or	If treatment fails, retreat with
	Alternatively, Metronidazole 2 g PO as a	Clotrimazole, 100 mg vaginal tablet for	metronidazole, 500 mg PO bid for
	single dose	7 days	7 days; if treatment fails again,
	or	*or*	metronidazole, 2 g PO qd for 3-5 days
	Clindamycin 300 mg PO bid for 7 days	Miconazole, 100 mg vaginal	
	or	suppository for 7 days	
	Clindamycin ovules 100 g intravaginally	*Oral agent:* fluconazole, 150 mg,	
	qhs for 3 days	single dose	
	Treatment of male sex partner does not	Complicated infections may require	
	prevent recurrence	10-14 days of topical therapy or	
		sequential oral fluconazole doses*	

KOH, Potassium hydroxide.

*Complicated candidiasis includes moderate to severe symptoms in patients with uncontrolled diabetes, those with immunosuppression, those who have had recurrent episodes of candidal vaginitis, or those taking antibiotics. [45] Sequential fluconazole dosage = 150 mg on days 1 and 4.

SEXUALLY TRANSMITTED DISEASES

IV. MANAGEMENT

A. PARENTERAL THERAPY

1. Before oral therapy is instituted, parenteral therapy should be continued for at least 24 hours after clinical improvement occurs.

2. Treatment is cefotetan 2 g IV q12h *or* cefoxitin 2 g IV q6h *plus* doxycycline 100 mg IV q12h. Doxycycline should be given orally whenever possible because it is painful to infuse and its bioavailability is similar in intravenous and oral forms. Doxycycline therapy should continue for a total of 14 days.

3. Clindamycin 900 mg IV q8h *plus* gentamicin 2 mg/kg IV or IM loading dose, followed by a maintenance dose of 1.5 mg/kg q8h. Single daily gentamicin doses may be substituted. With transition to oral therapy, doxycycline 100 mg PO bid and clindamycin 450 mg qid should continue for 14 days.

4. Alternatively, ofloxacin 400 mg IV q12h *or* levofloxacin 500 mg IV daily with or without metronidazole 500 mg IV q8h *or* ampicillin-sulbactam 3 g IV q6h *plus* doxycycline 100 mg PO or IV q12h can be given.

B. ORAL THERAPY

1. If no clinical response occurs within 72 hours, the diagnosis should be reevaluated and the need for parenteral therapy assessed.

2. Ofloxacin 400 mg PO bid for 14 days *or* levofloxacin 500 mg PO daily with or without metronidazole 500 mg PO bid for 14 days.

3. Ceftriaxone 250 mg IM as a single dose *or* cefoxitin 2 g IM *plus* probenecid 1 g PO as a single dose *or* third-generation cephalosporin *plus* doxycycline 100 mg bid for 14 days with or without metronidazole 500 mg PO bid for 14 days.

VAGINITIS

I. SPECIAL CONSIDERATIONS (Table 46-2[43-45])

1. Recurrent vulvovaginal candidiasis is defined as four or more episodes per year.

2. The pathogenesis of this problem is not well understood. *Candida glabrata* is responsible for 10% to 20% of recurrent vulvovaginal candidiasis. Vaginal cultures can confirm the diagnosis and identify unusual etiological agents.

3. After the episode is treated (Table 46-2), maintenance therapy should be instituted for 6 months with clotrimazole 600-mg vaginal suppositories every week *or* ketoconazole 100 mg PO each day *or* fluconazole 100 to 150 mg PO each week *or* itraconazole 400 mg PO each month or 100 mg PO each day.

REFERENCES

[c] 1. McCormack WM. Pelvic inflammatory disease. N Engl J Med 1994; 330:115.

[b] 2. Westrom L et al. Pelvic inflammatory disease and fertility: a cohort study of 1844 women with laparoscopically verified disease and 657 control women with normal laparoscopic results. Sex Transm Dis 1992; 9:185.

[c] 3. Whitley RJ, Kimberlin DW, Roizman B. Herpes simplex viruses. Clin Infect Dis 1998; 26:541.

[a] 4. Fife KH et al. Valacyclovir versus acyclovir in the treatment of first-episode genital herpes infection: results of an international, multicenter, double-blind randomized clinical trial. Sex Transm Dis 1997; 24:481.

[a] 5. Diaz-Mitona F et al. Oral famciclovir for the suppression of recurrent genital herpes—a randomized controlled trial. JAMA 1998; 280:928.

[c] 6. Wald A. Therapies and prevention strategies for genital herpes. Clin Infect Dis 1999; 28(suppl 1):S4.

[d] 7. Centers for Disease Control and Prevention. 2001 Guidelines for the treatment of sexually transmitted diseases. MMWR Morb Mortal Wkly Rep 2002; 51(no RR-6).

[b] 8. Augenbraun M et al. Increased genital shedding of herpes simplex virus type 2 in HIV-seropositive women. Ann Intern Med 1995; 123:845.

[d] 9. Division of STD Prevention. Sexually transmitted disease surveillance, 1999. Atlanta: US Department of Health and Human Services, Public Health Service, Centers for Disease Control and Prevention; 2000.

[c] 10. Quinn TC. Sexually transmitted diseases. In Stobo JD, ed. The principles and practice of medicine, 23rd ed. Stamford, Conn: Appleton & Lange; 1996.

[c] 11. Hart G. Syphilis tests in diagnosis and therapeutic decision making. Ann Intern Med 1986; 104:368.

[c] 12. Emmert DH, Kirchner JT. Sexually transmitted diseases in women. Postgrad Med 2000; 107(2):181.

[b] 13. Romanowski B et al. Serologic response to treatment of infectious syphilis. Ann Intern Med 1991; 114(12):1057.

[a] 14. Rolfs RT et al. A randomized trial of enhanced therapy for early syphilis in patients with and without human immunodeficiency virus infection. N Engl J Med 1997; 337:307.

[b] 15. Davis LE, Schmitt JW. Clinical significance of CSF tests for neurosyphilis. Ann Neurol 1989; 25:50.

[b] 16. Malone JL et al. Syphilis and neurosyphilis in human immunodeficiency virus type-1 seropositive population: evidence for frequent serologic relapse after therapy. Am J Med 1995; 99(1):55.

[c] 17. Augenbraun MH, Rolfs R. Treatment of syphilis, 1998: nonpregnant adults. Clin Infect Dis 1999; 28(suppl 1):S21.

[b] 18. Yinnon A et al. Serologic response to treatment of syphilis with HIV infection. Arch Intern Med 1996; 156:321.

[b] 19. Rompalo AM et al. Modification of syphilitic genital ulcer manifestations by coexistent HIV infection. Sex Transm Dis 2001; 28(8):448.

[b] 20. DiCarlo RP, Martin DH. The clinical diagnosis of genital ulcer disease in men. Clin Infect Dis 1997; 25:292.

[c] 21. Jessamine PG, Ronald AR. Chancroid and the role of genital ulcer disease in the spread of human retroviruses. Med Clin North Am 1990; 74:1417.

[a] 22. Stamm WE et al. Effect of treatment regimes for *Neisseria gonorrhoeae* on simultaneous infection with *Chlamydia trachomatis*. N Engl J Med 1984; 310:545.

[b] 23. Goodhart ME et al. Factors affecting the performance of smear and culture tests for the detection of *Neisseria gonorrhoeae*. Sex Transm Dis 1982; 9(2):63.

[c] 24. Koumans EH et al. Laboratory testing for *Neisseria gonorrhoeae* by recently introduced nonculture tests: a performance review in the clinical and public health considerations. Clin Infect Dis 1998; 27:1171.

[a] 25. Van Dyck E et al. Detection of *Chlamydia trachomatis* and *Neisseria gonorrhoeae* by enzyme immunoassay, culture, and three nucleic acid amplification tests. J Clin Microbiol 2001; 39(5):1751.

46

SEXUALLY TRANSMITTED DISEASES

[d] 26. Centers for Disease Control and Prevention. Recommendations for the prevention and management of *Chlamydia trachomatis* infections. MMWR Morb Mortal Wkly Rep 1993; 42(no RR-14):1.

[a] 27. McNagny SE et al. Urinary leukocyte esterase test: a screening method for the detection of asymptomatic chlamydial and gonococcal infections in men. J Infect Dis 1992; 165:573.

[b] 28. Rietmeijer CA et al. Unsuspected *Chlamydia trachomatis* infection in heterosexual men attending a sexual transmitted diseases clinic: evaluation of risk factors and screening methods. Sex Transm Dis 1991; 18:28.

[c] 29. Schachter J, Stoner E, Moncada J. Screening for chlamydial infections in women attending family planning clinics. West J Med 1983; 138:375.

[b] 30. Stamm WE, Cole B. Asymptomatic *Chlamydia trachomatis* urethritis in men. Sex Transm Dis 1986; 13:163.

[b] 31. Berg AO. Establishing the cause of genitourinary symptoms in women in a family practice. JAMA 1984; 251:620.

[b] 32. Jones RB et al. *Chlamydia trachomatis* in the pharynx and rectum of heterosexual patients at risk for genital infection. Ann Intern Med 1985; 102:757.

[c] 33. Black CM. Current methods of laboratory diagnosis of *Chlamydia trachomatis* infections. Clin Microbiol Rev 1997; 10(1):160.

[c] 34. McCormack WM, Rein MF. Urethritis. In Mandell GL, Bennett JE, Dolin R, eds. Principles and practice of infectious diseases, 5th ed. New York: Churchill Livingstone; 2000.

[b] 35. Janier M et al. Male urethritis with and without discharge: a clinical and microbiological study. Sex Transm Dis 1995; 22:244.

[b] 36. Horner PJ et al. Association of *Mycoplasma genitalium* with acute non-gonococcal urethritis. Lancet 1993; 342:582.

[c] 37. Burstein GR, Zenilman JM. Nongonococcal urethritis—a new paradigm. Clin Infect Dis 1999; 28(suppl 1):S66.

[a] 38. Stamm WE et al. Azithromycin for empirical treatment of NGU syndrome in men. JAMA 1995; 274:545.

[c] 39. Simms I, Stephenson JM. Pelvic inflammatory disease epidemiology: what do we know and what do we need to know? Sex Transm Infect 2000; 76:80.

[c] 40. Sweet R. Microbial etiology of pelvic inflammatory disease. In Landers D, Sweet R, eds. Pelvic inflammatory disease. New York: Springer-Verlag; 1996.

[b] 41. Hillis S et al. Delayed care of pelvic inflammatory disease as a risk factor for impaired fertility. Am J Obstet Gynecol 1993; 168:1503.

[b] 42. Wolner-Hanssen P et al. Decreased risk of symptomatic chlamydial pelvic inflammatory disease associated with oral contraceptive use. JAMA 1990; 263:54.

[c] 43. Thomason JL, Gelbart SM. *Trichomonas vaginalis*. Obstet Gynecol 1989; 74:536.

[c] 44. World Health Organization. An overview of selected curable sexually transmitted diseases. In Global program on AIDS. Geneva, Switzerland: World Health Organization; 1995.

[c] 45. Sobel JD. Vaginitis. N Engl J Med 1997; 337:1896.

Soft Tissue Infections and Osteomyelitis

Patrick R. Sosnay, MD, and Sara Cosgrove, MD

Fast Facts

- Cellulitis is infection of the superficial soft tissue. Osteomyelitis is infection of the bone. These infections are frequently seen in adult medicine.
- Gram-positive organisms are the pathogens that most commonly cause simple cellulitis; the most common of these are *Staphylococcus aureus* and *Streptococcus* species (groups A, B, C, G). Osteomyelitis is most frequently caused by *S. aureus*.
- Therapy for both involves administration of appropriate antimicrobials directed against the offending organisms, as well as modification of local or systemic risk factors. Chronic osteomyelitis also requires surgical débridement.
- Whereas cellulitis is most often treated empirically, microbiological data should guide therapy for osteomyelitis. Culture of the infected bone is the gold standard.
- Patients with a rapidly progressing infection or a systemic inflammatory response from their infection warrant imaging and consideration of a surgical evaluation. Gas gangrene, necrotizing fasciitis, and skin and soft tissue infections caused by toxin-producing strands of *S. aureus* and group A *Streptococcus* are emergencies that need immediate surgical débridement.

1. Evaluation of a patient with a soft tissue infection begins with a history and physical examination. Comorbid diseases should be noted. Risk factors for development of soft tissue infections are listed in Box 47-1.
2. The patient should be questioned and the medical record reviewed to determine whether prosthetic material is present in joints or other areas. Patients often have recurrence of cellulitis or osteomyelitis with the same organism; therefore prior culture data can be important to guide therapy. Osteomyelitis can recur if not fully treated originally. An occupational or recreational history often provides clues that suggest a source and a microorganism (Tables 47-1 and 47-2).
3. Most adult bone and soft tissue infections originate from a local source of microbiological invasion. Cellulitis at a surgical site and osteomyelitis underneath a diabetic foot ulcer are both examples of a break in the structural integrity that allows a direct route for infection.
4. Less commonly, osteomyelitis occurs via hematogenous spread from a primary bacteremia (common in children) or a vascular focus of

---

BOX 47-1

RISK FACTORS FOR DEVELOPMENT OF SOFT TISSUE INFECTIONS

Diabetes mellitus: impaired sensation, impaired circulation, dry skin resulting from sympathetic neuropathy, impaired immunity

Lower extremity edema: impaired lymphatic drainage, congestive heart failure, obesity, nephrotic syndrome, cirrhosis

Severe onychomycosis: provides portal of entry

Immune compromise

TABLE 47-1

CLINICAL SITUATIONS AND ASSOCIATED PATHOGENS IN CELLULITIS

Situation	Pathogenic Organism	Comments
Hot tub exposure, folliculitis	Pseudomonas	
Edema resulting from lymphatic obstruction, postvenectomy status	Streptococcus species	
Aquarium exposure, nodular cellulitis	Mycobacterium marinum	Antimycobacterial drugs
Freshwater exposure	Aeromonas species	
Saltwater exposure, especially in cirrhotic patients	Vibrio species	Treat with doxycycline
Fingertips of health care workers	Herpes simplex	Antivirals
Dermatomal distribution of rash, especially with vesicles	Herpes zoster	Antivirals
Cellulitis surrounding diabetic foot ulcer	Often polymicrobial	Perform wound care and evaluate vascular supply

Data from Hook WE et al. Arch Intern Med 1986; 146:295.

---

infection, such as endocarditis or catheter infection with subsequent secondary bacteremia.

5. Finding and treating the source (be it an ulcer or another type of compromised skin integrity) accompanies antibiotic therapy in the management of these infections.

Cellulitis

I. EPIDEMIOLOGY

1. The organisms most commonly seen in cellulitis are *S. aureus* and *Streptococcus* species (groups A, B, C, and G). Risk factors for cellulitis include both local factors, such as disruption of the cutaneous barrier and edema, and host factors, such as diabetes and morbid obesity. Associations between risk factors and organisms that cause cellulitis are reviewed in Box 47-1.[1]

2. Most cases of cellulitis are diagnosed and managed in the outpatient

TABLE 47-2

CLINICAL SITUATIONS AND ASSOCIATED PATHOGENS IN OSTEOMYELITIS

Situation	Pathogenic Organism	Comments
Any type of osteomyelitis	*Staphylococcus aureus*	Most common cause of any osteomyelitis
Foreign body, prosthetics	Coagulase-negative *Staphylococcus*	
Nosocomial infections	Enterobacteriaceae or *Pseudomonas aeruginosa*	Gram-negative coverage according to hospital resistance patterns
Bites,* fist injury, diabetic ulcers, decubitus ulcers	Streptococci, anaerobes, *Eikenella corrodens*	
Sickle cell disease	*Salmonella* or *Streptococcus pneumoniae*	Hematogenous seeding

*Data from Nedeiros I, Saconato H. Cochrane Database System Rev 2001, issue 2.

setting. Hospital admission should be considered for patients who have high fever or are systemically ill, are unresponsive to outpatient antibiotic therapy, or are unable to control factors that predisposed them to cellulitis (e.g., homelessness, uncontrolled diabetes).

II. CLINICAL PRESENTATION

1. The differential diagnosis of cellulitis is listed in Box 47-2.
2. Pain is the most common complaint of patients with cellulitis. Patients may also have other cardinal manifestations of inflammation: redness, warmth over the infected area, swelling, and loss of function. These complaints may not be as obvious if the patient has compromised sensation of the affected area, as occurs with diabetic patients or those with spinal cord injuries.
3. The timing of the onset of symptoms is important. The sudden development of a painful extremity is more suggestive of acute arterial insufficiency or venous occlusion. Infections that come on rapidly or spread quickly are worrisome and merit immediate attention.
4. Box 47-3 presents the differentiation between simple cellulitis and deeper soft tissue infections.

III. DIAGNOSTICS

1. A patient with soft tissue infection should undergo imaging if a deeper infection is suspected.
2. Simple cellulitis may show as swelling or haziness of subcutaneous fat on plain radiographs. Radiographs with radiolucent foci indicate the presence of gas.[2-8]
3. Ultrasound is most helpful when an abscess is suspected. If an abscess contains considerable debris, however, it may not be discernible from surrounding tissue.[9]

BOX 47-2

DIFFERENTIAL DIAGNOSIS OF CELLULITIS

Deep venous thrombosis

Arterial insufficiency

Venous stasis

Tinea corporis

Necrotizing fasciitis

Lymphedema

Erysipelas

Cutaneous anthrax

BOX 47-3

DIFFERENTIATING BETWEEN SIMPLE CELLULITIS AND DEEPER SOFT TISSUE INFECTIONS

SUPERFICIAL INFECTIONS (CELLULITIS)

Occasional fever

No signs of systemic inflammation

Tender, warm, erythematous area of interest

Well demarcated

Lymphangitic streaking may be present

Blood cultures unlikely to be positive*

Cutaneous fungal infection can be portal of entry†

DEEPER SOFT TISSUE INFECTIONS (ABSCESS, FASCIITIS)

Fever more common

Signs of systemic inflammation: tachycardia, hypotension

Tender, warm area of interest

Fluctuance in some cases

Less well demarcated

Blood cultures may be positive

Creatinine phosphokinase levels elevated if myonecrosis

*Data from Perl B et al. Clinic Infect Dis 1999; 29:1438.
†Data from Baddour LM, Bisno AL. JAMA 1984; 251:1049.

4. Computed tomography (CT) and magnetic resonance imaging (MRI) are the most helpful imaging modalities when deeper infection is suspected because of the increased resolution offered. CT with intravenous contrast can detect preabscess phlegmons or fluid accumulations. MRI delineates the soft tissue better than other modalities but can take longer to obtain and is more expensive.[9] Local preference and consultation with a radiologist about what imaging is available expeditiously should determine the modality used.

5. If gas gangrene or necrotizing fasciitis is strongly suspected, obtaining imaging studies should not delay surgical débridement.

TABLE 47-3

ANTIMICROBIAL THERAPY FOR CELLULITIS AND SOFT TISSUE INFECTIONS

Entity	Typical Organism	Antimicrobial Agent and Duration
"Community-acquired" cellulitis	*Staphylococcus, Streptococcus*	Cephalexin, clindamycin, dicloxacillin
"Hospital-acquired" cellulitis	Consider methicillin-resistant *Staphylococcus*	Vancomycin
Severe "community-acquired" cellulitis	*Staphylococcus, Streptococcus*	IV cefazolin, clindamycin, or oxacillin
Diabetic foot ulcer	Polymicrobial	Fluoroquinolone plus clindamycin or metronidazole; β-lactam/β-lactamase inhibitor; carbapenem

6. Establishment of a microbiological diagnosis in cellulitis can be challenging; therefore cellulitis is treated empirically. Culture of skin or soft tissue has a low yield in detecting a pathogenic organism.[10] If an intact bullous lesion is present, sterile aspiration at the bedside can yield a pathogenic organism.

7. Toxin-producing streptococcal species and gram-negative organisms are most likely to form bullae.

8. Erysipelas is a distinct type of cellulitis caused by group A *Streptococcus* with prominent lymphatic involvement. It commonly occurs in areas of lymphatic disruption and is a painful, often bright red area with peau d'orange appearance resulting from lymphatic obstruction.[11]

IV. MANAGEMENT

1. Antimicrobial therapy for soft tissue infections represents one arm of treatment. Cellulitis can be treated with intravenous or oral antibiotics, with the extent of infection and the general clinical status of the patient determining which mode of administration is appropriate (Table 47-3).

2. Local wound care is the other, sometimes overlooked, arm of treatment. Patients should elevate the affected extremity.

3. If the site of the break in the cutaneous barrier is an ulcer, débridement of devitalized tissue must be carried out. This can be performed surgically or with wound care preparations that have débriding qualities.

4. Diabetic patients should be educated in foot care and inspection. Proper footwear can prevent pressure ulcers. A bedbound patient can be put in a bed designed to prevent ulcers, and frequent positioning can augment this effort. Patients with intractable venous insufficiency ulcers can be helped with compression stockings.

5. Fungal infections around the toes in a leg with cellulitis should be treated with topical preparations.

47

SOFT TISSUE INFECTIONS AND OSTEOMYELITIS

Osteomyelitis

I. EPIDEMIOLOGY

1. The diagnosis and management of osteomyelitis depend on the etiology and the time course of the infection. Osteomyelitis can be acquired by hematogenous seeding of bone or by local spread of infection in an area of soft tissue breakdown. Hematogenous osteomyelitis occurs if the patient has bacteremia, which may or may not be recognized. Osteomyelitis has a bimodal distribution, with higher incidence in children and the elderly. It can occur in any bone but is most frequently seen in bones with large blood supply, such as the femur and the spine.

2. Hematogenous osteomyelitis usually occurs as an acute infection and is most commonly caused by *S. aureus*. Osteomyelitis caused by *Mycobacterium tuberculosis* (Pott's disease) has a predilection for the spine and should be considered in the differential diagnosis of any patient with spinal osteomyelitis.[1,2]

3. Osteomyelitis occurring secondary to local spread of soft tissue infection can be classified as acute or chronic. Acute infections of bone occur with penetrating trauma or as a result of a complex fracture.

4. A hospital internist is most likely to manage chronic osteomyelitis at an ulcer site. This occurs frequently in the feet of patients with diabetes or vascular insufficiency or as a consequence of relative vascular insufficiency at the site of a pressure ulcer in elderly or immobilized patients. Table 47-2 reviews some of the pathogens that are associated with osteomyelitis.

II. CLINICAL PRESENTATION

1. Presenting complaints in patients with osteomyelitis vary, depending on whether the infection is of hematogenous or local origin. Presenting symptoms of hematogenous osteomyelitis are pain associated with swelling and fever or chills.

2. Questioning the patient about intravenous catheters or injecting drug use helps in determining the source of bacteremia.

3. The physical examination can be unremarkable, but often the patient has localized swelling and tenderness. The suspicion of vertebral osteomyelitis mandates a thorough neurological examination, in which the clinician looks for evidence of spinal cord compromise caused by vertebral destruction.

III. DIAGNOSTICS

1. MRI is the image modality of choice in diagnosing hematogenous osteomyelitis because it detects marrow inflammation and has superior spatial resolution in imaging the spinal cord and nerve roots.

2. Blood cultures are occasionally positive with hematogenous osteomy-

elitis and should always be obtained because the results will guide therapy.

3. In patients with a known ulcer the clinician must determine whether bone infection is present beneath the soft tissue injury. A diabetic foot ulcer that is greater than 2 cm, or that the clinician can probe bone within, has very high specificity for osteomyelitis.[13]

4. When there is no obvious sign of bone involvement on examination, imaging modalities and surgical exploration with bone biopsy become the diagnostic choices.

5. Imaging in osteomyelitis is well studied,[14] but there is no consensus on the best modality. Table 47-4 reviews the options for imaging in osteomyelitis.[15]

6. In general all of these imaging modalities lack specificity diagnosing osteomyelitis in patients with contiguous inflammation. Nuclear medicine bone scans have been the recommended imaging modality to diagnose osteomyelitis.[16] However, MRI has superior specificity and adds the ability to characterize the surrounding soft tissue.[17,18]

7. In determining what test to order, the clinician should consult with the radiologist because local preference often dictates what study is performed.

8. Radiolabeled antigranulocyte monoclonal antibodies (sulesomab) are superior to white blood cell scans for detecting osteomyelitis in diabetic foot ulcers, with a sensitivity 91%, a specificity of 56%, and an accuracy of 80%. Availability of this agent and cost are important limiting factors.[19]

9. Erythrocyte sedimentation rate and C-reactive protein are useful markers of systemic inflammation that have been used in osteomyelitis, but the use of either test is complicated when soft tissue infection or any other cause of acute inflammation is present. Erythrocyte sedimentation rate and C-reactive protein are most helpful in assessing and monitoring the efficacy of treatment because of their sensitivity.

IV. MANAGEMENT

1. A longer treatment course is required in osteomyelitis, providing greater incentive to establish a microbiological diagnosis. Diagnostic culture specimens are obtained by bone biopsy, which is best performed by aiming the needle through healthy tissue, rather than going through the ulcer. Biopsy can also be performed if the patient is to undergo surgical débridement, which is necessary in chronic osteomyelitis.

2. Culture of an ulcer or drainage from a sinus tract has been shown not to be useful in determining a pathogenic organism.[20] Culturing an ulcer may be beneficial only to search for resistant organisms when empirical treatment is being used.

3. Osteomyelitis is traditionally treated with 4 to 6 weeks of parenteral

TABLE 47-4

IMAGING MODALITIES IN OSTEOMYELITIS

Imaging Modality	Findings	Advantages	Disadvantages	Sensitivity and Specificity (%)
Plain radiograph	No findings for first 10-21 days, then soft tissue swelling, periosteal elevation, and eventual cortical erosion	Inexpensive, readily available, well suited to following known infection, able to detect other pathological conditions (e.g., neuropathic joints)	Time needed to see pathological changes; periosteal reaction not specific for infection	Sensitivity 28-93 Specificity 50-92
Computed tomography	Similar to plain radiographs with greater resolution	Greater sensitivity than plain radiographs; better able to characterize soft tissue; can be used to direct biopsy; adjuvant once diagnosis of osteomyelitis made; able to detect sequestra (partially liquefied infected bone)	Beam-hardening effect from bone; radiological diagnosis lags behind pathological	
Magnetic resonance imaging	Low signal intensity on T1, high signal intensity (bright) on T2	Very sensitive because of ability to differentiate between normal and abnormal bone marrow; outstanding soft tissue resolution	Expense; contraindicated with pacemakers, defibrillators, and other metal hardware; claustrophobia	Sensitivity 77-99 Specificity 83-100
Technetium bone scan	Increased signal from osteoblastic activity and skeletal vascularity	Detects osteomyelitis earlier than plain film or computed tomography; allows imaging of entire skeleton	Expense; three- or four-phase procedure takes >24 hours; any bone turnover will yield false positive	Sensitivity 61-86 Specificity 25-45
Indium white blood cell scan	Increased signal from radiolabeled white blood cells	Specific for infection, as opposed to bone turnover	Expense; poor differentiation between osteomyelitis and overlying soft tissue infection	Sensitivity 80-89 Specificity 29-69 (staged technetium then indium scan improves sensitivity to 89-100)

Data from Levine SE et al. Foot Ankle Int 1994; 15:151; and Morrison WB et al. Radiology 1993; 189:251.

antibiotics directed against biopsy-proven pathogens. Unless the patient is unstable, antibiotics can wait until microbiological data are obtained. Hematogenous osteomyelitis is most often caused by a single organism and can be treated with antibiotics specific for that organism.

4. Diabetic foot ulcers with underlying osteomyelitis are frequently infected with gram-negative organisms and anaerobes, in addition to gram-positive organisms, and require broad coverage guided by culture information.[21]

5. Duration of therapy is once again subjective, but most clinicians agree on 4 to 6 weeks of parenteral treatment. Clinicians frequently substitute oral fluoroquinolones because they allow outpatient treatment of what used to be an inpatient disease. Reviews of the use of oral fluoroquinolones show that they have comparable cure rates in osteomyelitis caused by *Enterobacter* species. They are also efficacious when used in combination with rifampin for the treatment of *S. aureus*.[22,23]

6. Oral outpatient therapy should be considered only after the patient is fully evaluated with appropriate cultures, diagnostic imaging, and débridement, which usually requires in-hospital evaluation.

7. Osteomyelitis at ulcer sites may require surgical repair of the soft tissue defect with local tissue or a free flap. It is not realistic to cure chronic osteomyelitis at an ulcer site without healing the ulcer. Local and surgical débridement is usually necessary and should be considered in all cases of local osteomyelitis. In addition, patients should have evaluation of the vascular supply to the affected area with ankle-brachial indices and angiography.

8. Management of contiguous osteomyelitis is most effective when a multidisciplinary approach is taken, with involvement of vascular and plastic surgeons, infectious disease physicians, and wound care specialists. Amputation of a portion of the affected extremity deserves consideration when systemic infection is uncontrollable, when the vascular supply to the area cannot be improved with surgical or radiological intervention, or when the ulcer does not heal despite local wound care and appropriate antibiotics. Consideration of amputation also mandates thorough vascular evaluation. Débridement of necrotic tissue can be performed manually (sharp débridement). Alternatively, wound care preparations that have intrinsic débriding qualities may be used.

PEARLS AND PITFALLS

- Deeper soft tissue infections can be a surgical emergency.
  - Necrotizing fasciitis is an infection that occurs in a deeper tissue plane than with cellulitis and spreads rapidly along the fascial surface. This infection has high morbidity and mortality. Findings that raise the question of necrotizing fasciitis include tenderness out of proportion to

other clinic signs of inflammation, an indurated or brawny quality spreading beyond the area of superficial infection, and any unexplained vital sign abnormality. Fournier's gangrene is an equivalent deep tissue infection in the perineal region. Necrotizing fasciitis caused by group A *Streptococcus* is especially fulminant. Toxins produced by strains of group A *Streptococcus* up-regulate inflammatory cytokines, leading to a syndrome similar to staphylococcal toxic shock syndrome.

- Gas gangrene (or clostridial myonecrosis) is a deep tissue infection caused by *Clostridium* species. Any question of these deeper infections should warrant imaging if the patient is clinically stable. The treatment of deeper soft tissue infections is surgical, with empirical broad antibiotic coverage that should be narrowed according to intraoperative cultures. Use of clindamycin as an antimicrobial has a theoretical benefit because the inhibition of protein synthesis may decrease toxin production. Clindamycin has similar efficacy at high and low inoculum ("Eagle effect").[24]

- The treatment of infected prosthetic joints and other hardware is beyond the scope of this discussion and should be managed with infectious disease and orthopedic surgery consultations. (See two helpful review articles.[25,26])

- Periorbital and facial cellulitis can become severe, with extension to the central nervous system as a potential complication. An ear, nose, and throat surgeon and an ophthalmologist should be consulted.

- Infection of the joint space may occur as a result of hematogenous spread or direct inoculation. Typically movement of the joint evokes severe pain. Treatment involves antibiotics and surgical drainage.

- Osteomyelitis of the vertebral bodies occurs primarily from hematogenous source. A coexisting epidural abscess increases the risk of central nervous system extension of the infection. Osteomyelitis in the vertebral spine can destroy vertebrae and lead to cord compression. MRI is the imaging modality of choice because of its superior spatial resolution and its usefulness in assessment of the spinal cord and nerve roots.

- Cutaneous anthrax has become an entity of increased clinical importance. The clinical hallmarks of cutaneous anthrax, a primarily toxin-mediated reaction, include a painless papulovesicular lesion with massive surrounding edema that progresses to an eschar within 2 to 5 days. Systemic toxicity may be present. Antimicrobials sterilize the lesion within 24 hours but do not change the clinical course of edema and eschar formation.[27]

- Pyomyositis is a rare entity of deep muscle abscesses typically caused by *S. aureus.* Clinical hallmarks are mild systemic symptoms, normal creatine phosphokinase levels, and induration of muscle without fluctuance. CT or MRI shows deep muscle abscesses. Treatment consists of drainage and antistaphylococcal antibiotics.[28]

REFERENCES

[b] 1. Dupuy A et al. Risk factors for erysipelas of the leg (cellulitis): case-control study. Br Med J 1999; 318:1591.

[b] 2. Levine SE et al. Magnetic resonance imaging for the diagnosis of osteomyelitis in the diabetic patient with a foot ulcer. Foot Ankle Int 1994; 15:151.

[a] 3. Morrison WB et al. Diagnosis of osteomyelitis: utility of fat-suppressed contrast-enhanced MR imaging. Radiology 1993; 189:251.

[a] 4. Nepola JV et al. Diagnosis of infections in ununited fractures: combined imaging with indium-111 labeled leukocytes and technetium 99m methylene diphosphonate. J Bone Joint Surg Am 1993; 75:1816.

[d] 5. Eckman MH et al. Foot infections in diabetic patients: decisions and cost-effectiveness analysis. JAMA 1995; 273:713.

[c] 6. Newman LG. Imaging techniques in the diabetic foot. Clin Podiatr Med Surg 1995; 12:75.

[a] 7. Johnson JE. Prospective study of bone, indium-111-labeled white blood cell, and gallium-67 scanning for evaluation of osteomyelitis in the diabetic foot. Foot Ankle Int 1996; 17:10.

[b] 8. Newman LG et al. Unexpected osteomyelitis in diabetic foot ulcers: diagnosing and monitoring by leukocyte scanning with indium In 111 oxyquinoline. JAMA 1991; 266:1246.

[c] 9. Struk DW et al. Imaging of soft tissue infections. Radiol Clin North Am 2001; 39(2):277.

[c] 10. Ginsberg MB. Cellulitis: analysis of 101 cases and review of the literature. South Med J 1981; 74:530.

[c] 11. Swartz MN. Cellulitis and subcutaneous tissue infections. In Mandell GL, editor. Principles and practice of infectious disease 2001. Philadelphia: Churchill Livingstone; 2001.

[c] 12. Laughlin RT et al. Osteomyelitis. Curr Opin Rheumatol 1995; 7:315.

[a] 13. Grayson MC et al. Probing to bone in infected pedal ulcers: a clinical sign of underlying osteomyelitis. JAMA 1995; 273:721.

[d] 14. Tehranzadeh J et al. Imaging of osteomyelitis in the mature skeleton. Radiol Clin North Am 2001; 39(2):233.

[c] 15. Gold RH et al. Osteomyelitis: findings on plain radiography CT, MR, and scintigraphy. Am J Roentgenol 1991; 157:365.

[c] 16. Palestro CJ, Torres MA. Radionuclide imaging in orthopedic infections. Semin Nucl Med 1997; 27;334.

[b] 17. Morrison WB et al. Diagnosis of osteomyelitis: utility of fat suppressed contrast-enhanced MR imaging. Radiology 1993; 22:239.

[b] 18. Morrison WB et al. Osteomyelitis in the feet of diabetics: clinical accuracy, surgical utility and cost-effectiveness of MR imaging. Radiology 1995; 196:557.

[b] 19. Harwood SJ et al. Use of sulesomab, a radiolabeled antibody fragment, to detect osteomyelitis in diabetic patients with foot ulcers by leukoscintigraphy. Clin Infect Dis 1999; 28:1200.

[b] 20. Mackowiak PA et al. Diagnostic value of sinus tract cultures in chronic osteomyelitis. JAMA 1978; 239:2772.

[d] 21. Tomas MB et al. The diabetic foot. Br J Radiol 200; 73:443.

[d] 22. Lew DP, Waldvogel FA. Use of quinolones in osteomyelitis and infected orthopedic prosthesis. Drugs 1999; 58:85.

[c] 23. Rissing JP. Antimicrobial therapy for chronic osteomyelitis in adults: role of the quinolones. Clin Infect Dis 1997; 25:1327.

[b] 24. Stevens DL et al. Effect of antibiotics on toxin production and viability of *Clostridium perfringens*. Antimicrob Agents Chemother 1997; 31:213.

[b] 25. Fisman DN et al. Clinical effectiveness and cost-effectiveness of 2 management strategies for infected total hip arthroplasty in the elderly. Clin Infect Dis 2001; 32:419.

[c] 26. Gillespie WJ. Prevention and management of infection after total joint replacement. Clin Infect Dis 1997; 25:1310.

[b] 27. Freedman A et al. Cutaneous anthrax associated with microangiopathic hemolytic anemia and coagulopathy in a 7-month-old infant. JAMA 2002; 287:869.

[c] 28. Christin L, Sarosi GA. Pyomyositis in North America: case reports and review. Clin Infect Dis 1992; 15:668.

47

SOFT TISSUE INFECTIONS AND OSTEOMYELITIS

Urinary Tract Infections

Hossein Ardehali, MD, PhD, and Eric Nuermberger, MD

48

UTI is a common problem that leads to substantial morbidity and medical expenditure. An estimated 20% to 40% of American women receive medical treatment for a UTI at some point during their lifetime, resulting in up to 8 million visits to physicians' offices a year and more 1 million hospital admissions. The annual costs for uncomplicated acute cystitis surpass 1 billion dollars. About 250,000 cases of pyelonephritis occur annually in the United States.[1]

I. DEFINITIONS

1. **Bacteriuria:** Presence of bacteria in the urine.
2. **Asymptomatic bacteriuria:** Presence of significant bacteriuria in the absence of any symptoms.
3. **Acute cystitis:** Clinical syndrome caused by infection of the bladder epithelium or urethra.

4. **Complicated UTI:** UTI associated with an underlying condition (e.g., obstruction, foreign body, instrumentation, renal insufficiency, renal transplant, pregnancy, or [possibly] male gender) that may increase the risk of therapeutic failure.

5. **Relapse:** Recurrence of bacteriuria with the original isolate within 2 weeks after termination of therapy.

6. **Reinfection:** Recurrence of bacteriuria with a new organism.

7. **Acute pyelonephritis:** Clinical syndrome caused by infection of the renal parenchyma.

8. **Chronic pyelonephritis:** Inflammation and scarring of the kidney parenchyma caused by persistent or repeated infection. It occurs most commonly in children with severe vesicoureteral reflux and UTI. Interstitial nephritis, which is noninfectious renal interstitial inflammation, should be distinguished from chronic pyelonephritis.

9. **Acute bacterial prostatitis:** Infection of the prostate caused by uropathogens. Patients have a tender prostate and symptoms of cystitis, and the condition usually responds promptly to antibiotics.

10. **Chronic bacterial prostatitis:** Subacute process characterized by recurrent prostatic infection. It may manifest itself as dysuria or pelvic pain.

II. EPIDEMIOLOGY

1. The prevalence of bacteriuria is 3% to 7% in women younger than 60 years and 10% to 25% in women older than 60 years. The prevalence in younger adult men is much lower (<0.1%) but may increase to 4% to 15% in older age.

2. Box 48-1 lists conditions associated with an increased risk of UTI.

BOX 48-1

CONDITIONS THAT INCREASE THE RISK OF URINARY TRACT INFECTIONS

FEMALES

Older age

Diabetes mellitus

Sexual intercourse

Use of diaphragms

Use of spermicide

MALES

Older age

Anatomical abnormalities

?Sexual activity, particularly anal intercourse

Data from Platt R et al. Am J Epidemiol 1986; 124:977; and Bengtsson C et al. Scand J Urol Nephrol 1998; 32:284.

III. ETIOLOGY AND PATHOGENESIS

1. Most UTIs are caused by Enterobacteriaceae originating from the digestive tract. The most common organism in ambulatory patients is *Escherichia coli* (50%-80% of cases). Recurrent UTIs or UTIs associated with long-term catheterization or recent antibiotic use are increasingly associated with *Proteus, Pseudomonas,* and *Enterococcus* species. Another gram-positive organism, *Staphylococcus saprophyticus,* causes approximately 10% of cystitis in young women.[4] *Candida albicans* and other *Candida* species are occasionally found in diabetic women and in patients with indwelling catheters, but they usually represent colonization rather than invasive infection.

2. In women the most common route of infection is migration of the organism from the rectum to the vagina, followed by distal urethral colonization and subsequent bladder infection. Normal urinary flow and the antiadherent and antibacterial properties of the bladder mucosa are host defenses that aid in preventing infection. Pyelonephritis most commonly results from the ascension of organisms from the bladder but is occasionally caused by bacteremic spread (most commonly caused by *Staphylococcus aureus*).

IV. CLINICAL PRESENTATION

1. Symptoms of acute cystitis include dysuria (painful or difficult urination), urgency, frequency, suprapubic pain, and sometimes gross hematuria. In women, frequency and dysuria may also be caused by vaginitis, which may be accompanied by vaginal discharge or itching. The differential diagnosis of UTI also includes urethritis or acute urethral syndrome, which is the diagnosis in up to half of women with frequency and dysuria. The most common causative organisms of acute urethral syndrome are *Neisseria gonorrhoeae* and *Chlamydia trachomatis;* less commonly *E. coli* or other uropathogens are the cause. The etiology is unknown in some cases. Hematuria suggests cystitis rather than urethral syndrome or vaginitis.

2. Patients with acute pyelonephritis usually have a temperature above 38.5° C, chills, and flank pain, all of which may help distinguish this condition from acute cystitis. In addition to symptoms of lower tract infection, patients may have constitutional symptoms, including nausea, vomiting, diarrhea, headache, anorexia, malaise, and myalgia. If the flank pain radiates to the groin, ureteral obstruction by a calculus should be suspected. Older patients may have a paucity of symptoms, even with pyelonephritis and bacteremia.

V. DIAGNOSIS

1. In general, the diagnosis of acute uncomplicated UTI can be made in a young or middle-aged woman on the basis of the clinical presentation

48

URINARY TRACT INFECTIONS

and without a urinalysis. Similarly, pretreatment cultures do not improve outcomes and are not needed before therapy is started.

2. Urinalysis and culture are recommended for patients with an unclear diagnosis, recurrent or relapsing cystitis, pyelonephritis, or complicated UTIs. A clean-voided midstream urine specimen is preferable for diagnosis of UTI. For patients who cannot cooperate, straight catheterization or suprapubic aspiration should be performed. Quantitative cultures may help differentiate infection from contamination during collection. Because more than 90% of patients with acute pyelonephritis have bacteriuria ($>10^5$ bacteria/mL), this criterion has been established to indicate a UTI. However, in symptomatic women, more than 100 gram-negative bacteria per milliliter in the presence of pyuria is also considered to be consistent with UTI and should be treated. Any growth of a bacterial pathogen in urine obtained by suprapubic aspiration suggests infection.

3. Pyuria is defined as the presence of more than 5 WBCs per high-power field in centrifuged urine sediment, or more than 10 cells per milliliter of unspun urine. Pyuria is present in over 95% of symptomatic patients with UTI and over 90% of symptom-free patients with bacteriuria, whereas only 1% of asymptomatic nonbacteriuric patients have pyuria. Detection of leukocyte esterase by urine dipstick is less sensitive but may be used as an alternative. Dipstick leukocyte esterase has a sensitivity of 75% to 95% and a specificity of 65% to 95%. Although rarely used today, Gram's stain of unspun urine may aid in diagnosis before culture results are available, and the results may alter therapy if they reveal gram-positive cocci. Nitrites in the urine indicate the presence of Enterobacteriaceae. Although the differentiation between pyelonephritis and acute cystitis is important, clinical criteria are not always sufficient to make this distinction. Blood cultures are positive in 25% to 40% of patients with acute pyelonephritis. WBC casts are found in up to 60% of these patients on careful inspection of the urine, and when present they indicate infection of the renal parenchyma. Imaging should be considered in patients with severe UTI, recurrent pyelonephritis, relapsed cystitis, symptoms suggesting stone, symptoms or fever lasting longer than 72 hours despite therapy, and selected male patients (see section on acute cystitis in men in "Pearls and Pitfalls").

VI. MANAGEMENT

A. ACUTE UNCOMPLICATED BACTERIAL CYSTITIS

1. A 3-day course of TMP-SMX is standard therapy for acute uncomplicated bacterial cystitis. Treatment for 7 days gives no further benefit. Other 3-day regimens include trimethoprim alone (useful for patients intolerant of sulfa drugs) and the fluoroquinolones, including norfloxacin (Box 48-2).[1] Single-dose therapy is less effective.

2. In general, β-lactams are less effective in eradicating infection and

---

BOX 48-2

COMMON ANTIBIOTICS RECOMMENDED FOR THE TREATMENT OF UNCOMPLICATED URINARY TRACT INFECTION

WOMEN

Trimethoprim-sulfamethoxazole, one double-strength tablet bid for 3 days

Ciprofloxacin, 500 mg PO bid for 3 days

Nitrofurantoin, 100 mg PO qid for 3 days

Fosfomycin, 3 g PO as a single dose

MEN

As above, but for 7-10 days

Moxifloxacin is not excreted in the urine and should not be used for treatment of urinary tract infection. A single parenteral dose (1 mg/kg) of an aminoglycoside can eradicate a simple urinary tract infection.

preventing recurrence than TMP-SMX, trimethoprim alone, or the fluoroquinolones. β-Lactams are rapidly excreted and may reach adequate drug concentrations in urine for only a short period of the dose interval. Furthermore, because of increasing resistance among enteric uropathogens, ampicillin and amoxicillin can no longer be relied on for empirical treatment.[5]

3. Nitrofurantoin therapy for UTI has not been studied adequately. In one small study 3 days of nitrofurantoin therapy was found to be significantly less effective than the same duration of TMP-SMX.[5] In a larger study 7 days of nitrofurantoin therapy was found to be equivalent to 7 days of TMP-SMX therapy, but eradication rates were low for both treatments (77%-83%).[6]

4. In summary, TMP-SMX double strength given twice daily (or adjusted for renal function) for 3 days is highly effective therapy for uncomplicated acute cystitis in nonpregnant women. Greater than 90% eradication is expected with this regimen. The fluoroquinolones are also effective in treating cystitis, but because they are expensive and their widespread use may lead to increased resistance, they should not be used as first-line empirical therapy for uncomplicated cystitis. In areas where the prevalence of resistance to TMP-SMX among uropathogens is high (e.g., >20%), fluoroquinolones should be considered for empirical therapy because resistance is associated with clinical failure.

B. ACUTE PYELONEPHRITIS

1. Less severe episodes of acute pyelonephritis, characterized by low-grade fever and slightly elevated WBC count, no sign of sepsis, and no nausea or vomiting, in a compliant patient can be treated on an outpatient basis with 7 to 14 days of oral antibiotics. For empirical therapy, oral fluoroquinolones should be used. Oral TMP-SMX can be used if resistance rates in the community are low or the organism is known to be susceptible, although fluoroquinolones appear to be more

effective.[7] If the infecting agent is a gram-positive organism, amoxicillin or amoxicillin–clavulanic acid should be used.[1]

2. Patients with vomiting, high fever, high WBC count, or evidence of sepsis should be admitted and treated initially with an intravenous fluoroquinolone, aminoglycoside with or without ampicillin, or a second- or third-generation cephalosporin with or without an aminoglycoside. After clinical improvement and defervescence, the antibiotic can be changed to an oral regimen to complete treatment, even if the patient had bacteremia with gram-negative bacilli.[8]

PEARLS AND PITFALLS

- Acute cystitis in men.
  - Although UTI rarely affects men during youth and adulthood, the prevalence increases in men who are institutionalized or are past middle age. The increased incidence of UTI in these groups may be a consequence of prostatic hypertrophy or introduction of bacteria during instrumentation of the urinary tract, such as catheterization. Sexual intercourse may play an important role in causing UTIs in young men; studies have shown that male UTIs may be associated with the same pathogens found in the partner's vaginal flora. Furthermore, urethral stricture may develop in men with a history of urethritis and cause obstructive symptoms and postvoid residual urine, increasing the risk of UTI. Homosexual men have higher rates of UTI, probably because of anal intercourse and a higher incidence of sexually transmitted diseases.[9]
  - In men, more than 10^3 colony-forming units/mL of urine is a reliable measure for the diagnosis of UTI. Gram-negative bacilli, especially *E. coli,* are the most common causative organisms. Unlike women, men should have treatment for 7 to 10 days because of the increased likelihood of complicated infection.
  - Urological evaluations uncover a functional abnormality in approximately 30% of healthy young men and in most elderly men with UTI.[10] However, it is not clear whether these abnormalities are related to the UTI. In general, it is recommended that all young men without risk factors for UTI be evaluated for anatomical or functional abnormality. Older men with an enlarged prostate, men with a history of active anal intercourse, uncircumcised men, and HIV-infected men with a CD4+ count of less than 200/mm³ do not necessarily need further evaluation.
- Acute prostatitis in men.
  - About 25% of male genitourinary complaints are attributable to prostatitis. Acute bacterial prostatitis typically causes a tender prostate and may be associated with systemic symptoms and dysuria. It usually responds readily to antibiotic therapy.
  - Chronic bacterial prostatitis occurs more insidiously and is characterized by recurrent urinary tract infections.

- *E. coli* followed by *Proteus*, *Klebsiella*, *Pseudomonas*, *Serratia*, and *Enterobacter* are the most common causes of bacterial prostatitis. Diagnosis is based on clinical findings and localization cultures, also known as the "four-cup test." This test involves collecting the first 10 mL of voided urine (specimen 1), discarding the next 100 mL voided, collecting a midstream urine specimen (specimen 2), massaging the prostate and collecting any expressed prostatic secretion (specimen 3), and finally collecting the first 10 mL of urine voided after the massage (specimen 4). Cultures of the first two urine specimens should be negative, whereas specimens 3 and 4 should be positive to support a diagnosis of prostatitis. Greater than 15 leukocytes per high-power field in prostatic secretions further suggests inflammation.[9]

- Empirical treatment of acute bacterial prostatitis consists of ciprofloxacin or TMP-SMX for 4 weeks.[11] Ofloxacin and ampicillin plus gentamicin for 4 weeks are other options. Chronic bacterial prostatitis should be treated with a fluoroquinolone such as ciprofloxacin, TMP-SMX, or doxycycline for 6 to 12 weeks.

- Negative urine and prostatic fluid cultures and the presence of inflammatory cells in the prostatic fluid characterize nonbacterial prostatitis. Men with nonbacterial prostatitis usually have genitourinary, rectal, or perineal pain or dysuria. Treatment is not well defined, but conservative measures such as nonsteroidal antiinflammatory drugs, α-blockers, lifestyle changes (such as sexual practices and exercise), and prostatic massages have been suggested. Some physicians recommend a 14-week course of antibiotic therapy to help exclude occult bacterial prostatitis.

- Treatment of acute cystitis in patients with indwelling catheters.
  - Bacteria can adhere to the catheter surface and promote the growth of biofilms that may protect the bacteria from antibiotics. Therefore therapy frequently fails in patients with an indwelling catheter. The treatment of these patients must include removing the old catheter and inserting a new sterile catheter. Because bacteriuria develops in almost all patients with long-term indwelling catheters, treatment with antibiotics should be given only when symptoms occur with evidence of infected urine. Obtaining routine urine cultures in the absence of symptoms is discouraged.
  - Preventive measures include avoiding use of indwelling catheters when possible, changing catheters every 2 to 4 weeks, and using catheters with a closed drainage system. Up to 17% of nosocomial bacteremias are the result of UTIs caused by indwelling catheters, which makes prevention of infection a top priority.

- Candiduria.
  - The most common risk factors for candiduria include recent antibiotic therapy, instrumentation of the urinary tract, diabetes mellitus, and advanced age. *Candida* is the most frequent isolate from the urine of

48

URINARY TRACT INFECTIONS

patients in the surgical intensive care unit. *C. albicans* is the most frequently isolated organism, and *C. glabrata* is second.[11] In most patients candiduria represents colonization and does not require treatment.

- Discontinuation of indwelling urinary catheters will result in eradication of the organism in 40% of patients.[11] Although fluconazole 200 mg/day for 14 days may shorten the time to a negative urine culture, the frequency of negative urine cultures at the end of 2 weeks of therapy is similar to that occurring with discontinuation of indwelling catheters alone.[12] Neutropenic patients, patients who have urinary tract hardware, and renal transplant recipients are at higher risk of subsequent dissemination from candiduria and should probably be treated.[13]

- Patients with symptomatic disease and patients who will undergo urological manipulations should also be treated. Fluconazole 200 mg/day for 7 to 14 days is usually effective. Removal of urinary tract hardware should also be considered. Amphotericin B can be given intravenously for 7 to 14 days; however, this therapy is associated with more adverse effects. Bladder irrigation with amphotericin B (50-200 mg/mL) may transiently clear candiduria, but it is rarely indicated. Persistent candiduria warrants imaging of the kidneys to exclude parenchymal infection.[13]

- Asymptomatic bacteriuria.
  - Up to 5% of pregnant women have asymptomatic bacteriuria. It is more common in weeks 9 to 17 of pregnancy. Pyelonephritis develops in up to 40% of these subjects if they are not treated.[14] Asymptomatic bacteriuria is also common in elderly patients, especially nursing home patients. Long-term use of indwelling catheters significantly increases the risk of bacteriuria (100% at 4 weeks).
  - Asymptomatic bacteriuria does not appear to contribute to mortality in elderly patients, so unless it is symptomatic, bacteriuria should not be treated in this population. Treatment of asymptomatic bacteriuria is recommended for pregnant women, renal transplantation patients, neutropenic patients, patients who have had an indwelling catheter removed that was in place for less than a week, and those who are going to undergo a urological or orthopedic procedure.

- Sterile pyuria.
  - Sterile pyuria refers to pyuria in the absence of bacteriuria. It may indicate infection with bacteria requiring special media for cultivation (e.g., *Ureaplasma urealyticum* and *C. trachomatis*), *Mycobacterium tuberculosis*, or fungi. It can also occur in noninfectious urological conditions, such as calculi, interstitial nephritis, vesicoureteral reflux and other anatomical abnormalities, and polycystic kidney disease. Prostatitis may be another cause of sterile pyuria.

REFERENCES

[a] 1. Warren JW et al. Guidelines for antimicrobial treatment of uncomplicated acute bacterial cystitis and acute pyelonephritis in women. Clin Infect Dis 1999; 29:745.

[b] 2. Platt R et al. Risk factors for nosocomial urinary tract infection. Am J Epidemiol 1986; 124:977.

[c] 3. Bengtsson C et al. Bacteriuria in a population sample of women: 24-year follow up study; results from the prospective population-based study of women in Gothenburg, Sweden. Scand J Urol Nephrol 1998; 32:284.

[b] 4. Johnson JR, Stamm WE. Diagnosis and treatment of acute urinary tract infections. Infect Dis Clin North Am 1990; 4:12.

[a] 5. Hooton TM et al. Randomized comparative trial and cost analysis of 3-day antimicrobial regimens for treatment of acute cystitis in women. JAMA 1995; 273:41.

[a] 6. Spencer RC et al. Nitrofurantoin modified release versus trimethoprim or co-trimoxazole in the treatment of uncomplicated urinary tract infection in general practice. J Antimicrob Chemother 1994; 33(suppl A):121.

[a] 7. Talan DA et al. Comparison of ciprofloxacin (7 days) and trimethoprim-sulfamethoxazole (14 days) for acute uncomplicated pyelonephritis in women. JAMA 2000; 283:1583.

[a] 8. Mombelli G et al. Oral vs intravenous ciprofloxacin in the initial empirical management of severe pyelonephritis or complicated urinary tract infections: a prospective randomized clinical trial. Arch Intern Med 1999; 159:53.

[b] 9. Lipsky BA. Prostatitis and urinary tract infection in men: what's new; what's true? Am J Med 1999; 106:327.

[b] 10. Lipsky BA. Urinary tract infections in men. Ann Intern Med 1989; 110:138.

[b] 11. Kauffman CA et al. for the NIAID Mycoses Study Group. Prospective multicenter surveillance study of funguria in hospitalized patients. Clin Infect Dis 2000; 30:14.

[b] 12. Falagas ME, Gorbach SL. Practice guidelines: urinary tract infections. Infect Dis Clin Pract 1995; 4:241.

[a] 13. Rex JH et al. Practice guidelines for the treatment of candidiasis. Clin Infect Dis 2000; 30:662.

[c] 14. Sweet RL. Bacteriuria and pyelonephritis during pregnancy. Semin Perinatol 1997; 1:25.

48

URINARY TRACT INFECTIONS

Viral Hepatitis

John Clarke, MD, and David Thomas, MD

FAST FACTS

- Hepatitis A.
  - Hepatitis A is the most common form of acute viral hepatitis in the United States and worldwide.
  - Transmission is fecal-oral; the incubation period is 15 to 50 days.
  - Diagnosis is made by detection of hepatitis A virus (HAV) IgM antibody.
  - Intramuscular immune globulin should be offered to all household contacts.
  - The HAV vaccine is recommended for travelers to endemic areas, men who have sex with men, illicit drug users, recipients of clotting factor concentrates, and persons with chronic liver disease.
- Hepatitis B.
  - Approximately 400 million people worldwide and 1.25 million people in the United States are chronically infected with hepatitis B.
  - In developed nations, most infections result from sexual activity and injection drug use. In developing nations, perinatal and intrafamilial exposure and probably unsafe medical procedures dominate.
  - Diagnosis of hepatitis B virus (HBV) infection and determination of chronicity is based on serological testing (hepatitis B surface antigen [HBsAg]/antibody to hepatitis B surface antigen [anti-HBs], antibody to hepatitis B core antigen [anti-HBc], hepatitis B e antigen [HBeAg], anti-HBe) and HBV DNA detection.
  - Current options for treatment of chronic hepatitis B approved by the Food and Drug Administration (FDA) are lamivudine and interferon-alfa, with approximate HBeAg seroconversion rates of 30% in 1 year.
  - Universal infant immunization for HBV is now recommended in the United States.
- Hepatitis C.
  - Hepatitis C is the most common form of chronic hepatitis in the United States; an estimated 2.7 million people in the United States have chronic HCV infection.
  - Hepatitis C is the single leading indication for liver transplantation.
  - Intravenous drug abuse and blood transfusions before 1990 are the most common risk factors.
  - Acute HCV infection is usually clinically silent.
  - Approximately 85% of acutely infected individuals will develop chronic disease.

49

cont'd

FAST FACTS—CONT'D

- Cirrhosis develops in 15% to 20% of patients with chronic HCV infection.
- Current treatment is with interferon-alfa or pegylated interferon-alfa plus ribavirin. Sustained virological clearance rates are estimated to be approximately 50%.

Hepatitis A

I. VIROLOGY AND EPIDEMIOLOGY

1. HAV is a small nonenveloped RNA hepatovirus (picornavirus family) that is transmitted by the fecal-oral route. The incubation period is 15 to 50 days, with a mean period of approximately 30 days.[1]
2. Virus is excreted in feces for approximately 1 to 2 weeks before the onset of illness and for approximately 1 week thereafter, although longer periods of fecal excretion have been reported.
3. Most patients have complete clinical recovery and normalization of liver function tests within 3 to 6 months after onset of symptoms.[1]
4. Hepatitis A is particularly prevalent in the economically developing regions of Africa, Asia, and Latin America, where seroprevalence rates approach 100% and most infections occur by 5 years of age. In contrast, seroprevalence rates are approximately 33% in the United States and are estimated to be as low as 10% in regions of western Europe where the age of acquisition is also later.[1] Approximately 50% of clinically apparent acute viral hepatitis in the United States is attributed to hepatitis A.[2]
5. Enteric (fecal-oral) transmission via community contacts is the predominant method of HAV spread. Low socioeconomic status, large families, household crowding, poor education, inadequate human waste disposal systems, involvement with day care centers, involvement with mentally handicapped people, work associated with sewage, oral-anal homosexual practices, digital rectal intercourse, high numbers of sexual partners, and injection drug use have all been associated with hepatitis A transmission. Travel to developing nations is an important risk factor because hepatitis A is the most frequently diagnosed form of hepatitis imported into developed countries. In addition, occasional outbreaks have been linked to contaminated water supply or foods.
6. Transfusion-associated hepatitis A is documented but such a rare event that laboratory screening of blood donations for hepatitis A does not exist. No evidence of maternal-neonatal transmission has been found.[1]

II. CLINICAL PRESENTATION

1. Hepatitis A may begin with a nonspecific prodrome of fever, malaise, weakness, anorexia, nausea, vomiting, arthralgias, myalgias, and upper respiratory symptoms; this is often followed by dark urine, jaundice, mild pruritus, and slight liver enlargement and tenderness.

2. Laboratory studies are notable for normal to low white blood cell counts and markedly abnormal liver function tests, particularly serum aminotransferase levels, which may rise to between 500 and 5000 U/L.

3. Viral hepatitis usually has a benign course in young, healthy individuals, and the mortality rate from HAV infection is low.[3,4]

4. Atypical courses such as fulminant liver failure, cholestatic hepatitis, and relapsing hepatitis are uncommon or rare. Illness is usually more severe in adults than in children, in whom HAV infection is often asymptomatic. Those who are elderly, are immunosuppressed, or have chronic liver disease have more severe disease if they contract HAV infection.

5. Hepatitis A causes a self-limited infection; it does not cause chronic infection, and there is no carrier state.[1]

III. DIAGNOSTICS

1. Diagnosis of hepatitis A is obtained by detection of serum HAV IgM antibody during the acute phase of the illness. IgM antibody persists for 3 to 6 months after onset of symptoms. Detection of HAV IgG antibody without the presence of IgM antibody indicates past infection; it persists for decades after acute HAV infection and indicates recovery and resistance to subsequent HAV infections. Assays for saliva HAV antibodies are under development but are not yet readily available.[1] A typical serological course for HAV infection is shown in Fig. 49-1.

IV. MANAGEMENT

1. Given the generally benign nature of hepatitis A, most patients can be treated at home with symptomatic and supportive therapies.

2. No specific antiviral treatment is available for hepatitis A. Intake of alcohol, acetaminophen, and other potentially hepatotoxic substances should be avoided.

V. PROPHYLAXIS

1. Two forms of prophylaxis are available for hepatitis A: immune globulin and an inactivated HAV vaccine. A live, attenuated HAV vaccine is also available, but this is not used regularly in the United States.

2. Intramuscular immune globulin is used as postexposure prophylaxis for household contacts of infected individuals, as well as in hyperendemic areas or for interruption of communitywide outbreaks. The duration of

49

VIRAL HEPATITIS

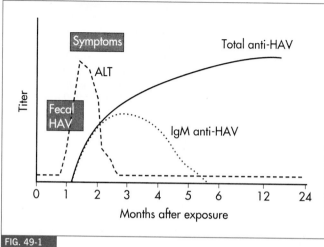

FIG. 49-1

Hepatitis A virus infection, typical serological course. *ALT,* Alanine aminotransferase; *HAV,* hepatitis A virus. *(From Centers for Disease Control and Prevention: Epidemiology and prevention of viral hepatitis A to E: an overview. www.cdc.gov. Accessed Jan. 15, 2003.)*

protection is dose dependent and no longer than 4 to 6 months. The safety profile is excellent.

3. Protective anti-HAV is detectable in the serum as early as 15 days after a single vaccination in 70% to 98% of those vaccinated.

4. Antibodies persist for at least 1 year after a single dose. Responses may be lower in individuals with HIV or immunocompromised status. Estimated duration of immunity after a two-dose vaccination is at least 10 years and perhaps as long as 50 years.

5. Current guidelines state that the HAV vaccine should be given to travelers to endemic areas, homosexual men, illicit drug users, recipients of clotting factor concentrates, and persons with chronic liver disease. These guidelines are heavily debated, and many experts believe that more liberal application of the HAV vaccine is necessary.[1,5] Administration of two doses of the vaccine is recommended.

Hepatitis B

I. VIROLOGY AND EPIDEMIOLOGY

1. HBV is a partially double-stranded DNA hepadnavirus that consists of a core (or nucleocapsid) and enclosed DNA.

2. The prevalence of HBV varies markedly worldwide; it is estimated that in parts of Southeast Asia and Africa more than 50% of the population are infected at some point in their lives and more than 8% are chronic carriers of the virus. The World Health Organization (WHO) estimates that 400 million people are infected worldwide. In the United States, where prevalence is markedly lower, an estimated 1.25 million people have chronic infection.[6]

3. Transmission is via parenteral routes. HBV is present in large quantities in serum and is also detectable in semen, saliva, cervical secretions, and leukocytes.

4. Most infections in developed countries occur via sexual activity or injection drug use. No clear risk factors are found in 20% to 30% of patients.

5. Neonatal transmission is a major route of infection in developing countries; however, routine infant immunoprophylaxis has greatly reduced the rate of transmission via this route in the United States.[6]

II. CLINICAL PRESENTATION

1. Clinical features of acute HBV are similar to that of hepatitis A infection; however, the acute infection is more likely to be subclinical.

2. In addition, chronic hepatitis B can be associated with extrahepatic features: polyarteritis nodosa, membranous or membranoproliferative glomerulonephritis, and leukocytoclastic vasculitis. The incubation period is 6 weeks to 6 months (average 12 to 14 weeks).[6]

3. Fulminant acute liver failure (coagulopathy, encephalopathy, cerebral edema) develops in 1% of patients with acute hepatitis B.[7]

4. The rate of clearance varies significantly based on age and immune response. Ninety-five percent of infected neonates will fail to clear the virus and become carriers. Similarly, 30% of children infected before the age of 6 (but after the neonatal period) will remain chronic carriers. However, only 3% to 5% of adults infected with HBV remain chronically infected.[6]

5. Rates of progression to cirrhosis and hepatocellular carcinoma vary according to the state of the immune system, the age of the patient, the serological stage of infection, and geographical and genetic factors.

6. The relative risk of death from cirrhosis in chronic HBV ranges from 12 to 79.[8] The relative risk of hepatocellular carcinoma ranges from 30 to 148. Without treatment, cirrhosis will eventually develop in an estimated 25% to 40% of patients with long-standing chronic hepatitis B.

III. DIAGNOSTICS

1. Infection with HBV is associated with characteristic changes in the serum levels of hepatitis B antigens and antibodies. These serological markers are used to diagnose HBV infection and to define different

49

VIRAL HEPATITIS

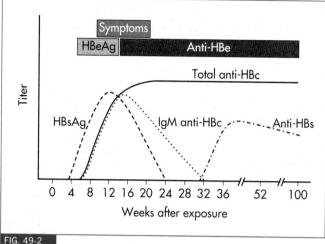

Acute hepatitis B virus infection with recovery, typical serological course. *Anti-HBc,* Antibody to hepatitis B core antigen; *anti-HBe,* antibody to hepatitis B e antigen; *anti-HBs,* antibody to hepatitis B surface antigen; *HBeAg,* hepatitis B e antigen; *HBsAg,* hepatitis B surface antigen. *(From Centers for Disease Control and Prevention: Epidemiology and prevention of viral hepatitis A to E: an overview. www.cdc.gov. Accessed Jan. 15, 2003.)*

clinical states; in addition, quantitative and qualitative tests for HBV DNA can be obtained. The major tests used for evaluation are listed below and illustrated in Figs. 49-2 and 49-3.

2. HBsAg (hepatitis B surface antigen): This is the serological hallmark of HBV infection and typically appears 1 to 10 weeks after acute exposure to HBV, before symptoms develop. Persistence of HBsAg for greater than 6 months defines chronic HBV infection.

3. HBsAb (anti-HBs) (antibody to hepatitis B surface antigen): This antibody is produced in response to exposure to the envelope antigen and confers protective immunity; the antibody is detectable in patients who have recovered from acute hepatitis B and in those immunized with HBV vaccine.

4. HBcAb (anti-HBc IgM/IgG; antibody to hepatitis B core antigen): Hepatitis B core antigen is expressed in infected hepatocytes but is not typically detectable in serum. IgM anti-HBc appears shortly after HBsAg is detected and may persist for 3 to 6 months (or more). IgM anti-HBc may also reappear during flares of chronic hepatitis B. IgG anti-HBc appears during acute hepatitis B and persists indefinitely. These antibodies are not protective.

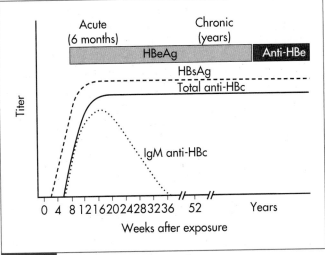

FIG. 49-3

Progression to chronic hepatitis B virus infection, typical serological course. *Anti-HBc,* Antibody to hepatitis B core antigen; *HBsAg,* hepatitis B surface antigen. *(From Centers for Disease Control and Prevention: Epidemiology and prevention of viral hepatitis A to E: an overview. www.cdc.gov. Accessed Jan. 15, 2003.)*

5. HBeAg/HBeAb (anti-Hbe; hepatitis B e antigen): This is a secretory protein that is processed from the precore protein and is generally considered to be a marker of HBV replication and infectivity. Seroconversion from HBeAg to HBeAb can occur and is usually associated with marked decline in HBV DNA in serum and remission of liver disease.

6. HBV DNA: The level of HBV DNA in serum generally parallels the presence of HBeAg; however, very sensitive tests can sometimes detect HBV DNA in persons without HBeAg in serum.[6]

IV. MANAGEMENT

1. Much like HAV, acute hepatitis B infection has no specific treatment. Current therapy consists of supportive measures.

2. Within the past several years two distinct treatments have been established for chronic hepatitis B infection: lamivudine and interferon. With both medications the goal is to reduce the chance that cirrhosis will develop, an outcome that correlates with seroconversion from HBeAg to anti-HBe. Because these drugs have similar efficacy but different delivery, dosage, and toxicity (according to guidelines of the

American Association for the Study of Liver Diseases), either is appropriate for first-line therapy among patients with chronic HBV. Research on additional therapies is ongoing.[9,10]

3. Lamivudine is an oral nucleoside analog that was first recognized to be effective in HBV in studies of human immunodeficiency virus (HIV)-infected patients who were coinfected with HBV. Lamivudine rapidly suppresses HBV DNA and leads to HBeAg seroconversion in 15% to 30% after 1 year of therapy. Histological improvement is seen in approximately 50%. Lamivudine is conveniently given as a daily pill, and side effects are minimal at the dosage used to treat chronic hepatitis.

4. Unfortunately, lamivudine therapy leads to the emergence of resistant variants (called YMDD mutants) in 14% to 45% of patients after 1 year of therapy. Lamivudine was FDA approved for treatment of chronic HBV in 1998.[11,12]

5. Interferon-alfa (both alfa-2a and alfa-2b) is a recombinant agent that has immunomodulatory and antiviral effects. Among carefully selected patients approximately 30% to 40% will seroconvert to anti-HBe and lose HBV DNA after a 4-month course.[13,14]

6. Interferon has significant side effects: flulike symptoms, fever, myalgia, bone marrow suppression, thyroid abnormalities, and depression. It is given as a subcutaneous injection either daily or three times per week. A new pegylated formulation of interferon can be taken once daily.

7. Unlike lamivudine therapy, interferon use does not result in the emergence of variant strains. However, it typically causes a transient increase in hepatic inflammation and transaminase levels. Interferon-alfa was FDA approved for treatment of chronic HBV in 1992.[6,10,15]

V. PROPHYLAXIS

1. The plasma hepatitis B vaccine was introduced in 1982 and results in antibody formation to HBsAg. It has largely been replaced in the United States by recombinant formulations.

2. Protective serum titers of anti-HBs (>10 mIU/mL) develop in 95% of healthy adults who receive a series of three intramuscular doses. Hepatitis B was initially recommended only for persons thought to be at high risk for acquisition of HBV infection; in 1991, however, this policy was changed because the U.S. incidence of HBV had not changed significantly with the prior strategy.

3. Currently WHO endorses the inclusion of hepatitis B vaccine series in routine childhood immunization programs.

4. In addition to vaccination, postexposure prophylaxis can be provided with HBV-specific immunoglobin (HBIG) administration. Within 12 hours of exposure of a susceptible person, the first HBV vaccine dose and HBIG should be given simultaneously in separate sites. Documented vaccine nonresponders require two doses of HBIG given 1 month apart after exposure.[5]

Hepatitis C

I. VIROLOGY AND EPIDEMIOLOGY

1. The hepatitis C virus is a single-stranded RNA flavivirus that infects an estimated 170 million persons worldwide. Prevalence is markedly varied among countries, with the highest recorded prevalence in Egypt (thought to result from use of parenteral antischistosomal therapy; prevalence ranges from 6% to 28%).[16]

2. In the United States approximately 1.8% of the population (4 million people) are HCV seropositive and 2.7 million people are estimated to have ongoing HCV infection.[17] The estimated U.S. incidence is approximately 30,000 new cases per year, and chronic HCV is the single leading cause of chronic liver disease.

3. HCV is the leading indication for liver transplantation.[18]

4. Transmission is parenteral. The major risk factors for acquisition of HCV appear to be intravenous drug use and blood transfusions before 1990. Hepatitis C has 6 genotypes and over 50 subtypes. Genotypes 1a and 1b are the most common in the United States and other Western countries.[18,19]

II. CLINICAL PRESENTATION

1. HCV infection is infrequently diagnosed during the acute phase of illness because the majority of infected persons have minimal or no symptoms at that time. Clinical manifestations, when they do occur, typically begin 7 to 8 weeks (range 2 to 26 weeks) after exposure to HCV and generally consist of jaundice, malaise, and nausea.[20] Acute fulminant hepatitis C infection is documented but rare.[21]

2. HCV is more likely than HBV to lead to chronic infection in exposed adults. An estimated 74% to 86% of exposed adults have persistent viremia.[17,22]

3. Spontaneous clearance of viremia once infection has been established is rare. In time, chronic inflammation and fibrosis associated with nonspecific symptoms such as fatigue develop in most patients. However, serious consequences such as hepatocellular carcinoma and death typically do not occur without the presence of cirrhosis.

4. Cirrhosis develops in approximately 15% to 20% of patients with chronic HCV. The period between inoculation and detection of cirrhosis is highly variable and may exceed 30 years.[20,23]

5. Risk factors associated with rapid progression of cirrhosis include alcohol use, coinfection with HIV or HBV, male sex, and older age.[18,19]

6. Once cirrhosis is established, the risk of hepatocellular carcinoma is approximately 1% to 4% per year.[24]

7. HCV infection is associated with several extrahepatic diseases. HCV is the chief cause of essential mixed cryoglobulinemia, and cryoglobulins can be found in up to half of persons with HCV infection (although few individuals have symptomatic disease).[25,26]

8. Hepatitis C has also been associated with membranoproliferative

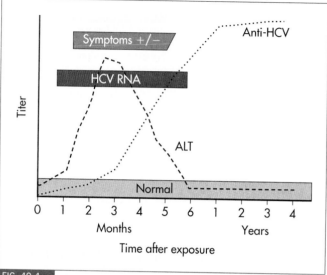

FIG. 49-4

Serological pattern of acute HCV infection with recovery. *ALT,* Alanine aminotransferase; *anti-HCV,* antibody to hepatitis C antigen; *HCV,* hepatitis C virus. *(From Centers for Disease Control and Prevention: Epidemiology and prevention of viral hepatitis A to E: an overview. www.cdc.gov. Accessed Jan. 15, 2003.)*

glomerulonephritis, lichen planus, sicca syndrome, porphyria cutanea tarda, and non-Hodgkin's lymphoma.[18]

III. DIAGNOSTICS

1. Antibodies to HCV (anti-HCV) indicate exposure to the virus and are not protective. In association with abnormalities in liver function tests, this finding is highly suggestive of chronic hepatitis C infection. However, anti-HCV is not diagnostic of ongoing hepatitis C infection.
2. HCV RNA testing is used to assess whether infection is ongoing. HCV RNA testing can be performed as a quantitative or qualitative study.
3. RNA level does not correlate with severity of infection or prognosis and is used chiefly to stratify response to therapy. Knowledge of the HCV genotype is not necessary for diagnosis but may be useful in predicting response to therapy.
4. Once the diagnosis is established, liver biopsy is considered to be the gold standard for assessing severity of infection.[18,19] Typical serological patterns of acute and chronic hepatitis C infection are shown in Figs. 49-4 and 49-5.

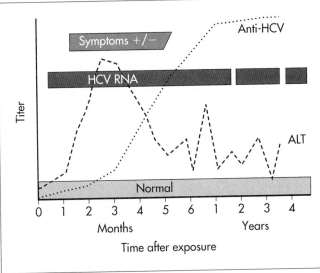

FIG. 49-5

Serological pattern of acute HCV infection with progression to chronic infection. *ALT,* Alanine aminotransferase; *anti-HCV,* antibody to hepatitis C antigen; *HCV,* hepatitis C virus. *(From Centers for Disease Control and Prevention: Epidemiology and prevention of viral hepatitis A to E: an overview. www.cdc.gov. Accessed Jan. 15, 2003.)*

IV. MANAGEMENT

1. Because of the significant prevalence and disease burden associated with HCV, considerable attention has been focused on possible treatment options.
2. Currently, treatment is recommended for patients with persistently elevated transaminase levels, detectable HCV RNA, and histological evidence of fibrosis or inflammation or for patients with significant extrahepatic manifestations of infection.[20,27]
3. Given the length of therapy and the side effects involved, however, the decision to treat HCV infection must be made on an individual basis, with consideration of such factors as age, genotype, and likelihood of progression.[28] Checking HCV quantitative viral load is recommended only if therapy is planned; following viral loads in the absence of active therapy is not predictive of disease course.
4. In initial studies of treatment of chronic HCV, interferon-alfa was used as monotherapy. When it was given in subcutaneous doses three times a week for 12 to 18 months, a biochemical response was seen

in approximately 46% of patients and a sustained virological response was seen in 15% to 20%.[29-31]

5. When interferon-alfa was used in combination with the nucleoside analog ribavirin, an improved rate of sustained virological response was noted.[32,33] In a large multicenter clinical trial the rate of virological response at 48 weeks was 48% with combination therapy and 13% with interferon-alfa alone.[34]

6. Pegylated interferon is created by the addition of a polyethylene glycol moiety to the interferon molecule. This addition extends the half-life and duration of therapeutic activity, resulting in a sustained serum concentration and the ability to use the medication on a once-a-week basis. In several large trials comparing pegylated interferon to standard interferon dosage, the pegylated form improved rates of virological clearance (30% versus 8%,[35] 39% versus 19%,[36] 23% versus 12%[37]).

7. To date, the highest reported rates of sustained virological clearance are with the combination therapy of pegylated interferon and ribavirin. A 54% rate of sustained virological clearance was recently reported in one large trial.[38] The combination was recently approved by the FDA and is the current standard of care (assuming there are no contraindications) for treatment of chronic HCV.[39]

8. Interferon is associated with significant side effects, including flulike symptoms, headache, rigors, fatigue, fever, myalgias, thrombocytopenia, depression, diarrhea, and leukocytopenia. Interferon is contraindicated for patients with psychosis, severe depression, neutropenia, thrombocytopenia, symptomatic heart disease, decompensated cirrhosis, uncontrolled seizures, or organ transplant.

9. Side effects of ribavirin include hemolysis, nausea, anemia, nasal congestion, and pruritus.

10. Ribavirin is contraindicated in pregnancy, end-stage renal disease, anemia, hemoglobinopathy, and severe heart disease.

11. Several factors were predictive of higher response rates to HCV treatment. Patients with mild histological disease had better outcomes than those with significant evidence of fibrosis or cirrhosis. Patients with genotypes 2 or 3 did significantly better than those with genotypes 1 or 4 (unfortunately, genotype 1 is the most common in the United States and western Europe). Patients with higher viral loads tended to have lower rates of sustained virological clearance.[15,18,40]

V. PROPHYLAXIS

1. No clinical benefit has been shown with immune globulin prophylaxis, and it is not recommended after exposure. No vaccine for hepatitis C is available.

2. Needle-stick transmission of HCV is an important concern for health

care workers. It is not possible to prevent infection after exposure to HCV, and HCV infection will develop in an estimated 2% to 10% of exposed individuals.

3. Since clinical symptoms may be slight, at a minimum the HCV antibody and alanine aminotransferase (ALT) levels should be measured within several days of exposure and 6 months thereafter.

4. Recent data suggest that treatment of acute HCV infection with interferon may be highly effective in preventing chronic HCV infection.[41] In one recent study viral clearance occurred in 98% of patients.[42]

PEARLS AND PITFALLS

- Hepatitis A.
  - Diagnosis of acute HAV infection is based on detection of IgM antibody; IgG antibody has no role in evaluation of acute HAV infection, and the test should not be ordered.
  - The HAV vaccine should be offered to all patients with HCV infection and should be administered in two doses scheduled 6 months apart.
- Hepatitis B.
  - Diagnosis of acute HBV infection is based on detection of HBsAg and IgM anti-HBc.
  - Chronic HBV infection is defined by persistence of HBsAg or HBV DNA for longer than 6 months.
  - Infectivity and replication of HBV correlate with the presence of HBeAg.
  - Treatment of chronic HBV infection is aimed at reducing the risk of cirrhosis and hepatocellular carcinoma, which correlates with seroconversion of HBeAg to anti-HBe.
- Hepatitis C.
  - Initial diagnosis of HCV infection should be based on levels of HCV-antibody rather than HCV RNA (because of the relative expense of the tests).
  - If acute HCV infection is suspected, HCV RNA should be measured as well as HCV-antibody.
  - If a patient with risk factors or an elevated ALT level is found to be HCV-antibody positive, first the patient should be counseled regarding the probability of infection, the potential risk of transmission, and cessation of alcohol. After that, the likelihood that treatment will be helpful and possible in the upcoming months should be assessed. HCV RNA testing, genotype studies, and liver biopsy can be deferred to the outpatient setting, given the expense and low clinical relevance if treatment is not anticipated.
  - HCV infection develops in 2% to 10% of people exposed by needlestick. Prophylaxis is not indicated; however, treatment of acute HCV with interferon has been shown to be remarkably effective, with one study reporting a 98% rate of viral clearance.[42]
- Hepatitis D.
  - The hepatitis D virus, or delta agent, is a defective, single-stranded

RNA-containing passenger virus that requires the presence of hepatitis B virus for its expression.[43]

- HDV infection occurs either as a simultaneous infection with hepatitis B virus or as a superinfection in an HBV carrier.
- HDV is an important consideration as the cause of hepatitis flare-up in a person with chronic hepatitis B infection or fulminant acute hepatitis B infection. HDV is most prevalent in the Mediterranean countries, the Middle East, and northern Africa. It is relatively uncommon in the United States except among intravenous drug users.
- HDV is detected by measurement of anti-HDV or HDV RNA. The combination of chronic HBV and HDV portends a poor prognosis with increased disease severity.[44,45]
- Clinical trials of combined treatment for HBV and HDV have been disappointing to date.[15,46]
- Hepatitis E.
  - Hepatitis E virus is a single-stranded RNA virus similar to the Caliciviridae family. It is transmitted by the fecal-oral route. Hepatitis E is rare in the United States but has been responsible for large outbreaks of waterborne hepatitis infection in India, Burma, Afghanistan, Algeria, and Mexico.[47,48] In the largest recorded outbreak more than 100,000 individuals were infected in the Xinjiang region of China.[49]
  - Illness is limited because there is no carrier state, and the mortality rate in nonpregnant patients is low. For reasons that are not understood, fulminant hepatic failure occurs more frequently during pregnancy, particularly in the third trimester, and results in a 15% to 25% mortality rate in this population.[50,51]
  - Diagnosis is confirmed by detection of anti-HEV IgM (this test is not commercially available but can be obtained from the Centers for Disease Control and Prevention through a research protocol). Treatment is supportive.
- Hepatitis G (hepatitis GB virus-C).
  - The hepatitis G virus (appropriately called hepatitis GB virus-C) is a flavivirus that is parenterally transmitted and associated with chronic viremia.
  - In several trials GB virus-C has been detected in more than 50% of intravenous drug users,[52] 20% of patients receiving hemodialysis,[53] 6% to 71% of hemophilic patients,[54] and approximately 2% of eligible blood donors.[55,56]
  - No causal relationship between GB virus-C and clinical hepatitis in humans has been established.[2,56]
- Acute viral hepatitis according to type is shown in Fig. 49-6. Table 49-1 provides estimates of the acute and chronic disease burden for viral hepatitis, and Table 49-2 gives an overview of viral hepatitis.

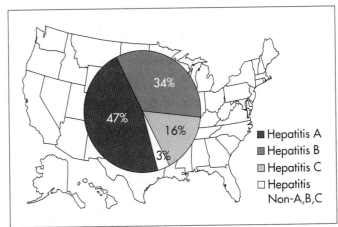

FIG. 49-6

Acute viral hepatitis by type, United States, 1982-1993. *(From Centers for Disease Control and Prevention: CDC Sentinel Counties Study on Viral Hepatitis. www.cdc.gov. Accessed Jan. 15, 2003.)*

TABLE 49-1

ESTIMATES OF ACUTE AND CHRONIC DISEASE BURDEN FOR VIRAL HEPATITIS, UNITED STATES

	Type of Hepatitis			
	A	B	C	D
Acute infections (×1000) per year*	125-200	140-320	35-180	6-13
Fulminant deaths per year	100	150	?	35
Chronic infections	0	1 million–1.25 million	3.5 million	70,000
Chronic liver disease deaths per year	0	5000	8000-10,000	1000

From Centers for Disease Control and Prevention: Epidemiology and prevention of viral hepatitis A to E: an overview. www.cdc.gov. Accessed Jan. 15, 2003.
*Range based on estimated annual incidence, 1984-1994.

TABLE 49-2
VIRAL HEPATITIS OVERVIEW

	Type of Hepatitis				
	A	B	C	D	E
Source of virus	Feces	Blood and blood-derived body fluids	Blood and blood-derived body fluids	Blood and blood-derived body fluids	Feces
Route of transmission	Fecal-oral	Percutaneous permucosal	Percutaneous permucosal	Percutaneous permucosal	Fecal-oral
Chronic infection	No	Yes	Yes	Yes	No
Prevention	Preexposure and postexposure immunization	Preexposure and postexposure immunization	Blood donor screening; risk behavior modification	Preexposure and postexposure immunization; risk behavior modification	Ensuring safe drinking water

From Centers for Disease Control and Prevention: Epidemiology and prevention of viral hepatitis A to E: an overview. www.cdc.gov. Accessed Jan. 15, 2003.

REFERENCES

[c] 1. Koff RS. Hepatitis A. Lancet 1998; 351:1643.
[b] 2. Alter MJ et al. Acute A-E hepatitis in the United States and the role of hepatitis G virus infection. N Engl J Med 1997; 336:741.
[b] 3. Lednar WM et al. Frequency of illness associated with epidemic hepatitis A virus infections in adults. Am J Epidemiol 1985; 122:226.
[b] 4. Tong MJ et al. Clinical manifestations of hepatitis A: recent experience in a community teaching hospital. J Infect Dis 1995; 171S1:S15.
[c] 5. Lemon SM, Thomas DL. Vaccines to prevent viral hepatitis. N Engl J Med 1997; 336:196.
[c] 6. Lee WM. Hepatitis B virus infection. N Engl J Med 1997; 337:1733.
[c] 7. Lee WM. Acute liver failure. N Engl J Med 1993; 329:1862.
[a] 8. McMahon BJ et al. Hepatitis B–related sequelae: prospective study in 1400 hepatitis B surface antigen positive Alaska native carriers. Arch Intern Med 1990; 150:1051.
[c] 9. Maddrey WC. Update in hepatology. Ann Intern Med 2001; 134:216.
[d 10. Malik AH, Lee WM. Chronic hepatitis B infection: treatment strategies for the next millennium. Ann Intern Med 2000; 132:723.
[a] 11. Dienstag JL et al. Lamivudine is a tolerable, effective therapy for hepatitis B. N Engl J Med 1999; 341:1256.
[a] 12. Lai CL et al. A one-year trial of lamivudine for chronic hepatitis B. N Engl J Med 1998; 339:61.
[a] 13. Hoofnagle JH et al. Randomized controlled trial of recombinant human alfa-interferon in patients with chronic hepatitis B. Gastroenterology 1988; 95:1318.
[a] 14. Wong DKH et al. Effect of alpha-interferon treatment in patients with hepatitis B e antigen-positive chronic hepatitis B: a meta-analysis. Ann Intern Med 1993; 119:312.
[c] 15. Hoofnagle JH, Di Bisceglie AM. The treatment of chronic viral hepatitis. N Engl J Med 1997; 336:347.
[c] 16. Frank C et al. The role of parenteral antischistosomal therapy in the spread of hepatitis C virus in Egypt. Lancet 2000; 355:887.
[b] 17. Alter MJ et al. The prevalence of hepatitis C virus infection in the United States, 1988 through 1994. N Engl J Med 1999; 341:556.
[c] 18. Lauer GM, Walker BD. Hepatitis C virus infection. N Engl J Med 2001; 345:41.
[c] 19. Di Bisceglie AM. Hepatitis C. Lancet 1998; 351:351.
[d] 20. National Institutes of Health Consensus Development Conference Panel statement: management of hepatitis C. Hepatology 1997; 26:2S.
[b] 21. Farci P et al. Hepatitis C virus–associated fulminant hepatic failure. N Engl J Med 1996; 335:631.
[b] 22. Conry-Cantilena C et al. Routes of infection, viremia, and liver disease in blood donors found to have hepatitis C virus infection. N Engl J Med 1996; 334:1691.
[d] 23. EASL International Consensus Conference on Hepatitis C: Paris, 26-28, February 1999, consensus statement. J Hepatol 1999; 30:956.
[c] 24. Di Bisceglie AM. Hepatitis C and hepatocellular carcinoma. Hepatology 1997; 26:34S.
[b] 25. Agnello V et al. A role for hepatitis C virus infection in type II cryoglobulinemia. N Engl J Med 1992; 327:1490.
[b] 26. Horcajada JP et al. Mixed cryoglobulinaemia in patients with chronic hepatitis C infection: prevalence, significance and relationship with different viral genotypes. Ann Med 1999; 31:352.
[c] 27. Liang TJ et al. Pathogenesis, natural history, treatment, and prevention of hepatitis C. Ann Intern Med 2000; 132:296.
[a] 28. Mathurin P. Slow progression rate of fibrosis in hepatitis C virus patients with persistently normal transaminase levels: a pilot randomized controlled study. Hepatology 1998; 27:868.
[a] 29. Poynard T et al. Meta-analysis of interferon randomized trials in the treatment of viral hepatitis C: effects of dose and duration. Hepatology 1996; 24:778.
[a] 30. Lindsay KL et al. Response to higher doses of interferon alfa-2b in patients with hepatitis C: a randomized multicenter trial. Hepatology 1996; 24:1034.
[a] 31. Shiffman ML. Use of high-dose interferon in the treatment of chronic hepatitis C. Semin Liver Dis 1999; 19S1:25.

49

VIRAL HEPATITIS

[a] 32. Poynard T et al. Randomized trial of interferon alfa-2b plus ribavirin for 48 weeks or for 24 weeks versus interferon alfa-2b plus placebo for 48 weeks for treatment of chronic infection with hepatitis C virus. Lancet 1998; 352:1426.

[a] 33. Davis GL et al. Interferon alfa-2b alone or in combination with ribavirin for the treatment of relapse from chronic hepatitis C. N Engl J Med 1998; 339:1493.

[a] 34. McHutchinson JG et al. Interferon alfa-2b alone or in combination with ribavirin as initial treatment for chronic hepatitis C. N Engl J Med 1993; 339:1485.

[a] 35. Heathcote EJ et al. Peginterferon alfa-2a in patients with chronic hepatitis C and cirrhosis. N Engl J Med 2000; 343:1673.

[a] 36. Zeuzem S et al. Peginterferon alfa-2a in patients with chronic hepatitis C. N Engl J Med 2000; 343:1666.

[a] 37. Lindsay KL et al. A randomized, double-blind trial comparing pegylated interferon alfa-2b to interferon alfa-2b as initial treatment for chronic hepatitis C. Hepatology 2001; 34:395.

[a] 38. Manns MP et al. Peginterferon alfa-2b plus ribavirin compared with interferon alfa-2b plus ribavirin for initial treatment of chronic hepatitis C: a randomised trial. Lancet 2001; 358:958.

[d] 39. National Institutes of Health Consensus Development Program Statement: management of hepatitis C: 2002. June 10-12, 2002 (draft statement via NIH website: http://consensus.nih.gov).

[c] 40. Sharieff KA et al. Advances in treatment of chronic hepatitis C: "pegylated" interferons. Cleve Clin J Med 2002; 69:155.

[b] 41. Sulkowski MS et al. Needlestick transmission of hepatitis C. JAMA 2002; 287:2406.

[b] 42. Jaeckel E et al. Treatment of acute hepatitis C with interferon alfa-2b. N Engl J Med 2001; 345:1452.

[c] 43. Rizzetto M, Verme G. Delta hepatitis—present status. J Hepatol 1985; 1:187.

[c] 44. Govindarajan S et al. Fulminant B viral hepatitis: role of delta agent. Gastroenterology 1984; 86:1417.

[b] 45. Smedile et al. Influence of delta infection on severity of hepatitis B. Lancet 1982; 2:945.

[a] 46. Farci P et al. Treatment of chronic hepatitis D with interferon alfa-2a. N Engl J Med 1994; 330:88.

[d] 47. Skidmore SJ. Hepatitis E. Br Med J 1995; 310:414.

[c] 48. Balayan MS. Epidemiology of hepatitis E virus infection. J Viral Hepat 1997; 4:155.

[c] 49. Zhuang H. Hepatitis E and strategies for its control. In Wen Y, editor. Viral hepatitis in China: problems and control strategies. Monogr Virol 1992; 19:126.

[b] 50. Khuroo MS et al. Incidence and severity of viral hepatitis in pregnancy. Am J Med 1981; 70:252.

[b] 51. Hussaini SH et al. Severe hepatitis E infection during pregnancy. J Viral Hepat 1997; 4:51.

[b] 52. Thomas DL et al. Association of antibody to GB virus C (hepatitis G virus) with viral clearance and protection from reinfection. J Infect Dis 1998; 177:539.

[c] 53. Alter HJ. The cloning and clinical implications of HGV and HGBV-C. N Engl J Med 1996; 334:1536.

[b] 54. Mauser-Bunschoten EP et al. Hepatitis G virus RNA and hepatitis G virus-E2 antibodies in Dutch hemophilia patients in relation to transfusion history. Blood 1998; 92:2164.

[c] 55. Linnen et al. Molecular cloning and disease association of hepatitis G virus: a transfusion-transmissible agent. Science 1996; 271:505.

[b] 56. Alter HJ et al. The incidence of transfusion-associated hepatitis G virus infection and its relation to liver disease. N Engl J Med 1997; 336:747.

Acute Renal Failure

John J. Friedewald, MD, and Michael J. Choi, MD

FAST FACTS

- Acute renal failure (ARF) is defined as a rise in creatinine level of greater than 0.5 over baseline or a decrease in glomerular filtration rate (GFR) by 50% over a period of days to weeks.
- ARF develops in 5% of hospitalized patients.[1]
- Approximately 30% of patients with ARF require dialysis.[2]
- Infection accounts for 75% of deaths in patients with ARF, followed by cardiopulmonary complications.[3]
- Depending on severity of patient illness, mortality from ARF can range from 7% to 80% in intensive care unit and postoperative patients.[4]
- The underlying cause of acute renal failure is prerenal in 60% to 70% of cases, intrinsic in 25% to 40% of cases, and postrenal in 5% to 10% of cases.[3]
- Associated electrolyte abnormalities (e.g., hyperkalemia) should be diagnosed rapidly and treated appropriately.

50

I. EPIDEMIOLOGY

1. ARF is a common condition, but because of varied definitions its incidence has proved difficult to quantify in large studies. The frequency among patients is 1% at admission, 2% to 5% during hospitalization, and up to 4% to 15% after cardiopulmonary bypass.[4]
2. ARF is characterized by a decline in renal function or the GFR over a period of hours to days. This decline leads to an inability of the kidney to excrete nitrogenous waste products and to maintain fluid and electrolyte balance.

II. CLINICAL PRESENTATION

1. Patients with ARF are often asymptomatic. However, certain clues in the history and physical examination can suggest the presence of ARF. A history of exposure to nephrotoxic medications, recent angiography, or findings associated with volume depletion can lead to a diagnosis. Anuria is an important clue that suggests a postrenal cause. Signs of tissue ischemia may suggest rhabdomyolysis. A rash may accompany allergic interstitial nephritis. Signs of emboli in the legs or livedo reticularis may suggest an atheroembolic cause of ARF, especially in patients with recent intravascular catheter manipulations. Signs of systemic vasculitis such as palpable purpura, pulmonary hemorrhage, and sinusitis might herald glomerulonephritis as a cause of ARF.
2. ARF can be divided into three categories: prerenal failure, intrinsic renal failure, and postrenal failure. A careful history and physical

examination should help focus the differential diagnosis (Table 50-1). Special attention should be paid to recent medications (Table 50-2).

III. DIAGNOSTICS (Fig. 50-1)

A. LABORATORY STUDIES

1. Measuring levels of serum creatinine and blood urea nitrogen (BUN) is crucial in making the diagnosis of ARF. In addition, all patients should have a basic metabolic panel; measurement of calcium, phosphorus, albumin, uric acid, and creatine kinase levels; complete blood cell count with differential; and liver function tests. Eosinophilia with a history of drug exposure may suggest allergic interstitial nephritis as a cause. An abnormal serum electrophoresis may suggest myeloma as the cause of ARF. A plasma BUN/creatinine ratio should be calculated. A BUN/creatinine ratio greater than 20 favors a prerenal cause, whereas ratios between 10 and 20 favor intrinsic or postrenal failure, with caveats as mentioned in the "Pearls and Pitfalls" section below. All patients should have a urinalysis with urine indices (urine sodium and creatinine levels with urine osmolality determination) in cases of oliguric renal failure.

2. The urine sediment should be examined by light microscopy. In prerenal ARF a bland urinary sediment is the norm with trace or no proteinuria and perhaps a few hyaline casts. Heme-positive urine in the absence of red blood cells suggests the presence of myoglobin or hemoglobin as seen in rhabdomyolysis or transfusion reaction. Pigmented granular casts are typically found in ischemic or toxic acute renal failure or acute tubular necrosis (ATN). White blood cell casts can be seen in interstitial nephritis and red blood cell casts in glomerulonephritis. Urine eosinophils may suggest AIN but can also be present in atheroembolic disease and pyelonephritis. Oxalate crystals may be seen in cases of ethylene glycol toxicity.

3. The fractional excretion of sodium ($Fe_{Na} - [P_{Cr}/U_{Cr}]/[P_{Na}/U_{Na}]$, where P is plasma and U is urine) should be calculated for all patients with oliguria. An Fe_{Na} of less than 1% is common in euvolemic subjects with normal sodium balance and renal function and moderate salt intake.[5] Clinically, a high Fe_{Na} (>1%) is most often due to ATN but may also be seen in volume depletion (up to 10% of the time) or in volume depletion with ongoing diuretic therapy (causing salt wasting). Conversely, a low Fe_{Na} (<1%) is more commonly associated with prerenal causes of ARF (with the exceptions stated in Box 50-1).

4. Hyperkalemia can complicate ARF and requires prompt therapy (see section on hyperkalemia).

5. Uremia can lead to several dangerous conditions and may be an indication for emergency dialysis (see later discussion). Encephalopathy, pericarditis, bleeding (resulting from platelet dysfunction caused by uremia), nausea and vomiting, and pruritus may all be seen with elevations in the serum urea nitrogen concentration. The history

TABLE 50-1
DIFFERENTIAL DIAGNOSIS OF ACUTE RENAL FAILURE

Type of Acute Renal Failure and Underlying Problem	Possible Disorders
Prerenal acute renal failure	
True intravascular depletion	Sepsis, hemorrhage, overdiuresis, poor fluid intake, vomiting, diarrhea
Decreased effective circulating volume to the kidneys	Congestive heart failure, cirrhosis or hepatorenal syndrome, nephrotic syndrome
Impaired renal blood flow because of exogenous agents	Angiotensin-converting enzyme inhibitors, nonsteroidal antiinflammatory drugs
Intrinsic acute renal failure	
Acute tubular necrosis	Ischemia
	Toxins: drugs (e.g., aminoglycosides), contrast agents, pigments (myoglobin or hemoglobin)
Glomerular disease	Rapidly progressive glomerulonephritis: systemic lupus erythematosus, small-vessel vasculitis (Wegener's granulomatosis or microscopic polyangiitis), Henoch-Schönlein purpura (immunoglobulin A nephropathy), Goodpasture's syndrome
	Acute proliferative glomerulonephritis: endocarditis, poststreptococcal infection, postpneumococcal infection
Vascular disease	Microvascular disease: atheroembolic disease (cholesterol plaque microembolism), thrombotic thrombocytopenic purpura, hemolytic-uremic syndrome, HELLP syndrome, or postpartum acute renal failure
	Macrovascular disease: renal artery occlusion, severe abdominal aortic disease (aneurysm)
Interstitial disease	Allergic reaction to drugs, autoimmune disease (systemic lupus erythematosus or mixed connective tissue disease), pyelonephritis, infiltrative disease (lymphoma or leukemia)
Postrenal acute renal failure	Benign prostatic hypertrophy or prostate cancer, cervical cancer, retroperitoneal disorders, intratubular obstruction (crystals or myeloma light chains), pelvic mass or invasive pelvic malignancy, intraluminal bladder mass (clot, tumor, or fungus ball), neurogenic bladder, urethral strictures

Modified from Agrawal M, Swartz R. Am Fam Phys 2000; 61(7):2077.
HELLP, Hemolysis, elevated liver enzymes, and low platelet count.

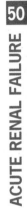

ACUTE RENAL FAILURE

50

TABLE 50-2

DRUGS ASSOCIATED WITH ACUTE RENAL FAILURE

Mechanism	Drug
Reduction in renal perfusion through alteration of intrarenal hemodynamics	NSAIDs, angiotensin-converting enzyme inhibitors, cyclosporine, tacrolimus (FK506), radiocontrast agents, amphotericin B, interleukin-2*
Direct tubular toxicity	Aminoglycosides, radiocontrast agents, cisplatin, cyclosporine, tacrolimus, amphotericin B, methotrexate, foscarnet, pentamadine, organic solvents, heavy metals, intravenous immune globulin†
Heme pigment–induced tubular toxicity (rhabdomyolysis)	Cocaine, ethanol, lovastatin‡
Intratubular obstruction by precipitation of the agent	Acyclovir, sulfonamides, ethylene glycol,§ chemotherapeutic agents,¶ methotrexate
Allergic interstitial nephritis‖	Penicillins, cephalosporins, sulfonamides, rifampin, ciprofloxacin, NSAIDs, thiazide diuretics, furosemide, cimetidine, phenytoin, allopurinol
Hemolytic-uremic syndrome	Cyclosporine, tacrolimus, mitomycin, cocaine, quinine, conjugated estrogens

Modified from Thadhani R, Pascual M, Bonventre JV. N Engl J Med 1996; 334:1448.
NSAIDs, Nonsteroidal antiinflammatory drugs.
*Interleukin-2 produces a capillary leak syndrome with volume contraction.
†Mechanism unclear; may be due to additives.
‡ARF most likely to occur when lovastatin is given in combination with cyclosporine.
§Ethylene glycol–induced toxicity can cause calcium oxalate crystals.
¶Uric acid crystals may form as a result of tumor lysis.
‖Many other drugs in addition to those listed here cause allergic interstitial nephritis.

and physical examination of a patient with ARF should include specific queries to rule out these conditions.

B. RADIOLOGICAL STUDIES

1. Urinary outlet obstruction must be ruled out early in the evaluation of ARF, particularly in patients with severe oliguria or anuria.
2. Bladder catheterization is simple and can rule out urethral obstruction.
3. Renal ultrasound is used to rule out obstruction, but its sensitivity may be only 80% to 85%.[4] False negative results caused by a nondilated collecting system may occur with acute obstruction, retroperitoneal fibrosis, or hypovolemia. Ultrasound also provides valuable information about renal size, echotexture, and vasculature. Small kidneys may indicate a more chronic renal failure.
4. A spiral computed tomography (CT) scan without contrast media can be performed to evaluate for urolithiasis. An important exception is that a CT scan cannot reliably detect indinavir calculi.[6]

C. RENAL BIOPSY

1. In most cases of ARF, renal biopsy is not necessary for diagnosis. If the aforementioned studies suggest an intrinsic cause of ARF that is

BOX 50-1

CLINICAL STATES IN WHICH FRACTIONAL EXCRETION OF SODIUM MAY BE LOW (<1%)

Nonazotemic: normal renal function, moderate sodium intake

Azotemic: volume depletion

Hepatic failure

   Congestive heart failure

   Acute glomerulonephritis

   Myoglobinuric or hemoglobinuric acute renal failure (oliguric phase)

   Contrast nephrotoxicity (oliguric phase)

   Polyuric renal failure with severe burns

   Renal transplant rejection

   Nonoliguric acute tubular necrosis (10% of cases)

   Early acute interstitial nephritis

   Acute urinary tract obstruction

Modified from Steiner RW. Am J Med 1984; 77:699.

50

ACUTE RENAL FAILURE

not toxic or ischemic tubular necrosis (ATN), a biopsy may be of value.

2. A study of patients with ARF who underwent renal biopsy showed that knowledge of the specific histological picture changed management in nearly three fourths of cases.[7]

IV. MANAGEMENT

1. Initial therapy of ARF is directed toward reversing the underlying cause and correcting fluid and electrolyte abnormalities.

2. Medications that are primarily eliminated by the kidney should be administered at appropriate dosage levels to avoid toxicity.

3. Hyperkalemia and other electrolyte abnormalities should be treated as previously discussed.

4. Relief of urinary obstruction should be addressed early in the evaluation, particularly in patients with anuria.

5. Metabolic acidosis, if severe (bicarbonate level <12 mEq/L or pH <7.2), can be treated with sodium bicarbonate in either oral or intravenous forms. The base deficit can be calculated to determine how much bicarbonate is needed, according to the following formula: bicarbonate deficit (mEq/L) = $0.5 \times$ weight (kg) $\times$ (24 − measured serum HCO_3^-). This formula is conservative and may underestimate the true deficit with serum bicarbonate levels below 10 mEq/L.[8]

6. Volume-depleted states should be treated with infusions of saline. However, patients with oliguria or anuria often have volume overload at presentation. Furosemide should initially be used to treat hypervolemia. A dose between 20 and 100 mg should be administered, and if an adequate response is not achieved in the first hour, the dose should be doubled. If the volume overload is life threatening and not

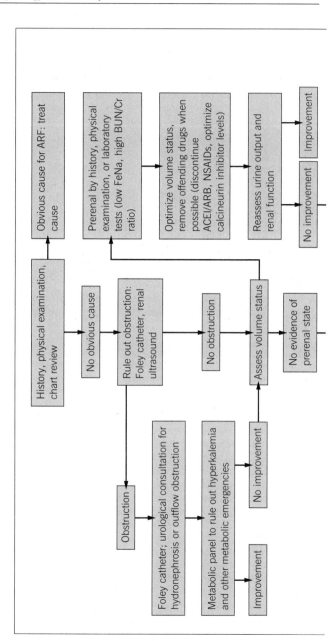

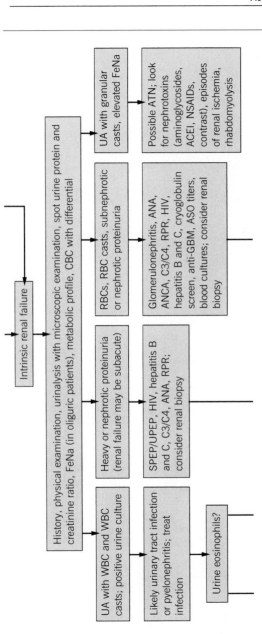

FIG. 50-1

Diagnosis and management of a patient with acute renal failure. *ACEI*, Angiotensin-converting enzyme inhibitor; *ANA*, antinuclear antibody; *ANCA*, antineutrophilic cytoplasmic antibody; *anti-GBM*, anti-glomerular basement membrane antibody; *ARB*, angiotensin receptor blocker; *ARF*, acute renal failure; *ASO*, antistreptolysin O; *ATN*, acute tubular necrosis; *BUN/Cr*, blood urea nitrogen/creatinine; *C3/C4*, complements 3 and 4; *CBC*, complete blood cell count; *FeNa*, fractional excretion of sodium; *FSGS*, focal segmental glomerulosclerosis; *HIV*, human immunodeficiency virus; *HSP*, Henoch-Schönlein purpura; *NSAIDs*, nonsteroidal antiinflammatory drugs; *RBC*, red blood cell; *RPR*, rapid plasma reagin; *SLE*, systemic lupus erythematosus; *SPEP*, serum protein electrophoresis; *UA*, urinalysis; *UPEP*, urine protein electrophoresis; *WBC*, white blood cell (count).

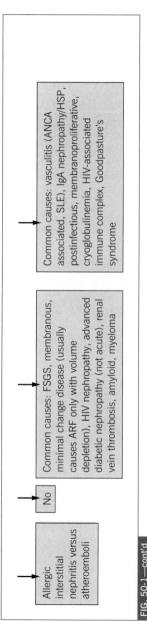

Allergic interstitial nephritis versus atheroemboli

No

Common causes: FSGS, membranous, minimal change disease (usually causes ARF only with volume depletion), HIV nephropathy, advanced diabetic nephropathy (not acute), renal vein thrombosis, amyloid, myeloma

Common causes: vasculitis (ANCA associated, SLE), IgA nephropathy/HSP, postinfectious, membranoproliferative, cryoglobulinemia, HIV-associated immune complex, Goodpasture's syndrome

FIG. 50-1—cont'd

Diagnosis and management of a patient with acute renal failure. *ACEI*, Angiotensin-converting enzyme inhibitor; *ANA*, antinuclear antibody; *ANCA*, antineutrophilic cytoplasmic antibody; *anti-GBM*, anti-glomerular basement membrane antibody; *ARB*, angiotensin receptor blocker; *ARF*, acute renal failure; *ASO*, antistreptolysin O; *ATN*, acute tubular necrosis; *BUN/Cr*, blood urea nitrogen/creatinine; *C3/C4*, complements 3 and 4; *CBC*, complete blood cell count; *FeNa*, fractional excretion of sodium; *FSGS*, focal segmental glomerulosclerosis; *HIV*, human immunodeficiency virus; *HSP*, Henoch-Schönlein purpura; *NSAIDs*, nonsteroidal antiinflammatory drugs; *RBC*, red blood cell; *RPR*, rapid plasma reagin; *SLE*, systemic lupus erythematosus; *SPEP*, serum protein electrophoresis; *UA*, urinalysis; *UPEP*, urine protein electrophoresis; *WBC*, white blood cell (count).

adequately treated with medication, ultrafiltration via dialysis may be necessary (see later discussion). No trials have studied the effectiveness of diuretics in modifying the course of ARF when used solely to change from an oliguric to a nonoliguric state. In a study of ICU patients with acute renal failure, an association was observed between the use of diuretics and both an increased risk of death and nonrecovery of renal function. Because of the design of the trial, however, a causal relationship between diuretic use and death or nonrecovery of renal function could not be established.[10]

7. Dopamine is commonly used in patients with ARF. When used in low, "renal" doses (1-3 $\mu g \cdot kg^{-1} \cdot min^{-1}$ IV), it is thought to selectively dilate splanchnic vasculature and increase renal blood flow. Although dopamine has been shown to be natriuretic and phosphaturic, no trials have demonstrated that dopamine has a favorable effect on the course of ARF.[2]

8. Renal replacement therapy with hemodialysis, peritoneal dialysis, or continuous dialysis and hemofiltration is recommended for severe derangements encountered in ARF. In any of the following settings consultation with a nephrologist is warranted. The mnemonic "AEIOU" can be used to help recall the indications for acute dialysis.

a. Acidosis: Life-threatening acidosis in the setting of ARF.

b. Electrolyte imbalances such as severe hyperkalemia.

c. Ingestions: Certain toxic ingestions can be cleared by dialysis (ethylene glycol, lithium, paraldehyde, phenytoin, and salicylates are commonly seen members of a long list).

d. Overload: Volume overload refractory to diuretic therapy.

e. Uremia: Some people use a BUN level greater than 100 mg/dL as the criterion, but also in the case of uremic pericarditis, encephalopathy, or nausea and vomiting caused by uremia.

PEARLS AND PITFALLS

• The evaluation of ARF among patients with renal allografts should not differ from that for other patients. Prerenal ARF in the setting of volume depletion is complicated by the vasoconstrictive effects of calcineurin inhibitors (cyclosporine and tacrolimus). ARF may develop in renal transplant recipients as a result of acute calcineurin inhibitor toxicity. When this occurs, trough levels of these medications should be followed closely and the patient should be asked about any recently started drugs. Medication interactions are a frequent cause of toxic levels of calcineurin inhibitors. Obstructive uropathy caused by trauma, ureteral stenosis, or compression by lymphocele is common and may necessitate evaluation of the graft by ultrasonography. Acute rejection is an intrinsic cause of ARF and may be suggested by subtherapeutic levels of immunosuppressive agents. Renal biopsy is often performed to assess for the presence and level of rejection.

• False elevations of serum creatinine (pseudoacute renal failure) may occur when substances (e.g., ketoacids, cefoxitin) are falsely analyzed as creatinine. Trimethoprim and cimetidine can inhibit renal tubular

50

ACUTE RENAL FAILURE

secretion of creatinine, and increased muscle protein breakdown (creatine) may increase creatinine production. Common elevations of BUN not associated with renal failure are seen in patients receiving corticosteroids, those with increased catabolism, or those with gastrointestinal tract bleeding.

- Use of radiocontrast agents commonly leads to acute reductions in renal function, especially in patients with preexisting renal dysfunction, diabetic nephropathy, or hypovolemia or those taking drugs that affect renal blood flow (e.g., angiotensin-converting enzyme inhibitors). Recent evidence suggests that in addition to hydration with saline before and after the procedure (in this study a contrast-enhanced CT scan), administration of the antioxidant *N*-acetylcysteine (Mucomyst 600 mg PO bid before and after the procedure) can prevent reductions in renal function in patients with preexisting renal insufficiency (patients had a mean serum creatinine level of 2.4 mg/dL).[9]
- In patients with ARF that will probably progress to chronic renal failure, long-term vascular access should be a priority from the outset. Because patients receiving long-term hemodialysis often have vascular access created in an upper extremity, care should be taken to protect the non-dominant arm. In particular, placement of indwelling catheters in the subclavian vein should be avoided to reduce the risk of stenosis of that vessel. Subclavian stenosis can lead to outflow problems from a vascular shunt created in that arm.

REFERENCES

[c] 1. Nolan CR, Anderson RJ. Hospital-acquired acute renal failure. J Am Soc Nephrol 1998; 9:710.

[c] 2. Albright RC. Acute renal failure: a practical update. Mayo Clin Proc 2001; 76:67.

[c] 3. Agrawal M, Swartz R. Acute renal failure. Am Fam Phys 2000; 61(7):2077.

[c] 4. Thadhani R, Pascual M, Bonventre JV. Acute renal failure. N Engl J Med 1996; 334:1448.

[c] 5. Steiner RW. Interpreting the fractional excretion of sodium. Am J Med 1984; 77:699.

[b] 6. Schwartz BF et al. Imaging characteristics of indinavir calculi. J Urol 1999; 161:1085.

[b] 7. Richards NT et al. Knowledge of renal histology alters patient management in over 40% of cases. Nephrol Dial Transplant 1994; 9:1255.

[c] 8. Fernandez PC, Cohen RM, Feldman GM. The concept of bicarbonate distribution space: the crucial role of body buffers. Kidney Int 1989; 36:747.

[a] 9. Tepel M et al. Prevention of radiographic-contrast-agent-induced reductions in renal function by acetylcysteine. N Engl J Med 2000; 343:180.

[b] 10. Mehta R et al. Diuretics, mortality, and nonrecovery of renal function in acute renal failure. JAMA 2002; 288(20):2547.

Magnesium and Phosphate Disorders

Peter V. Johnston, MD, and Milagros Samaniego, MD

51

FAST FACTS

- Disorders of magnesium.
  - Normal serum magnesium levels range between 1.3 and 2 mEq/L. Between 60% and 70% of the body's magnesium is stored in bone, 30% is stored intracellularly elsewhere in the body, and only the remaining 1% or less resides in the extracellular space.[1,2]
  - As with other primarily intracellular cations, the serum magnesium level often does not accurately reflect the intracellular magnesium content or total body magnesium.
  - The most common causes of hypomagnesemia are related to malabsorption in the gastrointestinal (GI) tract or decreased reabsorption in the kidneys.
  - The most common cause of hypermagnesemia is magnesium administration in the setting of renal insufficiency.
- Disorders of phosphate.
  - Of the body's phosphorus stores, 80% to 90% is stored in bone, 10% to 20% in the soft tissues, and less than 1% in the extracellular space.[1,2]
  - Because of the low percentage of phosphorus in the extracellular space, serum levels are not a reliable indicator of total body stores.
  - Phosphorus is critical for energy storage in the form of adenosine triphosphate (ATP) and for the formation of membranes. It plays an important role in many signaling pathways.
  - Hypophosphatemia most commonly results from a shift of phosphate from the extracellular to the intracellular space. Such shifts are often transient and do not accurately reflect systemic phosphate levels.
  - Hyperphosphatemia in renal failure generally occurs when the glomerular filtration rate is less than 20 mL/min. Chronic hyperphosphatemia is a major reason that secondary hyperparathyroidism often develops in the setting of chronic renal failure.[3]

Disorders of Magnesium

I. EPIDEMIOLOGY

1. Abnormalities in serum magnesium levels are common in hospitalized patients. Up to 65% of intensive care unit patients and 12% of regular floor patients have hypomagnesemia. Up to 30% of alcoholics admitted to the hospital have magnesium deficiency at presentation.[2]

2. Hypermagnesemia is less common in hospitalized patients, occurring primarily in cases of renal insufficiency in which magnesium has been administered exogenously in the form of laxatives (e.g., magnesium citrate or magnesium sulfate enemas) or antacids (aluminum and magnesium oxide).

HYPOMAGNESEMIA

I. DIAGNOSIS

1. Abnormalities in magnesium concentration are usually diagnosed when an abnormal serum level is found on routine testing. Hypomagnesemia is defined as a magnesium concentration of 1.3 mg/dL or less. Mild magnesium deficiency has vague symptoms such as anorexia, lethargy, and weakness, which are likely to go unrecognized in most cases. More severe deficiency can result in paresthesias, muscle cramps, and irritability. The most common physical findings in hypomagnesemia are those that actually result from hypocalcemia, which is commonly present in magnesium-deficient patients. These findings include tetany, as elicited by positive Trousseau's or Chvostek's signs, and spontaneous carpopedal spasm.[1,2]

2. In addition to hypocalcemia, hypomagnesemia is often associated with hypokalemia, hypophosphatemia, and metabolic alkalosis. When hypomagnesemia and hypokalemia occur together, the correction of hypomagnesemia is often necessary before the hypokalemia can be corrected. The mechanism behind this is not well understood, although magnesium repletion is needed to stop renal potassium wasting in some cases.

3. The most common concern about hypomagnesemia is the potential for cardiac arrhythmias, particularly ventricular tachycardia and torsades de pointes. In addition, hypomagnesemia decreases the threshold for development of digoxin toxicity and the arrhythmias that accompany this state. Electrocardiographic changes described with hypomagnesemia are similar to those in hypokalemia and include QT, PR, and QRS prolongation; T wave flattening and inversion; and in some cases pronounced U wave formation.[2,4] These changes may be seen as serum magnesium levels fall below 1.4 mEq/L and are thought to result indirectly from the effect of magnesium deficiency on the maintenance of intracellular potassium concentrations.

4. The differential diagnosis of hypomagnesemia is broad. The condition typically results from decreased intake, increased excretion, or increased utilization by the body, which are most often due to alterations in the GI, renal, and endocrine systems (Fig. 51-1). Magnesium is acquired via the GI tract, and GI malabsorption (e.g., caused by diarrhea, malabsorptive syndromes, or prolonged nasogastric suction) is one of the most common causes of magnesium deficiency. Patients with magnesium deficiency should be evaluated to rule out

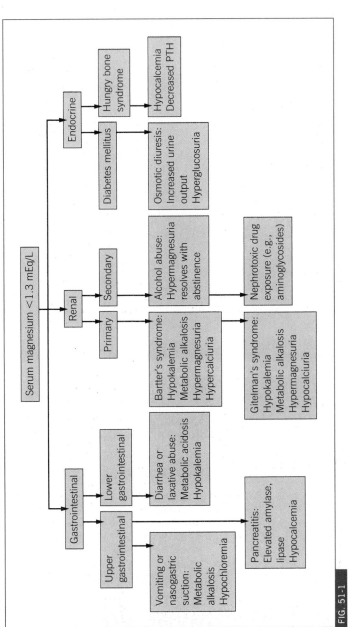

FIG. 51-1

Differential diagnosis of hypomagnesemia. *PTH,* Parathyroid hormone.

GI losses, and the magnesium level of patients with diarrhea or other evidence of malabsorption should be checked.

5. Renal losses of magnesium generally occur because of an alteration in magnesium reabsorption. This most often results from one of two mechanisms: an alteration of sodium reabsorption in the segments in which magnesium transport passively follows that of sodium (e.g., use of diuretics, osmotic diuresis, or high–urine output states) or a primary defect in renal tubular magnesium reabsorption (e.g., alcoholism, hereditary tubular defects). The majority of the filtered magnesium is reabsorbed in the loop of Henle, so both loop and thiazide diuretics can inhibit net magnesium reabsorption while the potassium-sparing diuretics (i.e., amiloride, spironolactone [Aldactone], and triamterene) tend to enhance magnesium transport and lower magnesium excretion. As a result, potassium-sparing diuretics can be used to counter renal magnesium wasting.[5]

6. Alcohol and drugs (Table 51-1) are common causes of hypomagnesemia because of their effect on renal magnesium handling. In chronic alcoholism a primary magnesium wasting state appears to result from alcohol-induced tubular dysfunction. Abstinence reverses this condition within 4 weeks.[6]

7. Hereditary renal tubular defects such as Gitelman's and Bartter's syndromes, while rare, should be considered in cases of chronic hypomagnesemia that are associated with hypokalemic metabolic alkalosis and are resistant to magnesium repletion. Hypomagnesemia is much more common in Gitelman's syndrome, in which the Na-Cl transporter function in the distal convoluted tubule is impaired. In Bartter's syndrome a defect in Na-Cl transport is present in the thick ascending limb of the loop of Henle.[7,8] Based on clinical findings, many of these patients are misdiagnosed as diuretic abusers because the electrolyte abnormalities associated with Gitelman's syndrome mimic those of patients taking thiazide diuretics and Bartter's syndrome mimics the electrolyte effects of loop diuretics.

TABLE 51-1

DRUGS COMMONLY ASSOCIATED WITH HYPOMAGNESEMIA AND MECHANISMS OF MAGNESIUM WASTING

Drug	Mechanism of Hypomagnesemia
Diuretics	Impairment of sodium reabsorption in the loop and distal nephron
Amphotericin B	Distal tubular injury
Aminoglycosides	Proximal tubular injury
Cyclosporine	Unclear
Tacrolimus	Unclear
Rapamycin	Unclear
Steroids	Mineralocorticoid activity
Cisplatinum and carboplatinum	Proximal tubular injury
Pentamidine	Proximal tubular injury
Foscarnet	Proximal tubular injury

8. Diabetes mellitus is the most common endocrine-related cause of hypomagnesemia, which results from the glycosuria and the osmotic diuresis that accompany this disease.[2] Endocrine-related hypomagnesemia also occurs as part of the "hungry bone" syndrome that follows parathyroidectomy in patients with primary or tertiary hyperparathyroidism.[9] In these patients magnesium uptake by renewing bone is increased after an acute decrease in parathyroid hormone (PTH) levels. Correction of hypomagnesemia is central to correction of the hypocalcemia that is part of this syndrome.

II. MANAGEMENT

1. The decision to replete magnesium in a hospitalized patient should be based on the clinical presentation. Asymptomatic mild hypomagnesemia in an otherwise healthy patient is of questionable clinical significance and does not require emergency intervention. In such patients a diagnostic workup should be pursued, and if magnesium replacement is deemed necessary, a sustained-release oral preparation should be administered. In patients with underlying or acute cardiovascular disease the common practice is to maintain serum magnesium levels in the high normal range to stabilize the myocardium against arrhythmias. A causal relationship between arrhythmias and hypomagnesemia is lacking, but hypomagnesemia is commonly associated with potassium and calcium abnormalities, which are believed to be proarrhythmic, and normal serum magnesium levels are important in the correction of these latter abnormalities.[4] The therapeutic role of magnesium administration is well known in torsades de pointes and digoxin toxicity–related arrhythmias despite normal serum levels.[10] It may also have benefit in multifocal atrial tachycardia and the arrhythmias associated with ischemic cardiomyopathy[11,12]; however, the need for replacement has been shown to be associated with worse outcomes in patients with acute myocardial infarction.[13] Magnesium repletion is often performed in acute asthma exacerbations, although most studies have not shown a benefit for this practice in adults.[14,15]

2. For symptomatic patients or those for whom magnesium correction is a pressing clinical need, magnesium sulfate may be given intravenously as a slow infusion. In patients with normal renal function, magnesium is readily handled and doses from 1 to 6 g IV may be safely given. Serum magnesium can be expected to increase 0.1 to 0.2 mg/dL for each gram of magnesium sulfate infused. Side effects of intravenously administered magnesium may include hypotension and flushing, although these can be minimized by a slow administration rate. In patients with renal insufficiency, magnesium repletion should generally be avoided unless absolute magnesium deficiency is documented or the patient is symptomatic. In such patients magnesium replacement should be carried out with great care by dose reduction to 25% to 50% of that given to a patient with normal renal function.

51

MAGNESIUM AND PHOSPHATE DISORDERS

HYPERMAGNESEMIA

I. DIAGNOSIS

1. Hypermagnesemia, defined as a serum magnesium concentration greater than 2.3 mEq/L, is relatively rare.[2,9] When it does occur, it is usually in the setting of renal insufficiency or after the administration of a high magnesium load (e.g., therapy for preeclampsia). At low levels of elevation, symptoms of hypermagnesemia are rare, but as serum levels increase to greater than 4 mEq/L, GI, neuromuscular, central nervous system, and cardiovascular effects may be seen. These may begin with nausea and paresthesias but can progress to muscle weakness, eventual loss of deep tendon reflexes, sedation, and central effects resulting in bradycardia, hypotension, and hypoventilation. Coma and respiratory paralysis may occur at levels greater than 30 mEq/L and may result in death.[1,16]

2. The differential diagnosis of hypermagnesemia is much narrower than that of hypomagnesemia. In hospitalized patients hypermagnesemia is usually iatrogenic. Noniatrogenic causes include rhabdomyolysis and tumor lysis syndrome, which generate magnesium release as muscle or tumor cells break down. Hypermagnesemia may occur in conjunction with hypercalcemia in adrenal insufficiency, probably owing to concomitant volume depletion and hemoconcentration. The same two electrolyte abnormalities are a feature of Dead Sea water poisoning caused by the very high concentrations of both magnesium and calcium in the ingested water.[17]

II. MANAGEMENT

1. The treatment of hypermagnesemia is generally based on addressing the underlying cause. When the etiology is iatrogenic, magnesium supplementation should be stopped. Hypermagnesemia of noniatrogenic origin usually responds to intravenous fluids, and as long as the hypermagnesemia is asymptomatic, it is safe to simply follow magnesium levels as they decline. In symptomatic hypermagnesemia, however, intravenous administration of calcium may be used to antagonize magnesium receptor activity and loop diuretics along with hypotonic intravenous fluids can be used to augment renal excretion. In grave situations hemodialysis may be used.[16]

Disorders of Phosphate

I. EPIDEMIOLOGY

1. Hypophosphatemia is common in hospitalized patients and in various studies has been found in 2% to 30% of inpatients.[2,18]

2. Up to 60% of patients receiving hemodialysis for end-stage renal disease have some degree of hyperphosphatemia, which puts them at risk for visceral and vascular calcification. Premature coronary artery

calcification is well known to occur in patients with end-stage renal disease and contributes to mortality in the nearly 50% of these patients who die of cardiovascular disease.[19]

HYPOPHOSPHATEMIA

I. DIAGNOSIS

1. Hypophosphatemia is defined as a serum phosphate level less than 2.7 mg/dL. Mild hypophosphatemia (1-2.7 mg/dL) is rarely symptomatic and more often reflects redistribution of phosphate from the extracellular to intracellular space than an underlying total body phosphate deficiency. In contrast, severe hypophosphatemia (<1 mg/dL) often reflects total body phosphate depletion and thus may have broad systemic manifestations because of a lack of intracellular ATP production.[2] This is especially true when an acute change in serum phosphate concentration occurs. Symptoms of severe, acute hypophosphatemia are severe themselves and may include respiratory failure resulting from diaphragmatic and intercostal muscle weakness, myopathy, rhabdomyolysis, and cardiac dysfunction resulting from altered contractility.[1,2] Chronic hypophosphatemia, as seen in malnourished patients, alcoholics, and patients with rickets, puts patients at high risk of episodes of severe symptomatic hypophosphatemia when serum phosphate levels change rapidly. This is due in part to these patients' limited ability to generate a compensatory shift of phosphate from the intracellular to the extracellular space.

2. The differential diagnosis of hypophosphatemia can be broken down into three general categories: compartmental phosphate shifts, decreased intestinal phosphate reabsorption, and increased renal phosphate excretion (Fig. 51-2). The most common of these is compartmental phosphate shifts. Intracellular shifts in phosphate are favored by metabolic states that favor glycolysis, which in turn results in the consumption of phosphate. A common example of this is hyperventilation (whether caused by sepsis, pain, or mechanical ventilation), in which the resultant respiratory alkalosis increases the activity of phosphofructokinase, which is the rate-limiting step in glycolysis.[1] Hyperinsulinemia, whether from an exogenous or an endogenous source, also favors the movement of phosphate into the intracellular space. This is commonly seen in patients being treated for diabetic ketoacidosis or those receiving intravenous carbohydrate solutions after severe malnutrition (the refeeding syndrome). Among other conditions that cause intracellular phosphate shifts that may result in hypophosphatemia are rapidly growing malignancies, which can consume large amounts of phosphate, and the "hungry bone syndrome" that results from a sudden fall in intact PTH levels after parathyroidectomy.[9]

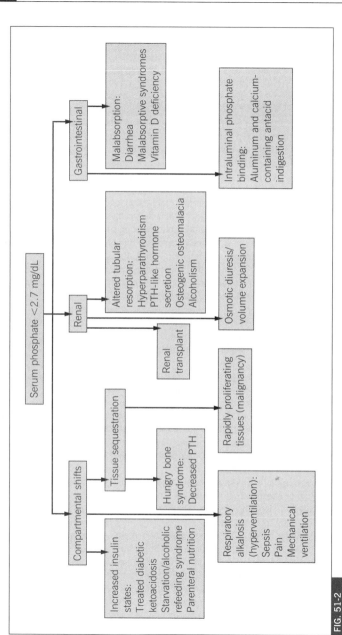

FIG. 51-2

Differential diagnosis of hyperphosphatemia. *PTH*, Parathyroid hormone.

3. The other two etiological categories of hypophosphatemia reflect the mechanisms by which the body acquires and excretes phosphate. A decrease in intestinal phosphate absorption may occur in the setting of chronic diarrhea or malabsorptive syndromes. Chronic malabsorption may also result in vitamin D deficiency, which in turn negatively affects phosphate absorption because 1,25-dihydroxyvitamin D stimulates active phosphate absorption in the gut.[18,20] Patients with steatorrhea are at high risk for this form of hypophosphatemia. In addition, hypophosphatemia may develop in patients with gastroesophageal reflux disease as a result of intraluminal phosphate binding by calcium- or aluminum-containing antacids, although this has become less common with the widespread use of histamine antagonists and proton pump inhibitors in place of antacids.[21]

4. The kidney exerts a major influence on phosphate balance, and thus alterations in renal phosphate handling can significantly affect phosphate stores. Renal phosphate reabsorption occurs primarily in the proximal tubule, where 80% or more of the filtered load is reabsorbed, and in the distal tubule, where another small amount is reabsorbed.[2,18] Phosphate reabsorption is linked to sodium reabsorption via a sodium-phosphate cotransporter on the luminal membrane of the nephron. This transporter uses the favorable inward concentration gradient for sodium to drive the active reabsorption of phosphate. Renal excretion of phosphate is under the control of PTH. Increased PTH inhibits the action of the sodium-phosphate cotransporter, thereby reducing the absorption of phosphate and causing phosphaturia. As a result, hypophosphatemia caused by renal losses often occurs in the setting of primary hyperparathyroidism.[2] In addition, hypophosphatemia may be seen in malignancies that produce PTH-like hormones (i.e., PTH-related peptide)[22] or in cases of oncogenic osteomalacia.[23,24] The latter condition is characterized by hypophosphatemia caused by selective renal phosphate wasting, low plasma calcitriol levels, and osteomalacia. It is a paraneoplastic syndrome that is associated with mesenchymal and vascular malignancies and resolves within weeks after removal of the tumor.[23,24] Increased renal phosphate excretion is more commonly seen in osmotic diuresis and acute volume expansion. In osmotic diuresis, phosphaturia occurs as the result of glucosuria, whereas in acute volume expansion phosphaturia is the result of natriuresis. Chronic alcoholism, in addition to causing hypophosphatemia as a result of malnutrition, causes a phosphaturic state through a direct effect of ethanol on the renal parenchyma.[6]

II. MANAGEMENT

1. Mild asymptomatic hypophosphatemia need not be treated, especially if the patient is otherwise healthy or there is reason to suspect a temporary intracellular shift of serum phosphate without underlying total body deficiency.

51

MAGNESIUM AND PHOSPHATE DISORDERS

2. Insulin induces a shift of phosphate from the extracellular to the intracellular space. As a result, hypophosphatemia is often encountered when large amounts of insulin are administered intravenously, as in the treatment of diabetic ketoacidosis (DKA). Such hypophosphatemia is usually temporary and resolves with resolution of the DKA and return to a regular diet. In such cases phosphate repletion is not generally recommended.[18]

3. If no underlying cause for hypophosphatemia is found or despite efforts to correct the underlying abnormality a patient remains hypophosphatemic, supplementation should begin with oral phosphate preparations. These are generally given as one packet or capsule (8 mmol) every 3 to 4 days.

4. Intravenous administration of phosphate should be avoided unless a patient has symptomatic hypophosphatemia. Intravenous phosphate should be given slowly, 0.08 to 0.16 mmol/kg in half normal saline over 6 hours. The electrolytes of a patient receiving intravenous phosphate should be carefully monitored. Such administration is most often complicated by hyperphosphatemia and hypocalcemia, so serum phosphate and calcium levels should be followed with great care.

HYPERPHOSPHATEMIA

I. DIAGNOSIS

1. Hyperphosphatemia is defined as a serum level greater than 4.5 mg/dL, which occurs most often in the setting of renal insufficiency. The symptoms of hyperphosphatemia are due primarily to the hypocalcemia that occurs as calcium-phosphate crystals precipitate and are deposited in the soft tissues. The risk for hypocalcemia and tissue deposition is greatest when the product of the serum calcium and phosphate levels exceeds 70, especially when this occurs acutely.[2] Vascular calcification occurs readily in the setting of hyperphosphatemia and probably explains the clear link between hyperphosphatemia and increased cardiovascular mortality risk in patients receiving dialysis.[20,25]

2. The most important and common cause of hyperphosphatemia is renal insufficiency, although alterations in renal handling of phosphate resulting from hypoparathyroidism (PTH inhibits renal phosphate absorption) or tumoral calcinosis (a rare inherited disorder in which renal phosphate absorption is increased) may cause hyperphosphatemia in the absence of primary renal insufficiency.[1,2] Hyperphosphatemia may also follow an increased phosphate load from either endogenous or exogenous sources. Increased phosphate from endogenous sources occurs in the setting of tissue breakdown (e.g., rhabdomyolysis and the tumor lysis syndrome). The tumor lysis syndrome (see Chapter 36 for more details) is seen after the initiation of chemotherapy in highly metabolically active tumors such as lymphomas

and leukemias. Phosphate overload from an exogenous source occurs most often in the setting of underlying renal insufficiency, and patients with end-stage renal disease or significant renal insufficiency should not be given phosphate-based laxatives or enemas. This fact should be recalled every time a patient with renal insufficiency is prepared for a colonoscopy or barium enema. The preferred bowel preparation for colonoscopy or barium enema in such patients is oral gastrointestinal lavage with polyethylene glycol (Golytely), which is electrolyte balanced and phosphate free.

3. Pseudohyperphosphatemia is an artifactual phenomenon in which the serum phosphate level is elevated because of an increase in other serum components. This most often occurs when high levels of paraproteins are present, as in the case of multiple myeloma, because such paraproteins can interfere with the colorimetric measurements used to determine phosphate levels. Other conditions thought to have a similar effect include hyperlipidemia, hyperbilirubinemia, and hemolysis (although only the effect of paraproteins has been well documented).[26] Because of this phenomenon, in cases of hyperphosphatemia that cannot be otherwise explained the presence of abnormal proteins should be ruled out.

II. MANAGEMENT

1. As mentioned previously, hyperphosphatemia is most problematic when the calcium-phosphate product (serum calcium × serum phosphate) is greater than 70. When this level is exceeded, the patient is at high risk for calcium deposition in tissues and at significantly increased risk of death.[19] Current guidelines for patients with chronic renal failure recommend maintaining serum phosphate levels between 3 and 5 mg/dL with a calcium-phosphate product less than 55.[19,25] The first management choice in hyperphosphatemia is to limit dietary phosphate to less than 1 g per day. Phosphate intake can be limited only by limiting protein intake. This may have additional benefits for patients with chronic renal failure because limiting renal protein load may slow the progression of renal failure, but patient adherence to such a diet is often difficult to maintain.[27] Strict limitation of dietary protein is not always advisable for patients receiving maintenance dialysis, since many of these patients have overt or borderline malnutrition and actually require protein supplementation rather than protein restriction. Such patients should be encouraged to avoid unnecessary dietary phosphate (e.g., dairy products, certain vegetables, and soft drinks) while increasing the intake of high–biological value sources of protein (e.g., meat and eggs).

2. If hyperphosphatemia is unresponsive to dietary modification alone or the urgency of correction necessitates other measures, oral phosphate binders should be instituted. These should always be administered with meals. The first choice is usually calcium carbonate (Tums,

Os-Cal, Caltrate) or calcium acetate (Phos-Lo), which are inexpensive and have relatively limited side effects compared with other available drugs. Calcium-containing phosphate binders should be given at starting doses of 500 to 1000 mg (calcium carbonate) or 667 to 1334 mg (calcium acetate) three times a day with meals. Administration with meals maximizes phosphate binding and minimizes calcium absorption,[28] but calcium-containing phosphate binders may be taken between meals if a dose is missed or a patient is on "no oral intake" (NPO) status. If the hyperphosphatemia is not adequately controlled with calcium salts, or if hypercalcemia is present, a non-aluminum-based oral phosphate binder such as sevelamer (Renagel) should be used. Sevelamer is a polymeric compound that binds phosphate within the intestinal lumen, limiting absorption and decreasing serum phosphate concentrations without altering calcium, aluminum, or bicarbonate concentrations. It is very effective but is currently much more expensive than calcium salts and therefore not often used as a first-line agent. Starting dosage is 800 mg tid with meals. Sevelamer is contraindicated for patients with bowel obstruction and should be used with caution for those with bowel motility disorders. It should not be taken between meals if a dose is missed. Aluminum- and magnesium-based phosphate binders (e.g., Amphojel), although once popular, have been largely abandoned because of the dangers of aluminum and magnesium accumulation in the setting of renal failure.[2,27]

3. If volume overload is not an issue, patients with acute severe hyperphosphatemia may be given isotonic or glucose-containing intravenous fluids to promote the urinary excretion of phosphate or compartmental phosphate shifts, respectively. If volume overload is an issue, hemodialysis or continuous hemofiltration can be used. Because of the multicompartmental distribution of phosphate, however, hemodialysis is not very efficient at removing it. Serum phosphate levels generally decrease rapidly during the first hour of hemodialysis but return to predialysis levels by the end of treatment. Continuous venovenous hemodialysis does provide a more efficient phosphate clearance than conventional intermittent hemodialysis and should be considered as the modality of choice for the management of acute severe hyperphosphatemia in patients with end-stage renal disease.[29]

4. The adequate treatment of hyperphosphatemia in patients with chronic renal insufficiency is of great importance to prevent the development of secondary hyperparathyroidism. The normal level of intact PTH (iPTH) is 10 to 65 pg/mL, but to avoid oversuppression of the parathyroid glands, the iPTH level of patients with end-stage renal disease should be maintained at two to four times the upper normal levels (150-200 pg/mL). In refractory cases parathyroidectomy may be performed.[30]

PEARLS AND PITFALLS

- Disorders of magnesium.
  - Because magnesium is primarily an intracellular cation, serum magnesium levels often do not reflect total body magnesium stores.
  - When hypomagnesemia and hypokalemia occur together, correction of hypomagnesemia is frequently necessary before the hypokalemia will respond to repletion.
  - The hypomagnesemia of chronic alcoholism generally resolves with 4 weeks of abstinence.
- Disorders of phosphate.
  - Phosphate-based laxatives or enemas may contribute to hyperphosphatemia in patients with end-stage renal disease and thus should be used only with caution. Golytely is the oral gastrointestinal lavage of choice in the setting of renal insufficiency.
  - Increased exogenous or endogenous insulin, as is seen with the treatment of DKA or the feeding of malnourished patients, may result in hypophosphatemia. It is important to remember, however, that this hypophosphatemia is caused by shifting of phosphate from the extracellular to the intracellular space and often does not reflect total body phosphate depletion. Repletion of phosphate in this setting should be undertaken cautiously and generally only in cases of symptomatic hypophosphatemia because of the risk of hyperphosphatemia.
  - In chronic renal insufficiency, limiting phosphate intake can be truly accomplished only by limiting protein intake. Unfortunately, dialyzed patients have overt or borderline malnutrition and thus require high-protein diets. Such patients should be encouraged to avoid other sources of unnecessary dietary phosphate, including dairy products, some vegetables, and cola drinks.
  - Hypophosphatemia is a common abnormality in renal transplant recipients. The potential mechanisms of transplant-related hypophosphatemia are varied and complex. Although persistent secondary or tertiary hyperparathyroidism may play a major role in the phosphaturia of transplantation, new research suggests that the mechanism is independent of PTH.[31]
  - Pseudohyperphosphatemia is an artifactual phenomenon that may occur in the setting of paraproteinemia (e.g., multiple myeloma), hyperlipidemia, hyperbilirubinemia, or hemolysis. In cases of hyperphosphatemia that cannot otherwise be explained, the coexistence of these conditions should be ruled out.

51

MAGNESIUM AND PHOSPHATE DISORDERS

REFERENCES

[c] 1. Fauci AS et al. Harrison's principles of internal medicine, 14th ed. New York: McGraw-Hill; 1998.

[c] 2. Weisinger JR, Ezequiel Bellorin-Font. Magnesium and phosphorus. Lancet 1998; 352:391.

[c] 3. Llach F, Velasquez Forero F. Secondary hyperparathyroidism in chronic renal failure: pathogenic and clinical aspects. Am J Kidney Dis 2001; 38(5 suppl):S20.

[c] 4. Gettes LS. Electrolyte abnormalities underlying lethal and ventricular arrhythmias. Circulation 1992; 85(1 suppl):I70.

[c] 5. Greenberg A. Diuretic complications. Am J Med Sci 2000; 319(1):10.

[b] 6. DeMarchi S et al. Renal tubular dysfunction in chronic alcohol abuse—effects of abstinence. N Engl J Med 1993; 329(26):1927.

[c] 7. Zarraga Larrondo S et al. Familial hypokalemia-hypomagnesemia or Gitelman's syndrome: a further case. Nephron 1992; 62(3):340.

[c] 8. Scheinman SJ et al. Genetic disorders of renal electrolyte transport. N Engl J Med 1999; 340(5):1177.

[c] 9. Wilson JD et al. Williams textbook of endocrinology, 9th ed. Philadelphia: WB Saunders; 1998.

[c] 10. Tzivoni D, Keren A. Suppression of ventricular arrhythmias by magnesium. Am J Cardiol 1990; 65(20):1397.

[a] 11. Ince C et al. Usefulness of magnesium sulfate in stabilizing cardiac repolarization in heart failure secondary to ischemic cardiomyopathy. Am J Cardiol 2001; 88(3):224.

[c] 12. McCord J, Borzak S. Multifocal atrial tachycardia. Chest 1998; 113(1):203.

[b] 13. Ziegelstein RC et al. Magnesium use in the treatment of acute myocardial infarction in the United States (observations from the Second National Registry of Myocardial Infarction). Am J Cardiol 2001; 87(1):7.

[a] 14. Rodrigo G, Rodrigo C, Burschtin O. Efficacy of magnesium sulfate in acute adult asthma: a meta-analysis of randomized trials. Am J Emerg Med 2000; 18(2):216.

[a] 15. Porter RS et al. Intravenous magnesium is ineffective in adult asthma, a randomized trial. Eur J Emerg Med 2001; 8(1):9.

[c] 16. Schelling JR. Fatal hypermagnesemia. Clin Nephrol 2000; 53(1):61.

[c] 17. Porath A et al. Dead sea water poisoning. Ann Emerg Med 1989; 18(2):187.

[c] 18. Hodgson SF, Hurley DL. Acquired hypophosphatemia. Endocr Metab Clin North Am 1993; 22(2):397.

[c] 19. Block GA, Port FK. Re-evaluation of risks associated with hyperphosphatemia and hyperparathyroidism in dialysis patients: recommendations for a change in management. Am J Kidney Dis 2000; 35(6):1226.

[c] 20. Subramanian R, Khardori R. Severe hypophosphatemia: pathophysiologic implications, clinical presentations, and treatment. Medicine 2000; 79(1):1.

[c] 21. Agus ZS. Causes of hypophosphatemia. UpToDate Online, 2002.

[c] 22. Warrell RP. Etiology and current management of cancer-related hypercalcemia. Oncology 1992; 6(10):37.

[c] 23. Clunie GP, Fox PE, Stamp TC. Four cases of acquired hypophosphataemic ("oncogenic") osteomalacia: problems of diagnosis, treatment and long-term management. Rheumatology 2000; 39(12):1415.

[c] 24. Cai Q et al. Inhibition of renal phosphate transport by a tumor product in a patient with oncogenic osteomalacia. N Engl J Med 1994; 330(23):1645.

[c] 25. Block GA. Prevalence and clinical consequences of elevated Ca x P product in hemodialysis patients. Clin Nephrol 2000; 54(4):318.

[c] 26. Larner AJ. Pseudohyperphosphatemia. Clin Biochem 1995; 28(4):391.

[c] 27. Malluche HH, Monier-Faugere MC. Understanding and managing hyperphosphatemia in patients with chronic renal disease. Clin Nephrol 1999; 52(5):267.

[c] 28. Ghazali A et al. Management of hyperphosphatemia in patients with renal failure. Curr Opin Nephrol Hypertens 1993; 2(4):566.

[b] 29. Tan HK et al. Phosphatemic control during acute renal failure: intermittent hemodialysis versus continuous hemodiafiltration. Int J Artif Organs 2001; 24(4):186.

[c] 30. Ifudu O. Care of patients undergoing hemodialysis. N Engl J Med 1998; 339(15):1054.

[c] 31. Heering P, Degenhardt S, Grabensee B. Tubular dysfunction following renal transplantation. Nephron 1996; 74(3):501.

Dialysis

Jennifer S. Myers, MD, and Milagros Samaniego, MD

Fast Facts

- The leading causes of end-stage renal disease (ESRD) in the United States are diabetes and hypertension.
- Blacks have a disproportionately high incidence of ESRD compared with whites: 758 compared with 180 per million population per year.[1]
- Life expectancy for adults with ESRD is approximately 10 years or less, similar to the life expectancy of patients with other serious illnesses such as cancer. The yearly mortality rate for patients on dialysis is close to 25%.[1]
- The estimated yearly cost (including hospitalizations, physicians' fees, medications, dialysis) to care for a patient with ESRD in the United States in 1989 was over $35,000.[2]
- Cardiovascular disease (i.e., coronary, cerebrovascular, and peripheral artery disease) and infection account for most deaths in the dialysis population.

52

I. TYPES OF DIALYSIS

A. HEMODIALYSIS

1. Hemodialysis (HD) is the most common form of renal replacement therapy in the United States. Diffusion of solutes between blood and a dialysis solution (dialysate) results in the removal of toxic metabolites (or drugs) and the replacement of essential body buffers.
2. The rate of volume removal (if indicated) can be adjusted by changing the transmembrane pressure across the dialyzer. Bicarbonate has replaced acetate as the dialysate buffer in the United States.[3]
3. The concentrations of potassium, calcium, and bicarbonate in the dialysate can be adjusted based on the predialysis levels of these plasma components.
4. HD is the preferred method of renal replacement therapy for patients with abdominal wall defects, intraperitoneal adhesions caused by multiple surgeries, intraabdominal malignancies, and active gastrointestinal (GI) disorders (e.g., inflammatory bowel disease), which preclude placement of an intraperitoneal catheter.
5. The most common complication during HD is hypotension. Dialysis-related hypotension is usually a result of volume depletion induced by the ultrafiltration process, but other causes of hypotension (bleeding, heart disease, pericardial effusion, sepsis, medications, autonomic neuropathy, adrenal insufficiency, and bioincompatibility) should not be overlooked.

6. Occasionally a systemic reaction consisting of hypotension, nausea, shortness of breath, and chest pain can be caused by a reaction to the dialysis membrane. This so-called first-use syndrome is more common with the use of nonbiocompatible cellulose membranes. It is a result of the activation of the complement system that occurs when blood comes in contact with a nonbiocompatible dialysis membrane.[4]

7. More biocompatible membranes (polysulfones) have been developed and are in common use today. Polysulfone membranes are used in HD of critically ill patients or in conditions in which clearance of middle-size molecules is critical.

8. Hypersensitivity reactions can also occur as a result of allergy to ethylene oxide (used to sterilize the dialyzer) or polyacrylonitrile (a synthetic noncellulose dialysis membrane). Reactions to polyacrylonitrile, the dialysis membrane used for continuous replacement therapy (i.e., continuous venovenous HD), occur in patients taking angiotensin-converting enzyme (ACE) inhibitors and are bradykinin-dependent reactions.

B. PERITONEAL DIALYSIS

1. Peritoneal dialysis (PD) is the preferred method of dialysis outside the United States. A plastic catheter (Tenckhoff catheter) is surgically implanted in the peritoneal cavity. Dialysate is then infused into the peritoneum, where it is left to dwell for several hours. Solute transport takes place by diffusion across the peritoneal membrane. Ultrafiltration is accomplished by the addition of glucose to the dialysate.

2. Two thirds of patients use continuous ambulatory PD in which the dialysate is exchanged four times each day. The other one third use automated PD in which a mechanical cycler infuses and drains dialysate at night. The latter method allows the patient more freedom during the day and can be augmented if necessary with one or two daytime exchanges.[5]

3. PD is the preferred method of renal replacement therapy for patients with extensive vascular disease limiting HD access sites, patients unable to tolerate the rapid blood pressure variation during HD (e.g., patients with severe congestive heart failure or unstable angina), and patients who want to avoid the lifestyle limitations imposed by HD sessions.

4. The most serious complication of PD is peritonitis. It should be suspected when abdominal pain, fever, or a cloudy dialysate develops in a patient receiving PD.

5. Peritonitis is diagnosed by examination of the dialysate for the presence of polymorphonuclear leukocytes (>50% polymorphonuclear leukocytes in a white blood cell count >100/mm^3 is compatible with a diagnosis of peritonitis).

6. The most common causative organisms are gram-negative rods, followed by gram-positive cocci and yeast.

7. Antibiotic selection is ultimately guided by the bacteria in the

peritoneal fluid, and the routes of administration are oral, intraperitoneal, or intravenous according to the severity of the infection.

8. A reasonable empirical regimen is one that includes a first-generation cephalosporin (e.g., cefazolin or cephalothin) and an antibiotic effective against most gram-negative rods (e.g., ceftazidime, aminoglycoside, or extended-spectrum fluoroquinolone). The use of aminoglycosides should be avoided if the patient has a residual urine output of 100 mL/day.[6]

9. As infection with vancomycin-resistant enterococci has become prevalent in outpatient dialysis units, the empirical use of vancomycin, formerly the antibiotic of choice for peritonitis, has decreased. At present the use of vancomycin is recommended only if methicillin-resistant *Staphylococcus epidermidis* or *Staphylococcus aureus* infection is suspected.

10. Fungal peritonitis is a more difficult infection to clear and often necessitates catheter removal.

11. Other complications are related to the small (1 mL/min) but steady absorption of peritoneal fluid through the diaphragmatic lymphatics. Excessive glucose absorption can result in hyperlipidemia or worsening of glycemic control in a diabetic patient. The addition of insulin to the dialysate is effective in controlling blood sugar levels.[7]

12. Pleural effusions can develop if dialysis fluid enters the pleural space in excess (either through lymphatics or through microscopic diaphragmatic defects). These are diagnosed on the basis of an extremely high glucose concentration in the pleural fluid.

C. CONTINUOUS RENAL REPLACEMENT THERAPIES

1. Continuous renal replacement therapy (CRRT) can be performed as dialysis (solute removal), filtration (convection-based solute and water removal), or both. Since the development of CRRT in 1977, its use has continued to grow and it is now commonplace in intensive care units.[8] The major advantage over "traditional" HD, which is conducted in 4- to 6-hour sessions, is its slower rate of volume removal, which is essential for hemodynamically unstable patients.

2. Considerable nomenclature is used to describe variations in the physical process of CRRT. Arteriovenous or continuous arteriovenous hemofiltration (CAVHD) refers to a process in which an arterial catheter pumps blood, by virtue of systemic arterial pressure, out of the body into an extracorporeal circuit. The blood is returned to the body through a central venous catheter. Disadvantages of this process include the risks involved with arterial puncture (bleeding, embolization, and peripheral ischemia) and the reliance on systemic arterial pressure to allow adequate volume and solute removal. In addition, patients with peripheral vascular disease or hypotension and high vasopressor requirements (common in the populations needing CRRT) may have unreliable blood flow.[9]

3. The placement of one dual-lumen catheter in a central vein, or alternatively two separate venous catheters, is needed to perform venovenous or continuous venovenous hemofiltration (CVVHD). An extracorporeal blood pump is then required to push blood through the dialysis circuit. Because of the inherent disadvantages with CAVHD described previously, CVVHD has become more popular.[10]

II. VASCULAR ACCESS

1. Native arteriovenous (AV) fistulas are the preferred form of vascular access because of their longer life span and lower incidence of thrombosis and infection.[11] The 2-year survival rate for the Cimino-Brescia fistula (surgically created between the radial artery and cephalic vein) is greater than 75%. Venipuncture should be avoided in the nondominant arm and the upper part of the dominant arm to preserve these sites for possible future vascular access.

2. AV grafts are made of polytetrafluoroethylene and are surgically interposed to connect an adjacent artery and vein (e.g., brachial artery to basilic vein, femoral artery to femoral vein) The most common complication is thrombosis or stenosis of the graft as a result of intimal hyperplasia. Stenosis can also result in less efficient dialysis because of the recirculation of blood.

3. A temporary dual-lumen cuffed catheter is used in patients recovering from acute renal failure or those awaiting maturation of a fistula. Half of these catheters are still functional at 1 year.[12]

4. Infection (e.g., epidural abscess, endocarditis, osteomyelitis) or thrombosis of the catheter eventually leads to its replacement or discontinuation. Dual-lumen cuffed catheters remain the access of choice for intravenous drug users whose anatomy does not allow the placement of a native AV fistula or AV graft.

5. A dual-lumen temporary catheter can be inserted into the femoral or internal jugular vein for urgent or emergency dialysis. Insertion into the subclavian vein is generally avoided because it is associated with a high incidence of central venous thrombosis. Central venous thrombosis may preclude future use of the ipsilateral arm for more permanent dialysis access.

III. CARE OF THE PATIENT RECEIVING HEMODIALYSIS

A. NUTRITION

1. Dietary restriction (the "renal diet" of low protein, potassium, and sodium) in the patients receiving dialysis is outdated. This concept stems from the early days of renal replacement therapy when inefficient HD was the rule. Amino acids are lost during the dialysis process. In addition, many patients who recently began dialysis are malnourished because of the catabolic state in progressive renal failure.

2. Protein intake should therefore be generous and equal to at least 1.5 g/kg of total body weight. The ideal renal diet or enteral or parenteral

supplementation is high in protein and calories but low in potassium and phosphate (see below).

B. ELECTROLYTES AND VITAMINS

1. Sodium restriction is not warranted unless dictated by comorbidities (e.g., congestive heart failure, liver disease, or excessive interdialytic weight gain). Diets high in sodium promote water retention and the inherent risks of volume overload, but routine dialysis sessions are usually efficient in removing the accumulated volume.

2. Although potassium supplements should not be given to patients receiving dialysis, strict dietary restriction is unnecessary. Dialyzed patients have a reduction in total body potassium, and the cardiac and neuromuscular response to hyperkalemia is less pronounced and less common than in non-ESRD patients.[13]

3. Hypokalemia immediately after an HD session is common because most of the body's potassium is intracellular. Potassium replacement is inappropriate at this time, however, because the potassium level gradually rises to normal levels between sessions. As a good practice, postdialysis electrolyte levels should not be used to prescribe replacement therapy.

4. Management of magnesium and phosphate levels is addressed in Chapter 51.

5. Water-soluble vitamins (B complex) are dialyzable and should be given in a replacement form on a daily basis. In contrast, fat-soluble vitamins (A, D, E, K) tend to accumulate.

6. Calcitriol, or 1,25-OH vitamin D, is commonly prescribed as a suppressant of parathyroid hormone. Intact parathyroid hormone levels should be monitored to prevent oversupplementation with calcitriol, which can lead to hypercalcemia.

C. ANEMIA

1. Normocytic, normochromic anemia is universal in the ESRD population. It is a consequence of the decline in erythropoietin production by the kidney.

2. Recombinant erythropoietin is efficient in correcting the anemia and improving anemia-related symptoms in patients with ESRD. The starting dose is 50 to 100 U/kg body weight three times a week as a subcutaneous injection. Iron deficiency should be evaluated and treated in each patient because it can blunt the response to erythropoietin.[14]

3. Intravenous iron replacement is the preferred method to replenish iron stores in dialyzed patients. A transferrin saturation of 40% or less and a ferritin level of 400 ng/mL or less indicate iron deficiency. Blood transfusion should be avoided when possible because it can result in sensitization of human leukocyte antigens, which would affect future kidney transplantation.

4. Anemia can be exacerbated by an acute bleeding episode in a patient with ESRD.

52

DIALYSIS

5. The bleeding may be recalcitrant because of the acquired platelet dysfunction that occurs in uremia. Bleeding time is prolonged in this population as a result of abnormal platelet adhesion, aggregation, and factor III release. The initial approach is to ensure adequate dialysis and appropriately identify and treat the underlying bleeding source. In addition, desmopressin (0.3 μg/kg IV or SQ), conjugated estrogens (0.6 mg/kg), and fresh frozen plasma or cryoprecipitate infusion may be helpful if bleeding persists.[15,16]

D. RENAL OSTEODYSTROPHY

1. There are several types of bone disease, which can occur in isolation or in combination in patients with chronic renal failure.

2. Secondary hyperparathyroidism caused by phosphate retention and calcitriol deficiency can lead to increased bone turnover and the histological disease osteitis fibrosa cystica.

3. Clinical manifestations are often subtle but include bone and joint pain, lytic lesions, and metastatic calcifications.

4. Secondary hyperparathyroidism is most commonly diagnosed on the basis of laboratory abnormalities, which include hyperphosphatemia, hypocalcemia, increased alkaline phosphatase, and elevated serum intact parathyroid hormone level (iPTH), which is usually at least 200 to 400 pg/mL in this disease.

5. Prophylaxis and treatment include phosphate binders, calcitriol supplementation, and careful monitoring of the iPTH level. The normal level of iPTH is 10 to 65 pg/mL, but to avoid oversuppression of the parathyroid glands, the iPTH level of patients with ESRD should be maintained at two to four times the upper normal levels (i.e., at ~150-200 pg/mL). Parathyroidectomy is performed in refractory cases.[13]

6. Defective bone mineralization and reduction in bone turnover characterize osteomalacia, or adynamic bone disease. Although it has several causes, aluminum intoxication is the most likely culprit in the ESRD population. Clinical manifestations include proximal muscle weakness, bone pain, and low iPTH levels. The disease is initially diagnosed by bone biopsy. Prevention and treatment include avoidance of long-term aluminum binders and selective use of desferoxamine in patients with documented aluminum toxicity.

7. A form of amyloidosis caused by the accumulation of β_2-microglobulin fibrils may occur in patients with ESRD.

8. Clinical manifestations vary but may include arthropathy, carpal tunnel syndrome, and fractures. Diagnosis is confirmed by bone biopsy with Congo red staining for amyloid and immunohistochemical staining for β_2-microglobulin. Treatment is supportive because no method of amyloid removal or mobilization is known. Interestingly, most forms of dialysis-related amyloidosis abate after renal transplantation.

E. CARDIOVASCULAR RISK FACTORS IN END-STAGE RENAL DISEASE

1. Cardiovascular disease accounts for approximately half of all deaths in the ESRD population. The relationship is complex because of the high

prevalence of comorbid conditions and underlying vascular disease in the ESRD population.

2. In addition to the usual cardiovascular risk factors common in patients with ESRD (i.e., advancing age, hypertension, hyperlipidemia, obesity, smoking), other factors such as hyperhomocysteinemia, accelerated atherosclerosis, and impaired oxygen delivery by uremia toxins may contribute to the increased incidence of coronary artery disease in this population.[13]

3. Because of abnormalities in baseline electrocardiograms (e.g., left ventricular hypertrophy pattern) and the usual inability of ESRD patients to perform adequately on exercise treadmill tests, noninvasive diagnosis of coronary artery disease is usually performed with chemical stress tests.

4. Hypertension is nearly universal during progressive renal failure. In a patient receiving dialysis, hypertension is defined as a predialysis mean arterial pressure above 106 mm Hg (i.e., 140/90 mm Hg) when the patient is believed to be at the so-called dry weight.[17]

5. Fluid retention and preexisting essential hypertension are the most common causes. Erythropoietin, arterial calcification, and increased activity of the sympathetic nervous system and renin-angiotensin system can also contribute to refractory hypertension.[18]

6. For new dialysis patients the most important initial goal in hypertension management is fluid removal and sodium restriction to achieve better control of blood pressure and an ideal dry weight.

7. The definition and determination of dry weight are difficult. In general the dry weight is the weight at which the blood pressure has normalized or at which the signs of hypervolemia are absent and the beginning signs of hypovolemia (muscle cramps, hypotension) appear.

8. The amount of excessive extracellular volume may not be enough to induce edema; therefore the absence of edema does not exclude volume overload. The dry weight must be recorded, frequently reassessed by clinical means, and altered as patients gain muscle mass because they are receiving adequate dialysis and nutrition.

9. Despite achievement of the dry weight and dietary adherence, a large proportion of patients receiving dialysis still require antihypertensive medications.

10. The choice of drug should be guided by the presence of comorbid conditions. Recent studies (HOPE, RENAAL, and AASK trials) have demonstrated the benefit of ACE inhibitors and angiotensin II receptor blockers in decreasing the cardiovascular morbidity and mortality of patients with renal insufficiency.[19-22]

11. Although these studies did not include patients with ESRD, the results can be extrapolated to this population. Furthermore, the blockade of aldosterone has been shown to provide cardiovascular protection in patients with renal insufficiency.

12. The use of ACE inhibitors and angiotensin II or aldosterone receptor blockers is usually impractical in patients with advanced renal

52

DIALYSIS

insufficiency because of the side effects of these drugs (hyperkalemia, further decline in glomerular filtration rate).

13. Once dialysis is initiated, these drugs should be the agents of choice for the treatment of hypertension, congestive heart failure (i.e., systolic dysfunction), or excessive interdialytic weight gain. ACE inhibitors and angiotensin II receptor blockers can elicit resistance to erythropoietin, so hematocrit values must be monitored closely.

14. Calcium channel blockers are usually effective and well tolerated in patients receiving dialysis.

15. Although the AASK trial showed a higher mortality among black patients treated with a calcium channel blocker as a single agent,[21] the use of these drugs in combination with an ACE inhibitor or a β-blocker can be beneficial.

16. Calcium channel blockers (e.g., nifedipine, amlodipine) are effective antihypertensive agents in patients receiving dialysis. Because HD does not remove calcium channel blockers, these agents are effective in controlling intradialytic hypertension, although they also account for intradialytic hypotension when given shortly before dialysis.

17. β-Blockers are indicated if the patient has coexistent coronary artery disease or congestive heart failure (i.e., diastolic dysfunction). Labetalol is often chosen because it lacks the potential bronchospastic and hyperlipidemic properties of other β-blockers.

18. Clonidine patches are also widely used.

19. If hypertension is still refractory despite adequate dialysis and compliance with antihypertensive medication regimens, consideration should be given to other contributing factors, such as erythropoietin, use of nonsteroidal antiinflammatory drugs, renovascular hypertension, and expanding cyst size in polycystic kidney disease.

20. Minoxidil can be effective in treating refractory hypertension, but it is associated with many side effects, the most important of which are hirsutism, reflex tachycardia, and pericardial effusion. In patients with advanced renal insufficiency, minoxidil can cause severe sodium retention and peripheral edema. This sodium retention is the direct result of peripheral arterial vasodilatation and can be controlled with the use of loop diuretics.

F. LABORATORY VALUES IN END-STAGE RENAL DISEASE

1. Serum enzyme levels and other laboratory values are frequently abnormal in advanced renal failure. Since the diagnosis of many conditions relies on such values, knowledge of the expected variations in these values in patients with ESRD is valuable.

2. Cardiac enzymes are frequently used to assess the presence of underlying myocardial damage. Nonspecific elevations in creatine kinase, creatine kinase isoenzyme, and troponin T levels are common in patients with ESRD and often lead to unnecessary cardiac evaluations when other indicators of myocardial damage are absent. At least one observational study has shown that cardiac troponin I is a

more specific indicator of myocardial damage in the renal failure population.[23]

3. Abnormalities in aminotransferase, alkaline phosphatase, and pancreatic enzyme levels in patients with renal failure also hinder the evaluation of GI disease. Concentrations of serum alanine aminotransferase (ALT [SGPT]) and aspartate aminotransferase (AST [SGOT]) tend to be lower than normal. A deficiency in pyridoxine, a necessary coenzyme for ALT and AST, is one proposed mechanism.[24]

4. In one study the use of standard reference values for aminotransferases was not a sensitive marker in hepatitis C–positive patients who were receiving dialysis. A lowering of the conventional upper limit of normal has been proposed as follows: from 40 to 24 IU/L for AST and from 40 to 17 IU/L for ALT.[25]

5. In most patients the majority of alkaline phosphatase arises from liver or bone. Serum levels of this enzyme are sometimes elevated in the dialysis population because of concurrent, untreated secondary hyperparathyroidism.

6. Both amylase and lipase levels may be elevated in patients with renal failure in the absence of pancreatic damage. This is due primarily to impaired renal clearance. The elevation usually does not exceed a threefold increase.[26]

7. The erythrocyte sedimentation rate (ESR), although not a serum enzyme level, is frequently elevated in patients with renal failure in the absence of another systemic inflammatory disease. The degree of elevation is most striking in patients with nephrotic range proteinuria. An increase in plasma factors, particularly fibrinogen, accounts for the elevation. Patients should be evaluated for other causes of an elevated ESR as clinically indicated.

PEARLS AND PITFALLS

- The HD process is important in the treatment of some poisonings and overdoses. It should be considered in the following circumstances.
  - When intoxication has occurred with a drug whose endogenous clearance is substantially lower than its HD clearance.
  - When a patient's condition is deteriorating despite the use of standard medical treatments and antidotes for the suspected drug in excess.
  - When life-threatening acidosis or electrolyte abnormalities accompany the poisoning.
- Dialysis is most useful in removing toxins with a low molecular weight, low amount of protein binding, and small volume of distribution. Lithium is the prototypic example. Other common agents for which HD can be a useful adjunct in elimination include barbiturates, bromides, chloral hydrate, alcohols, procainamide, theophylline, salicylates, and selected β_2-blockers.
- HP can remove selected toxins that are not efficiently removed by conventional HD. The process involves passing anticoagulated blood

52

DIALYSIS

TABLE 52-1

RECOMMENDED USE OF HEMODIALYSIS AND HEMOPERFUSION IN DRUG OVERDOSE AND POISONING

Drug	Procedure	Indications
Ethylene glycol	HD	Severe acidosis, serum level >20 mg/dL
Methanol	HD	Severe acidosis, serum level >50 mg/dL
Lithium	HD	Serum level >4 mEq/L; serum level >2.5 mEq/L with severe symptoms or renal insufficiency
Salicylates	HD	Severe acidosis, CNS symptoms, serum level >800 mg/L, fluid overload preventing sodium bicarbonate administration, deterioration despite adequate supportive care and alkaline diuresis
Theophylline	Hemoperfusion or HD	Serum level >40 μg/mL, severe acidosis, CNS symptoms, inability to tolerate repeated oral charcoal administration

Modified from Tierney LM et al. Current medical diagnosis and treatment. Stamford, Conn: Appleton & Lange; 1999.
CNS, Central nervous system; *HD,* hemodialysis.

through specifically designed columns containing adsorbent particles such as charcoal or polystyrene resin.[27]

- Peritoneal dialysis is much less effective than either HD or HP and is rarely used. Table 52-1 is a selected list of drugs that are effectively removed by HD or HP, along with the typical indications for such procedures.

- When a drug or substance is highly lipid soluble and not present in high concentrations in the plasma, both HD and HP are inefficient for substance removal. Common examples of such potentially toxic drugs are digoxin, tricyclic antidepressants, and calcium channel blockers.

REFERENCES

[d] 1. Renal Data System. USRDS 1997 annual data report. Bethesda, Md: National Institute of Diabetes and Digestive and Kidney Diseases; 1997.

[d] 2. Freidman EA. End-stage renal disease therapy: an American success story. JAMA 1996; 275:1118.

[d] 3. Diamond SM, Henrich WL. Acetate dialysis versus bicarbonate dialysate: a continuing controversy. Am J Kidney Dis 1987; 9:3.

[d] 4. Hakim RM et al. Complement activation and hypersensitivity reactions to dialysis membranes. N Engl J Med 1984; 311:878.

[c] 5. Pastan S, Bailey J. Dialysis therapy. N Engl J Med 1998; 338:1428.

[d] 6. Keane WF et al. Adult peritoneal dialysis related peritonitis treatment recommendations: update 2000. Perit Dial Int 2000; 20:396.

[d] 7. Scarpioni L et al. Peritoneal dialysis in diabetics: optimal insulin therapy on CAPD: intraperitoneal versus subcutaneous treatment. Perit Dial Int 1996; 16(suppl 1):S275.

[d] 8. Kramer P et al. Arteriovenous haemofiltration: a new and simple method for treatment of over-hydrated patients resistant to diuretics. Klin Wochenschr 1977; 55:1121.

[c] 9. Forni LG, Hilton PJ. Continuous hemofiltration in the treatment of acute renal failure. N Engl J Med 1997; 336:1303.

[c] 10. Manns M, Sigler MH, Teehan BP. Continuous renal replacement therapies: an update. Am J Kidney Dis 1998; 32:185.

[c] 11. Feldman HI, Kobrin S, Wasserstein A. Hemodialysis vascular access morbidity. J Am Soc Nephrol 1996; 7:523.

[d] 12. McLaughlin K et al. Long-term vascular access for hemodialysis using silicon dual-lumen catheters with guidewire replacement of catheters for technique salvage. Am J Kidney Dis 1997; 29:553.

[c] 13. Ifudu O. Care of patients undergoing hemodialysis. N Engl J Med 1998; 339:1054.

[c] 14. Fishbane S, Maesaka JK. Iron management in end-stage renal disease. Am J Kidney Dis 1997; 29:319.

[d] 15. Mannucci PM et al. Deamino-8-D-arginine vasopressin shortens the bleeding time in uremia. N Engl J Med 1983; 308:8.

[d] 16. Livio M et al. Conjugated estrogens for the management of bleeding associated with renal failure. N Engl J Med 1986; 315:731.

[d] 17. Daugirdas JT, Blake PG, Ing TS: Handbook of dialysis, 3rd ed. Philadelphia: Lippincott, Williams & Wilkins; 2001.

[c] 18. Zucchelli P, Santoro A, Zuccala A. Genesis and control of hypertension in hemodialysis patients. Semin Nephrol 1988; 8:163.

[a] 19. Yusuf S. Effects of an angiotensin-converting-enzyme inhibitor, ramipril, on cardiovascular events in high-risk patients. Heart Outcomes Prevention Evaluation Study Investigators. N Engl J Med 2000; 342:145.

[a] 20. Brenner BM et al. Effects of losartan on renal and cardiovascular outcomes in patients with type 2 diabetes and nephropathy. N Engl J Med 2001; 345:861.

[a] 21. Agodoa LY et al. Effect of ramipril vs amlodipine on renal outcomes in hypertensive nephrosclerosis: a randomized controlled trial. JAMA 2001; 285:2719.

[d] 22. Mann JF et al. Renal insufficiency as a predictor of cardiovascular outcomes and the impact of ramipril: the HOPE randomized trial. Ann Intern Med 2001; 134:629.

[d] 23. Martin GS, Becjer BN, Schulman G. Cardiac troponin-I accurately predicts myocardial injury in renal failure. Nephrol Dial Transpl 1998; 13:1709.

[d] 24. Cohen GA et al. Observations on decreased serum glutamic oxaloacetic transaminase (SGOT) activity in azotemic patients. Ann Intern Med 1976; 84:275.

[b] 25. Febrizi F et al. Influence of hepatitis C virus (HCV) viremia upon serum aminotransferase activity in chronic dialysis patients. Nephrol Dial Transplant 1997; 12:1394.

[d] 26. Royse VL, Jensen DM, Corwin HL. Pancreatic enzymes in chronic renal failure. Arch Intern Med 1987; 147:537.

[d] 27. Muirhead EE, Reid AF. Resin artificial kidney. Lab Clin Med 1948; 33:841.

52

DIALYSIS

Hyperkalemia

Patty P. Chi, MD, and Derek M. Fine, MD

FAST FACTS

- Potassium homeostasis is determined by potassium intake (39 mg of K^+ = 1 mEq), the distribution of potassium in cells and extracellular fluid, and urinary potassium excretion.
- Cardiac arrhythmia is the major complication of hyperkalemia. An electrocardiogram (ECG) should be obtained to look for peaked T waves, PR prolongation, ST segment depression, widening of QRS complexes, and flattening of P waves.
- Treatment options include the following.
  - Intravenous calcium gluconate or chloride to stabilize myocardium and counter arrhythmias.
  - $D_{50}W$, insulin, and sodium bicarbonate to cause temporary trans-cellular shifts.
  - Diuretics and sodium polystyrene sulfonate (Kayexalate) for permanent removal of potassium.
- Patients with severe hyperkalemia and ECG abnormalities and patients with renal failure should have dialysis to remove potassium more quickly and effectively.

I. EPIDEMIOLOGY AND CLINICAL PRESENTATION
A. MECHANISM OF POTASSIUM HOMEOSTASIS

1. The plasma potassium level is determined by potassium intake, equilibration of potassium across cell membranes, and urinary potassium excretion. Insulin and β-adrenergic agonists facilitate the movement of potassium into cells by activating the sodium-potassium adenosine triphosphatase pump (Na,K-ATPase) in the cell membrane after a potassium load. Most potassium is ultimately excreted in urine by potassium secretion in the cortical collecting tubule. This secretion is stimulated by increased plasma potassium concentration, aldosterone level, and sodium and water delivery to the distal site.[1]

B. PATHOPHYSIOLOGICAL EFFECTS OF HYPERKALEMIA

1. Hyperkalemia decreases the ratio of intracellular to extracellular K^+ concentration. Even though one would expect to see increased membrane excitability, a net decrease in membrane excitability occurs because of persistent depolarization that inactivates sodium channels in the cell membrane.[2]
2. **Cardiovascular:** Arrhythmia (e.g., ventricular fibrillation, asystole) is a potentially fatal complication of hyperkalemia.
   a. ECG manifestations: These do not necessarily occur in order; thus a

patient may progress from peaked T waves to the "sine-wave," skipping the intermediate changes.
(1) Peaked T waves.
(2) PR prolongation.
(3) ST segment depression.
(4) Loss of P waves.
(5) QRS widening to "sine-wave."
3. **Neuromuscular:** Muscle weakness, paralysis, and paresthesia.
4. **Gastrointestinal:** Nausea, vomiting, and ileus.
5. **Renal:** Natriuresis, decreased ammonia production.
6. **Endocrine:** Increased aldosterone and insulin secretion.[3]

II. DIAGNOSTICS (Fig. 53-1)

A. INITIAL DIAGNOSTIC TESTS
1. The serum potassium measurements should be repeated to ensure that no laboratory error has occurred and that hyperkalemia is not spurious (see section on pseudohyperkalemia below).
2. Obtaining an ECG is imperative in hyperkalemia. The ECG manifestations are not consistent among patients with the same numerical potassium value. For example, one patient with a potassium level of 6 mEq/L may have only peaked T waves on the ECG, whereas another patient with the same potassium level may have "sine-waves." Generally, however, peaked T waves are seen in mild hyperkalemia and "sine-wave" morphology is seen in severe hyperkalemia. Patients with chronic hyperkalemia (i.e., chronic renal failure) may have few or no ECG changes and can usually tolerate hyperkalemia better than those with acute hyperkalemia.

B. CAUSES OF HYPERKALEMIA
1. Increased potassium intake (39 mg K^+ = 1 mEq).
a. KCl-containing salt substitute (may contain as much as 2300 mg K^+ per teaspoon).
b. Potassium supplements.
c. Nutritional and herbal supplements.
d. Stored packed red blood cells (after >10 days in storage).
e. Penicillin G potassium (1.7 mEq/10^6 U).
2. Transcellular potassium shifts.
a. Pseudohyperkalemia caused by the following.
(1) Hemolysis during phlebotomy.
(2) Clotted sample.
(3) Leukocytosis (>100,000 cells/mm^3).[4,5]
(4) Thrombocytosis (>1 million cells/mm^3),[4,6,7] 0.15 mEq/L for every 100,000/mm^3 elevation in platelet count.[8]
(5) Hereditary spherocytosis and familial pseudohyperkalemia, when a temperature-dependent potassium leakage from red blood cells occurs after the sample is collected.[9,10]
b. Cell death: Rhabdomyolysis, burns, tumor lysis, massive hemolysis

(increased blood urea nitrogen, phosphate, and uric acid levels would be expected in a catabolic state).

c. Metabolic acidosis (excluding organic acidoses such as lactic acidosis or ketoacidosis): Causes transcellular shift of potassium out of cells.

d. Insulin deficiency, hyperglycemia, and hyperosmolality as in diabetic ketoacidosis (DKA) and hyperosmolar diabetic nonketotic coma. Patients in DKA lack sufficient insulin to facilitate potassium movement into cells through NA,K-ATPase. In addition, hyperosmolality promotes water movement from cells into the extracellular space. This raises the intra-cellular potassium concentration, which in turn promotes a gradient for passive potassium movement out of cells through potassium chan-nels. Some potassium is also carried along with water through the water pores in the cell membrane (solvent drag).[1]

e. Hyperkalemic periodic paralysis: Autosomal dominant point mutation in the skeletal muscle cell Na$^+$ channel gene. Episodes are precipitated by rest after exercise or the ingestion of potassium.

f. Drugs.[11]
   (1) β-Blockers.
   (2) Intravenously administered amino acids (arginine).
   (3) Succinylcholine.
   (4) Digoxin intoxication.

3. **Decreased urinary excretion.**

a. Renal failure: In acute tubular necrosis, oliguria and epithelial cell damage lead to decreased K$^+$ secretion.[4] In chronic renal failure, K$^+$ excretion is increased from functioning nephrons as long as urine output is adequate. In an oliguric state, however, little or no flow occurs to the distal potassium secretory site.[12]

b. Decreased effective circulating volume: For example, heart failure, cirrhosis, salt-wasting nephropathy.

c. Hypoaldosterone states: For example, adrenal insufficiency, hyporenine-mic hypoaldosteronism, type 4 renal tubular acidosis (RTA). The trans-tubular potassium concentration gradient (TTKG) is useful in distinguish-ing hypoaldosteronism from other causes of hyperkalemia.

TTKG = (Urine K/Plasma K) / (Urine osmolality/Plasma osmolality)
     = (Urine K)(Plasma osmolality) / (Plasma K)(Urine osmolality)

A TTKG greater than 10 suggests increased K$^+$ intake with appropriate K$^+$ excretion. TTKG less than 5 to 7 is suggestive of decreased K$^+$ secretion resulting from aldosterone deficiency or resistance.[3]

d. Type 1 RTA: Type 1 RTA is usually associated with hypokalemia, but in the hyperkalemic form, sodium reabsorption is impaired in the cortical collecting tubule, resulting in loss of electronegativity and decreased po-tassium secretion.[13]

e. Selective impairment of potassium secretion caused by a toxic effect on the potassium-secreting cells in the cortical and outer medullary collecting tubules: This is seen in a variety of tubulointerstitial diseases

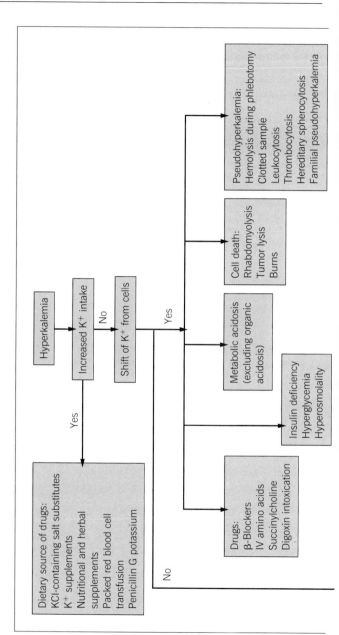

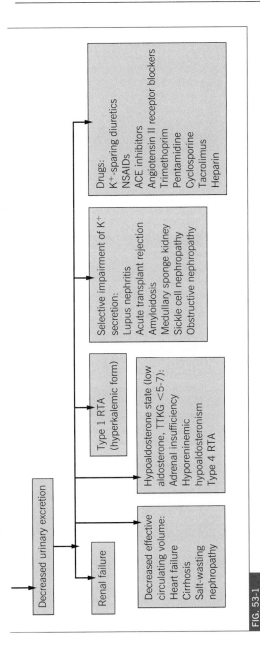

FIG. 53-1

Differential diagnosis of hyperkalemia. *ACE,* Angiotensin-converting enzyme; *K+,* potassium ion; *NSAIDs,* nonsteroidal antiinflammatory drugs; *RTA,* renal tubular acidosis; *TTKG,* transtubular potassium concentration gradient.

such as lupus nephritis, acute transplant rejection, amyloidosis, medullary sponge kidney, sickle cell nephropathy, and obstructive nephropathy.[14-19]

f. Ureterojejunostomy: Hyperkalemia is most likely caused by absorption of urinary potassium by the jejunum.[20]

g. Drugs.[11]

(1) Potassium-sparing diuretics (spironolactone, triamterene, amiloride).

(2) Nonsteroidal antiinflammatory drugs.

(3) Angiotensin-converting enzyme inhibitors.

(4) Angiotensin II receptor blockers.

(5) Trimethoprim.

(6) Pentamidine.

(7) Cyclosporine.

(8) Tacrolimus (FK506).

(9) Heparin.

III. MANAGEMENT (Fig. 53-2)

A. ANTAGONIZING MEMBRANE EFFECT

1. **Calcium chloride or calcium gluconate to avoid arrhythmia:** Hyperkalemia induces depolarization of the resting membrane potential, leading to inactivation of sodium channels and decreased membrane excitability. In this way calcium is thought to counteract the membrane effect of hyperkalemia, although the exact mechanism is not well understood. Administration of calcium is especially crucial in patients with ECG changes associated with hyperkalemia. At least 1 to 2 ampules of calcium gluconate or calcium chloride should be given. In general, 1 ampule of calcium gluconate contains 10 mL of 10% solution. Calcium chloride solution contains three times more elemental calcium than calcium gluconate. Therefore 3 to 4 mL of 10% $CaCl_2$ solution will yield 90 mg Ca^{2+}. The protective effect of calcium begins within minutes, but the effect is relatively short lived (30-60 minutes). Administration of calcium can be repeated as needed because of its short effect.

B. INCREASED POTASSIUM ENTRY INTO CELLS

1. **Insulin and glucose:** The patient should be given 1 to 2 ampules of $D_{50}W$ and 10 U of regular insulin to drive potassium into cells temporarily. Onset of action occurs in approximately 5 to 10 minutes, and duration is 4 to 6 hours.[21,22]

2. **Sodium bicarbonate:** The patient should be given 1 to 3 ampules (50-150 mmol) of sodium bicarbonate to increase the pH and drive potassium into cells. This is especially effective in the setting of metabolic acidosis. However, excessive use of sodium bicarbonate should be avoided because alkalosis may exacerbate arrhythmia by lowering the serum ionized calcium concentration. The effect of bicarbonate begins in 5 to 15 minutes and lasts for 1 to 2 hours.[4] For

unclear reasons, bicarbonate is generally not effective in patients with end-stage renal disease.[23,24]

3. **β_2-Adrenergic agonists:** These drugs increase potassium movement into cells by increasing Na,K-ATPase. Usually 20 mg of albuterol by nebulizer or 0.5 mg IV lowers serum K^+ by 0.5 to 1.5 mEq/L within 30 minutes. The effect lasts about 2 to 4 hours.[1,4,25]

C. REMOVAL OF EXCESS POTASSIUM

1. **Loop or thiazide diuretics:** These drugs are helpful in removing potassium permanently in patients with renal function.

2. **Cation exchange resin:** Sodium polystyrene sulfonate (Kayexalate) binds potassium in the gut and thereby permanently removes potassium. Sodium polystyrene sulfonate 30-60 g PO decreases K^+ by 0.5 mmol/L over 6 to 8 hours. When sodium polystyrene sulfonate is given as a retention enema every 30 to 60 minutes, it decreases K^+ by 0.5 to 0.75 mmol/hr.[3] Sodium polystyrene sulfonate should be used with caution, particularly in patients with impaired GI motility. Acute colonic necrosis has been associated with sodium polystyrene sulfonate use, especially in patients with uremia, hypovolemia, or peripheral vascular disease and in those on immunosuppressive therapy.[26-28]

3. Dialysis is used if the above therapies are not effective or in patients who have severe hyperkalemia, are at risk for cardiac arrhythmia, and need to have potassium removed more urgently and effectively.[23]

PEARLS AND PITFALLS

- Serum potassium level should be rechecked to rule out spurious results. In all cases an ECG should be obtained simultaneously.
- If the ECG prompts suspicion of hyperkalemia, therapy should begin before the result of the repeated laboratory test is available.
- In patients with preexisting heart disease, cardiac arrest may occur without premonitory ECG changes.[4]
- Increased potassium intake must be considered as a possible cause of hyperkalemia (39 mg K^+ = 1 mEq). Some fruits and vegetables contain large amounts of potassium. The patient's medications should be reviewed to ensure that they do not contain potassium. Penicillin G potassium contains 1.7 mEq/10^6 U.
- Administration of excessive sodium bicarbonate should be avoided because alkalosis may exacerbate arrhythmia.
- Bicarbonate may not be effective in patients with end-stage renal disease.
- Sodium polystyrene sulfonate should be given to patients with impaired GI motility or constipation, since it has been associated with acute colonic necrosis.
- Sodium polystyrene sulfonate exchanges 2 to 3 mEq Na^+ for each milliequivalent of K^+ absorbed. Volume overload may be a problem with sodium polystyrene sulfonate use.[4]

53

HYPERKALEMIA

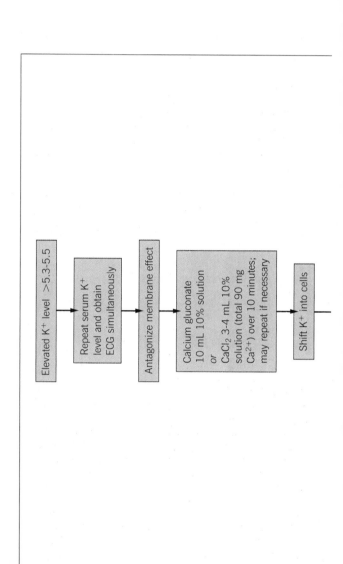

Elevated K+ level >5.3-5.5

↓

Repeat serum K+ level and obtain ECG simultaneously

↓

Antagonize membrane effect

↓

Calcium gluconate 10 mL 10% solution

or

CaCl₂ 3-4 mL 10% solution (total 90 mg Ca²⁺) over 10 minutes; may repeat if necessary

↓

Shift K+ into cells

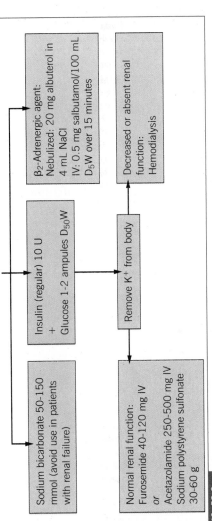

FIG. 53-2

Treatment of hyperkalemia. Ca^{2+}, Calcium ion; $CaCl_2$, calcium chloride; *ECG*, electrocardiogram; K^+, potassium ion; *NaCl*, sodium chloride. (*Data from Johnson RJ, Feehally J. Comprehensive clinical nephrology. St Louis: Mosby; 2000; and Brenner B. The kidney, 5th ed. Philadelphia: WB Saunders; 1995.*)

Within the figure:

- Sodium bicarbonate 50-150 mmol (avoid use in patients with renal failure)

- Insulin (regular) 10 U + Glucose 1-2 ampules $D_{50}W$

- β_2-Adrenergic agent:
  Nebulized: 20 mg albuterol in 4 mL NaCl
  IV: 0.5 mg salbutamol/100 mL D_5W over 15 minutes

- Remove K^+ from body

- Normal renal function:
  Furosemide 40-120 mg IV
  or
  Acetazolamide 250-500 mg IV
  Sodium polystyrene sulfonate 30-60 g

- Decreased or absent renal function:
  Hemodialysis

HYPERKALEMIA

53

REFERENCES

[c] 1. Rose BD, Post TW. Clinical physiology of acid-base and electrolyte disorders, 5th ed. New York: McGraw-Hill; 2001.

[c] 2. Berne RM, Levy, MN. Cardiovascular physiology, 4th ed. St Louis: Mosby; 1981.

[c] 3. Johnson RJ, Feehally J. Comprehensive clinical nephrology. St Louis: Mosby; 2000.

[c] 4. Brenner B. The kidney, 5th ed. Philadelphia: WB Saunders; 1995.

[b] 5. Ho AMH, Woo JCH, Chiu L. Spurious hyperkalemia with severe thrombocytosis and leukocytosis. Can J Anaesth 1991; 38(5):613.

[b] 6. Nijsten MW, de Smet BJ, Dofferhoff AS. Pseudohyperkalemia and platelet counts. N Engl J Med 1991; 325(15):1107.

[c] 7. Michiels JJ. Pseudohyperkalemia and platelet count in thrombocythemia. Am J Hematol 1993; 42(2):237.

[c] 8. Graber M et al. Thrombocytosis elevates serum potassium. Am J Kidney Dis 1988; 12(2):116.

[b] 9. Alani FS et al. Pseudohyperkalemia associated with hereditary spherocytosis in four members of a family. Postgrad Med J 1994; 70(828):749.

[b] 10. Iolascon A et al. Familial pseudohyperkalemia maps to the same locus as dehydrated hereditary stomatocytosis (hereditary xerocytosis). Blood 1999; 93(9):3120.

[c] 11. Perazella MA. Drug-induced hyperkalemia: old culprits and new offenders. Am J Med 2000; 109:307.

[c] 12. Schon DA, Silva P, Hayslett JP. Mechanism of potassium excretion in renal insufficiency. Am J Physiol 1974; 227(6):1323.

[c] 13. Batlle DC. Segmental characterization of defects in collecting tubule acidification. Kidney Int 1986; 30(4):546.

[c] 14. DeFronzo RA et al. Investigations into mechanisms of hyperkalemia following renal transplantation. Kidney Int 1977; 11(5):357.

[c] 15. DeFronzo RA et al. Impaired renal tubular potassium secretion in systemic lupus erythematosus. Ann Intern Med 1977; 86(3):268.

[b] 16. Luke RG et al. Hyperkalemia and renal tubular acidosis due to renal amyloidosis. Ann Intern Med 1969; 70(6):1211.

[b] 17. Green J et al. Renal tubular handling of potassium in patients with medullary sponge kidney. Arch Intern Med 1984; 144(11):2201.

[b] 18. DeFronzo RA et al. Impaired renal tubular potassium secretion in sickle cell disease. Ann Intern Med 1979; 90(3):310.

[b] 19. Batlle DC, Arruda JAL, Kurtzman MA. Hyperkalemic distal renal tubular acidosis associated with obstructive uropathy. N Engl J Med 1981; 304(7):373.

[c] 20. Agarwal R, Afzalpurkar R, Fordtran JS. Pathophysiology of potassium absorption and secretion by the human intestine. Gastroenterology 1994; 107(2):548.

[b] 21. Allon M, Takeshian A, Shanklin N. Effect of insulin-plus-glucose infusion with or without epinephrine on fasting hyperkalemia. Kidney Int 1993; 43(1):212.

[b] 22. Allon M, Copkney C. Albuterol and insulin for treatment of hyperkalemia in hemodialysis patients. Kidney Int 1990; 38(5):869.

[b] 23. Blumberg A et al. Effect of various therapeutic approaches on plasma potassium and major regulating factors in terminal renal failure. Am J Med 1988; 85(4):507.

[b] 24. Blumberg A, Weidmann P, Ferrari P. Effect of prolonged bicarbonate administration on plasma potassium in terminal renal failure. Kidney Int 1992; 41(2):369.

[a] 25. Liou HH et al. Hypokalemic effects of intravenous infusion or nebulization of salbutamol in patients with chronic renal failure: comparative study. Am J Kidney Dis 1994; 23(2):266.

[b] 26. Gerstman BB, Kirkman R, Platt R. Intestinal necrosis associated with postoperative orally administered sodium polystyrene sulfonate in sorbitol. Am J Kidney Dis 1992; 20(2):159.

[b] 27. Lillemoe KD et al. Intestinal necrosis due to sodium polystyrene (Kayexalate) in sorbitol enemas: clinical and experimental support for the hypothesis. Surgery 1987; 101(3):267.

[c] 28. Rogers FB, Li SC. Acute colonic necrosis associated with sodium polystyrene sulfonate (Kayexalate) enemas in a critically ill patient: case report and review of the literature. J Trauma 2001; 51(2):395.

Hyponatremia

Kerri L. Cavanaugh, MD, and Derek M. Fine, MD

FAST FACTS

- Hyponatremia is defined as a serum sodium concentration less than 135 mEq/L.[1]
- Severe hyponatremia occurs at a serum sodium concentration less than 120 mEq/L.
- Hyponatremia is almost always a problem with water balance.
- Treatment should be based on the severity of symptoms and the rate of development of hyponatremia.
- Too rapid correction of the serum sodium concentration may result in the development of central pontine myelinolysis.[2,3]

I. EPIDEMIOLOGY

1. The epidemiology of hyponatremia is summarized in Table 54-1.[4-10]
2. Populations at high risk for acute neurological symptoms are premenopausal women,[10] postoperative patients, patients taking thiazide diuretics, elderly hospitalized patients, ultradistance exercise participants, and patients with psychogenic polydipsia.[12]

II. CLINICAL PRESENTATION

1. Symptoms of hyponatremia are related to both the absolute concentration of sodium and the rate of development of the hyponatremia. Acute hyponatremia onset refers to onset within 48 hours (Table 54-2).[13]
2. Symptoms and physical findings are due to excess water entry into cells of the brain and other tissues.[3] Cerebral edema develops and can progress to intracranial hypertension. This occurs particularly if the rate of development of hyponatremia is rapid because the brain's ability to adapt by exporting solute takes time. If cerebral edema has developed, care must be taken not to correct the hyponatremia too quickly because of the risk that central pontine myelinolysis will develop.

III. DIAGNOSTICS

1. Diagnosis is based on laboratory assessment, specifically the serum sodium level. The next step is to measure the plasma osmolality (P_{osm}) (Box 54-1). It is important to evaluate initially for possible pseudohyponatremia, which represents reduced serum sodium caused by either a reduction in the component of plasma that is predominantly plasma water or a translocation of sodium from intracellular to extracellular by various osmotic gradients. Hyponatremia with a normal measured

---

TABLE 54-1

EPIDEMIOLOGY OF HYPONATREMIA

Population	Prevalence (%)
Hospitalized patients	2.5[4]
Surgical patients	2.2[5]
Oncology patients	3.7[6]
Emergency room patients	4.4[7]
Elderly residents of nursing homes	8-18[8]
Intensive care unit patients	30[9]
Overall: severe hyponatremia	1.1[10]

TABLE 54-2

SYMPTOMS OF HYPONATREMIA

Level of Hyponatremia	Serum Sodium Level (mEq/L)	Symptoms
Mild	125-135	Anorexia, apathy, restlessness, nausea, lethargy, muscle cramps
Moderate	120-125	Agitation, disorientation, headache
Severe	<120	Seizures, coma, depressed reflexes, Cheyne-Stokes breathing, incontinence, death

---

BOX 54-1

FORMULAS TO GUIDE THERAPY FOR HYPONATREMIA

Calculated plasma osmolality $(P_{osm}) = 2 \times [Na^+] + \dfrac{[Glucose]}{18} + \dfrac{BUN}{2.8}$

Osmolal gap = Measured P_{Osm} − Calculated P_{Osm} (Normal ≤10 mOsm/L)

Total body water (TBW) = 0.6 (men) or 0.5 (women) × Body weight (kg)

Sodium deficit (estimate) = TBW × (Desired [Na] − Plasma [Na])

BUN, Blood urea nitrogen.

P_{osm} can be associated with hyperlipidemia, hyperproteinemia, and state following transurethral resection of the prostate (TURP) or bladder.[13] Both hyperlipidemia and hyperproteinemia cause a reduction in the total plasma water by occupying a greater portion of the plasma. This reduction in plasma water leads to a measured reduction in serum sodium concentration without actual change in total body sodium content. After TURP the resulting hyponatremia is hypothesized to be due to the large volume of solution (hypotonic: glycine or sorbitol, or isotonic: mannitol) used during the procedure or secondary retained solutes.[1] If serum osmolality is measured early in the course, these patients will have an abnormal osmolal gap (measured P_{osm} − calculated P_{osm}) greater than 10 mOsm/L. Treatment is not usually

TABLE 54-3

APPROACH TO HYPOOSMOTIC HYPONATREMIA BY VOLUME STATUS

	Volume Status				
Hypovolemia		Euvolemia		Hypervolemia	
U_{Na} >20 mEq/L	U_{Na} <20 mEq/L	U_{Na} >20 mEq/L		U_{Na} >20 mEq/L	U_{Na} <20 mEq/L
RENAL LOSSES	EXTRARENAL LOSSES	Glucocorticoid deficiency		Renal failure	Cirrhosis
Diuretic losses	GI losses (vomiting, diarrhea)	Hypothyroidism			Heart failure
Mineralocorticoid deficiency		Drugs			Nephrotic syndrome
Salt-losing nephropathy	Burns	SIADH			Pregnancy
Bicarbonaturia with RTA and metabolic alkalosis	Pancreatitis Trauma Marathon runners	Reset osmostat			
Ketonuria					
Osmotic diuresis					
Cerebral salt-wasting syndrome					

GI, Gastrointestinal; *RTA*, renal tubular acidosis; *SIADH*, syndrome of inappropriate antidiuretic hormone secretion; U_{Na}, urinary sodium.

54

HYPONATREMIA

recommended unless the patient is symptomatic or has end-stage renal disease requiring hemodialysis.

2. Elevated P_{osm} can be associated with hyperglycemia, mannitol administration, or intravenous immune globulin administration with concurrent renal failure. Such cases are often classified as translocational hyponatremia.[13] The correction for hyperglycemia is a 1.6-mEq/L reduction in plasma sodium for every 100 mg/dL elevation in plasma glucose.[1]

3. More likely the P_{osm} will be low or hypoosmotic, representing a dysfunction of water excretion. An assessment of the patient's volume status can assist with identifying an etiology as illustrated in Table 54-3.

4. Other helpful laboratory tests include urine osmolality, a full chemistry panel, serum uric acid concentration, and urinary sodium concentration. The serum uric acid level can also be used in the evaluation of the patient's volume status. If the serum uric acid level is less than 4 mg/dL, the patient is most likely euvolemic and the syndrome of inappropriate secretion of antidiuretic hormone (SIADH) should be considered. If the uric acid level is elevated, the patient may be either hypovolemic or hypervolemic.[14]

IV. MANAGEMENT

Box 54-2 outlines the acute management of hyponatremia.

A. HYPERVOLEMIC HYPONATREMIA

1. The pathophysiology is related to excessive secretion of antidiuretic hormone, or vasopressin (ADH), caused by decreases in the effective circulating volume and glomerular filtration rate. Hypervolemic hyponatremia is often a hallmark of advanced systemic disease. It usually develops at a chronic rate.
2. Treatment.
a. Fluid restriction, especially free water to less than urine output.
b. Treatment of underlying disease.

BOX 54-2

ACUTE MANAGEMENT OF HYPONATREMIA

ACUTE DEVELOPMENT WITH ASSOCIATED SYMPTOMS

Risk of cerebral edema outweighs risk of rapid correction; thus act quickly.

The goal hourly correction rate is 1.5-2 mEq/L/hr for 3-4 hours until symptoms resolve.[13]

Administer 3% saline with intravenous furosemide.

Check the plasma sodium level every 2 hours.

Consider evaluation for intensive care unit placement.

CHRONIC DEVELOPMENT

Treatment is controversial, especially if the patient is only mildly symptomatic.

The goal hourly correction rate is 0.5 mmol/L, not to exceed a serum value of 126-130 mmol/L or the administration of more than 25 mmol/L per 48 hours.[13]

Restriction of free water intake is recommended.

UNKNOWN DURATION

Assess clinical symptoms; consider imaging to evaluate for edema.

If symptoms are severe, the goal hourly correction rate is 1-2 mmol/L for 3-4 hours.[13]

VOLUME DEPLETION

Recommend isotonic saline for replacement.

Hypertonic saline is reserved for patients with symptoms.

Dilute solutions have no role.

HYPOKALEMIA

Potassium should be repleted. Potassium is also an effective osmole, and as it shifts between intracellular and extracellular spaces, sodium will also shift.[13]

NOTE

If the plasma sodium concentration rises too quickly, water can be administered to reduce the risk of demyelinating disease.

B. HYPOVOLEMIC HYPONATREMIA

1. Losses of both solute and volume and subsequent replacement with water or other hypoosmotic solutions lead to this state. Losses can be either renal or extrarenal (e.g., GI tract, insensible losses such as skin or pulmonary) and can result from third spacing of fluid into tissue (burns, trauma, or pancreatitis).

2. When the volume loss is due to vomiting complicated by metabolic alkalosis, the urine sodium level may be greater than 20 mEq/L because of high urine bicarbonate losses. The urine chloride level is usually less than 10 mEq/L.[13]

3. Diuretic therapy can lead directly to acute development of severe hyponatremia. Patients who are being treated with thiazide diuretics and drink large amounts of water are at high risk for this state. Three mechanisms are at work: direct volume depletion, potassium depletion, and direct inhibition of urinary dilution by diminished NaCl absorption in the loop of Henle and distal tubule.[13] Thiazide diuretics may result in a loss of effective ions in excess of water. This effect usually occurs within 2 weeks of starting therapy.[15]

4. Treatment.
   a. Discontinuation of offending diuretic agent.
   b. Volume replacement, with fluid composition based on severity of symptoms and electrolytes needed.

5. Cerebral salt wasting is a controversial form of hyponatremia described in patients with cerebral insults, such as subarachnoid hemorrhage. In these patients hyponatremia similar to SIADH develops; they are usually volume depleted, however, and the measured elevation of urine sodium is due to urinary wasting. The mechanism is unknown.[16]

C. EUVOLEMIC HYPONATREMIA

1. Cortisol deficiency causes ADH release. In this state a component of effective volume depletion may be involved. In addition, ADH is cosecreted with corticotropin-releasing hormone by cells in the paraventricular nucleus, and in the deficient state the absence of a negative feedback control results in excessive ADH secretion.[13]

2. Severe hypothyroidism is part of the differential diagnosis but is quite rare as a cause of hyponatremia. The mechanism is unknown.[13]

3. Reset osmostat is a condition in which a patient's osmoreceptor responds to changes in plasma osmolality but the threshold for ADH release is reduced. Thus the plasma sodium concentration is below normal but usually stable (125-130 mEq/L).[13] Clinical conditions reported to place patients at risk for this state include quadriplegia, psychosis, chronic malnutrition, alcoholism, and pregnancy.[17] The diagnosis can be confirmed with normal excretion of a water load.

4. Treatment.
   a. Corticosteroid replacement if the cause is cortisol deficiency.
   b. Thyroid hormone replacement if the cause is hypothyroidism.
   c. Correction of the underlying disorder.

54

HYPONATREMIA

V. SPECIAL CASE: SYNDROME OF INAPPROPRIATE ANTIDIURETIC HORMONE SECRETION

Box 54-3 lists the causes and features of SIADH.

A. PATHOPHYSIOLOGY

1. Four types of osmoregulatory defect have been described in SIADH.[13]

a. (I) ADH secretion appears to be independent of osmoreceptor control or a nonosmotic stimulus is present.

b. (II) The osmostat is reset so that the urine is diluted maximally, but the threshold value for the stimulus is below the normal range.

BOX 54-3

SYNDROME OF INAPPROPRIATE ANTIDIURETIC HORMONE SECRETION*

CAUSES

Enhanced hypothalamic ADH production

Infections: meningitis, encephalitis, abscess, varicella-zoster virus

Vascular: subarachnoid hemorrhage, cerebrovascular accident, temporal arteritis

Neoplasm

Psychosis

Human immunodeficiency virus, Guillain-Barré syndrome, acute intermittent porphyria, hypothalamic sarcoidosis, multiple sclerosis

Drugs: intravenously administered cyclophosphamide, chlorpropamide

Pulmonary disease

Postoperative state

Severe nausea

Idiopathic

Ectopic ADH production: small cell carcinoma of lung

Oxytocin during labor

Prolactinoma

Waldenström's macroglobulinemia

Head trauma

Shy-Drager syndrome

Delirium tremens

FEATURES

Hyponatremia and hypoosmolality

Urinary osmolality >100 mOsm/kg

Urinary sodium level >20 mEq/L

Normovolemia

Normal renal, adrenal, and thyroid function

Normal acid-base and potassium balance

Hypouricemia in some cases

ADH, Antidiuretic hormone.

*Characterized by nonphysiological release of ADH and impaired water excretion with normal sodium excretion (volume).

c. (III) Urinary dilution is impaired because of a constant and nonsuppressible leak of ADH.

d. (IV) The osmoregulation response is normal, but the patient cannot excrete a water load. Possible reasons for this are increased renal sensitivity or another antidiuretic stimulus.

B. MANAGEMENT

1. Treatment of SIADH includes fluid restriction so that the total daily input of volume is less than the total urine output. The restriction includes free water. Acute management is recommended as previously described (Box 54-2). Initiation of a loop diuretic may also be helpful in correction of the hyponatremia of SIADH. If the SIADH is a chronic condition, in addition to fluid and free water restriction the treatment may include a high-salt, high-protein diet and other agents such as demeclocycline (300 mg bid) or lithium.[13]

2. Use of isotonic saline to treat hyponatremia caused by SIADH will result in sodium excretion in the urine and ultimately in water retention with worsening of the hyponatremia.[1]

3. For SIADH, U_{osm} remains approximately constant. The effective osmolality of the fluid given must be greater than that of the urine to raise the plasma sodium concentration.[13]

PEARLS AND PITFALLS

- Primary polydipsia is often associated with an underlying psychosis, such as schizoprenia.[1] Patients complain of polyuria and thirst. A central defect in thirst regulation is thought to be present.[13] Rarely, the intake of water exceeds the maximum dilutional ability of the kidney, resulting in severe hyponatremia. Management includes treatment of the underlying disorder and monitoring of water intake.

- Beer podomania or "tea and toast syndrome" is a phenomenon seen in patients who drink excessive amounts of beer or tea (hypotonic solution) and do not consume a protein- and solute-rich diet. If the patient does not take in enough solute, the maximal urine volume capacity is significantly reduced and the patient cannot excrete sufficient amounts of water.[1]

- Central pontine myelinolysis is a complication of therapy caused by overly rapid correction of serum sodium. This syndrome has been associated with central demyelinating lesions, particularly in the pons. Symptoms typically are neurological and include paraparesis or quadriparesis, dysarthria, dysphagia, coma, and seizures.[2] Diagnosis is usually confirmed by computed tomography or magnetic resonance imaging of the brain, although lesions may not be detectable for 4 weeks.[2] Risk factors include the following.[12]
  - More than a 12 mEq/L elevation in plasma sodium in the first 24 hours.
  - Overcorrection of plasma sodium level to greater than 140 mEq/L in the first 48 hours.

54

HYPONATREMIA

- Hypoxic or anoxic episodes.
- Hypercatabolism (burns).
- Malnutrition (alcoholism).
- Overcorrection sometimes occurs because of failure to recognize exogenous sources of sodium (e.g., fluid administered in the emergency room before admission) or an electrolyte shift caused by concomitant administration of potassium.[18]

REFERENCES

[c] 1. Adrogue JH, Madias NE. Hyponatremia. N Engl J Med 2000; 342:1581.

[c] 2. Laureno R, Karp BI. Myelinolysis after correction of hyponatremia. Ann Intern Med 1997; 126(1):57.

[b] 3. Arieff AI, Llach F, Massry SG. Neurological manifestations and morbidity of hyponatremia: correlation with brain water and electrolytes. Medicine 1976; 55:121.

[b] 4. Anderson RJ. Hyponatremia: a prospective analysis of its epidemiology and the pathogenetic role of vasopressin. Ann Intern Med 1985; 102:164.

[b] 5. Madiba TE, Haffejee AA, Mokoena TR. Hyponatraemia—a prospective analysis of surgical patients. S Afr J Surg 1998; 36:78.

[b] 6. Berghmans T, Paesmans M, Body JJ. A prospective study on hyponatraemia in medical cancer patients: epidemology, aetiology and differential diagnosis. Support Care Cancer 2000; 8:192.

[b] 7. Lee CT, Guo HR, Chen JB. Hyponatremia in the emergency department. Am J Emerg Med 2000; 18:264.

[b] 8. Miller M, Morley JE, Rubenstein LZ. Hyponatremia in a nursing home population. J Am Geriatr Soc 1995; 43:1410.

[b] 9. DeVita MV et al. Incidence and etiology of hyponatremia in an intensive care unit. Clin Nephrol 1990; 34:163.

[b] 10. Erasmus RT, Matsha TE. The frequency, aetiology and outcome of severe hyponatraemia in adult hospitalised patients. Cent Afr J Med 1998; 44:154.

[b] 11. Ayus JC, Wheeler JM, Arieff AI. Postoperative hyponatremia encephalopathy in menstruant women. Ann Intern Med 1992; 117:891.

[c] 12. Gross P. Treatment of severe hyponatremia. Kidney Int 2001; 60:2417.

[c] 13. Rose BD et al. Clinical physiology of acid-base and electrolyte disorders. New York: McGraw-Hill; 1994.

[c] 14. Maesaka JK. An expanded view of SIADH, hyponatremia, and hypouricemia. Clin Nephrol 1996; 46:79.

[b] 15. Ashraf N, Locksley R, Arieff AI. Thiazide-induced hyponatremia associated with death or neurologic damage in outpatients. Am J Med 1981; 70:1163.

[c] 16. Kumar S, Berl T. Sodium. Lancet 1998; 352:220.

[c] 17. Fried LF, Palevsky PM. Hyponatremia and hypernatremia. Med Clin North Am 1997; 81:585.

[c] 18. Phuong-Chi TP, Chen PV, Phuong-Thu TP. Overcorrection of hyponatremia: where do we go wrong? Am J Kidney Dis 2000; 36:1.

Delirium

Cynthia Brown, MD, and Gail V. Berkenblit, MD, PhD

FAST FACTS

- Delirium is a state of disturbed consciousness characterized by decreased attention and cognition. It develops over a short period and fluctuates in course.[1]
- Delirium affects 10% to 30% of hospital inpatients and is often unrecognized.[2-4]
- An episode of delirium during a hospitalization increases a patient's risk of complications during the hospitalization, as well as the long-term risk of institutionalization and death.[3,5]
- The most common risk factors for delirium are increasing age and underlying dementia.[6-8]
- Medication is implicated in 30% to 40% of delirium episodes.[9]
- Treatment should include identification and treatment of the underlying cause and environmental and pharmacological measures to ensure the patient's safety.[9-11]
- Antipsychotics alone or in combination with benzodiazepines are the primary medications used in treating delirium.[9,10]

55

I. EPIDEMIOLOGY

1. Delirium is underrecognized but extremely common.
2. Prevalence of delirium among hospitalized patients ranges from 10% to 30%.[2] The prevalence has remained unchanged over the past decade.[10]
3. Delirium develops in 30% to 40% of hospitalized patients with acquired immunodeficiency syndrome, approximately 25% of patients with cancer,[10] and up to 50% of patients after repair of a hip fracture.[2]
4. Health care professionals have been poor at recognizing delirium. In one study 10% of patients older than 64 years had delirium at presentation based on a screening examination.[4] In only one in five, however, was the condition recognized by an emergency department physician. Other studies support these data, with reported rates of nondetection from 33% to 66%.[12]

II. CLINICAL PRESENTATION

1. Delirium is defined as a disturbance of consciousness with an accompanying decline in cognition that cannot be better explained by an underlying dementia.[1]
2. Delirium develops over a short period, usually hours to days, and fluctuates during the course of the day.

3. The fourth edition of the *Diagnostic and Statistical Manual of Mental Disorders* (DSM-IV) lists four subcategories of delirium—due to General Medical Condition, due to Substance Abuse or Withdrawal, due to Multiple Etiologies, or Not Otherwise Specified.[1]

4. The disturbance in consciousness may be manifested as decreased or increased alertness, but it is frequently subtler with a patient demonstrating decreased attention. The patient may be easily distractible and have an impaired ability to focus, shift, or maintain attention.[1] Questions frequently have to be repeated, and the patient perseverates on a single answer.

5. The change in cognition has varied presentations. The patient may show a slight impairment in recent memory or disorientation to time. However, perceptual disturbances also occur and can range from misinterpretations of stimuli to frank hallucinations.[1]

6. Delirium is often associated with alterations in sleep-wake cycle and diurnal variation.[1] Patients may exhibit psychomotor agitation, retardation, or both during the course of the day. Agitation may range from lethargy and unresponsiveness to threatening behavior with staff or climbing out of bed. Emotional disturbances such as anxiety or fear may also accompany delirium.

7. The differential diagnosis for delirium includes dementia, psychotic disorders, and affective disorders such as depression (Box 55-1).[9]

8. Differentiating dementia from delirium can be difficult because they often overlap. Delirium develops in 25% to 50% of patients with dementia during their hospital stay.[2]

9. Delirium can be differentiated from dementia by its acute and fluctuating course. Patients with depression and psychotic disorders do not exhibit alterations in consciousness.

A. RISK FACTORS AND CAUSES

1. Some groups of patients have specific intrinsic factors in their history that place them at higher risk for delirium while in the hospital.

2. Age and underlying dementia are the strongest predictors for the development of delirium.[6,8]

3. Some other identified risk factors are comorbid medical condition, alcohol use, diminished ability to perform activities of daily living, treatment with multiple medications, and visual or hearing impairment (Box 55-2).[6]

BOX 55-1
DIFFERENTIAL DIAGNOSIS OF DELIRIUM
Dementia
Psychotic disorders
Affective disorders such as depression
Cerebrovascular accident

4. While the factors listed above predispose a patient to an episode of delirium, they alone are not causative. In several studies and reviews, medications have been the most common causative agent and are implicated in 20% to 40% of cases.[2,8,9]

5. Almost every class of medication has been reported to cause changes in mental status, but some groups of medications are frequently implicated (Box 55-3).[2,9,10]

6. Addition of more than three medications during a hospitalization has been associated with the development of delirium.[8]

BOX 55-2

RISK FACTORS FOR DELIRIUM

PATIENT FACTORS

Age

Independence with activities of daily living

Prior episode of delirium

Hearing or visual impairment

Multiple hospital admissions

Multiple medications

Immobility

COMORBID CONDITIONS

Dementia

Acquired immunodeficiency syndrome

Cancer

Liver disease

Fracture

Malnutrition

Alcohol or substance abuse

Renal insufficiency

Burns

Psychiatric illness

PERIOPERATIVE

Duration of operation

Emergency procedure

Type of operation

ENVIRONMENTAL FACTORS

Social isolation

Sensory deprivation

Sleep deprivation

Novel environment

Loss of day-night differentiation

BOX 55-3

MEDICATIONS AND SUBSTANCES THAT CAN CAUSE DELIRIUM

DRUGS OF ABUSE

Alcohol
Phencyclidine
Cocaine
Marijuana
Heroin, opioids
Hallucinogens
Amphetamines
Sedatives
Inhalants

NARCOTIC ANALGESICS

Meperidine
Morphine
Codeine
Hydromorphone
Oxycodone

BENZODIAZEPINES

Alprazolam
Chlordiazepoxide
Triazolam
Diazepam
Lorazepam

ANTICHOLINERGIC DRUGS

Diphenhydramine
Tricyclic antidepressants
Scopolamine
Quinidine
Thioridazine
Benztropine

PARKINSONIAN AGENTS

Levodopa, carbidopa
Dopamine agonists
Amantadine

MISCELLANEOUS

H_2 receptor blockers
Fluoroquinolones
Anticonvulsants
Corticosteroids
Lithium
β-Blockers

7. One study found infection to be the primary precipitating factor in 34% of cases of delirium.[7]
8. Myriad medical causes can be found (Box 55-4), and the clinician must be astute in looking for these causes.[10]
9. Local factors such as undertreated pain or a bladder catheter can lead to delirium.[8] Some interventions used in the behavioral management of delirious patients, including restraints, can worsen delirium.
10. Multiple factors are frequently implicated. Only 56% of cases have a single cause. On average, 2.8 causes per patient are identified.[10]

III. DIAGNOSTICS

1. The diagnosis of delirium is twofold. First the episode of delirium must be identified, and then a search for the precipitating factors should be made.
2. An astute health care professional should be able to identify delirium on the basis of a complete general, psychiatric, and neurological history and examination.
3. The DSM-IV criteria discussed previously provide guidelines for identifying an episode of delirium.

55

DELIRIUM

BOX 55-4

MEDICAL CAUSES OF DELIRIUM

Infection (e.g., urinary tract infection, pneumonia, sepsis, meningitis)
Drug intoxication (therapeutic or illicit substances)
Hypotension
Hypertensive emergency
Acute myocardial infarction
Exacerbation of chronic obstructive pulmonary disease
Hypoxia
Hypercarbia
Pulmonary embolism
Dehydration
Electrolyte disturbances (hyponatremia, hypercalcemia, hypernatremia)
Acid-base disturbances
Uremia
Seizures or postictal state
Vitamin deficiency (thiamine, niacin)
Cerebrovascular accident
Intracerebral hemorrhage
Subdural hemorrhage
Urinary retention
Hepatic encephalopathy
Hypoglycemia or hyperglycemia
Hypothyroidism or hyperthyroidism

4. More formal assessments for delirium are used primarily in research settings, but some of these can easily be used by clinicians. For example, the Confusion Assessment Method (CAM) introduced by Inouye and associates in 1990 has become the most widely used tool to screen for delirium and has a reported sensitivity of 94% to 100% and a specificity of 90% to 95%.[13]

5. The Confusion Rating Scale was designed to help nursing staff identify patients with delirium.[10]

6. No specific laboratory or diagnostic tests are available to diagnose delirium, although an electroencephalogram will frequently show diffuse slowing.[10]

7. Once the diagnosis of delirium has been established, identification of the precipitating factor becomes important for appropriate treatment.

8. When evaluating a patient with delirium, the clinician should review the medication list for potential causative agents. Vital signs, including temperature and pulse oximetry, should always be obtained.

9. Depending on the patient's individual factors, the physician should consider other tests based on clinical judgment (Box 55-5). For

---

BOX 55-5

WORKUP OF DELIRIUM

FOR ALL PATIENTS

Vital signs (blood pressure, pulse, temperature, pulse oximetry)
Review of all medications

FOR MOST PATIENTS

Electrolytes (sodium, potassium, calcium, magnesium, phosphate)
Fingerstick glucose
Complete blood cell count
Urinalysis
Blood urea nitrogen and creatinine

FOR SELECTED PATIENTS

Arterial blood gases
Therapeutic drug levels (digoxin, anticonvulsants, theophylline)
Blood and urine cultures
Electrocardiogram
Creatinine kinase, troponin
Chest radiography
Urine and blood toxicology
Lumbar puncture
Electroencephalogram
Computed tomography of head
Ammonia
Thyroid function tests

example, fingerstick glucose measurements should be performed for all diabetic patients with altered mental status.

10. Other tests to consider on an individual basis include electrocardiography, complete blood count, measurement of electrolyte and therapeutic drug levels, arterial blood gas assessment, and urine or serum toxicology screening.

IV. MANAGEMENT

1. Treatment of an episode of delirium should include multiple strategies.

2. Identification and treatment of the underlying cause of delirium is the first step, since delirium is unlikely to clear unless the precipitating factor is addressed. In some cases treatment of the underlying cause may be the only treatment necessary. For instance, correction of hypoglycemia in a diabetic patient should cause a return to a baseline level of mental functioning.

3. In many cases the underlying cause is not rapidly correctable or the mental status lags behind physical recovery. In this situation the treatment strategy focuses on providing supportive care through environmental and pharmacological measures.

4. Interventions that provide familiarity, orientation, and stimulation are the primary goals of environmental strategies.[10,14] Having a clock and a calendar in each patient room provides orientation, and staff should reinforce such information as day, location, and condition during interactions with patients. The presence of family or friends or having familiar objects in the room helps the patient maintain a connection to his or her usual environment.[14]

5. A sense of timelessness frequently pervades medical environments; providing clear day-night clues such as dimming hallway and room lights and minimizing ambient noise during the night helps to maintain usual sleep-wake cycles.[10]

6. Education of the patient and the family regarding the delirium and its cause is important to ensure a supportive therapeutic environment.

7. Mechanical restraints should be avoided unless the patient's behavior risks harm to self or others.

8. Correction of sensory impairments with glasses and hearing aids improves a patient's ability to interact with the environment and decreases the patient's risk of misinterpreting environmental clues.[9]

9. Participation in usual activities such as feeding and grooming provides stimulation and familiarity; early involvement in physical and occupational therapy is important to limit debilitation and provide stimulation.[9,10]

10. Pharmacological treatment of delirium should be limited to patients whose behavior may harm themselves or others and to medications specifically indicated for the underlying cause of delirium.[9]

11. Caution must be used when prescribing any medication because

55

DELIRIUM

almost all medication classes have been implicated as causes of delirium.

12. Antipsychotic medications have long been the primary class of drugs used for the treatment of delirium and have been shown to be superior to benzodiazepines except in cases of seizures or withdrawal from alcohol or sedatives.[10]

13. Within the antipsychotic class, haloperidol is the preferred drug because it has fewer anticholinergic effects, causes minimal depression of the cardiovascular system, and has no active metabolite.[10] Dosage is given in Box 55-6.

14. The recommended dose of haloperidol depends on individual patient factors and level of disturbance. The initial dose of haloperidol is usually between 0.5 and 10 mg intramuscularly or intravenously.

15. More extrapyramidal side effects are seen when haloperidol is given by the intramuscular route. Caution should be used with intravenous administration of haloperidol because QT prolongation and cardiac arrhythmia may occur. Doses may be repeated every 20 to 30 minutes until behavior has been adequately controlled and every 2 to 4 hours thereafter as needed.[9,10]

16. The onset of action of haloperidol is approximately 20 minutes. When a faster onset of action is required, droperidol may be used with the knowledge that greater hypotension and sedation are associated with its use.[10]

17. Newer antipsychotic medications such as risperidone and olanzapine have not been thoroughly enough studied to recommend their routine use, and they are not available in parenteral forms.[9] These compounds, however, are known to have less associated sedation and extrapyramidal side effects.[9]

BOX 55-6

PHARMACOLOGICAL TREATMENT OF DELIRIUM

ANTIPSYCHOTIC MEDICATIONS

Haloperidol (preferred) 0.5-10 mg IV or IM q2-4h as needed for agitation; maximum dose 100 mg q24h

Droperidol 0.625-2.5 mg IV or IM q8h as needed; patient requires cardiac monitoring to watch QT interval

Risperidone 0.5-2.5 mg PO q12h as needed; not well validated and has long dose interval

BENZODIAZEPINES

For use as adjunctive treatment with antipsychotics or in alcohol or sedative withdrawal

Lorazepam (preferred) 1-2 mg IV or IM q4h as needed, with monitoring for respiratory depression and sedation

18. The primary side effects to remember when prescribing antipsychotic medications are extrapyramidal symptoms, neuroleptic malignant syndrome, and prolongation of the QT interval, particularly at higher doses.[10]

19. Benzodiazepines are a second class of medications frequently used in treating delirium. As discussed in Chapter 74, they are the treatment of choice for seizures and alcohol or sedative withdrawal. Use of benzodiazepines is outlined in Box 55-6.

20. Benzodiazepines are not recommended as monotherapy for the treatment of delirium because studies have shown that they are less effective than antipsychotic medication.[10]

21. Benzodiazepines, however, may provide an important adjunctive treatment for delirium; with their use the antipsychotic dose can be reduced, limiting side effects of the neuroleptic medications.

22. An advantage of benzodiazepines is that flumazenil rapidly reverses their effects.

23. Caution must be used when prescribing benzodiazepines because of their effects on mental status. They can cause myriad side effects, including delirium, sedation, respiratory depression, and physical dependence with severe withdrawal symptoms such as seizures.[9,10] Patients with decreased metabolism resulting from hepatic insufficiency are at risk for accumulation of this class of medications.[10]

24. Lorazepam is a frequently used benzodiazepine for the treatment of delirium. It has several advantages, including a rapid onset and short duration of action and no major active metabolites.[9]

55

DELIRIUM

PEARLS AND PITFALLS

- Outcomes.
  - An episode of delirium during a hospital stay is a significant predictor of poor hospital and long-term outcomes.
  - Both medical and surgical patients in whom delirium develops have longer hospital stays because of an increased risk of complications such as aspiration pneumonia and decubitus ulcers.[10]
  - Multiple studies have shown delirium to be a risk factor for readmission or placement in a nursing home.[3,7,10]
  - Symptoms of delirium frequently are not completely resolved at the time of hospital discharge. Inouye and associates demonstrated significant long-term decline in performance of activities of daily living and increased nursing home placement.[3] After adjustment for confounding factors such as age, dementia, and APACHE score, the data showed an adjusted odds ratio for new nursing home placement of 3 at hospital discharge and at 3 months. A trend toward increased risk of death at hospital discharge and at 3 months was also noted.
  - In a more recent study delirium was shown to increase long-term mortality of all causes at 3 years with a risk ratio of 2.24,[5] supporting data reported by others.[2,3]

- Prevention.
  - In a recent article by Inouye,[11] an aggressive new strategy to prevent delirium was proposed. This intervention is a multidisciplinary tactic involving nursing staff, physical and occupational therapists, and physicians.
  - Several individual risk factors were targeted, including cognitive impairment, sleep deprivation, immobility, dehydration, and visual and hearing impairment.
  - Among the interventions made in regard to the targeted risk factors were cognitively stimulating activities and ambulation or range-of-motion exercises performed three times daily. In addition, many interventions focused on patient comfort, including strict noise reduction, warm drinks, relaxation tapes, and massage to promote good sleep hygiene.
  - The interventions were time consuming, but the program yielded encouraging results with a significant reduction (33%) in the number of patients in whom delirium developed. In addition, the total days of delirium and total number of episodes of delirium were significantly decreased in the intervention group.
  - If delirium developed, however, the multidisciplinary preventive strategy had no effect on its severity or likelihood of recurrence, which suggests that primary prevention is the best strategy.
- Comorbid conditions.
  - Multiple risk factors and comorbid conditions predispose a patient to delirium; some of these merit special consideration for treatment.
  - Patients with impaired liver function are at increased risk not only of delirium, but also of adverse effects from the treatment of delirium. This increased susceptibility is conferred through decreased albumin level and impaired metabolism.[10]
  - Many medications circulate in plasma bound to albumin or other plasma proteins; a decrease in albumin and other plasma proteins causes the level of unbound medication in the blood to rise.[10] This alteration can increase the tissue bioavailability of a drug, leading to therapeutic effects at less than usual doses and a greater potential for adverse side effects.[10]
  - Many of the medications used to treat delirium are metabolized by the liver, but no recommendations have been made for specific dosage alterations of most drugs because no test accurately measures the amount of liver impairment and pharmacodynamics cannot be readily assessed.[15] Haloperidol, however, is generally thought to have similar pharmacokinetics in patients with liver dysfunction and in normal patients because glucuronidation is important in its metabolism.[10]
  - The American Psychiatric Association recommends that only benzodiazepines undergoing glucuronidation be used in advanced liver disease to decrease difficulties with delayed oxidation and therefore

extended therapeutic effects. Benzodiazepines requiring only glucuronidation are lorazepam, temazepam, and oxazepam.[10]

- Treatment of elderly patients with delirium requires special attention. Elderly patients are particularly susceptible to delirium and also have more risk factors for the development of delirium, such as multiple medical problems, polypharmacy, sensory deficits, and age-related decline in hepatic metabolism.

- Lower doses of medication are recommended for treatment of the elderly.[10] For instance, 0.5 mg of haloperidol or lorazepam can be used as a starting dose rather than the usual 1- to 2-mg doses.

- Special consideration should be paid to medications having anticholinergic side effects, since these effects are especially prominent in the elderly.[10] Medications commonly used in clinical practice for nonpsychiatric indications are often culprits and include ranitidine, diphenhydramine, and digoxin.

55

DELIRIUM

REFERENCES

[d] 1. American Psychiatric Association. Diagnostic and statistical manual of mental disorders, 4th ed. Washington, DC: American Psychiatric Association; 1999.

[c] 2. Francis J. Delirium in older patients. J Am Geriatr Society 1992; 40:829.

[b] 3. Inouye SK et al. Does delirium contribute to poor hospital outcome? A three-site epidemiologic study. J Gen Intern Med 1998; 13:234.

[b] 4. Lewis LM. Unrecognized delirium in ED geriatric population. Am J Emerg Med 1995; 13:142.

[b] 5. Curyto KJ et al. Survival of hospitalized patients with delirium: a prospective study. Am J Geriatr Psychiatry 2001; 9:141.

[b] 6. Elie M et al. Delirium risk factors in elderly hospitalized patients. J Gen Intern Med 1998; 13:204.

[b] 7. George J, Bleasdale S, Singleton SJ. Causes of delirium in elderly patients admitted to a district general hospital. Age Ageing 1997; 26:423.

[b] 8. Inouye SK, Charpentier PA. Precipitating factors for delirium in hospitalized elderly persons. JAMA 1996; 275:852.

[c] 9. Meagher D. Delirium: optimizing management. Br Med J 2001; 322:144.

[d] 10. American Psychiatric Association. Practice guidelines for the treatment of patients with delirium. Washington, DC: American Psychiatric Association; 1999.

[a] 11. Inouye SK et al. A multicomponent intervention to prevent delirium in hospitalized older patients. N Engl J Med 1999; 340:669.

[c] 12. Inouye SK. The dilemma of delirium: clinical and research controversies regarding diagnosis and evaluation of delirium in hospitalized elderly medical patients. Am J Med 1994; 97:278.

[b] 13. Inouye SK et al. Clarifying confusion: the confusion assessment method, a new method for detecting delirium. Ann Intern Med 1990; 113:941.

[b] 14. Meagher DJ et al. Use of environmental strategies and psychotropic medication in the management of delirium. Br J Psychiatry 1996; 168:512.

[c] 15. Rodighiero V. Effects of liver disease on pharmacokinetics: an update. Clin Pharmacokinet 1999; 37:399.

Status Epilepticus

Andrew Mammen, MD, PhD, and Ronald Lesser, MD, PhD

FAST FACTS

- The estimated incidence of status epilepticus (SE) in the United States is 102,000 to 152,000 cases per year, and about 55,000 deaths are associated with SE each year.[1,2]
- SE occurs most often in younger age groups and in persons over 60 years of age.
- SE often occurs in one of three contexts.
  - In patients with an acute or chronic process affecting the brain (e.g., metabolic disturbances, head injury, central nervous system [CNS] infection, hypoxia, drug intoxication or withdrawal, stroke, brain tumor).
  - As an acute exacerbation in known epileptic patients, often as a consequence of poor compliance with antiepileptic drug (AED) regimens.
  - As the first seizure in a patient who will go on to develop epilepsy. About 12% to 30% of adult patients who develop epilepsy present with SE.
- The mortality rate associated with SE is 3% to 35%.[3] Young age is a favorable prognostic indicator. Patients with prolonged seizures and with severe physiological disturbances have higher mortality and morbidity rates.

56

I. CLINICAL PRESENTATION

A. TYPES OF SEIZURES

1. Seizures may be partial or generalized.
2. With partial seizures only limited areas of the brain are affected and dysfunction may likewise be limited (e.g., clonic movements and paresthesias of a single limb, aphasia, visual changes).
3. During simple partial seizures consciousness remains unimpaired.
4. If the patient experiences an alteration of consciousness, the seizures are complex partial.
5. In generalized seizures the entire brain is involved and the patient experiences loss of consciousness. During a convulsive generalized seizure the patient demonstrates tonic, clonic, or tonic-clonic movements.
6. Absence seizures also result from generalized seizure activity affecting both hemispheres of the brain. Absence seizures usually begin in childhood and are manifested as a brief lapse in awareness with generalized brain involvement on an encephalogram (EEG) at seizure onset.

7. Complex partial seizures are also manifested as decreased awareness but begin with more localized brain involvement at seizure onset.

8. Any type of seizure may evolve into a generalized seizure with impaired consciousness.

B. DEFINITIONS

1. Status epilepticus is defined as any seizure lasting longer than 30 minutes or when two or more seizures occur within 30 minutes and the patient does not return to a normal level of consciousness between seizures.

2. Prolonged SE may have significant long-term adverse effects on cognitive function. Therefore SE is regarded as a medical emergency, and most clinicians choose to treat seizures before 30 minutes is allowed to elapse.

3. Generalized tonic-clonic seizures are sometimes described as progressing through five phases, but it is unusual for all these phases to occur in a given patient (Table 56-1).

4. Classic generalized tonic-clonic seizures are easily recognized, and when they persist, the condition is termed overt generalized convulsive status epilepticus (overt GCSE).

5. As overt GCSE seizures evolve, the clonic activity may become less pronounced and patients may have only twitching movements in a restricted distribution. These patients are still having generalized seizures, as reflected in the electroencephalogram (EEG), and are said to be having subtle GCSE seizures.

6. At the extreme end of this spectrum, some patients with impaired consciousness and seizure activity on EEG have no observable repetitious movements. This state, termed nonconvulsive status epilepticus (NCSE), should be considered in patients with altered mental status that cannot be otherwise explained.

7. It is important to recognize that although subtle GCSE and NCSE

TABLE 56-1	
PHASES OF GENERALIZED TONIC-CLONIC SEIZURES	
Phase	Description and Symptoms
1. Premonitory	Headache, irritability; may precede seizures by hours to days
2. Myoclonic jerks, brief tonic-clonic seizures	Generally precede generalized tonic-clonic seizures by a few minutes
3. Tonic	Contraction of axial musculature and limbs, often with "epileptic cry" as respiratory muscles contract
4. Clonic	Jerking at a frequency of about four jerks per second; at end of clonic phase, which typically lasts less than 3 minutes, relaxation of sphincter muscles may result in bladder or bowel incontinence
5. Postictal	Patient may be asleep or confused at this time

seizures may be less alarming to onlookers, in some circumstances they may be just as harmful to the CNS as overt GCSE seizures.

II. DIAGNOSTICS
A. ELECTROENCEPHALOGRAPHY
1. Overt GCSE tonic-clonic seizures are easily recognized and do not require EEG confirmation before initiating treatment.
2. In contrast, subtle GCSE and NCSE seizures usually require EEG evaluation.
B. DIFFERENTIAL DIAGNOSIS (Box 56-1)

III. MANAGEMENT[4]
A. TREATMENT OF ONGOING SEIZURE (Fig. 56-1)
1. The patient should be maintained in a lateral decubitus position to prevent aspiration.
2. Oxygen should be administered.
3. If the seizure has just started, the physician should watch and wait for 3 minutes. Most seizures stop without intervention in this period. During the wait the following should be done.
   a. The fingerstick glucose level should be checked because hypoglycemia is a common cause of seizure.
   b. Two peripheral intravenous lines should be placed, avoiding the antecubital area because flexion of the arm may block intravenous access.
   c. Vital signs should be monitored, and a syringe with 0.1 mg/kg of lorazepam (or 5-10 mg of diazepam) should be prepared.
   d. Any additional relevant history should be obtained (e.g., whether the patient is taking an AED).
4. Blood tests should be ordered, including electrolytes, complete blood count, magnesium, calcium, ammonia, toxicology screen, and anticonvulsant levels (if applicable.)
5. If the fingerstick revealed a low glucose level, 100 mg of thiamine and then 1 ampule of 50% dextrose (D_{50}; D-glucose) should be administered.
6. If glucose levels are normal, or if the seizure persists after glucose is given, lorazepam, up to 0.1 mg/kg, should be administered at 2 mg/min. It should be administered 1 to 3 mg at a time, waiting a minute or two between infusions for the seizure to subside. The entire dose of benzodiazepine should be given only if the seizure persists. If no intravenous access can be obtained, lorazepam may be given intramuscularly. Diazepam is equally effective at terminating sei-

---

BOX 56-1

DIFFERENTIAL DIAGNOSIS OF STATUS EPILEPTICUS

Myoclonus secondary to metabolic compromise (hypercarbia, hypoxia)

Medication side effect (tardive dyskinesia)

Pseudoseizures

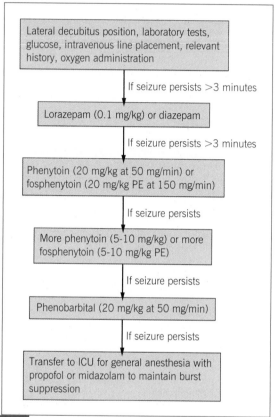

FIG. 56-1

Management approach for patients with status epilepticus.

zures,[5] although its antiseizure duration is only 15 to 30 minutes. In contrast, lorazepam's antiseizure duration is 12 to 24 hours. Respiratory depression is a possibility with either benzodiazepine. Additional doses of the benzodiazepine can be given, with the increasing risk of respiratory depression kept in mind.

7. Between 3 and 4 minutes should be allowed for the full dose of benzodiazepine to terminate the seizure. If the seizure stops and its cause (e.g., electrolyte imbalance) can be rapidly corrected, no further intervention may be necessary.

8. If the seizure persists, administer phenytoin 20 mg/kg IV at up to 50 mg/min or fosphenytoin 20 mg/kg phenytoin equivalents (PE) IV at

150 mg/min. In patients who have been taking phenytoin and whose blood levels are thought to be low, half this dose may be given. During infusion the electrocardiogram (ECG) should be continuously monitored and the blood pressure checked. If the ECG changes or the patient becomes hypotensive, the infusion rate should be slowed or the infusion stopped until these complications resolve.

9. If seizures persist after phenytoin or fosphenytoin infusion, an additional 5 to 10 mg/kg may be administered.

10. If the seizure continues, the patient should probably be transferred to an intensive care unit (ICU) because intubation will most likely be required.

11. Phenobarbital 20 mg/kg IV at 50 to 75 mg/min should be administered. The ECG and blood pressure should continue to be monitored. Intubation will probably be required, and blood pressure support may also be needed at this point. If seizures continue, an additional 5 to 10 mg/kg of phenobarbital may be given.

12. If the patient is already in an ICU setting, or if the seizures have persisted for more than 1 hour, anesthesia with midazolam or propofol should be started (see below).

B. REFRACTORY STATUS EPILEPTICUS

1. Seizures that do not respond to phenobarbital should be considered refractory, and the patient should be treated with anesthesia induction.

2. The patient should be intubated, ventilated, and in an ICU setting with cardiovascular monitoring.

3. Arterial and central venous catheters should be placed.

4. Continuous EEG monitoring should be initiated.

5. A loading dose of propofol, 1 to 2 mg/kg IV, should be administered, followed by infusion at a rate of 2 to 10 mg/kg/hr. Alternatively, midazolam at a loading dose of 0.2 mg/kg IV should be followed by 0.75 to 10 µg/min.

6. The rate of maintenance dose infusion should be titrated to maintain a burst-suppression EEG pattern.

7. Hypotension is treated with intravenous fluids, low-dose dopamine, and low-dose dobutamine. The rate of propofol/midazolam infusion can be reduced if necessary.

8. Anesthesia is maintained for 12 to 24 hours, then the infusion is tapered to assess for seizure activity. Repeated anesthesia administration may be needed if seizures recur.

PEARLS AND PITFALLS

- Usually about 90% of phenytoin is bound to albumin and other serum proteins, and only unbound drug crosses the blood-brain barrier and is pharmacologically active. The range of 10 to 20 µg/mL often listed on laboratory slips includes both bound and unbound drug. Thus the range of unbound phenytoin in otherwise healthy patients is likely to be 1 to 2 µg/mL. However, patients with hypoalbuminemia or renal failure or

56

STATUS EPILEPTICUS

those taking medications that compete for protein-binding sites may have a relatively higher proportion of unbound, active phenytoin. These patients may have adequate unbound levels and good seizure control with "subtherapeutic" total phenytoin levels. For this reason it is sometimes helpful to obtain at least one total and one free phenytoin level simultaneously to determine the correlation between total and free levels in an individual patient.

- The concept of "therapeutic range" is widely misunderstood. For example, a phenytoin level of 11 µg/mL is *not* equivalent to a level of 19 µg/mL. Some patients do well with levels below the ranges quoted on the laboratory slips. Others require levels above the ranges quoted on the laboratory slips. Therefore, for example, a patient whose seizures are not controlled with a phenytoin level of 19 µg/mL may have seizures controlled with a phenytoin level of 27 µg/mL.

- Fosphenytoin infusion does not carry the same risk of adverse cardiovascular events that phenytoin infusion does (e.g., hypotension.) The use of fosphenytoin should especially be considered for patients with known cardiovascular disease and the critically ill. Fosphenytoin is converted to phenytoin in the body and can be monitored in the same way as phenytoin.

- As many as one third of women with epilepsy have an increase in seizure frequency during pregnancy.[6] The physiological changes of pregnancy, stress, and sleep deprivation may all contribute to this. Furthermore, the rate of AED noncompliance has been found to increase during and after pregnancy, perhaps because of concerns regarding fetal AED exposure and breast-feeding. Because seizures in pregnancy can be harmful to both mother and fetus, SE should be treated as outlined previously. In pregnancy the total phenytoin level may decrease, whereas the unbound level remains stable. Obtaining both an unbound and a total phenytoin level initially in a pregnant patient is advisable. Once the percentage of unbound drug is known, total levels can be obtained while the SE is managed, with the unbound level inferred from the total level.

- NCSE should be considered in the differential diagnosis of patients with altered mental status that cannot be otherwise explained. Forced gaze deviation, episodic rhythmic movements, and acute changes in blood pressure may be signs of NCSE. When NCSE is suspected, an EEG should be obtained as soon as possible.

- After a generalized seizure, examination of the cerebrospinal fluid (CSF) may reveal a pleocytosis of about 9 to 80 white blood cells/µL. This pleocytosis is transitory and peaks about 24 hours after the seizure. Nonetheless, CSF pleocytosis should never be attributed to seizures until all cultures are negative.

- Serum prolactin levels often rise transiently (for only 15-30 minutes) after generalized tonic-clonic seizures and some complex partial seizures. Thus their measurement is occasionally used to help distinguish epileptic seizure activity from pseudoseizures. However, not all seizures are accompanied by a rise in serum prolactin. Furthermore, prolactin levels may rise after other "spells" that may be confused with seizures, such as vasovagal syncope.[7] For these reasons, the routine measurement of prolactin levels after seizures is unnecessary. In particular, a patient with an altered mental status and a normal serum prolactin level may still be in NCSE; an EEG must be obtained to make that determination.

REFERENCES

[c] 1. Bradley WG et al. Neurology in clinical practice. Newton, Mass: Butterworth-Heinemann; 2000.

[c] 2. DeLorenzo RJ et al. Epidemiology of status epilepticus. J Clin Neurophysiol 1995; 12:316.

[d] 3. Dodson WE et al. Treatment of convulsive status epilepticus: recommendations of the Epilepsy Foundation of America's Working Group on Status Epilepticus. JAMA 1993; 270:854.

[c] 4. Lowenstein DH, Allredge BK. Status epilepticus. N Engl J Med 1998; 338:970.

[a] 5. Leppik IE et al. Double-blind study of lorazepam and diazepam in status epilepticus. JAMA 1983; 249:1452.

[c] 6. Zahn CA et al. Management issues for women with epilepsy: a review of the literature. Neurology 1998; 51:949.

[b] 7. Lusic I et al. Serum prolactin levels after seizure and syncopal attacks. Seizure 1999; 8:218.

STATUS EPILEPTICUS

Nutrition Management

Dechen P. Surkhang, RD, LD, and Tricia Brusco, MS, RD, LD

FAST FACTS

- The prevalence of malnutrition in hospitalized patients is 20% to 50%.[1] Patients who are already malnourished tend to deteriorate further during hospitalization.[2,3]
- Malnutrition has been associated with poor wound healing, longer length of hospital stay, and increased morbidity and mortality rate.
- Patients with a normal albumin level can be malnourished; the weight history should be checked for a downward trend (e.g., anorexia nervosa).
- Patients with normal weight for height or even overweight can be malnourished; serum protein levels and diet history should be evaluated.
- The average 70-kg person has an energy reserve of approximately 191,000 kcal: 160,000 kcal in adipose tissues, 30,000 kcal in skeletal muscle, and 900 kcal in glycogen reserves.[4]
- The human body has no protein stores; all body protein serves vital functions, so any depletion without replacement will impair protein's functional role.

I. MALNUTRITION

1. Nutritional health is achieved when equilibrium is reached between nutrient requirements and nutrient intake. When an imbalance exists, with needs exceeding intake, malnutrition occurs.
2. Based on pathogenesis, biochemical parameters, and clinical findings, protein-calorie malnutrition in hospitalized patients can be divided into malnutrition with or without hypoalbuminemia, sometimes termed kwashiorkor or marasmus, respectively.

A. MARASMUS

1. Malnutrition without hypoalbuminemia (marasmus like) is characterized by gradual muscle wasting and loss of subcutaneous fat reserves resulting from inadequate intake of both protein and calories.
2. In prolonged starvation the basal metabolic rate (BMR) decreases by as much as 40%, and the brain and other tissues adapt to use ketone bodies as the predominant fuel, while visceral protein is preserved by a reduction in protein catabolism to approximately 20 g/day. Given small protein reserves and large adipose stores, this adaptation is critical for the individual's survival.
3. The malnourished patient appears thin and cachectic. Nourishing the patient to adequate nutrient intake immediately converts the patient to an anabolic state.

4. Special care must be taken when refeeding a severely malnourished person because severe fluid and electrolyte imbalances may occur ("refeeding syndrome").

B. HYPOALBUMINEMIC MALNUTRITION

1. Hypoalbuminemic malnutrition (kwashiorkor like) results from the body's metabolic response to injury, which contrasts sharply with the response to uncomplicated semistarvation.
2. Hypoalbuminemia is induced by increased production of catecholamine, glucocorticoid, and cytokines. These result in alterations in hepatic protein synthesis, increased degradation and catabolism, and changes in plasma concentration; therefore hypoalbuminemia should be viewed more as a marker of illness severity than as an indicator of impaired nutritional status.
3. BMR, core temperature, and nitrogen excretion increase.
4. Lacking the appropriate adaptive response, protein, fat, and glycogen reserves are mobilized at a rapid rate. The stressed patient uses glucose as a primary source of energy.
5. Because of the rapid onset of illness, malnourished patients tend to maintain their anthropometric measurements (e.g., weight and height, triceps skinfold) despite severe depression of visceral protein levels.
6. Nutritional support does not reduce the stress state but can minimize protein losses.
7. Only when the stress response mediator has resolved and the hormone levels begin to normalize will the patient convert from a catabolic to an anabolic state.

C. MEDICAL PROBLEM

1. In 1974, Butterworth first brought attention to the common occurrence of malnutrition in hospitals in the landmark article "The Skeleton in the Hospital Closet."[5]
2. Based on recent surveys, malnutrition continues to be an unrecognized and untreated problem.[6,7]

II. ASSESSMENT OF NUTRITION RISK

A. NUTRITION SCREEN

1. The nutrition screen is a simple tool that helps to identify patients who are at increased nutrition risk or who are already malnourished (Box 57-1).[8,9]
2. The screen uses readily available data in the clinical setting (e.g., height and weight) to identify patients in need of comprehensive nutrition assessment.

B. OBJECTIVES OF NUTRITION ASSESSMENT[10]

1. Identification of individuals who would benefit from nutrition support.
2. Restoration or maintenance of nutritional status based on the patient's nutritional requirements.
3. Identification of appropriate feeding modalities.
4. Monitoring of the effectiveness of these medical nutrition therapies.

BOX 57-1

NUTRITION RISK

Adults are considered at nutrition risk if any one of the following is present:

1. Involuntary weight loss or gain of the following:

   >10% of usual body weight in 6 months

   or

   >5% of usual body weight in 1 month

   or

   Weight of 20% over or under ideal body weight.

2. Presence of chronic disease or increased metabolic requirements.

3. Altered diets or diet schedule.

4. Inadequate nutrition intake, including not receiving food or nutrition products for longer than 7 days.

C. NUTRITION EVALUATION

1. Evaluation of a patient's nutritional status includes the basic medical history, diet history, physical observation, anthropometric data, weight, and biochemical data. This wide array of data must be integrated to achieve a complete assessment; no gold standard exists. Each assessment index has its limitations, with factors other than nutrition affecting results (e.g., weight changes from varying fluid status, and in liver disease with decreased synthetic function causing a decrease in visceral proteins).

2. Medical history.

a. Careful review of the patient's history, identifying disease and treatments that could adversely affect nutritional status, allows early detection of malnutrition and intervention with nutritional therapy.

b. Any conditions that alter intake, digestion, absorption, metabolism, and excretion will put the patient at increased nutrition risk (Table 57-1).[11]

3. Diet history.

a. Information is obtained from 24-hour recall and food frequency questionnaires.

b. History provides both qualitative and semiquantitative information about the patient's general intake pattern.

4. Physical observation.

a. By "eyeballing" the patient, the clinician can look for any overt signs of protein-calorie or micronutrient deficiencies (Table 57-2).[12,13]

5. Anthropometric data.

a. Measurements allow the evaluation of body composition.

b. Although specific and more reliable tools are available to determine body composition (e.g., underwater densitometry, bioelectric impedance analysis of fat and muscle, triceps skinfold measurements for fat store), in a clinical setting the more common and practical measurements used are height and weight.

TABLE 57-1

PATHOPHYSIOLOGICAL MECHANISMS OF MALNUTRITION

Mechanism	Pathophysiology and Disorders*	
Intake	Impairment or inability to regulate ingestion of nutrients	
	Anorexia nervosa	Inability to chew or swallow
	Bulimia	GI motility disorders
	Altered level of consciousness	Hyperemesis
	GI tract obstruction	Iatrogenic and self-imposed dietary restriction
Digestion	Impairment or inability to break down nutrients into absorbable entities	
	Disaccharidase deficiency	Cystic fibrosis
		Pancreatitis and biliary insufficiency
Absorption	Impairment or inability to assimilate nutrients	
	Inflammatory bowel disease	Short bowel syndrome
	Gastrectomy	Radiation enteritis
Excretion or increased losses	Impairment or inability to rid the body of waste products of metabolized nutrients, or increased losses of nutrients	
	Chronic renal disease	Dialysis
	Draining abscesses and wounds	Blood loss
	Fistulas	
Metabolism	Impairment or inability to assimilate nutrients	
	Inborn errors of metabolism	Chronic obstructive pulmonary disease
	Liver disease	
	Drug-nutrient interactions	Chronic renal disease
Requirements	Alteration in quantity of nutrients needed to obtain or maintain health that is beyond the individual's ability to consume	
	Trauma	Burns
	Sepsis	Hypermetabolic states
	Fever	

Modified from Burke MA, Liffrig T. In Nelson JK et al, editors. Mayo Clinic diet manual: a handbook of nutrition practices, 7th ed. St Louis: Mosby; 1994.

*Mechanisms are found in, but are not limited to, the diseases and disorders listed.

c. Height allows determination of ideal body weight (IBW)/desirable body weight (DBW) and usual body weight (UBW) to compare with current weight.

d. Height and weight measurements are also required for determining energy needs and body mass index (BMI).

6. Weight.

a. Weight is one of the most useful general parameters for identifying malnutrition and is easy to obtain.

b. It is easily confounded by a patient's varying fluid status, but with careful review, documented weights over time provide a crude measure of overall fat and muscle store.

c. Comparing a patient's current weight to IBW/DBW and UBW and determining the extent and duration of weight change provide important insight into the severity of the malnourished state (Table 57-3).[4,9]

TABLE 57-2

CLINICAL SIGNS AND SYMPTOMS OF NUTRITION INADEQUACY

	Clinical Signs and Symptoms	Nutrients
General	Wasted, skinny	Calorie
	Loss of appetite	Protein energy, zinc
Skin	Psoriasiform rash, eczematous scaling	Zinc, vitamin A, essential fatty acid
	Pallor	Folic acid, iron, vitamin B_{12}, copper
	Follicular hyperkeratosis	Vitamin A, vitamin C
	Perifollicular petechiae	Vitamin C
	Flaking dermatitis	Protein energy, niacin, riboflavin, zinc
	Bruising	Vitamin C, vitamin K
	Pigmentation changes	Niacin, protein energy
	Scrotal dermatosis	Riboflavin
	Skin thickening and dryness	Linoleic acid
Head	Temporal muscle wasting	Protein energy
Hair	Sparse and thin, dyspigmentation, easily pulled out	Protein
	Corkscrew hairs	Vitamin C
Eyes	History of night blindness	Vitamin A, zinc
	Photophobia, blurring, conjunctival inflammation	Riboflavin, vitamin A
	Corneal vascularization	Riboflavin
	Xerosis, Bitot's spots, keratomalacia	Vitamin A
Mouth	Glossitis	Riboflavin, niacin, folic acid, vitamin B_{12}, pyridoxine
	Bleeding gums	Vitamin C, riboflavin
	Cheilosis	Riboflavin, pyridoxine, niacin
	Angular stomatitis	Riboflavin, pyridoxine, niacin
	Hypogeusia	Zinc
	Tongue fissuring	Riboflavin, niacin, iron
	Tongue atrophy	Pyridoxine
	Nasolabial seborrhea	Iodine
Neck	Goiter	Iodine
	Parotid enlargement	Protein
Thorax	Thoracic rosary	Vitamin D
Abdomen	Diarrhea	Niacin, folate, vitamin B_{12}
	Distention	Protein energy
	Hepatomegaly	Protein energy
Blood	Anemia	Vitamin B_{12}, folic acid, pyridoxine
	Hemolysis	Phosphorus
Neurological	Tetany	Calcium, magnesium
	Paresthesia	Thiamine, vitamin B_{12}
	Loss of reflexes, wristdrop, footdrop	Thiamine
	Loss of vibratory and position sense	Vitamin B_{12}
	Dementia, disorientation	Niacin

cont'd

57

NUTRITION MANAGEMENT

TABLE 57-2

CLINICAL SIGNS AND SYMPTOMS OF NUTRITION INADEQUACY—cont'd

	Clinical Signs and Symptoms	Nutrients
Nails	Spooning	Iron
	Transverse lines	Protein
Extremities	Edema	Protein, thiamin
	Softening of bone	Vitamin D, calcium, phosphorus
	Bone tenderness	Vitamin D
	Bone ache, joint pain	Vitamin C
	Muscle wasting and weakness	Protein, calorie, vitamin D, selenium, sodium chloride
	Muscle tenderness, muscle pain	Thiamin
	Ataxia	Vitamin B_{12}

TABLE 57-3

EVALUATION OF BODY WEIGHT DATA

IBW (%) = Current weight/IBW × 100.
80%-90%: mild malnutrition.
70%-79%: moderate malnutrition.
≤69%: severe malnutrition.

UBW (%) = Current weight/UBW × 100.
85% to 95%: mild malnutrition.
75% to 84%: moderate malnutrition.
≤74%: severe malnutrition.
Recent weight loss (%) = (UBW − Current weight)/UBW × 100.

Time	Significant Weight Loss (%)	Severe Weight Loss (%)
1 week	1-2	>2
1 month	5	>5
3 months	7.5	>7.5
6 months	10	>10

Modified from Blackburn GL, Bistrain BR. J Parenter Enter Nutr 1977; 1:11. In Gottschlich MM et al, eds. A case based core curriculum of the American Society for Parenteral and Enteral Nutrition. Dubuque, Ia: Kendall/Hunt; 2001.
IBW, Ideal body weight; *UBW*, usual body weight.

d. Metropolitan Life Insurance tables and the Hamwi equation are two common reference methods for determining IBW/DBW (Table 57-4).
e. Body mass index (BMI).

$$\text{Weight (kg)/Height}^2 \text{ (m}^2\text{)}$$

(1) Also called the Quetlet index, BMI provides indirect measure of body fat, especially useful in identifying obesity.
(2) In cases of malnutrition it is difficult to distinguish between muscle and fat depletion.

TABLE 57-4

METROPOLITAN LIFE HEIGHT-WEIGHT TABLES AND HAMWI EQUATION

Height		Weight (lb)*		
Ft	In	Small Frame	Medium Frame	Large Frame
MEN				
5	2	128-134	131-141	138-150
5	3	130-136	133-143	140-153
5	4	132-138	135-145	142-156
5	5	134-140	137-148	144-160
5	6	136-142	139-151	146-164
5	7	138-145	142-154	149-168
5	8	140-148	145-157	152-172
5	9	142-151	148-160	155-176
5	10	144-154	151-163	158-180
5	11	146-157	154-166	161-184
6	0	149-160	157-170	164-188
6	1	160-164	160-174	168-192
6	2	155-164	164-178	172-197
6	3	158-172	167-182	176-202
6	4	162-176	171-187	181-207
WOMEN				
4	10	102-111	109-121	118-131
4	11	103-113	111-123	120-134
5	0	104-115	113-126	122-137
5	1	106-118	115-129	125-140
5	2	108-121	118-132	128-143
5	3	111-124	121-135	131-147
5	4	114-127	124-138	134-151
5	5	117-130	127-141	137-155
5	6	120-133	130-144	140-159
5	7	123-136	133-147	143-163
5	8	126-139	136-150	146-167
5	9	129-142	139-153	149-170
5	10	132-145	142-156	152-173
5	11	135-148	145-159	155-176
6	0	138-151	148-162	158-179

HAMWI EQUATION

Females

Weight = 100 lb for first 5 ft + 5 lb for each additional inch above 5 ft

Males

Weight = 106 lb for first 5 ft + 6 lb for each additional inch above 5 ft

Both: +10% for large frame; −10% for small frame.

*Weight according to frame (ages 25-59) for men wearing indoor clothing weighing 5 pounds and shoes with 1-inch heels and for women wearing indoor clothing weighing 3 pounds and shoes with 1-inch heels.

57

NUTRITION MANAGEMENT

TABLE 57-5

BODY MASS INDEX CLASSIFICATION

Classification	Body Mass Index (kg/m^2)
Underweight	<18.5
Normal	18.5-24.9
Overweight	25.0-29.9
Obesity	30.0-39.9
Extreme obesity	≥40

    (3) A BMI approaching 12 is usually associated with significant mortality.[14,15]

    (4) The National Institutes of Health (NIH)[16] has established BMI guidelines (Table 57-5).

    (5) Some cutoff points are not universally accepted; concerns remain over exact definitions of "overweight" and "obesity."

7. Biochemical data.

a. No single test exists that accurately assesses nutritional status.

b. Visceral protein measurements are the most widely used biochemical marker for measuring nutritional status (Table 57-6).[9,17,18]

c. Albumin, transferrin, and prealbumin are transport proteins that are influenced by both protein intake and calorie intake, as well as by hydration status, disease states, trauma, and liver function (site of these proteins' synthesis).

d. Half-life of serum proteins varies; therefore the lower the half-life, the more sensitive the proteins to acute changes in nutrient intake.

e. Understanding measurement limitations is essential in determining the reliability and utility of the data collected.

III. DETERMINATION OF NUTRITION REQUIREMENTS

A. ENERGY REQUIREMENT

1. Basal metabolic rate (BMR).

a. BMR is the minimum energy required for a person to maintain basic vital functions.

b. The term is used interchangeably with resting metabolic rate (RMR) and basal energy expenditure (BEE).

c. Body size, age, and gender contribute to energy requirements; many predictive equations use the variation in these factors to estimate energy requirements.

2. Harris-Benedict (HB) equation.

$$\text{Females: BEE} = 655.1 + 9.56W + 1.85H - 4.68A$$
$$\text{Males: BEE} = 66.5 + 13.75W + 5.0H - 6.78A$$

where W is weight in kilograms, H is height in centimeters, and A is age.

a. The HB equation is the most widely used method to determine BMR (BEE).

TABLE 57-6
SELECT LABORATORY TESTS FOR VISCERAL PROTEIN

Test	Functions	Half-Life (Days)	Clinical Interpretation	Increased Level	Decreased Level
Albumin (g/dL)	Transport protein; maintains plasma oncotic pressure	~20	Normal: 3.5-5.0 Mild depletion: 2.9-3.5 Moderate depletion: 2.1-2.8 Severe depletion: <2.1	Dehydration; administration of exogenous plasma products	Protein malnutrition; liver disease; infection; overhydration; malabsorption; nephrotic syndrome; catabolic stress
Transferrin (mg/dL)	Transport protein of iron	8-10	Normal: 200-400 Mild depletion: 150-199 Moderate depletion: 100-150 Severe depletion: <100	Iron deficiency anemia; pregnancy; acute hepatitis; chronic blood loss; dehydration	Protein malnutrition; acute catabolic status; end-stage liver disease; nephrotic syndrome
Prealbumin (mg/dL)	Transport protein for thyroxine and retinol-binding protein	2-3	Normal: 15.7-29.6 Mild depletion: 10-15 Moderate depletion: 5-10 Severe depletion: <5	Renal failure; corticosteroid therapy	Liver disease; zinc deficiency; acute stress; protein malnutrition

57

NUTRITION MANAGEMENT

b. Adjustments are made to the HB equation for a patient's condition by a stress factor ranging from 1.2 to 1.5, or as high as 2.0 for major stress such as burns.

3. **Quick initial assessment.**
a. Energy needs can be estimated by use of body weight alone: 25 to 35 kcal/kg of body weight.
b. Increased calories are reserved for patients with greater metabolic and physiological stress.

4. **Which weight to use.**
a. Current weight is preferred in the calculation of energy requirements for an underweight patient because with decreased lean body mass a concurrent lowering of BMR occurs.
b. Use of an "ideal body weight" may lead to overestimation of energy needs and a propensity to overfeed.
c. Current weight may be inappropriate to use in the determination of energy needs of obese patients, since a proportional relationship ceases to exist as body weight increases from increased adipose stores rather than from fat-free mass.
d. Use of adjusted body weight (ABW) is suggested if the body weight exceeds 125% of DBW.

$$ABW = (Current\ weight - IBW) \times 0.25 + IBW$$

5. **Indirect calorimetry.**
a. Indirect calorimetry is the most accurate method for determining energy requirements in the clinical setting.
b. Energy is expended in proportion to oxygen consumed.
c. The metabolic cart indirectly calculates energy expenditure by measuring the pulmonary gas exchange.
d. The ratio of carbon dioxide produced to oxygen consumed reflects the body's net substrate utilization, referred to as respiratory quotient (RQ).

RQ: carbohydrate	1.0
RQ: mixed diet	0.85
RQ: protein	0.82
RQ: fat	0.7

(1) Overfeeding generally increases the RQ to 1.0 or greater.
(2) With underfeeding or undernutrition the RQ is 0.7 or less, reflecting the use of ketones as an energy source.

B. PROTEIN REQUIREMENT

1. Based on the dietary reference intake (DRI), the protein needs of a healthy person are 0.8 g/kg body weight.
2. With the stress of illness leading to increased protein catabolism, the protein requirement increases as well.
3. A protein intake of 1.0 to 1.5 g/kg/day meets the needs of most hospitalized patients; those with severe stress may require as much as 2.0 g/kg/day.

4. **Urinary urea nitrogen (UUN).**

a. UUN is the most direct (24-hour) method of estimating protein need.

b. It is derived from the breakdown of both dietary protein and skeletal muscle.

c. UUN accounts for approximately 90% of the total urinary nitrogen.

5. **Nitrogen balance.**

a. Nitrogen balance is determined by measurement of 24-hour nitrogen excretion and concurrent assessment of 24-hour protein intake.

$$\text{Nitrogen balance} = (24\text{-hr protein intake}/6.25) - (\text{UUN [g/day]} + 4)$$
$$\text{Nitrogen intake} = \text{Protein intake}/6.25$$
$$4 = \text{Approximate correction factor for insensible nitrogen losses}$$

b. Measurement of nitrogen balance is unreliable for patients on oral diets because of difficulties in obtaining precise intake data.

c. For enterally and parenterally fed patients, proper intake can be calculated through intake and output (I&O) records.

6. **Percentage of total caloric intake.**

a. The percentage of total caloric intake provides an estimate of protein requirements.

b. Healthy, nonstressed individuals require about 10% to 12% of calories from protein.

c. The requirement increases to as much as 25% of total caloric intake in patients with increased metabolic demands.

IV. FEEDING MODALITIES (Fig. 57-1)[19-21]

A. FEEDING ROUTES

1. Two routes are available to meet patient's nutritional needs.

a. Patients can be fed through the gastrointestinal (GI) tract by means of volitional intake or by tube feeding.

b. Patients unable to use the GI tract can be fed intravenously (IV) through a peripheral or central vein.

B. ORAL NUTRITION

1. If patients' acceptance of the hospital diet is diminished, their diet can be augmented by the use of oral supplements.

2. Supplements currently available range from the basic lactose-containing milkshake (e.g., Carnation Instant Breakfast) to "elemental" drinks (e.g., Peptamen, Vivonex TEN), which are usually reserved for tube-fed patients. Familiarity with the nutrition department's formulary greatly assists in making the appropriate choice (Table 57-7).

3. In general, the more specialized the formula, the less palatable the product, and therefore the lower the patient's acceptance.

4. Underlying pathological conditions guide the selection of supplements (e.g., low-lactose supplement for patients with lactase deficiency; concentrated formulas for renal, hepatic, and heart failure; low-electrolyte supplement for renal impairment), but the best supplement undoubtedly is the one the patient is willing to consume.

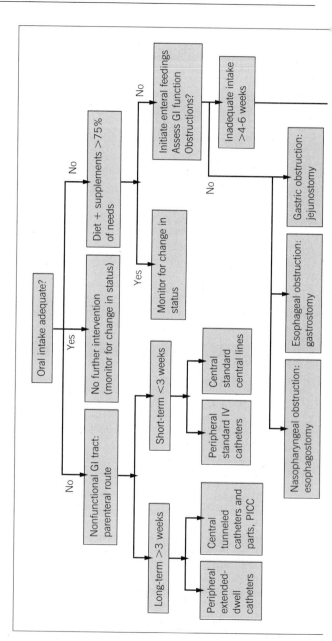

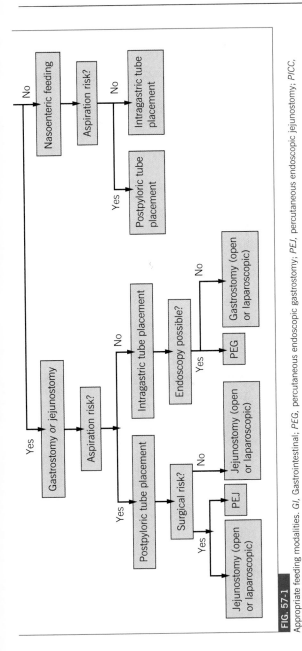

FIG. 57-1

Appropriate feeding modalities. *GI,* Gastrointestinal; *PEG,* percutaneous endoscopic gastrostomy; *PEJ,* percutaneous endoscopic jejunostomy; *PICC,* peripheral inserted central catheter.

TABLE 57-7

SELECT ORAL SUPPLEMENTS

Product/ Manufacturer	Portion	Protein (g)	Calories	Description
Instant Breakfast/ Nestles	9 oz with 2% milk	12	250	Milk based
NuBasic Juice/ Nestles	5.5 oz	6.5	163	Clear liquid, lactose free, low residue
Boost Drink/Mead Johnson	8 oz	10	240	Lactose free
Boost Pudding/ Mead Johnson	5 oz	7	240	Lactose free
Ensure Pudding/ Ross	4 oz	4	170	For volume-restricted diets, milk based
Ensure HP/Ross	8 oz	12	225	Extra protein per serving, lactose free
Resource Fruit Beverage/Novartis	8 oz	9	250	Fat free, clear liquid
Resource Shake Plus/Novartis	8 oz	15	480	Nutrient dense, high calorie, for volume-restricted patients

5. Providing patients with taste trials of supplements varying in consistency (e.g., pudding, juice, "milk like") and concentration is helpful in making the appropriate selection. Providing a variety of textures and tastes helps to minimize "taste fatigue."

6. When volitional intake consistently fails to meet 75% of nutritional needs, as determined by calorie counts, alternative nutrition support should be considered.

C. ENTERAL NUTRITION

1. Enteral nutrition entails the provision of nutrients through the GI tract. The term encompasses oral intake but is more synonymous with tube feeding.

2. Enteral nutrition is recommended when volitional intake is insufficient to meet nutritional needs and when the GI tract is functional and safely accessible.

3. Enteral nutrition has several advantages over parenteral nutrition.

a. Nutrient utilization is more effective through the normal physiological action of digestion and absorption.

b. Gut mucosal integrity is maintained.

c. Bacterial translocation into the systemic circulation is potentially decreased.

4. Once tube feeding is selected as therapy, the route of nutrient delivery is determined, based on the anticipated duration of tube-feeding therapy, accessibility and utility of the GI tract, and the patient's risk of aspiration (Fig. 57-1).

a. Nasoenteric (nasogastric, nasoduodenal, nasojejunal) tubes are intended for short-term therapy.

b. Percutaneous tubes (e.g., percutaneous endoscopic gastrostomy [PEG] and jejunostomy [PEJ]) and surgically placed feeding tubes (e.g., open gastrostomy) are for long-term management.

D. ENTERAL FORMULAS

1. A wide selection of enteral formulas are available, but generally the formulas are similar, with slight variations in macronutrients and micronutrients (Table 57-8). Formulas can be grouped into four categories according to their macronutrient composition: polymeric, monomeric, specialty, and modular.

2. Polymeric formulas.

a. Nutrients are intact, so normal GI function is required.

b. The formula is nutritionally complete when administered in adequate volume.

c. This group includes formulas that contain lactose, are lactose free, and contain fiber.

d. Fiber may be helpful in increasing stool bulk and trophic to the large bowel.

e. Polymeric formulas can also be used as oral supplements.

3. Monomeric formulas.

a. Monomeric formulas consist of partially or completely hydrolyzed nutrients; they are also referred to as "elemental."

b. They are appropriate for patients with compromised digestion and absorption.

c. They tend to have high osmolality because of low molecular weight of the hydrolyzed nutrients.

d. They are usually unpalatable and are typically reserved for tube feeding.

4. Specialty formulas.

a. Specialty formulas are designed for specific disease states.

b. This group includes formulas for respiratory disorders, diabetes, renal failure, hepatic disease, trauma, and compromised immune status.

c. Their effectiveness remains controversial; results of well-designed trials are still awaited.

d. They may be used if conventional therapy with standard formula fails.

5. Modular formulas.

a. Modular formulas provide a supplemental single-nutrient source.

b. They can be added to tube feeding to individualize the enteral regimen when standard polymeric formulas are unable to meet the patient's specific nutritional requirements.

6. Factors in selection.

a. The patient's digestive and absorptive capacity (intact versus hydrolyzed).

b. Caloric and protein density (based on needs, calories per milliliter, and grams of protein per milliliter).

57

NUTRITION MANAGEMENT

TABLE 57-8

SELECT ENTERAL FORMULAS

Product/Manufacturer	Kcal/mL	Protein (g/L)	Osmolality	Volume to Meet DRI* (mL)
1.0 TO 1.2 kcal/ml				
Ensure/Ross	1.06	60.0	590	948
Osmolite/Ross	1.06	67.2	300	1887
Promote/Ross	1.00	62.5	350	1250
Isocal/Mead Johnson	1.06	34.0	270	1890
Isocal HN Plus/Mead Johnson	1.20	54.0	390	1000
Ultracal/Mead Johnson	1.06	45.0	300	1120
Isosource Std/Novartis	1.20	43.0	490	1165
Nutren 1.0/Nestles	1.00	40.0	315	1500
1.5 TO 2.0 kcal/mL				
Ensure Plus HN/Ross	1.50	62.6	650	771
Nutren 1.5/Nestles	1.50	60.0	430	1000
Comply/Mead Johnson	1.50	60.0	460	830
Novasource 2.0/Novartis	2.00	90.0	790	948
TwoCal HN/Ross	2.00	83.5	730	948
Deliver 2.0/Mead Johnson	2.00	75.0	640	1000
Nutren 2.0/Nestles	2.00	80.0	745	750
FIBER CONTAINING				
Jevity/Ross	1.06	44.4	300	1321
Promote with fiber/Ross	1.00	62.5	380	1000
Nutren 1.0 with fiber/Nestles	1.00	40.0	320	1500
Fibersource Std/Novartis	1.2	43.0	490	1165
Fibersource HN/Novartis	1.2	53.0	490	1165
SPECIALIZED FORMULA (INTACT NUTRIENTS)				
NutriVent/Nestles	1.50	67.5	330	1000
Pulmocare/Ross	1.50	62.6	475	947
Novasource, Pulmonary/Novartis	1.50	70.0	650	933
Respalor/Mead Johnson	1.50	75.0	400	1000
Glucerna/Ross	1.00	41.8	355	1422
Glytrol/Nestles	1.06	45.0	380	1400
Diabeticsource/Novartis	1.00	50.0	360	1500
Choice DM/Mead Johnson	1.06	45.0	300	1120
NutraRenal/Nestles	2.00	70.0	650	750
Nepro/Ross	2.00	70.0	665	947
Magancal Renal/Mead Johnson	2.00	75.0	570	1000
Novasource Renal/Novartis	2.00	74.0	700	1000
SPECIALIZED FORMULA: INTACT NUTRIENTS				
Traumacal/Mead Johnson	2.00	82.0	560	2000
Impact/Novartis	1.00	56.0	375	1500

*Dietary reference intake.

cont'd

TABLE 57-8

SELECT ENTERAL FORMULAS—cont'd

Product/Manufacturer	Kcal/mL	Protein (g/L)	Osmolality	Volume to Meet DRI* (mL)
SPECIALIZED FORMULA: MONOMERIC HYDROLYZED NUTRIENTS				
Peptamen Diet/Nestle	1.06	40.0	270	1500
Alitraq/Ross	1.00	52.5	575	1500
Subdue/Mead Johnson	1.00	50.0	330	1180
Vivonex Plus/Novartis	1.00	45.0	650	1800
MODULAR FORMULA ANALYSIS				
Per Gram (g) of Product: Protein				

Product/Manufacturer	Kcal	Protein (g)
Casec/Mead Johnson	3.8	0.9
ProMod/Ross	5.6	1.0
Resource Protein Powder/Nestles	3.6	0.9
Per Milliliter (mL) of Product: Fat		

Product/Manufacturer	Kcal	Fat (g)
Mircolipid/Mead Johnson	4.5	0.51
MCT Oil/Mead Johnson	7.7	1.0
Per Gram (g) of Product: Carbohydrate (CHO)		

Product/Manufacturer	Kcal	CHO (g)
Moducal/Mead Johnson	3.8	1
Polycose/Ross	3.8	1

57

NUTRITION MANAGEMENT

  c. Fluid needs or limitations that meet patient's nutritional requirements (1.0 versus 1.5 versus 2.0 cal/mL).

7. Tube-feeding administration.

  a. The need for tube feeding is dictated by the patient's clinical status and feeding route.

  b. The three most common methods are continuous, intermittent, and bolus feeding.

  c. Continuous feeding.

    (1) Patients being fed through the small intestine, patients unable to tolerate large-volume infusion, and patients at increased aspiration risk need to be fed by continuous drip or by gravity over 18 to 24 hours.

    (2) Continuous feeding can be initiated at 30 mL/hr and increased as tolerated (based on gastric residuals and patient comments) by 30 to 50 mL q8-12h until the goal rate is achieved.

  d. Intermittent drip feeding and bolus feeding.

    (1) Intermittent drip feeding and bolus feeding are reserved for more stable patients.

    (2) They allow patients greater flexibility and autonomy.

    (3) These methods can mimic a daily meal regimen.

    (4) In intermittent feeding 200 to 400 mL can be infused over 30 to 40 minutes q3-4h.

(5) In bolus feeding a syringe is used to infuse up to 500 mL within a few minutes.

8. Complications (Table 57-9).[22]
  a. Gastrointestinal.
  b. Metabolic.
  c. Mechanical.

E. PARENTERAL NUTRITION

1. When the GI tract is not functional, accessible, or safe to use, parenteral nutrition (PN) is available to provide nutrients (dextrose, amino acids, fat, vitamins, minerals, trace elements, fluids) intravenously.

2. PN must be individualized according to the patient's needs and wishes.

3. PN can be infused peripherally or centrally.
  a. Central PN, which consistently provides complete nutrition, is termed total parenteral nutrition (TPN).
  b. Peripherally administered nutrition is termed peripheral parenteral nutrition (PPN).

4. The choice of PN therapy depends on the length of therapy, availability of IV access, and nutritional requirements, including fluids (Fig. 57-1).

5. PPN is usually reserved for short-term use (10-14 days) as a supplemental nutritional support.
  a. Peripheral veins are unable to tolerate hypertonic solutions with osmolarity greater than 900 mOsm/L, and thrombophlebitis is likely to occur.
  b. Dextrose and amino acids contribute to osmolarity, so limited nutrients are provided in PPN. Therefore, to meet a patient's needs, a large volume of solution (up to about 3 L) is required, which may exceed some patients' tolerance.

6. TPN is indicated for patients who have increased nutritional needs and require fluid restriction and long-term nutritional support (>3 weeks).
  a. Hypertonic TPN solutions fed into the central vein are diluted when mixed with the high blood flow.
  b. Osmolality may reach 1800 mOsm/L.

7. PN may be administered with all nutrients (dextrose, amino acids, fat) mixed together ("3 in 1"), also known as total nutrient admixture (TNA), or the dextrose–amino acid solution can be infused separately from the lipid emulsion.

8. Components.
  a. Carbohydrate (CHO).
    (1) In the form of dextrose monohydrate, CHO is mixed with amino acids to obtain PN solutions providing 3.4 kcal/g.
    (2) Solution is available in concentrations ranging from 2.5% to 70%, with concentrations greater than 10% reserved for TPN because of increased osmolarity.

(3) Providing 100 to 120 g of CHO minimizes the use of protein as an energy source.

(4) Excess CHO can have a deleterious effect, leading to fat synthesis and hepatic steatosis.

(5) Maximum glucose administration should not exceed 5 mg/kg/min.

b. Lipid emulsions.

    (1) Lipid emulsion is an isotonic concentrated source of calories providing 9 kcal/g.

    (2) It is a source of essential fatty acids.

    (3) A 2% to 4% amount of total calories from linoleic acid (or 10% of total fat calories) prevents essential fatty acid deficiency (EFAD).

    (4) Lipid emulsion is composed of soybean oil, sometimes in combination with safflower oil plus egg yolk phospholipid and glycerin.

    (5) It is available in concentrations of 10% (1.1 kcal/mL) and 20% (2 kcal/mL).

    (6) Intake should not exceed 60% of total calories or more than 2 g/kg/day.

c. Protein.

    (1) Protein is provided to maintain nitrogen balance or promote anabolism.

    (2) It is composed of essential, semiessential, and nonessential crystalline amino acids and provides 4 kcal/g.

    (3) Amino acid solution is available in concentrations of 3% to 15%.

    (4) As in enteral nutrition, specially formulated amino acid products are available, but their efficacy remains controversial.

d. Vitamins, minerals, and trace elements.

    (1) Standard vitamin and mineral preparations are added daily to PN solutions (Tables 57-10 to 57-12).

    (2) Requirements with PN are lower than the dietary reference intake (DRI) levels because normal digestion and absorption are bypassed.

    (3) Specific amounts must be adjusted as dictated by the patient's needs and nutritional status (e.g., vitamin K in patients undergoing anticoagulation).

9. Monitoring and complications.

a. Monitoring is particularly essential for patients receiving PN therapy (Table 57-13).

b. By adherence to protocols (e.g., line placement, line care) and by careful patient management, serious complications associated with PN therapy can be prevented.

c. Complications generally fall into three categories (Table 57-14).[23]

    (1) Technical or mechanical.

    (2) Metabolic.

    (3) Septic.

PEARLS AND PITFALLS

- Refeeding syndrome describes complications that occur when a chronically malnourished patient receives aggressive nutritional support,

57

NUTRITION MANAGEMENT

TABLE 57-9

COMPLICATIONS OF TUBE FEEDINGS

Complication	Possible Causes	Prevention and Therapy
MECHANICAL		
Pharyngeal irritation or erosion, otitis media	Large-bore vinyl or rubber tubes for prolonged periods	Small-bore polyurethane or silicone tubes
Obstruction of feeding tube lumen	Crushed medication, incompletely dissolved formula	Thoroughly crush medication and mix with water; flush tube after medication administration and after tube feeding is interrupted; flush tube three times daily
Tube placement	Coughing, vomiting, patient pulling	Replace tube and reconfirm by x-ray examination
GASTROINTESTINAL		
Gastric retention with pulmonary aspiration	Delayed gastric emptying; head of bed not elevated adequately; altered gag reflex; loss of lower esophageal sphincter integrity	Continuous infusion administration; head of bed elevated 3 to 45 degrees at all times; postpyloric feedings; gastric motility stimulants
Nausea and vomiting, abdominal distention, cramping	Inappropriate formula administration (rapid increase in volume, rate, concentration); lactose intolerance, cold formula; feeding infused with medications	Initiate and advance formula slowly; infuse isotonic formula for small bowel feedings
Diarrhea	Inappropriate formula administration (rapid increase in volume, rate, concentration); infusion of hyperosmolar formulation in small bowel	Initiate and advance formula slowly; infuse isotonic formula for small bowel feeding
	Antibiotic therapy	Obtain stool assay for *Clostridium difficile*
	Oral electrolyte solutions (hyperosmolar)	Distribute doses of KCI, Mg, and PO_4 throughout day and dilute well
	Lactose intolerance	Lactose-free formula
	Extended "nothing by mouth" status or starvation (GI mucosal atrophy)	Initiate and advance feedings slowly over several days to allow time for mucosal regeneration; use isotonic formula

	Malabsorption secondary to GI disease	Hydrolyzed chemically defined formula, pancreatic enzyme replacement if appropriate
	Contaminated formula	Change solutions and clean all equipment; do not administer formula for longer than 8 hours
Constipation	Inadequate water intake, reduced gastric motility, fecal impaction, inactivity, certain medications, inadequate fiber	Increase free water intake; stool softener or laxative; increase activity if possible; use fiber-containing formula
High gastric residuals	Reduced gastric motility; ileus; sedatives; hyperosmolar or high-fat formula	Maintain head of bed elevated; gastric motility stimulants; postpyloric feeding; lower osmolality or lower fat formula
METABOLIC		
Hyperglycemia/nonketotic dehydration/coma	Diabetes mellitus; stress (trauma or sepsis)	Insulin administration; use formula with 30%-50% kilocalories as fat; carbohydrate intake not exceeding 5 mg/kg/min
Hypertonic dehydration	Inadequate fluid administration, excessive fluid losses	Increase free water administration; replace fluid losses
Hypophosphatemia, hypomagnesemia, and hypokalemia (refeeding syndrome)	Rapid refeeding of malnourished patient	Slowly advance formula rate; monitor electrolytes daily for first week of feeding a malnourished patient; supplement if needed

GI, Gastrointestinal.

NUTRITION MANAGEMENT

57

TABLE 57-10

ADULT PARENTERAL NUTRITION FORMULATIONS: DAILY VITAMIN SUPPLEMENTATION*

Vitamin	Intake
Thiamin (B_1)	3.0 mg
Riboflavin (B_2)	3.6 mg
Niacin	40.0 mg
Folic acid	400.0 µg
Pantothenic acid	15.0 mg
Pyridoxine (B_6)	4.0 mg
Cyanocobalamin	5.0 µg
Biotin	60.0 µg
Ascorbic acid	100.0 mg
Vitamin A	3300.0 IU
Vitamin D	200.0 IU
Vitamin E	10.0 IU

Vitamin K supplementation of 2 to 4 mg/wk in TPN patients not receiving oral anticoagulation therapy.
*Assumes normal organ function.

TABLE 57-11

ADULT TOTAL PARENTERAL NUTRITION FORMULATIONS: DAILY TRACE ELEMENT SUPPLEMENTATION*

Trace Element	Intake
Chromium	10.0-15.0 µg
Copper	0.5-1.5 mg
Manganese	0.15-0.80 mg
Zinc	2.5-4.0 mg

*Assumes normal organ function.

TABLE 57-12

ADULT TOTAL PARENTERAL NUTRITION: DAILY ELECTROLYTE RECOMMENDATIONS

Electrolyte	Daily Range
Calcium	10-15 mEq
Magnesium	8-20 mEq
Phosphate	20-40 mmol
Sodium	1-2 mEq/kg *plus* replacement for losses
Potassium	1-2 mEq/kg *plus* replacement for losses
Acetate	As needed to maintain acid-base balance
Chloride	As needed to maintain acid-base balance

TABLE 57-13

TOTAL PARENTERAL NUTRITION MONITORING GUIDELINES

Variable	Suggested Frequency*	
	Initial Period	Later Period
Weight	Daily	Daily
Serum electrolytes	Daily	3/week
Blood urea nitrogen	3/week	1/week
Serum total calcium or ionized Ca^{++}, inorganic phosphorus, magnesium	3/week	1/week
Serum glucose	Daily	3/week
Serum triglycerides	Weekly	Weekly
Liver function enzymes	3/week	1/week
Hemoglobin, hematocrit	Weekly	Weekly
Prothrombin time	Weekly	Weekly
Platelet count	Weekly	Weekly
White blood cell count	As indicated	As indicated
Clinical status	Daily	Daily
Catheter site	Daily	Daily
Temperature	Daily	Daily
Intake and output†	Daily	Daily

*"Initial period" refers to time during which full glucose intake is being achieved. "Later period" implies that the patient has achieved a steady metabolic state. In the presence of metabolic instability, the more intensive monitoring under the initial period should be followed.

†"Intake and output" refers to all fluids entering the patient (e.g., oral, intravenous, medications) and all fluids leaving (e.g., urine, surgical drain, suctioning, vomitus, diarrhea).

whether orally, enterally, or parenterally (Box 57-2).[24] It is characterized by severe fluid and electrolyte shifts that may lead to cardiac, pulmonary, and neuromuscular complications. With the delivery of nutrients a nutritionally deprived patient shifts from fat to carbohydrate as an energy source. This shift results in increased insulin secretion, with increased cellular uptake of glucose, potassium, phosphorus, and magnesium and reduced excretion of sodium and water. At presentation the patient may have hypokalemia, hypophosphatemia, hypomagnesemia, and edema, all hallmarks of the refeeding syndrome. Recommendations to prevent the refeeding syndrome are as follows.[25]

- Be aware of the syndrome.
- Measure electrolytes before providing nutritional support and supplements as needed.
- Closely monitor electrolytes (at least the first week), I&O, and weight.
- Provide nutrition slowly (begin at 20 kcal/kg of current weight).
- In malnourished patients "a little nutrition support is good, too much is lethal."
- The use of therapeutic diets has been identified as one of the causes of malnutrition in elderly persons.[26] Based on clinical experience, therapeutic diets, especially the calorie-restricted "ADA" diet, "low-protein" diet, and "renal" diet, further restrict an already compromised oral intake. This situation largely results from limited food volume and restricted food

Text continued on p. 865

TABLE 57-14

MAJOR COMPLICATIONS WITH TOTAL PARENTERAL NUTRITION

TECHNICAL OR MECHANICAL: CATHETER INSERTION

Complication	Etiology	Signs and Symptoms	Treatment	Prevention
Pneumothorax	Subclavian venipuncture	Dyspnea; chest pain; cyanosis	Observation if small	Use internal jugular for high-risk patients
	Unusual anatomy			
	Improper training		Check tube if large or progressive	Trained and approved physician
	Multiple punctures			Stop after three to four attempts and find help
	Failure to remove respirator			Ambu bag during procedure except during thrust of needle
	Slow leak			Repeat chest film
Malposition	Anatomical	Pain or tingling in ear or neck area on side of insertion, or none	Reposition with guidewire or fluoroscopy or new puncture; catheter removal	Proper position if possible
	Needle passed through vein	None; no free reflux of blood		
Subclavian artery puncture	Incorrect insertion	Return of bright-red blood under high pressure; hematoma	Remove needle; elevate head of the bed; pressure to puncture site; close patient observation	Strict adherence to technique
Carotid artery puncture	Internal jugular catheterization	Untreated hematoma may lead to tracheal obstruction	Local application of direct pressure	
Catheter embolism	Shearing off of section of catheter	Cardiac irritability	Radiological or surgical removal	Never pull back catheter through needle

Complication	Cause	Signs	Treatment	Prevention
Air embolism	During catheter threading	Dyspnea; chest pain; tachycardia; tachypnea; cyanosis; paresis; cardiac arrest	Needle aspiration of heart; left side down in steep Trendelenburg's position	Trendelenburg's position during insertion; keep hub covered; Valsalva's maneuver each time catheter open to air
	Tubing disconnection	Dyspnea; chest pain; tachycardia; tachypnea	As above; reconnect tubing; contact physician	Tape tubing connections; use Luer-Lok syringes
Catheter obstruction	Patent tract after removal of catheter	Cyanosis; disorientation; paresis; cardiac arrest		Ointment and occlusive dressing for 12-24 hr
	Mechanical (pump) failure; kink in catheter	Solutions stop running; occlusion alarm	Adjust pump; reset alarm; aspiration of catheter	Hourly monitoring of solution; close observation during dressing change
Thrombosis	Mechanical irritation; patient's hypercoagulable state	Distended collateral veins and chest wall; acute unilateral edema of arm, neck, and face; pleuritic chest pain; inability to thread catheter	Catheter removal; intravenous heparin; venogram	Prevention not always possible; heparin in TPN solution; do not cycle TPN if low antithrombin III level
SEPTIC				
Catheter-related sepsis	Inadequate asepsis during catheter insertion; inadequate dressing care and solution maintenance or preparation; immunosuppression	Glucose intolerance; spiking temperature; elevated white blood cell count; hypotension; disorientation; inflammation or drainage from catheter exit site	Removal of catheter; culture of solution; chest film; cultures of urine and sputum; wound drainage; blood culture (central, peripheral); catheter removal with tip culture (new wire or guidewire); antimicrobial therapy when indicated	Rigid adherence to specific policies and procedures; inspection of catheter site for each dressing change procedure

Modified from Griggs BA et al. A basic nursing guide to providing TPN for the adult patient. Washington, DC: American Society for Parenteral and Enteral Nutrition; 1984.

GI, Gastrointestinal; *TPN,* total parenteral nutrition.

NUTRITION MANAGEMENT

57

TABLE 57-14

MAJOR COMPLICATIONS WITH TOTAL PARENTERAL NUTRITION—cont'd

Complication	Etiology	Signs and Symptoms	Treatment	Prevention
SEPTIC—cont'd				
Septic thrombosis	Untreated catheter sepsis; bacteremic seeding from unknown or other source	Same as for catheter-related sepsis plus unilateral pain and swelling in arm, shoulder, and neck area	Venogram; removal of catheter and culture of tip; IV heparin; antimicrobial therapy	Immediate response to suspected sepsis; periodic changes of catheter (new puncture, over guidewire) when other septic source
METABOLIC				
Hyperglycemia	Diabetes mellitus	Elevated blood glucose level; glycosuria	Regular insulin SQ or IV	Coordinate initiation and insulin requirement
	Too rapid initiation		Slow rate	Start slow with stepwise increments
	Infection or sepsis		Addition of regular insulin	
	Drug related (e.g., steroids)		Slow rate until blood glucose level stable (may increase fat source for calories)	Advance more slowly
	Stress from major surgery		Slow rate or stop infusion	Halve infusion rate during surgery; stop hypertonic solution and infuse dextrose solution or lactated Ringer's solution several hours to 24 hr preoperatively and postoperatively

Hyperglycemic hyperosmolar nonketotic dehydration	Uncontrolled hyperglycemia	Elevated blood glucose level; glycosuria; osmotic diuresis; metabolic imbalances; lethargy; coma; death	Stop hypertonic solution;hydration with free water; judicious doses of IV insulin or potassium; close laboratory and patient monitoring	Immediate and proper control of blood glucose level to <200 mg/L
Hypoglycemia	Sudden decrease or cessation of infusion owing to mechanical problem	Blood glucose level in range of 40 mg/dL; lethargy	Bolus dextrose infusion; monitoring of serum glucose	Accurate administration with hourly patient monitoring
Hyperkalemia	Inability to utilize administered potassium; decrease in renal function; low cardiac output; systemic sepsis	Cardiac arrythmias	Stop infusion; monitoring of serum glucose (see Chapter 53 for further details of management)	Close metabolic monitoring
Hypokalemia	Increased requirement with anabolism; excessive GI losses	Cardiac arrhythmias; muscle weakness; impaired respiratory function	Increased potassium in solution; measurement and replacement of losses	Close metabolic monitoring
Hypophosphatemia	Lack of phosphate supplementation; excessive use of phosphate binders; increased demand during anabolism	Lethargy; altered speech; peripheral paresthesias; increased respirations; coma	Add phosphate to solution; may require peripheral repletion; adjust amount per patient	Standardize solutions; close metabolic monitoring

Modified from Griggs BA et al. A basic nursing guide to providing TPN for the adult patient. Washington, DC: American Society for Parenteral and Enteral Nutrition; 1984.

GI, Gastrointestinal; TPN, total parenteral nutrition.

cont'd

NUTRITION MANAGEMENT

57

TABLE 57-14

MAJOR COMPLICATIONS WITH TOTAL PARENTERAL NUTRITION—cont'd

Complication	Etiology	Signs and Symptoms	Treatment	Prevention
METABOLIC—cont'd				
Hypocalcemia	Lack of or insufficient supplementation	Paresthesia twitching: positive Chvostek's sign	Add or adjust calcium in solution	Close metabolic monitoring
Hypomagnesemia	Lack of or insufficient amounts of magnesium in solution	Tingling sensation around mouth; paresthesias; dizziness; disorientation	Add or adjust magnesium in solution	Standardize solutions; close metabolic monitoring
Essential fatty acid deficiency	Lack of fat supplementation	Dry scaly skin; hair loss	IV administration of 10% or 20% fat emulsion	Routinely include fat emulsion each week
Vitamin K deficiency	Deficient oral intake; severe diarrhea; obstructive jaundice; prolonged antibiotic therapy	Hematuria; ecchymoses; bleeding; purpura; increased prothrombin time	Weekly PO or IM administration of vitamin K	Monitoring of prothrombin time
Iron deficiency	Excessive blood loss	Pallor; fatigue; listlessness; exertional dyspnea; headache; paresthesias	Iron dextran IM or whole blood	Serial determination of hemoglobin, mean cell volume, serum iron
Zinc deficiency	Chronic illness; diseases that predispose to excessive GI losses	Diarrhea; central nervous system disturbances; skin lesions; poor wound healing; alopecia; anorexia; growth retardation	Refeed and treat illness; addition of zinc to solution	Serial determination of serum zinc

Modified from Griggs BA et al. A basic nursing guide to providing TPN for the adult patient. Washington, DC: American Society for Parenteral and Enteral Nutrition; 1984.
GI, Gastrointestinal; *TPN,* total parenteral nutrition.

BOX 57-2

PATIENT RISK PROFILE FOR REFEEDING SYNDROME

Anorexia nervosa

Classic kwashiorkor

Classic marasmus

Chronic malnutrition and underfeeding

Chronic alcoholism

Morbid obesity with massive weight loss

Patient unfed for 7 to 10 days with evidence of stress and depletion

Prolonged fasting

Prolonged intravenous hydration

57

choices; in addition, the patient finds the diet unpalatable. When nutrition is provided to a patient identified as at nutritional risk or to an already malnourished patient, a less restrictive diet should be offered. Close monitoring of appropriate laboratory parameters, monitoring of oral intake by calorie counts (assessing both inadequacy and excesses, if any, such as sodium in the case of heart failure), and adjustment of medications are necessary for these patients.

- Postpyloric feedings have been recommended to prevent aspiration, but this tube placement does not eliminate the risk of aspiration.

NUTRITION MANAGEMENT

REFERENCES

[b] 1. Bistrain BR et al. Prevalence of malnutrition in general medical patients. JAMA 1976; 253:1567.

[b] 2. Weisner RL et al. Hospital malnutrition: a prospective evaluation of general medical patients during the course of hospitalization. Am J Clin Nutr 1979; 32:418.

[b] 3. McWhirter JP, Pennington CR. Incidence and recognition of malnutrition in hospital. Br Med J 1994; 308:945.

[c] 4. Blackburn GL, Bistrain BR. Nutritional and metabolic assessment of the hospitalized patient. J Parenter Enter Nutr 1977; 1:11.

[c] 5. Butterworth CE. The skeleton in the hospital closet. Nutr Today 1974; 9:4.

[b] 6. Edington J et al. Prevalence of malnutrition on admission to four hospitals in England. The Malnutrition Prevalence Group. Clin Nutr 2000; 19:191.

[b] 7. Kelly IE et al. Still hungry in hospital: identifying malnutrition in acute hospital admissions. Q J Med 2000; 93:93.

[d] 8. ASPEN Board of Directors. Clinical pathways and algorithms for delivery of parenteral and enteral nutrition support in adults. Silver Spring, Md: American Society for Parenteral and Enteral Nutrition; 1998.

[c] 9. Shopbell JM, Hopkins B, Shronts EP. Nutrition screening and assessment. In Gottschlich MM et al, eds. A case based core curriculum of the American Society for Parenteral and Enteral Nutrition. Dubuque, Ia: Kendall/Hunt; 2001.

[c] 10. Hammond KA. Dietary and clinical assessment. In Mahan LK, Escott-Stump S, eds. Krause's food, nutrition and diet therapy, 10th ed. Philadelphia: WB Saunders; 2000.

[c] 11. Burke MA, Liffrig T. Nutrition screening and assessment. In Nelson JK et al, eds. Mayo Clinic diet manual: a handbook of nutrition practices, 7th ed. St Louis: Mosby; 1994.

[c] 12. Bistrain B. Nutritional assessment. In Goldman L, Bennett JC: Cecil textbook of medicine, 21st ed. Philadelphia: WB Saunders; 2000.

[c] 13. Russell RM. Nutritional assessment. In Wyngaarden JB, Smith LH Jr, Bennett JC, eds. Cecil textbook of medicine, 19th ed. Philadelphia: WB Saunders; 1992.

[c] 14. Henry CJK. Body mass index and the limits of human survival. Eur J Clin Nutr 1990; 44:329.

[c] 15. Hoffer LJ. Starvation. In Shils ME, Olson JA, Shike M, eds. Modern nutrition in health and disease, 8th ed. Philadelphia: Lea & Febiger; 1994.

[d] 16. National Institutes of Health. Clinical guidelines on the identification, evaluation, and treatment of overweight and obesity in adults. The Obesity Education Initiative. NIH Pub No 98-4083, Bethesda, Md: National Institutes of Health; 1998.

[c] 17. Russell MK, McAdams MP. Laboratory monitoring of nutritional status. In Matarese LE, Gottschlich MM, eds. Contemporary nutrition support practice: a clinical guide. Philadelphia: WB Saunders; 1998.

[c] 18. Selected laboratory measurements in nutrition assessment. In Lysen LK. Quick reference to clinical dietetics. Gaithersburg, Md: Aspen; 1997.

[c] 19. Bloch AS, Mueller C. Enteral and parenteral nutrition support. In Mahan LK, Escott-Stump S, eds. Krause's food, nutrition and diet therapy, 10th ed. Philadelphia: WB Saunders; 2000.

[c] 20. Gorman RC, Morris JB. Minimally invasive access to the gastrointestinal tract. In Rombeau JC, Rolandelli RH, eds. Clinical nutrition: enteral and tube feeding. Philadelphia: WB Saunders; 1997.

[c] 21. Ali A et al. Nutrition support algorithms. Nutritional Support Services 1988; 8(7):13.

[c] 22. Mullan HD, Muscalli VL, eds. The Johns Hopkins Hospital nutrition reference manual. Baltimore: Johns Hopkins University Press; 2001.

[c] 23. Griggs BA et al. A basic nursing guide to providing TPN for the adult patient. Washington, DC: American Society for Parenteral and Enteral Nutrition; 1984.

[c] 24. Solomon SM, Kirby DF. The refeeding syndrome: a review. J Parenter Enter Nutr 1990; 14:90.

[b] 25. Abassi AA, Rudman D. Undernutrition in the nursing home: prevalence, consequences, causes and prevention. Nutr Rev 1994; 52(4):113.

Asthma

Tatiana M. Prowell, MD, and Mark C. Liu, MD

FAST FACTS

- Asthma occurs in 5% of the U.S. population; one half of these cases develop in childhood.
- The best predictor of the diagnosis of asthma is a history of atopy.
- Essential features of asthma are chronic airway inflammation, airway hyperresponsiveness, and episodes of reversible airway obstruction.
- Individual patient "triggers" should always be assessed. Intrinsic triggers include respiratory infections, heart failure, gastroesophageal reflux, and exercise; extrinsic triggers include tobacco smoke, pets, extreme weather, and other environmental antigens in the home or workplace.
- Symptoms of asthma are often worse at night and during early morning hours.

I. EPIDEMIOLOGY

A. PREVALENCE AND MORTALITY

1. Prevalence of asthma increased 58.6% between 1982 and 1996.
2. Cause-specific mortality from asthma is on the rise, especially among women and urban minority populations.[1]
3. Hospitalization is more common among blacks than in other races.
4. Blacks 15 to 24 years of age have the highest asthma-related mortality rate.[2]

B. PRIMARY CARE AND HOSPITALIZATION

1. Access to primary care and appropriate management by primary care physicians can preclude the need for hospitalization in asthmatic patients.[3,4]
2. Of asthmatic adults hospitalized for an asthma flare, approximately 50% are not receiving chronic antiinflammatory therapy.[5]
3. Approximately 75% of patients have no plan for treating an exacerbation.[6]

II. CLINICAL PRESENTATION

A. SYMPTOMS

1. Symptoms include intermittent wheezing, cough, chest tightness, and shortness of breath.
2. Symptoms are often are worse at night because of increased broncho-motor tone from 3 to 4 AM.
3. Common triggers, usually identifiable by the patient, include respiratory infections, exercise, emotional stress, pets, dust, pollen, cigarette smoke, and cold dry air.

4. Many patients have a personal or family history of allergic rhinitis, sinusitis, atopy (e.g., eczema, keratosis pilaris, ichthyosis vulgaris, lichen simplex chronicus), or asthma.

B. PHYSICAL FINDINGS

1. Physical examination findings are most helpful in the setting of an acute flare, when wheezing, coughing, a prolonged expiratory phase, hyperinflation, and decreased breath sounds may be noted.

2. Other important physical findings include nasal polyps; nasal mucosal edema, pallor, or erythema; rhinorrhea; and dry skin with lichenification or excoriation.

III. DIAGNOSTICS

A. PEAK EXPIRATORY FLOW

1. The most simple test to support the diagnosis of asthma is peak expiratory flow (PEF) monitoring using an inexpensive peak flow meter.

2. With normal diurnal variation, PEF reaches its nadir in the early morning and peaks in early afternoon, a pattern that is exaggerated in asthmatic patients.

3. Patients should be asked to keep a diary of PEF measurements on waking, before use of a β-agonist, and in the afternoon after use of a β-agonist. Variability of 20% or more between any two measurements strongly suggests asthma.[7]

B. SPIROMETRY

1. Spirometry is the gold standard test for diagnosing asthma (Fig. 58-1).

2. Measuring forced expiratory volume in 1 second (FEV_1), forced vital capacity (FVC), and the FEV_1/FVC ratio (fractional lung emptying in 1 second) may demonstrate an obstructive ventilatory defect.

3. Decreased FVC in a patient without restrictive lung disease reflects an elevated residual volume (RV), which may also suggest obstruction.

C. BRONCHIAL PROVOCATION TEST

1. The bronchial provocation test is also used to confirm the diagnosis of asthma.

2. FEV_1 is measured serially as the patient inhales increasing concentrations of a provocative agent such as methacholine or histamine.

3. Although a positive test (defined as a decrease in FEV_1 of 20% or more) is not specific for asthma, a negative test has a predictive value of greater than 95% and can exclude the diagnosis in most cases.

IV. MANAGEMENT

A. INPATIENT MANAGEMENT OF ACUTE EXACERBATION

1. Bronchodilator therapy.

a. The short-acting inhaled β_2-agonists (e.g., albuterol) are the mainstay of therapy for breakthrough symptoms and acute exacerbations of asthma.

b. Bronchodilators have onset of action within minutes and can be administered through metered-dose inhaler (MDI) or nebulizer. When equivalent doses are used, an MDI with spacer (used correctly) is equivalent to a nebulizer in terms of length of emergency department (ED) stay, hospitalization rate, and PEF,[8,9] except in cases of severe obstruction when the data are conflicting.[10,11]

c. No good data exist on the use of subcutaneous (SQ) terbutaline or epinephrine, and their routine use is discouraged because of potential cardiovascular side effects.

d. Because asthma causes ventilation-perfusion mismatch, hypoxemia may be transiently worsened by bronchodilators. Thus oxygen should always be given with bronchodilators during acute flares.

e. Several randomized trials have shown equivalent outcomes with intermittent and continuous nebulizer treatments, except in the subpopulation of patients with the most severe flares (PEF of <200 L/min or <50% of predicted), in whom continuous treatments decrease rate of admission, improve PEF, and shorten hospital stay.[12-14]

f. No evidence is available to guide the tapering of bronchodilator treatments.

(1) Patients should be evaluated frequently for signs of improvement or fatigue.

(2) In general, treatments should not be tapered until the PEF is 50% or greater of predicted, at which time treatments may be decreased to every 4 hours, with additional treatments every 2 hours on an as-needed basis.

2. **Corticosteroid therapy.**

a. Multiple studies have shown that systemic corticosteroids (e.g., methylprednisolone, prednisone), usually given in 7-day pulsed courses, decrease the rate of relapse after an acute exacerbation.[15] Subsequent studies failed to show benefit of steroid doses exceeding 40 mg/day. However, good evidence supports discharge of the patient with a short course of oral prednisone,[16] which need not involve tapering doses.[17]

b. Inhaled corticosteroids (e.g., fluticasone, beclomethasone) are equivalent to systemic corticosteroids in terms of relapse prevention after an exacerbation.[18]

c. The addition of inhaled corticosteroids to oral prednisone can further decrease β_2-agonist use, likelihood of relapse, and symptoms after an acute exacerbation.[19]

d. Current recommendations support initiation of an inhaled steroid at least 48 hours before discharge in addition to systemic corticosteroids; a general approach would be to start fluticasone 220 μg 1 puff bid or the equivalent.

3. **Anticholinergic therapy: ipratropium.**

a. The only available anticholinergic for asthma is ipratropium bromide (Atrovent).

b. It is preferred therapy for β-blocker–induced bronchospasm.

c. It may have a role in treatment of severe asthma exacerbations.

d. Data on the addition of ipratropium to standard therapy are contradictory and limited by small patient populations and short follow-up times.

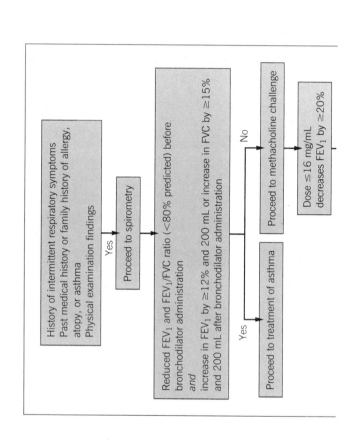

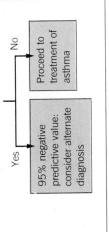

No

Yes

95% negative predictive value: consider alternate diagnosis

Proceed to treatment of asthma

FIG. 58-1

Management approach to the patient with a diagnosis of asthma. *FEV₁,* Forced expiratory volume in 1 second; *FVC,* forced vital capacity.

58

ASTHMA

e. Several studies have shown no clear clinical benefit of routine use of ipratropium for flares; however, subgroup analyses of the most severe asthma flares have shown statistically significant but clinically modest effects on PEF and hospitalization rate.[20-24]

f. No data support the use of ipratropium more frequently than every 6 hours.

4. **Emergency therapy: magnesium sulfate.**

a. Magnesium sulfate is often used in the ED for acute asthma flares.

b. Most studies and recent metaanalyses have found no clinically significant effects with routine use of magnesium in terms of PEF or hospitalization rate.[25]

c. Magnesium sulfate has possible benefit in a subgroup with the most severe exacerbations in whom an increase in PEF of approximately 50 L/min and a modest decrease in hospitalization rate have been shown.[26,27]

d. In extremely severe flares the clinician may consider giving an IV bolus of 2 g $MgSO_4$ over 20 minutes followed by a continuous drip of 2 g/hr, following blood pressure and serum magnesium levels.[28]

5. **Other acute therapy.**

a. Theophylline is a bronchodilator with a narrow therapeutic window and minimal efficacy in acute exacerbations.[29] Although new studies are under way to reevaluate theophylline's role in acute asthma flares, currently its routine use is discouraged.

b. Antibiotics do not play a role in the management of an acute asthma flare unless the patient has obvious pneumonia.

B. **OUTPATIENT MANAGEMENT OF CHRONIC ASTHMA** (Tables 58-1 and 58-2)

1. **Inhaled corticosteroids.**

a. Corticosteroids are the cornerstone of asthma management.

b. Corticosteroids have multiple beneficial effects.
   (1) Decrease in symptoms.[30]
   (2) Decrease in bronchial reactivity to provocative agents.[31]
   (3) Reduction in the need for β-agonist use.
   (4) Improvement in FEV_1 or PEF.[32]
   (5) Decrease in frequency and severity of exacerbations.[33]
   (6) Decrease in incidence of relapse after an exacerbation.[19]

c. It is important to advise patients to rinse the mouth and to use a spacer with these medications to minimize local side effects (e.g., thrush, hoarseness) and systemic absorption across the gastrointestinal (GI) tract.

d. Serious systemic side effects are uncommon in adults receiving moderate doses but may include adrenal suppression, cataracts, glaucoma, and decreased bone mineral density.

2. **Long-acting bronchodilators.**

a. Long-acting bronchodilators include $β_2$-adrenergic agonists, such as salmeterol, and phosphodiesterase inhibitors, such as theophylline and aminophylline.

TABLE 58-1
CLASSIFICATION SCHEME FOR CHRONIC ASTHMA

Category	Symptoms	Nocturnal Symptoms	Pulmonary Function
Mild intermittent	Symptoms less than twice a week; activity unlimited; flares brief and rare	Twice a month or less	FEV_1 or PEF ≥80% predicted; PEF varies by ≤20%
Mild persistent	Symptoms more than twice a week; activity mildly limited; flares once a week	Twice a month or less	FEV_1 or PEF >80% predicted; PEF varies by 20%-30%
Moderate persistent	Symptoms daily; activity moderately limited; flares twice a week or more	More than once a week	FEV_1 or PEF 60%-80% predicted; PEF varies by >30%
Severe persistent	Symptoms constant; activity severely limited; flares frequent and prolonged	Often	FEV_1 or PEF 60% predicted; PEF varies by >30%

Modified from National Heart, Blood and Lung Institute. Guidelines for the diagnosis and management of asthma. Expert Panel Report 2. National Asthma Education and Prevention Program. NIH Pub No 97-4051. Bethesda, Md: National Institutes of Health; 1997.
FEV_1, Forced expiratory volume in 1 second; *PEF*, peak expiratory flow.

58

ASTHMA

b. Salmeterol is well tolerated and has demonstrated superiority over albuterol taken on a scheduled[34] or as-needed (prn) basis,[35] in terms of symptom reduction and improvement in FEV_1 or PEF.

c. Theophylline is rarely used in adults except in cases of refractory asthma because of its narrow therapeutic window. Adverse reactions include GI intolerance, dose-related arrhythmias, seizures, and drug-drug interactions.

3. **Mast cell release inhibitors.**

a. Mast cell release inhibitors include cromolyn and nedocromil.

b. These drugs have few side effects.

c. They may be useful for exercise-induced bronchospasm and allergen-induced asthma.

4. **Leukotriene modifiers.**

a. Leukotriene modifiers decrease leukotriene production (e.g., zileuton).

b. These agents block leukotriene receptors (e.g., zafirlukast and montelukast).

c. Leukotriene modification has beneficial effects.

   (1) Prevention of airway smooth muscle contraction.

   (2) Decrease in vascular permeability.

   (3) Prevention of inflammatory cell migration.

d. Although leukotriene modifiers have a clear benefit in terms of symptoms and PEF compared with placebo,[25] inhaled corticosteroids produce greater improvement in symptoms, PEF, and frequency of

TABLE 58-2		
APPROACH TO CHRONIC MANAGEMENT OF ASTHMA BY SEVERITY		
Asthma Category	Preferred Controller Agents	Rescue Agents
Mild intermittent	None	Inhaled β_2-agonist prn*
Mild persistent	Low-dose inhaled steroid *or* Mast cell inhibitor *or* Leukotriene modifier†	Inhaled β_2-agonist prn*
Moderate persistent	Intermediate-dose inhaled steroid with or without long-acting inhaled β_2-agonist *or* Other controller‡	Inhaled β_2-agonist prn*
Severe persistent	High-dose inhaled steroid *and* Long-acting inhaled β_2-agonist *and* Other controllers‡	Inhaled β_2-agonist prn*

Modified from National Heart, Blood and Lung Institute. Guidelines for the diagnosis and management of asthma. Expert Panel Report 2. National Asthma Education and Prevention Program. NIH Pub No 97-4051. Bethesda, Md: National Institutes of Health; 1997.

prn, As needed.

*Daily or increasing use of short-acting inhaled β_2-agonist indicates suboptimal asthma control and the need to reevaluate environmental triggers (e.g., pets, cigarette smoke) and to advance to the next phase of controller agents.

†Other controllers would include sustained-release phosphodiesterase inhibitor.

‡Other controllers would include sustained-release phosphodiesterase inhibitor *or* long-acting oral β_2-agonist in lieu of long-acting inhaled β_2-agonist.

exacerbations[36,37] and are thus preferred except in cases of aspirin-sensitive asthma.

e. Reported side effects include hepatotoxicity, GI intolerance, angioedema or anaphylaxis, and rarely Churg-Strauss syndrome (controversial).

5. **Systemic corticosteroids.**

a. Systemic corticosteroids should be used as long-term controller medications only in patients with severe, persistent asthma after other therapies have been exhausted.

b. They have multiple benefits in asthma.[38]

(1) Decreased airway hyperresponsiveness.

(2) Improvement of symptoms.

(3) Decrease in frequency of exacerbations.

(4) Less need for β_2-agonist use.

c. These agents have significant long-term toxicities.[39]

(1) Osteoporosis.

(2) Cataracts.

(3) Weight gain.

(4) Diabetes.

(5) Adrenal suppression.

6. **Steroid-sparing agents.**

a. Steroid-sparing agents include methotrexate, cyclosporine, and gold.

b. Reduction in steroid dose is often clinically minimal.[40]

c. Steroid-sparing agents should be reserved for the rare patient with severe persistent asthma who remains symptomatic while receiving high-dose corticosteroids.

7. Short-acting bronchodilators.

a. Short-acting bronchodilators have less of a role in the long-term management of asthma and should be used only as rescue medications (see previous section on bronchodilator therapy).

b. Use of albuterol has been associated with an increase in fatal and near-fatal outcomes, even after adjustment for disease severity.[41]

c. Scheduled use of short-acting β_2-agonists has no role.

d. Albuterol on an as-needed basis is equivalent to scheduled dosage in terms of PEF, symptoms, and exacerbations in mild disease.[42]

C. NONPHARMACOLOGICAL MANAGEMENT OF ASTHMA

1. Allergy history.

a. All asthmatic patients should be screened for a history of allergies.

b. Common household allergens include dust mites (frequently found in carpets and bedding materials), pollen, cockroaches, molds, and pets.

c. Surprisingly, studies have failed to demonstrate a significant benefit of decreasing allergen exposure.[43]

d. Immunotherapy using identified patient-specific allergens has been shown to reduce symptoms and bronchial hyperreactivity significantly.[42]

e. Adverse reactions such as atopic dermatitis and rhinitis are common.

f. Anaphylactic reactions can occur.

2. Asthma triggers.

a. Nonspecific asthma triggers include sinusitis, exercise, weather changes, tobacco smoke, gastroesophageal reflux disease, and upper respiratory infections.

b. Asthma triggers frequently initiate asthma exacerbations.

c. Avoiding or modifying triggers appears to reduce symptoms but may not produce a significant improvement in measures of pulmonary function.[44]

3. Patient education and self-monitoring.

a. Patient education and self-monitoring are key components of asthma management.

b. Every patient should have a peak flow meter.

c. All patients should be educated about the differences between "controller" and "rescue" medications.

d. Staff should confirm correct technique with MDIs, spacer devices, and peak flow meters.

e. A written plan for the diagnosis of asthma and actions to take in exacerbations should be developed (Table 58-3).

   (1) The plan should be based on the patient's personal best PEF (or predicted PEF).

   (2) It should include specific values for each zone and specific directions on how to alter medications.

TABLE 58-3

GENERALIZED EXAMPLE OF ASTHMA FLARE ACTION PLAN

Zone	Interpretation	Action
Green zone 80%-100% predicted PEF	Good control	No change needed
Yellow zone 50%-79% predicted PEF	Inadequate control	Add rescue medications; increase dose of controllers
Red zone <50% predicted PEF	Medical emergency	Add or increase rescue medications; call physician immediately

Modified from National Heart, Lung and Blood Institute. Guidelines for the diagnosis and management of asthma. Expert Panel Report 2. National Asthma Education and Prevention Program. NIH Pub No 97-4051. Bethesda, Md: National Institutes of Health; 1997.
PEF, Peak expiratory flow.

PEARLS AND PITFALLS

- When to call the medical intensive care unit.
  - Tachypnea, tachycardia, diaphoresis, accessory muscle use, and inability to complete full sentences because of dyspnea characterize a severe asthma flare.
  - Other clinically established markers of a life-threatening flare include pulsus paradoxus of 25 mm Hg or more (inspiratory fall in systolic blood pressure ≥25 mm Hg, compared with normal decrease <10 mm Hg), bradycardia, hypotension, mental status changes, pneumothorax, diminishing respiratory effort, and cyanosis.[28]
  - Arterial blood gases should be assessed whenever the PEF is less than 50% of the predicted value or if there is any suspicion of carbon dioxide (CO_2) retention.
  - Early in an asthma flare, patients have respiratory alkalosis caused by dyspnea and hyperventilation. As respiratory muscles become fatigued, pseudonormalization of CO_2 tension and pH occurs as CO_2 retention and respiratory acidosis develop. Although oxygenation may still be normal, this is worrisome for impending respiratory failure.
  - In overt respiratory failure, patients have frank respiratory acidosis with hypercapnia and hypoxemia. They usually require immediate endotracheal intubation, mechanical ventilation, sedation, and possibly pharmacological paralysis.
  - Because intubation is always preferable on an elective rather than an emergency basis, any patient with evidence of respiratory muscle fatigue deserves early evaluation by the intensive care unit staff and frequent reevaluation by a physician.
- Exercised-induced asthma (EIA).
  - Exercise-induced bronchospasm may be an isolated problem or only one trigger of asthma in a given patient.
  - Patients generally report cough, shortness of breath, wheezing, or chest

tightness, which begins during exercise and peaks approximately 10 minutes after cessation of activity.

- Symptoms usually resolve spontaneously within 30 minutes of activity.
- EIA is most commonly a clinical diagnosis but may be confirmed by a decrease of greater than 15% in PEF or FEV_1 after exercise.
- Therapeutic options include albuterol or salmeterol taken 30 minutes before exercise; salmeterol has a more prolonged effect.[45]
- Nedocromil can be taken shortly before exercise for a 1- to 2-hour effect.[46]
- An inhaled steroid may be used on a regular basis in an attempt to reduce use of short-acting agents.[31]
- When appropriately managed, EIA should not prevent an athlete from participating in recreational or competitive sports.[47]

- Asthma and pregnancy.
  - Asthma is managed the same way in pregnant women as in nonpregnant patients.
  - Nedocromil, cromolyn, zafirlukast, and montelukast are pregnancy class B agents (chance of fetal harm is remote, but possible).
  - Most of the remaining drugs used to treat asthma, such as albuterol, salmeterol, zileuton, theophylline, and systemic or inhaled corticosteroids, are pregnancy class C agents (chance of fetal harm exists, but risks and benefits must be weighed).
  - Some experts consider beclomethasone and budesonide the inhaled steroids of choice to initiate during pregnancy, but a change to these agents is unnecessary for a pregnant woman whose asthma is well controlled by other agents.
  - Use of any of these agents in pregnancy is preferable to suboptimal asthma control.
  - Poor control of asthma during pregnancy has been associated with a number of adverse fetal outcomes, including increased risk of prematurity, low birth weight, and increased mortality in the perinatal period.[5]

- Allergic bronchopulmonary aspergillosis (ABPA).
  - ABPA is a complex hypersensitivity disorder often seen in patients with severe asthma and cystic fibrosis when their airways become colonized with *Aspergillus*.
  - ABPA should be suspected when asthma patients have recurrent fever, malaise, eosinophilia, and pulmonary infiltrates.
  - With increasing recognition of the prevalence of ABPA among asthmatic patients, many experts now recommend routine screening with a skin test for *Aspergillus fumigatus,* especially for atopic patients.
  - Diagnostic criteria for ABPA include the presence of asthma, positive skin test for *Aspergillus*, elevated total serum IgE level (>1000 ng/mL), *Aspergillus*-specific immunoglobulin E (IgE) or IgG antibodies, and pulmonary infiltrates or central bronchiectasis seen on computed tomography (CT).

58

ASTHMA

- In one prospective study of asthmatic patients, skin testing for *Aspergillus* and chest CT scans were performed on atopic asthmatic patients. A negative skin test for *Aspergillus* was found to rule out ABPA. The test was cost effective and permitted early treatment for this steroid-responsive condition.[48]
- Limited studies also suggest a benefit from the antifungal itraconazole.[49]

REFERENCES

[c] 1. American Lung Association. http://www.lungusa.org/data/asthma/; 2000.

[c] 2. McFadden ER Jr, Warren EL. Observations on asthma mortality. Ann Intern Med 1997; 127(2):142.

[c] 3. Pappas G et al. Potentially avoidable hospitalizations: inequalities in rates between US socioeconomic groups. Am J Public Health 1997; 87:811.

[c] 4. Gibson PG, Coughlan J, Wilson AJ, et al. The effects of self-management education and regular practitioner review in adults with asthma. (Cochrane Review, latest version 26 Feb 98). In The Cochrane Library. Oxford: Update Software.

[d] 5. National Heart, Lung and Blood Institute. Guidelines for the diagnosis and management of asthma. Expert Panel Report 2. National Asthma Education and Prevention Program. NIH Pub No 97-4051. Bethesda, Md: National Institutes of Health; 1997.

[b] 6. Hartert TV et al. Inadequate outpatient medical therapy for patients with asthma admitted to two urban hospitals. Am J Med 1996; 100:386.

[c] 7. Tierney LM Jr et al. Current medical diagnosis and treatment 2000. New York: Appleton & Lange; 2000.

[a] 8. Idris AH et al. Emergency department treatment of severe asthma: metered-dose inhaler plus holding chamber is equivalent in effectiveness to nebulizer. Chest 1993; 103:665.

[a] 9. Colacone A et al. A comparison of albuterol administered by metered dose inhaler (and holding chamber) or wet nebulizer in acute asthma. Chest 1993; 104:835.

[a] 10. Rudnitsky GS et al. Comparison of intermittent and continuously nebulized albuterol for treatment of asthma in an urban emergency department. Ann Emerg Med 1993; 22:1842.

[c] 11. Marin MG. Low-dose methotrexate spares steroid usage in steroid-dependent asthmatic patients: a meta-analysis. Chest 1997; 112:29.

[a] 12. Lin RY et al. Continuous versus intermittent albuterol nebulization in the treatment of acute asthma. Ann Emerg Med 1993; 22:1847.

[a] 13. Colacone A et al. Continuous nebulization of albuterol in acute asthma. Chest 1990; 97:693.

[a] 14. Papo M et al. A prospective, randomized study of continuous versus intermittent nebulized albuterol for severe status asthmaticus in children. Crit Care Med 1993; 21:479.

[c] 15. Rowe BH et al. The effectiveness of corticosteroids in the treatment of acute exacerbations of asthma: a meta-analysis of their effect on relapse following acute assessment. In Cates C et al, eds. Airway Review Group Module—Cochrane Library. Cochrane Collaboration; May 1997.

[a] 16. Chapman KR et al. Effect of a short course of prednisone in the prevention of early relapse after emergency room treatment of acute asthma. N Engl J Med 1991; 324:788.

[a] 17. O'Driscoll B et al. Double blind trial of steroid tapering in acute asthma. Lancet 1993; 341:324.

[a] 18. FitzGerald JM et al. A randomized, controlled trial of high dose, inhaled budesonide versus oral prednisone in patients discharged from the emergency department following an acute asthma exacerbation. Can Respir J 2000; 7:61.

[a] 19. Rowe BH et al. Inhaled budesonide in addition to oral corticosteroids to prevent asthma relapse following discharge from the emergency department: a randomized controlled trial. JAMA 1999; 281:2119.

[c] 20. Rodrigo G, Rodrigo C, Burschtin O. A meta-analysis of the effects of ipratropium bromide in adults with acute asthma. Am J Med 1999; 107:363.

[c] 21. Stoodley R et al. The role of ipratropium bromide in the emergency management of acute asthma exacerbation: a meta-analysis of randomized controlled trials. Ann Emerg Med 1999; 34(1):8.

[c] 22. Lin RY et al. The role of ipratropium bromide in the emergency management of acute asthma exacerbations: a meta-analysis of randomized controlled trials. Ann Emerg Med 1998; 31(2):208.

[a] 23. Karpel J et al. A comparison of ipratropium and albuterol versus albuterol alone for the treatment of acute asthma. Chest 1996; 110(3):611.

[a] 24. Patrick D et al. Severe exacerbations of COPD and asthma: incremental benefit of adding ipratropium to usual therapy. Chest 1990; 98:295.

[c] 25. Rowe BH et al. Intravenous magnesium sulfate treatment for acute asthma in the emergency department: a systematic review of the literature. Ann Emerg Med 2000; 36(3):181.

[c] 26. Rodrigo G et al. Efficacy of magnesium sulfate in acute adult asthma: a meta-analysis of randomized trials. Am J Emerg Med 2000; 18(2):216.

[c] 27. Alter et al. Intravenous magnesium as an adjuvant in acute bronchospasm: a meta-analysis. Ann Emerg Med 2000; 36(3):191.

[c] 28. Abou-Shala N, MacIntyre N. Obstructive lung diseases. II. Emergent management of acute asthma. Med Clin North Am 1996; 80:678.

[a] 29. Self T et al. Inhaled albuterol and oral prednisone therapy in hospitalized adult asthmatics: does aminophylline add any benefit? Chest 1990; 98:1317.

[a] 30. van Essen-Zandvliet EE et al. Effects of 22 months of treatment with inhaled corticosteroids and/or beta-2-agonists on lung function, airway responsiveness, and symptoms in children with asthma. The Dutch Chronic Non-specific Lung Disease Study Group. Am Rev Respir Dis 1992; 146:547.

[a] 31. Vathenen AS et al. Effect of inhaled budesonide on bronchial reactivity to histamine, exercise, and eucapnic dry air hyperventilation in patients with asthma. Thorax 1991; 46:811.

[a] 32. Haahtela T et al. Comparison of a beta 2-agonist, terbutaline, with an inhaled corticosteroid, budesonide, in newly detected asthma. N Engl J Med 1991; 325:388.

[b] 33. Dompeling E et al. Slowing the deterioration of asthma and chronic obstructive pulmonary disease observed during bronchodilator therapy by adding inhaled corticosteroids: a 4-year prospective study. Ann Intern Med 1993; 118(10):770.

[a] 34. D'Alonzo GE et al. Salmeterol xinafoate as maintenance therapy compared with albuterol in patients with asthma. JAMA 1994; 271:1412.

[a] 35. Pearlman DS et al. A comparison of salmeterol with albuterol in the treatment of mild-to-moderate asthma. N Engl J Med 1992; 327:1420.

[a] 36. Malmstrom K et al. Oral montelukast, inhaled beclomethasone, and placebo for chronic asthma: a randomized, controlled trial. Montelukast/Beclomethasone Study Group. Ann Intern Med 1999; 130:487.

[a] 37. Malmstrom K et al. Oral montelukast, inhaled beclomethasone, and placebo for chronic asthma: a randomized, controlled trial. Ann Intern Med 1995; 30(6):487.

[a] 38. Juniper EF et al. Effect of long-term treatment with an inhaled corticosteroid (budesonide) on airway hyperresponsiveness and clinical asthma in nonsteroid-dependent asthmatics. Am Rev Respir Dis 1990; 142:832.

[c] 39. Lipworth BJ. Systemic adverse effects of inhaled corticosteroid therapy: a systematic review and meta-analysis. Arch Intern Med 1999; 159:941.

[a] 40. Raimondi A et al. Treatment of acute severe asthma with inhaled albuterol delivered via jet nebulizer, metered dose inhaler with spacer, or dry powder. Chest 1997; 112(1):24.

[b] 41. Spitzer WO et al. The use of β-agonists and the risk of death and near death from asthma. N Engl J Med 1992; 326:501.

[a] 42. Drazen JM et al. Comparison of regularly scheduled with as-needed use of albuterol in mild asthma. N Engl J Med 1996; 335:841.

[c] 43. Gotzsche PC, Hammarquist C, Burr M. House dust mite control measures in the management of asthma: meta-analysis. Br Med J 1998; 317:1105.

[c] 44. Field SK, Sutherland LR. Does medical antireflux therapy improve asthma in asthmatics with gastroesophageal reflux? A critical review of the literature. Chest 1998; 114:275.

58

ASTHMA

[a] 45. Kemp JP et al. Prolonged effect of inhaled salmeterol against exercise-induced broncho-spasm. Am J Respir Crit Care Med 1994; 150:1612.

[b] 46. Albazzaz MK et al. Dose-response study of nebulized nedocromil sodium in exercise induced asthma. Thorax 1989; 44:816.

[c] 47. Nastasi KJ et al. Exercise-induced asthma and the athlete. J Asthma 1995; 32:249.

[b] 48. Eaton T et al. Allergic bronchopulmonary aspergillosis in the asthma clinic: a prospective evaluation of CT in the diagnostic algorithm. Chest 2000; 118(1):66.

[a] 49. Stevens DA et al. A randomized trial of itraconazole in allergic bronchopulmonary aspergillosis. N Engl J Med 2000; 342:756.

Chronic Obstructive Pulmonary Disease

Majd Mouded, MD, David Zaas, MD, and Robert Wise, MD

FAST FACTS

- Chronic obstructive pulmonary disease (COPD) is the fourth leading cause of death in the United States.
- Mortality from COPD is increasing, especially in women.
- Inhaled bronchodilators are the mainstay of management for both acute exacerbations and management of chronic stable COPD.
- The optimal dose and duration of steroids in the treatment of acute COPD exacerbations is not known, but steroids do hasten the recovery from exacerbations, which are characterized by worsening dyspnea or gas exchange.
- Antibiotics may be useful when exacerbations are characterized by an increase in volume and purulence of sputum, but the optimal agent has not yet been defined.
- Oxygen is the only treatment, which has been shown to reduce mortality in advanced COPD.
- Smoking cessation is the only intervention that has been shown to slow the progression of COPD.

I. EPIDEMIOLOGY

A. DEFINITIONS

1. According to the American Thoracic Society (ATS),[1] COPD is progressive airflow obstruction resulting from chronic bronchitis or emphysema.
2. Chronic bronchitis is defined as a chronic productive cough for longer than 3 months in 2 successive years, not resulting from another identifiable cause.
3. Emphysema is an abnormal permanent enlargement of airspaces distal to the terminal bronchioles with destruction of the airway walls.

B. MORBIDITY AND MORTALITY[2]

1. COPD is a major cause of morbidity and mortality.
2. The exact number of individuals with COPD is unknown.
3. In 1994 an estimated 14 million individuals in the United States had COPD.
   a. This includes 12.5 million with primary chronic bronchitis and 1.6 million with primary emphysema.
   b. The vast majority show a combination of both processes.

4. COPD is still the fourth leading cause of death in the United States, where 112,584 deaths were caused by COPD in 1998.
5. In 1995 the age-adjusted death rates per 100,000 population ranged from 15.6 in black women to 54.7 in white men.
6. The mortality rate in men has been stable since the 1980s.
7. The mortality rate in women has doubled since the 1980s.
8. The mortality rate is higher in whites than nonwhites and inversely related to socioeconomic status for unclear reasons.

C. CIGARETTE SMOKING

1. Cigarette smoking is by far the most important risk factor for development of COPD.
2. Lung capacity of a normal individual decreases progressively with age, which is reflected in a decreasing 1-second forced expiratory volume (FEV_1) of approximately 30 mL per year.
3. Smoking increases the rate of decline in FEV_1 to approximately 45 mL per year.
4. Rate of decline is proportional to the quantity of tobacco use.
5. About 15% of smokers show declines in FEV_1 of two to three times those of nonsmokers, and clinically symptomatic COPD develops in these smokers.
6. The reason that progressive lung disease develops only in certain patients is unclear.
7. Occupational exposures, airway hyperreactivity (AHR), and air pollution may interact with tobacco use to affect the development and severity of COPD.

D. α_1-ANTITRYPSIN DEFICIENCY

1. α_1-Antitrypsin deficiency is the most common genetic cause of COPD.
2. It accounts for less than 1% of COPD cases.
3. α_1-Antitrypsin normally inhibits neutrophil elastase and leads to basilar panacinar emphysema.
4. Numerous phenotypes of α_1-antitrypsin deficiency exist.
5. PiZZ is the most common subtype.
   a. PiZZ accounts for 95% of cases.
   b. It is found most often whites of Northern European descent.
   c. PiZZ affects 50,000 to 100,000 Americans.
   d. α_1-Antitrypsin deficiency often leads to mild COPD, with a late age of presentation in nonsmokers.

II. CLINICAL PRESENTATION

The clinical presentation of COPD is initially subtle and progresses with the deterioration of pulmonary function. Patients have often smoked more than one pack per day for over 20 years at the time of clinical presentation.

A. MILD CHRONIC OBSTRUCTIVE PULMONARY DISEASE

1. Mild COPD is often manifested as intermittent cough, especially in the morning.
2. Patients have recurrent respiratory infections.

BOX 59-1

PHYSICAL EXAMINATION FINDINGS IN CHRONIC OBSTRUCTIVE PULMONARY DISEASE

Hyperinflation with increased anteroposterior diameter

Prolonged expiratory phase

Expiratory wheezing and basilar crackles

Accessory muscle use and pursed-lip breathing

Cyanosis

Jugular venous distention and tender pulsatile liver

Loud P_2 and murmur of tricuspid regurgitation

Lower extremity edema

Drowsiness

Asterixis

Modified from American Thoracic Society. Am J Respir Crit Care Med 1995; 152:S77.

3. Dyspnea occurs only with vigorous exertion.

4. Presentation is usually in the fifth decade of life.

5. In some patients severe airflow obstruction develops without a predominant cough.

6. Many patients have variability in their symptoms from day to day.

B. PROGRESSION OF CHRONIC OBSTRUCTIVE PULMONARY DISEASE

1. As COPD progresses, the interval between respiratory infections and disease exacerbations decreases.

2. Dyspnea on exertion becomes more prominent with less vigorous activity.

C. SEVERE CHRONIC OBSTRUCTIVE PULMONARY DISEASE

1. Patients may lose weight.

2. Lower extremity edema is caused by cor pulmonale.

3. Morning headache and drowsiness are caused by hypercapnia.

D. PHYSICAL EXAMINATION (Box 59-1)

1. Decreased breath sounds are the most sensitive and specific physical examination findings in the identification of patients with COPD.[3]

III. DIAGNOSTICS

Tests useful in diagnosing COPD and assessing its progression include chest radiography, computed tomography (CT), pulmonary function tests (PFTs), α_1-antitrypsin screening, and arterial blood gas (ABG) analysis.

A. RADIOGRAPHY AND COMPUTED TOMOGRAPHY

1. Chest x-ray findings can demonstrate hyperinflation with flattened diaphragms, increased retrosternal airspace, and narrow cardiac silhouette.

2. Emphysematous changes may cause the lung parenchyma to be hyperlucent, with rapid tapering of the pulmonary vasculature.

59

CHRONIC OBSTRUCTIVE PULMONARY DISEASE

3. In advanced disease cor pulmonale may be evident, with right ventricular hypertrophy and enlarged pulmonary arteries.
4. High-resolution chest CT is the most sensitive and specific study for the bullous changes associated with emphysema.

B. α_1-ANTITRYPSIN SCREENING[4]

1. Patients with COPD before age 45 years.
2. Patients without a smoking history.
3. Patients with a strong family history of COPD.

C. PULMONARY FUNCTION TESTS

1. PFTs are essential in the diagnosis, prognosis, and staging of COPD.
2. Evidence of airway obstruction is reflected in a FEV_1/FVC (forced vital capacity) ratio less than 72%.
3. FEV_1 is the single most important variable in quantifying COPD severity and long-term prognosis.
4. FEV_1 has been shown to predict long-term mortality from all causes.[5,6]
5. Air trapping from COPD may cause an increased total lung capacity (TLC), residual volume (RV), and RV/TLC ratio.
6. Alveolar destruction associated with emphysema decreases the area for gas exchange. As a result a gas transfer defect occurs that is reflected in a decreased diffusing capacity for carbon monoxide (DLCO).[7]

D. CLASSIFICATION OF DISEASE SEVERITY

1. Classification of disease severity varies among the ATS,[1] European Respiratory Society (ERS),[8] and British Thoracic Society (BTS),[9] with the BTS including clinical features as well as FEV_1 (Table 59-1).
2. Variation in COPD severity classification has led to a newer system and consensus statement by the U.S. National Heart, Lung and Blood Institute (NHLBI) and World Health Organization (WHO), known as the Global Initiative for Chronic Obstructive Lung Disease (GOLD) summary.[4]
a. The GOLD recommendation is that initial PFT testing be performed both before and after bronchodilator therapy to exclude the diagnosis of asthma and to evaluate the degree of AHR.
b. All further PFT testing should then be done only after bronchodilator therapy, to standardize the nonreversible component of the FEV_1.

IV. MANAGEMENT

A. ACUTE EXACERBATIONS

1. Etiological considerations.
a. An environmental irritant, gastroesophageal reflux, heart failure, and viral or bacterial infection may exacerbate COPD.
b. When a patient cannot be managed as an outpatient or has a poor response to emergency department therapy, hospital admission is necessary for continued management.

TABLE 59.1

STAGING SYSTEMS FOR CHRONIC OBSTRUCTIVE PULMONARY DISEASE

Staging System	Mild	Moderate	Severe
ATS[1]: FEV_1	≥50% predicted	35%-49% predicted	<35% predicted
ERS[8]: FEV_1	≥70% predicted	50%-69% predicted	<50% predicted
BTS[9]: FEV_1	60%-79% predicted	40%-59% predicted	<40% predicted
Cough	"Smoker's cough"	With or without sputum	Prominent
Dyspnea	Minimal	On exertion	On exertion or at rest
Lung examination findings	Normal	With or without wheeze	Hyperinflation, wheeze
Other findings	Normal	Normal	Cyanosis, edema
NHLBI/WHO GOLD Summary[4]: FEV_1 after bronchodilator	≥80% predicted	IIa: 50%-79% predicted IIb: 30%-49% predicted	<30% predicted, *or* Presence of respiratory failure or clinical signs of right-sided heart failure
	With or without chronic symptoms	With or without chronic symptoms	

Modified from Bach PB et al. Ann Intern Med 2001; 134:600.

CHRONIC OBSTRUCTIVE PULMONARY DISEASE   59

c. Treatment strategies for COPD vary from patient to patient and among institutions (Box 59-2).[1]

d. The cause of the exacerbation should be treated when possible.

e. Pharmacotherapy should then be initiated (see below).

2. β_2-Adrenergic agonists.

a. β_2-Adrenergic agonists act to bronchodilate the airways directly through the sympathetic nervous system.

b. They are first-line treatment during an acute COPD exacerbation.

c. These agents are usually delivered by metered-dose inhaler (MDI) with a spacer or in nebulized form.

d. Many studies have shown equivalence between the two delivery methods, but not all the studies used equal doses or medications.[10-13]

e. Initial use of a nebulizer may improve pulmonary function earlier than with an MDI.[14]

BOX 59-2

EMERGENCY DEPARTMENT EVALUATION OF PATIENT WITH ACUTE EXACERBATIONS OF CHRONIC OBSTRUCTIVE PULMONARY DISEASE

HISTORY

Baseline respiratory status

Sputum volume and characteristics

Duration and progression of symptoms

Dyspnea severity

Exercise limitations

Sleep and eating difficulties

Home care resources

Home therapeutic regimen

Symptoms of comorbid acute or chronic conditions

PHYSICAL EXAMINATION

Evidence of:

   Cor pulmonale

   Bronchospasm

   Pneumonia

   Hemodynamic instability

   Altered mentation

   Paradoxical abdominal retractions

   Use of accessory respiratory muscles

   Acute comorbid conditions

STANDARD DIAGNOSTIC TESTS

Arterial blood gases

Pulse oximetry

Chest radiograph

Electrocardiogram

f. If the patient's ability to coordinate an MDI is a concern, the nebulized solution should be used, especially in the setting of an acute exacerbation.

g. Short-acting β_2-agonists such as albuterol may be used every 30 to 60 minutes as required during an acute exacerbation.

h. Once the patient's condition has stabilized, the frequency of treatments may be gradually decreased to the recommended doses of 1 or 2 puffs q4-6h or 0.5 mL (2.5 mg) of nebulized solution.[1]

i. Continuous nebulization is not usually recommended because its safety and value have not been demonstrated; however, it may be used in the setting of impending respiratory failure to avoid mechanical ventilation.

j. Long-acting β_2-agonists have been shown to be beneficial in the long-term management of COPD.[15]

k. Safety of long-acting β_2-agonists in an acute exacerbation has not been demonstrated, and no evidence of clinical benefit in a COPD exacerbation has been shown.

3. **Anticholinergic agents.**

a. Anticholinergic agents act to reduce the parasympathetic tone of the airways.

b. They may be more effective than β-agonists for bronchodilation in stable COPD.[12]

c. These agents should be used early in the management of an acute COPD exacerbation.

d. Underdosage is common; these agents may be used in doses substantially higher than the usual dose, up to 8 to 12 MDI inhalations q4h.[16]

e. Ipratropium.

   (1) Ipratropium has been shown to improve gas exchange and symptoms.

   (2) Long-term use does not prevent the progression of underlying lung disease.[17]

   (3) Ipratropium is often used in combination with a β_2-agonist, resulting in more potent, synergistic bronchodilation than with either agent alone.[18]

f. Inhaled anticholinergics are poorly soluble in lipids and thus have few systemic side effects.[19]

g. Similar to β-agonists, inhaled anticholinergics may be used in either an MDI or a nebulized solution.

   (1) Recommended doses for MDI are 2 puffs (36 μg of ipratropium) approximately q6h.

   (2) In nebulized form, approximately 500 μg of ipratropium is given in each 2.5 mL of solution.

h. Anticholinergics are often used concurrently for convenience.

4. **Corticosteroids.**

a. Systemic corticosteroids, in either oral or intravenous formulations, are often used for acute exacerbations of COPD.

b. Earlier studies of systemic steroids were equivocal.

   c. More recent, randomized clinical trials show that during an acute exacerbation, steroids help to reduce the duration of the exacerbation and improve FEV_1.[7]

     (1) Benefit is shown from high-dose methylprednisolone (125 mg IV q6h for 72 hours), followed by a 2-week steroid taper; a more prolonged 6-week taper offers no benefit.[20]

     (2) Similar benefit is obtained from prednisone 30 mg/day PO for 2 weeks for patients with pH greater than 7.26.[21]

     (3) Although recent clinical trials appear to support the empirical use of systemic corticosteroids for acute exacerbations of COPD, the most effective dose and duration of therapy have not been established.

   d. High-dose steroids are associated with complications,[22] so it appears reasonable initially to follow the GOLD recommendation of giving 30 to 40 mg of prednisone for 10 to 14 days,[4] with the understanding that the course may have to be tailored to various clinical situations.

   e. It is important to avoid high-dose, prolonged steroid treatment whenever possible.

   f. Inhaled corticosteroids have no role in an acute COPD exacerbation, although they may be beneficial in outpatient management.

  5. Theophylline.

   a. ATS and ERS guidelines recommend that theophylline be given in severe COPD exacerbations if other immediate bronchodilators are ineffective.[1,8]

   b. BTS guidelines are more equivocal about the use of theophylline.[9]

   c. Theophylline can be used for maintenance therapy when other bronchodilators do not provide adequate relief.[1]

   d. Theophylline may have several beneficial effects.[18]

     (1) Causes bronchodilation.

     (2) Improvement in peripheral ventilation and mucociliary clearance.

     (3) Blunting of airway reactivity.

     (4) Decrease in mucus secretion.

     (5) Reduction in pulmonary vascular resistance.

     (6) Improvement of right-sided heart contractility.

     (7) Improvement of effectiveness of respiratory muscles.

   e. Patients may have clinical improvements that are not detected by changes in FEV_1 but that may be detected by measurements of lung volumes. Serum goals in this setting are 8 to 12 µg/mL of theophylline, but the correlation between serum levels and symptom relief may vary considerably among patients.

   f. A level of 20 µg/mL may optimize bronchodilation in severe COPD exacerbations but may place the patient at risk for significant side effects with its narrow therapeutic index.

   g. Doses should be adjusted for patients with congestive heart failure (CHF), hypoxia, or liver dysfunction because of alterations in drug clearance.

h. Drug-drug interactions must be monitored because many other agents interfere with the metabolism of theophylline.

i. Common toxicities of theophylline include (in order of increasing serum concentrations) anxiety, nervousness, and tremor; palpitations, tachycardia, and arrhythmias; gastrointestinal upset; dangerous arrhythmias; headaches; seizures; and death. If any toxicity is noted, levels should be checked and doses then reduced or held.

6. **Antibiotics.**

a. Bacterial colonization is difficult to distinguish from active infection in patients with COPD.

b. Limited evidence has shown that antibiotics are effective.

c. The ATS, BTS, and ERS have advocated antibiotic use for patients who have an exacerbation characterized by an increase in the volume or purulence of sputum.[1,8,9,23]

d. Benefit appears to be greater for more severe attacks.[8]

e. *Haemophilus influenzae, Moraxella catarrhalis,* and *Streptococcus pneumoniae* account for more than 70% of the bacteria isolated from the sputum of patients with COPD exacerbations.

f. Other bacteria include *Staphylococcus aureus, Pseudomonas aeruginosa,* chlamydiae, and Enterobacteriaceae.[24]

g. When choosing an antibiotic, the physician should consider spectrum of activity, tissue penetration, duration of therapy, frequency of administration, local resistance patterns, and mechanisms of excretion.

7. **Oxygen therapy.**

Proper tissue oxygenation is always the goal in COPD management. Oxygen (O_2) is essential for tissues and can relieve pulmonary vasoconstriction, which reduces right-sided heart strain and ischemia.

a. For long-term management, O_2 has been shown to decrease mortality.[25,26]

b. The management goal is a Pao_2 greater than 60 mm Hg, usually corresponding to an O_2 saturation of 90% to 93%.

c. O_2 delivery with nasal cannulae (NC) can be estimated as 20% + ($4 \times O_2$ flow [L]).

   (1) NC deliver up to a 44% fraction of inspired oxygen (Fio_2) with 6 L.

   (2) Venturi masks deliver a fixed Fio_2 of 24%, 28%, 31%, 35%, or 40%.

   (3) Simple face masks deliver an Fio_2 of 35% to 55% at 6 to 10 L.

   (4) Nonrebreather masks deliver approximately 60% to 90% Fio_2.

d. Most COPD exacerbations do not necessitate a large amount of oxygen supplementation.

e. If hypoxemia is not corrected by low-flow O_2, other causes of hypoxia should be considered, including pneumonia, pulmonary embolus, or shunting across a patent foramen ovale.

f. Close monitoring of oxygenation in patients with COPD and carbon dioxide (CO_2) retention is important in preventing hypercapnia, respiratory acidosis, and possible respiratory failure.[1]

    (1) Patients with a history of CO_2 retention should be treated with a known concentration of O_2 by Venturi mask to prevent respiratory depression.

    (2) ABG monitoring is indicated after changes in O_2 concentration until a stable Pao_2 greater than 60 mm Hg with a pH greater than 7.3 is achieved.

    (3) O_2 concentration delivered by an NC increases as the minute ventilation falls, potentially initiating a cycle of worsening ventilatory failure.

    (4) If a patient is at risk for respiratory acidosis, a Venturi mask, which provides a fixed Fio_2, is preferred.

    (5) If the patient remains acidemic, either noninvasive or mechanical ventilation must be considered.

8. **Mucolytic agents.**[1,7]

  a. Mucolytic agents have no proven benefit for management of COPD exacerbation.

  b. They are not currently recommended by ATS, BTS, or ERS guidelines.

  c. They may worsen bronchospasm in patients with AHR.

9. **Chest physical therapy.**[1,7]

  a. Chest physical therapy has not been shown to be effective in the treatment of COPD exacerbation.

  b. Resulting chest disruption may further increase bronchoconstriction.

  c. The role of postural drainage is unclear, but it may have some benefit for patients with lobar atelectasis and mucus plugging or with concomitant bronchiectasis.

10. **Noninvasive positive-pressure ventilation (NIPPV).**

  a. NIPPV provides ventilatory support without use of endotracheal airway.[27]

  b. Several delivery methods are available.

    (1) Volume ventilation.

    (2) Pressure-controlled ventilation.

    (3) Bilevel positive airway pressure ventilation (BiPAP).

    (4) Continuous positive airway pressure ventilation (CPAP).

  c. Four studies comparing the NIPPV delivery methods found no difference in gas exchange, need for intubation, adverse side effects, or mortality.[7]

  d. NIPPV requires the patient's cooperation. If a patient is anxious, uncooperative, or combative, successful NIPPV is unlikely.

  e. In alert patients with severe COPD exacerbations, use of noninvasive ventilation to improve hypercapnia is associated with lower rates of intubation and shorter hospitalizations.[28]

  f. Once started on NIPPV, the patient must be closely monitored for dyspnea, respiratory rate, oxygen saturation, respiratory secretions, hemodynamic instability, fatigue, mental status, and asynchrony with the ventilator.

  g. Monitoring of Pao_2, Pco_2, and pH is essential to determine whether the patient is improving.

h. Complications include gastric distention, eye irritation, and skin breakdown, especially at the bridge of the nose.

i. If the patient is unable to tolerate NIPPV or worsens clinically, endotracheal intubation is indicated.

j. NIPPV is contraindicated in the setting of cardiovascular instability, craniofacial injury, or inability to protect the airway.

11. **Mechanical ventilation (see Chapter 63).**

a. Patients with severe respiratory compromise may require intubation for ventilatory support.

b. Indications.
   (1) Respiratory muscle fatigue.
   (2) Worsening acidosis or hypoxemia.
   (3) Cardiovascular instability.
   (4) Worsening mental status.

c. Known complications.
   (1) Ventilator-associated pneumonia.
   (2) Pulmonary barotrauma.
   (3) Laryngotracheal damage.

B. STABLE SYMPTOMATIC CHRONIC OBSTRUCTIVE PULMONARY DISEASE

1. Once the acute COPD exacerbation has been resolved, the patient will need to be placed back on a stable regimen. The detailed management of stable COPD is beyond the scope of this chapter; a brief overview is presented below.

2. **"Step-up" approach.**

a. Management recommendations entail a "step-up" approach (Box 59-3).[1,8,9]

b. Smoking cessation is a major component.

c. Short-acting β_2-agonists are used initially on an as-needed basis.

d. Regular use of β_2-agonists and anticholinergics is instituted if better control is needed.

e. Theophylline may be added if tolerated by the patient.

f. Oral and inhaled steroids may also be added when exacerbations are frequent and severe.

g. Pulmonary rehabilitation and exercise training have demonstrated benefit.

h. Patients should be evaluated for home O_2 therapy.

3. **Pharmacological management.**

a. The mainstay of treatment for chronic COPD management continues to be inhaled bronchodilators.

b. Both β_2-agonists and anticholinergics are effective in improving pulmonary function and decreasing dyspnea. These agents have an additive benefit when used together.[19]

c. Long-acting β_2-agonists are also beneficial and may be more convenient for the patient with COPD.

BOX 59-3

STEP-UP PHARMACOLOGICAL THERAPY FOR COPD PATIENTS

MILD, VARIABLE SYMPTOMS

Selective β_2-agonist MDI aerosol, 1 or 2 puffs q2-6h prn; not to exceed 8-12 puffs/24 hr

MILD TO MODERATE CONTINUING SYMPTOMS

Ipratropium MDI aerosol, 2-6 puffs q6-8h; not to be used more frequently, *plus* selective β_2-agonist MDI aerosol, 1-4 puffs prn qid when needed or as regular supplement

Consider sustained-release (SR) β_2-agonist, 2 puffs bid

If response to the above is unsatisfactory or a mild to moderate increase in symptoms occurs, consider doing one or more of these:

    Adding SR theophylline 200-400 mg bid or 400-800 mg hs for nocturnal bronchospasm

    Using SR β_2-agonist 2 puffs bid if not done

SUBOPTIMAL CONTROL OF SYMPTOMS

Consider course of PO steroids (e.g., prednisone), up to 40 mg/day for 10-14 days
If improvement occurs, wean to low daily dose or alternate-day dose
Consider use of inhaled corticosteroid

SEVERE EXACERBATION

Increase β_2-agonist dose; consider nebulized solution.
Increase ipratropium dose; consider nebulized solution.
Add antibiotic if indicated.
Refer patient to the emergency department if not improving rapidly.

Modified from American Thoracic Society. Am J Respir Crit Care Med 1995; 152:S77.
MDI, Metered-dose inhaler.

d. Salmeterol is more effective than ipratropium in improving pulmonary function, and both agents are more effective than placebo in improving dyspnea.[15]

e. Use of inhaled corticosteroids continues to be controversial.
   (1) They may improve pulmonary function (FEV$_1$) in patients with COPD.[22]
   (2) They may have some benefit in airway reactivity, patient symptoms, and prevention of exacerbations.[29,30]
   (3) Side effects (e.g., decreased bone density, increased skin bruising) must be weighed against the benefits.[30]

f. Long-term use of oral steroids has no role in COPD.
   (1) They may be more harmful in the long term.
   (2) In most patients long-term oral steroid therapy can be tapered off without difficulty.

BOX 59-4

INDICATIONS FOR LONG-TERM OXYGEN THERAPY

ABSOLUTE INDICATIONS

Pao_2 ≤55 mm Hg *or*

Sao_2 ≤88%

PRESENCE OF COR PULMONALE

Pao_2 55-59 mm Hg *or* Sao_2 ≤89%

ECG evidence of "P" pulmonale

Hematocrit >55%

Congestive heart failure

ONLY IN SPECIFIC SITUATIONS

Pao_2 ≥60 mm Hg *or* Sao_2 ≥90%

With lung disease and other clinical needs (e.g., sleep apnea with nocturnal desaturation) not corrected by CPAP ventilation:

If patient meets criteria at rest, O_2 should also be prescribed during sleep and exercise

If patient is normoxemic at rest but desaturates during exercise or sleep (Pao_2 ≤55 mm Hg), O_2 should be prescribed; consider nasal CPAP or BiPAP ventilation

Modified from American Thoracic Society: Am J Respir Crit Care Med 1995; 152:S77.
BiPAP, Bilevel positive airway pressure; *CPAP*, continuous positive airway pressure; *ECG*, electrocardiogram; *Pao₂*, arterial oxygen partial pressure (tension); *Sao₂*, arterial oxygen saturation.

4. **Pulmonary rehabilitation.**
   a. Pulmonary rehabilitation involves education and exercise programs that help patients with COPD perform activities of daily living.
   b. It is an important aspect of outpatient management that should not be disregarded.
   c. Improvements in quality of life, well-being, and health status have been reported.
   d. Patients report improved exercise tolerance, reduced respiratory symptoms, increased independence, less anxiety, and increased feelings of hope and self-esteem.[1]

5. **Long-term O_2 therapy** (Box 59-4).
   a. O_2 therapy improves survival in patients with severe COPD and hypoxia.[25,26]
   b. Beneficial effects can result.
      (1) Reversal of secondary polycythemia.
      (2) Increase in body weight.
      (3) Improvement in right-sided heart function, neuropsychological functioning, and activities of daily living.

6. **Immunizations.**
   a. The ATS, ERS, and BTS recommend yearly influenza immunization.[1,8,9]

b. The ATS recommends pneumococcal vaccination.
   (1) Evidence supporting benefit is less convincing.[4]
   (2) Use seems reasonable because there are few adverse outcomes.

7. **Smoking cessation.**
a. Smoking cessation is the most effective preventive treatment for COPD.
b. It is the only treatment shown to alter the progression of COPD.[17]
c. Once a patient stops smoking, the rate of decline in lung function returns to the original rate.
d. Damage is not reversed.
e. The most effective strategy to date has been bupropion paired with use of nicotine replacement by transdermal patch, gum, inhaler, or nasal spray and smoking cessation counseling.[31]

8. **Lung volume reduction surgery.**
a. Lung volume reduction surgery has been offered as an intervention in advanced disease.[32-34]
b. Improvement in FEV_1 and lung mechanics is seen in most but not all surgical patients.
c. Some patients benefit greatly, but lung function appears to deteriorate more quickly in the 5 years after lung volume reduction despite initial improvement.
d. Surgical mortality is prohibitive.
e. Benefits of surgery are minimal for patients with an FEV_1 less than 20% of the predicted value and either a DLCO less than 20% of the predicted value or homogeneous emphysema seen on CT.
f. Questions about long-term mortality and duration of benefit remain.

9. **Lung transplantation.**
a. COPD is the leading cause of lung transplant referrals: 45.1% for single-lung transplant and 19.4% for double-lung transplant.[35-38]
b. Much debate surrounds the optimal time for referral, given the high variability in survival for patients with COPD.
c. Current indications.
   (1) FEV_1 less than 25% of predicted (without reversibility).
   (2) $Paco_2$ of 55 mm Hg or higher.
   (3) Elevated pulmonary artery pressure with progressive deterioration (e.g., cor pulmonale).
d. A referral should be given to patients who are willing and qualified, have an elevated $Paco_2$ and progressive deterioration, and are receiving long-term O_2 therapy because they have a poor prognosis.
e. Current statistics show that 1-, 3-, and 5-year survival rates after transplantation are 80.6%, 62.5%, and 41.8%, respectively.
f. With high variability of survival among patients with COPD, whether identifiable subgroups of patients with COPD are more likely to benefit from transplantation than other groups is still unclear.
g. Further research to identify the best surgical candidates is needed.

PEARLS AND PITFALLS

- Oxygen delivery and hypercarbia.
  - Oxygen administration in patients with COPD can cause an increase in P_{CO_2}.
  - The mechanism was previously thought to be a decreased respiratory drive when P_{O_2} was increased.
  - The Haldane effect is a possible contributor because oxygenated hemoglobin does not bind CO_2 as well.
  - Some suggest that a major contributor to the hypercarbia may be ventilation-perfusion mismatching with hyperoxia, leading to increased physiological dead space.[39] These changes result partly from the shallow, rapid breathing adopted when patients with COPD are in respiratory failure.
  - Review of four randomized trials on O_2 supplementation showed increases in P_{CO_2} with administration of O_2 concentrations as low as 24% and 28%. Most of the increases were not clinically significant. The patients most at risk were those with concurrent hypercarbia and hypoxemia.[7]
  - Titration of O_2 during a COPD exacerbation must be closely monitored.
- β-Blockers and COPD.
  - COPD is thought to be a relative contraindication to the use of β-blockers.
  - Because β-blockers offer significant reduction in mortality in certain conditions (e.g., coronary artery disease, CHF), their use in COPD should be further defined.
  - Studies of patients with asthma seem to indicate the safety of the selective β-blockers, especially metoprolol, atenolol, and esmolol. When AHR did occur, it seemed to be easily reversible with the use of inhaled β-agonists and ipratropium. Nonselective β-blockers, however, seemed to produce more bronchoconstriction, which was not as easily reversed.[40]
  - Although patients with COPD often have airway reactivity, the degree is not usually as great as in asthmatic patients.
  - Data suggest that patients with mild COPD not requiring frequent bronchodilators benefit from β-blockade after myocardial infarction.
  - β-Blockade in moderate to severe COPD does not confer the same mortality benefit, presumably because of bronchospasm.[41]
  - If β-blockers are to be administered, selective β_1-blocking agents should be used, started at the lowest possible dose and titrated under close medical supervision.
- β-Agonists and arrhythmias.
  - No large clinical studies have analyzed cardiac function and arrhythmia potential in patients taking β-agonists.
  - Previous small-scale studies have shown conflicting results with regard to arrhythmias induced by β-agonist bronchodilators. Many of these

studies either were not controlled or used only a one-time β-agonist dose. The studies also did not comment on patients' previous cardiovascular status.

- One study of patients with severe COPD (FEV_1 <1 L) showed no difference in either supraventricular tachycardia or ventricular ectopy in patients using placebo or salbutamol four times a day. However, asymptomatic arrhythmias were common in both groups.[42]
- Whether acute COPD exacerbation increases the potential for arrhythmia is unknown, but this seems likely. Therefore no good recommendation can be made with regard to the use of β-agonists in the setting of arrhythmias.
- If a β-agonist is needed and an arrhythmia is noted or suspected or the patient is at high risk, the patient should undergo cardiac monitoring.
- Hypoxia should be corrected because it may contribute to arrhythmias.
- Anticholinergic dosage should be maximized because these agents have less arrhythmogenic potential.

REFERENCES

[d] 1. American Thoracic Society. Standards for the diagnosis and care of patients with chronic obstructive pulmonary disease. Am J Respir Crit Care Med 1995; 152:S77.

[c] 2. Hurd S. The impact of COPD on lung health worldwide: epidemiology and incidence. Chest 2000; 117:1S.

[b] 3. Badgett RG et al. Can moderate chronic obstructive pulmonary disease be diagnosed by historical and physical findings alone? Am J Med 1993; 94(2):188.

[d] 4. Pauwels RA et al. Global strategy for the diagnosis, management, and prevention of chronic obstructive pulmonary disease. NHLBI/WHO Global Initiative for Chronic Obstructive Lung Disease (GOLD) Workshop Summary. Am J Respir Crit Care Med 2001; 163:1256.

[b] 5. Schunemann HJ et al. Pulmonary function is a long-term predictor of mortality in the general population: 29-year follow-up of the Buffalo Health Study. Chest 2000; 118(3):656.

[b] 6. Peto R et al. The relevance in adults of air-flow obstruction, but not of mucus hypersecretion, to mortality from chronic lung disease: results from 20 years of prospective observation. Am Rev Respir Dis 1983; 128(3):491.

[c] 7. Bach PB et al. Management of acute exacerbations of chronic obstructive pulmonary disease: a summary and appraisal of published evidence. Ann Intern Med 2001; 134:600.

[d] 8. Siafakas NM et al. Optimal assessment and management of chronic obstructive pulmonary disease (COPD). European Respiratory Society Task Force. Eur Respir J 1995; 8:1398.

[d] 9. British Thoracic Society Standards of Care Committee COPD Guideline Group. BTS guidelines for the management of chronic obstructive pulmonary disease. Thorax 1997; 52(suppl 5):1.

[b] 10. Summer WS et al. Aerosol bronchodilator delivery methods. Arch Intern Med 1989; 149:618.

[a] 11. Salzman GA et al. Aerosolized metaproterenol in the treatment of asthmatics with severe airflow obstruction: comparison of two delivery methods. Chest 1989; 95:1017.

[a] 12. Braun SR et al. A comparison of the effect of ipratropium and albuterol in the treatment of chronic obstructive airway disease. Arch Intern Med 1989; 149:544.

[b] 13. Turner MO et al. Bronchodilator delivery in acute airflow obstruction: a meta-analysis. Arch Intern Med 1997; 157:1736.

[a] 14. Morley TF et al. Comparison of β-adrenergic agents delivered by nebulizer vs. metered dose inhaler with Inspirease in hospitalized asthmatic patients. Chest 1988; 94:1205.

[a] 15. Mahler DA et al. Efficacy of salmeterol xinafoate in the treatment of COPD. Chest 1999; 115:957.

[b] 16. Gross NJ et al. Dose response to ipratropium as a nebulized solution in patients with chronic obstructive pulmonary disease. Am Rev Respir Dis 1989; 139:1188.

[b] 17. Anthonisen NR et al. Effect of smoking intervention and the use of an inhaled anticholinergic bronchodilator on the rate of decline of FEV_1. The Lung Health Study. JAMA 1994; 272:1497.

[c] 18. Gross NJ, Skorodin MS. Anticholinergic, antimuscarinic bronchodilators. Am Rev Respir Dis 1984; 129:856.

[c] 19. Zimet I. Pharmacologic therapy of obstructive airway disease. Clin Chest Med 1990; 11:461.

[c] 20. Niewoehner DE et al. Effect of systemic glucocorticoids on exacerbations of chronic obstructive pulmonary disease. N Engl J Med 1999; 340:1941.

[a] 21. Davies L, Angus RM, Calverley PMA. Oral corticosteroids in patients admitted to hospital with exacerbations of chronic obstructive pulmonary disease: a prospective randomized controlled trial. Lancet 1999; 354:456.

[b] 22. Van Grunsven PM et al. Long-term effects of inhaled corticosteroids in chronic obstructive pulmonary disease: a meta-analysis. Thorax 1999; 54:7.

[b] 23. Anthonisen NR et al. Antibiotic therapy in exacerbations of chronic obstructive pulmonary disease. Ann Intern Med 1987; 106:196.

[c] 24. Schelentag JJ, Tillotson GS. Antibiotic selection and dosing for the treatment of acute exacerbations of COPD. Chest 1997; 112:314S.

[b] 25. Medical Research Council Working Party. Long-term domiciliary oxygen therapy in chronic hypoxic cor pulmonale complicating chronic bronchitis and emphysema. Lancet 1981; 1:681.

[b] 26. Nocturnal Oxygen Therapy Trial Group. Continuous or nocturnal oxygen therapy in hypoxemic chronic obstructive lung disease. Ann Intern Med 1980; 93:391.

[c] 27. Hillberg RE, Johnson DC. Current concept: noninvasive ventilation. N Engl J Med 1997; 337:1746.

[c] 28. Brochard L et al. Noninvasive ventilation for acute exacerbations of chronic obstructive pulmonary disease. N Engl J Med 1995; 333:817.

[a] 29. Paggiaro PL et al. Multicenter randomised placebo-controlled trial of fluticasone propionate in patients with chronic obstructive pulmonary disease. Lancet 1998; 351:773.

[b] 30. Lung Health Study Research Group. Effect of inhaled triamcinolone on the decline in pulmonary function in chronic obstructive pulmonary disease. N Engl J Med 2000; 343:1902.

[a] 31. Jorenby DE et al. A controlled trial of sustained-release bupropion, a nicotine patch, or both for smoking cessation. N Engl J Med 1999; 340:685.

[b] 32. Gelb RF et al. Lung function 5 yr after lung volume reduction surgery for emphysema. Am J Respir Crit Care 2001; 163:1562.

[a] 33. National Emphysema Treatment Trial Research Group. Patients at high risk of death after lung volume reduction surgery. N Engl J Med 2001; 345:1075.

[c] 34. Fessler HE, Wise RA. Lung volume reduction surgery: is less really more? Am J Respir Crit Care Med 1999; 159:1031.

[c] 35. Housenpud JD et al. The Registry of the International Society for Heart and Lung Transplantation: sixteenth official report—1999. J Heart Lung Transplant 1999; 18:611.

[c] 36. Studer SM, Orens JB. Optimal timing of lung transplantation in end-stage lung disease. Clin Pulm Med 2000; 7(2):97.

[d] 37. Maurer JR et al. International guidelines for the selection of lung transplant candidates. J Heart Lung Transplant 1998; 17(7):703.

[b] 38. United Network for Organ Sharing (UNOS). 1998 SR & OPTN annual report. http://www.unos.org. Accessed February 2002.

[b] 39. Aubier M et al. Effects of the administration of O_2 on ventilation and blood gases in patients with chronic obstructive pulmonary disease during acute respiratory failure. Am Rev Respir Dis 1980; 122:747.

[c] 40. Tafreshi MJ, Wienacker AB. β-Adrenergic blocking agents in bronchospastic diseases: a therapeutic dilemma. Pharmacotherapy 1999; 19(8):974.

59

CHRONIC OBSTRUCTIVE PULMONARY DISEASE

[b] 41. Chen J et al. Effectiveness of beta-blocker therapy after acute myocardial infarction in elderly patients with chronic obstructive pulmonary disease or asthma. J Am Coll Cardiol 2001; 37(7):1950.

[a] 42. Hall IP, Woodhead MA, Johnston IDA. Effect of high-dose salbutamol on cardiac rhythm in severe chronic airflow obstruction: a controlled study. Respiration 1994; 61:214.

Adult Cystic Fibrosis

Christian A. Merlo, MD, and Michael P. Boyle, MD

60

I. EPIDEMIOLOGY

CF is the most common lethal autosomal recessive disorder in those of European descent, affecting 1 in every 3500 births.[1]

A. INCIDENCE AND CARRIER FREQUENCY

1. Incidence varies among other ethnic groups and is much lower in Asians and blacks, occurring in 1 in 10,000 and 1 in 15,300 live births, respectively.[2]
2. Frequency of early death has kept the total number of individuals with CF in the United States to approximately 30,000.
3. Carrier frequency varies with ethnic group as well.
   a. In whites, 1 in 25 is a carrier for defective CFTR, but such carriers are not clinically affected.
   b. Carrier frequency is also much lower in blacks, Asians, and Hispanics.
4. CF is caused by mutations in the CFTR gene located on the long arm of chromosome 7.
   a. Because CF is an autosomal recessive disease, an individual must have two CF mutations to develop CF.
   b. More than 1000 mutations have been identified since the gene was cloned in 1989.[3]
   c. The most common mutation in CFTR, accounting for more than 71% of alleles, is a three-base pair (bp) deletion resulting in the deletion of phenylalanine at position 508 (ΔF508).
   d. Frequency of mutations varies among populations.[4,5]

(1) Mutation W1282X has a higher prevalence in Ashkenazi Jews.

(2) Mutation S1255X is more prevalent in blacks.

B. AGE AND SURVIVAL

1. Full range of age is seen in CF, from newborns to late adulthood.

2. The severity of lung disease in CF results in a median survival of only 32.3 years.

3. Advances in antibiotics, airway clearance, and nutrition have contributed to an increase in survival.

a. Improvement in survival has resulted in a rapidly growing adult CF population.

b. Clearly, CF is no longer a disease primarily of children.

c. Survival of patients with CF has increased steadily during the past 50 years.

d. Median predicted survival for a child with CF in 1960 was less than 10 years.

e. By 2000, median survival had increased to more than 32 years.

f. Current estimates suggest that by 2005, there will be more than 10,000 individuals with CF over age 18 years, more than 40% of the total CF population.

g. The oldest current living individuals with CF are in their seventies.

II. CLINICAL PRESENTATION

A. CYSTIC FIBROSIS TRANSMEMBRANE CONDUCTANCE REGULATOR

1. CFTR protein acts as a cyclic adenosine monophosphate (cAMP)–regulated chloride channel in the apical membrane of epithelial cells.

2. Abnormalities in CFTR lead to disruption in ion transport in epithelium-lined organs (lungs, sinuses, pancreatic ducts, sweat glands, intestines, vas deferens).

3. Abnormal ion transport promotes excessive salt and water absorption and results in the plugging of ducts with thick, tenacious, and difficult-to-clear secretions.

4. Secretions in the lungs combined with chronic infection lead to lung scarring and progressive loss of lung function that is characteristic of CF.

B. AGE AT DIAGNOSIS AND PATIENT HISTORY

1. In the majority of patients with CF the disease is diagnosed early in childhood.

2. In 5% to 10% the diagnosis is made in adulthood.

3. When the diagnosis not made until adulthood, individuals are often labeled with a diagnosis of asthma, bronchiectasis, or chronic sinusitis.

4. A history of failure to thrive as a child, persistent respiratory infections, nasal polyposis, sinusitis, intestinal obstruction, malabsorption, recurrent pancreatitis, hepatobiliary disease, and male infertility is suggestive of CF.

BOX 60-1

COMMON CLINICAL CHARACTERISTICS OF CYSTIC FIBROSIS

Chronic sinusitis

Nasal polyposis

Chronic cough and sputum production

Colonization with *Staphylococcus aureus, Haemophilus influenzae, Pseudomonas aeruginosa,* or *Burkholderia cepacia*

Bronchiectasis

Hemoptysis

Airway obstruction

History of allergic bronchopulmonary aspergillosis

History of meconium ileus

Distal intestinal obstruction syndrome

Pancreatic insufficiency

Recurrent pancreatitis

Appendicitis

Cirrhosis

Vitamin A, D, E, and K deficiencies

Clubbing

Male infertility with obstructive azoospermia

---

5. Inquiry about a family history of CF is important, although many patients with CF do not have a family history of the disease.

C. PHYSICAL EXAMINATION

1. Chest examination may demonstrate increased anteroposterior (AP) diameter and upper lung field crackles, consistent with the chronic airway obstruction and upper lobe bronchiectasis seen with CF lung disease.

2. A loud P_2 may be a clue to secondary pulmonary hypertension.

3. Nasal examination may demonstrate generalized erythema and the presence of nasal polyps.

4. Digital clubbing is common, although its severity is not predictive of the extent of lung disease.

5. Hepatomegaly can be seen in patients with associated liver disease.

6. Diagnosis of CF is based on clinical characteristics (Box 60-1) and evidence of CFTR dysfunction by sweat chloride testing, CFTR genotyping, or direct measurement of ion transport by nasal potential difference.

III. DIAGNOSTICS

The diagnosis of CF requires *both* clinical and laboratory findings. An individual must demonstrate some of the clinical criteria and also have laboratory evidence of dysfunction of CFTR. This dysfunction can be demonstrated in one of three ways: pilocarpine sweat chloride test, genotyping, or nasal potential difference (NPD).

A. SWEAT CHLORIDE CONCENTRATION

1. Sweat chloride concentration is the best initial diagnostic test for CF when a patient has a suggestive clinical picture.
2. Sweat is collected from the skin after stimulation by pilocarpine iontophoresis, and the chloride concentration is determined.
3. Normal sweat chloride concentration is less than 40 mmol/L and for most individuals is approximately 20 mmol/L.
4. CF is suggested when the chloride concentration is greater than 60 mmol/L; most patients with CF have a sweat chloride concentration in excess of 80 mmol/L.
5. A very small percentage of patients with CF have normal or borderline sweat chloride values (40-60 mmol/L).

B. GENOTYPING

1. Genotyping is screening for the presence of two CFTR mutations known to cause CF when a patient has a suggestive clinical picture but a nondiagnostic sweat test.
2. Sensitivity depends on the number of mutations tested for and the patient's ethnic background.[4,6]
3. The most common test screens for approximately 80 of the 1000 mutations. These 80 mutations account for more than 90% of all CF cases.
4. Because most genotyping screens do not test for all mutations, patients with a convincing clinical picture but equivocal sweat test and genotyping results can be offered a direct measurement of their CFTR function with NPD.

C. NASAL POTENTIAL DIFFERENCE

1. NPD directly measures CFTR function by measuring ion transport in the epithelial cells, which line the interior of the nose.
2. Individuals without CF generally show a brisk response in chloride transport after stimulation of CFTR with low-chloride and isoproterenol solutions.
3. Patients with CF demonstrate little or no chloride transport.
4. NPD measurements are performed at only a limited number of specialized centers that have experience in the procedure's technical aspects.

D. RADIOGRAPHY AND COMPUTED TOMOGRAPHY

1. The most common radiographic finding of the chest is bronchiectasis.
2. Hyperinflation, bronchial dilation, and increased interstitial markings of the upper lobes are frequently seen on plain films.
3. A high percentage of patients with normal posteroanterior (PA) films have a distinctly outlined orifice to the right upper lobe bronchus, which helps to distinguish these patients from asthmatic patients.[7]
4. Nodules or branching opacities often represent plugging or mucoid impaction of the airways.
5. Advanced disease may lead to atelectasis, pneumothorax, or enlargement of the pulmonary arteries with cor pulmonale.

BOX 60-2

DIFFERENTIAL DIAGNOSIS OF BRONCHIECTASIS

Postinfectious (measles, mycoplasma, pertussis)

Allergic bronchopulmonary aspergillosis

Hyper–immunoglobulin E syndrome (Job's syndrome)

Common variable immunodeficiency

Immunoglobulin A deficiency

Rheumatoid arthritis

Sjögren's syndrome

Sarcoidosis

Cystic fibrosis

Young's syndrome

Kartagener's syndrome

Primary ciliary dyskinesia

6. Chest computed tomography (CT) often reveals pathological findings not readily apparent on chest films.
7. High-resolution CT is much better for detecting peribronchial thickening, mucoid impaction, and early bronchiectasis (Box 60-2).[8]

IV. MANAGEMENT

A. PULMONARY DISEASE

1. **Severity.**

a. Airway obstruction, impaired mucociliary clearance of secretions, bronchiectasis, and chronic infection are characteristic of CF and lead to progressive loss of lung function.

b. Patients demonstrate an average decline in FEV_1 of about 1.5% to 4% per year.

c. A wide spectrum of severity of lung disease is seen in CF.

   (1) Some patients demonstrate a rapid decline in lung function.

   (2) Other patients reach adulthood with near-normal lung function.

d. Therapy is directed at airway clearance, management of airflow obstruction, and treatment of infection.

2. **Chronic infection.**

a. Infection is present in the airways of most patients with CF.

b. The clinical course is marked by periods of stability interrupted by exacerbations, characterized by increased sputum production, dyspnea, fatigue, weight loss, and decline in FEV_1.

c. Exacerbations most often result from bacterial infections.

d. *Staphylococcus aureus* and *Haemophilus influenzae* are common pathogens in children.

e. Prevalence of *Pseudomonas aeruginosa* rises during childhood and adolescence so that 80% of CF patients are infected with *Pseudomonas* by age 18 years.

f. Aggressive treatment of infection is the recommended approach.

(1) In adults the typical antimicrobial regimen consists of tobramycin IV and antipseudomonal penicillin or cephalosporin.

(2) Antibiotics are tailored to the results of sputum culture.

g. Hospitalization is warranted for severe exacerbations and failure of outpatient therapy.

3. **Tobramycin.**

a. Even without frequent exacerbations, chronic infection leads to a progressive loss of lung function.

b. Inhaled tobramycin (TOBI) 300 mg bid every other month in nebulized form is recommended for long-term therapy.[9]

(1) TOBI slows the decline in FEV_1.

(2) It decreases sputum concentration of *Pseudomonas*.

(3) It decreases the frequency of hospitalizations.

c. Tobramycin is generally well tolerated and usually not associated with nephrotoxicity or ototoxicity.

d. It should be started on an alternate-month basis when the FEV_1 falls below 70% of predicted value, although the treatment strategy may be tailored to each individual.

4. **Airway clearance.**

a. Dornase-α, recombinant human deoxyribonuclease (DNase), helps to decrease the viscosity of expectorated sputum in CF.[10]

(1) Given at a dose of 2.5 mg nebulized each day, dornase-α improves FEV_1 in patients with mild to moderate lung disease in CF.

(2) Dornase-α should be offered to patients with daily cough, sputum production, and evidence of airflow obstruction.

b. Along with DNase, regular airway clearance is a cornerstone of CF therapy. Methods include the following.

(1) Chest percussion.

(2) Aerobic exercise.

(3) "Flutter" valves.

(4) External percussive vests.

c. Treatment of bronchospasm can also decrease airway obstruction.

(1) More than 50% of patients with CF have asthma symptoms.

(2) Asthmatic CF patients benefit from inhaled corticosteroids and bronchodilators.

5. **Lung transplantation.**

a. Bilateral lung transplantation remains an option for severe progressive pulmonary disease.

b. An FEV_1 less than 30% of predicted value, frequent hospitalizations, declining functional status, and pulmonary hypertension should prompt referral for transplant evaluation.

c. For patients with end-stage CF, transplantation is often the only therapy with potential for significant improvement in quality of life.

d. The procedure carries risks, and 5-year survival is slightly less than 50%.[11]

B. SINUS DISEASE
1. Dysfunction of nasal epithelial cells in CF leads to formation of thick mucus that occludes the nasal sinuses and predisposes to infection.
2. Sinus disease is almost universal in patients with CF, although not all patients have significant symptoms.
3. Sinus disease is characterized by chronic sinusitis and nasal polyposis.
4. Treatment consists of antimicrobial therapy and saline lavage for sinusitis.
5. Nasal steroids have been used for polyposis, but data on effectiveness are largely anecdotal.
6. Surgery is often necessary for patients with recurrent symptoms despite medical treatment.

C. GASTROINTESTINAL DISEASE
1. Pancreatic dysfunction.
   a. Approximately 90% of patients with CF have pancreatic exocrine dysfunction and require treatment with oral pancreatic enzymes.
   b. When untreated, patients have frequent bulky, foul-smelling stools and malabsorption of fat, protein, and the fat-soluble vitamins A, D, E, and K.
   c. Because adequate nutrition is crucial, patients are treated with pancreatic enzymes at a dose of 1000 to 2000 lipase units/kg/meal.
   d. Treatment includes high-fat, high-salt diets with fat-soluble vitamin supplementation.
2. Distal intestinal obstruction syndrome (DIOS).
   a. Pancreatic-insufficient patients are at risk for DIOS.
   b. Bowel obstruction is caused by thickened mucus and impacted fecal matter.
   c. DIOS is characterized by right lower quadrant pain, decreased appetite, constipation, and often a palpable mass.
   d. Plain films of the abdomen demonstrate air-fluid levels and large amounts of stool.
   e. Primary treatment is with oral GoLytely, although complete obstruction may require therapeutic meglumine diatrizoate (Gastrografin) enemas.
   f. Medications should be reviewed, and narcotics and other agents that slow gastric motility should be avoided.
   g. Surgery is rarely required.
3. Pancreatitis.
   a. The 10% of CF patients who do not have exocrine pancreatic insufficiency are at increased risk for pancreatitis.
   b. Recent studies demonstrate that any patient with chronic idiopathic pancreatitis is at increased risk for carriage of CFTR mutations.[12]
   c. Treatment is similar to that for non-CF pancreatitis.
4. Liver involvement.
   a. Almost all patients with CF have liver involvement.
   b. Clinically significant disease is not uniformly present.

60

ADULT CYSTIC FIBROSIS

c. Patients with chronically elevated liver function tests are treated with ursodeoxycholic acid to decrease biliary sludging.

d. More serious liver involvement is relatively infrequent but can result in focal biliary or multilobular cirrhosis.

e. Liver transplantation is an option for patients with progressive liver disease, cirrhosis, and portal hypertension.

D. ENDOCRINE DISEASE

More than 22% of adults with CF have abnormalities in glucose regulation. These abnormalities range from impaired glucose tolerance to CF-related diabetes (CFRD) with fasting hyperglycemia requiring intermittent or chronic insulin therapy.

1. CFRD.

a. CFRD is similar to insulin-dependent diabetes and is associated with pancreatic islet cell destruction and insulin deficiency.

b. CFRD is therefore best managed with insulin therapy.

c. The use of oral hypoglycemics in CF is still under investigation.

2. Osteoporosis and osteopenia.

a. Approximately 65% of CF patients over age 18 years have evidence of either osteoporosis or osteopenia by bone densitometry studies.

b. Etiology of bone loss is multifactorial; likely causes include calcium and vitamin D malabsorption, use of corticosteroids, and chronic infection.

c. Treatment includes calcium and vitamin D supplementation and weight-bearing exercise.

d. Bisphosphonates are often added to the treatment regimen in patients with significant osteoporosis.

E. INFERTILITY

1. Men with CF.

a. CFTR dysfunction causes congenital bilateral atresia of the vas deferens (CBAFD).

b. Among men with CF, 98% are infertile because of obstructive azoospermia.

c. These men produce normal spermatozoa.

d. Sperm-harvesting procedures with in vitro fertilization allow them to father children.[13]

2. Women with CF.

a. Women with CF are usually fertile.

b. They have only a slight reduction in their ability to conceive compared with non-CF women, which should be emphasized, particularly when women with CF are taking antibiotics that may decrease the efficacy of oral contraceptives.

c. Neonatal outcomes in pregnant CF patients are generally favorable.

d. Perinatal complications are more likely in mothers with CF and severe lung disease, diabetes, or poor nutritional status.[14]

PEARLS AND PITFALLS

- Correct dosage of antibiotics.
  - Patients with CF require higher than usual doses of aminoglycosides because of increased clearance.
  - One recommended approach to dosage of tobramycin is 5 mg/kg bid IV. Checking tobramycin peak and trough levels is imperative because volume of distribution and clearance may vary substantially among individuals.[15]
  - Bactericidal effects of tobramycin are based on peak serum concentration. A peak of 12 µg/mL and a trough of less than 2 µg/mL are accepted goal levels.
- Resistant and unusual organisms.
  - Multidrug-resistant *Pseudomonas* may infect patients with CF and advanced lung disease.
  - Resistant organisms can slow the patient's clinical response to antibiotic therapy.
  - Synergy studies are often used to identify combinations of antimicrobial agents that have added activity against specific pathogens, although effect on clinical outcomes requires further study.
  - Infections with *B. cepacia*, *S. maltophilia*, or nontuberculous mycobacteria may cause a patient with CF to fail to respond to antipseudomonal antibiotics.
  - Most of the above infections are not as responsive to aminoglycoside or cephalosporin therapy and may require treatment with trimethoprim-sulfamethoxazole, minocycline, or antituberculous medications.
  - An experienced microbiology laboratory is vital to the detection of these organisms.
  - *B. cepacia* is of particular concern in CF because it can be associated with rapid decline in pulmonary function and poor clinical outcome.[16] *Burkholderia* strains can also be easily passed between individuals with CF, causing local epidemics.[17] Hospitalized patients with *Burkholderia* should therefore be separated geographically from other hospitalized patients with CF.
- Allergic bronchopulmonary aspergillosis (ABPA).
  - Up to 15% of CF patients acquire ABPA.[18]
  - Classic diagnostic criteria in patients who do not have CF include asthma, eosinophilia, pulmonary infiltrates, central bronchiectasis, elevated serum IgE levels, positive skin prick test for *Aspergillus fumigatus*, and elevated serum specific IgE and IgG levels for *A. fumigatus*.
  - A new diagnosis of ABPA may be missed in patients with CF because many have coincident asthma, infiltrates, and bronchiectasis. The diagnosis is generally suggested when serum IgE level is greater than 500 IU/mL, *Aspergillus*-specific IgE or IgG is present, or the serum IgE level decreases by 50% with treatment.[19]

- Systemic corticosteroids remain the mainstay in therapy for ABPA in patients with CF.
- If no contraindications exist, itraconazole may be added in an effort to reduce fungal burden and lower prednisone doses.
- Pneumothorax.
  - Secondary spontaneous pneumothorax is a frequent complication of CF in patients with advanced lung disease.
  - Pneumothorax is usually manifested as dyspnea and sudden onset of pleuritic chest pain.
  - Because of previous pleural scarring, pneumothoraces may be loculated and difficult to assess on chest radiograph. CT scan may help in detection and treatment planning.
  - Tube thoracostomy remains the initial treatment of choice.
  - Pleurodesis for persistent pneumothorax may complicate subsequent lung transplantation and should not be performed without consultation with CF and lung transplant caregivers.
- Pulmonary hypertension.
  - Although mild to moderate pulmonary hypertension is common in patients with CF, severe pulmonary hypertension is relatively uncommon.[20]
  - History of progressive shortness of breath, increased jugular venous pressure, increased pulmonic component of the second heart sound, and peripheral edema suggests the diagnosis.
  - Sudden dramatic increase in the O_2 requirement without a change in the chest radiograph in a patient with end-stage CF lung disease should alert the clinician to the possibility of pulmonary hypertension with right-to-left shunt through a patent foramen ovale.

REFERENCES

[b] 1. Kosorok MR, Wei WH, Farrell PM. The incidence of cystic fibrosis. Stat Med 1996; 15:449.

[c] 2. Mickle JE, Cutting GR. Clinical implications of cystic fibrosis transmembrane conductance regulator mutations. Clin Chest Med 1998; 19:443.

[b] 3. Kerem B et al. Identification of the cystic fibrosis gene: genetic analysis. Science 1989; 245:1073.

[b] 4. Abeliovich D et al. Screening for five mutations detects 97% of cystic fibrosis (CF) chromosomes and predicts a carrier frequency of 1:29 in the Jewish Ashkenazi population. Am J Hum Genet 1992; 51:951.

[b] 5. Macek M Jr et al. Identification of common cystic fibrosis mutations in African-Americans with cystic fibrosis increases the detection rate to 75%. Am J Hum Genet 1997; 60:1122.

[b] 6. Macek M Jr et al. Sensitivity of the denaturing gradient gel electrophoresis technique in detection of known mutations and novel Asian mutations in the CFTR gene. Hum Mutat 1997; 9:136.

[b] 7. Grum CM, Lynch III JP. Chest radiographic findings in cystic fibrosis. Semin Respir Infect 1992; 7:193.

[b] 8. Demirkazik FB et al. High resolution CT in children with cystic fibrosis: correlation with pulmonary functions and radiographic scores. Eur J Radiol 2001; 37:54.

[a] 9. Ramsey BW et al. Intermittent administration of inhaled tobramycin in patients with cystic fibrosis. Cystic Fibrosis Inhaled Tobramycin Study Group. N Engl J Med 1999; 340:23.

[a] 10. Fuchs HJ et al. Effect of aerosolized recombinant human DNase on exacerbations of respiratory symptoms and on pulmonary function in patients with cystic fibrosis. The Pulmozyme Study Group. N Engl J Med 1994; 331:637.

[b] 11. 2000 annual report. Addison, Tex: International Registry for Heart and Lung Transplantation: 2000.

[b] 12. Cohn JA et al. Relation between mutations of the cystic fibrosis gene and idiopathic pancreatitis. N Engl J Med 1998; 339:653.

[d] 13. McCallum TJ et al. Fertility in men with cystic fibrosis: an update on current surgical practices and outcomes. Chest 2000; 118:1059.

[b] 14. Gilljam MM et al. Pregnancy in cystic fibrosis: fetal and maternal outcome. Chest 2000; 118:85.

[b] 15. Touw DJ. Clinical pharmacokinetics of antimicrobial drugs in cystic fibrosis. Pharm World Sci 1998; 20:149.

[b] 16. Ledson MJ et al. Outcome of *Burkholderia cepacia* colonisation in an adult cystic fibrosis centre. Thorax 2002; 57:142.

[b] 17. Isles A et al. *Pseudomonas cepacia* infection in cystic fibrosis: an emerging problem. J Pediatr 1984; 104:206.

[b] 18. Geller DE et al. Allergic bronchopulmonary aspergillosis in cystic fibrosis: reported prevalence, regional distribution, and patient characteristics. Epidemiologic Study of Cystic Fibrosis. Chest 1999; 116:639.

[a] 19. Nepomuceno IB, Esrig S, Moss RB. Allergic bronchopulmonary aspergillosis in cystic fibrosis: role of atopy and response to itraconazole. Chest 1999; 115:364.

[b] 20. Fraser KL et al. Pulmonary hypertension and cardiac function in adult cystic fibrosis: role of hypoxemia. Chest 1999; 115:1321.

60

ADULT CYSTIC FIBROSIS

Hemoptysis

Sarah B. Noonberg, MD, PhD, and Edward Haponik, MD

FAST FACTS

- Hemoptysis refers to the expectoration of blood or blood-tinged sputum.
- Pseudohemoptysis refers to the expectoration of blood arising from the nasal passages, oropharynx, sinuses, or gastrointestinal (GI) tract.
- Volume of blood expectorated does not correlate with severity of underlying cause of hemoptysis but is the strongest predictor of short-term mortality.
- Cause of death in massive hemoptysis is almost always asphyxiation rather than exsanguination.
- Initial management of massive hemoptysis should focus on ensuring adequate airway protection and oxygenation, protecting the nonbleeding lung, and monitoring hemodynamic status.
- Appropriate selection and timing of diagnostic tests are determined by the clinician's appraisal of risk factors and most likely cause of bleeding.

61

I. EPIDEMIOLOGY AND ETIOLOGY

A. OCCURRENCE AND MORTALITY

1. Hemoptysis is a relatively common and important clinical problem in both inpatient and outpatient settings.
2. Most cases are caused by minor mucosal erosions arising from respiratory infections, are self-limited, and have favorable outcomes.
3. In less than 5% of cases the hemoptysis is massive and carries a mortality risk of up to 80%.[1-3]
4. Massive or life-threatening hemoptysis has been variably defined as 100 to 1000 mL blood/24 hr, leading to large discrepancies in reported mortality rates.[4,5]

B. CAUSES

1. Recent studies indicate that the epidemiology and etiology of hemoptysis have changed greatly over the past 50 years.[6,7]
2. Literature up to the 1960s demonstrated that hemoptysis resulted from tuberculosis (TB), lung abscess, or bronchiectasis in 90% of patients.[8]
3. More recently, because of increases in antimicrobial use, smoking rates, and numbers of immunocompromised patients, conditions such as bronchogenic carcinoma, fungal infections, and chronic bronchitis have become the more frequent causes of hemoptysis.
4. Differences among studies in publication date, geography, patient demographics, TB prevalence, availability of diagnostic testing, and

inpatient/outpatient percentages all contribute to the wide variation in reported frequencies.

5. Impact of the human immunodeficiency virus (HIV) epidemic on the etiology of hemoptysis has not been well studied.

a. One report of HIV-positive patients described a 1.9% incidence of hemoptysis with primarily infectious causes.[9]

b. *Pneumocystis carinii* pneumonia and Kaposi's sarcoma have only rarely been reported to cause significant hemoptysis.

C. CRYPTOGENIC HEMOPTYSIS

1. In 10% to 30% of patients with hemoptysis the cause is not determined despite radiological and bronchoscopic evaluation.

2. Cases are challenging to both patient and physician.

3. The prognosis appears excellent; in one series of 67 patients with non-massive hemoptysis and normal bronchoscopy and chest computed tomography (CT) scans, 90% of cases resolved spontaneously without intervention.[10]

4. Seasonal variation in the incidence of hemoptysis may occur, with a peak incidence in late winter and a nadir in late summer,[10,11] which suggests a link to respiratory infections.

5. Cryptogenic causes are less common when bleeding is massive, estimated at up to 15% of cases.[1,12]

6. Prognosis has not been well studied in this subgroup of patients, although spontaneous resolution of bleeding and good prognosis in all patients have been reported.[12]

II. CLINICAL PRESENTATION AND PATHOPHYSIOLOGY

The clinical presentation of patients with hemoptysis depends largely on the rate, degree, and source of blood loss. Understanding of the blood supply to the lungs has important diagnostic and therapeutic implications.

A. ANATOMICAL CONSIDERATIONS

1. Lungs are served by a dual blood supply with anastomoses at several levels.

2. Pulmonary arteries arise from the right ventricle, branch into smaller vessels, and interact with only terminal bronchioles before branching into a capillary network that surrounds the alveoli for gas exchange.

3. The pulmonary vascular bed is extremely compliant and can normally accommodate the entire cardiac output with pressures of only 15 to 20/5 to 10 mm Hg.

4. The bronchial circulation has substantial anatomical variation.

a. It generally arises from the aorta or intercostal arteries.

b. It supplies nutrients to the tracheobronchial tree to the level of terminal bronchioles.

c. Intercostal arteries have extensive anastomoses and form both peribronchial and submucosal plexuses under systemic pressures.

5. Beyond the terminal bronchioles are anastomoses with the pulmonary capillaries.

6. Blood then feeds back to the left atrium, causing the physiological 5% right-to-left cardiac shunt.

B. CHRONIC PULMONARY DISEASE

1. Bronchial arteries become dilated, tortuous, and hypertrophied, with the following results.
   a. Increased pressures within bronchopulmonary anastomoses.
   b. Increased propensity for bleeding.
2. Although this high-pressure systemic circuit represents only a fraction of total pulmonary blood flow, it is the source of bleeding in most patients with hemoptysis.
3. Under conditions of chronic inflammation, collateral systemic vessels can be recruited from subclavian, axillary, intercostal, and phrenic arteries to the bronchopulmonary circulation.
4. One angiographic study demonstrated that up to 45% of cases of hemoptysis involved these nonbronchial systemic collaterals,[13] making arteriographic diagnosis and treatment challenging.

C. MASSIVE VERSUS NONMASSIVE HEMOPTYSIS

1. No standard definition of "massive" or "nonmassive" hemoptysis.
2. Some advocate that hemoptysis be classified by its clinical effect rather than by an arbitrary cutoff volume of blood expectorated.[14,15]
3. Patients often have difficulty quantifying blood loss, especially when blood is mixed with sputum or is swallowed.
4. In diffuse alveolar hemorrhage the amount of blood expectorated is often only a fraction of blood lost.
   a. Compliance of distal airspaces is high.
   b. Cough reflex is diminished.
5. Clots in central airways may pose a major threat in patients with notably less blood loss.
6. Evaluation of the degree of hemoptysis in the context of the patient's overall clinical status is important, especially when pulmonary reserve is limited.
7. A small bleed may herald a much larger, life-threatening bleed, a scenario that is extremely unpredictable.

D. APPROACH TO THE PATIENT

1. Despite the magnitude and frequency of hemoptysis as a clinical problem, no consensus exists on diagnostic or treatment algorithms.
2. Few prospective trials have been conducted to guide management in outpatient or inpatient settings.
3. Approaches vary substantially with institutional resources.
4. In life-threatening cases when cardiovascular or airway patency is at risk, initial goals are therapeutic rather than diagnostic (see "Management").
5. When bleeding has stopped or stabilized, with no evidence of cardiopulmonary compromise, a more elective diagnostic workup is appropriate (see "Diagnostics").

61

HEMOPTYSIS

III. DIAGNOSTICS

A. SOURCE OF BLEEDING

1. Bleeding can result from a variety of pulmonary, cardiovascular, hematological, infectious, and systemic disorders (Box 61-1).[1,3,8]
2. The first step in evaluating a stable patient with hemoptysis is to rule out an upper airway or GI source.
3. Several quick historical, clinical, and laboratory findings can assist in differentiating hemoptysis from hematemesis (vomiting of blood) (Table 61-1).[16]
4. Once a pulmonary source of bleeding is confirmed, a detailed history can often reveal clues to the possible etiology and contributing factors (Table 61-2).

B. PHYSICAL EXAMINATION

Although physical examination may provide clues to a possible diagnosis, it is notoriously unreliable for detecting the site of bleeding.[12]

1. **General appearance:** Well appearing versus chronically ill.
2. **Vital signs:** Tachypnea, tachycardia, orthostasis, hypoxia.
3. **Head and neck:** Presence or absence of oropharyngeal and nasopharyngeal sites of bleeding, lymphadenopathy, jugular venous distention.
4. **Chest:** Trauma, consolidation, wheezes, crackles, bruits.
5. **Cardiac:** Ventricular heaves, murmurs, opening snap, split or pronounced S_2 or S_3.
6. **Abdominal:** Stigmata of liver disease, splenomegaly.
7. **Extremities:** Clubbing, cyanosis, edema, splinter hemorrhages, telangiectasias.

C. LABORATORY STUDIES

1. Initial laboratory studies should help clarify the presence of the following.
   a. Infection: White blood cell count (WBC) with differential.
   b. Blood loss: Serial hematocrits.
   c. Coagulopathy: Platelet count, prothrombin time, partial thromboplastin time.
   d. Renal dysfunction: Electrolyte panel with blood urea nitrogen (BUN) and creatinine.
2. Arterial blood gas (ABG) analysis.
   a. ABG analysis is not mandatory for all patients.
   b. It should be considered for patients with tachypnea, altered mental status, or lower extremity swelling and those in whom hypoxia is suspected.
3. Sputum.
   a. If easily obtainable, samples should be sent for bacterial, fungal, and mycobacterial culture as well as cytological tests.
   b. Sputum induction or chest percussion may exacerbate bleeding and should be avoided during initial evaluation.
4. Urinalysis (UA) is useful in patients with suspected pulmonary-renal syndrome.

BOX 61-1

COMMON AND UNCOMMON CAUSES OF HEMOPTYSIS

PULMONARY

Bronchiectasis*
Bronchitis (acute or chronic)*
Cystic fibrosis*
Bullous emphysema
Lipoid pneumonia
Bronchiolitis obliterans with organizing pneumonia
Sarcoidosis
Hypersensitivity pneumonitis

INFECTIOUS

Necrotizing bacterial pneumonia*
Lung abscess
Fungal infections*
Parasitic infections
Tuberculosis*
Septic embolism
Pneumocystis carinii pneumonia

CARDIAC

Mitral stenosis*
Eisenmenger's syndrome
Congestive heart failure*
Severe pulmonary hypertension

HEMATOLOGICAL

Coagulopathy*
Thrombocytopenia*
Platelet dysfunction
Disseminated intravascular coagulation

IATROGENIC

Bronchoscopy*
Transbronchial or percutaneous biopsy*
Pulmonary artery rupture (Swan-Ganz catheter trauma)
Tracheostomy
Transtracheal aspiration

TRAUMA

Blunt or penetrating chest injury*
Fat embolism
Foreign body aspiration

cont'd

61

HEMOPTYSIS

BOX 61-1

COMMON AND UNCOMMON CAUSES OF HEMOPTYSIS—cont'd

NEOPLASTIC

Bronchogenic carcinoma*
Bronchial adenoma*
Angiosarcoma
Kaposi's sarcoma
Metastatic carcinoma or sarcoma

COLLAGEN-VASCULAR DISORDERS

Systemic lupus erythematosus*
Wegener's granulomatosis*
Microscopic polyarteritis
Goodpasture's syndrome*
Mixed connective tissue disorder
Idiopathic pulmonary hemosiderosis
Churg-Strauss syndrome
Nonspecific vasculitis

VASCULAR

Pulmonary arteriovenous malformation*
Pulmonary embolism with infarction*
Aortic aneurysm
Bronchovascular fistula

DRUGS AND TOXINS

Anticoagulants
Antiplatelet agents
Thrombolytics
D-Penicillamine
Solvents
Cocaine
Amiodarone
Phenytoin

OTHER

Amyloidosis
Broncholithiasis
Catamenial (pulmonary endometriosis)
Munchausen syndrome
Cryptogenic*

*More common cause of hemoptysis.

TABLE 61-1	
PATIENT HISTORY AND EXAMINATION CLUES DIFFERENTIATING HEMOPTYSIS FROM HEMATEMESIS	
Hemoptysis	**Hematemesis**
History of cardiac or pulmonary disease	History of gastrointestinal or liver disease
Chest pain	Abdominal pain
History of cough	History of nausea and vomiting
Blood frothy (air bubbles)	Blood not frothy (no air bubbles)
Blood liquid or clotted	Blood liquid or "coffee grounds"
Blood with alkaline pH	Blood with acidic pH
Sputum in blood	Food particles in blood
Presence of alveolar macrophages	Absence of parenchymal cells

Data from Camacho J, Prakash U. Mayo Clin Proc 1995; 70:83.

61

HEMOPTYSIS

5. Chest radiograph.
  a. Chest x-ray examination is mandatory for all patients with significant hemoptysis.
  b. Hemoptysis is frequently nonlateralizing.
  c. The radiograph may be misleading in the presence of prolonged bleeding and cough.
6. Purified protein derivative (PPD) and respiratory isolation for all patients with TB risk factors.

D. FURTHER EVALUATION

1. No standard algorithms have been established for the workup of patients whose bleeding site is still unknown after the initial assessment.
2. The pressure to make a diagnosis and possibly detect an early neoplasm must be weighed against the substantial cost of evaluation and low likelihood of serious illness in this patient population.[10]
3. The list of possible causes is extensive (Box 61-1) and can be pursued with a variety of laboratory and imaging studies, as well as more invasive testing.
4. The clinician's task is to use the initial history, physical examination, laboratory data, and chest radiograph to stratify patients with regard to their risk and to guide further evaluation (Fig. 61-1).

E. MALIGNANCY AND BRONCHOSCOPY

1. In most cases of cryptogenic hemoptysis, both patient and clinician are most concerned about underlying malignancy, but the risk is generally less than 5%.[7,8,17]
2. Age over 40 years, male gender, smoking history greater than 40 pack-years, and hemoptysis of more than 1 week's duration have predictive value in detecting a neoplasm by bronchoscopy.[7,8,17-20]
3. In the absence of these risk factors, likelihood of malignancy is extremely low and lends weight to a more conservative, watchful approach.

TABLE 61-2

IMPORTANT CLUES TO DIAGNOSIS IN PATIENTS WITH PULMONARY HEMOPTYSIS

Clue	Etiology and Contributing Factors
History of present illness	
Acute onset of cough and fever; ill contacts	Bacterial or viral bronchitis or pneumonia
Acute onset of chest pain	Trauma, embolism, aortic aneurysm
Fever, night sweats, weight loss	Bronchogenic carcinoma, TB, fungal infection, endocarditis, lung abscess
Shortness of breath	Any cardiac, pulmonary, infectious, or embolic source
Cyclical recurrence	Catamenial
Past medical history	
Pulmonary disorders	Bronchiectasis, cystic fibrosis, chronic bronchitis, bronchovascular fistula
TB	Reactivation, lung abscess, broncholithiasis, bronchogenic carcinoma, aspergilloma
Cardiac disorders	Congestive heart failure, mitral stenosis, congenital heart disease
Neoplasm	Metastatic disease, fungal disease
Medications	Amiodarone, nitrofurantoin, aspirin, nonsteroidal antiinflammatory drugs, anticoagulants
Family history	
Bleeding diathesis	Coagulopathy, pulmonary arteriovenous malformations, Osler-Weber-Rendu disease
Pulmonary disease	Cystic fibrosis
Thrombophilia	Systemic lupus erythematosus, pulmonary thromboembolism
Social history	
Smoking	Bronchitis, emphysema, neoplastic disease
Drug use	Cocaine-induced endocarditis, embolic disease
Exposures	Hypersensitivity reaction, neoplastic disease
Travel	Paragonimiasis, ascariasis, amebiasis, coccidioidomycosis, histoplasmosis, TB, pulmonary embolism
Illnesses associated with human immunodeficiency virus	Bacterial pneumonia, *Pneumocystis carinii* pneumonia, Kaposi's sarcoma, TB, thrombocytopenia
Review of systems	
Rash, arthralgias, hematuria	Collagen-vascular disorder, amyloidosis

TB, Tuberculosis.

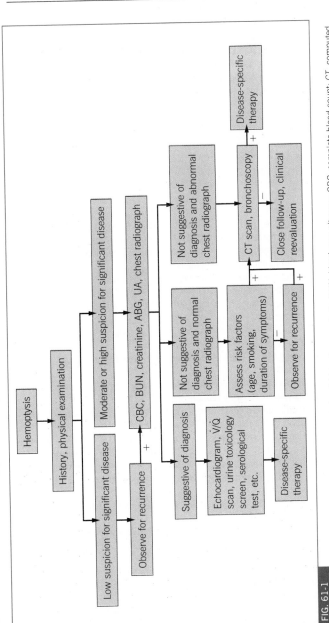

FIG. 61-1

Diagnostic algorithm for evaluation of hemoptysis. *ABG*, Arterial blood-gas analysis; *BUN*, blood urea nitrogen; *CBC*, complete blood count; *CT*, computed tomography; *UA*, urinalysis; *V/Q*, ventilation-perfusion.

61

HEMOPTYSIS

    4. Conversely, presence of one or more of these risk factors should prompt a more vigorous, urgent evaluation.

F. COMPUTED TOMOGRAPHY

1. Optimal role and timing of CT for patients with hemoptysis have evolved substantially over the past two decades.
2. Early retrospective studies demonstrated that CT could increase diagnostic yield but rarely altered management.
3. More recent studies have shown CT to be complementary to bronchoscopy.[8,21,22]

    a. The combination of bronchoscopy and CT led to a diagnosis in 93% of patients, whereas each study alone was diagnostic in only 42% and 67% of patients, respectively.[23]

    b. Higher diagnostic yield of CT in this study compared with older studies probably reflects increased use of higher resolution imaging techniques.

4. In only one small prospective study did CT imaging before bronchoscopy increase the diagnostic yield of detecting lung cancer by bronchoscopy and decrease the total number of invasive studies needed to establish a diagnosis.[24]
5. Despite the paucity of data, obtaining CT scans before bronchoscopy should be considered for all patients.

    a. If CT shows widespread metastatic disease, bronchiectasis, or another benign process, an invasive procedure may be avoided.

    b. If a peripherally located lesion is found, percutaneous biopsy would be a more appropriate initial invasive study.

    c. If bronchoscopy shows malignancy, staging CT scans would be needed regardless.

6. Multiple studies show that CT will identify a small proportion of tumors not detected by bronchoscopy.
7. Underlying medicolegal risks and the relative ease of access lend support to the use of the CT scan as an initial diagnostic modality for patients with risk factors and no abnormalities on initial evaluation.
8. The type of CT scan (high-resolution versus spiral CT versus conventional CT) should be chosen based on clinical suspicion of underlying disease (bronchiectasis versus pulmonary embolism versus lung abscess).
9. Dialog with the radiologist before the test can be helpful in increasing diagnostic yield.
10. If CT does not provide a diagnosis and risk factors are present, bronchoscopy is generally indicated.

G. OTHER STUDIES

1. Echocardiography, ventilation-perfusion imaging, and urine and serum toxicology may be useful but are cost effective only when pretest probability is sufficiently high.
2. Serological tests (e.g., ANA, ANCA, anti–glomerular basement antibodies) are expensive and should be ordered only if the diagnosis

of diffuse alveolar hemorrhage or a pulmonary renal syndrome is strongly considered.

3. Radionuclide imaging with technetium 99m/sulfur colloid or labeled red blood cells is rarely of benefit.[25]

IV. MANAGEMENT

The expectoration of large quantities of frank blood (>200 mL/day) can be terrifying for both patient and physician. Such an event is life threatening and should be treated as a medical emergency in an intensive care setting. Because the clinical course can be unpredictable, pulmonologists, anesthesiologists, interventional radiologists, and thoracic surgeons should be consulted early.

A. INITIAL MANAGEMENT

1. Objectives.
   a. Assessment of airway patency.
   b. Oxygenation.
   c. Ventilation.
   d. Hemodynamic status.
2. Early elective intubation is required for all patients in whom an adequate airway cannot be ensured, with use of an 8.0 or larger endotracheal tube to allow subsequent bronchoscopy.
3. If the bleeding lung is known, patient should be placed with that lung in a dependent position to avoid compromise of the nonbleeding lung.
4. Selective lung intubation versus double-lumen intubation.[1,3,26]
   a. These are technically challenging and potentially dangerous procedures.
   b. The decision should be deferred to an experienced intensivist.
5. Large-bore intravenous access is imperative.
6. Blood should be sent immediately for complete blood count (CBC), type and screen, and coagulation studies.
7. Any significant thrombocytopenia or coagulopathy should be corrected.

B. MASSIVE HEMOPTYSIS (Fig. 61-2)

1. No prospective clinical trials have defined an ideal management algorithm for massive hemoptysis.
2. Bronchoscopy should be performed first in almost all patients because it can be both diagnostic and therapeutic.
3. Adequate bleeding control is provided by topical thrombin or fibrinogen, iced saline, epinephrine injections, laser photocoagulation, balloon tamponade, cryotherapy, or electrocautery, as indicated by endobronchial findings.[27-29]
4. If these measures are unsuccessful, bronchial arteriography with embolization can usually result in cessation of bleeding, although rebleeding rates as high as 46% are seen in patients with bronchiectasis, cystic fibrosis, aspergilloma, and carcinoma.[15,26,30]
5. If bleeding continues despite these measures, surgical intervention may be warranted.

61

HEMOPTYSIS

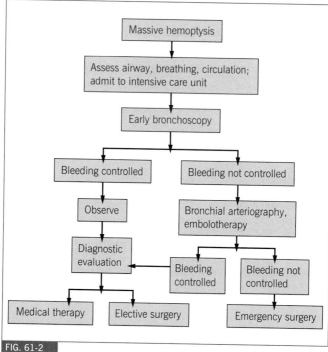

FIG. 61-2

Emergency management of hemoptysis.

6. Every effort should be made to stabilize the patient before surgery; data show that perioperative mortality is much higher when bleeding remains active.[14,31]

7. Initial surgical intervention was once advocated over medical (nonsurgical) therapy. Data supported this conclusion, but inoperable (and therefore sicker) patients biased these results in favor of the surgical group.[4,26,31]

8. No large prospective trial has compared surgical and medical therapy for patients who are surgical candidates.

9. Overall mortality in massive hemoptysis ranges from 7% to 80%.[1-4,26]

C. ADJUNCTIVE MEASURES

Although occasionally advocated, data to support adjunctive measures are limited.

1. Vasopressin IV.

a. Vasopressin constricts bronchial vessels.

b. Its use is advocated in the treatment of massive hemoptysis.

c. Contraindications include coronary artery disease and severe hypertension.

d. Vasopressin may lower the diagnostic and therapeutic value of subsequent bronchial arteriography and embolization.

2. Besides cardiopulmonary supportive care, judicious use of cough suppressants can help prevent rebleeding in patients with normal or nonlateralizing chest radiographs and scant hemoptysis.

3. With larger bleeds it is important that the patient maintain ability to cough blood from the airways to prevent an obstructing clot.

4. Use of a stool softener is recommended because straining can increase intrathoracic pressure and exacerbate bleeding.

D. DIFFUSE ALVEOLAR HEMORRHAGE

1. Patients with hemorrhage from pulmonary capillaritis syndromes may have rapid clinical deterioration despite only modest blood loss, necessitating rapid diagnosis and initiation of treatment.

2. Most patients require pulsed methylprednisolone followed by oral prednisone.

3. Second-line immunosuppressants include cyclophosphamide (Cytoxan) and azathioprine (Imuran), with limited data on their effectiveness.

4. Plasmapheresis has been used with success in Goodpasture's syndrome but has not proven effective in other diffuse hemorrhagic syndromes.

5. Prompt treatment is important in reducing the probability of progression to pulmonary fibrosis and in preventing irreversible renal damage.

6. Despite treatment, morbidity and mortality are still high, from both the disease and the complications of immunosuppressive therapy.

PEARLS AND PITFALLS

- Criteria for hospital admission.
  - No established guidelines define which patients with hemoptysis require admission.
  - It is reasonable to admit all patients with documented hemoptysis of frank blood of at least 50 to 100 mL for observation when the etiology is unknown.
  - Patients with coagulopathy, serious cardiopulmonary conditions, or hypoxia should also be strongly considered for admission.
  - For patients with blood-streaked sputum and evidence of pneumonia, the PORT study can be used to guide decisions.[32]
  - Public health concerns mandate that when TB is strongly suspected, patients should be placed in isolation until the sputum is analyzed.
  - Homeless patients and patients who are less likely to follow up on therapy should be given special consideration and an expedited evaluation.
- Allaying fears.
  - Even when hemoptysis is scant and probably the result of a bronchitic

infection, most patients need extra reassurance because of the known association of hemoptysis with TB and cancer.

- For patients who smoke, hemoptysis may represent a unique opportunity to intervene with cessation efforts.

REFERENCES

[c] 1. Cahill BC, Ingbar DH. Massive hemoptysis: assessment and management. Clin Chest Med 1994; 15:147.

[c] 2. Crocco JA et al. Massive hemoptysis. Arch Intern Med 1968; 121:495.

[c] 3. Thompson AB, Teschler H, Rennard SI. Pathogenesis, evaluation, and therapy for massive hemoptysis. Clin Chest Med 1992; 13:69.

[b] 4. Bobrowitz ID, Ramakrishna S, Shim YS. Comparison of medical vs. surgical treatment of major hemoptysis. Arch Intern Med 1983; 143:1343.

[b] 5. Corey R, Hla KM. Major and massive hemoptysis: reassessment of conservative therapy. Am J Med Sci 1987; 294:301.

[c] 6. Santiago S, Tobias J, Williams AJ. A reappraisal of the causes of hemoptysis. Arch Intern Med 1991; 151:2449.

[b] 7. Johnston H, Reisz G. Changing spectrum of hemoptysis: underlying causes in 148 patients undergoing diagnostic flexible fiberoptic bronchoscopy. Arch Intern Med 1989; 149:1666.

[c] 8. Ingbar DH. Causes and management of massive hemoptysis. www.utdol.com version 10.3. Accessed Jan. 29, 2003.

[c] 9. Nelson JE, Forman M. Hemoptysis in HIV-infected patients. Chest 1996; 110:737.

[b] 10. Adelman M et al. Cryptogenic hemoptysis: clinical features, bronchoscopic findings, and natural history in 67 patients. Ann Intern Med 1985; 102:829.

[b] 11. Boulay F et al. Seasonal variation in cryptogenic and noncryptogenic hemoptysis hospitalizations in France. Chest 2000; 118:1.

[b] 12. Pursel SE, Lindskog GE. Hemoptysis: a clinical evaluation of 105 patients examined consecutively on a thoracic surgical service. Am Rev Respir Dis 1961; 84:329.

[b] 13. Keller FS et al. Nonbronchial systemic collateral arteries: significance in percutaneous embolotherapy for hemoptysis. Radiology 1987; 164:687.

[c] 14. Garzon AA, Cerruti MM, Golding ME. Exsanguinating hemoptysis. J Thorac Cardiovasc Surg 1982; 84:829.

[b] 15. Mal H et al. Immediate and long-term results of bronchial artery embolization for life-threatening hemoptysis. Chest 1999; 115:996.

[c] 16. Camacho J, Prakash U. Resident's clinic: 46-year-old man with chronic hemoptysis. Mayo Clin Proc 1995; 70:83.

[d] 17. O'Neil KM, Lazarus AA. Hemoptysis: indications for bronchoscopy. Arch Intern Med 1991; 151:171.

[d] 18. Jackson CV, Savage PJ, Quinn DL. Role of fiberoptic bronchoscopy in patients with hemoptysis and a normal chest roentgenogram. Chest 1985; 87:142.

[a] 19. Gong H, Salvatierra C. Clinical efficacy of early and delayed fiberoptic bronchoscopy in patients with hemoptysis. Am Rev Respir Dis 1981; 124:221.

[b] 20. Weaver LJ, Solliday N, Cugell DW. Selection of patients with hemoptysis for fiberoptic bronchoscopy. Chest 1979; 76:7.

[b] 21. Haponik EF et al. Computed chest tomography in the evaluation of hemoptysis: impact on diagnosis and treatment. Chest 1987; 91:80.

[b] 22. McGuinness G et al. Hemoptysis: prospective high resolution CT/bronchoscopic correlation. Chest 1994; 105:1155.

[b] 23. Hirschberg B, Glazer BI, Kramer MR: Hemoptysis: etiology, evaluation and outcome in a tertiary referral hospital. Chest 1997; 112:440.

[b] 24. Laroche C et al. Role of computed tomographic scanning of the thorax prior to bronchoscopy in the investigation of lung cancer. Thorax 2000; 55:359.

[b] 25. Haponik EF et al. Radionuclide localization of massive pulmonary hemorrhage. Chest 1984; 86:208.

[c] 26. Dweik RA, Stoller JK. Flexible bronchoscopy in the 21st century: role of bronchoscopy in massive hemoptysis. Clin Chest Med 1999; 20:89.

[b] 27. Edmonstone WM et al. Life-threatening hemoptysis controlled by laser photocoagulation: short report. Thorax 1983; 38:788.

[b] 28. Saw EC et al. Flexible fiberoptic bronchoscopy and endobronchial tamponade in the management of massive hemoptysis. Chest 1976; 70:589.

[b] 29. Tsukamoto T, Sasaki H, Nakamura H. Treatment of hemoptysis patients by thrombin and fibrinogen-thrombin infusion therapy using a fiberoptic bronchoscope. Chest 1989; 96:473.

[b] 30. Remy J et al. Traitement, par embolisation, des hemoptysies graves ou repetees liees a une hypervascularisation systemique. Nouv Presse Med 1973; 2:231.

[c] 31. Conlan AA et al. Massive hemoptysis: review of 123 cases. J Thorac Cardiovasc Surg 1983; 85:120.

[b] 32. Fine MJ et al. A prediction rule to identify low-risk patients with community acquired pneumonia. N Engl J Med 1997; 336:243.

61

HEMOPTYSIS

Interstitial Lung Disease

Kerry Dunbar, MD, and Albert J. Polito, MD

Fast Facts

- The interstitial lung diseases are a group of lung disorders characterized pathologically by interstitial inflammation and fibrosis and physiologically by a restrictive pattern on pulmonary function tests (PFTs) and a gas transfer defect.
- The most common interstitial lung disease is idiopathic pulmonary fibrosis (IPF), which requires the presence of usual interstitial pneumonia (UIP) on biopsy.
- Distinct from UIP are the other interstitial lung diseases, including desquamative interstitial pneumonia (DIP), acute interstitial pneumonia (AIP), and nonspecific interstitial pneumonia (NSIP).
- Surgical lung biopsy is the diagnostic gold standard in determining the pathological subtype of idiopathic interstitial pneumonia.
- Response to treatment and prognosis are related to the pathological characteristics seen on biopsy.

62

I. EPIDEMIOLOGY

A. PREVALENCE AND INCIDENCE

1. The prevalence of IPF is estimated to be 3 to 20 cases/100,000 population.[1,2]
2. The incidence of IPF is reported as 10.7 cases/100,000 males and 7.4 cases/100,000 females.[2]
3. IPF is most common in adults 50 to 70 years of age.
4. Familial forms of IPF are transmitted in an autosomal dominant pattern.[3]

B. CAUSES

1. No clear environmental or infectious links have been found.
2. Cigarette smoking may increase the risk of IPF.
3. Odds ratio of 2.3 (95% confidence interval [CI] 1.3-3.8) has been reported for 21 to 40 pack-years of tobacco use.[4]
4. Investigation into medications, infectious agents, environmental dusts, and other causes continues, although none is definitively linked to development of IPF.

C. TYPES, AGE, AND GENDER

1. UIP is the most common of the idiopathic interstitial pneumonias.
2. In a lung biopsy series of 102 patients[5]:
   a. 62% had UIP.
   b. 8% had DIP.
   c. 14% had NSIP.
   d. 2% had AIP.

e. The remaining patients had other diagnoses after lung biopsy.
3. UIP affects middle-aged adults, with a mean age of onset of 57 years.
4. DIP also occurs in middle-aged patients, at a slightly younger mean age of 45 years.
5. AIP and NSIP both have mean age of onset of 49 years.
6. UIP and DIP occur predominantly in men, with a male/female ratio of 2:1.[6]
7. Gender distribution is equal in AIP.
8. NSIP more frequently affects females, with a male/female ratio of 1:1.4.[6]

II. CLINICAL PRESENTATION

A. IDIOPATHIC PULMONARY FIBROSIS
1. Also called cryptogenic fibrosing alveolitis, IPF is the most common interstitial lung disease and serves as the prototype.
2. In general, patients complain of progressive dyspnea on exertion and nonproductive cough and have dry, basilar crackles on examination.
3. Presentation varies somewhat depending on whether the patient has IPF or one of the other idiopathic interstitial pneumonias (see below).

B. PATHOPHYSIOLOGICAL FEATURES
1. Inflammation and fibrotic changes in the interstitium are characteristic.
2. PFTs show a restrictive pattern.
3. The gas transfer defect is characterized by a low carbon dioxide lung diffusing capacity (DLCO).

C. DIFFERENTIAL DIAGNOSIS
1. More than 150 agents and clinical situations can cause interstitial lung disease.
2. Most fall into several large groups (Box 62-1).
a. Occupational and environmental causes.
b. Connective tissue disease.
c. Drug toxicity.
d. Idiopathic disorders.

D. HISTORICAL STUDIES
1. Hamman and Rich provided the first pathological description of idiopathic interstitial lung disease in four patients in 1944.[7]
2. Subsequent years brought many more reports of what came to be termed IPF, but one of the most perplexing aspects of this literature was the wide range of responses to therapy.
a. Many patients progressed despite all interventions.
b. Some stabilized and even showed improvement and resolution.
3. To explain the differences in IPF disease progression, Liebow promoted a classification system for interstitial pneumonia based on pathology. His initial description of five categories in 1975 was revised to four major categories based on histopathological analysis of lung biopsy specimens.[8]

BOX 62-1
DIFFERENTIAL DIAGNOSIS OF INTERSTITIAL LUNG DISEASE

ENVIRONMENTAL AND OCCUPATIONAL

Organic dusts (e.g., farmer's lung, grain handler's lung)

Asbestosis

Silicosis

Pneumoconiosis of coal workers

Berylliosis

Hard metal pneumoconiosis

Talcosis

COLLAGEN-VASCULAR DISEASE AND VASCULITIS

Rheumatoid arthritis

Systemic lupus erythematosus

Scleroderma

Polymyositis and dermatomyositis

Sjögren's syndrome

Mixed connective tissue disease

Goodpasture's syndrome

Wegener's granulomatosis

Churg-Strauss syndrome

SYSTEMIC DISEASES (OTHER THAN COLLAGEN-VASCULAR DISEASE)

Histiocytosis X

Lymphangioleiomyomatosis

Tuberous sclerosis

Gaucher's disease

Amyloidosis

DRUGS AND THERAPIES

Radiation

Nitrofurantoin

Methotrexate

Gold

Penicillamine

Amiodarone

Bleomycin

Melphalan

Chlorambucil

Phenytoin

Heroin

IDIOPATHIC PULMONARY DISORDERS

Sarcoidosis

Bronchiolitis obliterans with organizing pneumonia

Chronic eosinophilic pneumonia

Idiopathic pulmonary fibrosis

E. IDIOPATHIC INTERSTITIAL PNEUMONIA

The four patterns seen on biopsy have implications for prognosis and response to treatment (Table 62-1). The most important lesson from this classification system is that the clinical term "idiopathic pulmonary fibrosis" (IPF) should be used only when there is a pathological diagnosis of *usual* interstitial pneumonia (UIP). All the other pathological conditions described below have a course that differs from that of the typical patient with IPF.[6]

1. Usual interstitial pneumonia.
   a. True diagnosis of IPF requires UIP on pathological examination.
   b. The hallmark of UIP is temporal heterogeneity of the biopsy specimen.
   c. On low-power view the involvement is patchy, with different degrees of disease seen.
      (1) Normal lung tissue is seen.
      (2) Interstitial inflammation and fibrotic changes.
      (3) End-stage honeycombing.
      (4) Fibroblast foci, or collections of proliferating fibroblasts thought to be the "leading edge" of fibrosis formation, are also prominent.
   d. Subpleural and basal areas are most involved early in the disease.

2. Desquamative interstitial pneumonia.
   a. More uniform appearance on a low-power view (temporally homogeneous).
   b. "Desquamative" is a misnomer in that the macrophages were originally thought to be desquamated pneumocytes.
   c. Biopsy specimens show the following.
      (1) Alveolar spaces contain increased numbers of macrophages with yellow-brown pigment.
      (2) Fibroblast foci are absent.
      (3) Little or no honeycomb change is present.
   d. Respiratory bronchiolitis interstitial lung disease (RBILD) is a subtype of DIP characterized by accumulation of macrophages in peribronchiolar airspaces.

3. Acute interstitial pneumonia.
   a. Patients originally described by Hamman and Rich had acute onset of symptoms; thus AIP is also called Hamman-Rich syndrome.
   b. Pathological examination shows the following.
      (1) Interstitial fibrosis with active fibroblast proliferation throughout the lung.
      (2) AIP resembles the diffuse alveolar damage seen with acute respiratory distress syndrome (ARDS).
   c. Changes are uniform across the biopsy specimen.

4. Nonspecific interstitial pneumonia.[9]
   a. Nonspecific interstitial pneumonia is characterized by a mixed picture.
      (1) Diffuse chronic inflammatory cell infiltrate is present in the alveolar septa, often with plasma cells and lymphocytes.
      (2) Infiltrate is mixed with areas of fibrosis.

TABLE 62-1
FEATURES OF IDIOPATHIC INTERSTITIAL PNEUMONIA

	UIP	DIP	AIP	NSIP
Male/female	2:1	2:1	1:1	1:1.4
Average age at onset	59	45	49	49
High-resolution computed tomography scan	Patchy bilateral reticular infiltrates; subpleural and basal predilection; traction bronchiectasis; honeycombing	Bilateral patchy ground-glass infiltrates in a mosaic pattern; basal predominance	Diffuse bilateral ground-glass infiltrates with or without consolidation	Bilateral patchy ground-glass infiltrates with interlobular interstitial thickening; rare honeycombing
Biopsy findings	Fibroblast foci; patchy inflammation; honeycomb changes; areas of normal lung; subpleural	Macrophages with yellow-brown pigment in alveolar spaces; no fibroblast foci; no honeycombing	Interstitial fibrosis; active fibroblast proliferation diffusely; resembles diffuse alveolar damage	Chronic inflammatory cell infiltrate in alveolar septa; rare areas of BOOP or fibroblast foci; normal lung may be seen
Temporal heterogeneity?	Yes	No	No	No
Mortality (%)	59-70	27.5	62	16
Mean survival time	2.8-5.6 years	12 years	1-2 months	13 years
Response to treatment	Poor	Good	Poor	Good

AIP, Acute interstitial pneumonia; *BOOP,* bronchiolitis obliterans with organizing pneumonia; *DIP,* desquamative interstitial pneumonia; *NSIP,* nonspecific interstitial pneumonia; *UIP,* usual interstitial pneumonia.

INTERSTITIAL LUNG DISEASE

62

(3) Rare fibroblast foci and rare areas of bronchiolitis obliterans organizing pneumonia (BOOP) may be present.

(4) Normal lung is often seen on the slide, but diseased areas are affected to the same degree.

b. The insult probably occurred at one point in time, so the damage is temporally uniform.

F. ONSET AND COURSE

1. Patients with UIP complain of slow but steady development of exertional dyspnea and dry cough over at least 6 months and more often over 1 year or more. Fatigue and weight loss may also occur.

2. DIP and NSIP also cause the indolent onset of dyspnea and cough.

3. AIP has an acute onset.

a. Dyspnea, cough, and fever progress rapidly, frequently culminating in respiratory failure.

b. A viral-like prodrome precedes the development of AIP in approximately 50% of patients.[6]

4. In patients with any of these diagnoses, it is important to rule out other causes of interstitial lung disease by questioning about occupational or environmental exposures, extrapulmonary symptoms, and medications.

G. PHYSICAL EXAMINATION

1. Basilar inspiratory crackles, described as "sounding like Velcro," are heard.

2. Clubbing is present in 25% to 50% of patients.[5,10]

3. Presence of rashes, joint pain, or arthritis suggests that connective tissue disease might be the cause of interstitial lung disease.

III. DIAGNOSTICS

A specific diagnosis of interstitial lung disease is made through composite assessment of the history, physical examination, PFTs, high-resolution computed tomography (HRCT), and lung biopsy.

A. LABORATORY STUDIES

1. Few laboratory studies are useful for the diagnosis of IPF, but laboratory tests may help rule out other causes of lung disease.

2. Up to 20% of patients with IPF have a positive rheumatoid factor or a low positive antinuclear antibody (ANA) titer (<1:160).[11] Higher titers suggest an autoimmune cause of interstitial lung disease.

3. The lactate dehydrogenase (LDH) level may be elevated, but this is a nonspecific finding seen in many pulmonary diseases.

B. PULMONARY FUNCTION TESTS[10]

1. In patients with any of pathological conditions listed earlier, PFTs show a restrictive pattern.

2. Vital capacity and total lung capacity are decreased.

3. DLCO is also reduced, often out of proportion to the degree of restriction.

4. In early disease, arterial oxygen levels may be normal at rest and may decline during exercise.

5. End-stage patients show resting hypoxemia.[10]

C. CHEST RADIOGRAPHY[12,13]

1. The chest radiography typically shows bilateral, interstitial, reticulonodular infiltrates, particularly in the lung bases and periphery.

2. The pattern of involvement may be asymmetrical.

3. Lung volumes may be reduced.[10]

4. Lymphadenopathy, pleural changes, and effusions are not found in IPF.

5. A normal chest radiograph does not exclude IPF.

6. Based on chest radiography, a "confident" diagnosis of IPF has 64% to 76% accuracy.[12]

D. HIGH-RESOLUTION COMPUTED TOMOGRAPHY

In the past decade, HRCT has become the best radiographic technique for evaluating interstitial lung disease. When trained observers made a confident diagnosis of IPF on HRCT, 80% to 90% of the time a subsequent biopsy indeed showed UIP.[12,13] Of all biopsies that showed UIP, however, in only two thirds was a confident diagnosis made from HRCT and clinical presentation. In the other one third, the diagnosis could have been missed without biopsy.[14] Each type of idiopathic interstitial pneumonia has particular features on HRCT suggesting the diagnosis.

1. **Usual interstitial pneumonia.**[10]

a. Reticular markings are found in the lung bases, typically in subpleural or peripheral regions.

b. Involvement is bilateral and patchy.

c. Traction bronchiectasis, honeycombing, and linear bands are present.

d. Much less often, ground-glass infiltrates are found.[10]

2. **Desquamative interstitial pneumonia.**[15]

a. Bilateral ground-glass infiltrates in mosaic pattern are seen, with infiltrates abutting normal areas of lung.

b. Lower lung zones are affected most.

c. Honeycombing is absent.

3. **Acute interstitial pneumonia.**[6]

a. Diffuse bilateral ground-glass infiltrates or consolidation or both are present throughout the lungs.

b. The appearance is similar to ARDS.

4. **Nonspecific interstitial pneumonia.**[9]

a. Patients have bilateral patchy, diffuse ground-glass infiltrates.

b. Intralobular interstitial thickening and rare honeycombing are seen.

E. LUNG BIOPSY

1. Lung biopsy is the most definitive way to diagnose idiopathic interstitial pneumonia.

2. It allows the identification of different pathological subtypes.

3. Lung biopsy can rule out other, more easily treated disorders (e.g., sarcoidosis).

62

INTERSTITIAL LUNG DISEASE

4. Knowing the pathological type on biopsy helps to generate a prognosis and predict the patient's response to treatment.
5. Unfortunately, transbronchial biopsies obtained by fiberoptic bronchoscopy are too small to permit identification of the diseases discussed here.[16]
6. Video-assisted thoracoscopic surgery and open lung biopsy provide larger pieces of tissue and are the standard biopsy techniques for interstitial lung disease.

IV. MANAGEMENT

Optimal therapy for IPF has been difficult to determine for several reasons. Historically, biopsies were not routinely performed, and studies on patients with "IPF" probably included diseases other than UIP. Because the various diseases demonstrate different responses to therapy, with NSIP and DIP responding better than UIP and AIP, the quoted response rates for patients with "IPF" from older studies must be questioned. There are very few randomized, placebo-controlled trials of treatment, even in the newer literature.

A. THERAPEUTIC RESPONSE AND PROGNOSIS

1. Mortality and survival.
   a. Mortality rate is 59% to 70% in patients with UIP, with mean survival of 2.8 to 5.6 years.[5,17]
   b. Mortality rate is 27.5% in DIP, with average survival of 12 years.[17]
   c. Average mortality is 62% in AIP, with mean survival of 1 to 2 months.[6]
   d. Average mortality is 16% in NSIP[9]; mean survival was 13 years in one study.[5]
2. DIP is more responsive to steroid therapy than is UIP.[17]
3. AIP is rapidly progressive.[6]
4. NSIP has a better prognosis because of good response to therapy.[9]
5. Of patients with IPF, 40% die of respiratory failure.
6. Other causes of death include infection, bronchogenic carcinoma, pulmonary emboli, heart failure, and coronary artery disease.[18]

B. CORTICOSTEROIDS AND IMMUNOSUPRESSANTS[10]

The American Thoracic Society and European Respiratory Society (ATS/ERS) issued an international consensus statement on IPF in 2000 recommending a combination of corticosteroids and other immunosuppressants as first-line therapy for IPF.[10]

1. The patients is given prednisone 0.5 mg/kg/day with azathioprine 2 to 3 mg/kg/day or cyclophosphamide 2 mg/kg/day.
2. Therapy is continued for 3 to 6 months and is then adjusted or discontinued if the patient has not responded.
3. Changes in dyspnea, PFTs, and HRCT are used to gauge response.
4. Therapy continues if the patient's symptoms and objective tests are stable or improved.
5. ATS/ERS recommendations are based more on theoretical benefits of individual drugs than on true evidence-based medicine.

6. Corticosteroids are traditionally used in treatment of IPF to reduce inflammation and development of fibrosis.

7. Historical studies, with significant limitations noted earlier, suggest that 10% to 30% of patients treated with steroids improve.[10,19]

8. Few controlled trials of corticosteroid therapy in IPF are available, and several studies showed little or no improvement in patients treated with steroids.[20]

9. Azathioprine used with corticosteroids may be steroid sparing and may improve survival, but these data come from only one small trial.[21]

10. Cyclophosphamide has been used with corticosteroids as a steroid-sparing agent and may improve survival, although results of studies are mixed.[22,23]

C. OTHER MEDICATIONS

1. When the antifibrotic agents colchicine and d-penicillamine were used in combination with steroids, neither showed any benefit over steroids alone.[24,25]

2. A pilot study of patients treated with interferon-γ1b combined with low-dose prednisolone demonstrated improved total lung capacity and arterial oxygenation at rest and with exertion compared with patients receiving prednisolone alone.[26]

3. Results from a large, multicenter, randomized placebo-controlled trial of interferon-γ1b in patients with IPF, started in late 2000, are anticipated.

4. Other cytotoxic agents, including cyclosporine and methotrexate, have not shown benefit.

5. Antioxidants such as glutathione and N-acetylcysteine are also being studied.[10]

D. LUNG TRANSPLANTATION

1. Single-lung transplantation for IPF and UIP is another treatment option.

2. Definitive criteria for the timing of transplant referral are still lacking.

3. Oxygen dependence, clinical deterioration, and functional limitation should prompt transplant evaluation.

4. Because patients with IPF have the highest mortality of all patients on the waiting list for lung transplant, evaluation should begin early.[27]

PEARLS AND PITFALLS

- If all the clinical data support a diagnosis of IPF, a surgical lung biopsy may not be necessary. However, if data are atypical for IPF (e.g., lack of subpleural distribution of infiltrates on HRCT, lack of honeycombing, development of symptoms over <6 months), early surgical lung biopsy is crucial to differentiate between UIP and the other interstitial lung diseases.

- The most useful objective way to track response to treatment in patients with IPF is pulmonary function testing. In particular, the DLCO is often the most sensitive indicator of a change in the patient's pulmonary status.

62

INTERSTITIAL LUNG DISEASE

- Adverse effects of treatment for IPF are a major cause of morbidity and should be monitored, with appropriate prophylaxis instituted, as follows.
  - Administer *Pneumocystis carinii* prophylaxis for all patients treated with steroids.
  - Obtain a baseline dual energy x-ray absorptiometry scan for all patients treated with steroids to evaluate for osteoporosis, and institute treatment if it is present.
  - Monitor fasting blood glucose levels to evaluate for steroid-induced diabetes mellitus.
  - Check the complete blood count and liver function tests every 2 to 4 weeks in patients treated with cyclophosphamide or azathioprine.
  - Monitor the urinalysis every 2 to 4 weeks in patients treated with cyclophosphamide to evaluate for hemorrhagic cystitis.
- Patients with IPF have an increased risk of lung cancer. What appears to be dense fibrosis on chest radiograph may actually be a mass.

REFERENCES

[b] 1. Iwai K et al. Idiopathic pulmonary fibrosis: epidemiologic approaches to occupational exposure. Am J Respir Crit Care Med 1994; 150:670.

[b] 2. Coultas DB et al. The epidemiology of interstitial lung diseases. Am J Respir Crit Care Med 1994; 150:967.

[b] 3. Bitterman PB et al. Familial idiopathic pulmonary fibrosis: evidence of lung inflammation in unaffected family members. N Engl J Med 1986; 314:1343.

[b] 4. Baumgartner KB et al. Cigarette smoking: a risk factor for idiopathic pulmonary fibrosis. Am J Respir Crit Care Med 1997; 155:242.

[b] 5. Bjoraker JA et al. Prognostic significance of histopathologic subsets in idiopathic pulmonary fibrosis. Am J Respir Crit Care Med 1998; 157:199.

[c] 6. Katzenstein AL, Myers JL. Idiopathic pulmonary fibrosis: clinical relevance of pathologic classification. Am J Respir Crit Care Med 1998; 157:1301.

[c] 7. Hamman L, Rich A. Acute diffuse interstitial fibrosis of the lungs. Bull Johns Hopkins Hosp 1944; 74:177.

[c] 8. Liebow AA. Definition and classification of interstitial pneumonias in human pathology. Prog Respir Res 1975; 8:1.

[c] 9. Katzenstein AL, Myers JL. Nonspecific interstitial pneumonia and the other idiopathic interstitial pneumonias: classification and diagnostic criteria. Am J Surg Pathol 2000; 24:1.

[d] 10. American Thoracic Society. Idiopathic pulmonary fibrosis: diagnosis and treatment: international consensus statement. American Thoracic Society (ATS) and European Respiratory Society (ERS). Am J Respir Crit Care Med 2000; 161:646.

[b] 11. Chapman JR et al. Definition and clinical relevance of antibodies to nuclear ribonucleoprotein and other nuclear antigens in patients with cryptogenic fibrosing alveolitis. Am Rev Respir Dis 1984; 130:439.

[b] 12. Grenier P et al. Chronic diffuse interstitial lung disease: diagnostic value of chest radiography and high-resolution CT. Radiology 1991; 179:123.

[b] 13. Wells AU et al. The predictive value of appearances on thin-section computed tomography in fibrosing alveolitis. Am Rev Respir Dis 1993; 148:1076.

[b] 14. Raghu G et al. The accuracy of the clinical diagnosis of new-onset idiopathic pulmonary fibrosis and other interstitial lung disease: a prospective study. Chest 1999; 116:1168.

[b] 15. Hartman TE et al. Desquamative interstitial pneumonia: thin-section CT findings in 22 patients. Radiology 1993; 187:787.

[c] 16. Raghu G. Interstitial lung disease: a diagnostic approach. Are CT scan and lung biopsy indicated in every patient? Am J Respir Crit Care Med 1995; 151:909.

[b] 17. Carrington CB et al. Natural history and treated course of usual and desquamative interstitial pneumonia. N Engl J Med 1978; 298:801.

[c] 18. Panos RJ et al. Clinical deterioration in patients with idiopathic pulmonary fibrosis: causes and assessment. Am J Med 1990; 88:396.

[b] 19. Flaherty KR et al. Steroids in idiopathic pulmonary fibrosis: a prospective assessment of adverse reactions, response to therapy, and survival. Am J Med 2001; 110:278.

[c] 20. Mapel DW, Samet JM, Coultas DB. Corticosteroids and the treatment of idiopathic pulmonary fibrosis: past, present, and future. Chest 1996; 110:1058.

[a] 21. Raghu G et al. Azathioprine combined with prednisone in the treatment of idiopathic pulmonary fibrosis: a prospective double-blind, randomized, placebo-controlled clinical trial. Am Rev Respir Dis 1991; 144:291.

[a] 22. Johnson MA et al. Randomised controlled trial comparing prednisolone alone with cyclophosphamide and low dose prednisolone in combination in cryptogenic fibrosing alveolitis. Thorax 1989; 44:280.

[b] 23. Zisman DA et al. Cyclophosphamide in the treatment of idiopathic pulmonary fibrosis: a prospective study in patients who failed to respond to corticosteroids. Chest 2000; 117:1619.

[a] 24. Douglas WW et al. Colchicine versus prednisone in the treatment of idiopathic pulmonary fibrosis. A randomized prospective study. Members of the Lung Study Group. Am J Respir Crit Care Med 1998; 158:220.

[a] 25. Selman M et al. Colchicine, D-penicillamine, and prednisone in the treatment of idiopathic pulmonary fibrosis: a controlled clinical trial. Chest 1998; 114:507.

[a] 26. Ziesche R et al. A preliminary study of long-term treatment with interferon gamma-1b and low-dose prednisolone in patients with idiopathic pulmonary fibrosis. N Engl J Med 1999; 341:1264.

[b] 27. Hosenpud JD et al. Effect of diagnosis on survival benefit of lung transplantation for end-stage lung disease. Lancet 1998; 351:24.

Mechanical Ventilation

David N. Hager, MD, Michael J. McWilliams, MD, and Landon S. King, MD

63

I. EPIDEMIOLOGY

The need for intubation and ventilator management is one of the most common reasons for admission to the intensive care unit (ICU).

A. REASONS FOR INTUBATION[2]

1. **Acute respiratory failure.**
a. Acute respiratory failure may result from sepsis, adult respiratory distress syndrome (ARDS), cardiogenic pulmonary edema, pneumonia, trauma, burns, and surgical complications.
b. It accounts for 66% of intubations.
2. **Coma:** 15%.
3. **Chronic obstructive pulmonary disease (COPD):** 13%.
4. **Neuromuscular weakness:** 5%.

B. GOALS OF MECHANICAL VENTILATION

1. Reduce the work of breathing.
2. Improve oxygenation.
3. Correct acute progressive respiratory acidosis.

II. CLINICAL PRESENTATION

The decision to initiate mechanical ventilation is often difficult and lacks clearly defined parameters.

A. POSSIBLE INDICATIONS FOR VENTILATOR SUPPORT

1. Indications for ventilator support include the following.
   a. Use of accessory muscles of breathing.
   b. Inability to speak in full sentences.
   c. RR >30 breaths/min.
2. ABG analysis may be helpful in the assessment.

B. PATIENT CATEGORIES

Most patients requiring mechanical ventilation fall into one of three categories.

1. Failure of ventilation.
   a. Elevated partial pressure of carbon dioxide (P_{CO_2}).
   b. Severe airway obstruction: asthma, COPD, mass, vocal cord paralysis, laryngeal edema.
   c. Muscle failure: muscle weakness, paralysis, exhaustion, or absent central nervous system (CNS) signal.
2. Ineffective gas exchange despite supplemental oxygen (O_2).
   a. Injury of blood-gas interface: ARDS, pneumonia, sepsis.
   b. Congested blood-gas interface: cardiogenic pulmonary edema.
3. Inability to protect airway: mental state changes, fear of aspiration.

III. MANAGEMENT

A. SEDATION

1. Both intubation and mechanical ventilation are unpleasant and typically associated with agitation and anxiety.
2. Most mechanically ventilated patients require some sedation and analgesia.
3. Many ICUs have standardized sedation protocols for this purpose; two strategies follow.
   a. Narcotic-benzodiazepine combination.
      (1) Better analgesia, anxiolysis, and sedation.
      (2) See Table 63-1.
   b. Sedative-free interval.[3]
      (1) Minimizes duration of intubation and morbidities associated with sedation.
      (2) Used daily, even when extubation is not part of immediate plan.
      (3) Decreases duration of ICU admission and helps avoid oversedation.

B. PARALYSIS

1. Most mechanically ventilated patients are managed adequately without paralytic agents (Table 63-2).[4-8] These patients require paralytics only during ETT placement.
2. Patients requiring continuous paralysis.
   a. These patients are monitored with an electrical stimulating device placed

TABLE 63-1
SEDATIVE DRUGS

Sedative	Recommended Dose	Action	Adverse Effects
Benzodiazepine (midazolam, lorazepam; these short-acting agents are preferred)	Midazolam: bolus (5 mg) before intubation, then 1-2 mg/hr continuous infusion Lorazepam: 1-2 mg/hr continuous infusion	Anxiolytic; amnestic; sedation; acts as antiepileptic; treatment for alcohol withdrawal	Numerous drug interactions; no analgesic properties; prolonged use can lead to withdrawal on discontinuation
Narcotic (morphine, fentanyl)	Morphine: 1-2 mg/hr continuous infusion Fentanyl: 25-50 µg/hr continuous infusion	Pain relief; sedation	Respiratory depressant; can cause hypotension (fentanyl less than morphine); depressed gastrointestinal motility
Propofol	5-50 µg/kg/min continuous infusion	Sedative with extremely rapid onset of action and patient recovery on discontinuation	Should not be used for longer than 48 hours; hypertriglyceridemia; pancreatitis; high caloric load that may contribute to elevated CO_2; increased incidence of infection; hypotension most common adverse effect; expensive
Haloperidol	2.5-20 mg IV push as needed	Antipsychotic with sedative properties; especially effective in delirious patients; no cardiac or respiratory depression	Prolongs QT interval; rarely, causes neuroleptic malignant syndrome; no analgesia

MECHANICAL VENTILATION

63

TABLE 63-2

NEUROMUSCULAR BLOCKING AGENTS (PARALYTICS)

Drug	Dose	Onset and Duration	Uses	Adverse Effects
Succinylcholine	1-1.5 mg/kg	Onset in 30 seconds; lasts only 10 minutes	Intubation	Increases serum potassium level; prolonged paralysis possible; hypertension; arrhythmias; elevated ICP; malignant hyperthermia
Nondepolarizing blockers (vecuronium, atracurium, pancuronium)	Vecuronium: 0.1 mg/kg Atracurium: 0.4-0.5 mg/kg Pancuronium: 0.1 mg/kg	Onset not as rapid as succinylcholine, but effects longer lasting: 45-90 minutes	Intubation; maintaining neuromuscular blockade for ventilatory support; atracurium is tolerated by patients with liver or renal failure; vecuronium has the fewest adverse cardiac effects	Pancuronium: vagolytic; increases HR and BP Atracurium: can cause increased histamine release; contraindicated in asthmatic patients and those in anaphylactic shock

BP, Blood pressure; *HR,* heart rate; *ICP,* intracranial pressure.

over the ulnar or orbicularis oculi nerve, set to deliver a "train of four" stimulus.

b. The goal is to allow the least possible neuromuscular blockade while retaining the beneficial effects of paralysis in patients undergoing mechanical ventilation.

c. Heavy sedation and analgesia are required with paralysis.

d. Thromboembolism prophylaxis is also required.

C. INTUBATION

1. ETT placement is one of the most complication-ridden aspects of mechanical ventilation.

2. Complications include tube malposition, esophageal intubation, difficult intubation (which can lead to tooth damage), significant aspiration, laryngeal damage, pneumothorax, and death.[9-11]

3. Tube malposition can be identified shortly after intubation by auscultation of bilateral axillae.

4. End-tidal carbon dioxide ($ETco_2$) measurement and chest radiography ensure proper tube placement, minimizing the catastrophic complications of esophageal intubation.

5. A seemingly positive $ETco_2$ may be observed with esophageal intubation after vigorous positive-pressure ventilation via bag-mask as exhaled gas from the pharynx is forced into the stomach. A capnogram tracing in this case will taper to zero after a few breaths.[12]

D. CHOICE OF VENTILATION MODE

1. The ventilation mode selected depends on multiple dynamic variables, including indicators of the following:

a. Gas exchange: ABGs.

b. Airway pressure: peak, plateau, auto-PEEP.

c. Breathing patterns: spontaneous V_t, RR, minute ventilation.

d. Hemodynamics: blood pressure, cardiac output, pulmonary capillary wedge pressure (PCWP), urine output.

e. Historical or radiographic information regarding lung parenchyma: pneumonia, COPD, asthma, interstitial fibrosis, ARDS, barotrauma.

2. Clinical judgment and experience have a prominent role in selecting the mode of ventilation.[13]

3. Assist-control ventilation (ACV).

a. ACV is the simplest and most frequently used mode.

b. The clinician sets a baseline rate and a baseline tidal volume. In this case a minimum minute ventilation is established.

c. Additional inspiratory efforts by the patient above the set rate result in delivery of a full V_t.

d. Example: Set RR of 10 breaths/min, set V_t of 500 mL to equal or exceed a minute ventilation of 5000 mL. If the patient is "breathing over the ventilator," a patient-initiated respiratory rate of 13 breaths/min will result in a minute ventilation of 6500 mL (RR = 13 breaths/min, V_t = 500 mL).

   e. Advantages and uses.
     (1) Adequate minute ventilation is guaranteed.
     (2) Full support is provided to patients with respiratory muscle weakness, as in neuromuscular blockade or muscle fatigue.
     (3) ACV is often used to "rest" a patient between continuous positive airway pressure (CPAP) or T-piece weaning trials.
   f. Problems.[14,15]
     (1) Rapidly breathing patients trigger the ventilator to administer a "full" breath, which can lead to respiratory alkalosis and hyperinflation if adequate time is not given for the lungs to empty.
     (2) This "breath stacking" may lead to the development of auto-PEEP, also known as dynamic hyperinflation.
     (3) Auto-PEEP may inhibit venous return, decrease cardiac output, and decrease blood pressure.
     (4) Pneumothorax or pneumomediastinum, or in extreme cases cardiac arrest, may also occur.

4. Synchronized intermittent mandatory ventilation (SIMV).
   a. The clinician determines a baseline RR and Vt.
   b. As in the above example (RR = 10, $V_t = 500$), the "baseline" minute ventilation is 5000 mL.
   c. The feature distinguishing SIMV from ACV is what happens when the patient attempts to breathe at a rate greater than the set rate.
     (1) As noted above, additional breaths in the ACV mode result in a full V_t.
     (2) Patient-initiated breaths above the set rate in SIMV result in a V_t dependent on patient effort.
   d. Example: Set RR of 10 breaths/min, set V_t of 500 mL to equal or exceed minimum minute ventilation of 5000 mL. If the patient is "breathing over the ventilator," supplemental breaths will probably have variable impact on the minute ventilation. A patient-initiated rate of 13 breaths/min results in a minute ventilation of (5000 + a + b + c), where *a, b, c* might be 300, 145, and 605 mL. Resulting minute ventilation is therefore 6050 mL.
   e. SIMV is often used in conjunction with pressure support (see below) in an effort to overcome the resistance of the ETT and minimize the risk of breath stacking.
   f. Advantages and uses.
     (1) Each spontaneous breath results in the delivery of variably sized V_ts, decreasing the risk of respiratory alkalosis.
     (2) SIMV has historically been an attractive mode for initial stages of weaning, allowing the patient to gradually assume responsibility for the work of breathing. Although appealing in concept, this approach has not been consistently effective.
   g. Problems.
     (1) SIMV may increase the work of breathing.
     (2) This may be by design for the purpose of exercise, but in a fatiguing

patient, adding pressure support or changing to ACV would be appropriate.

5. **Pressure-support ventilation (PSV).**

a. In PSV the patient determines RR, inspiratory flow rate, and V_t.

b. If spontaneous inspiratory effort by the patient is adequate (-2 cm H_2O), the ventilator is triggered to generate a peak positive airway pressure chosen by the clinician.[16]

c. This positive pressure in the airway decreases the work required by patient to inflate the lungs.

d. At a minimum, chosen PSV should decrease the work of breathing by reducing the impact of resistance to airflow through the ETT.

e. PSV for a given breath is stopped when the inspiratory flow rate falls below 25% of its peak.

f. Initial settings are usually 5 to 10 cm H_2O.

g. PSV is then titrated to patient comfort and effective oxygenation and ventilation, as indicated by ABG analysis and the patient's clinical appearance.

h. Advantages and uses.

   (1) PSV is useful by itself or in conjunction with PEEP as a weaning mode (see below).

   (2) Most alert patients are more comfortable on PSV than SIMV or ACV because PSV allows for natural variance in RR and V_t.

i. Problems.

   (1) There is no guaranteed ventilation with PSV. Therefore, if the patient stops breathing for any reason (neuromuscular blockade, fatigue, weakness), ventilation ceases.

   (2) SIMV set at a low rate (6-8 breaths/min) is sometimes used as a precaution to avoid this problem.

6. **Extrinsic positive end-expiratory pressure (PEEP).**

a. PEEP is pressure applied by the mechanical ventilator to the airways at the end of expiration.

b. Extrinsic PEEP is separate and distinct from auto-PEEP (see later).

c. It has two primary uses.

   (1) Extrinsic PEEP is used to decrease the work of breathing in patients with obstructive airway disease.

   (a) By applying extrinsic PEEP, as defined below, the clinician can decrease the negative inspiratory pressure the patient must generate to pull air into the lungs.

   (b) Example: If 5 cm H_2O of auto-PEEP is present, and if negative 2 cm H_2O of pressure is needed to trigger ventilator support, the total negative pressure the patient must generate to trigger ventilator assistance is 7 cm H_2O.[17] Application of 5 cm H_2O of extrinsic PEEP would reduce patient-dependent negative inspiratory pressure to 2 cm H_2O, making it easier to trigger ventilator support and decrease the work of breathing.

63

MECHANICAL VENTILATION

(2) Extrinsic PEEP is used to increase arterial oxygen partial pressure (Pao_2) by minimizing atelectasis, decreasing intrapulmonary shunting, and pushing intraalveolar water into the interstium.[18]

(a) It allows reduction in Fio_2 and avoidance of O_2 toxicity.

(b) It can be used in conjunction with ACV, SIMV, and PSV modes.

(c) As with auto-PEEP, high levels may decrease venous return and therefore cardiac output. Hypotension occurs more often in hypovolemic patients.

E. WEANING

1. General considerations before withdrawal of ventilator support.

a. Resolution of respiratory failure.

b. Discontinuation of sedatives and neuromuscular blockers.

c. Hemodynamic stability.

d. Optimization of metabolic and electrolyte disorders.

e. Good gas exchange.

2. Parameters used to assess patient's readiness for weaning.[19]

a. Pao_2 greater than or equal to 60 mm Hg, with Fio_2 less than or equal to 0.4.

b. PEEP less than or equal to 5 cm H_2O.

c. Pao_2/Fio_2 ratio greater than 200.

3. Other parameters to note are blood pressure, heart rate, and RR, although their predictive value is generally poor.

4. Maximal inspiratory pressure (MIP).

a. MIP is a useful index; MIP greater than 20 cm H_2O has been associated with a 60% success rate.

b. MIP of 20 cm H_2O or less predicted failure 100% of the time.

5. Tobin index (RR/V_t in liters).[20]

a. Index less than 105 breaths/min/L suggested a 78% success rate.

b. Index of 105 or greater predicted failure 95% of the time.

6. Once a patient is deemed appropriate for weaning, the clinician can pursue either gradual or rapid withdrawal of ventilator support. Generally it is reasonable to attempt rapid withdrawal first.

a. Modes include T-piece and CPAP trials.

b. CPAP and PEEP are often used interchangeably in mechanically ventilated patients. If the patient fails the trial based on hemodynamic or respiratory factors, or if the Tobin index is greater than 105, factors compromising weaning should be sought. These include poor respiratory center output from sedation or intrinsic central depression, a peripheral neuromuscular disorder, metabolic and electrolyte abnormalities (e.g., hypophosphatemia, malnutrition), overfeeding with resulting hyperventilation, phrenic nerve abnormality, and poor cardiac function.

c. For patients who fail rapid withdrawal of support, repeated T-piece or CPAP trials on a daily basis are recommended, rather than tapering of SIMV from full assistance to minimal assistance.[21,22]

7. Daily weaning trials for all ICU patients decrease duration of intubation and ICU stay.[23]

F. COMPLICATIONS

1. Intubation and mechanical ventilation are necessary for many critically ill patients, but complications can affect morbidity and mortality. Barotrauma and volutrauma are complications affecting the lung parenchyma, as is oxygen toxicity. It is also important to be aware of complications associated with the ETT itself: sinusitis, soft tissue necrosis, tracheal stenosis, laryngeal damage, esophageal perforation, and aspiration.

2. Barotrauma has traditionally referred to the rupture of small airways and alveolar walls by high pressure.
   a. The result is extravasation of air into the bronchovascular sheath, pleural cavity, mediastinum, pericardium, soft tissue of the head and neck, or some combination.[24]
   b. Along with abnormalities on chest radiography, the patient with barotrauma is likely to have pain and tachypnea, if not hypotension and hypoxia.

3. Volutrauma has been described as pulmonary edema, diffuse alveolar damage, and epithelial and microvascular permeability resulting from overdistention of airspaces rather than actual rupture.[25] Volutrauma tends to suggest a compromise of the blood gas interface.

4. Chest radiography is helpful in delineating macroscopic lung damage.

5. To minimize lung trauma resulting from excessive airway and alveolar pressure and volume, two measurements are noted.
   a. Plateau pressure (P_{plat}).
      (1) P_{plat} is static pressure measured at end inspiration.
      (2) It is obtained by occlusion of the expiratory flow valve on the ventilator for a few seconds to allow a given V_t to distribute evenly throughout all patent airways and alveoli.
      (3) It is a more accurate reflection of intrapulmonary pressures and associated parenchymal injury than peak pressure (P_{pk}) because P_{plat} represents the pressure imposed on distended alveoli.
   b. Auto-PEEP.
      (1) Auto-PEEP is the pressure remaining in airways and alveoli at the instant before inspiration.
      (2) It is found in patients with obstructive lung disease: COPD, asthma, obliterative bronchiolitis, bronchiectasis, cystic fibrosis.
      (3) This pressure must be overcome either by the patient's inspiratory effort or by positive-pressure ventilation for lung inflation to take place.
      (4) Auto-PEEP is measured by occlusion of the exhalation port immediately before inspiration, which allows equalization of pressures between the alveoli and the ETT, thereby allowing the machine to measure pressure remaining in the system (lungs and tubing) at end expiration.[26]
   c. Previous discussion describes auto-PEEP as an entity primarily associ-

63

MECHANICAL VENTILATION

ated with obstructive airway disease. Auto-PEEP may also occur if the patient is delivered excessively high V_t at a high RR, in which case the lungs are not given adequate time to deflate between breaths. The result is excessive intraalveolar pressures at both end inspiration and end expiration, with an increased likelihood of barotrauma and volutrauma.

d. High P_{pk} is sometimes erroneously related to barotrauma and volutrauma. Peak pressure represents the pressure measured in the large airways while V_t is being administered and does not reflect the stress on the alveoli, where barotrauma and volutrauma occur.

6. **Oxygen toxicity.**

a. Toxic effects of high Fio_2 on the lung include tracheobronchitis with decreased mucociliary clearance, absorption atelectasis, acute lung injury, altered ventilatory drive, and bronchopulmonary dysplasia.[14]

b. Observational animal and human studies suggest that the mechanism of this damage is the result of increased free radical production.[27-31]

c. For this reason O_2-conservative strategies are routinely used for mechanically ventilated patients to minimize the risk of O_2 toxicity. A common goal is to decrease Fio_2 to less than 0.5 by increasing PEEP.

7. **Acute respiratory distress and hypoxemia.**

a. Causes of hypoxemia in ventilated patients can be categorized into those associated with the ventilator, advancing disease, new medical problem, procedures, and medications.[32]

b. First the patient should be disconnected from the ventilator and bag-mask ventilated with 100% O_2 because the mechanical ventilator itself is responsible for decompensation in one third of cases.[33]

c. If symptoms are not corrected shortly, the problem is with either the ETT or the patient.

d. Hemodynamic trends over the preceding several hours may suggest the cause of acute decompensation.

e. The ETT should be suctioned.

f. Focused physical examination and chest radiograph are important at this point.

g. If the ventilator is not implicated in decompensation, measurement of P_{pk} and P_{plat} may be helpful.[34]

   (1) Low or declining P_{pk} and hyperventilation suggest an air leak in the ventilator system.

   (2) Unchanged P_{pk} is consistent with progressive pulmonary hypertension, pulmonary emboli, and evolution of right-to-left cardiac shunts.

h. When the P_{pk} is elevated, P_{plat} is obtained and compliance (V_t/P_{plat}) is calculated.

i. P_{plat} will be unchanged in obstructive processes such as aspiration, bronchospasm, and ETT tube kinking or obstruction, provided significant auto-PEEP has not developed.

j. P_{plat} will increase when compliance has decreased, as in pneumothorax, ARDS, cardiogenic pulmonary edema, auto-PEEP, patient-ventilator asynchrony, and extrathoracic processes.

PEARLS AND PITFALLS

- Prone ventilation.
  - Placing a patient face down improves systemic oxygenation by increasing functional residual capacity (FRC) and thereby decreasing shunt. It directs blood toward the better-aerated ventral lung regions, improving cardiac output, and promotes secretion clearance.
  - Better oxygenation allows use of less toxic levels of Fio_2 and lower intraalveolar pressures (less need for extrinsic PEEP).[35]
  - The prone position is therefore an appealing technique for critically ill hypoxic patients but has never been proved to benefit mortality.[36]
- ARDS and low tidal volume ventilation.
  - The ARDS Network demonstrated a 22% reduction in mortality and fewer ventilator days by using low-V_t ventilation (6 mL versus 12 mL/kg ideal body weight), permissive hypercapnia, and a goal P_{plat} less than 30 cm H_2O in treatment of ARDS.[37]
  - ARDS was defined in these patients as (1) Pao_2/Fio_2 ratio less than 300, (2) bilateral pulmonary infiltrates, and (3) no clinical evidence of left atrial hypertension, or PCWP less than 18 mm Hg.
  - Benefit is thought to result from decreased V_t-induced barotrauma and volutrauma.
  - Special considerations include the following.
    - Increased RR is necessary to maintain adequate minute ventilation, which often requires increased levels of sedation.
    - Permissive hypercapnia results from increased anatomical dead space per tidal volume. Continuous bicarbonate infusion may be used to treat mild to moderate respiratory acidosis.
  - A second investigation is examining a high-PEEP versus a low-PEEP protocol using low V_t.
- Noninvasive positive-pressure ventilation (NPPV).
  - NPPV refers to ventilatory support that does not involve intubation.
  - NPPV is delivered most frequently through a face mask or nasal mask as CPAP or bilevel positive airway pressure (BiPAP).
  - Originally designed as a method of treating chronic respiratory failure, NPPV has shown promise in the treatment of acute respiratory failure.
  - In patients with COPD and hypercarbic respiratory failure, NPPV has been associated with improvement in vital signs, decreased Pco_2, and decreased need for endotracheal intubation compared with control groups not originally given ventilatory support.[38-40]
  - In hypoxic respiratory failure, data are conflicting on whether NPPV is associated with reduced need for endotracheal intubation.[41,42]
  - When NPPV was compared with conventional mechanical ventilation in 64 patients with hypoxemic respiratory failure, NPPV was as

effective in improving gas exchange and was associated with fewer complications and shorter length of ICU stay.[43]

- Studies suggest that NPPV is an acceptable treatment for both hypercarbic and hypoxemic respiratory failure and in certain situations may be substituted for intubation and conventional mechanical ventilation.
- NPPV is not for all patients. The patient must be awake, cooperative enough to wear the mask, and able to protect the airway.
- In general, NPPV should be set at the lowest O_2 level and pressure support that correct the oxygenation or ventilation defect.
- BiPAP is more physiological, but comparative data are insufficient to recommend it over CPAP.
- Local preference will often govern choice, and the clinician should consult with the respiratory therapy department to determine what is available and typically used in the given institution. Initial settings might be CPAP of 3 to 5 mm H_2O and pressure support of 7 to 10 mm H_2O.
- As with traditional mechanical ventilation, the patient should be assessed frequently and appropriate adjustments made.

REFERENCES

[b] 1. Sasse SA et al. Arterial oxygenation time after an Fi_{O_2} increase in mechanically ventilated patients. Am J Respir Crit Care Med 1995; 152:148.
[c] 2. Esteban A et al. How is mechanical ventilation employed in the intensive care unit? An international utilization review. Am J Respir Crit Care Med 2000; 161:1450.
[a] 3. Kress JP et al. Daily interruption of sedative infusions in critically ill patients undergoing mechanical ventilation. N Engl J Med 2000; 342:1471.
[c] 4. Hunter JM. New neuromuscular blocking drugs. N Engl J Med 1995; 332:1691.
[c] 5. Whittaker M. Plasma cholinesterase variants and the anesthetist. Anaesthesia 1980; 35:174.
[c] 6. Yentis SM. Suxamethonium and hyperkalemia. Anaesth Intensive Care 1990; 18:91.
[c] 7. Elliot JM, Bion JF. The use of neuromuscular blocking drugs in intensive care practice. Acta Anaesthesiol Scand 1995; 39:70.
[d] 8. Shapiro BA et al. Practice parameters for sustained neuromuscular blockade in the adult critically ill patient: an executive summary. Crit Care Med 1995; 23:1601.
[b] 9. Schwartz DE, Lieberman JA, Cohen NH. Women are at greater risk than men for malpositioning of the endotracheal tube after emergent intubation. Crit Care Med 1994; 22:1127.
[b] 10. Schwartz DE, Matthay MA, Cohen NH: Death and other complications of emergency airway management in critically ill adults: a prospective investigation of 297 tracheal intubations. Anesthesiology 1995; 82:367.
[b] 11. Kollef MH, Legare EJ, Damiano M. Endotracheal tube misplacement: incidence, risk factors, and impact of a quality improvement program. South Med J 1994; 87:248.
[c] 12. Szaflarski NL, Cohen NH. The use of capnography in critically ill adults. Heart Lung 1991; 20:363.
[c] 13. Tobin MJ. Mechanical ventilation. N Engl J Med 1994; 330:1056.
[c] 14. Almog Y, Brower R. Complications of mechanical ventilation. In Complications in the medical intensive care unit. New York: Chapman & Hall; 1997.
[d] 15. Rogers PL et al. Auto-PEEP during CPR: an "occult" cause of electromechanical dissociation. Chest 1991; 99:492.
[c] 16. Sassoon CSH, Gruer SE. Characteristics of the ventilator pressure- and flow-trigger variables. Intensive Care Med 1995; 21:159.
[b] 17. Rossi A et al. Measurement of static compliance of mechanical ventilation: the effect of intrinsic positive end-expiratory pressure. Am Rev Respir Dis 1985; 131:672.

[b] 18. Malo J, Ali J, Wood LDH. How does positive end-expiratory pressure reduce intrapulmonary shunt in canine pulmonary edema? J Appl Physiol 1984; 57:1002.

[c] 19. Lessard MR, Brochard LJ. Weaning from ventilatory support. Clin Chest Med 1996; 17:475.

[b] 20. Yang K, Tobin MJ. A prospective study of indexes predicting the outcome of weaning from mechanical ventilation. N Engl J Med 1991; 324:1445.

[a] 21. Brochard L et al. Comparison of three methods of gradual withdrawal from ventilatory support during weaning from mechanical ventilation. Am J Respir Crit Care Med 1994; 150:896.

[a] 22. Esteban A et al. A comparison of four methods of weaning patients from mechanical ventilation. N Engl J Med 1995; 332:345.

[a] 23. Ely EW et al. Effect on the duration of mechanical ventilation of identifying patients capable of breathing spontaneously. N Engl J Med 1996; 335:1864.

[c] 24. Macklin CC. Transport of air along sheaths of pulmonic blood vessels from alveoli to mediastinum. Arch Intern Med 1939; 64:913.

[c] 25. Parker JC, Hernandez LA, Peevy KJ. Mechanisms of ventilator-induced lung injury. Crit Care Med 1993; 21:131.

[c] 26. Pepe PE, Marini JJ. Occult positive end-expiratory pressure in mechanically ventilated patients with airflow obstruction: the auto-PEEP effect. Am Rev Respir Dis 1982; 126:166.

[b] 27. Royer F et al. Increase in pulmonary capillary permeability in dogs exposed to 100% O_2. J Appl Physiol 1988; 65:1140.

[b] 28. Royston BD, Webster NR, Nunn JF. Time course of changes in lung permeability and edema in the rat exposed to 100% oxygen. J Appl Physiol 1990; 69:1532.

[b] 29. Fox RB et al. Pulmonary inflammation due to oxygen toxicity: involvement of chemotactic factors and polymorphonuclear leukocytes. Am Rev Respir Dis 1981; 123:521.

[b] 30. Barber RE, Hamilton WK. Oxygen toxicity in man. N Engl J Med 1970; 283:1478.

[b] 31. Hyde RW, Rawson AJ. Unintentional iatrogenic oxygen pneumonitis: response to therapy. Ann Intern Med 1969; 71(3):517.

[c] 32. Glauser FL, Polatty RC, Sessler CN. Worsening oxygenation in the mechanically ventilated patient: causes, mechanisms, and early detection. Am Rev Respir Dis 1988; 138:458.

[b] 33. Zwillich CW et al. Complications of assisted ventilation: a prospective study of 354 consecutive episodes. Am J Med 1974; 57:161.

[d] 34. Marino PL. The ICU book, 2nd ed. Baltimore: Williams & Wilkins; 1997.

[c] 35. Albert RK. Prone ventilation. Clin Chest Med 2000; 21:511.

[a] 36. Gattinoni L et al. Effect of prone positioning on the survival of patients with acute respiratory failure. N Engl J Med 2001; 345:568.

[a] 37. Ventilation with lower tidal volumes as compared with traditional tidal volumes for acute lung injury and the acute respiratory distress syndrome. Acute Respiratory Distress Syndrome Network. N Engl J Med 2000; 342:1301.

[a] 38. Bott J et al. Randomised controlled trial of nasal ventilation in acute ventilatory failure due to chronic obstructive airways disease. Lancet 1993; 341:1555.

[a] 39. Kramer N et al. Randomized, prospective trial of noninvasive positive pressure ventilation in acute respiratory failure. Am J Respir Crit Care Med 1995; 151:1799.

[a] 40. Brochard L et al. Noninvasive ventilation for acute exacerbations of chronic obstructive pulmonary disease. N Engl J Med 1995; 333:817.

[a] 41. Wysocki M et al. Noninvasive pressure support ventilation in patients with acute respiratory failure: a randomized comparison with conventional therapy. Chest 1995; 107:761.

[a] 42. Confalonieri M et al. Acute respiratory failure in patients with severe community-acquired pneumonia: a prospective randomized evaluation of noninvasive ventilation. Am J Respir Crit Care Med 1999; 160:1585.

[a] 43. Antonelli et al. A comparison of noninvasive positive-pressure ventilation and conventional mechanical ventilation in patients with acute respiratory failure. N Engl J Med 1998; 339:429.

63

MECHANICAL VENTILATION

Pulmonary Embolism and Deep Venous Thrombosis

David Zaas, MD, and David Pearse, MD

FAST FACTS

- Of patients with a lower extremity deep venous thrombosis (DVT), 30% will develop symptomatic pulmonary embolism (PE) and another 30% will develop asymptomatic PE.[1]
- Between 40% and 60% of patients with venous thromboembolism (VTE) have an identifiable clinical risk factor for DVT.[2]
- About 20% of patients with PE have a normal arterial oxygen partial pressure (Pao_2 >80 mm Hg).[3]
- Combination of the lack of (1) pleuritic chest pain, (2) dyspnea, and (3) tachypnea has a high specificity (97%) for the absence of PE.[3]
- Duplex lower extremity ultrasound is 95% sensitive and 96% specific for symptomatic proximal DVT, but only 30% to 60% sensitive for asymptomatic proximal DVT.[4]
- Normal or high-probability ventilation-perfusion ($\dot{V}/\dot{Q}$) scans have good predictive value but are uncommon; each occurred in less than 15% of the $\dot{V}/\dot{Q}$ scans in the Prospective Investigation of Pulmonary Embolism Diagnosis (PIOPED) study.[5]
- Angiography is a relatively safe procedure with a morbidity less than 2% and a mortality less than 0.5%.[4]

64

I. EPIDEMIOLOGY

A. INCIDENCE

1. VTE is frequently unrecognized because of its nonspecific clinical presentation and is often not diagnosed until autopsy.
2. VTE is reported to affect 1 in 1000 people in the United States and Europe every year.
3. In the United States each year there are approximately 600,000 cases of PE, leading to 50,000 to 200,000 deaths per year.
4. In only 33% of these patients was PE diagnosed before death.[1,6]

B. SOURCE OF THROMBUS

1. Thrombi most often form in the venous system of the lower extremities, specifically the deep venous system of the calf.
2. Approximately 20% of untreated calf DVTs extend into the proximal veins of the lower extremity.
3. Among patients with lower extremity VTE, symptomatic PE develops in approximately 30% and asymptomatic PE develops in another 30%.
4. Other, less common sources of thrombus include the pelvic, renal, and axillary veins, as well as the inferior vena cava (IVC).[1]

5. It is often erroneously stated that upper extremity thrombosis in the internal jugular, subclavian, axillary, or brachial veins rarely causes PE; however, 36% of upper extremity DVTs may lead to PE.[7]

C. RISK FACTORS

1. Risk factors include both clinical risk factors and inherited or acquired blood clotting abnormalities (Box 64-1).[1,2]

2. Virchow's classic triad of VTE includes venous stasis, vascular endothelial damage, and hypercoagulability.

3. Risk of DVT increases with age; for every 10-year increase in age, the risk has been shown to double.[8]

4. All types of malignancies are associated with an increased risk of thrombosis; however, hypercoagulability is most pronounced with visceral adenocarcinomas.

5. Multiple abnormalities of the coagulation pathway cause an increased tendency for thrombosis.

a. Most common is the factor V Leiden mutation, leading to resistance to activated protein C. Approximately 5% of Caucasians and 1% of African-Americans are heterozygous for this defect.

BOX 64-1

RISK FACTORS FOR VENOUS THROMBOEMBOLISM

CLINICAL RISK FACTORS

Trauma
Prior venous thromboembolism
Malignancy, especially adenocarcinoma
Age over 40 years
Heart failure
Immobilization
Obesity
Oral contraceptives
Smoking
Pregnancy and parturition

BLOOD CLOTTING ABNORMALITIES

Factor V Leiden–activated protein C resistance
Protein C deficiency
Protein S deficiency
Antithrombin III deficiency
Anticardiolipin-antiphospholipid antibody
Heparin-induced thrombocytopenia
Hyperhomocysteinemia
Prothrombin 20210A
Elevated factor VIII levels

b. Other, less common defects of the clotting cascade, such as protein C, protein S, or antithrombin III deficiency, induce a greater relative risk of thrombosis.[6]

II. CLINICAL PRESENTATION

PE can have a variety of presentations, and the manifestations are nonspecific and often missed. Only 25% of patients with suspected PE at presentation truly have PE.

A. THREE TYPES[6]

1. Dyspnea with or without pleuritic chest pain and hemoptysis.
2. Hemodynamic instability and syncope.
3. Indolent pulmonary complaints mimicking congestive heart failure (CHF) or pneumonia.

B. SYMPTOMS

1. Dyspnea and pleuritic chest pains are the most frequently reported symptoms, present in 73% and 66% of patients, respectively.
2. Other symptoms, such as cough, hemoptysis, leg pain and swelling, palpitations, and wheezing, are present in a minority of patients.
3. Lack of the combination of pleuritic chest pain, dyspnea, and tachypnea is 97% specific for the absence of PE.[3]

C. PHYSICAL SIGNS

1. The most common physical signs of PE are tachypnea, crackles, and tachycardia, present in 70%, 51%, and 30% of patients, respectively.
2. Signs present in less than 25% of patients with PE include an S_4, a loud P_2, diaphoresis, fever, Homans' sign, pleural friction rub, an S_3, and cyanosis.[3]

D. DIFFERENTIAL DIAGNOSIS

1. The differential diagnosis is extensive, involving a wide range of pulmonary processes that can cause many of the nonspecific symptoms cited previously.
2. The presence of unexplained dyspnea and risk factors for thrombosis should raise suspicion of a PE.
3. Diagnosis can be especially difficult in elderly patients or patients with underlying lung disease because PE may mimic heart failure, pneumonia, or an exacerbation of underlying lung disease.

III. DIAGNOSTICS

The diagnosis of PE is often difficult because the gold standard diagnostic test, pulmonary angiography, is invasive, expensive, and not available at all hospitals. All other tests have limited sensitivities and specificities when used alone. Thus a series of diagnostic algorithms have been proposed. To make the diagnosis accurately, these algorithms depend on the pretest probability of PE, as determined by the physician's clinical assessment (Fig. 64-1).[3] Evaluation of PE includes several of the tests described below combined to "rule in" or "rule out" a suspected PE.

64

PULMONARY EMBOLISM AND DVT

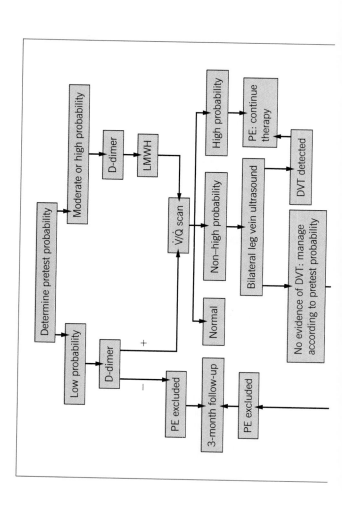

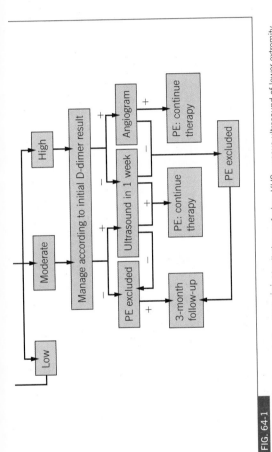

FIG. 64-1

Diagnosis of pulmonary embolism (PE). $\dot{V}/\dot{Q}$, Ventilation-perfusion; *VUS*, venous ultrasound of lower extremity. *(From Rodger M, Wells P. Thromb Res 2001; 103:221.)*

64

PULMONARY EMBOLISM AND DVT

A. ARTERIAL BLOOD GAS ANALYSIS[9]

1. Arterial blood gases (ABGs) should be measured in any patient undergoing evaluation for a suspected PE.
2. Obstruction of pulmonary arteries by thrombus causes impaired diffusion of both carbon dioxide (CO_2) and oxygen (O_2).
3. Obstruction of pulmonary arteries increases dead space ventilation, which is usually compensated for by an increase in minute ventilation. Because of this compensatory hyperventilation, patients with PE are rarely hypercapnic at presentation.
4. Hypercapnia is found in patients unable to increase their minute ventilation, either those with massive often-fatal PE or those undergoing fixed ventilation, such as controlled mechanical ventilation.
5. Hypoxemia has a multifactorial etiology.
   a. Although animal and human studies have documented diffusion impairments after PE, this explains less than 15% of the observed hypoxemia.
   b. Hypoxemia results from a combination of shunt from atelectasis and a patent foramen ovale, $\dot{V}/\dot{Q}$ mismatch, low mixed-venous oxygen partial pressure (Pvo_2), or diffusion impairment.
6. The most common ABG findings in patients with PE are respiratory alkalosis with hypocapnia, hypoxemia, and an elevated alveolar-to-arterial oxygen (A-ao$_2$) gradient.
7. Unfortunately, ABG analysis alone is neither sensitive nor specific for PE diagnosis.
8. Approximately 20% of patients with PE have a normal Pao_2 (>80 mm Hg).
9. A-ao$_2$ gradient is more sensitive than hypoxemia alone in the evaluation of PE because it takes into account the hyperventilation and hypocapnia.
   a. Even a normal A-ao$_2$ gradient does not rule out a diagnosis of PE.[3]
   b. Normal A-ao$_2$ gradient in the setting of PE can often be found in younger patients with either no preexisting cardiopulmonary disease or limited vascular obstruction.[4]

B. CHEST RADIOGRAPH

1. Hypoxemia in a patient with a clear chest radiograph is a common clinical setting in which the diagnosis of PE is entertained.
2. Findings on chest radiography are most helpful in excluding other causes of hypoxemia.
3. The most common radiographic abnormalities are atelectasis, small pleural effusions, and peripherally based infiltrates.
4. Classic chest x-ray findings include Westermark's sign (prominent central pulmonary artery with decreased pulmonary vascularity), Hampton's hump (wedge-shaped peripheral-based infiltrates just above the diaphragm), and Palla's sign (enlargement of the right descending pulmonary artery). These are found in less than 7% of patients.[3]

C. ELECTROCARDIOGRAM

1. The electrocardiogram (ECG) is not very helpful in the diagnosis of PE.
2. The ECG is often abnormal, but the changes are nonspecific.
3. The most common abnormalities are nonspecific ST segment and T wave changes, along with sinus tachycardia.[3]
4. ECG findings indicative of elevated right-sided heart pressures, such as P-pulmonale, right ventricular hypertrophy, right axis deviation, right bundle branch block, and $S_1Q_3T_3$, are found in less than 6% of patients with PE; therefore their absence is not helpful in the diagnostic evaluation of PE.[3]
5. A nonspecific ECG finding is T wave inversion in V_1-V_4 caused by inferoposterior ischemia as a result of right coronary artery compression from right ventricular overload.[10]

D. LOWER EXTREMITY DUPLEX ULTRASOUND

1. Although still considered the diagnostic gold standard, venography has been replaced under most circumstances by ultrasound (US) for the diagnosis of DVT.
2. US is 95% sensitive and 96% specific for detecting symptomatic DVT in the popliteal or more proximal veins. Unfortunately, sensitivity for asymptomatic proximal DVT is only 30% to 60%.
3. US is also less useful for diagnosis of calf DVT.
   a. Isolated calf DVT infrequently causes PE.
   b. When the initial study is negative, serial US at 7-day interval is useful to rule out propagation of calf DVT.[4]
4. US is also useful in identifying other causes of leg swelling that may be mistaken for lower extremity DVT, such as a hematoma, Baker's cyst, and abscess.
5. US is limited when access to the desired area of the extremity is difficult, as in obese, edematous, or immobile patients.
6. Utility of US of the internal jugular, subclavian, axillary, and brachial veins for upper extremity DVT is similar to that of the lower extremities.
7. Upper extremity US is 78% to 100% sensitive for symptomatic thrombosis but only 36% sensitive for asymptomatic upper extremity DVT.[7]

E. VENOGRAPHY

1. Venography should be considered if clinical suspicion differs from the results of venous US (a very high clinical suspicion and negative US results, or a low clinical suspicion and positive US results).
2. Diagnosis of recurrent DVT by means of venous US is more difficult; 1 year after an initial lower extremity DVT, 50% of patients have persistently abnormal venous compression on US.[4]
3. For documentation of a new thrombosis, a larger area of venous involvement or an increase in venous diameter of greater than 4 mm in that same area must be present.
4. Therefore venography may be helpful to distinguish acute thrombosis from chronic residual changes.

64

PULMONARY EMBOLISM AND DVT

F. MAGNETIC RESONANCE IMAGING AND MAGNETIC RESONANCE VENOGRAPHY

1. Preliminary data indicate that magnetic resonance imaging (MRI) and magnetic resonance venography (MRV) may prove to be valuable noninvasive techniques for the diagnosis of lower extremity DVT.
2. These modalities have a sensitivity and specificity of almost 100% for symptomatic proximal DVT, as well as increased sensitivity for asymptomatic DVT.
3. MRI can also be used to diagnose pelvic thrombosis and distinguish acute from chronic VTE.
4. Large-scale randomized studies to evaluate both the efficacy and the cost effectiveness of MRV are ongoing.
5. MRV may be used instead of venography when US results are inadequate or inconclusive.[7]
6. Use of MRI for evaluation of PE is still mostly experimental.
   a. Preliminary small studies found MRI to have high sensitivity and specificity.[7]
   b. MRI can be performed rapidly, without the risks associated with contrast material used for spiral computed tomography (CT) and pulmonary angiography.

G. VENTILATION-PERFUSION SCAN

1. The $\dot{V}/\dot{Q}$ scan is the most common noninvasive test used for diagnosis of PE.
2. It has limited sensitivity and specificity when used alone.
3. The value of the $\dot{V}/\dot{Q}$ scan was investigated in the multicenter prospective PIOPED study.[5]
   a. Almost 1000 patients who underwent $\dot{V}/\dot{Q}$ scanning were followed, and approximately 800 of those underwent pulmonary angiography.
   b. Prevalence of PE was 33%.
   c. Combining scan findings with pretest assessment of clinical likelihood improved overall diagnostic accuracy.
   d. Results led the conclusions below.
4. High-probability scan.
   a. Helpful to diagnose PE, with positive predictive value of 88%.
   b. Less helpful when clinical suspicion was low.
   c. Less accurate in patients with previous history of PE.
5. Normal scan.
   a. Useful to rule out PE.
   b. Negative predictive value of 91%.

   Note: Unfortunately, high-probability and normal lung scans comprised only a small percentage of $\dot{V}/\dot{Q}$ scans in the PIOPED study—13% and 14%, respectively.
6. Low-probability scan.
   a. Makes PE unlikely when clinical suspicion is low.
   b. Negative predictive value of about 86%.

7. Intermediate-probability scan.
   a. Not helpful to rule in or rule out PE.
8. PE is often present in patients with a high clinical pretest probability and nondiagnostic V̇/Q̇ scan.
9. Utility of the V̇/Q̇ scan is decreased in individuals with underlying lung disease; almost 60% of patients with chronic obstructive pulmonary disease (COPD) had intermediate-probability scans.
10. Most pulmonary disease processes affect not only airspaces but also the vasculature, compromising the specificity of V̇/Q̇ scanning.
11. In a majority of patients, clinical assessment and V̇/Q̇ scanning alone are not adequate to diagnose PE and further testing is required.

H. SPIRAL COMPUTED TOMOGRAPHY

1. Use of spiral CT to evaluate for PE has increased over the past several years.
2. Many small studies advocate spiral CT as the initial diagnostic modality for PE.
3. Only four studies at this time have compared spiral CT with pulmonary angiography.
4. Studies report a wide range of sensitivities, from 53% to 100%, with great interobserver variability.[7]
5. Spiral CT is a technically challenging study to read, especially for an inexperienced radiologist.
6. It appears useful for identifying a large central PE, especially in unstable patients, because of the ease and rapidity in obtaining the study.
7. It is also useful for simultaneous examination of the lung parenchyma, which may help delineate other pulmonary disease (e.g., pneumonia, emphysema).
8. Spiral CT is less sensitive for subsegmental PE, although the significance of this type of PE is unknown, and false-positive results can result from lymph nodes compressing the vasculature.
9. Disadvantages of spiral CT include the contrast dye load, with the risk of allergic reactions and nephrotoxicity.
10. Spiral CT is a promising tool for future evaluation of PE, although data are still incomplete and its exact role in the diagnostic algorithm of PE evaluation is undefined.

I. D-DIMER

1. D-dimers are specific degradation products of cross-linked fibrin that are found in the blood.
2. Two common assay systems are used to detect D-dimers.
   a. Enzyme-linked immunosorbent assay (ELISA)-based system.
      (1) Many studies report high sensitivity (>95%) of D-dimer ELISA assays and therefore a useful negative predictive value (>95%).[11]
      (2) Unfortunately, D-dimer ELISA assays are time consuming and are not used clinically at many institutions.

64

PULMONARY EMBOLISM AND DVT

b. Latex agglutination assay.
   (1) The latex agglutination assay is more widely available because it is easier and less time consuming to perform.
   (2) Sensitivity is variable, however, and the test is of questionable clinical value.

3. A study comparing latex agglutination and ELISA D-dimer assays in 103 patients undergoing pulmonary angiography found that both assays were similar, with sensitivities of 97% to 100% and negative predictive values greater than 94%.[12]

4. In contrast, another study discovered that 8 of 98 patients had normal D-dimer levels by latex agglutination and angiographic evidence of acute PE.[13]

5. D-dimer data based on ELISA assays are promising.

6. The clinical utility of latex agglutination assays is yet to be determined and probably varies among assays.

7. Utility of any D-dimer assay will continue to be limited by a high percentage of false-positive D-dimer assays in hospitalized patients.

8. The negative predictive value of a negative D-dimer assay depends on the patient population. For example, oncology patients have an increased pretest probability of a positive D-dimer test, and the negative predictive value is decreased compared with the general population.[14]

J. PULMONARY ANGIOGRAPHY

1. Pulmonary angiography is the gold standard for the diagnosis of PE.

2. Morbidity and mortality of pulmonary angiography are often incorrectly overstated; in the PIOPED study, morbidity was less than 2% and mortality less than 0.5%.[5]

3. Limitations include the high cost of the procedure and the requirement for a skilled and experienced interventional radiologist.

4. Pulmonary angiography is an invasive diagnostic test that exposes patients to the risks of nephrotoxic contrast dye (typically 120 mL).

5. Pulmonary angiography should be performed when the diagnosis is in doubt after a workup with noninvasive modalities.

K. DIAGNOSTIC ALGORITHM

1. The diagnostic workup for PE depends on the clinical pretest probability of low, intermediate, or high likelihood of PE.

2. Assessment of pretest probability is based on the physician's clinical assessment of the risk factors, symptoms, and physical examination and the likelihood of an alternative diagnosis.

3. Assessment of cardiopulmonary reserve depends on the patient's underlying health and the severity of the presentation, including hemodynamic stability and oxygenation.

4. An example of a diagnostic PE algorithm is detailed in Fig. 64-1.[13]

IV. MANAGEMENT

A. ANTICOAGULATION

1. Anticoagulation is used to prevent new clot formation in patients with PE while the body degrades existing clot.

2. Both proximal DVT and PE are treated in the same manner.

3. Indication for anticoagulation in lower leg DVT is more controversial because it is unlikely to cause PE without extension into the proximal venous system.

4. Symptomatic calf DVT is usually treated with 3 months of anticoagulation.

5. Alternatively, lower leg DVT can be monitored with serial US over 10 to 14 days to watch for signs of progression.[6]

6. The classic regimen of anticoagulation for DVT above the popliteal fossa or for PE consists of intravenous administration of unfractionated heparin followed by orally administered warfarin.

   a. When the diagnosis of VTE is suspected and no contraindications to anticoagulation are present, heparin should be started. An example of a heparin dosage algorithm is included in Part IV of the book.

   b. Activated partial thromboplastin time (aPTT) must be measured initially every 6 to 8 hours to obtain an aPTT of 45 to 70 seconds (ratio 1.5-2.3). Studies examining the efficacy of unfractionated heparin found near-complete reduction in significant morbidity and mortality associated with PE. An untreated control population had a 25% mortality rate, as well as an additional 25% incidence of nonfatal, recurrent episodes of PE.[6]

   c. Low molecular weight heparin (LMWH) is a recent alternative to unfractionated heparin.[15] Weight-based dosage of LMWH has been studied only in patients with near-normal renal function (creatinine level <2 mg/dL) and in patients who were not extremely underweight or obese (i.e., in those whose weight was between 50 and 120 kg). The use of LMWH for the treatment of DVT with or without PE may allow outpatient management of a clinically stable patient.

   d. Warfarin (Coumadin) is started at the same time as heparin or after heparin is therapeutic to avoid the very low risk of warfarin-induced skin necrosis in protein C– and protein S–deficient patients.

   e. Warfarin should be started at 5 mg/day. A loading dose increases the complications of anticoagulation without decreasing the time needed to reach a therapeutic prothrombin time (PT). The dosage should be adjusted to reach an international normalized ratio (INR) of 2.5 ± 0.5.

   f. Once the goal INR has been obtained, heparin should be continued for an additional 48 hours to achieve therapeutic anticoagulation with warfarin.

7. The American Thoracic Society has issued recommendations on the duration of anticoagulation for three major risk groups (Table 64-1).

64

PULMONARY EMBOLISM AND DVT

TABLE 64-1

DURATION OF ANTICOAGULATION IN MAJOR RISK GROUPS

Risk Group*	Duration of Anticoagulation
1. First event, reversible risk factor, age <60 years	3-6 months
2. First event, reversible risk factor, age >60 years *or* First event with idiopathic disease	6-12 months
3. Recurrent event or first event, irreversible risk factor	12 months–life

From American Thoracic Society. Am J Respir Crit Care Med 1999; 160:1043.
*Reversible risk factors include surgery, trauma, and immobility; irreversible risk factors include factor V Leiden and antithrombin III deficiency.

B. THROMBOLYTIC AGENTS

1. Treatment of PE with thrombolytic therapy has been studied for more than three decades.
2. Urokinase, streptokinase, and tissue plasminogen activator (t-PA, TPA) have been shown to cause more rapid clot lysis and quicker resolution of hemodynamic changes, but no convincing evidence of morbidity or mortality benefits that would justify an increased bleeding risk has been shown.[16]
3. The only widely accepted indication is shock in a patient with a large, hemodynamically significant PE.
   a. Data supporting use of thrombolytic agents in a patient with shock are mostly anecdotal.
   b. In a randomized study eight patients with PE and shock received streptokinase or heparin; all four heparin-treated patients died, whereas all four patients who received streptokinase survived.[17]
4. Thrombolytic agents may play a larger role in the treatment of PE once a subset of patients can be defined who would receive clinical benefit from these drugs rather than heparin.
5. The utility of echocardiography to evaluate for evidence of right-sided heart failure as a marker for patients who may benefit from thrombolytic agents is being investigated.

C. INFERIOR VENA CAVA FILTERS

1. Inferior vena cava filters are used to prevent the progression of lower extremity DVT to PE.
2. Traditional indications include an inability to tolerate anticoagulation and the failure of anticoagulation.
3. Few randomized trials have evaluated the efficacy of IVC filters; in 400 patients randomly assigned to filters plus at least 3 months of anticoagulation or to anticoagulation alone, IVC filters decreased the incidence of PE within the first year.[18]
   a. No significant benefit in either incidence of PE or mortality was seen after 1 year.
   b. Initial benefits of IVC filters were offset by an increase in recurrent deep venous thromboembolism, possibly resulting from thrombosis at the filter site.

4. Based on this study, anticoagulation is still the first choice in treatment of VTE and the use of IVC filters should be limited to patients in whom anticoagulation is either contraindicated or ineffectual.

5. Patients who have an IVC filter in place may benefit from anticoagulation to prevent thrombus formation below the filter. Removable IVC filters are under investigation and may be useful for high-risk patients in the future.

PEARLS AND PITFALLS

- Oncology patients: The value of the D-dimer assay in a group of oncology patients was diminished because of an increased pretest probability, with negative predictive value of only 78% in oncology patients versus greater than 90% in the general population.[14]

- Pregnant patients: Warfarin is contraindicated in pregnancy.

- Renal failure: Use of LMWH is not recommended for patients with reduced creatinine clearance unless the clinician can rapidly monitor anti–factor Xa levels.

- Heparin-induced thrombocytopenia: Platelet counts are monitored every 3 to 5 days to evaluate for thrombocytopenia while patients are receiving heparin.[19]

- Consideration for intensive care unit monitoring: The mortality and morbidity in patients with PE are manifestations of extreme hemodynamic compromise and right-sided heart failure. Intensive monitoring of patients during the initial 24 hours of therapy is a reasonable approach.

64

PULMONARY EMBOLISM AND DVT

REFERENCES

[c] 1. Hull RD, Pineo GF. Prophylaxis of deep venous thrombosis and pulmonary embolism: current recommendations. Med Clin North Am 1998; 82(3):477.

[c] 2. Lensing AW et al. Deep-vein thrombosis. Lancet 1999; 353:479.

[b] 3. Stein PD et al. Clinical, laboratory, roentgenographic, and electrocardiographic findings in patients with acute pulmonary embolism and no pre-existing cardiac or pulmonary disease. Chest 1991; 100(3):598.

[c] 4. Kearon C, Ginsberg J, Hirsch J. The role of venous ultrasound in diagnosis of suspected deep venous thrombosis and pulmonary embolism. Ann Intern Med 1998; 128(12):1044.

[a] 5. PIOPED Investigators. Value of the ventilation/perfusion scan in acute pulmonary embolism. JAMA 1990; 263(20):2753.

[d] 6. Myers TM. State of the art: venous thromboembolism. Am J Respir Crit Care Med 1999; 159:1.

[d] 7. American Thoracic Society. The diagnostic approach to acute venous thromboembolism: official statement. Am J Respir Crit Care Med 1999; 160:1043.

[b] 8. Wells P et al. Use of a clinical model for safe management of patients with suspected pulmonary embolism. Ann Intern Med 1998; 129:997.

[b] 9. Eliot CG. Pulmonary physiology during pulmonary embolism. Chest 1992; 101(4):163S.

[c] 10. Goldhaber S. Pulmonary embolism. N Engl J Med 1998; 339(2):93.

[c] 11. Bounameaux H et al. Plasma measurement of D-dimer as diagnostic aid in suspected thromboembolism: an overview. Thromb Haemost 1994; 71:1.

[b] 12. Quinn DA et al. D-dimers in the diagnosis of pulmonary embolism. Am J Respir Crit Care Med 1999; 159:1445.

[b] 13. Kutinsky I, Roche V. Normal D-dimer levels in patients with pulmonary embolism. Arch Intern Med 1999; 159:1569.

[b] 14. Lee A et al. Clinical utility of a rapid whole blood D-dimer assay in patients with cancer who present with suspected acute deep venous thrombosis. Ann Intern Med 1999; 131:417.

[a] 15. Simonneau G et al. A comparison of low-molecular-weight heparin with unfractionated heparin for acute pulmonary embolism. Tinzaparine ou Heparine Standard: Evaluations dans l'Embolie Pulmonaire (THESEE) Study Group. N Engl J Med 1997; 337:663.

[c] 16. Arcasoy S, Kreit J. Thrombolytic therapy of pulmonary embolism: a comprehensive review of current evidence. Chest 1999; 115:1695.

[a] 17. Jerges-Sanchez C et al. Streptokinase and heparin versus heparin alone in massive pulmonary embolism: a European multi-center double blind trial. J Thromb Thrombolysis 1995; 2:227.

[a] 18. Descous H et al. A clinical trial of vena caval filters in the prevention of pulmonary embolism in patients with proximal deep vein thrombosis. N Engl J Med 1998; 338(7):409.

[c] 19. Brieger DB et al. Heparin-induced thrombocytopenia, J Am Coll Cardiol 1998; 31:1339.

Pulmonary Function Tests

Anna Hemnes, MD, Michael J. McWilliams, MD, and Charles Wiener, MD

FAST FACTS

- Obstructive ventilatory defect is defined by a forced expiratory volume in 1 second/forced vital capacity (FEV_1/FVC) ratio of 70% or less.
- Restrictive ventilatory defect is defined by total lung capacity (TLC) of 80% or less of the predicted value.
- Postbronchodilator FEV_1 and age are the most important mortality predictors in chronic obstructive pulmonary disease.[1]
- A diffusion capacity of the lung for carbon monoxide (DLCO) of less than 50% of predicted is predictive of oxygen desaturation with exercise.[2]
- The airways of asthmatic people are 100 to 1000 times more sensitive to bronchoconstricting agents than the airways of normal subjects.[3]

Frequently Used Tests

1. Many pulmonary function tests (PFTs) are available, but this chapter focuses on those most commonly used. A full set of PFTs generally consists of spirometry, helium lung volume measurements, and measurement of the DLCO. Individual values are compared with those predicted by patient height, age, sex, and race. Fig. 65-1 and Table 65-1 illustrate and define the various lung volumes and capacities important in pulmonary function tests.

2. Other tests are available to evaluate the strength of respiratory muscles. The "sniff test" involves the use of fluoroscopy to assess diaphragmatic movement. By having patients inspire or expire against a closed valve, the clinician can assess maximal inspiratory pressure and maximal expiratory pressure. Exercise cardiopulmonary testing is helpful in assessing the functional capacity of the patient and differentiating cardiac from pulmonary causes of dyspnea.[4]

3. The most common indications for PFTs include the evaluation of dyspnea, the evaluation of known lung injury, the monitoring of disease progression, the assessment of response to therapy, preoperative risk assessment, and prognostication. PFTs are not indicated for routine screening of asymptomatic healthy patients.[5] They may have a role in screening certain populations, such as cigarette smokers, for subclinical disease or accelerated progression of lung injury.[6] Daily spirometry has been shown to be useful in the management of acute asthma exacerbations.

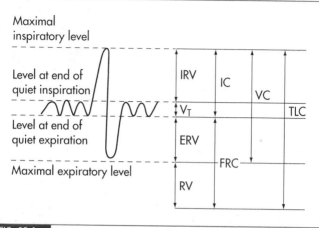

FIG. 65-1

Inspired and expired volumes during normal quiet breathing. Most lung volumes and capacities can be measured by spirometry. (Total lung capacity, functional reserve capacity, and residual volume are not determined by spirometry.) *ERV*, Expiratory reserve volume; *FRC*, functional residual capacity; *IC*, inspiratory capacity; *IRV*, inspiratory reserve capacity; *RV*, residual volume; *TLC*, total lung capacity; *VC*, vital capacity; *V_T*, tidal volume. (From Honig EG, Ingram RH Jr. Functional assessment of the lung and diagnostic techniques. Sci Am WebMD [www.samed.com]. Accessed Jan. 29, 2003.)

I. INTERPRETATION

The basic interpretation of PFTs aims to identify the presence of obstructive ventilatory defects, restrictive ventilatory defects, or gas exchange defects.

A. OBSTRUCTION

1. The hallmark of an obstructive defect is a decrease in the expiratory flow rate; thus spirometry is the best test for its evaluation. First the FEV_1/FVC ratio should be considered. A consensus statement on spirometry put forth in 1994 by the American Thoracic Society (ATS) dictates that establishment of normal values and standardization of interpretation are the job of the director of a PFT laboratory.[7] Therefore, at Johns Hopkins, if the measured ratio is less than 5% of the predicted ratio, obstruction is present. Once obstruction is detected, it must be quantified by a determination of the absolute value of FEV_1 in liters. If the FEV_1 is greater than 2 L, the obstruction is mild; between 1 and 2 L, it is moderate; and less than 1 L, it is severe. If obstruction is present, total lung capacity (TLC) may be greater than normal because of hyperinflation. Vital capacity may be diminished as residual volume (RV) is significantly enlarged because of

TABLE 65-1

PULMONARY FUNCTION TESTS

Test	Technique	Data Obtained
Spirometry	Maximal inhalation followed by maximal exhalation, measuring volume of air and time	FVC, FEV_1, FEV_1/FVC, VC
Flow-volume loops	Same as spirometry, but data are recorded in a graph of flow versus volume	Graphic evaluation of inspiration and expiration
Diffusing capacity of CO	Inhalation of fixed concentration of CO and helium, breath holding for 10 seconds, then expiration with measurement of end tidal CO and helium	Uptake and diffusing capacity of CO
Helium lung volumes	Maximal expiration, then inhalation of a known concentration of helium until steady state is reached	RV, ERV, IRV, TV with calculation of TLC, VC, FRC, IC
Methacholine challenge	Inhalation of increasing doses of methacholine (a bronchoconstrictor) followed by forced exhalation	Effects of a bronchoconstrictor on FEV_1

CO, Carbon monoxide; *ERV*, expiratory reserve volume; *FEV₁*, forced expiratory volume in 1 second; *FRC*, functional reserve capacity; *FVC*, forced vital capacity; *IC*, inspiratory capacity; *IRV*, inspiratory reserve volume; *RV*, residual volume; *TLC*, total lung capacity; *TV*, tidal volume; *VC*, ventilatory capacity.

65

PULMONARY FUNCTION TESTS

air trapping. On flow-volume loops patients with obstruction appear to have a concave expiratory flow pattern with relatively normal inspiration as compared with normal subjects (Fig. 65-2). Frequent causes of obstruction are chronic obstructive pulmonary disease, asthma, cystic fibrosis, and bronchiolitis obliterans.

2. Bronchodilators can be used to differentiate fixed obstruction (e.g., emphysema) from reversible obstruction (e.g., asthma). If FEV_1 or FVC increases by 12% or more *and* an absolute improvement of 200 mL occurs in response to bronchodilation, the obstruction has a reversible component.[8] Most patients who respond to bronchodilators during this test also respond clinically, but many people who have no response to bronchodilators in the pulmonary function laboratory do demonstrate some clinical improvement; thus the decision to treat a patient with bronchodilators remains a clinical one.[9]

3. Intermittent obstruction from bronchospasm may not be manifested as a decrease in FEV_1/FVC if the test is performed at a time when no bronchospasm is present. In this situation methacholine challenge testing is used to assess airway hyperreactivity. If FEV_1 decreases by 20% or more in response to methacholine, bronchial hyperreactivity is present. Not all persons with bronchial hyperreactivity have asthma: up to 50% of people with allergic rhinitis but no asthma symptoms have a positive methacholine challenge test result.[10] However, a

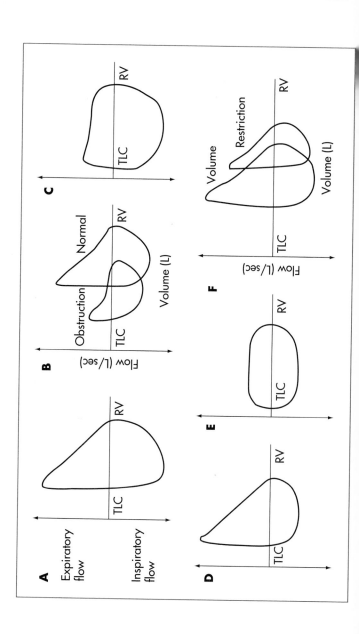

FIG. 65-2

Flow-volume curves. Flow is shown on the ordinate with expiration above and inspiration below the intercept. Volume is shown on the abscissa from left to right from total lung capacity to residual volume. **A,** Normal expiratory flow-volume curve. **B,** In variable extrathoracic obstruction the expiratory flow-volume curve has a scooped-out appearance resulting from progressive decreases in flow as lung volume becomes smaller. Obstruction is volume dependent. Flow rates at any given lung volume (isovolumic flow) are reduced. Because of air trapping, the entire curve may be shifted to a higher lung volume (leftward). This pattern is typical of chronic obstructive pulmonary disease of asthma. **C,** Expiratory flow-volume curve showing a decreased flow that is the same at all lung volumes. Obstruction, which is not dependent on lung volume, is caused by upper airway obstruction, not disease of the lung parenchyma. **D,** Disproportionate reduction of inspiration airflow is indicative of variable extrathoracic upper airway obstruction. **E,** Fixed airway obstruction, the site of which is undetermined, shows volume-independent reduction of flow in both inspiration and expiration. **F,** Expiratory flow-volume curve in a patient with a restrictive disorder. Isovolumic flow rates are increased, whereas the volume axis is compressed and shifted toward lower volume (rightward). *RV,* Residual volume; *TLC,* total lung capacity. *(From Honig EG, Ingram RH Jr. Functional assessment of the lung and diagnostic techniques. Sci Am WebMD [www.samed.com]. Accessed Jan. 29, 2003.)*

PULMONARY FUNCTION TESTS

65

normal methacholine test result has a negative predictive value of 95% if no bronchodilators were used before the test.

4. Flow-volume loops can be helpful in localizing and characterizing an obstruction. Extrathoracic obstructions can be differentiated from intrathoracic obstructions by the presence of truncated inspiratory curves. Comparisons of various curves can help to differentiate fixed from variable obstructions. Fig. 65-2 illustrates examples of variable and fixed intrathoracic and extrathoracic obstructive flow-volume loops.

B. RESTRICTION

1. The hallmark of a restrictive defect is decreased lung volumes. To evaluate a patient for restriction, the physician should first look at TLC. If the TLC is less than 80% of the predicted value, restriction is present. Between 65% and 80% the restrictive ventilatory defect is mild, between 50% and 65% it is moderate, and at less than 50% it is severe. The other lung volume measurements (RV, FRC) may suggest cause of the restriction. A decrease in FRC suggests either a noncompliant lung or a chest wall pathological condition (e.g., morbid obesity or kyphoscoliosis). RV, which mainly measures airway closure in adults, is normal in association with chest wall disease, decreased with parenchymal lung disease and large pleural effusions, and increased with neuromuscular disease (e.g., amyotrophic lateral sclerosis). In cases of parenchymal lung disease causing restriction (e.g., interstitial lung disease), TLC, RV, and FRC generally all decrease proportionally. A restrictive ventilatory defect with a normal FRC should raise suspicion for neuromuscular disease.

C. GAS TRANSFER

1. Carbon monoxide (CO) has a high affinity for hemoglobin, so it has a virtually unlimited reservoir in the pulmonary vascular bed and the pressure gradient for CO diffusion depends solely on the partial pressure of CO in the alveolus. Thus resistance to diffusion depends on the resistance across the alveolar-capillary membrane. Common causes of low DLCO include interstitial lung disease (hypothetically as the result of scarring of alveolar-capillary units with loss of alveolar architecture) and emphysema (because of the loss of gas transfer surface area). Other causes of decreased DLCO include congestive heart failure with pulmonary edema, pulmonary hypertension, and pulmonary embolism. DLCO can be increased in patients with polycythemia (because of increased volume for diffusion of CO), pulmonary hemorrhage (because of increased extravascular blood volume), early congestive heart failure (because of increased pulmonary blood volume), and left-to-right cardiac shunts.[11]

PEARLS AND PITFALLS

- Abnormal PFT results in obese patients have been shown to be indicative of intrinsic respiratory dysfunction and not merely secondary to obesity, except in the morbidly obese.[12]

- Based on the test descriptions, it is clear that patient effort greatly affects the results of PFTs and is an important determinant of accuracy and reproducibility. In general, patients need to be alert and cooperative for the measurements to be obtained. Standards put forth by the ATS are used by the technicians in the PFT laboratory, and each test result will be accompanied by a statement about the quality of the test: good, fair, or poor.[13] Fair- and poor-quality tests should be interpreted with caution. To obtain a high-quality test, the examiner should encourage patients to participate to the best of their ability.
- Since age, gender, race, and especially height affect normal values, selection of the appropriate reference values is imperative. The ATS has published guidelines for selecting such values,[5] and in general the lower limit of normal ranges should be used.[8]

REFERENCES

[b] 1. Anthonisen NR et al. Prognosis in chronic obstructive pulmonary disease. Am Rev Respir Dis 1986; 133:14.

[b] 2. Owens GR. The diffusing capacity as a predictor of arterial oxygen desaturation during exercise in patients with COPD. N Engl J Med 1984; 310:1218.

[c] 3. Braman SS, Corrao WM. Bronchoprovocation testing. Clin Chest Med 1989; 10:165.

[c] 4. McKelvie RS, Jones NL. Cardiopulmonary exercise testing. Clin Chest Med 1989; 10:277.

[d] 5. Screening for adult respiratory disease: official American Thoracic Society statement, March 1983. Am Rev Respir Dis 1983; 128:768.

[b] 6. Camilli AE et al. Longitudinal changes in forced expiratory volume in one second in adults: effects of smoking and smoking cessation. Am Rev Respir Dis 1987; 135:794.

[d] 7. American Thoracic Society. Standardization of spirometry. Am J Respir Crit Care Med 1995; 152:1107.

[d] 8. American Thoracic Society. Lung function testing: selection of reference values and interpretative strategies. Am Rev Respir Dis 1991; 144:1202.

[c] 9. Crapo RO. Pulmonary-function testing. N Engl J Med 1994; 331:25.

[a] 10. Braman SS et al. Airway hyperresponsiveness in allergic rhinitis. Chest 1987; 91:671.

[c] 11. Weinberger SE et al. Use and interpretation of the single-breath diffusing capacity. Chest 1980; 78:483.

[b] 12. Ray CA et al. Effects of obesity on respiratory function. Am Rev Respir Dis 1983; 128:501.

[d] 13. American Thoracic Society. Standardization of spirometry—1987 update: statement of the American Thoracic Society. Am Rev Respir Dis 1987; 136:1285.

Pulmonary Hypertension

*Hunter C. Champion, MD, PhD, Reda Girgis, MD,
and Sean P. Gaine, MD, PhD*

FAST FACTS

66

- Pulmonary hypertension can be divided into five categories.
  - Pulmonary hypertension associated with disorders of the respiratory system or hypoxemia.
  - Pulmonary venous hypertension.
  - Chronic thromboembolic disease.
  - Pulmonary arterial hypertension.
  - Pulmonary hypertension caused by disorders directly affecting the pulmonary vasculature.
- All forms of pulmonary hypertension have similar characteristic pathological changes, including in situ thrombosis, smooth muscle hypertrophy, and intimal proliferation.
- In the diagnostic workup of pulmonary hypertension, initial testing should include the following.
  - Echocardiogram.
  - Chest radiograph.
  - Ventilation-perfusion ($\dot{V}/\dot{Q}$) scan or pulmonary angiogram.
  - Sleep study.
  - Serological testing to rule out secondary forms of pulmonary hypertension.
  - Catheterization of the right side of the heart is essential to confirm diagnosis, determine prognosis, and assign therapy.
- Therapy.
  - Calcium channel blocker therapy.
  - Continuous intravenous epoprostenol in patients with advanced pulmonary hypertension.
  - Lung transplantation in patients in whom maximal medical therapy fails.
- Management of patients with advanced pulmonary hypertension on the ward can be difficult. Great care should be taken to avoid agents that can lower systemic arterial pressure, such as sedatives, especially benzodiazepines, and sympatholytic drugs.
- Maintenance therapy with calcium channel blockers or prostacyclin infusion must not be interrupted.

I. EPIDEMIOLOGY

1. Pulmonary hypertension comprises a relatively rare group of diseases that result in elevated pulmonary arterial pressure and right-sided heart failure. With the recent awareness of the disease entity, the

widespread use of less invasive diagnostic techniques, and the improvements in treatment modalities, however, the diagnosis of pulmonary hypertension is being made more frequently at the primary care level. The World Symposium on Primary Pulmonary Hypertension in 1998 divided the causes of pulmonary hypertension into five distinct categories (Box 66-1).

2. Disorders of the respiratory system and hypoxemia result in pulmonary hypertension, either because of parenchymal destruction or because

---

BOX 66-1

CLASSIFICATION OF PULMONARY HYPERTENSION

PULMONARY ARTERIAL HYPERTENSION

Primary pulmonary hypertension
  Sporadic
  Familial
Pulmonary arterial hypertension related to the following:
  Collagen-vascular disease (scleroderma, lupus, rheumatoid arthritis)
  Congenital systemic-to-pulmonary shunts (Eisenmenger's syndrome)
  Portoprimary hypertension
  Human immunodeficiency virus infection
  Drugs and toxins (fenfluramine, L-tryptophan, indomethacin, H_2 inhibitors, oral contraceptives, bush tea, ragwort)

PULMONARY HYPERTENSION ASSOCIATED WITH DISORDERS OF THE RESPIRATORY SYSTEM OR HYPOXEMIA

Parenchymal lung disease
  Chronic obstructive pulmonary disease
  Interstitial pulmonary fibrosis
  Cystic fibrosis
Chronic alveolar hypoxemia
  Exposure to long-term low oxygen tension such as at high altitudes

PULMONARY HYPERTENSION CAUSED BY CHRONIC THROMBOTIC OR EMBOLIC DISEASE

Thromboembolic obstruction of proximal pulmonary arteries
Obstruction of distal pulmonary arteries

PULMONARY VENOUS HYPERTENSION

Mitral valve disease
Chronic left ventricular dysfunction
Pulmonary venoocclusion disease

PULMONARY HYPERTENSION CAUSED BY DISORDERS DIRECTLY AFFECTING THE PULMONARY VASCULATURE

Inflammation
Pulmonary capillary hemangiomatosis

of $\dot{V}/\dot{Q}$ mismatching and chronic alveolar hypoxia. An elevation in left atrial pressure would be expected to cause a similar rise in the upstream pulmonary artery pressure simply by backward transmission resulting in pulmonary venous hypertension.

3. Pulmonary hypertension can result when chronic thrombotic or embolic disease, including a variety of emboli, such as thromboemboli, tumor emboli, or *Schistosoma mansoni* ova, leads to pulmonary vascular occlusion. Although the vast majority of patients who survive an acute pulmonary embolism recover completely, chronic thromboembolic pulmonary hypertension occurs in some patients (<1%) whose vascular obstruction is not effectively removed. In these patients recanalized residua remain, narrowing or obstructing the pulmonary vascular bed, which results in chronic pulmonary hypertension.

4. Disorders directly affecting the pulmonary vasculature, such as capillary hemangiomatosis, or inflammatory conditions, such as sarcoidosis, can also lead to pulmonary hypertension. Recently a form of familial pulmonary hypertension was shown to be related to mutations in the bone morphogenic protein-II gene, which is related to the TGF-β family.[1]

5. Pulmonary arterial hypertension (PAH) produces characteristic abnormalities in the wall of small distal pulmonary arteries. These abnormalities involve narrowing of the vessel lumen, smooth muscle hypertrophy, and intimal proliferation.[2-6]

II. CLINICAL PRESENTATION

1. Patients with pulmonary hypertension generally have nonspecific symptoms. Symptoms directly attributable to pulmonary hypertension, however, include dyspnea on exertion, fatigue, chest pain, syncope with exertion, and lethargy. Fatigue, lethargy, and syncopal symptoms generally reflect the inability to increase cardiac output in order to overcome the vascular obstruction of the pulmonary arterioles during stress or exercise. Less common symptoms include cough, hemoptysis, and hoarseness caused by impingement on the left recurrent laryngeal nerve by a dilated main pulmonary artery.[5]

2. Physical examination findings can detect the presence of pulmonary hypertension and right ventricular hypertrophy in early disease, as well as right ventricular failure in more advanced forms of disease. As pulmonary arterial pressure increases, a more pronounced pulmonic component to the second heart sound (P_2) is manifested. This P_2 can be palpable in advanced disease. Auscultation usually reveals a systolic ejection murmur consistent with tricuspid regurgitation. With more advanced disease a diastolic regurgitation murmur is sometimes detected. A prominent A wave in the jugular venous pulse, associated with the right-sided fourth heart sound, characterizes the right ventricular hypertrophy. In the right-sided heart failure of advanced

66

PULMONARY HYPERTENSION

disease, systemic venous hypertension is characterized by more significant tricuspid regurgitation, a resulting prominent V wave of the jugular pulsation, peripheral edema, and hepatic congestion. The jugular venous pressure may be difficult to determine in patients with advanced, decompensated disease because the top of the internal jugular vein may be present above the level of the jawline.[2,5]

III. DIAGNOSIS

1. The diagnostic evaluation of a patient with suspected pulmonary hypertension seeks to categorize patients into one of the five distinct categories (Box 66-2). In this treatment-based classification system the underlying causes of the pulmonary hypertension are ascertained to guide therapy.

A. ELECTROCARDIOGRAPHY

1. The electrocardiogram may demonstrate signs of right ventricular hypertrophy or strain.
2. Findings in patients with chronic right ventricular overload may include right axis deviation, an R/S ratio greater than 1 in lead V_1, increased P wave amplitude in lead II (P pulmonale) as a result of right atrial enlargement, incomplete or complete right bundle branch block, or any combination of these.
3. These findings tend to have high specificity but low sensitivity.

BOX 66-2

STUDIES TO EVALUATE SUSPECTED PULMONARY HYPERTENSION AND RULE OUT SECONDARY CAUSES

Echocardiogram
    Estimation of right ventricular systolic pressure
    Left ventricular function
    Systemic-to-pulmonary shunt
Chest radiograph and pulmonary function tests
    Chronic obstructive pulmonary disease
    Interstitial pulmonary fibrosis
    Abnormalities of the thoracic cage
Ventilation-perfusion scan or pulmonary angiogram
    Chronic thromboembolic disease
Sleep study
    Obstructive sleep apnea
Blood tests
    Serological tests (antinuclear antibodies, human immunodeficiency virus)
        Lupus, scleroderma, rheumatoid arthritis, human immunodeficiency virus–associated pulmonary hypertension
    Liver function tests
        Portopulmonary hypertension

B. TWO-DIMENSIONAL ECHOCARDIOGRAPHY

1. An echocardiogram provides an estimate of pulmonary artery pressure and reveals left ventricular dysfunction, mitral valve disease, or evidence of congenital heart disease as a cause for the pulmonary hypertension. Stress on the right side of the heart initially results in hyperkinesis. As the disease progresses, however, right ventricular hypokinesis ensues.

2. Tricuspid regurgitation, a secondary manifestation of dilation of the right ventricle and tricuspid annulus, is used to estimate right ventricular systolic pressure by Doppler examination.

3. The use of echocardiography and Doppler imaging is a sensitive method of diagnosing pulmonary hypertension, since right ventricular systolic pressure (RVSP) generally approximates pulmonary artery pressure. However, RVSP estimation by this method usually underestimates the RVSP (by as much as 20%) when correlated with pressures obtained during catheterization of the right side of the heart.

C. CHEST RADIOGRAPHY

1. The chest radiographs of patients with pulmonary hypertension usually show enlargement of the central pulmonary arteries and attenuation of the peripheral vessels, resulting in oligemic lung fields.

2. Right ventricular and right atrial dilation are observed on chest radiographs in later stages of disease and result in a decrease in the retrosternal space on the lateral view.

3. Other signs of chronic obstructive pulmonary disease and thoracic cage abnormalities can also be observed on chest radiographs.

D. PULMONARY FUNCTION TESTS

1. A full set of pulmonary function tests (spirometry, lung volumes, and diffusing capacity) demonstrates parenchymal lung diseases, pulmonary fibrosis, emphysema, or thoracic cage abnormalities as a cause for the pulmonary hypertension.

2. Only severe interstitial lung disease (lung volume <50% of predicted) results in pulmonary hypertension. Moreover, a mildly restrictive pattern can be caused by pulmonary hypertension itself.

E. SLEEP STUDY

1. In patients who are overweight and have a history of loud snoring and hypersomnolence, a sleep study is performed to rule out obstructive sleep apnea, a potentially reversible cause of pulmonary hypertension.

F. PULMONARY VENTILATION/PERFUSION SCAN

1. All patients with pulmonary hypertension should have a $\dot{V}/\dot{Q}$ scan to rule out thromboembolic disease.

2. If the results of the $\dot{V}/\dot{Q}$ scan are abnormal, pulmonary angiography and spiral chest computed tomography (CT) with contrast dye are obtained to define the extent of the disease and explore the feasibility of thromboendarterectomy surgery. Spiral chest CT with contrast

66

PULMONARY HYPERTENSION

media alone is not adequate to rule out chronic thromboembolic disease.

G. LUNG BIOPSY AND SEROLOGICAL TESTING

1. Lung biopsy is rarely necessary, generally poorly tolerated by patients with severe pulmonary hypertension, and reserved for cases in which the clinical diagnosis is unclear.
2. A number of blood tests, including those for antinuclear antibody, rheumatoid factor, and human immunodeficiency virus (HIV), are performed to look for causes of PAH. HIV infection is associated with the development of PAH, with a frequency estimated at 0.5%, that is clinically and pathologically indistinguishable from primary pulmonary hypertension (PPH).
3. Portal hypertension is associated with the development of pulmonary hypertension, a condition called portopulmonary hypertension. The presence of portal hypertension may be demonstrated on abdominal imaging using Doppler ultrasonography or by obtaining the hepatic wedge pressure at the time of catheterization.[2,5]

IV. MANAGEMENT

A. SECONDARY PULMONARY HYPERTENSION

1. The diagnostic evaluation for patients with suspected pulmonary hypertension (Box 66-2) allows for the categorization of patients based on the treatment-oriented classification (Box 66-1). Once the pulmonary hypertension has been classified, attention can be focused on treating the underlying disease in an effort to attenuate the pulmonary hypertension.
2. In patients with a disorder of the respiratory system, such as emphysema, the underlying disease is treated with long-term oxygen therapy, steroids, and bronchodilator therapy when appropriate to reduce the pulmonary artery pressure. Similarly, if a patient has pulmonary venous disease caused by left ventricular dysfunction, afterload reduction and diuretics are administered in an effort to reduce left atrial pressure and thus pulmonary artery pressure.
3. Patients with mitral valve disease are considered for valve repair or replacement to reduce the chronically elevated left atrial pressure. In patients with long-standing mitral valve disease, however, repair or replacement of the valve might not correct the pulmonary hypertension. The mechanism for this retained pulmonary hypertension phenotype is not well understood.
4. Chronic thromboembolic pulmonary hypertension requires lifelong anticoagulation therapy, an inferior vena cava filter, and possibly a thromboendarterectomy to restore luminal patency and reduce pulmonary vascular resistance.[2-6]

B. PULMONARY ARTERIAL HYPERTENSION

1. Early in the course of PAH the pathological features of the predominant lesion are smooth muscle hypertrophy and vasoconstriction.

During this stage of the disease, treatment with oral vasodilator therapy relaxes the vascular smooth muscle and reduces pulmonary vascular resistance. Later in the disease the proliferative features predominate, leaving no room for conventional vasodilator therapy. Unfortunately, more than 75% of individuals with PAH are in the proliferative or irreversible stage at the time of presentation, probably because of delayed diagnosis. Right-sided heart catheterization and a trial with a short-acting pulmonary vasodilator are used to determine into which of these treatment category patients should fall.[2]

2. Right-sided heart catheterization yields three important pieces of information. First, it confirms the presence of elevated pressure and the absence of pulmonary venous hypertension by demonstrating a normal pulmonary capillary wedge pressure (~15 mm Hg). Second, hemodynamic measurements can predict survival in patients with PPH. For example, an individual with PPH and a right atrial pressure greater than 20 mm Hg has a median survival of 4 weeks without treatment, according to the National Institutes of Health registry. Similarly, if the cardiac index is less than 2 L/min, median life expectancy is about 1 year. This information is used to predict a patient's life expectancy by combining the right atrial pressure, cardiac index, and mean pulmonary artery pressure. Right-sided heart catheterization allows determination of the most appropriate therapy when performed in conjunction with a vasodilator trial. A safe, short-acting vasodilator should be used for the trial. The most ideal vasodilator is inhaled nitric oxide (NO). Inhaled NO is specific for the pulmonary vascular bed and has no effect on the systemic circulation because once the inhaled NO reaches the bloodstream, its actions are quenched by hemoglobin. Adenosine or intravenously administered epoprostenol can also be used in this diagnostic test.[2]

3. The right-sided heart catheterization and vasodilator trial help determine whether a patient is an acute responder, with decreased pulmonary vascular tone because of vasodilation, or a nonresponder, with more fixed and irreversible disease. What constitutes a positive acute response is controversial, but it is generally agreed that a drop in the mean pulmonary artery pressure by greater than 10 mm Hg with either no change or an increase in cardiac output suggests a significant degree of reversibility. A reduction in pulmonary vascular resistance (PVR) of more than 20% is also used as a measure of response to the vasodilator trial. However, the implications of an acute reduction in PVR resulting from an increased cardiac output without a decrease in pulmonary artery pressure is controversial. Therefore the definition of a responder in terms of pressure change rather than PVR is currently favored. For patients who demonstrate a positive response during the vasodilator trial, long-term oral vasodilator therapy with calcium channel blockers (i.e., amlodipine, diltiazem, or nifedipine) may be carefully initiated (Fig. 66-1). Treatment is started

66

PULMONARY HYPERTENSION

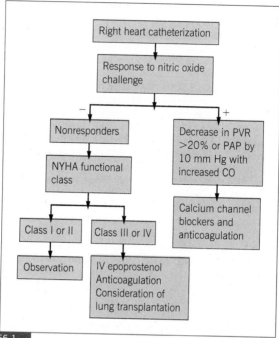

FIG. 66-1

Treatment of pulmonary arterial hypertension. *CO,* Cardiac output; *NYHA,* New York Heart Association; *PAP,* pulmonary artery pressure; *PVR,* pulmonary vascular resistance.

with a low dose and cautiously advanced to higher doses as tolerated, often to very high doses, with close monitoring of patient symptoms and systemic blood pressure. The systemic blood pressure should remain stable in responders while the decrease in pulmonary vascular resistance improves filling of the left side of the heart and restores the cardiac output.[2]

4. Patients with New York Heart Association (NYHA) class III or IV symptoms, who are found to be nonresponders during the acute vasodilator trial, are considered for continuous epoprostenol therapy. Intravenous prostacyclin therapy has been evaluated in several key trials, with follow-up of 16 months in the second trial. Benefits were seen in exercise capacity and pulmonary vascular resistance.[7,8] The paradox of epoprostenol therapy is that patients who do not respond to it during acute testing may respond to it over the long term, resulting in improved survival and hemodynamics in PPH. Epoprostenol slowly

decreases the pulmonary vascular resistance in pulmonary arteries previously believed to be "irreversible" and stiff as the result of proliferation. A recent randomized trial confirmed the benefits of epoprostenol therapy in patients with pulmonary hypertension associated with the scleroderma spectrum of disease, although a beneficial effect on mortality was not demonstrated.[9] However, epoprostenol therapy is currently approved by the Food and Drug Administration only for patients with a diagnosis of PPH and PAH associated with the scleroderma spectrum of diseases.[2]

5. Epoprostenol therapy is not suitable for pulmonary hypertension caused by conditions other than those listed under the classification "pulmonary artery hypertension" (Box 66-1). In patients with significant parenchymal lung disease, considerable shunting and increased oxygen requirements may develop during continuous epoprostenol therapy as blood flow to poorly ventilated regions improves. Acute pulmonary edema may develop during epoprostenol therapy in patients with pulmonary venous hypertension; therefore this treatment is contraindicated when the pulmonary capillary wedge pressure is elevated (>15 mm Hg). Generally, epoprostenol therapy is reserved for patients with PAH with normal lung parenchyma and left-sided heart function.

6. Inhaled iloprost has been studied for the treatment of PPH with good effect on exercise tolerance and NYHA class. The endpoint of this trial was 12 weeks, so long-term data are not yet available.[10]

7. Sildenafil is an emerging treatment for pulmonary hypertension. In a small randomized trial its use led to acute hemodynamic benefits in pulmonary hypertension. Sildenafil is not FDA approved for this indication.[11]

8. Bosentan, an endothelin-1 antagonist, is under intense investigation as a therapy for pulmonary hypertension. Because endothelin-1 is a potent vasoconstrictor, inhibition of this substance could lead to hemodynamic improvement in constricted pulmonary vasculature. A placebo-controlled trial has demonstrated the effectiveness of this oral medication in pulmonary hypertension (primary or associated with connective tissue disease).[12]

9. A number of adjunctive therapies are used in pulmonary hypertension. A retrospective analysis and a nonrandomized, prospective study suggest that anticoagulation increases survival in patients with PPH. Unless a contraindication exists, patients should undergo anticoagulation with warfarin in doses adjusted to achieve an international normalized ratio of approximately 2.0. Diuretics are important in the treatment of right ventricular dilation and failure. Although acute right ventricular failure in the setting of a right-sided myocardial infarct requires aggressive volume resuscitation, the high-pressure loaded right ventricle generally responds well to a cautious reduction in its volume. The dilated, pressure- and volume-loaded right ventricle com-

66

PULMONARY HYPERTENSION

presses the intraventricular septum, resulting in a reduction in left ventricular volume. In general the diuresis should be slow, 1 to 2 pounds (0.5-1.0 kg) a day, with close attention to renal function. Cardiac glycosides may produce a modest increase in cardiac output in patients with PPH and right ventricular failure, as well as a significant reduction in circulating norepinephrine levels. In patients with borderline systemic blood pressure, low-dose dopamine can maintain systemic blood pressure while enhancing natriuresis and also may be administered on a long-term basis as a bridge to lung transplantation.[2,5,6]

10. Single or bilateral lung transplantation is performed for patients who have not responded to medical therapy for pulmonary hypertension. Right ventricular dysfunction improves significantly on restoration of normal pulmonary vascular resistance. Heart-lung transplantation is reserved for patients with significant heart disease on the left side or complicated structural abnormalities associated with congenital heart disease. The 5-year survival rate after lung transplantation is between 45% and 50%.[2]

PEARLS AND PITFALLS

- Patients with pulmonary hypertension can pose a special problem to the house officer. Since the physiology and pathophysiology in pulmonary hypertension are reversed (i.e., the right ventricle is the dominant ventricle), great care must be taken because conventional treatment for congestive heart failure may prove disastrous in this patient population. The perils of negatively inotropic systemic vasodilators in patients with pulmonary hypertension are important to emphasize. There is a significant chance that in the majority of patients (approximately 75%) with PAH the pulmonary artery pressure will not respond to an acute vasodilator trial because of the advanced proliferative, irreversible pathological feature that is prevalent at presentation. On the other hand, the systemic blood pressure can be predicted with certainty to decrease eventually in all patients given a sufficient dose of these systemic vasodilators. Right ventricular coronary perfusion will be compromised as the systemic blood pressure drops while pulmonary pressures remain elevated, resulting in right ventricular ischemia. Moreover, in the confines of the pericardium, both ventricles are vying for dominance. The marked right ventricular dilation seen in severe pulmonary hypertension is in sharp contrast to the small underfilled and compressed left ventricle. Furthermore, the intraventricular septum moves paradoxically to the left during systole, so a decrease in left ventricular afterload and reduction in systemic blood pressure must be avoided. Therefore an abrupt decrease in left ventricular pressure by the empirical use of a calcium channel blocker can be disastrous.[2]

- Great care must be exercised when adding concomitant medications to the treatment of patients with pulmonary hypertension. Use of vasoconstricting agents, such as nasal decongestants, should be avoided. Sedation, when required, should be administered with caution, avoiding any agents known to decrease systemic blood pressure. Transfusion with platelets or fresh frozen plasma is often poorly tolerated because of the combination of a significant volume load and the presence of vasoactive compounds, such as thromboxane and serotonin, in these products. Use of agents that interfere with warfarin or potentiate the degree of anticoagulation should be avoided.[2]

- As important as caution is with regard to instituting new therapies, equal care must be taken when patients are already receiving treatment for pulmonary hypertension at presentation. Once calcium channel blockers have been successfully initiated in a patient with pulmonary hypertension, abrupt discontinuation can result in syncope and death because of rebound pulmonary hypertension. Therefore this pharmacotherapeutic regimen must be maintained and not abruptly stopped. This is especially true with patients receiving intravenous prostacyclin therapy. Abrupt discontinuation of the drug, even if only for a few seconds, can lead to syncope and death. Should central access be lost while the patient is in the hospital ward, intravenous prostacyclin can be administered via a peripheral vein until central access is again achieved.[2]

REFERENCES

[a] 1. Lane KB et al. Heterozygous germline mutations in BMPR-II are the cause of familial primary pulmonary hypertension. Nature Genet 2000; 26:81.

[a] 2. Gaine S. Pulmonary hypertension. JAMA 2000; 284:3160.

[b] 3. Gailie N et al. Primary pulmonary hypertension: insights into pathogenesis from epidemiology. Chest 1998; 114:184S.

[a] 4. Gaine S, Rubin L. Primary pulmonary hypertension. Lancet 1998; 352:719.

[b] 5. Brij S, Peacock AJ. Pulmonary hypertension: its assessment and treatment. Thorax 1999; 54:S28.

[a] 6. Rubin LJ. Primary pulmonary hypertension. N Engl J Med 1997; 336:111.

[b] 7. McLaughlin VV et al. Reduction in pulmonary vascular resistance with long-term epoprostenol (prostacyclin) therapy in primary pulmonary hypertension. N Engl J Med 1998; 338:273.

[a] 8. Barst RJ et al. A comparison of continuous intravenous epoprostenol (prostacyclin) with conventional therapy for primary pulmonary hypertension. N Engl J Med 1996; 334:296.

[a] 9. Badesch DB et al. Continuous intravenous epoprostenol for pulmonary hypertension due to the scleroderma spectrum of disease: a randomized, controlled trial. Ann Intern Med 2000; 132(6):425.

[a] 10. Hoeper MM et al. Long-term treatment of primary pulmonary hypertension with aerosolized iloprost, a prostacyclin analogue. N Engl J Med 200; 342:1866.

[a] 11. Ghofrani HA et al. Sildenafil for treatment of lung fibrosis and pulmonary hypertension: a randomized controlled trial. Lancet 2002; 360(9337):895.

[a] 12. Rubin LJ, Badesch DB, Barst RJ. Bosentan therapy for pulmonary arterial hypertension. N Engl J Med 2002; 346:896.

Pulse Oximetry and Arterial Blood Gas Interpretation

Majd Mouded, MD, Todd C. Pulerwitz, MD, and Henry E. Fessler, MD

Fast Facts

- Oxygen (O_2) content is determined mainly by hemoglobin (Hb) concentration and saturation.
- Pulse oximetry is a useful clinical tool as long as its limitations are understood.
- Cooximetry is the gold standard for determining Hb saturation.
- Blood analysis provides the most comprehensive evaluation of the effectiveness of gas exchange.
- Venous samples may be useful in certain clinical situations.

Blood is involved in the transport of both O_2 and carbon dioxide (CO_2) to and from the tissues and lungs. It is the disturbance of this process that results in many cardiopulmonary diseases. Understanding the differences between O_2-carrying capacity, O_2 saturation, partial pressure of O_2 (Po_2), and partial pressure of CO_2 (Pco_2) is a prerequisite to understanding how successfully O_2 is delivered to and CO_2 is removed from the tissues. This chapter explains how O_2-carrying capacity is determined and how its components are measured. In addition, we briefly discuss CO_2 transport in the blood. Pertinent clinical situations are discussed that may affect the accuracy of measured O_2 saturation and arterial partial pressure of O_2 (Pao_2). Issues regarding the specific causes of hypoxia, hypercarbia, and acid-base status are beyond the scope of this chapter and are discussed elsewhere.

I. OXYGEN TRANSPORT

1. O_2 is carried in the blood by two main mechanisms. The first involves plasma, in which O_2 can be dissolved, although its solubility in plasma is quite low. The concentration of O_2 in plasma can be calculated with the following equation:

   Concentration of O_2 (mL O_2/L plasma) = 0.03 (mL/L mm Hg) × Po_2 (mm Hg) = 0.003 (mL/dL mm Hg) × Po_2 (mm Hg)

2. Thus at a Pao_2 of 100 mm Hg each liter of blood will carry approximately 3 mL of O_2 in solution. Obviously this is inadequate to meet the O_2 demands of the body (resting O_2 consumption is approximately 250 mL/min). Therefore the second and more important means of O_2 transportation is by Hb.

3. Hb is a tetrameric protein found in red blood cells. It consists of four iron (Fe^{2+})-containing heme groups (two α- and two β-chains), which

can each bind one molecule of O_2. Three physiological properties of Hb are important.

a. Reversible binding with O_2: Ferrous iron would normally irreversibly oxidize into a ferric iron group (Fe^{3+}) in air (rust). However, the globin chains in Hb prevent this from occurring.

b. O_2 can associate and dissociate quickly. This enables complete transfer in the short time that the red blood cells are in the capillaries.

c. Cooperative binding: The binding of O_2 to one heme group facilitates binding of subsequent O_2 molecules.[1,2] In its deoxygenated state, Hb is in a T (tense) form. The binding of O_2 breaks salt bridges in the Hb molecule and changes Hb to a lower energy or R (relaxed) form.[3] This change facilitates O_2 binding to the Hb molecule. Conversely, O_2 has more difficulty binding Hb when no heme groups are bound. This results in a sigmoid oxyhemoglobin dissociation curve as illustrated in Fig. 67-1.

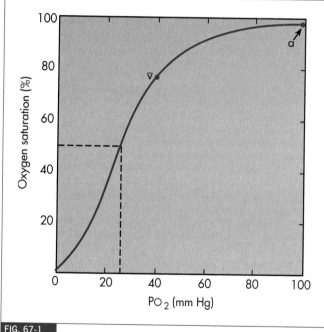

FIG. 67-1

Hemoglobin (Hb) dissociation curve. The dotted line represents the P_{50}, or the value at which Hb is 50% saturated. This curve applies for hemoglobin A at $[H^+] = 40$ nmol/L (pH = 7.40), temperature = 37° C, and 2,3-DPG = 15 μmol/g Hb. (From Berne RM, Levy MN: Physiology, 4th ed. St Louis: Mosby; 1998.)

4. The pressure of O_2 in its solvent serves as the driving force for O_2 binding. At a Pao_2 of 100 mm Hg the O_2 saturation of Hb molecules is approximately 97.4%. Since Hb is nearly completely saturated, little additional O_2 can be bound to Hb with a further increase in Po_2 (Fig. 67-1).

5. Temperature, hydrogen ion concentration, Pco_2, and 2,3-diphosphoglycerate (a by-product of anaerobic metabolism) influence the affinity of O_2 for Hb.[4] If the levels of any of these variables increase in the blood, the curve shifts to the right. This results in a decreased affinity of O_2 for the Hb molecule, releasing more O_2 to the tissue. If these levels decrease, the dissociation curve moves leftward and O_2 is more tightly bound to Hb. Therefore less O_2 is released at the systemic capillary beds. The relative effect of pH fluctuations is more significant than comparable changes in CO_2.[5] All these factors combine to shift the dissociation curve without altering its basic shape (Fig. 67-2).

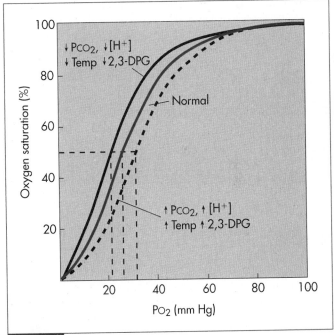

FIG. 67-2

Hemoglobin (Hb) dissociation curve changes in affinity. Increased Pco_2, H^+, temperature, and 2,3-DPG decrease Hb affinity and cause a shift to the right. Lowered levels increase Hb affinity and shift the curve to the left. *(From Berne RM, Levy MN: Physiology, 4th ed. St Louis: Mosby; 1998.)*

67

PULSE OXIMETRY AND ABG INTERPRETATION

6. Blood O_2 concentration is the sum of both dissolved and bound O_2. When 100% saturated, each gram of Hb in an adult can bind 1.34 mL of O_2.[6] Therefore the total concentration of O_2 in blood is derived by the following equation:

$$Cao_2 \text{ (mL/dL)} = (1.34 \times Hb \text{ [g/dL]} \times Sao_2) + (0.003 \times Pao_2 \text{ [mm Hg]})$$

7. Hb concentration is expressed in units of g/dL, while the saturation of Hb is calculated from the O_2 desaturation curve and expressed as a percentage. The impact of 50% reduction in each factor is illustrated in Table 67-1.

8. Both Hb quantity (Table 67-1) and saturation (Table 67-2) are more important for determining O_2 concentration than is Pao_2 because of the relative insignificance of dissolved O_2 in plasma. Changes in Hb concentration or saturation change the O_2 concentration by almost an equal magnitude. In contrast to the situation with Sao_2, relatively little change in the O_2 concentration occurs with changes in Pao_2 until the steep slope of the equilibrium curve is reached and significant Hb desaturation occurs (Table 67-2).

TABLE 67-1

INFLUENCE OF ANEMIA ON OXYGEN CONCENTRATION

Parameter	Normal	Hypoxemia	Anemia
Pao_2 (mm Hg)	90.0	45.0	90.0
Sao_2 (%)	98.0	80.0	98.0
Hemoglobin (g/dL)	15.0	15.0	7.50
Cao_2 (mL/dL)	20.0	16.3	10.1
Percent change in Cao_2		18.6	49.5

Data from Marino PL. The ICU book, 2nd ed. Baltimore: Williams & Wilkins; 1998.

TABLE 67-2

INFLUENCE OF SATURATION ON OXYGEN CONCENTRATION

Parameter	Decrease in Pao_2 Without Desaturation	Decrease in Pao_2 with Desaturation
Initial Pao_2 (mm Hg)	100.00	60.00
Pao_2 after decrease (mm Hg)	90.00	50.00
Initial Sao_2 (%)	0.99	0.92
Sao_2 after decrease (%)	0.98	0.84
Hemoglobin (g/dL)	15.00	15.00
Initial Cao_2 (mL/dL)	20.12	18.67
Cao_2 after decrease (mL/dL)	19.97	17.03
Percent change in Cao_2	0.70	8.80

II. CARBON DIOXIDE TRANSPORT

1. Three major mechanisms of transport exist in the blood: (1) dissolved CO_2, accounting for approximately 5% to 10% of the CO_2 content of blood (CO_2 is 20-fold more soluble in water than is O_2, with some of this undergoing conversion to carbonic acid [H_2CO_3])[7]; (2) bicarbonate ion (HCO_3^-), the major form of serum CO_2 (formed from rapid dissociation of carbonic acid); and (3) CO_2 bound to Hb and plasma proteins. Its first two forms are best illustrated by the following equation:

$$CO_2 + H_2O \xleftarrow{\text{CA}} \rightarrow H_2CO_3 \leftarrow \rightarrow H^+ + HCO_3^-$$

where CA is carbonic anhydrase. Of note, deoxygenated Hb is a weaker acid and has a higher affinity for CO_2 than does oxygenated Hb. Thus in the capillaries, as O_2 is released from Hb, CO_2 binds to the deoxygenated Hb. After transport to the lungs the binding of O_2 to Hb reverses the process and accelerates the removal of CO_2. The increased CO_2 affinity that occurs in deoxygenated blood is termed the Haldane effect[8] and accounts for approximately 50% of CO_2 elimination (Figs. 67-3 and 67-4).

III. ARTERIAL BLOOD GAS ANALYSIS

1. Arterial blood gas (ABG) analysis is the most effective method for assessing oxygenation and ventilation.
2. Blood sample analysis is performed by an automated blood gas analyzer, which can measure pH, P_{CO_2}, P_{O_2}, and cooximetry.
3. CO_2 tension (P_{CO_2}) is determined by chemical reaction: CO_2 consumed with resultant H^+ production.
4. P_{CO_2} is calculated based on the difference in pH change compared with a control value.
5. P_{O_2} is measured by an oxidation/reduction reaction.
6. O_2 saturation is calculated from a standard algorithm or measured separately by cooximetry as described later.[9]
7. An important secondary calculation from arterial blood gases is the arterial-alveolar gradient (A-a gradient). Its use in determining causes of hypoxia and hypercarbia is discussed in those sections.
8. The ABG analysis is essential in evaluating acid-base status.

A. ERRONEOUS RESULTS

1. Arterial blood gases can be drawn from multiple sites, including the radial, brachial, axillary, and femoral and dorsalis pedis arteries.
2. Excluding a rare mechanical error in the analyzer, technical and timing errors may cause faulty results. The four main causes of erroneous results are as follows.
a. Type of syringe: Plastic syringes are more convenient than glass because they are disposable, safer, and preheparinized. They allow gas diffusion through the walls of the syringe, however. Rapid

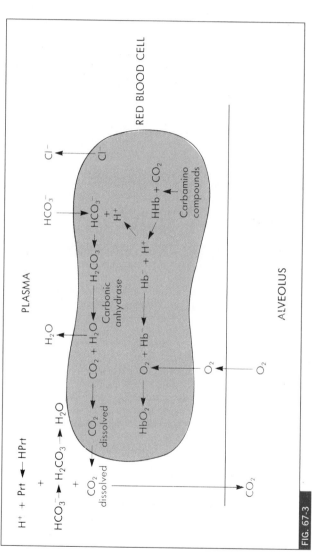

FIG. 67-3

Chemical reactions involving CO_2, O_2, and hemoglobin. *(From Berne RM, Levy MN: Physiology, 4th ed. St Louis: Mosby; 1998.)*

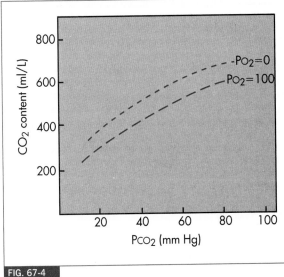

FIG. 67-4

Demonstration of the CO_2 equilibrium curve. The Haldane effect is illustrated by the increased CO_2 content in deoxygenated blood. *(From Berne RM, Levy MN: Physiology, 4th ed. St Louis: Mosby; 1998.)*

transport (<15 minutes) and transport on ice appear to negate this potential error.[10,11]

b. Air bubbles: Air in the syringe, even at 1% to 2% of the blood volume, may falsely alter both Po_2 and Pco_2. If a patient is hypoxic, a diffusion gradient of O_2 from the air in the syringe into the blood exists. CO_2 will follow a similar gradient and diffuse from blood into the air. Thus the Pao_2 and saturation would be falsely elevated while the Pco_2 would be falsely lowered. The error is exaggerated if the area of exposure is increased (e.g., via agitation) and the time allowed for diffusion is prolonged.[12]

c. Heparin-related changes: Heparin itself is slightly acidic and may slightly alter the pH. Liquid heparin may dilute the CO_2 in the sample, causing a significant Pco_2 reduction. Obtaining at least 2 mL of blood can minimize this error.[9]

d. Specimen handling: Leukocyte metabolism may falsely decrease Po_2 (especially in patients with marked leukocytosis). Thus, as discussed previously, rapid transport, on ice, of specimens to the laboratory will decrease errors.[10]

IV. VENOUS BLOOD GASES

1. At rest the difference in pH and P_{CO_2} between arterial and mixed venous blood gases is minimal. The $Paco_2$ usually differs by only 4 to 6 mm Hg, and the pH difference is about 0.03 to 0.05.[13]

2. Conditions of extreme stress may alter the relationship between arterial and venous blood gases. Patients after cardiopulmonary resuscitation have a significant difference between the arterial and venous pH and P_{CO_2}; venous gases may more accurately illustrate the acid-base status in tissue.[14] Pao_2 from an arterial sample generally differs significantly from a venous source (may vary by >40 mm Hg at Fio_2 of 21%).

3. Blood samples from exercising patients or those in shock or hypermetabolic states also show poor correlation between arterial and venous Po_2, Pco_2, and pH. Therefore an ABG should be performed to evaluate O_2 saturation, Pco_2, and pH in critically ill patients.

V. PULSE OXIMETRY

1. Pulse oximetry is a helpful and simple bedside test that gives important information about the O_2 saturation.

2. To interpret the data that pulse oximetry provides and recognize its limitations, the clinician must understand its working principles.

A. HISTORICAL BACKGROUND

1. **1865:** Hoppe-Seyler observed that the colored pigment he named "haemoglobin" changed color when agitated in the air.[15]

2. **1935:** Matthes was the first to develop a system of transillumination to measure O_2 saturation.[16]

3. **1974:** Aoyagi recognized that pulsatile variations affect the absorbance ratios, depending on the O_2 saturation.[17] The change occurs because of the introduction of fresh arterial blood with each cardiac ejection. This observation led to the invention of pulse oximeters that consist of two light-emitting diodes positioned opposite a photodetector on the other side of the interposed tissue (Fig. 67-5).

B. WORKING PRINCIPLES

1. The central principle of pulse oximetry is that all molecules absorb a specific wavelength of light. As Hb undergoes a structural change when binding to O_2, a different absorbance occurs, depending on the number of O_2 molecules bound (Hb is a tetramer with four separate sites to bind).

2. The pulse oximeter measures two wavelengths of transmitted light: 660 nm (red) and 940 nm (near infrared) (Fig. 67-5).

3. Oxyhemoglobin absorbs best at 940 nm, whereas deoxyhemoglobin absorbs 10 times more at 660 nm.[18]

4. Light transmitted several hundred times a minute locates a pulsatile signal (arterial). Computer mathematical equation compares the ratio of the red signal (660 nm, pulsatile/venous) to ratio of the infrared signal (940 nm, pulsatile/venous).

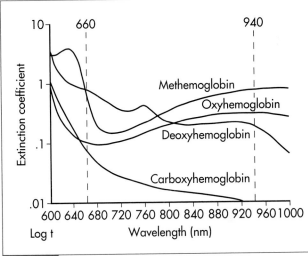

FIG. 67-5

Absorption spectra for the different types of hemoglobin in the wavelength range between 600 and 1000 nm. The wavelengths for the light-emitting diodes used in pulse oximetry are shown (660 and 940 nm). *(Redrawn from Wahr JA et al. Respir Care Clin North Am 1995; 1:77.)*

5. Ratios are compared with curves derived from studies of hypoxia on healthy volunteers. (Ratio 660/940 = 0.43, for which pulse oximeter registers 100% O_2 saturation; ratio of 3.4 will theoretically represent 0% saturation.[18])

C. LIMITATIONS

1. Although pulse oximetry is a simple test, many factors may confound the results. Its accuracy should always be considered when the physician is basing clinical decisions on the data obtained.

2. **Hypoxia:** The computer uses an experimentally derived curve to calculate the O_2 saturation (Spo_2). According to the manufacturers, if the true arterial oxygenation (Sao_2) is greater than 70%, the accuracy of Spo_2 compared with Sao_2 is 98% (differs less than 3%). For O_2 saturation lower than 75%, the computer extrapolates data and therefore O_2 saturation may be less accurate.[17]

3. **Optical interference:** Optical interference, both exogenous and endogenous, can significantly affect Spo_2.

a. Skin pigmentation: Darker skin pigmentation, although theoretically canceled out as part of the background absorbance, has been described to falsely elevate O_2 saturation.[19]

b. Nail polish: Blue and black hues (but not red) may artificially lower Sp_{O_2} up to 5%. The polish should be removed, or an alternative finger or the ear can be used.

c. Anemia: Although anemia has been mentioned to affect accuracy, severe anemia (Hb level of <3 g/dL) by itself does not appear to be a confounder.[20] When moderate anemia is combined with hypoxia (Sa_{O_2} <80%), some evidence suggests that pulse oximetry may underestimate Sa_{O_2}.[20,21]

d. Signal artifact: Can be caused by a false signal or low signal-to-noise ratio. A false signal may result from ambient light artifact or incomplete probe placement (most probes are covered with an opaque shield and should be checked for appropriate placement), or nonarterial sources of alternating signal such as cardiopulmonary resuscitation, repetitive coughing, or venous congestion caused by tricuspid valvular regurgitation or cardiomyopathy.[22,23] Magnetic resonance imaging machines have also been mentioned as a source of interference, as well as a potential cause of burns at the probe site. Low signal-to-noise ratio may be caused by peripheral vasoconstriction (e.g., hypothermia, hypotension, peripheral vascular disease) or may be iatrogenic (e.g., blood pressure cuff or arterial line on the same limb) and result in the inability to find a consistent and reliable pulse.

e. Intravenous dyes: Intravenous dyes (e.g., methylene blue for the treatment of methemoglobinemia) may profoundly lower measured O_2 saturations (high absorbance at 660 nm) to as low as 1% within 30 to 45 seconds of intravenous delivery, but only transiently, since return to baseline O_2 saturation occurs within 3 minutes.[24]

f. Dyshemoglobinemias: Potentially deadly are causes such as methemoglobinemia and carboxyhemoglobinemia. Oxygen saturations measured in these settings do not reflect oxygen delivery. Methemoglobinemia classically causes an oxygen saturation of approximately 82% to 86%, whereas carboxyhemoglobinemia classically causes oxygen saturations of 100%. In both situations, oxygen delivery is impaired.

4. Cooximetry is considered the gold standard for O_2 saturation because it provides accurate results in patients with dyshemoglobinemias. This apparatus calculates the O_2 saturation based on the absorption of four separate wavelengths. The extra two wavelengths entered into the appropriate mathematical equation allow the measurement of both methemoglobin and carboxyhemoglobin. This provides a fractional Hb saturation as compared with only a functional saturation with the pulse oximeter.

5. Owing to the shape of the O_2-Hb dissociation curve, large changes in Pa_{O_2} (e.g., from 150 to 60 mm Hg) may not significantly alter the O_2 saturation. Therefore, when hypoxia develops acutely, a delay of several minutes may occur before pulse oximetry recognizes the worsening hypoxia. In addition, oximetry should never be used to eval-

uate ventilation because hypoventilation may result in severe hypercarbia while supplemental oxygenation maintains a "reassuring" O_2 saturation of 95%. In this case an ABG measurement is required.

VI. CLINICAL CONSIDERATIONS

A. METHEMOGLOBIN

1. Methemoglobin (MHb) is formed when iron is oxidized from its ferrous to its ferric state.

2. Protective enzymatic pathways that reduce MHb (i.e., cytochrome-b_5 and indirectly glutathione and glucose-6-phosphate dehydrogenase) may be overwhelmed or blocked.

3. Common medications that may cause methemoglobinemia include benzocaine (topical spray), chloroquine, dapsone, lidocaine, methylene blue, nitrates, phenytoin, smoke inhalation, and sulfonamide antibiotics.[25]

4. Symptoms and signs are based on the percentage of total Hb affected.

5. Cyanotic skin discoloration may progress to anxiety, headache, tachycardia, confusion, seizure, and death.

6. Anemia or cardiopulmonary disease may result in earlier deterioration.

7. MHb fools both the pulse oximeter and the ABG assessment (Fig. 67-6). The pulse oximeter measures only two wavelengths (660 and 940 nm), and since MHb equally absorbs light, a ratio of 1.0 corresponds to a saturation of 82% to 86%.[20] The ABG assessment is also inaccurate, measuring only the dissolved O_2 concentration (it assumes the Hb molecules are in equilibrium with dissolved O_2).

8. Bedside test: MHb may have a chocolate brown color, and blowing 100% O_2 over 1 drop of blood on white filter paper will brighten deoxyhemoglobin, whereas methemoglobin will not change color.[25]

9. Cooximetry, which measures four wavelengths, can be used to detect MHb. Peak absorbance of MHb is 630 nm.

10. Treatment is recommended if the patient is symptomatic or if the MHb percentage is greater than 30% in an asymptomatic patient. Intravenous administration of methylene blue 1% solution 1 to 2 mg/kg over 3 minutes should result in a reduction of methemoglobin to Hb.[21]

11. Dapsone and benzocaine may cause a relapse of MHb formation. MHb levels should also be followed after treatment.[25]

12. If the patient's condition worsens, exchange transfusion or a hyperbaric chamber should be considered.

13. Alternative treatments under investigation include direct reducing agents (e.g., N-acetylcysteine) and cytochrome P450 inhibitors such as cimetidine.[23]

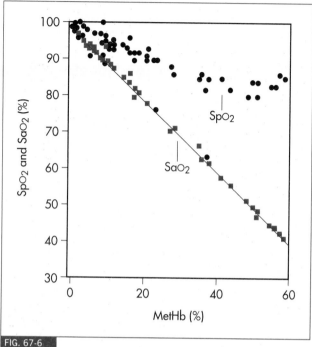

FIG. 67-6

Effect of methemoglobin on measured oxygen saturation by pulse oximetry. Spo_2 and Sao_2 versus methemoglobin (MetHb) at an Fio_2 of 1.0. Oxygen saturation consistently overestimated by Spo_2 is about 50% percent of Spo_2. *(Redrawn from UpToDate 9.1. www.utdol.com. Accessed Jan. 25, 2003.)*

B. CARBOXYHEMOGLOBIN

1. Common causes of carboxyhemoglobin formation include smoke inhalation from fire, poorly vented stove heaters, and suicide attempts by means of car exhaust.
2. Carbon monoxide (CO) toxicity results from CO binding to Hb with an affinity 240 times greater than that with O_2.
3. Binding impairs tissue oxygenation by interfering with the formation of oxyhemoglobin, as well as the release of O_2 to the tissues.
4. Clinical findings include headache, nausea, confusion, malaise, congestive heart failure, seizures, and death.
5. "Cherry red" lips may be seen because carboxyhemoglobin has absorbance characteristics similar to those of oxyhemoglobin.
6. As with MHb, the pulse oximeter provides an incorrectly high Spo_2 because the COHb is confused with O_2Hb (Fig. 67-7).

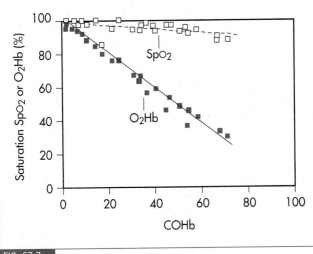

FIG. 67-7

Effect of carboxyhemoglobin on measured oxygen saturation by pulse oximetry. O_2Hb and Spo_2 versus carboxyhemoglobin (COHb) at an Fio_2 of 1.0. Oxygen saturation is consistently overestimated by Spo_2 in the presence of COHb. At high COHb levels of 70%, Spo_2 is close to 90%, while the actual O_2Hb has decreased to 30%. *(Redrawn from UpToDate 9.1. www.utdol.com. Accessed Jan. 25, 2003.)*

7. ABG measurement is also inaccurate, and a cooximeter is needed to document the CO level.

8. Treatment requires aggressive displacement of CO and maximal oxygenation (half-life of COHb reduced from 4 hours at Fio_2 of 0.21 to 75 to 80 minutes at Fio_2 of 1.0 and to 20 minutes with hyperbaric oxygenation at 2.0 atm).

9. Hyperbaric oxygenation remains controversial and is recommended only for patients with a COHb greater than 40% or loss of consciousness or for pregnant women with a COHb greater than 20% or evidence of fetal distress.[19]

10. Less common causes of dyshemoglobinemias are genetic variations in the Hb structure that may alter light absorption and provide spurious data (e.g., hemoglobin Koln).[19]

REFERENCES

[c] 1. Hill AV. The possible effects of the aggregation of the molecules of hemoglobin on its oxygen dissociation curve. J Physiol (Lond) 1910; 40:4.

[c] 2. Adair GS. The hemoglobin system. VI. The oxygen dissociation curve of hemoglobin. J Biol Chem 1925; 63:529.

67

PULSE OXIMETRY AND ABG INTERPRETATION

[c] 3. Crystal RG, West JB. The lung: scientific foundations, New York: Raven Press; 1991.

[c] 4. Benesch R, Benesch RE. The effect of organic phosphates from the human erythrocytes on the allosteric properties of hemoglobin. Biochem Biophys Res Commun 1967; 26:162.

[c] 5. Kilmartin JV, Rossi-Bernardi L. Interaction of hemoglobin with hydrogen ions, carbon dioxide, and organic phosphates. Physiol Rev 1973; 53:836.

[c] 6. Marino PL: The ICU book, 2nd ed. Baltimore: Williams & Wilkins; 1998.

[c] 7. West JB. Respiratory physiology, the essentials, 6th ed. Philadelphia: Lippincott, Williams & Wilkins; 2000.

[c] 8. Christiansen JC, Douglas G, Haldane JS. The absorption and dissociation of carbon dioxide by human blood. J Physiol (Lond) 1914; 48:244.

[d] 9. Williams AJ. ABC of oxygen: assessing and interpreting arterial blood gases and acid-base balance. Br Med J 1998; 317:1213.

[b] 10. Smeenk FW et al. Effect of four different methods of sampling arterial blood and storage time on gas tensions and shunt calculation in the 100% oxygen test. Eur Respir J 1997; 10:910.

[b] 11. Evers W, Racz GB, Levy AA. A comparative study of plastic (polypropylene) and glass syringes in blood-gas analysis. Anesth Analg 1972; 51:92.

[b] 12. Mueller RG. Lang GE, Beam JM. Bubbles in samples for blood gas determinations: a potential source of error. Am J Clin Pathol 1976; 65:242.

[b] 13. Adrogue HJ et al. Assessing acid-base status in circulatory failure: differences between arterial and central venous blood. N Engl J Med 1989; 320:1312.

[b] 14. Weil MH et al. Differences in acid-base status between venous and arterial blood during cardiopulmonary resuscitation. N Engl J Med 1986; 315:153.

[b] 15. Stoneham MD, Saville GM, Wilson IH. Knowledge about pulse oximetry among medical and nursing staff. Lancet 1994; 344:1339.

[c] 16. Grace R. Pulse oximetry: gold standard or false sense of security? Med J Aust 1994; 160:638.

[c] 17. Kelleher JF. Pulse oximetry. J Clin Monit 1989; 5:37.

[c] 18. Sinex JE. Pulse oximetry: principles and limitations. Am J Emerg Med 1999; 17:59.

[c] 19. UptoDate, Online 9.2. www.utdol.com. Accessed Aug. 25, 2002.

[b] 20. Jay GD, Hughes L, Renzi FP. Pulse oximetry is accurate in acute anemia from hemorrhage. Ann Emerg Med 1994; 24:32.

[b] 21. Severinghaus JW, Koh SO. Effect of anemia on pulse oximeter accuracy at low saturation. J Clin Monit 1990; 6:85.

[d] 22. Schnapp LM, Cohen NH. Pulse oximetry—uses and abuses. Chest 1990; 98:1244.

[d] 23. Moorthy SS, Dierdorf SF, Schmidt SI. Erroneous pulse oximetry data during CPR [letter]. Anesth Analg 1990; 70:339.

[b] 24. Kessler MR et al. Spurious pulse oximeter desaturation with methylene blue injection. Anesthesiology 1986; 65:550.

[c] 25. Wright RO, Lewander WJ, Woolf AD. Methemoglobinemia: etiology, pharmacology, and clinical management. Ann Emerg Med 1999; 34:646.

Acute Respiratory Failure

*J. Lucian Davis, Jr., MD, Anna Hemnes, MD, Majd Mouded, MD,
Michael J. McWilliams, MD, and Landon S. King, MD*

FAST FACTS

- Respiratory failure can be divided into hypoxic respiratory failure and hypercarbic ventilatory failure.
- When diagnosing respiratory failure, the physician should complete a focused history and physical examination and draw an arterial blood gas (ABG) sample.
- Respiratory effort and fatigue may provide more important clues to the presence of impending respiratory failure than ABG analysis.

68

Respiratory failure can be divided into oxygenation failure and ventilatory failure. Hypoxemia characterizes the former, whereas hypercarbia (also called hypercapnia) characterizes the latter. In many patients ventilatory and oxygenation failure are present simultaneously. However, oxygenation failure often occurs despite good ventilation (e.g., in patients with pulmonary embolism). In other patients (e.g., those with obstructive airways disease), ventilatory failure has only modest effects on arterial oxygenation. This chapter is meant to establish a framework for evaluating patients with respiratory failure. Clinical presentation, diagnosis, and management of the various disorders that may cause respiratory failure are addressed in subsequent chapters.

I. CLINICAL PRESENTATION

1. The clinical presentation of respiratory failure varies widely depending on cause and timing. A patient with drug overdose may be unconscious and hypopneic, whereas one with obesity hypoventilation may be sleepy with a normal respiratory rate; an asthmatic patient is likely to be agitated and tachypneic. The vital signs of a patient with suspected respiratory failure require the utmost attention. In addition to pulse, blood pressure, and respiratory rate, the patient's respiratory effort should be observed for clues to the cause of the respiratory failure and to the rapidity with which the clinician must act to correct this process. Often the simple question "Are you tiring out?" is the most astute diagnostic test for impending respiratory failure.

2. Table 68-1 provides guidelines for evaluating respiratory failure based on respiratory rate and oxygen saturation as measured by pulse oximetry.

GUIDELINE FOR EVALUATION OF RESPIRATORY FAILURE

Vital Signs	Suggested Diagnosis	Comments
RR decreased, any Sao_2	Hypoventilation	Generally seen with central nervous system alterations such as drug overdose
RR normal; Sao_2 decreased	Chronic hypoxia	Common in patients with chronic bronchitis ("blue bloaters") or obesity hypoventilation with chronic hypercapnia
RR increased, Sao_2 normal	Hypercarbia, hypoxia, metabolic acidosis	Common in pulmonary embolism, asthma, and sepsis; calculate A-a gradient (see Box 68-1) to detect hypoxemia that is unrecognized from pulse oximetry
RR increased, Sao_2 decreased	Complicated respiratory failure	Arterial blood gas measurement indicates whether hypoxia or hypercarbia is primarily driving increased RR; when both hypoxemia and hypercarbia represent changes from the patient's baseline, the clinician should look for a single disease process that is causing both

RR, Respiratory rate; *Sao_2*, oxygen saturation in arterial blood.

Hypoxia

I. DIAGNOSTICS

1. The ABG measurement is used to evaluate the degree of hypoxemia, arterial carbon dioxide (CO_2), and acid-base status and to calculate an arterial-alveolar (A-a) gradient. An excellent indicator of oxygenation is to divide the partial pressure of arterial oxygen (Pao_2) by the fraction of inspired oxygen (Pao_2/Fio_2). A ratio less than 300 reflects significant impairment in oxygenation (the normal ratio is 500). Arterial CO_2, the A-a gradient, and the response of these values to supplemental oxygen help determine the cause of hypoxia.

2. The A-a gradient is a calculated approximation of oxygenation in an idealized lung model. A-a gradients increase with age, with underlying lung disease, and with increasing Fio_2. An age-adjusted A-a gradient equation is presented in Box 68-1.[1] Given individual variability in A-a gradients, comparison to previous ABG measurements is the best means to assess changes in the A-a gradient.

3. Insufficient oxygen to meet metabolic demands can cause organ dysfunction and can occur despite oxyhemoglobin saturations (Sao_2) greater than 90%. Arterial oxygen content depends on total hemoglobin, the percent hemoglobin saturation, and a small component of dissolved oxygen. An additional factor, cardiac output, determines tissue oxygen delivery (Box 68-2).

4. Hypoxemia has a limited differential diagnosis. The five physiological causes of hypoxia include decreased Fio_2, hypoventilation, dif-

---

BOX 68-1

ALVEOLAR-ARTERIAL (A-a) OXYGEN GRADIENT EQUATION

A-a gradient = $Fio_2 \times (pAtm - pH_2O) - (Pco_2/R) - Paco_2$

At sea level on room air, this equation is A-a gradient = 150 −

$(1.25 \times Paco_2) - Pao_2$

Age-adjusted A-a gradient = $2.5 + (0.21 \times Age)$

A normal room air A-a gradient is 7 to 14. Atmospheric pressure (pATM) is 760 mm Hg at sea level; partial pressure of water vapor (pH_2O) is 47 mm Hg at sea level. The respiratory quotient (R) is equal to approximately 0.8. Fio_2, Fraction of inspired oxygen; PAo_2, alveolar oxygen pressure; Pao_2, arterial oxygen pressure; $Paco_2$, arterial carbon dioxide pressure used to approximate alveolar carbon dioxide pressure.

68

BOX 68-2

DETERMINATION OF ARTERIAL OXYGEN CONTENT

Arterial oxygen content (CaO_2) = $(1.39 \times Sao_2 \times Hb) + (0.0031 \times Pao_2)$

Normal values range from 18 to 21 mL O_2 per deciliter. Tissue oxygen delivery = cardiac output × Cao_2.
Hb, Hemoglobin concentration in milligrams per deciliter; *Sao_2*, percent of hemoglobin saturated.

fusion impairment, ventilation-perfusion ($\dot{V}/\dot{Q}$) mismatch, and shunt. Fig. 68-1 illustrates a diagnostic algorithm for approaching hypoxia, and Table 68-2 presents specific details of diagnosis and management of the specific causes.

II. MANAGEMENT

1. The goal of supplemental oxygen is to correct hypoxia using the simplest delivery system the patient can tolerate.
2. Nasal prongs provide oxygen in a way that allows speech, eating, and mobility. For each 1 L of oxygen, Fio_2 increases by 3% to 4%, although this varies depending on the respiratory rate and whether the patient's mouth is open (which allows room air to dilute the nasal oxygen flow).
3. Venturi masks predictably deliver specified oxygen concentrations. They allow oxygen flow to be titrated safely to oxygen saturations in patients who have chronic obstructive pulmonary disease (COPD) and are known to retain CO_2 with supplemental oxygen.
4. The nonrebreather mask maintains inhaled Fio_2 of approximately 80% to 90% through the use of a one-way valve that allows exhaled gases to exit the mask but prevents the entrainment of room air. If the valve is removed, the concentration of oxygen delivered is lower.
5. Oxygen flow from wall regulators is approximately 15 L/min and may be inadequate in some circumstances (e.g., tachypnea).
6. If these options are inadequate to improve oxygenation, ventilatory support in the form of noninvasive positive-pressure ventilation or

ACUTE RESPIRATORY FAILURE

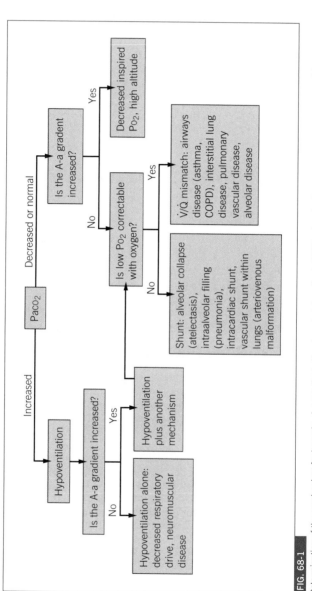

FIG. 68-1

Determination of the mechanism for hypoxia. *A-a gradient*, Alveolar-arterial gradient; *COPD*, chronic obstructive pulmonary disease; *V̇/Q̇*, ventilation-perfusion. (*Modified from Fauci AS et al. Harrison's principles of internal medicine, 14th ed. New York: McGraw-Hill; 1997.*)

TABLE 68-2
DIFFERENTIAL DIAGNOSIS OF HYPOXEMIA

Cause of Hypoxemia	Mechanism of Hypoxemia	Associated Diseases	Comments
Decreased FiO_2	Lower atmospheric pressure at high altitude or on airplanes decreases alveolar oxygen tension		Seldom clinically significant
Hypoventilation	Increased alveolar carbon dioxide concentration decreases alveolar oxygen concentration	See Table 68-3 for a detailed list of causes of hypercarbic ventilatory failure	Should correct with a small amount of supplemental oxygen
Diffusion impairment	Increased time for oxygen to cross the alveolar-capillary membrane decreases oxygen delivery to hemoglobin	Interstitial lung diseases	Desaturation with minimal exertion; pulmonary function tests with carbon monoxide diffusion capacity confirm the diagnosis
$\dot{V}/\dot{Q}$ mismatch	Altered ratio of ventilation to perfusion reduces efficiency of gas exchange and decreases oxygen delivery to hemoglobin	Airways disease (asthma, chronic obstructive pulmonary disease, bronchitis, pneumonia); interstitial lung disease; pulmonary vascular disease (pulmonary embolus, pulmonary hypertension)	Increased A-a gradient; normal or low PCO_2; PO_2 corrects with supplemental oxygen
Shunt	Mixed venous blood bypasses functional lung and lowers systemic oxygen tension	Intrapulmonary: alveolar disease (adult respiratory distress syndrome, atelectasis, pulmonary edema, pneumonia); vascular disease (arteriovenous malformation, hepatopulmonary syndrome); intracardiac (septal defects)	Increased A-a gradient; normal or mildly elevated PCO_2; PO_2 does not correct with supplemental oxygen

A-a gradient, Arterial-alveolar gradient; *FiO_2,* fraction of inspired oxygen; *PCO_2,* partial pressure of carbon dioxide; *$\dot{V}/\dot{Q}$,* ventilation-perfusion.

ACUTE RESPIRATORY FAILURE

68

TABLE 68-3

APPROACH TO HYPERCAPNIC RESPIRATORY FAILURE

Disease or Syndrome	Diagnostic Aids	Specific Therapy
DECREASED VENTILATORY DRIVE		
Narcotic or benzodiazepine overdose	Constricted pupils with narcotics; slow heart rate; flaccid muscles; decreased tendon reflexes	Naloxone or flumazenil
Central nervous system: medullary tumor, infarction, or other lesion	Ataxic breathing; no dyspnea; sudden respiratory arrest	
Myxedema	History of hypothyroidism; hypothermia; slow relaxation-phase tendon reflexes	Intravenous thyroxine
Severe metabolic alkalosis	History of loop diuretic use or protracted vomiting	Ammonium chloride or acetazolamide
Sleep apnea, obstructive or central	Morning headaches; loud snoring; periods of apnea, then arousal and hyperpnea; daytime somnolence	Nocturnal continuous positive airway pressure; medroxyprogesterone for obesity; hypoventilation
Multiple sclerosis	Waxing and waning course; cranial nerve deficits	
Encephalitis and postviral Reye's syndrome	Abnormal cerebrospinal fluid; increased serum NH_4^+ in Reye's syndrome	Appropriate antibiotics and antiviral drugs; neurosurgical measures to normalize intracranial pressures
CORTICOSPINAL TRACTS AND ANTERIOR HORN CELLS		
Poliomyelitis	Fever and muscle spasms; asymmetrical weakness; absent tendon reflexes; postpolio syndrome can develop 20-30 years after initial infection	
Amyotrophic lateral sclerosis	Men 50-70 years old; progressive, ascending weakness; bilateral peripheral muscle involvement; fasciculations	
Tetanus	Involuntary painful muscle spasms	Wound débridement; penicillin; human immune globulin
Traumatic cervical cordotomy	Trauma with acute quadriplegia	Immobilization of the neck

PERIPHERAL NERVE		
Guillain-Barré syndrome	Progressive ascending motor weakness; absent deep tendon reflexes	Plasmapheresis; intravenous immune globulin
Diphtheria	Recent history of pharyngitis or severe skin infection	Penicillin; diphtheria antitoxin
Idiopathic or postzoster phrenic neuropathy	Dyspnea in supine position; abdominal retraction on inspiration	Upright position
Porphyria	Young adult; abdominal pain; central nervous system or psychiatric signs; paradoxical diaphragmatic movement	Chlorpromazine; specific porphyria treatment
NEUROMUSCULAR JUNCTION		
Myasthenia gravis	History of fatigue; ptosis and diplopia	Edrophonium
Cholinergic crisis	History of myasthenia gravis; acetylcholinesterase therapy; abdominal pain; diarrhea; fasciculations	Atropine
Organophosphate poisoning	Insecticide exposure	Atropine and pralidoxime
Botulism	History of eating home-canned foods; dizziness; dry mouth; initial facial nerve paresthesias	Botulism antitoxin; penicillin
Aminoglycoside toxicity	Aminoglycoside therapy	Avoid use of aminoglycosides
Tick paralysis	Residence in southern or southwestern United States; progressive motor weakness	Remove tick
MUSCLE DISORDERS		
Muscular dystrophies	Symmetrical proximal muscular weakness; normal tendon reflexes	
Periodic paralysis	Familial inheritance; early morning weakness; high or low serum potassium level	Correct potassium level; intravenous saline
Inflammatory (polymyositis, dermatomyositis)	Muscle weakness and tenderness; can cause interstitial lung disease	Corticosteroids

cont'd

ACUTE RESPIRATORY FAILURE

68

TABLE 68-3

APPROACH TO HYPERCAPNIC RESPIRATORY FAILURE—cont'd

Disease or Syndrome	Diagnostic Aids	Specific Therapy
METABOLIC DISORDERS		
Hypercalcemia	Short QT interval	Intravenous saline and loop diuretic (see Chapter 36)
Hypophosphatemia		Intravenous or oral phosphate
CONDITIONS OF INCREASED IMPEDANCE		
Obstructive lung disease	History; radiographic hyperinflation	Inhaled bronchodilators; pulmonary toilet; treatment of specific disorder as indicated
Massive obesity	Body mass index >30	Upright position; tracheostomy
Massive ascites	Tense, protuberant abdomen	Paracentesis
Kyphoscoliosis	Hunched back	
Pneumothorax or pleural effusion	Chest radiograph	Chest tube or therapeutic thoracentesis

endotracheal intubation and mechanical ventilation must be considered. Mechanical ventilation is covered in Chapter 63.

Hypercarbia

1. Hypercarbia reflects either excessive CO_2 production or inadequate CO_2 elimination. Exercise, overfeeding, hyperthyroidism, burns, fever, and sepsis all increase CO_2 production by increasing the body's metabolic rate. Excessive CO_2 production, however, rarely causes ventilatory failure without some compromise in the ability to clear, or "blow off," this excess CO_2.

2. The purpose of ventilation is to allow the elimination of acid products of cellular respiration in the form of CO_2. The kidney helps the lung maintain pH by regulating serum bicarbonate concentration over time. Because the kidney does this slowly, the body must rely on ventilation when acidosis develops acutely.

I. DIAGNOSTICS

1. Ventilatory failure is also called hypercapnic respiratory failure. Strictly speaking, hypercapnia exists whenever the partial pressure of carbon dioxide (Pco_2) is greater than 45 mm Hg. Acute ventilatory failure occurs only when the patient has concurrent acidemia, implying that the change in Pco_2 has been too rapid or too extreme for metabolic processes to compensate and buffer the pH change. Thus an elevated Pco_2 associated with alkalemia, as seen in a patient who is volume contracted from vomiting or overdiuresis, reflects not ventilatory failure but appropriate respiratory compensation for a metabolic derangement of pH. Similarly, many patients with COPD or neuromuscular disease chronically retain CO_2 at supranormal levels because the Pco_2 has risen slowly enough for the kidney to compensate for the respiratory acidosis. In these and other patients the pH helps determine whether the hypercarbia is acute or chronic, as do past ABG results. Nevertheless, in any patient an elevated Pco_2 with a pH below 7.3 reflects an acute respiratory or metabolic acidosis for which the patient is failing to compensate. A pH below 7.2 is alarming because it suggests that respiratory or cardiovascular collapse is imminent.

2. Ventilation depends on respiratory rate and tidal volume. Control over the first resides in the brainstem alone. Regulation of the second, by contrast, is shared among the central and peripheral nervous systems, the chest wall, and the respiratory muscles. The respiratory mechanical pump fails when the "load" of CO_2 exceeds the removal capacity of its component parts.[2] These parts include the spinal cord, the peripheral nerves, the neuromuscular junction, the diaphragm and other respiratory muscles, the chest wall, the lung parenchyma, and the airways. Moving conceptually from head to lung, one can

easily evaluate at each level what diseases and syndromes can reduce the capacity of each component of the pump.[2]

II. MANAGEMENT

Table 68-3 outlines management options for hypercapnic respiratory failure.

PEARLS AND PITFALLS

- Pulse oximetry depends on pulse-coordinated receipt of the light wavelengths transilluminated by oxyhemoglobin through the tissues. Readings may be inaccurate in the absence of an observed arterial waveform, as may be seen with vasoconstriction or nail polish. Pulse oximetry is covered further in Chapter 67.
- Low Sao_2 of proportion to Pao_2 suggests methemoglobinemia. Low Pao_2 out of proportion to high Sao_2 suggests carboxyhemoglobinemia. Four-channel cooximetry confirms these diagnoses.
- When interpreting an ABG, the physician must document the amount of supplemental oxygen at the time of sampling and obtain previous ABG results for comparison.
- The half-lives of naloxone and flumazenil are substantially shorter than those of most opiates and benzodiazepines, and repeat doses or a naloxone drip may be necessary.

REFERENCES

[c] 1. Mellemgaard K. The alveolar-arterial oxygen difference: size and components of normal man. Acta Physiol Scand 1966; 67:10.
[c] 2. Bone RC et al. Pulmonary and critical care medicine. St Louis: Mosby; 1998.

Sleep-Disordered Breathing

Laura B. Herpel, MD, Carolyn Wong Simpkins, MD, PhD, and Philip L. Smith, MD

FAST FACTS

- Sleep-disordered breathing (SDB) refers to the presence of apneas or hypopneas during sleep that result in either electroencephalographic (EEG) evidence of arousal or decreased oxygen saturation (Sao_2).
- Apnea refers to the absence of airflow or breathing for 10 seconds or more.
- Hypopnea refers to inspiratory flow limitation (IFL) with either decreased Sao_2 or arousal.
- SDB is most often a result of obstructive sleep apnea (OSA) or obesity hypoventilation syndrome (OHS).
- Obesity with a body mass index (BMI) greater than 30 is the greatest risk factor for OSA or OHS, and weight reduction can dramatically improve symptoms.
- SDB is diagnosed by a polysomnogram (PSG) or "sleep study," which includes overnight monitoring of EEG, electrocardiography (ECG), Sao_2, respiratory effort, and eye, chin, and leg movements.
- Long-term consequences of OSA and OHS include systemic and pulmonary hypertension, right-sided heart failure, neurocognitive deficits, and decreased quality of life.
- The mainstay of treatment for OSA and OHS is nasal continuous positive airway pressure (CPAP), which can reverse some of the cardiovascular and neurological consequences and improve quality of life.

69

I. EPIDEMIOLOGY

1. SDB is a serious and underappreciated problem associated with substantial cardiovascular and neurocognitive sequelae and decreased quality of life. Given its strong association with obesity in the United States, it is likely to become more common over time. Recent estimates suggest that 24% of men and 9% of women in the United States have five or more SDB events per hour, but only 4% of men and 2% of women have these events with associated daytime hypersomnolence and meet diagnostic criteria for OSA.[1] This chapter focuses primarily on OSA, with discussions of other SDB syndromes in the "Pearls and Pitfalls" section.

2. The mechanism for OSA is pharyngeal collapse. OSA begins during sleep when the pressure surrounding the airway increases above the atmospheric pressure, causing apnea or hypopnea. Obesity (BMI >30) is the most common predisposing factor for OSA, although unusual oropharyngeal anatomy such as enlarged tonsils, retrognathia, and

1011

other craniofacial abnormalities are lesser risk factors. Hypothyroidism, acromegaly, congestive heart failure (CHF), acquired immunodeficiency syndrome, end-stage renal disease requiring hemodialysis, and being overweight (BMI 25-30) are also conditions associated with increased risk of OSA. OSA is seen more commonly in men and postmenopausal women. When seen in premenopausal women, it is usually in association with higher BMI.

3. The major morbidities associated with OSA are cardiovascular sequelae (including systemic and pulmonary hypertension, cor pulmonale, coronary artery disease, ventricular arrhythmias, and congestive heart failure) and neurocognitive sequelae (decreased cognition, decreased memory, and excessive daytime hypersomnolence). OSA may also result in personality changes, work-related difficulties, impotence, and motor vehicle accidents. The mortality rate associated with OSA is still unknown.

II. CLINICAL PRESENTATION AND PATHOPHYSIOLOGY

1. Patients with nearly all forms of SDB suffer from excessive daytime sleepiness as a result of disrupted and insufficient sleep. The next two paragraphs give an overview of the pathophysiology of OSA, which causes the frequent nighttime arousals. Subsequent paragraphs describe historical and clinical features of OSA.

2. The sleep-wake cycle is determined by homeostatic mechanisms and the body's intrinsic circadian rhythm. Normal sleep has two distinct forms: rapid eye movement (REM) and non-REM (consisting of four progressively deeper stages of sleep). REM sleep is notable for fluctuations in heart rate, blood pressure, and breathing, with paralysis of skeletal muscle, decreased respiratory drive, and dreams. Non-REM sleep is notable for stability of vital signs, including decreased heart rate, respiratory rate, and blood pressure and is seen as slow wave sleep on EEG.[2] Normal patterns of sleep progress through several cycles or REM and non-REM sleep per night, with intermittent brief arousals between cycles.

3. In patients with OSA, narrowing in the pharynx and hypopharynx results from increased surrounding pharyngeal pressure. The pressure at which upper airways collapse and airflow is halted is referred to as the critical pressure, or Pcrit. Muscle tone, sleep stage, increased adipose tissue, tonsillar hypertrophy, craniofacial abnormalities, and genetic factors all influence Pcrit.[3] The normal Pcrit during sleep approximates -13 cm H_2O. In normal individuals who snore the Pcrit is -8 cm H_2O. In patients with SDB the Pcrit ranges from -4 cm H_2O to as high as $+5$ to $+10$ cm H_2O. Upper airway collapse leads to obstruction, apnea, and arousal. The upper airway resistance syndrome represents a form of SDB that is similar to hypopnea, is characterized by inspiratory flow limitation, and is associated with either decreased Sao_2 or arousal.[4]

4. Patients with OSA typically have daytime fatigue that initially occurs

during passive activity but progresses to affect conversations, meal-times, and driving. Bed partners classically report years of loud snoring that often ends in choking, apnea, or awakening. Snoring that drives a partner to another bed is extremely specific but not sensitive for OSA. Patients may also report symptoms of fatigue, memory loss, difficulty concentrating, personality changes, and sexual dysfunction. Morning headaches are common, especially with pronounced nighttime hypoxia. When OSA is severe, patients may report symptoms of right- and left-sided heart failure.

5. On examination the majority of patients have obesity without other physical findings. In 5% to 10% of patients anatomical abnormalities such as retrognathia can be found, in addition to small upper airways and large tonsils.[5] Hypertension is seen in approximately 50% of patients with OSA and correlates with the number of SDB events per hour.[6,7] Lower extremity edema in men without a history of cardiac, renal, or hepatic dysfunction is common and specific for OSA.[5] Other signs of right- and left-sided heart failure can be seen with long-standing severe OSA (see Chapters 8 and 66).

III. DIAGNOSTICS (Fig. 69-1)

A. POLYSOMNOGRAM OR SLEEP STUDY

1. The PSG or sleep study is the definitive diagnostic test for OSA and involves continuous monitoring of ECG; EEG; Sao_2; respiratory rate; effort; airflow; eye, chin, and leg movements; and often $PAco_2$.
2. The following guidelines are used to diagnose and grade the severity of OSA (Table 69-1).
a. SDB events are characterized by apnea, hypopnea, and IFL resulting in either decreased Sao_2 or arousal on EEG.
b. PSG is interpreted, and summation of the number of apneas and hypopneas per hour of sleep is reported as the Sleep-Disordered Breathing Index, Apnea-Hypopnea Index, or Respiratory Disturbance Index, depending on the sleep center.[5]

SLEEP-DISORDERED BREATHING **69**

TABLE 69-1

DIAGNOSIS AND CLASSIFICATION OF OBSTRUCTIVE SLEEP APNEA

Degree of Obstructive Sleep Apnea	Number of Sleep-Disordered Breathing Events per Hour	Symptoms and Signs
Mild	5-30	Daytime hypersomnolence
Moderate	31-60	Severe daytime hypersomnolence and onset of systemic consequences
Severe	>60	Severe daytime hypersomnolence and progressive systemic and neurological consequences*

*Data from Nieto FJ et al. JAMA 2000; 283:1829.

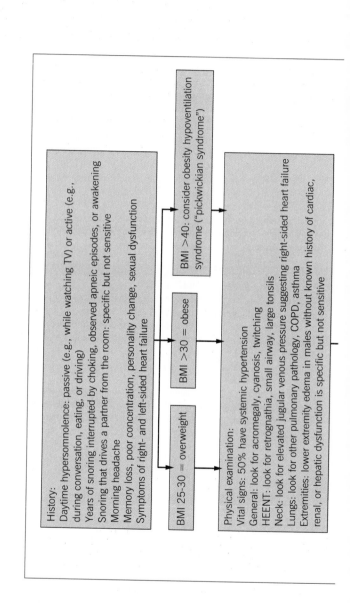

History:
Daytime hypersomnolence: passive (e.g., while watching TV) or active (e.g., during conversation, eating, or driving)
Years of snoring interrupted by choking, observed apneic episodes, or awakening
Snoring that drives a partner from the room: specific but not sensitive
Morning headache
Memory loss, poor concentration, personality change, sexual dysfunction
Symptoms of right- and left-sided heart failure

BMI 25-30 = overweight

BMI >30 = obese

BMI >40: consider obesity hypoventilation syndrome ("pickwickian syndrome")

Physical examination:
Vital signs: 50% have systemic hypertension
General: look for acromegaly, cyanosis, twitching
HEENT: look for retrognathia, small airway, large tonsils
Neck: look for elevated jugular venous pressure suggesting right-sided heart failure
Lungs: look for other pulmonary pathology, COPD, asthma
Extremities: lower extremity edema in males without known history of cardiac, renal, or hepatic dysfunction is specific but not sensitive

Blood work:
CBC looking for secondary polycythemia
ABGs looking for hypercapnia and hypoxia
TSH to rule out hypothyroidism

Other tests:
Echocardiogram will help define severity; pulmonary hypertension and right- and left-sided heart failure indicate systemic effects of moderate to severe SDB
PFTs usually reveal normal FEV_1; restrictive pattern is suggestive but not definitive or necessary; can rule out other pulmonary disease, e.g., asthma, COPD

Polysomnogram (gold standard):
Measures EEG; ECG; Sao_2; respiratory effort, rate, and flow; and eye, chin, and leg movements with or without $Paco_2$
5-30 SDB events per hour with daytime hypersomnolence = mild OSA
31-60 events per hour = moderate OSA
>60 events per hour = severe OSA
Obesity hypoventilation syndrome is a subset of OSA; consider it when hypercapnia, hypoxia, and BMI >40 are present

SLEEP-DISORDERED BREATHING 69

FIG. 69-1

Evaluation of patients with suspected sleep apnea. *ABGs*, Arterial blood gases; *BMI*, body mass index; *CBC*, complete blood cell count; *COPD*, chronic obstructive pulmonary disease; *ECG*, electrocardiogram; *EEG*, electroencephalogram; FEV_1, forced expiratory volume in 1 second; *HEENT*, head, eyes, ears, nose, and throat; *OSA*, obstructive sleep apnea; $Paco_2$, arterial partial pressure of carbon dioxide; *PFTs*, pulmonary function tests; Sao_2, oxygen saturation; *SDB*, sleep-disordered breathing; *TSH*, thyroid-stimulating hormone.

c. More than five SDB events per hour in association with daytime hypersomnolence is diagnostic of obstructive sleep apnea.[1]

d. The degree of daytime hypersomnolence has been shown in some studies to correlate with the severity of the SDB and degree of hypoxemia.[8]

e. Sleep studies are ideally performed in a hospital setting or laboratory environment, which requires referral to a center with such a facility.[2]

f. Certified sleep centers can be located through the American Academy of Sleep Medicine Website at www.aasmnet.org.

B. OTHER STUDIES

1. In addition to PSG, appropriate studies should be done to rule out other reversible medical conditions that may be contributing to the patient's symptoms and to assess the severity of disease.

2. Studies include the following.

a. Pulmonary function tests: These are performed to differentiate restrictive from obstructive lung disease. Patients with OSA have a normal FEV_1. The physician may see a restrictive defect in patients with severe obesity, which raises suspicion of OSA. Flow-volume curves may show a variable extrathoracic obstruction, which is neither sensitive nor specific for OSA.

b. Arterial blood gas (ABG) analysis: ABG analysis should be performed if patients have suspected OHS and a BMI greater than 40. It may be valuable in determining chronicity and severity and assessing for other confounding disorders. ABG values during waking hours could be normal (OSA) or demonstrate hypercarbia and hypoxemia (OHS).

c. Echocardiogram: The echocardiogram is used to assess for effects of SDB on cardiac function and severity of disease.

d. Thyroid function studies: Thyroid function is studied to assess for hypothyroidism as a contributing factor.

IV. MANAGEMENT

A. GENERAL TREATMENT

1. General treatment strategies in patients with OSA should focus on correcting the obstruction to prevent hypoxia, as well as correcting underlying medical conditions that may be contributing to the obstruction.

2. Patients should be educated to avoid alcohol and other sedating medications.

3. Patients should be strongly encouraged to lose weight. Weight reduction of 10% to 15% may dramatically improve symptoms and decrease Pcrit by as much as 6 cm H_2O. Some patients, however, require weight loss of up to 25% to see clinical improvement.[9-11]

B. NASAL CONTINUOUS AIRWAY PRESSURE

1. Nasal CPAP has been the mainstay of therapy since the 1980s[12] and works by increasing the intraluminal pharyngeal and hypopharyngeal pressure 5 to 10 cm H_2O above the Pcrit. The device consists of a

small machine that provides positive pressure through a tube leading to a tightly fitting nasal mask that is strapped to the face. In some cases chin straps to prevent mouth opening may be necessary.[13]

2. The following guidelines are useful in initiating and titrating nasal CPAP.

a. The range of nasal CPAP is usually 5 to 15 cm H_2O but may need to be as high as 20 cm H_2O, although higher pressures are less well tolerated. Settings are titrated by a technician in the sleep laboratory with the goal of eliminating IFL and thereby eliminating SDB.[2]

b. Relative contraindications include bullous lung disease and recurrent sinus and ear infections. There are no absolute contraindications.[13]

c. Adherence rates vary widely and can be increased with education and minimization of side effects. Adherence is more likely in patients who experience reduction in hypersomnolence, whereas nonadherence may be indicative of other underlying sleep disorders.[2,13]

d. Side effects include local skin irritation and dry mucosa (50%), sinus congestion and rhinorrhea (25%), eye irritation (25%), and sleep disturbance. Humidification of the air, nasal prongs or pillows, and correct mask size can eliminate these problems.

e. Routine outpatient follow-up is recommended for monitoring of response to treatment.

C. ORAL DEVICES

1. Oral devices are a second-line therapy for patients intolerant of nasal CPAP. They are 55% to 100% effective for patients who snore but less effective for patients with OSA.[3] Obtaining such a device requires a dental consultation.

2. Four potential surgical interventions are available for patients with OSA. Data on their efficacy are variable.

a. Uvulopalatopharyngoplasty: This involves removal of uvula, tonsils, rim of soft palate, and redundant posterior pharyngeal mucosa. Overall cure rates of 40% to 50% can be achieved, but rates may be higher in patients with abnormal upper airways (e.g., large tonsils, redundant tissue).[12]

b. Laser-assisted uvulopalatoplasty: This procedure involves the use of a laser device to remove part of the uvula and associated soft palate tissue. Snoring is decreased after the procedure, but no data on OSA are available. The procedure can be performed in an office setting with the patient under local anesthesia.[3]

c. Maxillofacial surgery: Maxillofacial surgery involves genioglossal advancement, resuspension of the hyoid bone with or without uvulopalatopharyngoplasty, or maxillomandibular advancement. It is used more often for patients with craniofacial abnormalities and has had varying success.[3]

d. Tracheostomy: Tracheostomy involves bypass of the source of obstruction and is 100% effective. It should be considered in severe cases when other treatments fail, but it is associated with risk of granuloma formation, speech impairment, and stoma infections.

D. NEWER OPTIONS

1. A variety of advances are under development for the diagnosis and treatment of OSA, but data on their efficacy are limited.
2. The following are some of the new techniques being investigated.

a. Automatic nasal CPAP devices have the capability to monitor airflow and pressure and respond by adjusting the mask pressure. These devices are currently being used, but few studies are available. They may be used diagnostically in the future; however, studies have not shown the devices to be effective in the diagnosis of mild to moderate OSA as compared with PSG. Concerns exist regarding the lack of diagnosis for other sleep disorders and the lack of safety without direct observation by a technician during titration.[14]

b. Oral CPAP devices are also being studied. Pressure is applied through the mouth, and no head gear is required.

c. Hypoglossal nerve stimulation is still being investigated. Stimulation of the hypoglossal nerve activates the genioglossus muscle and restores upper airway patency and muscle tone.[14]

d. New surgical techniques, including base of tongue and soft palate somnoplasty, are under investigation as alternatives to traditional, more invasive procedures. These techniques involve the generation of scar tissue to reduce the bulk of pharyngeal tissue.

PEARLS AND PITFALLS

- SDB encompasses OHS or the Pickwickian syndrome. This disorder is named after the 19th century novel *The Pickwick Papers,* in which Charles Dickens perfectly describes the characteristics of this disorder in the character of Mr. Wardle's boy Joe. OHS is a clinical syndrome characterized by more severe obesity (BMI >40) in association with the usual presentation of OSA to a more severe degree. OHS differs from OSA in that patients have a blunted respiratory drive, leading to hypercarbia and hypoxia that can persist into waking hours. Patients often manifest cyanosis, twitching, periodic respirations, secondary polycythemia, cor pulmonale, and right-sided heart failure in addition to daytime hypersomnolence.

- Treatment emphasizes weight loss, which may improve the ventilatory response to hypercarbia and hypoxia. Bariatric surgery or gastric stapling may be considered in severe cases. Treatment for OHS-associated sleep apnea is the same as for OSA with the addition of supplemental oxygen for daytime decreased Sao_2.[15] Limited data are available on the use of respiratory stimulants such as medroxyprogesterone and theophylline, but these medications have substantial side effects and patients need to be monitored closely.

- Central sleep apnea is distinguished from obstructive sleep apnea in that patients have cessation of respiratory effort as a result of decreased respiratory drive rather than obstruction. Central sleep apnea is rare in healthy individuals and is occasionally seen in patients with brainstem lesions or congestive heart failure. Treatment entails supplemental oxygen for hypoxemia and nasal CPAP for patients with Cheyne-Stokes respirations.[16]

- Narcolepsy is a disorder of excessive daytime sleepiness associated with cataplexy (loss of muscle tone and strength while awake, often associated with emotion), sleep paralysis (loss of muscle tone at the beginning or end of sleep), and hypnagogic hallucinations (vivid sensory experiences before the onset of sleep). It is a rare disorder (prevalence of 0.05% to 0.09%) with a peak incidence in the second decade of life. It is diagnosed with a sleep latency test demonstrating an abnormal sleep latency of less than 5 minutes and is often treated with stimulants.

- Insomnia is the most common sleep-related complaint and occurs at some point in 33% of individuals, with increased incidence in older age. It is characterized by an inability to fall asleep or stay asleep and can be transient, short term (<3 weeks), or chronic (>3 weeks). Underlying causes may include stress, medications, daytime napping, pain, and depression. Insomnia is common in hospitalized patients, and treatment is aimed at correcting the underlying cause (see Chapter 3).

- Restless leg syndrome (RLS) and periodic leg movement (PLM) are seen in 25% to 35% of individuals by 65 years of age. RLS is characterized by sensations of akathisia (inability to stay still) and sensory discomfort that is relieved with movement. It is treated with dopamine agonists. Semiinvoluntary leg movements while awake and semirhythmic leg movements while asleep characterize PLM. It is diagnosed by PSG and treated with antidepressants.

- Alcohol, narcotics, and benzodiazepines may increase OSA severity, perhaps in part by decreasing tone in pharyngeal muscles, which could increase upper airway collapsibility. Patients with severe OSA receiving these medications during procedures should receive nasal CPAP to prevent complications.

- About 1% to 2% of people with asthma have OSA. OSA should be considered when patients suffer from nocturnal asthma exacerbations. Nasal CPAP is effective and safe for patients with both asthma and OSA but interrupts sleep in patients with nocturnal asthma alone.[17]

- When treated with nasal CPAP, patients with CHF and OSA have been shown to have fewer events of nocturnal angina and increases in cardiac output and ejection fraction even in waking hours, as shown by echocardiogram.[12]

- Patients with moderate to severe hypersomnolence should be informed of increased driving risk. Patients with sleep apnea have automobile crash rates two to four times higher than in the normal population.[18]

69

SLEEP-DISORDERED BREATHING

REFERENCES

[b] 1. Young T et al. The occurrence of sleep disordered breathing among middle aged adults. N Engl J Med 1993; 328:1230.

[c] 2. Neubauer DN, Smith PL, Earley CJ. Sleep disorders. In Barker LR, Burton JR, Zeive PD, eds. Principles of ambulatory medicine, 5th ed. Baltimore: Williams & Wilkins; 1998.

[c] 3. Strollo PJ, Rogers RM. Obstructive sleep apnea. N Engl J Med 1996; 334:99.

[c] 4. Winakur SJ, Smith PL, Schwartz AR. Pathophysiology and risk factors for obstructive sleep apnea. Semin Respir Crit Care Med 1998; 19:99.

[c] 5. Neubauer DN et al. Sleep disorders. In Barker LR, Burton JR, Zeive PD, eds. Principles of ambulatory medicine, 4th ed. Baltimore: Williams & Wilkins; 1994.

[b] 6. Nieto FJ et al. Association of sleep disordered breathing, sleep apnea, and hypertension in a large community-based study. JAMA 2000; 283:1829.

[b] 7. Peppard PE et al. Prospective study of the association between sleep-disordered breathing and hypertension. N Engl J Med 2000; 342:1378.

[b] 8. Punjabi NM et al. Modeling hypersomnolence in sleep-disordered breathing. Am J Respir Crit Care Med 1999; 15:1703.

[c] 9. Levitzky MG. The control of breathing. In Houston MJ, Sheinis LA, eds. Pulmonary physiology, 4th ed. New York: McGraw-Hill; 1995.

[b] 10. Smith PL et al. Weight loss in mildly to moderately obese patients with obstructive sleep apnea. Ann Intern Med 1985; 103:850.

[b] 11. Schwartz AR et al. Effect of weight loss on upper airway collapsibility in obstructive sleep apnea. Am Rev Respir Dis 1991; 144:494.

[c] 12. Bradley TD, Phillipson EA. Sleep disorders. In Murray JF et al, eds. Textbook of respiratory medicine. Philadelphia: WB Saunders; 2000.

[d] 13. Smith PL et al. ATS guidelines: indications and standards for use of nasal continuous positive airway pressure (CPAP) in sleep apnea syndromes. Am J Respir Crit Care Med 1994; 150:1793.

[c] 14. Loube ED. Technologic advances in the treatment of obstructive sleep apnea syndrome. Chest 1999; 111:1426.

[b] 15. Burwell CS et al. Extreme obesity associated with alveolar hypoventilation: a Pickwickian syndrome. Am J Med 1956; 21:811.

[a] 16. Smith PL et al. The effects of protriptyline in sleep-disordered breathing. Am Rev Respir Dis 1983; 127:8.

[c] 17. Martin RJ. Alterations in airways disease during sleep: asthma and chronic obstructive pulmonary disease. In Tierney DF, ed. Current pulmonology, vol 16. St Louis: Mosby; 1995.

[d] 18. Strohl KP et al. ATS guidelines: sleep apnea; sleepiness; and driving risk. Am J Respir Crit Care Med 1994; 150:1463.

Approach to the Rheumatic Disorders

Philip Seo, MD

FAST FACTS

- The rheumatic disorders are an important cause of morbidity and mortality.
- The history and physical examination are more important than laboratory studies in diagnosing the underlying disorder.
- Many patients who complain of joint pain actually do not have inflammation of the joint.
- A useful approach to the diagnosis of arthritis is to consider the number of joints involved and the pattern of involvement, which can be used to narrow the differential diagnosis.

I. EPIDEMIOLOGY

1. By 2020, rheumatic diseases will affect 60 million Americans.[1] Rheumatic diseases already represent the leading cause of disability in the United States,[2] resulting in a total cost, in terms of expenditures and lost wages, equivalent to 2.5% of the gross national product,[3] a figure that fails to take into account the associated loss in quality of life.
2. Rheumatology encompasses a wide spectrum of disorders, from osteoarthritis to vasculitis, all of which have in common the presence of pain and inflammation. From a practical standpoint these diseases may be divided into two groups: those that are predominantly articular, with some systemic manifestations (such as the crystalline arthropathies), and those that are predominantly systemic syndromes, with some articular manifestations (such as systemic lupus erythematosus [SLE]).

II. CLINICAL PRESENTATION

1. The majority of the evaluation of the patient with rheumatic complaints takes place during the clinical history and physical examination. Laboratory abnormalities in the absence of appropriate clinical suspicion are notoriously unhelpful and misleading for this group of diseases.
2. The first step in the evaluation is to determine whether the patient truly has joint pain. Many patients who experience musculoskeletal discomfort localize their complaints to their joints, even when the primary process is not articular. Neuropathies, myopathies, periostitis, tendonitis, hypothyroidism, and fibromyalgia may all be interpreted by a patient as "arthritis," and a careful history and physical

examination can do much to exclude these mimics from the differential diagnosis.

3. The physical examination provides multiple clues for determining whether a patient has true joint pain. Patients with a true synovitis complain of pain on both active and passive range-of-motion exercises. Pain that is reproduced only on active range of motion (i.e., only when the patient moves the joint) implies that the periarticular structures, such as the tendons or the surrounding soft tissue (as in cellulitis), are the cause of pain, and not the joint itself. In addition, complaints that localize to a specific joint are less likely to be caused by diffuse musculoskeletal pain syndromes, such as fibromyalgia.

III. DIAGNOSTICS

A. HISTORY AND PHYSICAL EXAMINATION

1. Once it has been determined that a patient has true joint pain, the next step is to determine whether the complaints are noninflammatory or inflammatory (Fig. 70-1). This may be accomplished by asking about morning stiffness. Typically, patients with noninflammatory joint conditions note morning stiffness that lasts for less than 30 minutes and pain that is worst at the end of the day. Patients with inflammatory joint complaints, on the other hand, report morning stiffness that lasts for more than an hour and improves with activity during the day. Patients in this latter category frequently have systemic symptoms as well, including fatigue, malaise, low-grade fever, easy fatigability, unintentional weight loss, and occasionally depression.

2. The most common cause of noninflammatory joint pain is osteoarthritis (which typically affects the knees, the hips, and the carpometacarpal joints in the hands), but other common causes include avascular necrosis (occurring in patients with sickle cell disease or a history of chronic glucocorticoid use) and trauma to the joint. Patients who report their joints "locking" may have a torn meniscus or articular cartilage.

3. The presence of inflammatory joint pain is frequently confirmed by evidence of an active synovitis: on examination the involved joints are swollen, warm, and tender to palpation and feel like foam rubber, a sensation frequently described as "boggy." Examination of the small joints of the hands is best performed with the use of one hand to isolate the joint and the other to palpate for tenderness and evaluate range of motion. The inability of the patient to make a tight fist is a good clue to the presence of arthritis in a hand that looks normal at first glance.

4. Patients who have an inflammatory, active synovitis may be categorized in terms of the number of joints involved: a monoarthritis involves one joint; an oligoarthritis involves two to four joints; and a polyarthritis affects multiple joints.

5. The origin of the monoarthritis is limited to two major categories: infection (as in septic arthritis or Lyme disease) and crystalline arthritis

(as in gout or pseudogout). Examination of synovial fluid is crucial in determining the cause of the monoarthritis. However, the clinical picture and laboratory values associated with crystalline and septic arthritis have a considerable amount of overlap and may be difficult to separate in any particular patient.

6. An oligoarthritis may be caused by a crystalline arthritis or one of the seronegative spondyloarthropathies. The latter are associated with HLA-B27 and include ankylosing spondylosis, Reiter's disease, psoriatic arthritis, and enteropathic arthritis, all of which may be associated with lower back pain, enthesopathy (inflammation at the insertions of ligaments and tendons, classically seen as heel pain), and dactylitis (diffuse swelling of the entire digit). When gout presents as an oligoarthritis, it typically affects the joints in the lower extremities in an asymmetrical pattern. Pseudogout tends to involve the wrists, knees, and shoulders.

7. Polyarthritis with asymmetrical joint involvement has the same differential diagnosis as oligoarthritis. Causes of symmetrical polyarthritis, however, include rheumatoid arthritis, SLE, and the vasculitides. Rheumatoid arthritis generally affects the metacarpophalangeal and proximal interphalangeal joints and the wrists, and on examination the physician may find rheumatoid nodules on the extensor surfaces of the arms. SLE is more frequently associated with arthralgias than with arthritis, and the joint examination may be relatively benign. When considering vasculitis, the physician must simultaneously consider the mimickers of vasculitis (such as the hypercoagulable states and infective endocarditis), which require very different treatment.

8. The vasculitides are classified in terms of the vessels involved. The category of small vessel vasculitis includes the antineutrophilic cytoplasmic antibody (ANCA)-associated vasculitides (i.e., Wegener's granulomatosis, microscopic polyangiitis, and the Churg-Strauss syndrome), as well as other causes, including SLE, rheumatoid vasculitis, hypersensitivity vasculitis, mixed essential cryoglobulinemia, Henoch-Schönlein purpura, and Behçet's disease. Small vessel vasculitis may be associated with palpable purpura, periungual infarcts, peripheral neuropathy, splinter hemorrhages, and an active urinary sediment from glomerulonephritis.

9. The classic medium vessel vasculitis is polyarteritis nodosa, which may be associated with digital gangrene, severe Raynaud's phenomenon, intestinal ischemia, limb claudication, and mononeuritis multiplex. Involvement of the renal arteries may lead to hypertension and renal insufficiency. Symptoms develop in a stepwise fashion as individual vessels are affected. Approximately 10% of cases of polyarteritis nodosa are associated with hepatitis B infection, and treatment of the infection may lead to resolution of the arteritis.

10. Takayasu's arteritis and giant cell arteritis are examples of large

70

APPROACH TO THE RHEUMATIC DISORDERS

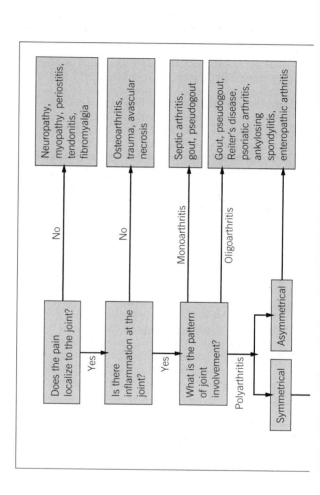

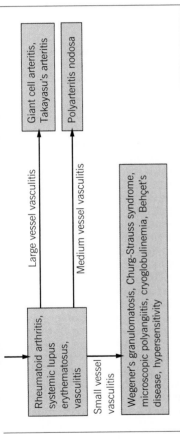

FIG. 70-1
Diagnosis of rheumatic disorders.

70

APPROACH TO THE RHEUMATIC DISORDERS

vessel vasculitis. Takayasu's arteritis is classically a disease of Asian women, and it causes inflammation, dilatation, or thrombosis of the arch of the aorta and the great vessels, leading to its nickname, the "pulseless disease." Giant cell arteritis, also known as temporal arteritis, rarely affects the aorta; classically, it is associated with temporal headache, visual change, and jaw claudication. Giant cell arteritis is a common cause of fever of unknown origin in the elderly.

B. LABORATORY ANALYSIS

1. Routine laboratory tests can provide multiple clues to the origin of a patient's rheumatic symptoms. An active sediment in a urine specimen may be consistent with lupus nephritis or one of the small vessel vasculitides. Renal insufficiency may also be seen in association with SLE, polyarteritis nodosa, or the hyperuricemia found with long-standing gout. Pseudogout is associated with hypercalcemia and hypophosphatemia.

2. Laboratory studies are frequently helpful to confirm the clinical assessment but are rarely sufficient by themselves. For example, 20% of patients with rheumatoid arthritis do not have detectable rheumatoid factor (although this does generally predict a more benign disease course); in contrast, rheumatoid factor may be seen in association with mixed essential cryoglobulinemia, chronic infections, and malignancy, as well as rheumatoid arthritis. In fact, the test for rheumatoid factor is frequently used to screen patients with hepatitis C infection for mixed essential cryoglobulinemia, since it is a technically easier and more reproducible test than the cryoglobulin assay itself.

3. The detection of antinuclear antibody (ANA) at low titer is by itself unhelpful. Up to 30% of normal individuals have ANA that is detectable at a titer of 1:40. The assays used by different institutions demonstrate different sensitivities (and the absolute titers may not correlate between laboratories), but titers less than 1:320 generally are not indicative of rheumatic disease. Very high titers are more specific for the presence of rheumatic disease but can be found not only with SLE, but also with Sjögren's syndrome, systemic sclerosis (or scleroderma), limited scleroderma (including CREST syndrome [calcinosis, Raynaud's phenomenon, esophageal involvement, sclerodactyly, and telangiectasia]), and polymyositis and even in some patients with rheumatoid arthritis.

4. The ANA is, however, very helpful in excluding the diagnosis of SLE, which is generally not seen in the absence of ANA. Similarly, if ANA is not detected, testing for antibodies to the extractable nuclear antigens (such as anti-double-stranded DNA, anti-Smith, anti-Ro, and anti-La) is unnecessary because these are rarely found in the absence of ANA (Table 70-1).

C. SYNOVIAL FLUID ANALYSIS

1. A diagnostic arthrocentesis may provide a great deal of information as to the origin of joint pain and has relatively few contraindications.

TABLE 70-1

AUTOANTIBODIES IN RHEUMATIC DISEASE

Disease	Antibody	Sensitivity (%)
Systemic lupus erythematosus	Antinuclear	95-100
Sjögren's disease	SSA/Ro	75
Systemic sclerosis	Scl 70	26-76
CREST syndrome	Centromere	80
Polymyositis	JO-1	20-30
Wegener's granulomatosis	c-ANCA	>90 (for active disease)
Microscopic polyangiitis	p-ANCA	>75
Mixed connective tissue disease	Ribonucleoprotein	100 (by definition)
Drug-induced systemic lupus erythematosus	Antihistone	90
Rheumatoid arthritis	Rheumatoid factor	80

ANCA, Antineutrophilic cytoplasmic nodules. *CREST,* calcinosis, Raynaud's phenomenon, esophageal involvement, sclerodactyly, and telangiectasia.

Synovial fluid should be evaluated for cell count with differential, presence of crystals, and culture. Occasionally on gross examination the fluid appears purulent, consistent with infectious arthritis.

2. When the diagnosis is less clear, the number of white blood cells in the synovial fluid can be helpful. Fewer than 200 white blood cells per microliter is generally considered to be noninflammatory and may be associated with degenerative joint disease, trauma, and nonarticular diseases. Between 200 to 500 white blood cells per microliter is consistent with an inflammatory effusion and may be seen with the crystalline arthropathies, the seronegative spondyloarthropathies, rheumatoid arthritis, and other causes. Septic arthritis is generally associated with more than 50,000 white blood cells per microliter, although lower numbers of cells may be seen in patients with human immunodeficiency virus infection or tuberculous arthritis.

D. **RADIOGRAPHIC ANALYSIS**

1. Radiographs can be helpful in the assessment of the patient with joint complaints. Osteoarthritis is accompanied radiographically by the presence of osteophytes, subchondral cysts, and joint space narrowing. Pseudogout is frequently accompanied by chondrocalcinosis, which is caused by the deposition of calcium pyrophosphate crystals in bone cartilage and leaves a telltale linear radiodensity at the articular surfaces. Patients with long-standing rheumatoid arthritis usually show evidence of erosions in the bones of the hands and feet. The presence of ulnar deviation in the hands in the absence of erosions should alert the examiner to the possibility of a Jaccoud-like arthropathy, which is associated with SLE.

2. Magnetic resonance imaging may be useful to confirm the presence of a lesion not apparent on plain films, such as a torn meniscus or a

small fracture. It is also useful for the detection of synovitis when the physical examination is equivocal.

IV. MANAGEMENT

1. Specific elements of the management of rheumatic disease depend on the underlying diagnosis and are discussed in greater detail in the following chapters. However, a few important common themes merit mention here.

2. Septic arthritis generally should be considered a medical emergency and deserves aggressive treatment with intravenous antibiotics to prevent long-term sequelae. Patients with septic arthritis frequently have to undergo arthrocentesis multiple times because antibiotics cannot penetrate a joint filled with pus.

3. A patient with monoarthritis not caused by infection (such as osteo-arthritis or the crystalline arthropathies) frequently experiences consid-erable relief from aspiration of the joint (which removes pressure on the joint capsule) and injection of the joint with corticosteroids. Many practitioners use a solution of triamcinolone acetate (40 g for a large joint, such as a knee; 20 g for a smaller joint, such as a wrist or ankle), mixed with an equivalent volume of 1% lidocaine. The latter provides rapid, albeit transient, relief of the patient's symptoms, allow-ing the corticosteroids time to work.

4. For any patient with arthritis, pain control is important and may be as simple as prescribing nonsteroidal antiinflammatory drugs, which are excellent at relieving the pain associated with inflammation and generally are well tolerated as long as the physician monitors for gastrointestinal and renal toxicity. These medications work better when taken on a fixed schedule, rather than only when the patient feels that he or she is experiencing enough pain to merit treatment with an analgesic.

5. Despite their long-term toxicity, corticosteroids are excellent anti-inflammatory and immunosuppressant agents. Patients who have severe symptoms of a rheumatic illness are commonly treated with corticosteroids, which are used in doses proportional to the severity of the illness. For example, a patient with acute monoarthritis caused by crystalline arthropathy or with polyarthritis from newly diagnosed rheumatoid arthritis might be treated initially with prednisone 40 mg PO qd to achieve immediate relief and to give other, less toxic medications time to work. In contrast, a patient with a life-threatening complication of SLE merits more aggressive treatment with intrave-nous corticosteroids, such as methylprednisolone in doses up to 1000 mg IV qd for 3 days.

PEARLS AND PITFALLS

- More patients are harmed than helped by a premature diagnosis of rheumatoid arthritis or SLE. When the diagnosis is not completely clear, the prudent approach is to treat the patient's symptoms and follow up clinically until the disease process manifests itself more clearly.

- A positive ANA alone does not establish the diagnosis of SLE.
- Most of the rheumatic diseases are difficult to diagnosis or exclude based on serological tests alone. The history is the most valuable tool for diagnosis of a rheumatic illness.
- Arthritis at the distal interphalangeal joints is commonly noted in only a handful of diseases: the seronegative spondyloarthropathies (especially psoriatic arthritis), osteoarthritis, and gout.
- Migratory arthritis (i.e., involvement of new joints as other joints improve) is seen in association with disseminated gonococcal infection.
- Osteoarthritis generally spares the wrists and the metacarpophalangeal joints; involvement of these joints should raise the suspicion of rheumatoid arthritis.

REFERENCES

[c] 1. Arthritis prevalence and activity limitations—United States, 1990. MMWR Morb Mortal Wkly Rep 1994; 43(24):433.

[c] 2. Prevalence of disabilities and associated health conditions—United States, 1991-1992. MMWR Morb Mortal Wkly Rep 1994; 43(40):730.

[c] 3. Yelin E, Callahan LF. The economic cost and social and psychological impact of musculoskeletal conditions. National Arthritis Data Work Groups. Arthritis Rheum 1995; 38(10):1351.

70

APPROACH TO THE RHEUMATIC DISORDERS

Crystalline Arthropathies

Megan E. Bowles Clowse, MD, MPH, and Alan Matsumoto, MD

FAST FACTS

- Acute gout and pseudogout typically appear in a single joint with abrupt onset of swelling, erythema, and severe pain with joint motion.
- The frequency of crystalline arthropathies increases with age. If a patient is young, secondary causes of gout or pseudogout should be considered.
- Treatment for an acute attack should be started promptly—the time until treatment is more important than the choice of treatment. Nonsteroidal antiinflammatory drugs (NSAIDs) work well for most patients.

71

I. EPIDEMIOLOGY

A. GOUT

1. The most common patient with gout is a man older than 40 years of age with hypertension, obesity, and a history of excessive alcohol use. The cumulative lifetime incidence of gout in men is around 6% to 10%.[1,2] Gout rarely develops in women before menopause. When it does, it is frequently associated with an identifiable cause, such as thiazide diuretics. Gout is rare in patients younger than 30 years; the diagnosis of gout in a young person should prompt a search for a metabolic disease that might lead to gout, such as an inherited enzyme deficiency or urate underexcretion.
2. An increased incidence in gouty attacks in the spring has been noted.[3,4] This goes against the conventional teaching that winter, with its increased likelihood for cold extremities, is more likely to lead to exacerbations of gout.
3. Many more patients have hyperuricemia (i.e., a serum uric acid level >7 mg/dL) than gout (Table 71-1). A uric acid elevation increases the risk for gout significantly but by itself generally does not merit treatment.[5]
4. Gout flare-ups can be triggered by alcohol consumption, nitrate-rich foods, and trauma or illness. Gout commonly develops in patients hospitalized for an acute illness or surgery.

B. PSEUDOGOUT

1. Pseudogout has equal gender distribution, but men are more likely to have acute attacks and women are more likely to have a chronic pseudoosteoarthritis.
2. The incidence of pseudogout increases with age. It is rare in patients younger than 50 years; therefore a diagnosis of pseudogout in a patient younger than 50 years merits an evaluation for secondary

TABLE 71-1

RELATIONSHIP BETWEEN URIC ACID LEVEL AND INCIDENCE OF GOUT

Serum Uric Acid Level (mg/dL)	Annual Incidence of Gout (%)	5-Year Incidence of Gout (%)
>9.0	4.9	22.0
8.0-8.9	4.1	9.8
7.0-7.9	0.9	6.0
<7.0	0.8	5.0

TABLE 71-2

TIME BETWEEN FIRST AND SECOND ATTACKS OF GOUT

Duration Between Initial Attack and Second Attack	Patients (%)
1 year	62
1-2 years	16
2-5 years	11
5-10 years	6
No recurrence in 10 years	7

causes, including hemochromatosis, hyperparathyroidism, hypomagnesemia, hypophosphatemia, hypothyroidism, and hypercalcemia.[6,7] In one study chondrocalcinosis from calcium pyrophosphate dihydrate (CPPD) deposition was found in radiographs of 15% of patients from 65 to 75 years old and 50% of patients over 85 years old, although, like hyperuricemia, chondrocalcinosis in the absence of symptoms associated with pseudogout does not merit therapy.[8]

II. CLINICAL PRESENTATION

A. GOUT

1. The acute gout attack is abrupt in onset and may be accompanied by fever. The affected joint is swollen and fluctuant and demonstrates exquisite pain on motion and palpation. Untreated, the attack resolves in 7 to 10 days; treatment leads to more rapid resolution of symptoms. After the resolution of an acute gouty attack, a pain-free interlude called the intracritical period typically occurs. The previously affected joint may continue to have urate crystals but is asymptomatic. Although some patients never have a second episode, most have subsequent attacks. The average time between the first and second attack is 11 months, although this varies widely (Table 71-2). Over time, the intracritical period shortens and the number of joints affected and the severity of systemic symptoms increase.[9]

2. With time, chronic gout may develop. Patients with chronic gout never have symptom-free periods. In these patients a deforming, symmetrical polyarthritis that can be confused with rheumatoid arthritis develops.

3. Some patients have tophaceous gout, characterized by subcutaneous deposits of urate crystals called tophi, which start as firm nodules that have mild erythema and form over affected joints, digits, the olecranon bursa, or ears. With time they harden and turn yellowish. Tophi develop in 15% to 22% of patients with gout, usually after it has been poorly controlled for years. In elderly women, however, the first manifestation of gout may be digital tophi that develop around osteoarthritic joints with little inflammation.[10]

4. Uric acid nephrolithiasis may develop in patients with hyperuricemia, with or without gout. Only 25% of patients with these stones have gout, and only 20% of patients with gout will have stones. The risk that stones will develop is sufficiently low to preclude significant benefit from treatment of hyperuricemia until after a stone has been recognized.[11] Chronic urate nephropathy results from a mild chronic inflammatory response to urate deposits in the kidney. This can lead to fibrosis and a mild worsening of renal function. Renal dysfunction seen with gout is more likely caused by coexisting hypertension, diabetes, obesity, or lead intoxication.[12]

B. PSEUDOGOUT

1. An acute pseudogout attack may be clinically identical to an attack of gout. It typically manifests with a single erythematous, swollen, and painful joint. More than 50% of pseudogout attacks affect the knee; the wrist, shoulder, and smaller joints are involved less frequently. An attack can be precipitated by surgery, trauma, or severe illness. Although patients with a pseudogout attack generally have fewer systemic symptoms than are seen with a gouty flare-up, fever, malaise, and a leukocytosis can all occur.

2. Some patients have intermittent acute attacks of pseudogout, which most commonly affect the knees, wrists, metacarpophalangeal joints, hips, shoulders, elbows, and spine. Recurrent attacks of pseudogout can mimic other forms of arthritis. Chronic CPPD deposition can promote progressive degeneration in multiple joints, creating a pseudoosteoarthritis. In a small number of patients CPPD deposition causes chronic inflammatory arthritis, sometimes referred to as pseudorheumatoid arthritis. CPPD crystals can be deposited in the spine, causing stiffness and ankylosis similar to that seen in patients with spondyloarthropathies. This manifestation is most frequently seen in patients with familial CPPD crystal deposition disease.

III. DIAGNOSTICS

A. HISTORY

1. The crystalline arthropathies frequently recur, so patients often recall similar attacks. Attacks of both gout and pseudogout are characterized by a rapid onset of joint pain and swelling, accompanied by systemic evidence of inflammation (including fever), which can last for several days if not treated.

71

CRYSTALLINE ARTHROPATHIES

2. Gout is associated with several medical conditions, including hypertension, diabetes, nephrolithiasis, renal transplantation, osteoarthritis, and heavy alcohol use, and may be precipitated by the initiation of allopurinol or thiazide diuretics. Pseudogout is associated with hemachromatosis or electrolyte imbalance and occasionally occurs after hyaluronate injection, intravenous pamidronate administration, or parathyroidectomy. Both gout and pseudogout can be precipitated by recent trauma, surgery, or illness.

B. PHYSICAL EXAMINATION

1. The classic presentation of gout is podagra, or inflammation of the first metatarsal joint. The initial joint affected by gout, however, is more often the ankle (39%) or the knee (27%).[13,14] Ninety percent of initial gout attacks are in a single joint, but recurrent bouts can present as an oligoarthritis.[15] Pseudogout most commonly affects the knees, followed by the wrists, shoulders, and smaller joints.

2. Both gout and pseudogout are associated with joint erythema and swelling, but the pain of gout is typically more severe and is out of proportion to the appearance of the joint. In addition, gout is sometimes accompanied by tophi, which appear hard and yellowish and may be found on digits, elbows, or ears or anywhere on the skin.

C. LABORATORY ANALYSIS

1. During an acute gout or pseudogout attack, patients often have a leukocytosis and neutrophilia. They may also have an elevation in erythrocyte sedimentation rate or other inflammatory markers.

2. The uric acid level during an acute attack is not useful in many cases. A normal uric acid level does not rule out gout; 40% of patients during a gout attack have a normal uric acid level, since the circulating level of uric acid can fall during an attack.[16,17]

3. Secondary gout can come from overproduction or underexcretion of uric acid. High cell turnover from tumor lysis or hemolytic anemia can cause gout. Associated disorders include obesity, hypertension, alcohol use, diabetes mellitus, and hypertriglyceridemia. Checking for these disorders may be worthwhile when a diagnosis of gout is made.

4. Deposition of calcium pyrophosphate crystals is associated with several diseases and electrolyte abnormalities. A diagnosis of pseudogout in a younger person should prompt an evaluation of the serum calcium, phosphorus, magnesium, alkaline phosphatase, ferritin, and thyroid-stimulating hormone levels, since abnormalities in any one of these may provide a clue to an underlying disorder.

D. SYNOVIAL FLUID ANALYSIS

1. Arthrocentesis is the gold standard for the diagnosis of gout and may be helpful in diagnosing pseudogout as well. The probability of infecting a sterile joint during arthrocentesis is low.[18]

2. Synovial fluid should be examined with a microscope under polarized light. Urate crystals are needlelike with negative birefringence. They are two to three times larger than a neutrophil and during an acute

attack may be found within neutrophils. When the polarized light is parallel to the crystal, it appears yellow. When it is perpendicular, it is blue. CPPD crystals are rhomboid in shape, with weakly positive birefringence. Under polarized light they are blue when the light is parallel and yellow when it is perpendicular.

3. Reproducibility of CPPD crystal identification between laboratories is poor, possibly because the crystals can be quite small and often are not birefringent, the crystals may degrade in an older sample, and dust on the slide can be mistaken for CPPD crystals (Table 71-3).[19,20]

E. RADIOGRAPHIC ANALYSIS

1. Radiographic studies are not diagnostic for early gout. In cases of chronic gout, however, soft tissue tophi, punched-out erosions with sclerotic margins near affected joints, and a relative preservation of the joint space are typical.[21] Periarticular erosions caused by chronic gout take on a "rat bite" appearance with a sharp overhang characteristic of the disease.

2. Radiographs may be useful in confirming the diagnosis of pseudogout. Anteroposterior radiographs of the knees and symphysis pubis and posteroanterior radiographs of the wrists may demonstrate chondrocalcinosis, which manifests as radiodensities in the cartilage of the joint, ligaments, or joint capsule. Once degenerative changes have developed, however, chondrocalcinosis in a collapsed joint space can be difficult to see.

IV. MANAGEMENT

A. GOUT

1. No benefit in renal function has been identified with treating asymptomatic hyperuricemia.[5,22] However, men in the Framingham study who had gout (but were not taking diuretics) had twice the incidence

71

CRYSTALLINE ARTHROPATHIES

TABLE 71-3
SYNOVIAL FLUID CHARACTERISTICS

Type of Arthritis	White Blood Cell Count (per cubic millimeter)	Differential Count	Type of Crystal	Other
Acute gout	>20,000	>70% neutrophils	Negative birefringence, needle shaped	Crystals are within the neutrophils
Chronic gout	<2000		Urate crystals as above, but fewer	Crystals are *not* in neutrophils
Pseudogout	15,000-30,000	90% neutrophils	Weakly positive birefringence, rhomboid	Crystals are within the neutrophils

of angina and 60% more cardiac disease than men without gout. This increased risk associated with gout appeared to be independent of hypertension, alcohol use, obesity, and diabetes.[23] No studies have shown a decreasing cardiac risk with improved uric acid control.

2. The most important factor in the treatment of the acute gout attack is the time to treatment; rapid initiation of therapy is much more important than the type of therapy used. Nonsteroidal antiinflammatory drugs (NSAIDs) are the treatment of choice. Indomethacin 50 mg PO qid has been used in trials, ketorolac 60 mg IM once has been shown to be effective in an emergency department setting,[24,25] and ibuprofen 800 mg PO tid can be effective as well. Cyclooxygenase-2 inhibitors are presumed to be effective, although they have not been well studied for this indication.

3. For patients with contraindications to NSAIDs (e.g., allergies, recent gastrointestinal hemorrhage, or significant renal dysfunction), corticosteroids are efficacious. Prednisone may be started at 30 to 50 mg PO every day for several days and then tapered over the next 10 days. This regimen is effective in achieving pain control, preventing rebound arthropathy, and reducing side effects.[26,27]

4. The side effects of diarrhea and abdominal pain frequently preclude the use of colchicine in treating acute gouty flare-ups. The dose required for relief uniformly produces diarrhea and does not provide faster or superior relief from pain compared with NSAIDs or corticosteroids. Intravenously administered colchicine has significant, possibly lethal, side effects, and its use is not recommended.

5. Intermittent therapy with NSAIDs or corticosteroids is sufficient for many patients with gout, since many do not have frequent attacks. Indications for long-term prophylactic medications are tophaceous gout, radiographic erosions, uric acid nephrolithiasis, urate nephropathy, recurrent episodes of acute gout that impair lifestyle, and patient preference.

6. Allopurinol is the drug of choice for long-term control of hyperuricemia and gout. It is generally well tolerated but should not be started during an acute gout attack because the rapid decrease in uric acid in the blood can actually worsen the attack. When allopurinol is started, a prophylactic medication (e.g., colchicine or an NSAID) should be given concomitantly for at least 6 months after the normalization of uric acid level is achieved. Allopurinol should be started at 100 mg PO qd and then increased by 100 mg every 2 to 4 weeks until the serum uric acid level is less than 6 mg/dL. In patients with renal insufficiency, allopurinol should be given every other day. Starting allopurinol at a higher dose increases the risk for allopurinol hypersensitivity reaction, with possibly lethal consequences. This syndrome is characterized by fever, rash, eosinophilia, and liver and renal dysfunction.

7. Colchicine works by decreasing the neutrophil reaction in the synovial fluid; it has no effect on uric acid levels. It is most effective when used as a prophylactic medication, not to treat an acute attack. Most patients need between 0.6 and 1.2 mg PO every day to prevent gout. In cases of mild gout colchicine can be used alone; however, the chronic effects of hyperuricemia, such as tophi and urate nephropathy, will not be prevented. In cases of more severe gout it can be used when allopurinol is initiated until the serum uric acid level has been normal for at least 6 months. It has been shown to be safer and less expensive than NSAIDs as prophylaxis during the initiation of allopurinol therapy.[27] Some patients benefit from lifelong use of the combination of colchicine and allopurinol to prevent flare-ups. Colchicine can have more diarrheal side effects in patients with impaired renal function.

8. Probenecid increases renal excretion of uric acid. It cannot be used, however, in patients who have renal insufficiency or a history of renal calculi.

B. PSEUDOGOUT

1. Asymptomatic chondrocalcinosis does not require therapy. An evaluation for the underlying cause of the joint changes may be warranted, however, because it may be the first clue to a systemic disease or metabolic abnormality.

2. The treatment of an acute pseudogout attack is the same as the treatment for an acute gout attack. Arthrocentesis and joint immobilization may lessen the pain of the attack. Colchicine may be helpful for patients with recurrent attacks of pseudogout, but nothing has been proved to decrease progressive crystal deposition. Even reversing the underlying cause rarely changes the course of the disease.

PEARLS AND PITFALLS

- Gout can have a different presentation in older women, who are more likely to have gout initially in the small joints of the hands, where osteoarthritis coexists.
- Urate and CPPD crystals can be found in the same joint.
- Finding crystals in a joint does not rule out an infectious cause.
- Laboratory examination for crystals can be falsely negative. If gout or pseudogout is strongly suspected but the aspirate is reported to be negative for crystals, the aspirate should be reexamined or empirical therapy should be considered.
- Allopurinol should never be started during an acute episode. When it is started, colchicine or an NSAID should be started as well to avoid worsening an attack.
- Colchicine should not be administered intravenously, and vigilance for the allopurinol hypersensitivity reaction should be maintained.
- Serum uric acid levels do not help in the diagnosis of gout; they may be low, elevated, or normal during an acute attack.

71

CRYSTALLINE ARTHROPATHIES

REFERENCES

[b] 1. Hochberg MC et al. Racial differences in the incidence of gout: the role of hypertension. Arthritis Rheum 1995; 38:628.

[b] 2. Roubenoff R et al. Incidence and risk factors for gout in white men. JAMA 1991; 266:3004.

[b] 3. Schlesinger N et al. Acute gouty arthritis is seasonal. J Rheumatol 1998; 25:342.

[b] 4. Gallerani M et al. Seasonal variation in the onset of acute microcrystalline arthritis. Rheumatology (Oxford) 1999; 38:1003.

[b] 5. Campion EW, Glynn RJ, DeLabry LO. Asymptomatic hyperuricemia: risks and consequences in the Normative Aging Study. Am J Med 1987; 82:421.

[c] 6. Jones AC et al. Diseases associated with calcium pyrophosphate deposition disease. Semin Arthritis Rheum 1992; 22:188.

[b] 7. Chaisson CE et al. Lack of association between thyroid status and chondrocalcinosis or osteoarthritis: the Framingham Osteoarthritis Study. J Rheumatol 1996; 23:711.

[b] 8. Wilkins E et al. Osteoarthritis and articular chondrocalcinosis in the elderly. Ann Rheum Dis 1983; 42:280.

[c] 9. Gutman AB. Gout. In Beeson PB, McDermott W, eds. Textbook of medicine, 12th ed. Philadelphia: WB Saunders; 1958.

[b] 10. Meyers OL, Monteagudo FS. Gout in females: an analysis of 92 patients. Clin Exp Rheumatol 1985; 3:105.

[c] 11. McGill NW. Gout and other crystal-associated arthropathies. Baillieres Best Pract Res Clin Rheumatol 2000; 14:445.

[b] 12. Berger L, Yu TF. Renal function in gout. IV. An analysis of 524 gouty subjects including long-term follow-up studies. Am J Med 1975; 59:605.

[b] 13. Koh WH, Seah A, Chai P. Clinical presentation and disease associations of gout: a hospital-based study of 100 patients in Singapore. Ann Acad Med Singapore 1998; 27:7.

[b] 14. Garcia CO, Kutzbach AG, Espinoza LR. Characteristics of gouty arthritis in the Guatemalan population. Clin Rheumatol 1997; 16:45.

[b] 15. Lawry GV 2nd, Fan PT, Bluestone R. Polyarticular versus monoarticular gout: a prospective, comparative analysis of clinical features. Medicine (Baltimore) 1988; 67:335.

[b] 16. Schlesinger N, Baker DG, Schumacher HR Jr. Serum urate during bouts of acute gouty arthritis. J Rheumatol 1997; 24:2265.

[b] 17. Logan JA, Morrison E, Mcgill PE. Serum uric acid in acute gout. Ann Rheum Dis 1997; 56:696.

[c] 18. Sack K. Monarthritis: differential diagnosis. Am J Med 1997; 102:30S.

[a] 19. Ivorra J, Rosas J, Pascual E. Most calcium pyrophosphate crystals appear as non-birefringent. Ann Rheum Dis 1999; 58:582.

[a] 20. Schumacher HR Jr et al. Reproducibility of synovial fluid analyses: a study among four laboratories. Arthritis Rheum 1986; 29:770.

[c] 21. Cornelius R, Schneider HJ. Gouty arthritis in the adult. Radiol Clin North Am 1988; 26:1267.

[b] 22. Langford HG et al. Is thiazide-produced uric acid elevation harmful? Analysis of data from the Hypertension Detection and Follow-up Program. Arch Intern Med 1987; 147:645.

[b] 23. Abbott RD et al. Gout and coronary heart disease: the Framingham Study. J Clin Epidemiol 1988; 41(3):237.

[a] 24. Shrestha M et al. Randomized double-blind comparison of the analgesic efficacy of intramuscular ketorolac and oral indomethacin in the treatment of acute gouty arthritis. Ann Emerg Med 1995; 26:682.

[b] 25. Shrestha M et al. Treatment of acute gouty arthritis with intramuscular ketorolac tromethamine. Am J Emerg Med 1994; 12:454.

[a] 26. Alloway JA et al. Comparison of triamcinolone acetonide with indomethacin in the treatment of acute gouty arthritis. J Rheumatol 1993; 20:111.

[b] 27. Groff GD, Franck WA, Raddatz DA. Systemic steroid therapy for acute gout: a clinical trial and review of the literature. Semin Arthritis Rheum 1990; 19:329.

Infectious Monoarthritis

Stuart M. Levine, MD, and Allan C. Gelber, MD, PhD

FAST FACTS

- Nongonococcal bacterial arthritis is a medical emergency.
- Crystal-induced arthritis is much more common than septic arthritis.
- Polyarticular septic arthritis occurs in 15% of patients and carries a 30% mortality rate.
- The physician should be aware of the possibility of sternoclavicular joint septic arthritis in intravenous drug users.
- Patients who are elderly, have rheumatoid arthritis, are immunosuppressed, or have prosthetic joints are at increased risk.
- Human immunodeficiency virus infection can manifest itself as an acute painful monoarthritis or oligoarthritis with bland synovial fluid.
- Arthrocentesis and synovial fluid analysis should be performed for all patients with an acutely inflamed, painful joint.
- After initial drainage, empirical antimicrobial therapy should begin immediately based on the likely pathogen.

72

I. OVERVIEW

1. The differential diagnosis of acute monoarthritis includes infectious arthritis (20%), crystal-induced arthritis (up to 80%), trauma, osteoarthritis, atypical rheumatoid arthritis, seronegative spondyloarthropathy, ischemic necrosis, foreign body synovitis, tumor, and systemic disease.[1]
2. Most diagnoses are suggested by the medical history, but differentiation between infectious and crystal-induced arthritis remains a clinical challenge.

II. CLINICAL PRESENTATION

1. In the assessment of a patient with presumed septic arthritis, the distribution of joint inflammation is important to note. Between 80% and 90% of nongonococcal bacterial joint infections are monoarticular,[1] whereas approximately 15% show polyarticular involvement.[2,3] Polyarticular septic arthritis is seen predominantly in patients with previous joint damage or with rheumatoid arthritis, in the elderly, and in other systemic inflammatory diseases associated with a destructive synovitis. It is associated with a mortality rate of up to 30% (compared with a 4% rate for monoarticular septic arthritis) despite adequate antimicrobial therapy.[3]
2. Most cases of septic arthritis develop as a result of hematogenous spread in older patients with underlying joint abnormalities[4,5]; a

primary source should always be sought in patients with atraumatic monoarthropathies.

3. Nongonococcal bacterial septic arthritis is the most destructive intraarticular infectious process encountered in clinical practice. Table 72-1 lists the most common etiological agents.

4. Disseminated gonococcal infections are more common, less destructive, and more responsive to treatment than other bacterial arthritides. They are usually seen in healthy, younger, sexually active patients. In one series 83% of patients were female and the mean age was 23 years. The most common physical examination findings were migratory polyarthritis and arthralgias (66%), knee synovitis (54%), dermatitis (39%), and genitourinary symptoms (63%).[6]

5. Gram-negative infections are more frequently seen in immunocompromised patients who have severe comorbid illness, extraarticular infections, or a history of intravenous drug abuse. (*Salmonella* causes septic arthritis in patients with systemic lupus erythematosus and sickle cell anemia, and *Pseudomonas* infections are more common in patients who are intravenous drug users.)

6. Tuberculosis should always be considered if patients have periarticular bony lesions and synovitis in the appropriate clinical setting. Lyme arthritis occurs months after the initial infection in about 60% of untreated patients; large joints are more swollen than painful, and attacks are usually intermittent. *Ureaplasma urealyticum* infection (hypogammaglobulinemia), *Pasteurella multocida* infection (dog bites), *Mycobacterium marinum* infection (freshwater or saltwater exposure), and fungal infections (immunocompromised patients) represent other causes of infectious arthritis.

III. DIAGNOSTICS
A. HISTORY AND PHYSICAL EXAMINATION

1. The patient should be asked about a history of systemic symptoms (fever, weight loss, night sweats), immunosuppression, sexual history, tick bites, travel, intravenous drug use, recurrence of symptoms, trauma, and presence of a prosthetic joint.

TABLE 72-1

MICROBIOLOGICAL PATHOGENS IN NONGONOCOCCAL SEPTIC ARTHRITIS

Agent	Prevalence (%)
Aerobic gram-positive bacteria	80
Staphylococcus aureus	60
Non–group A, β-hemolytic streptococci	15
Streptococcus pneumoniae	3
Aerobic gram-negative bacteria	18
Anaerobic infections	1
Other (e.g., mycobacteria)	1

Data from N Engl J Med 1993; 329:1013.

2. The sudden onset of pain and swelling in a joint should never be ignored. Any painful limitation of motion on physical examination should be noted; if flexion is maintained, the inflammatory process is unlikely to involve the joint space. In such a circumstance, cellulitis, bursitis, tendonitis, or damage to other periarticular structures should be considered.

3. A specific search for oral ulcers (Behçet's syndrome and systemic lupus erythematosus), skin rashes, and signs of peripheral embolization should be undertaken.

4. The presence of fever is not sensitive for the diagnosis of septic arthritis. A number of series of patients with nongonococcal bacterial arthritis have reported sensitivities for fever of less than 60%.[7,8]

B. ARTHROCENTESIS AND SYNOVIAL FLUID ANALYSIS

1. Arthrocentesis and synovial fluid analysis should be performed for all patients with an acute monoarthritis. All tests can be performed on 1 to 2 mL of fluid; 1 drop is enough for crystal analysis.

2. Cell count, Gram's stain and culture, and wet prep examination for crystals should be performed. Normal synovial fluid contains fewer than 200 cells/mm^3. In a prospective study of 100 consecutive patients undergoing arthrocentesis, only fluid white blood cell (WBC) counts greater than 2000/mm^3 (sensitivity 84%) and percentage of polymorphonuclear neutrophil leukocytes (PMNs) greater than 75% (sensitivity 75%) reliably distinguished inflammatory from noninflammatory causes. In an accompanying retrospective analysis of 28 patients with culture-positive septic arthritis, the median WBC count was 60,000/mm^3 (89% PMNs).[9] No absolute cutoff value has been established; a WBC count greater than 100,000/mm^3 is usually considered to reflect sepsis, but septic joints can have WBC counts as low as 2000/mm^3. These generally have profound neutrophilia (>85% PMNs).[7]

3. The algorithm in Fig. 72-1 can be used for initial management of patients with suspected septic arthritis.

C. RADIOGRAPHIC ANALYSIS

1. Radiographic features of septic arthritis include uniform cartilage loss, juxtaarticular osteoporosis, and loss of the white cortical line at the joint margin. Radiographs of the joint may add information to the history and physical examination. They can be used to visualize fractures, osteomyelitis, osteoarthritis, chondrocalcinosis, and tumors but cannot differentiate septic from inflammatory joints.

2. Magnetic resonance imaging can be useful in detecting soft tissue inflammation, osteomyelitis, meniscal tears, and ligamentous damage but also fails to discriminate between septic and inflamed joints.[10]

3. Radionuclide bone scans are very sensitive (up to 100%) for septic arthritis but lack specificity. They have little role in the routine clinical evaluation of an inflamed joint.[11]

72

INFECTIOUS MONOARTHRITIS

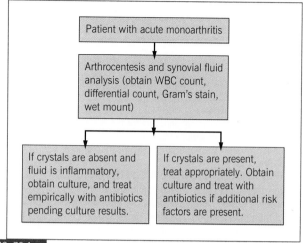

FIG. 72-1

Initial management of patients with suspected septic arthritis. *WBC,* White blood cell.

D. LABORATORY ANALYSIS

1. The importance of synovial fluid analysis is outlined in a previous section.
2. Gram-positive organisms were seen in approximately 50% to 60% of synovial fluid cultures in one study.[5] In this same series, synovial fluid or blood cultures were positive in 82% of cases.
3. WBC count may be normal in up to 40% of cases. The diagnosis of septic arthritis should never be excluded on the basis of absence of leukocytosis.
4. C-reactive protein level may be elevated in up to 98% of cases and may be useful in monitoring the response to therapy.[8]
5. Urethral, pharyngeal, and rectal culture samples should be obtained when gonococcal arthritis is being considered. One study noted the frequency of positive cultures as follows: urogenital, 86%; synovial fluid, 44%; rectal, 39%; blood, 13%; pharyngeal, 7%.[6]
6. When considering gout in the differential diagnosis, the physician should remember that serum uric acid levels during acute attacks may not be diagnostic; they may be low, elevated, or normal. Examination on the synovial fluid establishes the diagnosis of crystal-induced arthritis. Septic and crystal-induced arthritis can coexist in the same joint.

IV. MANAGEMENT

1. The goal of treatment in patients with septic arthritis is synovial fluid sterilization. This may be accomplished with a combination of par-

TABLE 72-2

RECOMMENDATIONS FOR EMPIRICAL ANTIMICROBIAL COVERAGE
IN SEPTIC ARTHRITIS

Gram's Stain	Antibiotic	Alternative	Comments
Gram-positive cocci (can be in pairs, chains, singly, or in clusters)	Vancomycin 1 g IV q12h; adjust for renal function	Third-generation cephalosporin	Alter antibiotic regimen once sensitivities are known; use oxacillin or nafcillin for methicillin-sensitive *Staphylococcus aureus,* third-generation cephalosporin for *Streptococcus pneumoniae*
Gram-negative cocci	Ceftriaxone 2 g IV qd	Imipenem 0.5 g IV q6h	Usually *Neisseria*
Gram-negative bacilli	Third-generation cephalosporin	Imipenem 0.5 g IV q6h	If patient is at risk for *Pseudomonas* infection, can add aminoglycoside, extended spectrum penicillin

72

INFECTIOUS MONOARTHRITIS

enteral antimicrobial therapy and arthrocentesis. Intraarticular antibiotics have no role.

2. Elderly patients, patients undergoing hemodialysis, and those with rheumatoid arthritis, a history of intravenous drug use, or prosthetic joints are especially prone to *Staphylococcus aureus* infections. Adequate drainage is particularly important in these patients.

3. Patients with prosthetic joints are at increased risk for infections with *Staphylococcus epidermidis* and methicillin-resistant *S. aureus,* and untreated infections can lead to joint loosening and the development of chronic osteomyelitis. Drainage, culture, and treatment with vancomycin are recommended. Repeat arthroplasty after débridement and 4 to 6 weeks of parenteral antibiotics can then be accomplished safely.[12]

4. Table 72-2 provides general recommendations for empirical antimicrobial coverage in cases of septic arthritis. Most studies recommend at least 2 weeks of parenteral treatment followed by 2 to 3 more weeks of oral treatment.[4,8,13]

5. One large retrospective review found slightly better joint outcomes in patients who underwent arthrocentesis (66%) rather than arthrotomy or arthroscopy (57%).[14] Arthrocentesis can be repeated as necessary to reduce discomfort and assess synovial fluid sterilization. Surgical drainage is indicated, however, if no clinical response is seen after 5 days of antimicrobial therapy; if the patient has septic arthritis in the hip, shoulder, or other areas that are difficult to aspirate; or if extensive soft tissue and extracapsular spread suggests the presence of abscess formation.

PEARLS AND PITFALLS

- Patients with low baseline WBC counts (e.g., those with acquired immunodeficiency disease or other immunosuppressive conditions) may have a septic joint with a low WBC count. These patients are prone to the development of fungal septic arthritis as well.
- Even in the setting of a crystal-proven arthritis, the possibility of concomitant septic arthritis should be considered.

REFERENCES

[c] 1. Baker DG, Schumacher HR. Acute monoarthritis. N Engl J Med 1993; 329:1013.

[b] 2. Goldenberg DL, Cohen AS. Acute infectious arthritis: a review of patients with nongonococcal joint infections (with emphasis on therapy and prognosis). Am J Med 1976; 60:369.

[b] 3. Dubost JJ et al. Polyarticular septic arthritis. Medicine (Baltimore) 1993; 72:296.

[b] 4. Martens PB, Ho G. Septic arthritis in adults: clinical features, outcome, and intensive care requirements. J Intensive Care Med 1995; 10:246.

[b] 5. Weston VC et al. Clinical features and outcome of septic arthritis in a single UK Health District 1982-1991. Ann Rheum Dis 1999; 58:214.

[b] 6. Wise CM et al. Gonococcal arthritis in an era of increasing penicillin resistance: presentations and outcomes in 41 recent cases (1985-1991). Arch Intern Med 1994; 154:2690.

[b] 7. Schlapbach P et al. Bacterial arthritis: are fever, rigors, leucocytosis and blood cultures of diagnostic value? Clin Rheum 1990; 9:69.

[c] 8. Gupta MN, Sturrock RD, Field M. A prospective 2-year study of 75 patients with adult-onset septic arthritis. Rheumatology (Oxford) 2001; 40:24-30.

[b] 9. Shmerling RH et al. Synovial fluid tests: what should be ordered? JAMA 1990; 264:1009.

[b] 10. Graif M et al. The septic versus nonseptic inflamed joint: MRI characteristics. Skeletal Radiol 1999; 28:616.

[b] 11. Mudun A et al. Tc-99m nanocolloid and Tc-99m MDP three-phase bone imaging in osteomyelitis and septic arthritis: a comparative study. Clin Nucl Med 1995; 20:772.

[b] 12. Hirakawa K et al. Results of 2-stage reimplantation for infected total knee arthroplasty. J Arthroplasty 1998; 13:22.

[c] 13. Smith JW, Piercy EA. Infectious arthritis. Clin Infect Dis 1995; 20:225.

[b] 14. Broy SB, Schmid FR. A comparison of medical drainage (needle aspiration) and surgical drainage (arthrotomy or arthroscopy) in the initial treatment of infected joints. Clin Rheum Dis 1986; 12:501.

Systemic Lupus Erythematosus

Traci Thompson Ferguson, MD, and Michelle Petri, MD, MPH

FAST FACTS

- Triggers of systemic lupus erythematosus (SLE) flare-ups include exposure to ultraviolet light, trimethoprim-sulfamethoxazole, *Echinacea*, infections, and possibly emotional stress.
- In the Hopkins Lupus Cohort the most common causes of hospitalization were active SLE (35%), infection (14%), and medical complications of SLE (13%). More than 90% of infections in this cohort were bacterial, and the most common medical complication was coronary artery disease.
- Sepsis is the most common cause of death in patients with end-stage renal disease caused by lupus nephritis.
- Women with SLE are two to three times more likely than women without SLE to be hospitalized for an acute myocardial infarction or stroke.
- Almost 50% of patients with SLE make antiphospholipid antibodies, which increase their risk of thrombosis.

73

I. EPIDEMIOLOGY

1. SLE is a chronic, systemic, autoimmune disease. Four other forms of lupus include drug-induced lupus (associated with hydralazine, procainamide, isoniazid, chlorpromazine, methyldopa, quinidine, sulfasalazine, and various other drugs and characterized by the resolution of symptoms after the offending agent is withdrawn),[1] chronic cutaneous (discoid) lupus (skin lesions present without any systemic manifestations), subacute cutaneous lupus, and neonatal lupus (manifesting as congenital heart block or skin lesions).
2. SLE is predominantly a disease of women of childbearing age. Women are nine times more likely to be affected by SLE than men, and the disease onset generally occurs during the second to fourth decades of life.
3. Ethnicity plays an important role in the natural history of SLE. African-Americans have a higher incidence and prevalence of SLE,[2] with more neurological disease, renal disease, and higher Systemic Lupus Activity Measure (SLAM) scores.[3] Native Americans have a twofold increase in SLE prevalence as compared with European Americans, with higher SLE Disease Activity Index (SLEDAI) scores at the time of diagnosis and a higher rate of vasculitis, renal involvement, and fatality.[4] Hispanics in the LUMINA Study Group were more likely to have cardiac and renal disease.[3]

4. The incidence of SLE has nearly tripled over the past four decades, from 1.51 per 100,000 in the 1950-1979 Rochester, Minnesota, cohort to 5.56 per 100,000 in the 1980-1992 cohort. The 1980-1992 cohort had a statistically significant improvement in survival rate over time ($p = .035$),[5] but the overall 10-year survival rate was still only approximately 80%.[6]

5. Over the past four decades the survival rate of patients with SLE has significantly increased.[5] A large multicenter European prospective trial showed a 5-year overall survival rate of 95%.[7] In a southern Chinese population, thrombocytopenia and high-dose steroids were independent risk factors for mortality.[8] Other predictors of mortality are the presence of nephritis (relative risk, 2.34), seizures (relative risk, 1.77), and thrombocytopenia,[9] along with disease activity, disease damage, and poverty.[10]

II. CLINICAL PRESENTATION

1. The diagnosis of SLE should be based on a combination of subjective and objective information, including the clinical presentation, results of standard blood analyses (e.g., a complete blood cell count, electrolyte balance, and urinalysis), the presence of autoantibodies (including antinuclear antibodies [ANA], anti-dsDNA, anti-Sm, anti-RNP, anti SS-A [Ro], anti SS-A [La]), and other data (e.g., results of a renal biopsy or low serum complement levels).

2. The updated 1982 revised criteria for the classification of SLE include new immunological criteria to enable the practitioner to classify SLE for research purposes (Table 73-1).[11,12]

3. According to the criteria, a patient is classified as having SLE if any four or more of the 11 criteria are present, either serially or simultaneously. The revised criteria published in 1982 (which included the identification of the LE cell and did not include the presence of anticardiolipin antibodies) have a sensitivity of 96% and a specificity of 96%.[11]

4. When evaluating a patient who may have signs or symptoms characteristic of SLE, the physician should exclude other rheumatic diseases, including mixed connective tissue disease, Sjögren's syndrome, polymyositis, dermatomyositis, scleroderma, and rheumatoid arthritis.

5. The diagnosis of SLE is based on characteristic objective symptoms and signs of autoimmunity, often in the setting of confirmatory laboratory tests such as a complete blood cell count, urinalysis, and creatinine. Autoantibodies that are specific for SLE (anti-dsDNA and anti-Sm), along with low complement levels, are also helpful. The presence of antinuclear antibodies (ANA) is not sufficient to diagnose SLE. A patient with a positive ANA assessment and pain is much more likely to have fibromyalgia than SLE.

TABLE 73-1
CRITERIA FOR THE CLASSIFICATION OF SYSTEMIC LUPUS ERYTHEMATOSUS

Criterion	Definition
Malar rash	Fixed erythema over the malar eminences, sparing the nasolabial folds
Discoid rash	Erythematous raised patches with adherent keratotic scaling and follicular plugging; atrophic scarring may occur in older lesions
Photosensitivity	Skin rash as a result of unusual reaction to sunlight
Oral ulcers	Oral or nasopharyngeal ulceration, usually painless
Arthritis	Nonerosive arthritis involving two or more peripheral joints
Serositis	Pleuritis or pericarditis
Renal disorder	Persistent proteinuria greater than +3 or presence of cellular casts
Neurological disorder	Seizures or psychosis in the absence of other explanation
Hematological disorder	Hemolytic anemia, or leukopenia ($<4000/mm^3$), or lymphopenia ($<1500/mm^3$), or thrombocytopenia ($<100,000/mm^3$)
Immunological disorder	Presence of antiphospholipid antibodies, or antibodies to native DNA or to Sm nuclear antigen
Antinuclear antibody	An abnormal titer of antinuclear antibody in the absence of drugs known to be associated with "drug-induced lupus" syndrome

III. DIAGNOSTICS
A. HISTORY AND PHYSICAL EXAMINATION

1. Many of the most common signs and symptoms associated with SLE are nonspecific. For example, patients with SLE may complain of constitutional symptoms, such as fatigue, fever, and weight loss. Similarly, they may complain of polyarthralgias or, somewhat less commonly, polyarthritis. More specific for the diagnosis of SLE is the presence of Jaccoud's arthropathy, which is a hand deformity caused by ligamentous laxity and easily reduced on physical examination. Other musculoskeletal manifestations of SLE include osteonecrosis, tenosynovitis, myositis, and corticosteroid-induced myopathy.

2. In a retrospective study of 702 women with SLE the morbidity ratio for fracture in women with SLE was 4.7 (95% CI, 3.8-5.8) when compared with age-matched women in the general population. Older age at the time of diagnosis and longer duration of corticosteroid use were independent determinants of time to a patient's first fracture.[13] Each 2-month exposure to higher daily prednisone doses confers a 1.2-fold increase in the risk of osteonecrosis.[14]

3. Cutaneous manifestations of SLE are common and typically include the presence of a malar rash, discoid lesions, alopecia, or oral and

nasal ulcerations. Less commonly, vasculitic lesions, urticarial lesions, panniculitis, and livedo reticularis may be seen.

4. SLE has multiple pulmonary signs, including pneumonitis, pleuritis, pleural effusions, pulmonary alveolar hemorrhage, and acute and chronic interstitial lung disease (which may lead to pulmonary hypertension). Pulmonary embolism may be seen in association with the antiphospholipid antibody syndrome.

5. Gastrointestinal signs and symptoms are comparatively less common and might include abdominal pain, anorexia, nausea, vomiting, pancreatitis, mesenteric vasculitis, serositis, ascites, and a protein-losing enteropathy.

6. The most common neuropsychiatric manifestations of SLE are seizure and psychosis; SLE has a number of reported neurological sequelae, however, such as brainstem dysfunction, stroke, major depression, encephalopathy, cognitive impairment, chorea, transverse myelitis, aseptic meningitis, peripheral neuropathy, cranial neuropathy, mononeuritis multiplex, pseudotumor cerebri, optic neuritis, uveitis, episcleritis, and scleritis.

7. Pericarditis and pericardial effusion are not uncommon cardiac manifestations of SLE. In addition, systolic or diastolic dysfunction, myocarditis, and Libman-Sacks endocarditis (sterile verrucous vegetations on the mitral valve, highly associated with antiphospholipid antibodies) all occur disproportionately in patients with SLE. The cardiovascular manifestation of SLE that is of most concern is coronary arteritis.

8. Patients with SLE have premature atherosclerosis with increased prevalence of coronary atherosclerosis,[15] carotid arthrosclerosis (41% versus 9%, $p < .005$), and left ventricular hypertrophy (32% versus 5%, $p < .005$) as compared with matched control subjects,[16] and peripheral vascular disease. In the Hopkins Lupus Cohort, risk factors for coronary artery disease (defined as angina or myocardial infarction) included duration of prednisone use, hypertension, hyperlipidemia, obesity, age, male sex, homocysteine level greater than 14.1 μmol/L, renal insufficiency, and the presence of antiphospholipid antibodies.[17-19]

B. LABORATORY ANALYSIS

1. Hematological abnormalities are common and include anemia, leukopenia, lymphopenia, and thrombocytopenia. Patients with SLE have a higher incidence of antiphospholipid antibody syndrome, which may manifest with a false-positive finding on a test for syphilis, a prolonged partial thromboplastin time, or the presence of anticardiolipin antibodies. Elevated results on liver function tests are a relatively uncommon, but recognized, manifestation of SLE.

2. Renal involvement in the form of lupus nephritis may be manifested as the presence of proteinuria or an active sediment and is associated with an overall poor prognosis. The World Health Organization classifies lupus nephritis in terms of five categories: type I (normal),

type II (mesangial abnormalities), type III (focal proliferative), type IV (diffuse proliferative glomerulonephritis), and type V (membranous). In a 1989 study of 148 patients, 42% had type II, 15% had type III, 25% had type IV, 7% had type V (membranous), and only 2% had a normal renal biopsy finding.[20]

3. Lupus nephritis is a common manifestation of SLE. A Singapore cohort of 335 patients with lupus showed a 23.8% incidence of lupus nephritis more than 6 months after lupus diagnosis. Hypertension, thrombocytopenia, and leukopenia confer an adjusted relative risk of 2.5 to 4.3 for the development of lupus nephritis more than 6 months after diagnosis.[21] Lupus nephritis is significantly more common in African-Americans than Caucasians[22] and correlates with the presence of antibodies to double-stranded DNA.

4. Significant baseline predictors of the development of renal insufficiency (defined as serum creatinine ≥1.6 mg/dL in men and ≥1.4 mg/dL in women) are extremes of age at baseline (<19 or >40 years of age) and longer duration of SLE before referral to an academic center.[23]

5. In a 10-year follow-up study of patients treated for severe lupus nephritis, predictors of remission included lower baseline creatinine level, white race, stable renal function after 4 weeks of treatment (of high-dose prednisone with cyclophosphamide), and type IV glomerulonephritis on biopsy; predictors of end-stage renal disease included higher baseline creatinine level, anti-Ro antibodies, and failure to attain remission with aggressive treatment.[24] A national collaborative network study and a recent review both revealed worse prognosis and poor response to treatment in African-Americans with lupus nephritis.[25,26]

6. Although the standardized incidence rate of end-stage renal disease caused by lupus nephritis has increased from 1.16 per million person-years in 1982 to 3.08 per million person-years in 1995 with approximately 60% of cases in patients 20 to 44 years of age, this increase in rate may not take into account the newer treatment options available, such as cyclophosphamide and mycophenolate mofetil.[27]

IV. MANAGEMENT

1. The management of a patient with SLE who is admitted to the hospital hinges on determining whether the patient's symptoms are a manifestation of a lupus flare-up or a manifestation of one of the complications of SLE (e.g., infection or chronic progressive anemia). For example, the origin of chest pain in a patient with SLE may be musculoskeletal, serositis from an active lupus flare-up, or ischemia from coronary arteritis.

2. Lupus patients may not be febrile when infected. Invasive studies (e.g., lumbar puncture, arthrocentesis, bronchoalveolar lavage, or

73

SYSTEMIC LUPUS ERYTHEMATOSUS

biopsy) may be necessary, depending on the organ presentation, to determine the presence or absence of infection.

3. Serological test results (such as anti-dsDNA, C3, or C4) are not predictive of later flares.[28] The most common pattern on the day of a flare-up is a reduction in anti-dsDNA levels.[29]

4. Most of the manifestations of SLE flare-ups respond readily to corticosteroids. Intravenously administered corticosteroids are commonly used to treat the more serious manifestations of SLE, such as nephritis, cerebritis, hematological abnormalities, and vasculitis. Methylprednisolone is administered in intravenous boluses of up to 1000 mg/day for 3 days in the treatment of life-threatening SLE flare-ups. Patients receiving intravenous methylprednisolone showed a trend toward overall improvement in the first weeks after administration in a double-blind, controlled trial of 25 patients with active SLE.[30] A small clinical trial of 21 patients reported that higher pulse doses of methylprednisolone for 3 days (1000 mg/day) offer no significant clinical improvement over lower doses (100 mg/day).[31] However, use of methylprednisolone pulse therapy for moderate to severe SLE flare-ups is very helpful in achieving quick control of disease activity and allowing slower agents a chance to take effect.

5. Oral corticosteroids are unfortunately a mainstay in maintenance treatment for many patients with SLE. One goal of combination therapy (steroids plus antimalarials or other immunosuppressants) is to limit the cumulative toxicity of long-term steroid use, such as cataract formation, avascular necrosis of bone, myopathy, osteoporosis, dyslipidemia, and glucose intolerance.[14]

6. Hydroxychloroquine is generally used to treat cutaneous lesions, arthritis, and serositis. A study of 47 patients who were receiving hydroxychloroquine for clinically stable SLE and were randomized to continuation of the antimalarial or to placebo (withdrawal of hydroxychloroquine) showed an increase in the severity of symptoms (relative risk of 2.5) and a shorter time to flare-up ($p = .02$) in the placebo group.[32] It is recommended that patients receiving hydroxychloroquine for stable SLE be maintained on this antimalarial drug not only to prevent flare-ups, but also to reduce the risk of later thrombosis.[33] A low risk of retinopathy is associated with hydroxychloroquine.

7. Dehydroepiandrosterone (DHEA) 200 mg PO qd has been shown to be steroid sparing and beneficial in stabilizing disease over a 1-year period.[34] In addition, DHEA is helpful in treating steroid-induced osteoporosis.[35]

8. Multiple immunosuppressive drugs can be used for the long-term management of SLE. For example, azathioprine is commonly used as a corticosteroid-sparing drug in patients with SLE and arthritis, serositis, nephritis, or the hematological or neurological manifestations of SLE. Cyclosporine is effective in limiting disease activity[36] but is rarely used

as a corticosteroid-sparing agent in patients with SLE because of its toxicity profile. Weekly doses of methotrexate (15-20 mg) can significantly control mild cutaneous and articular symptoms associated with SLE and can permit the gradual decrease in daily prednisone dose.[37] Similar results were found in patients with moderate symptoms of SLE, excluding renal or central nervous system disease.[38]

9. Cyclophosphamide is considered the standard of care in the treatment of lupus nephritis. In a randomized controlled clinical trial of 107 patients with active lupus nephritis with a median 7-year follow-up, intravenously administered cyclophosphamide plus low-dose prednisone was shown to be superior ($p = .027$) to high-dose prednisone alone in reducing the risk of end-stage renal disease.[39] Patients with lupus nephritis treated with either intravenous or oral administration of cyclophosphamide can achieve long-term preservation of renal function.[40] In the United States the National Institutes of Health cyclophosphamide regimen (750 mg/m^2 body surface area monthly for 6 months, followed by quarterly infusions for 2 years) is usually followed to treat diffuse proliferative glomerulonephritis.

10. The use of cyclophosphamide for the treatment of SLE has dramatically increased, especially among patients with lupus nephritis. The surge in use raises the concern for potential complications of this cytotoxic drug, including ovarian failure, later malignancy, and hemorrhagic cystitis. The last complication is reduced if mesna is given with each cyclophosphamide infusion.

11. A retrospective study of 70 premenopausal women with lupus treated with cyclophosphamide showed a 26% incidence rate of ovarian failure. Independent risk factors associated with ovarian failure included older age at time of cyclophosphamide treatment ($p = .001$) and increasing cumulative cyclophosphamide dose ($p = .02$).[41] The incidence of permanent amenorrhea after cyclophosphamide treatment ranges from 11% to 59%, dependent on age and cumulative dose of cyclophosphamide.[41,42] Recent studies suggest that luprolide (Lupron) may be helpful in protecting ovarian function.

12. A randomized controlled study of 42 patients with diffuse proliferative lupus nephritis revealed that a 12-month course of prednisolone and mycophenolate mofetil is less toxic and as effective as a regimen of prednisolone plus cyclophosphamide for 6 months followed by 6 months of prednisolone and azathioprine in achieving an approximate 80% complete remission rate (81% and 76%, respectively).[43]

PEARLS AND PITFALLS
- Renal insufficiency and proteinuria.
  - Monitor the quantity of excreted protein with monthly 24-hour urine collections.

73

SYSTEMIC LUPUS ERYTHEMATOSUS

- Add an angiotensin-converting enzyme inhibitor or angiotensin receptor blocker, or both, if significant proteinuria is present, both to optimize blood pressure control and to minimize renal sclerosis.[44,45]
- Accelerated atherosclerosis.
  - Control hypertension.
  - Check homocysteine level and institute folic acid repletion, if necessary.
  - Control hyperlipidemia.
  - Counsel regarding smoking cessation and weight loss.
  - Adjust the medical regimen to minimize corticosteroid doses. An increase in prednisone dose of 10 mg will increase the cholesterol level by 7.5 ± 1.46 mg/dL, the mean arterial blood pressure by 1.1 mm Hg, and the mean weight by 5.5 ± 1.23 pounds.[46]
- Thrombotic risk.
  - If the patient has moderate- to high-titer anticardiolipin antibody or lupus anticoagulant, evidence has shown that low-dose aspirin[47] or hydroxychloroquine[33] can reduce thrombotic risk.
  - Estrogen should not be given to patients with antiphospholipid antibodies unless the patient is already receiving anticoagulants.
  - If a patient with antiphospholipid antibodies has a thrombotic event, the target international normalized ratio is 3.
- Infection.
  - Monitor for signs and symptoms of infection at each clinical visit (obtain a chest radiograph for suspected pulmonary infection and urinalysis with culture for suspected urinary tract infection even if the patient is afebrile).
  - Institute *Pneumocystis carinii* pneumonia prophylaxis with dapsone (avoiding use of trimethoprim-sulfamethoxazole) if the patient requires high-dose cyclophosphamide.
- Health care maintenance.
  - Offer annual influenza vaccinations and ensure that pneumococcal vaccinations are up to date.

REFERENCES

[c] 1. Solinger AM. Drug-related lupus: clinical and etiologic considerations. Rheum Dis Clin North Am 1988; 14(1):187.

[b] 2. Petri M. The effect of race on incidence and clinical course in systemic lupus erythematosus: the Hopkins Lupus Cohort. JAMWA 1998; 53:9.

[b] 3. Reveille JD et al. Systemic lupus erythematosus in three ethnic groups. I. The effects of HLA class II, C4, and CR1 alleles, socioeconomic factors, and ethnicity at disease onset. LUMINA Study Group. Lupus in minority populations, nature versus nurture. Arthritis Rheum 1998; 41(7):1161.

[b] 4. Peschken CA, Esdaile JM. Systemic lupus erythematosus in North American Indians: a population based study. J Rheumatol 2000; 27:1884.

[b] 5. Uramoto KM et al. Trends in the incidence and mortality of systemic lupus erythematosus, 1950-1992. Arthritis Rheum 1999; 42:46.

[b] 6. Abu-Shakra M et al. Mortality studies in systemic lupus erythematosus: results from a single center. I. Causes of death. J Rheumatol 1995; 22:1259.

[b] 7. Cervera R et al. Morbidity and mortality in systemic lupus erythematosus during a 5-year period: a multicenter prospective study of 1,000 patients. European Working Party on Systemic Lupus Erythematosus. Medicine (Baltimore) 1999; 78:167.

[b] 8. Mok CC et al. A prospective study of survival and prognostic indicators of systemic lupus erythematosus in a southern Chinese population. Rheumatology (Oxford) 2000; 39:399.

[b] 9. Ward MM, Pyun E, Studenski S. Mortality risks associated with specific clinical manifestations of systemic lupus erythematosus. Arch Intern Med 1996; 156:1337.

[b] 10. Alarcon GS et al. Systemic lupus erythematosus in three ethnic groups. VII [correction of VIII]. Predictors of early mortality in the LUMINA cohort. LUMINA Study Group. Arthritis Rheum 2001; 45:191.

[d] 11. Tan EM et al. The 1982 revised criteria for the classification of systemic lupus erythematosus. Arthritis Rheum 1982; 25:1271.

[d] 12. Hochber MC. Updating the American College of Rheumatology revised criteria for the classification of systemic lupus erythematosus. Arthritis Rheum 1997; 40:1725.

[b] 13. Ramsey-Goldman R et al. Frequency of fractures in women with systemic lupus erythematosus: comparison with United States population data. Arthritis Rheum 1999; 42:882.

[b] 14. Zonana-Nacach A et al. Damage in systemic lupus erythematosus and its association with corticosteroids. Arthritis Rheum 2000; 43:1801.

[b] 15. Esdaile JM et al. Traditional Framingham risk factors fail to fully account for accelerated atherosclerosis in systemic lupus erythematosus. Arthritis Rheum 2001; 44:2331.

[b] 16. Roman MJ et al. Prevalence and relation to risk factors of carotid atherosclerosis and left ventricular hypertrophy in systemic lupus erythematosus and antiphospholipid antibody syndrome. Am J Cardiol 2001; 87:663.

[b] 17. Petri M et al. Plasma homocysteine as a risk factor for atherothrombotic events in systemic lupus erythematosus. Lancet 1996; 348:1120.

[b] 18. Petri M et al. Risk factors for coronary artery disease in patients with systemic lupus erythematosus. Am J Med 1992; 93:513.

[c] 19. Petri M. Detection of coronary artery disease and the role of traditional risk factors in the Hopkins Lupus Cohort. Lupus 2000; 9:170.

[b] 20. Gladman DD et al. Kidney biopsy in SLE. I. A clinical-morphologic evaluation. Q J Med 1989; 73:1125.

[b] 21. Thumboo J et al. Clinical predictors of nephritis in systemic lupus erythematosus. Ann Acad Med Singapore 1998; 27:16.

[b] 22. Petri M et al. Morbidity of systemic lupus erythematosus: role of race and socioeconomic status. Am J Med 1991; 91:345.

[b] 23. Rzany B et al. Risk factors for hypercreatinemia in patients with systemic lupus erythematosus. Lupus 1999; 8:532.

[b] 24. Korbet SM et al. Factors predictive of outcome in severe lupus nephritis. Lupus Nephritis Collaborative Study Group. Am J Kidney Dis 2000; 35:904.

[b] 25. Dooley MA et al. Cyclophosphamide therapy for lupus nephritis: poor renal survival in black Americans. Glomerular Disease Collaborative Network. Kidney Int 1997; 51:1188.

[c] 26. Austin HA, Balow JE. Natural history and treatment of lupus nephritis. Semin Nephrol 1999; 19:2.

[c] 27. Ward MM. Changes in the incidence of end-stage renal disease due to lupus nephritis, 1982-1995. Arch Intern Med 2000; 160:3136.

[b] 28. Ho A et al. A decrease in complement is associated with increased renal and hematologic activity in patients with systemic lupus erythematosus. Arthritis Rheum 2001; 44:2350.

[b] 29. Ho A et al. Decreases in anti-double-stranded DNA levels are associated with concurrent flares in patients with systemic lupus erythematosus. Arthritis Rheum 2001; 44:2342.

[a] 30. Mackworth-Young CG et al. A double blind, placebo controlled trial of intravenous methylprednisolone in systemic lupus erythematosus. Ann Rheum Dis 1988; 47:496.

[a] 31. Edwards JC, Snaith ML, Isenberg DA. A double blind controlled trial of methylprednisolone infusions in systemic lupus erythematosus using individualised outcome assessment. Ann Rheum Dis 1987; 46:773.

73

SYSTEMIC LUPUS ERYTHEMATOSUS

[a] 32. A randomized study of the effect of withdrawing hydroxychloroquine sulfate in systemic lupus erythematosus. The Canadian Hydroxychloroquine Study Group. N Engl J Med 1991; 324:150.

[c] 33. Petri M. Thrombosis and systemic lupus erythematosus: the Hopkins Lupus Cohort perspective. Scand J Rheumatol 1996; 25:191.

[b] 34. van Vollenhoven RF et al. Treatment of systemic lupus erythematosus with dehydroepiandrosterone: 50 patients treated up to 12 months. J Rheumatol 1998; 25:285.

[a] 35. van Vollenhoven RF et al. A double-blind, placebo-controlled, clinical trial of dehydroepiandrosterone in severe systemic lupus erythematosus. Lupus 1999; 8:181.

[a] 36. Dammacco F et al. Cyclosporine-A plus steroids versus steroids alone in the 12-month treatment of systemic lupus erythematosus. Int J Clin Lab Res 2000; 30:67.

[a] 37. Carneiro JR, Sato EI. Double blind, randomized, placebo controlled clinical trial of methotrexate in systemic lupus erythematosus. J Rheumatol 1999; 26:1275.

[b] 38. Gansauge S et al. Methotrexate in patients with moderate systemic lupus erythematosus (exclusion of renal and central nervous system disease). Ann Rheum Dis 1997; 56:382.

[a] 39. Austin HA 3rd. Therapy of lupus nephritis: controlled trial of prednisone and cytotoxic drugs. N Engl J Med 1986; 314:614.

[a] 40. Steinberg AD, Steinberg SC. Long-term preservation of renal function in patients with lupus nephritis receiving treatment that includes cyclophosphamide versus those treated with prednisone only. Arthritis Rheum 1991; 34:945.

[b] 41. Mok CC, Lau CS, Wong RW. Risk factors for ovarian failure in patients with systemic lupus erythematosus receiving cyclophosphamide therapy. Arthritis Rheum 1998; 41:831.

[b] 42. Boumpas DT et al. Risk for sustained amenorrhea in patients with systemic lupus erythematosus receiving intermittent pulse cyclophosphamide therapy. Ann Intern Med 1993; 119:366.

[a] 43. Chan TM et al. Efficacy of mycophenolate mofetil in patients with diffuse proliferative lupus nephritis. Hong Kong-Guangzhou Nephrology Study Group. N Engl J Med 2000; 343:1156.

[b] 44. Gonzalez-Gay MA et al. Successful response to captopril in severe nephrotic syndrome secondary to lupus nephritis. Nephron 1998; 80:353.

[b] 45. Ruggenenti P, Brenner BM, Remuzzi G. Remission achieved in chronic nephropathy by a multidrug approach targeted at urinary protein excretion. Nephron 2001; 88:254.

[b] 46. Petri M et al. Effect of prednisone and hydroxychloroquine on coronary artery disease risk factors in systemic lupus erythematosus: a longitudinal data analysis. Am J Med 1994; 96:254.

[b] 47. Erkan D et al. High thrombosis rate after fetal loss in antiphospholipid syndrome: effective prophylaxis with aspirin. Arthritis Rheum 2001; 44:1466.

Alcohol Withdrawal in the Inpatient Setting

Micol Rothman, MD, and Thomas O'Toole, MD

FAST FACTS

- Alcohol abuse and withdrawal are common and can have severe consequences.
  - More than 1 million patients are discharged from hospitals each year with an alcohol-related diagnosis. Alcohol dependence occurs in 15% to 20% of primary care and hospitalized patients.[1]
  - The lifetime prevalence of alcohol abuse in the United States is 13.7% to 23.5%, and the mortality rate of people who consume more than six drinks a day is 50% higher than that of matched control subjects.[2,3]
  - Patients who are hospitalized for alcohol withdrawal and receive no treatment have life-threatening occurrences such as seizures and delirium tremens.
- The diagnosis of alcohol withdrawal can be easily missed in patients admitted for reasons unrelated to alcohol abuse.

I. CLINICAL PRESENTATION

A. PATHOPHYSIOLOGY

1. Alcohol potentiates the inhibitory chloride influx mediated by γ-aminobutyric acid (GABA), leading to clinical sedation. As tolerance develops, GABA receptor function is down-regulated and thus withdrawal from alcohol can lead to hyperactivity.
2. Ethanol acts at the *N*-methyl-D-aspartate receptor as an inhibitor and diminishes the excitatory effects of glutamate. Over time an increase in neuroexcitatory tone develops; once alcohol is withdrawn, the hyperexcitable neurons cause the symptoms of withdrawal.
3. Alcohol causes α_2-receptors to inhibit norepinephrine release, and norepinephrine levels have been shown to be elevated during withdrawal.
4. Other neurotransmitters such as serotonin, dopamine, the hypothalamic-pituitary-adrenal axis, and opioid receptors have been implicated in craving for alcohol and withdrawal symptoms.[4]

II. DIAGNOSIS

A. INITIAL EVALUATION OF THE PATIENT WITH SUSPECTED ALCOHOL ABUSE OR WITHDRAWAL

1. History (may be limited; the physician should try to talk with the patient's family or other witnesses, read the ambulance report, and

speak with emergency room physicians or emergency medical services personnel).

2. Screening of all patients (including patients without known alcohol abuse) with the CAGE questionnaire,[5] which has been proved to be reliable.

a. Have you ever felt you ought to Cut down on your drinking?

b. Have people Annoyed you by criticizing your drinking?

c. Have you ever felt bad or Guilty about your drinking?

d. Have you ever had a drink first thing in the morning to steady your nerves or get rid of a hangover (Eye-opener)?

3. One "yes" response on the CAGE questionnaire suggests an alcohol problem; three or more correlate highly with alcohol abuse. If the person responds affirmatively to two or more questions, studies on medical inpatients have shown the sensitivity to be between 75% and 81% and the specificity to be between 89% and 96%.[3] The CAGE questionnaire has been faulted for implying that more people have alcohol problems than actually do, but the sensitivity and specificity improve with a greater number of affirmative answers.

4. Physical examination.

a. Assessment of vital signs: One of the key determinants of severity of withdrawal is vital sign instability, and patients often require monitoring in the intensive care unit.

b. Assessment of level of consciousness: Patients who require heavy sedation may need to be intubated for airway protection.

c. Assessment of the possibility of other acute events related to alcohol abuse: Evaluation includes a full trauma survey, abdominal examination, and rectal examination.

d. Assessment of signs of long-term alcohol abuse: If the physician suspects alcohol withdrawal but the history is unclear, signs of long-term alcohol abuse, such as testicular atrophy, gynecomastia, telangiectasias, and palmar erythema, should be sought.

5. Laboratory and radiological tests.

a. Patients with altered mental status should be assessed by measurement of the ammonia and electrolyte levels, including potassium, magnesium, and phosphorus. The anion gap should be calculated to assess for ketoacidosis, and if necessary serum and urine ketone assessment should be ordered. Calculation of the osmolar gap and blood and urine toxicology screening are needed, since patients may be abusing multiple substances.

b. The hematocrit and coagulation studies are performed to evaluate for acute gastrointestinal bleeding. If indicated, the amylase/lipase or lactate level should be checked.

c. Chest radiographs can be used to look for infiltrate or aspiration. A chest radiograph may also show "bar-stool fractures" or cardiomegaly.

d. An electrocardiogram can be used to evaluate arrhythmias.

e. If the medical history is unclear, liver function tests with aspartate aminotransferase and alanine aminotransferase assessment, coagulation studies, and hematocrit with indices can reveal clues of alcohol abuse.

6. Computed tomography of the head and lumbar puncture are indicated for patients with a temperature greater than 38° C, known head trauma, or new-onset focal seizures. They may not be necessary for patients with known alcohol withdrawal seizures and a consistent clinical picture. Low numbers of cells can be seen in the cerebrospinal fluid of postictal patients.

B. RANGE OF WITHDRAWAL

1. The *Diagnostic and Statistical Manual of Mental Disorders,* edition 4, gives the following criteria for a diagnosis of withdrawal.[6]

a. History of cessation or reduction in heavy and prolonged alcohol use.

b. Presence of two or more of the following: autonomic hyperactivity, hand tremor, insomnia, nausea or vomiting, tactile visual or auditory hallucinations, psychomotor agitation, anxiety, and seizures.

c. These symptoms cause clinically significant distress or impairment in social, occupational, or other important areas of functioning.

d. Symptoms are not due to a general medical condition and not accounted for by another mental disorder.[6]

C. SYMPTOMS OF WITHDRAWAL

1. Symptoms of alcohol withdrawal run the gamut from the mild (tremulousness, anxiety) to the moderate (seizures and hallucinations) to the most serious and life threatening (delirium tremens). The key features that will help a clinician differentiate among the stages are the degree of hyperarousal and the level of consciousness.

2. **Minor withdrawal:** Minor withdrawal consists of insomnia, vivid dreams, tremulousness, mild anxiety, gastrointestinal (GI) upset, headache, diaphoresis, and palpitations. On physical examination patients are frequently tachycardic and hypertensive with a coarse tremor. Minor withdrawal tends to occur soon after the cessation of alcohol consumption and may even begin while the blood alcohol level is still elevated. Therefore, in the emergency room setting, withdrawal remains important in the differential diagnosis of a patient who still has alcohol in the bloodstream. Mild symptoms often resolve in 24 to 48 hours without intervention. Many patients have similar symptoms each time they go through withdrawal, and as they recognize the signs, they self-medicate by consuming more alcohol to prevent withdrawal.

3. **Seizures:** Seizures usually originate 24 hours after the most recent drink but can also occur while alcohol remains in the bloodstream. The seizures are often generalized and can recur successively; however, less than 3% of seizures become status epilepticus.[7] Seizures frequently become more severe with each episode of withdrawal. This has been hypothesized to be similar to the "kindling" that occurs when neural sites are repeatedly stimulated in a low-intensity fashion.[8] As mentioned earlier, a workup for seizures should be pursued if a patient has a temperature greater than 38° C, known head trauma, and focal seizures or if

seizures began after the patient became delirious, since none of these features are typical for alcohol withdrawal seizures. Alcohol-related seizures occur more frequently in patients with underlying seizure disorders, often complicating the choice of optimal treatment. Benzodiazepines are the treatment of choice. The treatment options are outlined further in the following sections.

4. **Hallucinations:** Alcoholic hallucinations tend to develop within 12 to 24 hours of consumption of the last alcoholic drink and usually resolve by 24 to 48 hours. However, hallucinations occurring several days later in the course have been reported. The hallucinations are most often visual but can be auditory and can be accompanied by paranoia. A crucial point to understand is that alcoholic hallucinations are not equivalent to delirium tremens and in fact do not necessarily predict whether delirium tremens will develop. The key distinction is that patients with hallucinations are alert and often aware that the images are not real, whereas patients with delirium tremens have an altered sensorium.

5. **Delirium tremens:** Delirium tremens is the most life-threatening complication of alcohol withdrawal. As mentioned earlier, patients become delirious, with altered sensorium and hyperactive vital signs. Delirium tremens generally occurs 48 to 96 hours after the last drink but can appear later and last as long as 5 days. It can also occur after a period of mild withdrawal has seemingly resolved. The late onset of delirium tremens contributes to the difficulty of making the diagnosis in patients who are already hospitalized. It should be considered whenever hypertension, tachycardia, fever, sweating, and dehydration develop in an inpatient. Currently delirium tremens occurs in approximately 5% of patients undergoing withdrawal and carries a 1% mortality rate; in the past, however, the mortality rate was as high as 20%, generally from arrhythmias or concomitant illnesses. Studies have shown that delirium tremens is more common in older patients with a concomitant medical or surgical illness, in those with severe alcohol dependence, and in those whose last drink was further in the past.[9] Clinicians can also look for clues such as prior history of elevated blood alcohol level, aspartate aminotransferase elevation, or GI illness related to alcohol, since these can help predict more serious withdrawal episodes.

III. MANAGEMENT

A. TREATMENT OPTIONS FOR WITHDRAWAL

1. **Benzodiazepines:** Benzodiazepines have been studied since the 1950s and are currently recommended as first-line treatment for alcohol withdrawal. They have been proved to reduce signs and symptoms of withdrawal and prevent the onset of delirium. They alleviate the effect of withdrawal of ethanol by binding to the GABA receptor and enhancing

transmission of inhibitory ions. Although other classes of medications have a role in adjunctive therapy, only benzodiazepines have been recommended for monotherapy.[1]

2. Other agents.

a. Carbamazepine is used widely in Europe. It is an anticonvulsant and has been proved to be better than placebo in cases of mild to moderate withdrawal. No trials are available to demonstrate its effect in the prevention of human seizures or delirium.

b. Barbiturates are also used in Europe and are quite effective in treating seizures and delirium tremens, since they carry the advantage of long half-lives. They also act at the GABA receptor with a mechanism similar to benzodiazepines but are not generally used, since they have higher potential for abuse and cause respiratory depression more frequently than benzodiazepines.

c. Phenytoin is not helpful for alcohol withdrawal seizures and should be used only for patients with known seizure history or history of head trauma.[7] A randomized placebo-controlled double-blind study compared phenytoin with placebo and found no difference between the two in preventing recurrent seizures related to alcohol.[10]

d. Alcohol itself has been used for treatment of withdrawal. There are obvious concerns about furthering addiction with a potentially toxic medication that would require close monitoring of drug levels.

e. Sympatholytic drugs such as β-blockers can alleviate tachycardia and hypertension but may mask the clinical picture of withdrawal and thus delay diagnosis. β-Blockers have not been shown to stop seizures or delirium, although in one study they were shown to reduce the length of hospital stay.[11]

f. Clonidine acts on α_2-receptors to alleviate the excess of norepinephrine that can contribute to withdrawal. It can be used to control blood pressure and pulse in cases of minor withdrawal, but it has not been studied for delirium.[7]

g. Neuroleptics have been used for patients with marked hallucinations, generally to treat severe agitation, but the incidence of seizure is higher in patients treated with phenothiazines than in those given placebo.[1] Death from hyperthermia and cardiovascular collapse has also been reported.[4]

h. Thiamine should be administered to all patients with known alcohol abuse and dependence. Given before glucose, it can prevent the triad of Wernicke's encephalopathy—cognitive impairment, ocular dysfunction, and ataxia—but it has no particular role in the treatment of withdrawal.

i. Low magnesium level was thought to be crucial for the development of alcohol withdrawal in studies in the 1960s, but this has not been supported in follow-up studies.[7] Magnesium repletion has a role in patients with alcohol dependence, since they tend to have impaired

74

ALCOHOL WITHDRAWAL IN THE INPATIENT SETTING

nutrition and low magnesium levels. Left uncorrected, a low magnesium level can lead to dysrhythmias and weakness and exacerbate hypokalemia. Since serum values are unreliable as indices of total body stores, all patients with alcohol withdrawal should be given magnesium supplements.

B. DOSAGE OF BENZODIAZEPINES

1. **Three methods of dosage of benzodiazepines have been studied.**

a. Fixed-schedule dosage: This is the best regimen for patients who are at high risk for seizures or delirium tremens (i.e., those with a history of these conditions), since they should be treated regardless of symptoms. Generally a schedule of medication with taper dosages is written out by the house officer at the time of admission. The patient is assessed by nurses and physicians, and the taper dose and interval are adjusted.

> *EXAMPLE:* (1) Chlordiazepoxide 50-100 mg q6h on day 1 with chlordiazepoxide 25-100 mg q2h as needed. On day 2 adjustments are made to taper or keep the same dose. (2) Diazepam 5-10 mg PO 4-6h for 1 to 3 days with taper following.

b. Front-loading dosage: This involves delivering a large dose of a long-acting medication early on, which leads to an "auto-taper." Front loading has been proved to prevent seizures.

> *EXAMPLE:* Diazepam 10-20 mg PO q2h while the patient is awake until symptoms resolve.

c. Symptom-triggered dosage: This is the favored treatment among some clinicians and has been the subject of recent clinical trials; however, it requires high levels of nursing and physician care. It involves evaluation with the Clinical Institute Withdrawal Assessment (CIWA), a scale developed to grade the severity of alcohol withdrawal symptoms. Patients are assessed at fixed intervals for withdrawal symptoms and treated accordingly. Generally a score of less than 8 or 10 indicates that a patient does not require pharmacological treatment. A score of 10 to 20 may indicate the need for treatment, and a score greater than 20 indicates a higher chance of delirium tremens and merits immediate pharmacological intervention.

2. A randomized double-blind trial published in *JAMA* compared fixed-schedule chlordiazepoxide administration with symptom-triggered therapy. Patients admitted for alcohol withdrawal were selected at random for assessment of their withdrawal symptoms using the CIWA. Patients with seizure history or concurrent medical illness were excluded, which may limit the ability to generalize from this study, but patients with a history of delirium tremens were included. The patients treated via the symptom-triggered regimen re-

quired less medication overall (100 mg over a mean time of 9 hours, compared with 425 mg over a mean time of 68 hours) and had shorter hospital stays with faster recoveries. No differences were seen between the two groups with regard to entry into rehabilitation, discharges against medical advice, seizures, delirium tremens, lethargy, or hallucinations.[12]

3. A recent retrospective analysis at the Mayo Clinic compared two groups of patients: those admitted to the general medical service before and those admitted after the implementation of a symptom-triggered approach to treatment. Patients with a history of seizures or delirium tremens were included. The study demonstrated a decrease in delirium tremens in the group with the symptom-triggered approach but no change in the duration of treatment.[13] For practical purposes, however, the CIWA is time consuming for busy nurses or housestaff to administer.

> *EXAMPLE:* If CIWA is less than 8, monitor symptoms. If CIWA is 8 or greater, administer chlordiazepoxide 25 to 100 mg PO q1h.

4. House officers and attending physicians must take into account the feasibility of the various delivery methods and the prior withdrawal symptoms of the patient when deciding how to choose a method of benzodiazepine delivery. All regimens must be tailored to meet individual patient needs.

C. CHOOSING A BENZODIAZEPINE

1. The best medications for treating seizures and preventing delirium tremens are those with long half-lives, such as chlordiazepoxide and diazepam. They have the advantage of active metabolites that provide an automatic taper. However, oxazepam and lorazepam are better for patients with hepatic synthetic dysfunction, since they are shorter acting.

2. Medications that have a rapid onset may be more addictive and have a higher potential for abuse.

3. Table 74-1 lists the half-lives and frequently used dosages for various medications. The oral route is preferred when feasible.

PEARLS AND PITFALLS

- Asking outpatients about alcohol use patterns before elective surgery can help anesthesiologists and surgeons judge the likelihood of alcohol withdrawal in surgical settings.
- Alcohol withdrawal seizures can occur in the absence of autonomic instability; seizures can be focal or generalized.
- Fever is not generally a manifestation of delirium tremens.
- Oxazepam requires only glucuronidation (as opposed to glucuronidation and conjugation) by the liver for metabolism. This theoretically makes oxazepam a preferred agent in patients with hepatic synthetic dysfunction.

TABLE 74-1
CHARACTERISTICS OF BENZODIAZEPINES

Drug	Half-Life (hr)	Dosage	Active Metabolite?	Rapid Onset?	Caveats
Oxazepam (Serax)	8 ± 2.4	15-60 mg PO q6-8h	No		Better in hepatic dysfunction and elderly
Lorazepam (Ativan)	14 ± 5	2-4 mg PO q8-12h		Yes	Better in hepatic dysfunction and elderly
Diazepam (Valium)	43 ± 13	5-20 mg PO q6-8h		Yes	Longer acting; may provide smoother withdrawal
Chlordiazepoxide (Librium)	10 ± 3.4, although may be longer as a result of metabolites	50-100 mg PO q6-24h	Yes		Longer acting; may provide smoother withdrawal

REFERENCES

[c] 1. Mayo-Smith M et al. Pharmacological management of alcohol withdrawal. JAMA 1997; 278:144.

[c] 2. O'Connor P, Schottenfield R. Patients with alcohol problems. N Engl J Med 1998; 338:592.

[c] 3. Kitchens J. The rational clinical examination: does this patient have an alcohol problem? JAMA 1994; 272:1782.

[c] 4. Olmedo R, Hoffman RS. Withdrawal syndromes. Emerg Med Clin North Am 2000; 18:273.

[d] 5. Lohr R. Treatment of alcohol withdrawal in hospitalized patients. Mayo Clinic Proc 1995; 70:777.

[c] 6. American Psychiatric Association: Diagnostic and statistical manual of mental disorders, 4th ed. Washington, DC: American Psychiatric Association; 1994.

[c] 7. Turner R et al. Alcohol withdrawal syndromes: a review of the pathophysiology, clinical presentation and treatment. J Gen Intern Med 1989; 4:435.

[c] 8. Gonzalez L et al. Alcohol withdrawal kindling: mechanisms and implications for treatment. Alcohol Clin Exp Res 2001; 25:197S.

[b] 9. Ferguson J et al. Risk factors for delirium tremens development. J Gen Intern Med 1996; 11:410.

[b] 10. Chance J. Emergency department treatment of alcohol withdrawal seizures with phenytoin. Ann Emerg Med 1991; 20:520.

[a] 11. Kraus M et al. Randomized clinical trial of atenolol in patients with alcohol withdrawal. N Engl J Med 1985; 313:905.

[a] 12. Saitz R et al. Individualized treatment for alcohol withdrawal: a randomized, double-blind controlled trial. JAMA 1994; 272:519.

[a] 13. Jaeger TM, Lohr RH, Pankratz VS. Symptom-triggered therapy for alcohol withdrawal syndrome in medical inpatients. Mayo Clinic Proc 2001; 76:695.

74

ALCOHOL WITHDRAWAL IN THE INPATIENT SETTING

PART III

Formulary

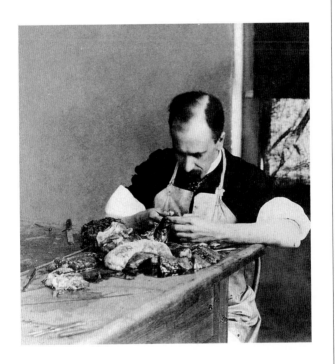

Formulary

Susan Arnold, PharmD, and Jeffrey Brewer, PharmD

I. NOTE TO THE READER

We have made every attempt to check dosages and medical content for accuracy. Because of the dynamic nature of medical information, the content in this section is frequently modified by drug companies and evolving clinical practice. The medications section is to be used as a guide only. Health care professionals should use sound clinical judgment to individualize therapy for every patient. We recommend that the reader check the package insert and published literature for changes in content, especially for newer medicines.

We would like to thank Lois Reynolds, PharmD, and Richard Muffoletto, RPh, for their significant contributions in writing two of the original sections. We also acknowledge the contribution of the many pharmacists at The Johns Hopkins Hospital who provided editorial assistance to ensure that the medication section was as complete as possible.

II. SAMPLE ENTRY

Pregnancy: Refer to explanation of pregnancy categories (on facing page).

Breast: Refer to explanation of breast-feeding categories (on facing page).

Kidney: Indicates need for caution or need for dose adjustment in renal failure.

How supplied

AMIKACIN ← Generic name
Amikin ← Trade name and other names
Inj: 50, 250 mg/mL
Solution, inj: 500 mg/100 mL in 0.9% NS
Antimicrobials ← Drug category

YES   3   C

Indication: Susceptible gram-negative organisms
Initial dose: 15 mg/kg IV daily divided q8-12h
Max dose: 1.5 g daily
15 mg/kg
Renal dose: CrCl 10-50 mL/min: 30%-70% dose q12-18h or 100% dose q24-48h
CrCl <10 mL/min: 20%-30% dose q24-48h or 100% dose q48-72h

Drug dosing

Adverse drug reaction: Rare: nausea, vomiting, weakness, eosinophilia, tremor, arthralgia, dyspnea, hypotension, neuromuscular blockade.
Comments:
Sodium = 1.3 mEq/g.
Poor CNS penetration unless meninges inflamed.
Pharmacokinetics altered in cystic fibrosis, burns, febrile neutropenia.
Drug/drug: Use caution with other nephrotoxic and ototoxic agents.
Use ideal body weight to determine dosage for most patients or dosing body weight for obese patients.
Monitor levels: Peak <15-35 μg/mL, trough <10 μg/mL.
Class side effects: Neurotoxicity, ototoxicity, nephrotoxicity, hypersensitivity reactions, azotemia.
Class contraindications: Hypersensitivity to the medication.

Brief remarks about side effects, drug interactions, precautions, therapeutic monitoring, and other relevant information

III. EXPLANATION OF BREAST-FEEDING CATEGORIES
See sample entry.
1 Compatible.
2 Use with caution.
3 Unknown with concerns.
X Contraindicated.
? Safety not established or unknown.

IV. EXPLANATION OF PREGNANCY CATEGORIES
A Adequate studies in pregnant women have not demonstrated a risk to the fetus in the first trimester of pregnancy, and there is no evidence of risk in later trimesters.
B Animal studies have not demonstrated a risk to the fetus, but there are no adequate studies in pregnant women; or animal studies have shown an adverse effect, but adequate studies in pregnant women have not demonstrated a risk to the fetus during the first trimester of pregnancy, and there is no evidence of risk in later trimesters.
C Animal studies have shown an adverse effect on the fetus, but there are no adequate studies in humans; or there are no animal reproduction studies and no adequate studies in humans.
D There is evidence of human fetal risk, but the potential benefits from the use of the drug in pregnancy women may be acceptable despite its potential risks.
X Studies in animals or humans demonstrate fetal abnormalities or adverse reaction; reports indicate evidence of fetal risk. The risk of use in pregnant women clearly outweighs any possible benefit.

V. EXPLANATION OF RENAL DOSAGE CATEGORIES
See sample entry.

VI. CATEGORIES
ANTIMICROBIALS
Aminoglycoside Agents, 1071
Antiviral Agents, 1073
Antifungal Agents, 1076
Cephalosporin Agents, 1081
Macrolide Agents, 1087
Penicillin Agents, 1089
Fluoroquinolone Agents, 1096
Tetracycline Agents, 1100
Other Agents, 1101
CARDIOVASCULAR
ACE Inhibitors, 1111
Angiotensin Receptor Blockers, 1117
Antiadrenergic, 1120
β-Blockers, 1123

CATEGORIES

ANTIMICROBIALS
Aminoglycoside Agents

AMIKACIN

Amikin
Inj: 50 mg/mL, 250 mg/mL
Solution, inj: 500 mg/100 mL in 0.9% NS
Antimicrobials

YES   3   C

Indication: Susceptible gram-negative organisms
Initial dose: 15 mg/kg IV daily divided q8-12h
Max dose: 1.5 g daily
      15 mg/kg
Renal dose: CrCl 10-50 mL/min: 30%-70% dose q12-18h or 100% dose
      q24-48h
      CrCl <10 mL/min: 20%-30% dose q24-48h or 100% dose
      q48-72h

Adverse drug reaction: Rare: nausea, vomiting, weakness, eosinophilia, tremor,
    arthralgia, dyspnea, hypotension, neuromuscular blockade.
Comments:
Sodium = 1.3 mEq/g.
Poor CNS penetration unless meninges inflamed.
Pharmacokinetics altered in cystic fibrosis, burns, febrile neutropenia.
Drug/drug: Use caution with other nephrotoxic and ototoxic agents.
Use ideal body weight to determine dosage for most patients or dosing body
  weight for obese patients.
Monitor levels: Peak <15-35 µg/mL, trough <10 µg/mL.
Class side effects: Neurotoxicity, ototoxicity, nephrotoxicity, hypersensitivity
    reactions, azotemia.
Class contraindications: Hypersensitivity to the medication.

GENTAMICIN

Garamycin
Inj: 10 mg/mL, 40 mg/mL
Antimicrobials

YES   3   C

Indication: Susceptible gram-negative organisms, adjunct agent for gram-
      positive synergy
Initial dose:
  Traditional dosage: 1.7-2 mg/kg IV q8-12h
  Extended-interval dosage: 5 mg/kg IV q24h
  Gram-positive synergy: 1 mg/kg IV q8h

Continued

For explanation of icons, see p. 1068.

GENTAMICIN *continued*

Renal dose: CrCl 10-50 mL/min: 30%-70% dose q12h, or 100% dose q24-48h
CrCl <10 mL/min: 20%-30% dose q24-48h, or 100% dose
q48-72h

Adverse drug reaction: Rare: anorexia, dyspnea, leukopenia, thrombocytopenia,
granulocytopenia, nausea, seizures, vomiting, neuromuscular blockade.
Comments:
Pharmacokinetics altered in cystic fibrosis, burns, febrile neutropenia.
Use ideal body weight in determining dosage for most patients or dosing body
weight for obese patients.
Monitor levels: Peak <4-10 µg/mL, trough <2 µg/mL.
Drug/drug: Use caution with other nephrotoxic and ototoxic agents.
Class side effects: Neurotoxicity, ototoxicity, nephrotoxicity, hypersensitivity
reactions, azotemia.
Class contraindications: Hypersensitivity to the medication.

STREPTOMYCIN

Inj: 1 g/2.5 mL
Antimicrobials

YES   1   D

Indication: Tuberculosis, tularemia
Initial dose:
    Tuberculosis: 15 mg/kg IM q24h
    Tularemia: 1-2 g IM divided q12h
Max dose: 2 g daily
Renal dose: CrCl 10-50 mL/min: 100% dose q24-72h
CrCl <10 mL/min: 100% dose q72-96h

Adverse drug reaction: CNS depression; rare: myocarditis, serum sickness,
leukopenia, thrombocytopenia, apnea, neuromuscular blockade, exfoliative
dermatitis.
Comments:
Approved for deep IM administration *only*.
Monitor levels: Peak <20 µg/mL, trough <5 µg/mL.
Drug/drug: Use caution with other nephrotoxic and ototoxic agents.
Contraindicated in labyrinthine disease.
Class side effects: Neurotoxicity, ototoxicity, nephrotoxicity, hypersensitivity
reactions, azotemia.
Class contraindications: Hypersensitivity to the medication.

TOBRAMYCIN

Nebcin, TOBI
Inj: 40 mg/mL
Solution, inhaled: 300 mg/5 mL
Antimicrobials

YES 3 C

Indication: Susceptible gram-negative organisms, cystic fibrosis with
  Pseudomonas aeruginosa
Initial dose:
  Traditional dosage: 1.7-2 mg/kg IV q8h
  Extended-interval dosage: 5 mg/kg IV q24h
  Cystic fibrosis: 300 mg via nebulizer q12h
Renal dose: CrCl 10-50 mL/min: 30%-70% dose q12h, or 100% dose
      q24-48h
      CrCl <10 mL/min: 20%-30% dose q24-48h, or 100% dose
      q48-72h

Adverse drug reaction: Tremor, lethargy, hallucinations, phlebitis; rare:
  seizures, dyspnea, nausea, vomiting, headache, weakness, hypotension.
Comments: Pharmacokinetics altered in cystic fibrosis, burns, febrile
  neutropenia.
Use ideal body weight in determining dosage for most patients or dosing body
  weight for obese patients.
Monitor levels: peak 4-10 μg/mL, trough <2 μg/mL.
No adjustment for renal dysfunction or weight with inhaled TOBI.
Drug/drug: Use caution with other nephrotoxic or ototoxic agents.
Class side effects: Neurotoxicity, ototoxicity, nephrotoxicity, hypersensitivity
  reactions, azotemia.
Class contraindications: Hypersensitivity to the medication.

Antiviral Agents

ACYCLOVIR

Zovirax
Caps: 200 mg
Tabs: 400, 800 mg
Oral liquid: 200 mg/5 mL
Inj: 500, 1000 mg
Antiviral agents

YES 1 B

Indication: Varicella zoster, herpes simplex virus (HSV)
Initial dose:
  Varicella zoster: 800 mg PO q4h (5 times daily) or 5-10 mg/kg IV q8h
  Genital HSV—initial treatment: 200 mg PO q4h (5 times daily)

Continued

ACYCLOVIR *continued*

Genital HSV—recurrent: 200 mg PO q4h, 400 mg PO q8h, 800 mg
PO q12h
Genital HSV—long-term suppressive therapy: 400 mg bid
HSV—severe infection: 5-10 mg/kg IV q8h
Max dose: 3200 mg daily
20 mg/kg q8h
Renal dose: CrCl 10-50 mL/min: 100% dose q12-24h
CrCl <10 mL/min: 100% dose q24h

Adverse drug reaction: Tremor, lethargy, hallucinations, phlebitis,
gastrointestinal irritation, rash, urticaria; rare: thrombocytopenia, leukopenia,
seizures, coma, vertigo, insomnia.
Comments:
Initiate within 48 hr of onset of shingles.
Use ideal body weight when determining dosage for obese patients.
Drug/drug: Probenecid and zidovudine may increase serum levels.
Class side effects: Headache, dizziness, confusion, nausea.
Class contraindications: Hypersensitivity to the medication.

AMANTADINE
Symmetrel
Caps, tabs: 100 mg
Oral liquid: 50 mg/5 mL
Antiviral agents

YES   3   C

Indication: Parkinson's disease, drug-induced extrapyramidal reactions,
influenza A virus
Initial dose:
Parkinsonism, drug-induced extrapyramidal reactions: 100-300 mg bid
Influenza A virus: 200 mg PO daily or divided bid (preferred)
Max dose: 200 mg daily because of adverse central nervous system reactions
Renal dose: CrCl 10-50 mL/min: q48-72h
CrCl <10 mL/min: q7 days

Adverse drug reaction: Orthostatic hypotension, anxiety, nervousness, nausea,
irritability, insomnia; rare: heart failure, depression, mental status change,
urinary retention.
Comments:
Drug/drug: Additive effect with other central nervous system stimulants.
Class side effects: Headache, dizziness, confusion, nausea.
Class contraindications: Hypersensitivity to the medication.

GANCICLOVIR

Cytovene
Inj: 500 mg
Caps: 250 mg
Antiviral agents

YES 3 C

Indication: Cytomegalovirus (CMV) retinitis, prevention of CMV disease
Initial dose:
  CMV retinitis:
    Induction: 5 mg/kg IV q12h
    Maintenance: 5 mg/kg IV daily × 7 days/wk or 6 mg/kg IV daily × 5 days/wk
  Prevention of CMV disease: 1 g PO tid
Renal dose: CrCl 25-50 mL/min: 2.5 mg/kg IV q12-24h
           CrCl 10-24 mL/min: 1.25 mg/kg IV q24h
           CrCl <10 mL/min: 1.25 mg/kg IV 3 × wk

Adverse drug reaction: Neutropenia, thrombocytopenia; rare: granulocytopenia, leukocytopenia, coma, vomiting, diarrhea, confusion, seizures.
Comments:
Oral ganciclovir has poor bioavailability (5%). Consider using oral valganciclovir.
Monitor complete blood cell count: baseline and within 2 weeks of initiation.
IM/SC administration contraindicated (pH = 11).
Drug/drug: Additive effect with other cytotoxic agents. Probenecid may increase serum levels.
Do not administer if absolute neutrophil count <500/mm^3 or platelets <25,000/mm^3.
Class side effects: Headache, dizziness, confusion, nausea.
Class contraindications: Hypersensitivity to the medication.

VALACYCLOVIR

Valtrex
Caplet: 500, 1000 mg
Antiviral agents

YES 1 B

Indication: Herpes zoster, episodic treatment and suppression of genital herpes
Initial dose:
  Herpes zoster: 500 mg PO tid x 7 days
  Genital herpes—episodic treatment: 500 mg–1 g PO bid × 10 days
  Genital herpes—suppression: 500 mg–1 g PO daily
Renal dose: CrCl 10-50 mL/min: 100% dose q12-24h
           CrCl <10 mL/min: 500 mg q24h

Continued

For explanation of icons, see p. 1068.

VALACYCLOVIR *continued*

Adverse drug reaction: Rare: thrombotic thrombocytopenic purpura, hemolytic-uremic syndrome, headache, nausea.
Comments:
Initiate dosage increment within 48 hr of development of rash.
Class side effects: Headache, dizziness, confusion, nausea.
Class contraindications: Hypersensitivity to the medication.

VALGANCICLOVIR

Valcyte
Tabs: 450 mg
Antiviral agents

YES   3   C

Indication: Cytomegalovirus retinitis
Initial dose:
   Induction: 900 mg PO bid
   Maintenance: 900 mg PO daily
Renal dose: CrCl 40-60 mL/min: 50% dose
   CrCl 25-40 mL/min: 50% dose, 50% frequency
   CrCl < 25 mL/min: 50% dose
   Induction: Every other day
   Maintenance: Twice weekly

Adverse drug reaction: Rare: thrombocytopenia, granulocytopenia, leukocytopenia, coma, vomiting, diarrhea, confusion, seizures.
Comments:
Monitor complete blood count: baseline and within 2 weeks of initiation.
Do not administer if absolute neutrophil count <500/mm^3 or platelets <25,000/mm^3.
Drug/drug: Additive effect with other cytotoxic agents. Probenecid may increase serum levels.
Class side effects: Headache, dizziness, confusion, nausea.
Class contraindications: Hypersensitivity to the medication.

Antifungal Agents

AMPHOTERICIN B DESOXYCHOLATE

Fungizone, Amphocin
Inj: 50 mg
Antifungal agents

NO   ?   B

Indication: Susceptible fungi
Initial dose: 0.25-1 mg/kg IV daily
Max dose: 1.5 mg/kg daily

Continued

AMPHOTERICIN B DESOXYCHOLATE *continued*

Adverse drug reaction: Headache, malaise, anorexia, nausea, vomiting,
diarrhea, fever, chills, cramping, anemia, hypokalemia, thrombophlebitis,
azotemia, renal tubular acidosis, rigors, hypomagnesemia: rare: seizures,
acute liver failure, arrhythmias, thrombocytopenia, leukocytopenia,
gastrointestinal hemorrhage, bronchospasm.

Comments:

Administer over 4-6 hr.

Salt loading with 10-15 mL/kg NS may decrease nephrotoxicity.

Monitor potassium and magnesium levels, renal function, liver function,
complete blood cell count.

Monitor 1-3 hr after dose for acute infusion-related reaction.

Drug/drug: Additive effects with other nephrotoxic and hypokalemic agents.

Class contraindications: Hypersensitivity to the medication.

AMPHOTERICIN B LIPID COMPLEX

Abelcet

NO ? B

Inj, solution: 100 mg/20 mL

Antifungal agents

Indication: Susceptible fungi in patient refractory to or intolerant of
conventional amphotericin B

Initial dose: 5 mg/kg IV daily

Max dose: 5 mg/kg daily

Adverse drug reaction: Fever, chills, rigors, renal insufficiency, hypokalemia,
hypomagnesemia; rare: renal failure, thrombocytopenia, leukocytopenia,
respiratory failure, hypotension, gastrointestinal hemorrhage.

Comments:

Monitor potassium and magnesium levels, renal function, liver function,
complete blood cell count.

Monitor 1-3 hr after dose for acute infusion-related reaction.

Class contraindications: Hypersensitivity to the medication.

AMPHOTERICIN B LIPOSOMAL

AmBisome

NO ? B

Inj: 50 mg

Antifungal agents

Indication: Susceptible fungi in patient refractory to or intolerant of
conventional amphotericin B; neutropenic fever

Continued

AMPHOTERICIN B LIPOSOMAL *continued*

Initial dose:
Susceptible fungi: 5 mg/kg IV daily
Neutropenic fever: 3 mg/kg IV daily

Adverse drug reaction: Anxiety, confusion, headache, asthenia, hypotension, fever, chills, rigors, nausea, vomiting, abdominal pain, diarrhea, renal insufficiency, azotemia, elevated liver function test results, bilirubinemia, hypomagnesemia, hypokalemia, dyspnea, tachycardia, epistaxis, hypocalcemia; rare: gastrointestinal hemorrhage.
Comments:
Monitor potassium and magnesium levels, renal function, liver function, complete blood cell count.
Monitor 1-3 hr after dose for acute infusion-related reaction.
Class contraindications: Hypersensitivity to the medication.

AMPHOTERICIN B CHOLESTERYL SULFATE COMPLEX

Amphotec   NO   ?   B
Inj: 50, 100 mg
Antifungal agents

Indication: Susceptible fungi in patient refractory to or intolerant of conventional amphotericin B
Initial dose: 3-4 mg/kg IV daily

Adverse drug reaction: Seizures, hypotension, tachycardia, hypokalemia, renal insufficiency, bilirubinemia, nausea, vomiting, pulmonary edema, fever, chills; rare: arrhythmias, bradycardia, heart failure, hemorrhage, renal failure, thrombocytopenia, leukocytopenia, hepatic failure.
Comments:
Monitor 1-3 hours after dose for acute infusion-related reaction.
Monitor potassium and magnesium levels, renal function, liver function, complete blood cell count.
Class contraindications: Hypersensitivity to the medication.

FLUCONAZOLE

NO   ?   C

Diflucan
Solution, inj: 200 mg/100 mL in 0.9% NS or D5W,
400 mg/200 mL in 0.9% NS or D5W
Tabs: 50, 100, 150, 200 mg
Oral liquid: 50 mg/5 mL
Antifungal agents

Indication: Candidal infections, cryptococcal meningitis
Initial dose:
 Oropharyngeal and esophageal candidiasis: 200 mg PO/IV load; then
100-200 mg PO daily

 Systemic candidiasis: 400 mg PO/IV
 Vaginal candidiasis: 150 mg PO × 1 dose
 Cryptococcal meningitis: 200-400 mg PO/IV daily

Adverse drug reaction: Nausea; rare: hepatotoxicity, Stevens-Johnson
 syndrome, anaphylaxis, alopecia.
Comments:
Drug/drug: Inhibits metabolism of cyclosporin A, warfarin, phenytoin,
 tacrolimus, rifampin.
Class contraindications: Hypersensitivity to the medication.

FLUCYTOSINE

YES   3   C

Ancobon
Caps: 250, 500 mg
Antifungal agents

Indication: Adjunct treatment of susceptible fungi
Initial dose: 50-150 mg/kg PO divided q6h
Max dose: 150 mg/kg daily
Renal dose: CrCl 10-50 mL/min: q12h
 CrCl <10 mL/min: q24h

Adverse drug reaction: Eosinophilia; rare: agranulocytosis, aplastic
 anemia, toxic epidermal necrolysis, respiratory arrest, leukopenia,
 bone marrow suppression, myocardial toxicity, hemorrhage, renal failure,
 thrombocytopenia.
Comments:
Use with extreme caution in patients with renal impairment, bone marrow
 suppression, AIDS.
Monitor serum levels; keep <100 µg/mL to prevent toxicity.
Class contraindications: Hypersensitivity to the medication.

ITRACONAZOLE

Sporanox
Caps: 100 mg
Oral liquid: 100 mg/10mL
Inj: 250 mg/25 mL
Antifungal agents

NO   3   C

Indication: Susceptible fungi, aspergillosis, histoplasmosis, blastomycosis, onychomycosis
Initial dose:
  Susceptible fungi: 200-400 mg PO daily
  Aspergillosis, histoplasmosis, blastomycosis: 200 mg IV bid × 2 days, then 200 mg IV daily
  Onychomycosis: 200 mg daily × 12 wk
Max dose: 400 mg daily
Renal dose: CrCl <30 mL/min: Avoid administration by injection

Adverse drug reaction: Nausea; rare: headache, rash, hypokalemia, increases in liver function test parameters.
Comments:
Liquid more bioavailable than caps.
Drug/drug: Many interactions with medications metabolized through the cytochrome P450 system, including increase in cyclosporin A and digoxin levels. Phenytoin, rifampin, and isoniazid may reduce itraconazole levels.
Class contraindications: Hypersensitivity to the medication.

KETOCONAZOLE

Nizoral
Tabs, scored: 200 mg
Antifungal agents

NO   ?   C

Indication: Uncomplicated vulvovaginal *Candida* infections
Initial dose: 200-400 mg PO daily/bid
Max dose: 800 mg

Adverse drug reaction: Nausea, vomiting; rare: suicidal tendencies, thrombocytopenia, leukopenia, hepatotoxicity, fever, headache, adrenal insufficiency.
Comments:
Drug/drug: Separate from drugs that increase pH. Avoid alcohol because of disulfiram-like effect. Use caution with other hepatotoxic agents. May increase cyclosporin A, tacrolimus, and warfarin levels. Phenytoin and rifampin may reduce ketoconazole levels.
Class contraindications: Hypersensitivity to the medication.

Cephalosporin Agents

CEFAZOLIN

Kefzol, Ancef
Inj: 500 mg, 1 g
Cephalosporin agents

YES   1   B

 Indication: Severe skin, soft tissue, respiratory, genitourinary, septicemia, bone, joint, and biliary tract infections
Initial dose: 250 mg–1 g IV/IM q8h
Max dose: 12 g daily
Renal dose: CrCl 11-34 mL/min: 50% dose q12h
CrCl <10 mL/min: 50% dose q24h

Adverse drug reaction: Urticaria, sterile abscess, phlebitis; rare: neutropenia, hemolytic anemia, thrombocytopenia, Stevens-Johnson syndrome.
Comments:
First-generation cephalosporin.
Sodium = 2 mEq/g.
Drug/drug: 10%-15% cross-reactivity with penicillin allergy.
Class side effects: Hypersensitivity reaction, local reaction, nausea, vomiting, diarrhea, rare: *Clostridium difficile* diarrhea, anaphylaxis.
Class contraindications: Hypersensitivity to the medication or other cephalosporins.

CEFEPIME

Maxipime
Inj: 500 mg, 1, 2 g
Cephalosporin agents

YES   1   B

 Indication: Urinary tract infection (UTI), pneumonia, skin and skin structure infections, empirical treatment in febrile neutropenia
Initial dose:
UTI, pneumonia, skin infection: 1-2 g IV q12h
Empirical for febrile neutropenia: 2 g IV q8h
Renal dose: CrCl 10-30 mL/min: 50% dose q24h
CrCl <10 mL/min: 25% dose q24h

Adverse drug reaction: Rare: thrombocytopenia.
Comments:
Fourth-generation cephalosporin.
10%-15% cross-reactivity with penicillin allergy.
Class side effects: Hypersensitivity reaction, local reaction, nausea, vomiting, diarrhea; rare: *Clostridium difficile* diarrhea, anaphylaxis.
Class contraindications: Hypersensitivity to the medication or other cephalosporins.

For explanation of icons, see p. 1068.

CEFIXIME
Suprax
Tabs: 200, 400 mg
Inj: 100 mg/5 mL
Cephalosporin agents

YES   1   B

Indication: Urinary tract infection (UTI), otitis media, pharyngitis, tonsillitis, chronic bronchitis, uncomplicated gonorrhea.
Initial dose:
  UTI, otitis media, pharyngitis, tonsillitis, chronic bronchitis: 400 mg PO daily or divided q12h
  Uncomplicated gonorrhea: 400 mg PO × 1 dose
Renal dose: CrCl 10-50 mL/min: 75% dose
           CrCl <10 mL/min: 50% dose

Adverse drug reaction: Rare: thrombocytopenia, leukocytopenia, Stevens-Johnson syndrome.
Comments:
Third-generation cephalosporin.
10%-15% cross-reactivity with penicillin allergy.
Class side effects: Hypersensitivity reaction, local reaction, nausea, vomiting, diarrhea; rare: *Clostridium difficile* diarrhea, anaphylaxis.
Class contraindications: Hypersensitivity to the medication or other cephalosporins.

CEFOTAXIME
Claforan
Inj: 500 mg, 1, 2 g
Cephalosporin agents

YES   1   B

Indication: Lower respiratory, central nervous system (CNS), urinary, skin, bone, joint, intraabdominal infections; uncomplicated gonorrhea
Initial dose:
  Lower respiratory, CNS, urinary, skin, bone, joint, intraabdominal infections: 1 g IV q8-12h
  Uncomplicated gonorrhea: 1 g IM × 1 dose
Max dose: 12 g daily
Renal dose: CrCl <10 mL/min: q24h

Adverse drug reaction: Urticaria, sterile abscess, phlebitis; rare: agranulocytosis, transient neutropenia, thrombocytopenia.
Comments:
Third-generation cephalosporin.

Continued

CEFOTAXIME *continued*

Sodium = 2.2 mEq/g.
10%-15% cross-reactivity with penicillin allergy.
Class side effects: Hypersensitivity reaction, local reaction, nausea, vomiting, diarrhea; rare: *Clostridium difficile* diarrhea, anaphylaxis.
Class contraindications: Hypersensitivity to the medication or other cephalosporins.

CEFOTETAN

Cefotan
Inj: 1, 2 g   YES   1   B
Solution, inj: 1, 2 g in 50 mL of D5W
Cephalosporin agents

Indication: Lower respiratory, urinary, skin, intraabdominal, bone, joint, gynecological infections
Initial dose: 500 mg–2 g IV q12h
Max dose: 6 g daily
Renal dose: CrCl 10-30 mL/min: 50% dose or 100% dose q24h
          CrCl <10 mL/min: 25% dose

Adverse drug reaction: Urticaria, sterile abscess, phlebitis; rare: agranulocytosis, nephrotoxicity, transient neutropenia, thrombocytopenia, hypoprothrombinemia.
Comments:
Second-generation cephalosporin.
Sodium = 1.5 mEq/g.
10%-15% cross-reactivity with penicillin allergy
Drug/drug: Avoid alcohol because of disulfiram-like effect. Probenecid may increase serum levels.
Class side effects: Hypersensitivity reaction, local reaction, nausea, vomiting, diarrhea; rare: *Clostridium difficile* diarrhea, anaphylaxis.
Class contraindications: Hypersensitivity to the medication or other cephalosporins.

CEFOXITIN

Mefoxin
Inj: 1, 2 g   YES   1   B
Solution, inj: 1, 2 g in 50 mL of D5W
Cephalosporin agents

Indication: Respiratory, skin, soft tissue, gynecological, bone, joint, intraabdominal, blood, genitourinary infections

Continued

For explanation of icons, see p. 1068.

CEFOXITIN *continued*

Initial dose: 1-2 g IV q6-8h
Max dose: 12 g daily
Renal dose: CrCl 10-50 mL/min: q8-12h
CrCl <10 mL/min: q24-48h

Adverse drug reaction: Urticaria, sterile abscess, phlebitis; rare: acute renal failure, neutropenia, hemolytic anemia, thrombocytopenia.
Comments:
Second-generation cephalosporin.
Sodium = 2.3 mEq/g.
10%-15% cross-reactivity with penicillin allergy.
Class side effects: Hypersensitivity reaction, local reaction, nausea, vomiting, diarrhea; rare: *Clostridium difficile* diarrhea, anaphylaxis.
Class contraindications: Hypersensitivity to the medication or other cephalosporins.

CEFTAZIDIME

Fortaz, Tazidime
Inj: 500 mg, 1, 2 g
Solution, inj: 1, 2 g in 50 mL of D5W
Cephalosporin agents

YES 1 B

Indication: Respiratory, urinary, gynecological, bone, joint, intraabdominal, central nervous system, skin, blood infections
Initial dose: 1 g IV q8-12h
Max dose: 6 g daily
Renal dose: CrCl 10-50 mL/min: q24-48h
CrCl <10 mL/min: q48h

Adverse drug reaction: Urticaria, sterile abscess, phlebitis; rare: seizures, leukopenia, agranulocytosis, thrombocytopenia.
Comments:
Third-generation cephalosporin.
10%-15% cross-reactivity with penicillin allergy.
Sodium = 2.3 mEq/g.
Drug/drug: Probenecid may increase serum levels.
Class side effects: Hypersensitivity reaction, local reaction, nausea, vomiting, diarrhea; rare: *Clostridium difficile* diarrhea, anaphylaxis.
Class contraindications: Hypersensitivity to the medication or other cephalosporins.

CEFTRIAXONE

Rocephin
Inj: 250, 500 mg, 1, 2 g
Cephalosporin agents

YES　1　B

 Indication: Respiratory, urinary, gynecological, bone, joint, intraabdominal, skin, blood infections; gonorrhea and sexual assault prophylaxis; meningitis

Initial dose:
　Respiratory, urinary, gynecological, bone, joint, intraabdominal, skin, blood infections: 1-2 g IV/IM daily or divided bid.
　Gonorrhea and sexual assault prophylaxis: 125-250 mg IM × 1 dose
　Meningitis: 2 g q12h
Max dose: 4 g daily

Adverse drug reaction: Rare: leukopenia, reversible cholelithiasis.
Comments:
Third-generation cephalosporin.
Sodium = 3.6 mEq/g.
10%-15% cross-reactivity with penicillin allergy.
Class side effects: Hypersensitivity reaction, local reaction, nausea, vomiting, diarrhea; rare: *Clostridium difficile* diarrhea, anaphylaxis.
Class contraindications: Hypersensitivity to the medication or other cephalosporins.

CEFUROXIME

Ceftin, Zinacef
Oral liquid: 750 mg, 1.5 g
Tabs: 125, 250, 500 mg (Ceftin)
Oral liquid: 125 mg/5 mL, 250 mg/5 mL (Ceftin)
Inj: 750 mg, 1.5 g
Cephalosporin agents

YES　1　B

 Indication: Urinary, lower respiratory, skin and skin structure, intraabdominal, blood infections; meningitis; upper and lower respiratory tract, urinary tract infections

Initial dose:
　Moderate to severe urinary, lower respiratory, skin and skin structure, intraabdominal, blood infections; meningitis: 750 mg–1.5 g
　　　　　　　　　　　　　　　　　　　　　　　　　　　IM/IV q8h

　Mild to moderate: 125-500 mg PO bid

Continued

For explanation of icons, see p. 1068.

CEFUROXIME *continued*

Max dose: 3 g q8h
Renal dose: CrCl 10-20 mL/min: q12h
CrCl <10 mL/min: q24h
PO dose not altered in renal failure

Adverse drug reaction: Urticaria, sterile abscess, phlebitis; rare: transient neutropenia, thrombocytopenia, hemolytic anemia.
Comments:
Second-generation cephalosporin.
10%-15% cross-reactivity with penicillin allergy.
Drug/drug: Probenecid may increase serum levels.
Sodium = 2.4 mEq/g.
Class side effects: Hypersensitivity reaction, local reaction, nausea, vomiting, diarrhea; rare: *Clostridium difficile* diarrhea, anaphylaxis.
Class contraindications: Hypersensitivity to the medication or other cephalosporins.

CEPHALEXIN

Keflex, Keftab
Caps: 250, 500 mg (Keflex)
Oral liquid: 125 mg/5 mL, 250 mg/5 mL (Keflex)
Tabs (monohydrate): 250, 500, 1000 mg (Keflex)
Tabs: 500 mg (Keftab)
Cephalosporin agents

YES 1 B

Indication: Respiratory, skin, soft tissue, bone, joint, genitourinary infections; otitis media
Initial dose: 250 mg–1 g PO q6h
Max dose: 4 g daily
Renal dose: CrCl <50 mL/min: 250-500 mg q12h

Adverse drug reaction: Anorexia, urticaria; rare: neutropenia, thrombocytopenia.
Comments:
First-generation cephalosporin.
10%-15% cross-reactivity with penicillin allergy.
Class side effects: Hypersensitivity reaction, local reaction, nausea, vomiting, diarrhea; rare: *Clostridium difficile* diarrhea, anaphylaxis.
Class contraindications: Hypersensitivity to the medication or other cephalosporins.

Macrolide Agents

AZITHROMYCIN

NO 3 B

Zithromax
Tabs: 250, 600 mg
Inj: 500 mg
Oral liquid: 100 mg/5 mL, 200 mg/5 mL
Macrolide agents

Indication: Acute exacerbation of chronic obstructive pulmonary disease (COPD), skin and soft tissue infection, uncomplicated *Chlamydia* sexually transmitted disease (STD), community-acquired pneumonia, pelvic inflammatory disease, prophylaxis against *Mycobacterium avium-intracellulare* (MAC) infection

Initial dose:

Acute COPD exacerbation, skin and soft tissue infection: Load: 500 mg PO × 1, then 250 mg PO daily × 4 days

Uncomplicated *Chlamydia* STD: 1 g PO × 1 dose

Community-acquired pneumonia: 500 mg IV daily × 2 days, then 500 mg PO daily

Pelvic inflammatory disease: 500 mg IV daily × 1-2 days, then 250 mg PO daily

Prophylaxis against MAC infection: 1.2 g PO q wk

Adverse drug reaction: Rare: angioedema, cholestatic jaundice.
Comments:
Drug/drug: Theophylline clearance decreased. Separate from aluminum- and magnesium-containing antacids.
Class side effects: Nausea, vomiting, diarrhea, abdominal pain.
Class contraindications: Hypersensitivity to the medication or other macrolides, hepatic failure.

CLARITHROMYCIN

YES 3 C

Biaxin, Biaxin XL
Tabs: 250, 500 mg
Tabs, sustained-release: 500 mg
Oral liquid: 125 mg/5 mL, 250 mg/5 mL
Macrolide agents

Indication: *Helicobacter pylori* treatment, *Mycobacterium avium-intracellulare* (MAC) prophylaxis and treatment, community-acquired pneumonia

Continued

CLARITHROMYCIN *continued*

Initial dose:
H. pylori treatment: 500 mg PO q8-12h depending on combination used
× 14 days
MAC prophylaxis and treatment, community-acquired pneumonia:
500 mg PO bid
Renal dose: CrCl <30 mL/min: 50% dose or 100% dose q24h

Adverse drug reaction: Abnormal taste.
Comments:
Drug/drug: Decreases metabolism of cyclosporin A, phenytoin, triazolam,
warfarin.
Class side effects: Nausea, vomiting, diarrhea, abdominal pain.
Class contraindications: Hypersensitivity to the medication or other macrolides,
hepatic failure.

ERYTHROMYCIN

Erythrocin, E-Mycin, EES, EryPed
Tabs: 250, 500 mg (base, stearate)
Tabs, delayed-release: 250, 333, 500 mg (base)
Oral liquid: 125 mg/5 mL, 250 mg/5 mL (estolate)
Inj: 500 mg, 1 g (lactobionate)
Tabs, chewable, scored: 200 mg (ethylsuccinate)
Oral liquid: 200 mg/5 mL, 400 mg/5 mL (ethylsuccinate)
Tabs: 250, 500 mg (stearate)
Macrolide agents

YES 1 B

Indication: Mild-moderate respiratory tract, skin, soft tissue infection;
uncomplicated urethral, endocervical, rectal infection with serious
tetracycline allergy; bowel preparation
Initial dose:
Mild-moderate respiratory tract, skin, soft tissue infection:
Base/estolate/stearate: 250-500 mg PO q6-12h
**Uncomplicated urethral, endocervical, rectal infection with serious
tetracycline allergy:** Ethylsuccinate: 400-800 mg PO q6-12h; lactobionate:
15-20 mg/kg IV divided q6h
Bowel preparation: Base: 1 g PO at 1 PM, 2 PM, and 11 PM the day before
the procedure
Renal dose: CrCl <10 mL/min: 50%-75% dose

Adverse drug reaction: Thrombophlebitis (IV), dryness, pruritus; rare:
ventricular arrhythmias, hypersensitivity reactions, cholestatic jaundice.
Comments:
Drug/drug: Decreases metabolism of cyclosporin A, phenytoin, triazolam,
warfarin.

Continued

ERYTHROMYCIN *continued*

Class side effects: Nausea, vomiting, diarrhea, abdominal pain.
Class contraindications: Hypersensitivity to the medication or other macrolides, hepatic failure.

Combination Agents

ERYTHROMYCIN/SULFISOXAZOLE

Pediazole
Oral liquid: 200/600 mg/5 mL
Combination agents

 Indication: Acute otitis media

Penicillin Agents

AMOXICILLIN

Amoxil, Polymox, Trimox
Caps: 250, 500 mg (Amoxil)
Oral liquid: 125, 200, 250, 400 mg/5 mL
Tabs, chewable, scored*: 125, 200, 250*, 400 mg
Tabs, scored*: 500, 875* mg
Penicillin agents

YES   1   B

 Indication: Urinary, respiratory, systemic infections (non-β-lactamase producers); endocarditis prophylaxis; *Helicobacter pylori* treatment
Initial dose:
  Urinary, respiratory, systemic infections (non-β-lactamase producers): 250-500 mg PO q8h or 500-875 mg PO q12h
  Endocarditis prophylaxis: 2 g 1 hr before procedure
  H. pylori treatment: 1 g PO bid × 14 days as part of a multidrug therapy
Max dose: 3 g daily
Renal dose: CrCl <10 mL/min: q24h

 Comments:
Aminopenicillin.
Drug/drug: Probenecid may increase serum levels. Amoxicillin may increase serum levels of methotrexate.
Monitor persistent diarrhea for *Clostridium difficile*.
Class side effects: Nausea, vomiting, diarrhea, rash, QT prolongation, tendonitis; rare: anaphylaxis, phlebitis, seizures, pseudomembranous colitis.
Class contraindications: Hypersensitivity to the medication or other penicillins.

For explanation of icons, see p. 1068.

AMOXICILLIN/CLAVULANIC ACID

Augmentin
Tabs, scored*: 250, 500, 875*/125 mg
Tabs, chewable: 125/31.25, 200/28.5, 250/62.5, 400/57 mg
Oral liquid: 125, 200, 250, 400, 600 mg/5 mL
Penicillin agents

YES   ?   B

Indication: Upper and lower respiratory tract, skin and skin structure, urinary infections
Initial dose: 250-500 mg PO q8h, or 875 mg PO q12h
Max dose: 2 g daily
Renal dose: CrCl 10-50 mL/min: q8-12h
CrCl <10 mL/min: q24h

Adverse drug reaction: Rare: thrombocytopenia, leukopenia, agranulocytosis, hemolytic anemia.
Comments:
Aminopenicillin.
Drug/drug: Probenecid may increase serum levels. Amoxicillin/clavulanic acid may increase serum levels of methotrexate.
Monitor persistent diarrhea for *Clostridium difficile*.
Contraindicated in cholestatic jaundice, hepatic dysfunction.
Class side effects: Nausea, vomiting, diarrhea, rash, QT prolongation, tendonitis; rare: anaphylaxis, phlebitis, seizures, pseudomembranous colitis.
Class contraindications: Hypersensitivity to the medication or other penicillins.

AMPICILLIN

Omnipen, Principen
Caps: 250, 500 mg
Inj: 125, 250, 500 mg, 1, 2 g
Oral liquid: 150, 250/5 mL
Penicillin agents

YES   ?   B

Indication: Urinary, systemic infections (non-β-lactamase producer); meningitis
Initial dose:
Urinary, systemic infections (non-β-lactamase producer): 250-500 mg PO q6h
Meningitis: 2 g IV q4h
Renal dose: CrCl 10-50 mL/min: q6-12h
CrCl <10 mL/min: q12-24h

Continued

AMPICILLIN *continued*

Adverse drug reaction: Rare: thrombocytopenia, leukopenia, agranulocytosis, hemolytic anemia.
Comments:
Aminopenicillin.
Sodium = 3 mEq/g.
Drug/drug: Probenecid may increase serum levels. Ampicillin may increase serum levels of methotrexate.
Monitor persistent diarrhea for *Clostridium difficile*.
Infuse >30 min to minimize the risk of seizures.
Class side effects: Nausea, vomiting, diarrhea, rash, QT prolongation, tendonitis; rare: anaphylaxis, phlebitis, seizures, pseudomembranous colitis.
Class contraindications: Hypersensitivity to the medication or other penicillins.

AMPICILLIN/SULBACTAM

Unasyn
Inj: 1.5, 3 g
Penicillin agents

YES ? B

Indication: Intraabdominal, gynecological, skin and skin structure infections
Initial dose: 1.5-3 g IV/IM q6h
Renal dose: CrCl 10-50 mL/min: q12h
CrCl <10 mL/min: q24h

Adverse drug reaction: Rare: thrombocytopenia, leukopenia, agranulocytosis, hemolytic anemia.
Comments:
Aminopenicillin.
Sodium = 10 mEq/3 g.
Drug/drug: Probenecid may increase serum levels. Ampicillin/sulbactam may increase serum levels of methotrexate.
Monitor persistent diarrhea for *Clostridium difficile*.
Class side effects: Nausea, vomiting, diarrhea, rash, QT prolongation, tendonitis; rare: anaphylaxis, phlebitis, seizures, pseudomembranous colitis.
Class contraindications: Hypersensitivity to the medication or other penicillins.

FORMULARY

Antimicrobials—Penicillins

For explanation of icons, see p. 1068.

DICLOXACILLIN

Dynapen, Pathocil
Caps: 125, 250, 500 mg
Oral liquid: 62.5 mg/5 mL
Penicillin agents

YES ? B

Indication: Penicillinase-producing staphylococci
Initial dose: 125-250 mg PO q6h

Adverse drug reaction: Rare: thrombocytopenia, leukopenia, agranulocytosis, hepatitis.
Comments:
Penicillinase-resistant penicillin.
Sodium = 0.6 mEq/250 mg cap.
Drug/drug: Probenecid may increase serum levels.
Monitor persistent diarrhea for *Clostridium difficile.*
Class side effects: Nausea, vomiting, diarrhea, rash, QT prolongation,
tendonitis; rare: anaphylaxis, phlebitis, seizures, pseudomembranous colitis.
Class contraindications: Hypersensitivity to the medication or other penicillins.

NAFCILLIN

Unipen, Nallpen
Inj: 500 mg, 1, 2 g
Penicillin agents

NO ? B

Indication: Methicillin-sensitive *Staphylococcus aureus*
Initial dose: 1-2 g IV q4-6h

Adverse drug reaction: Thrombophlebitis; rare: thrombocytopenia, transient leukopenia, granulocytopenia, neutropenia.
Comments:
Penicillinase-resistant penicillin.
Sodium = 2.9 mEq/g.
Drug/drug: May decrease cyclosporin A levels; use caution with other hepatotoxic agents.
Monitor persistent diarrhea for *Clostridium difficile.*
Class side effects: Nausea, vomiting, diarrhea, rash, QT prolongation,
tendonitis; rare: anaphylaxis, phlebitis, seizures, pseudomembranous colitis.
Class contraindications: Hypersensitivity to the medication or other penicillins.

OXACILLIN

Bactocil
Inj: 500 mg, 1, 4 g
Penicillin agents

M ? B

 Indication: Methicillin-sensitive *Staphylococcus aureus*
Initial dose: 1-2 g IV q4-6h

 Adverse drug reaction: Thrombophlebitis, hepatitis; rare: thrombocytopenia, hemolytic anemia, agranulocytosis, neutropenia.
Comments:
Penicillinase-resistant penicillin.
Sodium = 3.1 mEq/g.
Drug/drug: Probenecid may increase serum levels. Use caution with other hepatotoxic agents; may falsely decrease aminoglycoside level.
Monitor liver function tests and persistent diarrhea for *Clostridium difficile*.
Class side effects: Nausea, vomiting, diarrhea, rash, QT prolongation, tendonitis; rare: anaphylaxis, phlebitis, seizures, pseudomembranous colitis.
Class contraindications: Hypersensitivity to the medication or other penicillins.

PENICILLIN G

Bicillin LA (benzathine)
Inj: 1, 5, 10 MU (potassium)
Inj: 1.5 MU (sodium)
Inj: 300,000 U/mL, 600,000 U/mL
Penicillin agents

YES ? B

 Indication: Systemic infections, syphilis
Initial dose:
    Systemic infections: 2-4 MU IM/IV q4h
    Syphilis: 2.4 MU IM × 1 dose
Renal dose: CrCl 10-50 mL/min: 75% dose
             CrCl <10 mL/min: 20%-50% dose

 Adverse drug reaction: Rare: thrombocytopenia, agranulocytosis, exfoliative dermatitis.
Comments:
Sodium = 0.3 mEq/MU.
Potassium = 1.7 mEq/MU.
Monitor liver function tests, Jarisch-Herxheimer reaction after treatment, and persistent diarrhea for *Clostridium difficile*.
Penicillin G benzathine *must* be given intramuscularly.
Class side effects: Nausea, vomiting, diarrhea, rash, QT prolongation, tendonitis; rare: anaphylaxis, phlebitis, seizures, pseudomembranous colitis.
Class contraindications: Hypersensitivity to the medication or other penicillins.

For explanation of icons, see p. 1068.

PIPERACILLIN

Pipracil
Inj: 2, 3, 4 g
Penicillin agents

YES   ?   B

Indication: Moderate systemic infections; severe systemic and intraabdominal infections
Initial dose:
Moderate systemic infections: 2-3 g IV q6-12h
Severe systemic and intraabdominal infections: 2-3 g IV q4-6h
Max dose: 24 g daily
　　　　　2 g/IM site
Renal dose: CrCl 10-50 mL/min: q6h
　　　　　CrCl <10 mL/min: q8h

Adverse drug reaction: Bleeding, hypokalemia; rare: thrombocytopenia, hemolytic anemia.
Comments:
Extended-spectrum penicillin.
Sodium = 1.85 mEq.
Drug/drug: Probenecid may increase serum levels. Piperacillin may falsely decrease aminoglycoside level.
Monitor liver function tests and persistent diarrhea for *Clostridium difficile*.
Class side effects: Nausea, vomiting, diarrhea, rash, QT prolongation, tendonitis; rare: anaphylaxis, phlebitis, seizures, pseudomembranous colitis.
Class contraindications: Hypersensitivity to the medication or other penicillins.

PIPERACILLIN/TAZOBACTAM

Zosyn
Inj: 2.25, 3.375, 4.5 g
Penicillin agents

YES   ?   B

Indication: Moderate and severe systemic infections
Initial dose:
Moderate systemic infection: 2.25 g IV q6-8h
Severe systemic infection: 3.375 g IV q4-6h
Renal dose: CrCl 20-40 mL/min: 2.25 g q6h
　　　　　CrCl <20 mL/min: 2.25 g q8h

Adverse drug reaction: Headache, insomnia; rare: thrombocytopenia, hemolytic anemia.

Continued

PIPERACILLIN/TAZOBACTAM *continued*

Comments:
Extended-spectrum penicillin.
Sodium = 2.35 mEq (54 mg)/g.
Drug/drug: Probenecid may increase serum levels.
Monitor persistent diarrhea for *Clostridium difficile*.
Class side effects: Nausea, vomiting, diarrhea, rash, QT prolongation,
  tendonitis; rare: anaphylaxis, phlebitis, seizures, pseudomembranous colitis.
Class contraindications: Hypersensitivity to the medication or other penicillins.

TICARCILLIN

Ticar
Inj: 1, 3, 6 g
Penicillin agents

YES 1 B

 Indication: Lower respiratory, urinary, bone, joint, skin and skin structure,
  blood infections
Initial dose: 1-4 g IV q4-6h
Renal dose: CrCl 10-50 mL/min: 1-2 g q8h
  CrCl <10 mL/min: 1-2 g q12h

 Adverse drug reaction: Rare: leukopenia, neutropenia, thrombocytopenia,
  bleeding.
Comments:
Extended-spectrum penicillin.
Sodium = 5.2 mEq/g.
Drug/drug: Probenecid may increase serum levels.
Monitor persistent diarrhea for *Clostridium difficile*.
Class side effects: Nausea, vomiting, diarrhea, rash, QT prolongation,
  tendonitis; rare: anaphylaxis, phlebitis, seizures, pseudomembranous colitis.
Class contraindications: Hypersensitivity to the medication or other penicillins.

TICARCILLIN/CLAVULANIC ACID

Timentin
Inj: 3 g/100 mg
Penicillin agents

YES 1 B

 Indication: Lower respiratory, urinary, bone, joint, skin and skin structure,
  blood infections
Initial dose: 3.1 g IV q4-6h
Renal dose: CrCl 10-30 mL/min: 2 g q8h
  CrCl <10 mL/min: 2 g q12h

Continued

For explanation of icons, see p. 1068.

TICARCILLIN/CLAVULANIC ACID *continued*

Adverse drug reaction: Rare: leukopenia, neutropenia, thrombocytopenia, bleeding.
Comments:
Extended-spectrum penicillin.
Sodium = 4.75 mEq/g.
Drug/drug: Probenecid may increase serum levels.
Monitor persistent diarrhea for *Clostridium difficile.*
Class side effects: Nausea, vomiting, diarrhea, rash, QT prolongation, tendonitis; rare: anaphylaxis, phlebitis, seizures, pseudomembranous colitis.
Class contraindications: Hypersensitivity to the medication or other penicillins.

Combination Agents

AMOXICILLIN/LANSOPRAZOLE/ CLARITHROMYCIN
Prevpac
Caps, tabs: 500 mg × 4/ 30 mg × 2/ 500 mg × 2
Combination agents

Indication: *Helicobacter pylori* treatment

Fluoroquinolone Agents

CIPROFLOXACIN
Cipro
Tabs: 250, 500, 750 mg
Oral liquid: 250 mg/5 mL, 500/5 mL
Solution, inj: 200 mg/100 mL in D5W, 400 mg/200 mL in D5W
Fluoroquinolone agents

YES   X   C

Indication: Mild to moderate urinary tract infection (UTI); severe urinary, upper respiratory, intraabdominal infection; infectious diarrhea; prostatitis; nosocomial pneumonia; complicated bone and joint infection
Initial dose:
   Mild to moderate UTI: 250 mg PO q12h or 200 mg IV q12h
   Severe urinary, upper respiratory, intraabdominal infection; infectious diarrhea; prostatitis: 500-750 mg PO q12h or 400 mg IV q12h
   Nosocomial pneumonia; complicated bone and joint infection: 750 mg PO q12h or 400 mg IV q8h
Renal dose: CrCl 10-50 mL/min: 50%-75% dose
         CrCl <10 mL/min: 50% dose

Continued

CIPROFLOXACIN *continued*

Adverse drug reaction: Rash; rare: seizures, Stevens-Johnson syndrome.
Comments:
Use with caution in children under 18 years of age.
Drug/drug: Avoid using with magnesium-, aluminum-, or calcium-containing
  products or separate by several hr. Probenecid may increase serum levels.
  Ciprofloxacin may increase warfarin, theophylline levels. Sucralfate
  decreases absorption 50%.
Class side effects: Headache, nausea, diarrhea, vomiting, dizziness,
  photosensitivity; rare: hypersensitivity reaction.
Class contraindications: Hypersensitivity to the medication or other
  fluoroquinolones.

GATIFLOXACIN

Tequin
Tabs: 200, 400 mg   YES   3   C
Solution, inj: 200 mg/100 mL in D5W, 400 mg/200 mL in D5W
Fluoroquinolone agents

Indication: Moderate to severe urinary, upper respiratory infection
Initial dose: 400 mg PO/IV daily
Max dose: 400 mg daily
Renal dose: CrCl <40 mL/min: 400 mg × 1, then 200 mg q24h

Adverse drug reaction: Rare: seizures, psychoses.
Comments:
Use with caution in children under 18 years of age.
Drug/drug: Use caution with magnesium-, aluminum-, or calcium-containing
  products or separate by several hr. Avoid drugs that prolong QT interval.
Dosage increment IV = PO.
Class side effects: Headache, nausea, diarrhea, vomiting, dizziness,
  photosensitivity; rare: hypersensitivity reaction.
Class contraindications: Hypersensitivity to the medication or other
  fluoroquinolones.

For explanation of icons, see p. 1068.

LEVOFLOXACIN

Levaquin
Tabs: 250, 500 mg/100 mL in D5W, 750 mg/150 mL in D5W
Solution, inj: 250 mg/50 mL in D5W, 500, 750 mg
Fluoroquinolone agents

YES   X   C

Indication: Moderate to severe urinary, skin and skin structure, upper respiratory infections
Initial dose: 250-500 mg IV/PO q24h
Max dose: 750 mg daily
Renal dose: CrCl 10-50 mL/min: 500 mg × 1, then 250 mg q24-48h
CrCl <10 mL/min: 500 mg × 1, then 250 mg q48h

Adverse drug reaction: Rare: seizures, Stevens-Johnson syndrome, hypersensitivity reactions, pseudomembranous colitis.
Comments:
Use caution with children under 18 years of age.
Drug/drug: Avoid using with magnesium-, aluminum-, or calcium-containing products or separate by several hr. Avoid use of drugs that prolong QT interval.
Dosage increment IV = PO.
Class side effects: Headache, nausea, diarrhea, vomiting, dizziness, photosensitivity; rare: hypersensitivity reaction.
Class contraindications: Hypersensitivity to the medication or other fluoroquinolones.

MOXIFLOXACIN

Avelox
Solution, inj: 400 mg/5 mL in 0.9% NS
Tabs: 400 mg
Fluoroquinolone agents

NO   3   C

Indication: Moderate to severe upper and lower respiratory tract infections
Initial dose: 400 mg PO/IV daily
Max dose: 400 mg daily

Adverse drug reaction: Rare: Seizures, psychoses, abnormal liver function test results.
Comments:
Drug/drug: Avoid using with magnesium-, aluminum-, or calcium-containing products or separate by several hr. Avoid use of drugs that prolong QT interval.
Class side effects: Headache, nausea, diarrhea, vomiting, dizziness, photosensitivity; rare: hypersensitivity reaction.
Class contraindications: Hypersensitivity to the medication or other fluoroquinolones.

NORFLOXACIN

Noroxin
Tabs: 400 mg
Fluoroquinolone agents

YES   X   C

Indication: Moderate to severe urinary infection
Initial dose: 400 mg PO bid
Max dose: 800 mg daily
Renal dose: CrCl <30 mL/min: 400 mg q24h

Adverse drug reaction: Rare: seizures, anaphylactoid reaction.
Comments:
Drug/drug: Avoid using with magnesium-, aluminum-, or calcium-containing
products or separate by several hr. Norfloxacin may increase warfarin levels.
Class side effects: Headache, nausea, diarrhea, vomiting, dizziness,
photosensitivity; rare: hypersensitivity reaction.
Class contraindications: Hypersensitivity to the medication or other
fluoroquinolones.

OFLOXACIN

Floxin
Solution, inj: 200 mg/50 mL in D5W, 400 mg/100 mL in D5W
Tabs: 200, 300, 400 mg
Fluoroquinolone agents

YES   X   C

Indication: Moderate respiratory, skin and skin structure infection; gonorrhea;
urinary tract infection (UTI)
Initial dose:
Respiratory, skin and skin structure infection: 400 mg PO/IV q12h
Gonorrhea: 400 mg PO/IV × 1
UTI: 200-400 mg PO/IV q12h
Renal dose: CrCl 10-50 mL/min: 100% q12-24h
CrCl <10 mL/min: 50% q24h

Adverse drug reaction: Transient ocular discomfort (ophthalmic use); rare:
seizures, anaphylactoid reaction, pseudomembranous colitis.
Comments:
Dosage increment IV = PO.
Drug/drug: Avoid using with magnesium-, aluminum-, or calcium-containing
products or separate by several hr.
Class side effects: Headache, nausea, diarrhea, vomiting, dizziness,
photosensitivity; rare: hypersensitivity reaction.
Class contraindications: Hypersensitivity to the medication or other
fluoroquinolones.

For explanation of icons, see p. 1068.

Tetracycline Agents

DOXYCYCLINE

Vibramycin, Monodox
Inj: 100, 200 mg
Caps: 50, 100 mg
Caps, delayed-release: 100 mg
Oral liquid: 25 mg/5 mL, 50 mg/5 mL
Tetracycline agents

NO   ?   D

 Indication: Uncomplicated *Chlamydia*, urethral, endocervical, rectal infections; gonorrhea in patient with serious penicillin allergy
Initial dose: 100-200 mg PO/IV daily or divided bid

Adverse drug reaction: Epigastric distress, rash, increased pigmentation, urticaria; rare: anaphylaxis.
Comments:
Drug/drug: Phenytoin, barbiturates, carbamazepine may decrease levels.
Dosage increment: Infuse IV over 1 hr; IV = PO.
Class side effects: Photosensitivity, nausea, vomiting, diarrhea, anorexia, thrombophlebitis (IV), intracranial, hypertension, pseudotumor cerebri, neutropenia, thrombocytopenia.
Class contraindications: Hypersensitivity to the medication or tetracycline antibiotics.

MINOCYCLINE

Minocin
Caps: 50, 100 mg
Caps, pellet-filled: 50, 100 mg
Inj: 100 mg
Oral liquid: 50 mg/5 mL
Tetracycline agents

NO   ?   D

Indication: Susceptible organisms
Initial dose: Load: 200 mg PO/IV, then 100 mg PO/IV q12h

Adverse drug reaction: Anorexia, epigastric distress, oral candidiasis, rash, increased pigmentation, urticaria; rare: anaphylaxis.
Comments:
Do not take with milk or dairy products or divalent cations.
Dosage increment: IV = PO.
Class side effects: Photosensitivity, nausea, vomiting, diarrhea, anorexia, thrombophlebitis (IV), intracranial, hypertension, pseudotumor cerebri, neutropenia, thrombocytopenia.
Class contraindications: Hypersensitivity to the medication or tetracycline antibiotics.

TETRACYCLINE

Tetrachel, Sumycin
Caps: 100, 250, 500 mg
Tabs: 250, 500 mg
Oral liquid: 125 mg/5 mL
Tetracycline agents

 YES 1 D

Indication: *Chlamydia* infection, acne
Initial dose:
   ***Chlamydia* infection:** 500 mg PO qid
   Acne: 500 mg–1 g PO divided qid, then 125-500 mg PO daily
Renal dose: CrCl 10-50 mL/min: q12-24h
          CrCl <10 mL/min: q24h
          Avoid in end-stage renal disease

Adverse drug reaction: Epigastric distress, oral candidiasis, rash, increased
   pigmentation, urticaria, enamel defects; rare: anaphylactoid reaction, status
   asthmaticus, respiratory arrest, arrhythmias.
Comments:
Do not take with milk or dairy products or divalent cations.
Administer on empty stomach.
Class side effects: Photosensitivity, nausea, vomiting, diarrhea, anorexia,
   thrombophlebitis (IV), intracranial, hypertension, pseudotumor cerebri,
   neutropenia, thrombocytopenia.
Class contraindications: Hypersensitivity to the medication or tetracycline
   antibiotics.

Other Agents

AZTREONAM

Azactam
Inj: 500 mg, 1, 2 g
Other agents

 YES 1 C

Indication: Moderate to severe urinary, respiratory, intraabdominal,
        gynecological infection; urinary tract infection (UTI); severe
        infection
Initial dose:
   **Moderate to severe urinary, respiratory, intraabdominal,
   gynecological infection; UTI:** 1-2 g IV q8-12h
   Severe infection: 2 g IV q6h
Max dose: 8 g daily
Renal dose: CrCl 10-50 mL/min: Full dose × 1, then 50%-75% dose
          CrCl <10 mL/min: Full dose × 1, then 25% dose

Continued

For explanation of icons, see p. 1068.

AZTREONAM *continued*

Adverse drug reaction: Rare: seizures, neutropenia, pancytopenia, thrombocytopenia.
Comments:
Monobactam antibiotic.
Rare cross-sensitivity to penicillin or cephalosporin.
Contraindicated in patients with hypersensitivity to the medication.

CHLORAMPHENICOL

Chloromycetin
Inj: 1 g
Other agents

NO   3   C

Indication: Severe meningitis, blood infections
Initial dose: 50-100 mg/kg IV divided q6h
Max dose: 100 mg/kg daily for short-term only

Adverse drug reaction: Rare: aplastic anemia, hypoplastic anemia, agranulocytosis, thrombocytopenia, angioedema, anaphylaxis, Gray's syndrome in neonates, nausea, vomiting, hepatotoxicity.
Comments:
Sodium = 2.3 mEq/g.
Monitor complete blood cell, platelet, reticulocyte counts and iron levels; measure at baseline and q2 days.
Use with caution in glucose-6 phosphate dehydrogenase deficiency. Serious and fatal blood dyscrasias have occurred after short- and long-term administration.
Rare cross-sensitivity to penicillin or cephalosporin.
Contraindicated in patients with hypersensitivity to the medication.

CLINDAMYCIN

Cleocin
Inj: 900 mg/6 mL
Caps: 75, 150, 300 mg
Solution, inj: 300 mg/50 mL in D5W, 600 mg/50 mL in D5W
Other agents

NO   1   B

Indication: Skin and soft tissue infection, osteomyelitis, respiratory disease, pelvic inflammatory disease
Initial dose: 150-450 mg PO q6-8h
                  600-900 mg IV q6-8h
Max dose: 1.8 g PO daily
              4.8 g IV daily

Continued

CLINDAMYCIN *continued*

Adverse drug reaction: Nausea, cervicitis, vaginitis, *Candida albicans* infection, vulvar irritation, redness, diarrhea, pseudomembranous colitis; rare: transient leukopenia, thrombocytopenia, anaphylaxis.
Comments:
Lincosamide antibiotic.
Do not infuse faster than 30 mg/min.
Contraindicated in ulcerative colitis, enteritis, antibiotic-associated colitis, hepatic impairment, hypersensitivity to lincomycin or this medication.

COLISTIMETHATE

Coly-Mycin M, Colistin
Inj: 150 mg
Other agents

YES   ?   C

Indication: Susceptible organisms
Initial dose: 2.5-5 mg/kg IM/IV divided in 2-4 doses
Max dose: 5 mg/kg daily
Renal dose: Serum creatinine 1.6-2.5 mg/dL: 2.5 mg/kg q12-24h
Serum creatinine 2.6-4 mg/dL: 1.5 mg/kg q36h

Adverse drug reaction: Dose-related nephrotoxicity and neurotoxicity.
Comments:
Polymixin antibiotic.
Use ideal body weight in determining dosage increment.
Drug/drug: Use caution with other nephrotoxic and neurotoxic agents.
Contraindicated in patients with hypersensitivity to the medication.

DAPSONE

Tabs, scored: 25, 100 mg
Other agents

NO   1   C

Indication: Leprosy, prophylaxis against toxoplasmosis and *Pneumocystis carinii (jiroveci)* pneumonia (PCP)
Initial dose:
  Leprosy: 100 mg daily as part of a multidrug therapy
  Toxoplasmosis prophylaxis: 50 mg PO daily
  PCP prophylaxis: 100 mg PO daily
Max dose: 100 mg daily

Continued

For explanation of icons, see p. 1068.

DAPSONE *continued*

Adverse drug reaction: Rare: pancreatitis, hemolytic anemia (dose related), agranulocytosis, aplastic anemia, exfoliative dermatitis, toxic erythema, erythema multiforme, toxic epidermal necrolysis, morbilliform and scarlatiniform reactions, urticaria, erythema nodosum, sulfone syndrome.
Comments:
Sulfone antibiotic.
Use with caution in patients with glucose-6 phosphate dehydrogenase deficiency.
Dosage increment may need to be higher for high acetylators (35%-50% of African-Americans, Caucasians, and Mexicans, 80% of Japanese, Chinese, and Inuit).
Contraindicated in patients with hypersensitivity to the medication.

QUINUPRISTIN/DALFOPRISTIN

Synercid
Inj: 150/350 mg (10 mL)
Other agents

NO   ?   B

Indication: Vancomycin-resistant *Enterococcus* infections, skin and skin structure infections
Initial dose: 7.5 mg/kg IV q8-12h

Adverse drug reaction: Elevated bilirubin levels, infusion site reaction, arthralgia, myalgia.
Comments:
Streptogramin antibiotic.
Not active against *Enterococcus faecalis*.
Drug/drug: Avoid use of drugs that prolong QT interval. Quinupristin/dalfopristin decreases levels of cyclosporin A, midazolam, tacrolimus, verapamil, lovastatin.
Infuse over 60 minutes.
Contraindicated in patients with hypersensitivity to the medication and other streptogramin antibiotics.

IMIPENEM/CILASTATIN

Primaxin
Inj: 500 mg/500 mg in 0.9% NS, 250 mg/250 mg in 0.9% NS
Other agents

YES   ?   C

Indication: Moderate lower respiratory tract infections, moderate or severe gynecological infections and infections of skin and skin structures

Continued

IMIPENEM/CILASTATIN *continued*

> **Initial dose:**
> **Moderate infections:** 500-750 mg IM q12h
> **Severe infections:** 250 mg–1 g IV q6-8h
> **Max dose:** 2 g daily
> **Renal dose:** CrCl 10-50 mL/min: 50% dose
>   CrCl <10 mL/min: 25% dose

Adverse drug reaction: Pseudomembranous colitis, dose-related nausea; rare: seizures, agranulocytosis, hypersensitivity reactions, increases in liver function test parameters.
Comments:
Thienamycin antibiotic. Cilastatin reduces imepenem metabolism.
Use with caution in patients with β-lactam allergy.
Dosage increment: Adjust dose if patient <70 kg. The manufacturer has complicated nomograms for dosage changes based on weight and creatinine clearance.
Contraindicated in patients with hypersensitivity to the medication.

LINEZOLID

NO 3 C

Zyvox
Tabs: 400, 600 mg
Oral liquid: 100 mg/5 mL
Inj: 200 mg/100 mL in D5W, 600 mg/300 mL in D5W
Other agents

Indication: Vancomycin-resistant *Enterococcus* (VRE) infections, methicillin-resistant *Staphylococcus aureus* (MRSA) pneumonia, uncomplicated skin and skin structure infection
Initial dose:
VRE infection, MRSA pneumonia: 600 mg PO/IV q12h
Uncomplicated skin and skin structure infection: 400 mg PO q12h

Adverse drug reaction: Diarrhea, headache, nausea, vomiting, rash, insomnia, constipation, dizziness, thrombocytopenia.
Comments:
Oxazolidinone antibiotic.
Drug/drug: Additive effect with sympathomimetic agents. Avoid high-tyramine foods.
Contraindicated in patients with hypersensitivity to the medication.

For explanation of icons, see p. 1068.

MEROPENEM

Merrem IV
Inj: 500 mg, 1 g
Other agents

YES ? B

Indication: Severe infection, meningitis
Initial dose: 1-2 g IV q8h
Max dose: 6 g IV daily
Renal dose: CrCl 10-50 mL/min: 500 mg–1 g q12h
CrCl <10 mL/min: 500 mg q24h

Adverse drug reaction: Rare: seizure, bleeding events, nausea, vomiting, abdominal pain, diarrhea, headache, kidney and liver failure.
Comments:
Carbapenem antibiotic.
Sodium = 3.92 mEq/g.
Contraindicated in patients with hypersensitivity to other β-lactam antibiotics.
Class contraindications: Hypersensitivity to the medication.

METRONIDAZOLE

Flagyl, Flagyl ER
Tabs, scored: 250, 500 mg
Tabs, extended-release: 750 mg
Caps: 375 mg
Inj: 500 mg
Other agents

NO 3 B/C

Indication: Amebiasis, trichomoniasis, anaerobic infections, pseudomembranous colitis, *Helicobacter pylori* infection
Initial dose:
  Amebiasis: 500-750 mg PO q8h
  Trichomoniasis: 2 g PO × 1 dose
  Anaerobic infections: Load: 15 mg/kg, then 7.5 mg/kg (500 mg) IV/PO q6-8h
  Pseudomembranous colitis: 250 mg PO qid or 500 mg PO qid
  ***H. pylori* infection:** 500-750 mg PO tid or qid, as part of a multidrug therapy
Max dose: 4 g daily
Renal dose: CrCl <10 mL/min: 50% dose

Continued

METRONIDAZOLE *continued*

Adverse drug reaction: Candidiasis; rare: seizure, transient leukopenia, neutropenia.
Comments:
5-Nitroimidazole antibiotic.
Avoid use in first trimester of pregnancy.
Pregnancy category: C in first trimester.
Sodium = 2.8 mEq/g.
Do not administer by IV push.
Drug/drug: Avoid use of alcohol because of disulfiram-like effect.
Contraindicated in patients with hypersensitivity to this medication or other nitroimidazole derivatives.

NITROFURANTOIN

Macrodantin, Macrobid
Tabs: 25, 50, 100 mg   YES   1   B
Tabs, dual-release: 100 mg (25 mg macrocrystals, 75 mg monohydrate)
Oral liquid: 25 mg/5 mL
Other agents

Indication: Urinary tract infection (UTI), prophylaxis and long-term suppressive therapy for UTI
Initial dose:
  UTI: 50-100 mg PO q6h or 100 mg PO bid (dual-release)
  Prophylaxis and long-term treatment of UTI: 50-100 mg PO qhs
Renal dose: CrCl <50 mL/min: Avoid use

Adverse drug reaction: Ascending polyneuropathy (dose dependent), anorexia, nausea, vomiting, diarrhea, exfoliative dermatitis; rare: peripheral neuropathy, agranulocytosis, thrombocytopenia, hepatitis, pulmonary sensitivity reactions, Stevens-Johnson syndrome, anaphylaxis, hemolysis (glucose-6 phosphate dehydrogenase [G6PD] deficiency), methemoglobinemia.
Comments:
Nitrofuran antibiotic.
Use caution in patients with G6PD deficiency.
Contraindicated in patients with anuria or oliguria, pregnancy at term (38-42 weeks' gestation), and hypersensitivity to the medication.

RIFAMPIN

Rifadin, Rimactane
Caps: 150, 300 mg
Inj: 600 mg
Other agents

YES   1   C

Indication: Treatment of pulmonary tuberculosis, meningococcal carrier state
Initial dose:
    Treatment of pulmonary tuberculosis: 10-20 mg/kg (600 mg) PO/IV daily as part of a multidrug therapy
   Meningococcal carrier state: 600 mg q12h × 2 days
  Renal dose: CrCl 10-50 mL/min: 50%-100% dose
            CrCl <10 mL/min: 50%-100% dose

Adverse drug reaction: Transient abnormal liver function test parameters; rare: acute renal failure, thrombocytopenia, hepatotoxicity, shock.
Comments:
Drug/drug: Avoid concomitant use of hepatotoxic drugs. Decreases effectiveness oral contraceptives. Induces metabolism of warfarin, digoxin, cyclosporin A, verapamil.
Dosage increment: Adjust in renal failure.
Class contraindications: Hypersensitivity to the medication.

SULFAMETHOXAZOLE/ TRIMETHOPRIM

Bactrim, Bactrim DS, Cotrimoxazole
Tabs: 400/80 mg (SS), 800/160 mg (DS)
Oral liquid: 200/40 mg in 5 mL
Inj: 80/16 mg per mL
Other agents

YES   1   C/D

Indication: Urinary tract infection (UTI), bronchitis, prophylaxis and treatment of *Pneumocystis carinii (jeroveci)* pneumonia (PCP), toxoplasmic encephalitis prophylaxis
Initial dose:
  UTI, bronchitis: 1 DS PO q12h
  PCP/toxoplasmic encephalitis prophylaxis: 1 DS PO daily
  PCP treatment: 5 mg/kg (trimethoprim) IV/PO q6-8h
 Max dose: 960 mg (trimethoprim) daily
 Renal dose: CrCl 15-30 mL/min: 50%
           CrCl <15 mL/min: Not recommended

Continued

SULFAMETHOXAZOLE/TRIMETHOPRIM *continued*

Adverse drug reaction: Nausea, vomiting, diarrhea, toxic nephrosis with oliguria or anuria, serum sickness, drug fever; rare: seizures, pancreatitis, blood dyscrasias, hepatic necrosis, erythema multiforme, Stevens-Johnson syndrome, anaphylaxis, urolithiasis.

Comments:

Drug/drug: increases warfarin, methotrexate levels.

Use with caution in patients with glucose-6 phosphate dehydrogenase (G6PD) deficiency.

Contraindicated in patients with porphyria, folate-deficient megaloblastic anemia, renal failure, or hypersensitivity to sulfonamides.

Pregnancy category: D in third trimester.

VANCOMYCIN

Vancocin
Inj: 500 mg, 1 g
Caps: 125, 250 mg
Oral liquid: 1 g
Other agents

YES ? C

Indication: Methicillin-resistant *Staphylococcus aureus* (MRSA) infection, meningitis, other gram-positive infection with serious penicillin allergies, *Clostridium difficile* colitis

Initial dose:

MRSA infection, meningitis, other gram-positive infection with serious penicillin allergies: 10-15 mg/kg/dose IV q12h

***C. difficile* colitis:** 125 mg PO q6h

Renal dose: CrCl 10-50 mL/min: 1 g q24-48h
CrCl <10 mL/min: 1 g, treat again per levels

Adverse drug reaction: Rare: nephrotoxicity, ototoxicity, anaphylaxis, neutropenia, leukopenia.

Comments:

Glycopeptide antibiotic.

Drug/drug: Avoid concomitant use of ototoxic and nephrotoxic drugs.

Monitor complete blood cell count, drug levels.

Dosage increment based on actual body weight; trough level measured immediately before next dose, or 72 hr after first dose when glomerular filtration rate <15 mL/min.

Contraindicated in patients with previous hearing loss or hypersensitivity to the medication.

For explanation of icons, see p. 1068.

Combination Agents

OXYTETRACYCLINE/ PHENAZOPYRIDINE/ SULFAMETHIZOLE
Urobiotic
Caps: 250/50/250 mg
Combination agents

TETRACYCLINE/BISMUTH SUBSALICYLATE/METRONIDAZOLE
Helidac
Kit: 500 mg × 4/ 262.4 mg × 8/ 250 mg × 4
Combination agents

Indication: Treatment of *Helicobacter pylori* infection

RIFAMPIN/ISONIAZID
Rifamate
Caps: 300/150 mg
Combination agents

Indication: Tuberculosis

RIFAMPIN/ISONIAZID/PYRAZINAMIDE
Rifater
Tabs: 120/50/300 mg
Combination agents

Indication: Tuberculosis

CARDIOVASCULAR
ACE Inhibitors

BENAZEPRIL

Lotensin
Tabs: 5, 10, 20, 40 mg
ACE inhibitors

YES   ?   C/D

Indication: Hypertension
Initial dose: 10 mg PO daily
Max dose: 80 mg daily
Renal dose: CrCl 10-50 mL/min: 50%-75% dose
CrCl <10 mL/min: 25%-50% dose

Comments:
Usual maintenance dose is 20-40 mg daily.
Dosage increment q1-2 wk.
Divided dosage may be more effective in controlling blood pressure than same dose given once daily.
Drug/drug: In patients undergoing aggressive diuresis, halve initial dose. Additive effects with potassium-sparing diuretics. Increased lithium levels may be seen with coadministration.
Monitor potassium level and renal function at baseline and after dosage adjustments.
Pregnancy category: D in second and third trimesters.
Class side effects: Dry persistent nonproductive cough, rash, hypotension, hyperkalemia; rare: neutropenia, leukopenia, angioedema.
Class contraindications: Hypersensitivity to ACE inhibitors, bilateral renal artery stenosis.

CAPTOPRIL

Capoten
Tabs, scored: 12.5, 25, 50, 100 mg
ACE inhibitors

YES   ?   C/D

Indication: Hypertension, heart failure, left ventricular dysfunction after myocardial infarction, diabetic nephropathy
Initial dose: 25 mg PO bid/tid
Max dose: 450 mg daily
Renal dose: CrCl 10-50 mL/min: 75% dose q12-18h
CrCl <10 mL/min: 50% dose q24h

Continued

CAPTOPRIL *continued*

Adverse drug reaction: Rare: leukocytopenia, agranulocytosis, pancytopenia, thrombocytopenia.

Comments:

Dosage increment: 25 mg bid/tid q 1-2 wk, may increase sooner in monitored setting.

Drug/drug: In patients undergoing aggressive diuresis, halve initial dose. Additive effects with potassium-sparing diuretics. Increased lithium levels may be seen with coadministration.

Monitor potassium level and renal function at baseline and after dosage adjustment.

Pregnancy category: D in second and third trimesters.

Class side effects: Dry persistent nonproductive cough, rash, hypotension, hyperkalemia; rare: neutropenia, leukopenia, angioedema.

Class contraindications: Hypersensitivity to ACE inhibitors, bilateral renal artery stenosis.

ENALAPRIL, ENALAPRILAT

Vasotec, Vasotec IV
Tabs, scored*: 2.5*, 5*, 10, 20 mg
Inj: 1.25 mg/mL (2 mL)
ACE inhibitors

YES ? C/D

Indication: Hypertension
Initial dose: 2.5-5 mg PO daily/bid
1.25 mg IV over 5 min, may repeat in 1 hr
Maintenance: 1.25 mg IV q6h
Max dose: 40 mg daily
Renal dose: CrCl 10-50 mL/min: 75%-100% dose
CrCl <10 mL/min: 50% dose

Comments:

1.25 mg IV q6h roughly equivalent to 5 mg PO daily.

Dosage increment q 1-2 wk, may be divided.

Drug/drug: In patients undergoing aggressive diuresis, halve initial dose. Additive effects with potassium-sparing diuretics. Increased lithium levels may be seen with coadministration.

Monitor potassium level and renal function at baseline and after dosage adjustment.

Pregnancy category: D in second and third trimesters.

Class side effects: Dry persistent nonproductive cough, rash, hypotension, hyperkalemia; rare: neutropenia, leukopenia, angioedema.

Class contraindications: Hypersensitivity to ACE inhibitors, bilateral renal artery stenosis.

FOSINOPRIL

Monopril
Tabs, scored*: 10*, 20, 40 mg
ACE inhibitors

YES   ?   C/D

Indication: Hypertension, heart failure
Initial dose: 10 mg PO daily
Max dose: 80 mg daily
Renal dose: CrCl <10 mL/min: 75%-100% dose

Comments:
Usual maintenance dosage range is 20-40 mg daily.
Dosage increment q 1-2 wk.
Divided dosage may be more effective in controlling blood pressure than same
   dose given once daily.
Drug/drug: In patients undergoing aggressive diuresis, halve initial dose.
   Additive effects with potassium-sparing diuretics. Increased lithium levels
   may be seen with coadminstration.
Monitor potassium level and renal function at baseline and after dosage
   adjustment.
Pregnancy category: D in second and third trimesters.
Class side effects: Dry persistent nonproductive cough, rash, hypotension,
   hyperkalemia; rare: neutropenia, leukopenia, angioedema.
Class contraindications: Hypersensitivity to ACE inhibitors, bilateral renal artery
   stenosis.

LISINOPRIL

Zestril, Prinivil
Tabs: 2.5, 5, 10, 20, 30, 40 mg
ACE inhibitors

YES   ?   C/D

Indication: Hypertension, acute myocardial infarction, heart failure
Initial dose:
   Hypertension: 10 mg PO daily
   Acute myocardial infarction,
      heart failure: 5 mg PO daily within 24 hr, 5 mg after 24 hr, 10 mg
         after 48 hr
Max dose: 80 mg daily
Renal dose: CrCl 10-50 mL/min: 50%-75% dose
            CrCl <10 mL/min: 25%-50% dose

Comments:
Usual maintenance dosage range is 20-40 mg daily.
Dosage increment q1-2 wk.

Continued

For explanation of icons, see p. 1068.

LISINOPRIL *continued*

> Divided dosage may be more effective in controlling blood pressure than same dose given once daily.
>
> Drug/drug: In patients undergoing aggressive diuresis, halve initial dose. Additive effects with potassium-sparing diuretics. Increased lithium levels may be seen with coadministration.
>
> Monitor potassium level and renal function at baseline and after dosage adjustment.
>
> Pregnancy category: D in second and third trimesters.
>
> Class side effects: Dry persistent nonproductive cough, rash, hypotension, hyperkalemia; rare: neutropenia, leukopenia, angioedema.
>
> Class contraindications: Hypersensitivity to ACE inhibitors, bilateral renal artery stenosis.

MOEXIPRIL
Univasc
Tabs, scored: 7.5, 15 mg
ACE inhibitors

YES   ?   C/D

Indication: Hypertension
Initial dose: 7.5 mg PO daily
Max dose: 30 mg daily

Comments:
Dosage increment q 1-2 wk.

> Divided dosage may be more effective in controlling blood pressure than same dose given once daily.
>
> Drug/drug: In patients undergoing aggressive diuresis, halve initial dose. Additive effects with potassium-sparing diuretics. Increased lithium levels may be seen with coadministration.
>
> Monitor potassium level and renal function at baseline and after dosage adjustment.
>
> Pregnancy category: D in second and third trimesters.
>
> Class side effects: Dry persistent nonproductive cough, rash, hypotension, hyperkalemia; rare: neutropenia, leukopenia, angioedema.
>
> Class contraindications: Hypersensitivity to ACE inhibitors, bilateral renal artery stenosis.

QUINAPRIL

YES   ?   C/D

Accupril
Tabs, scored*: 5*, 10, 20, 40 mg
ACE inhibitors

Indication: Hypertension, heart failure
Initial dose: 10 mg PO daily
Max dose: 80 mg daily
Renal dose: CrCl 10-50 mL/min: 75%-100% dose
            CrCl <10 mL/min: 75% dose

Adverse drug reaction: Exfoliative dermatitis (rare).
Comments:
Divided dosage may be more effective in controlling blood pressure than same
    dose given once daily.
Drug/drug: In patients undergoing aggressive diuresis, halve initial dose.
    Additive effects with potassium-sparing diuretics. Increased lithium levels
    may be seen with coadministration.
Monitor potassium level and renal function at baseline and after dosage
    adjustment.
Pregnancy category: D in second and third trimesters.
Class side effects: Dry persistent nonproductive cough, rash, hypotension,
    hyperkalemia; rare: neutropenia, leukopenia, angioedema.
Class contraindications: Hypersensitivity to ACE inhibitors, bilateral renal artery
    stenosis.

RAMIPRIL

YES   ?   C/D

Altace
Caps: 1.25, 2.5, 5, 10 mg
ACE inhibitors

Indication: Hypertension, heart failure post myocardial infarction, reduction in
            risk of myocardial infarction and stroke from cardiovascular causes
Initial dose:
   Hypertension: 2.5 mg PO daily
   Heart failure: 2.5 mg PO bid
Max dose: 20 mg daily
Renal dose: CrCl 10-50 mL/min: 50%-75 % dose (hypertension)
            CrCl <10 mL/min: 25%-50% dose (heart failure)

Adverse drug reaction: Seizures (rare).
Comments:
Dosage increment q 1-2 wk.

Continued

RAMIPRIL *continued*

Divided dosage may be more effective in controlling blood pressure than same dose given once daily.

Drug/drug: In patients undergoing aggressive diuresis, halve initial dose. Additive effects with potassium-sparing diuretics. Increased lithium levels may be seen with coadministration.

Monitor potassium level and renal function at baseline and after dosage adjustment.

Pregnancy category: D in second and third trimesters.

Class side effects: Dry persistent nonproductive cough, rash, hypotension, hyperkalemia; rare: neutropenia, leukopenia, angioedema.

Class contraindications: Hypersensitivity to ACE inhibitors, bilateral renal artery stenosis.

TRANDOLAPRIL
Mavik
Tabs, scored*: 1*, 2, 4 mg
ACE inhibitors

YES ? C/D

Indication: Hypertension, heart failure, post myocardial infarction
Initial dose: 1-2 mg PO daily
Max dose: 8 mg daily

Comments:

Usual dosage range is 2-4 mg daily.

Dosage increment q 1-2 wk.

Divided dosage may be more effective in controlling blood pressure than same dose given once daily.

Drug/drug: In patients undergoing aggressive diuresis, halve initial dose. Additive effects with potassium-sparing diuretics. Increased lithium levels may be seen with coadministration.

Monitor potassium level and renal function at baseline and after dosage adjustment.

Pregnancy category: D in second and third trimesters.

Class side effects: Dry persistent nonproductive cough, rash, hypotension, hyperkalemia; rare: neutropenia, leukopenia, angioedema.

Class contraindications: Hypersensitivity to ACE inhibitors, bilateral renal artery stenosis.

Angiotensin Receptor Blockers

CANDESARTAN

Atacand
Tabs: 4, 8, 16, 32 mg
Angiotensin receptor blockers

NO   3   C/D

Indication: Hypertension
Initial dose: 16 mg PO daily
Max dose: 32 mg daily

Comments:
Significant blood pressure lowering is seen in 2 wk, maximal blood pressure
    lowering is usually seen in 4-6 wk.
Drug/drug: In patients undergoing aggressive diuresis, halve initial dose.
Pregnancy category: D in second and third trimesters.
Class side effects: Hypotension, dizziness, nasal congestion, muscle cramps;
    rare: cough, angioedema.
Class contraindications: Hypersensitivity to the medication, history of
    angioedema in response to an ACE inhibitor.

EPROSARTAN

Teveten
Tabs, scored*: 400*, 600 mg
Angiotensin receptor blockers

NO   3   C/D

Indication: Hypertension
Initial dose: 600 mg PO daily
Max dose: 800 mg daily

Comments:
Maximal blood pressure lowering seen in 2-3 wk.
Divided dosage may be more effective in controlling blood pressure than same
    dose given once daily.
Drug/drug: In patients undergoing aggressive diuresis, halve initial dose.
Pregnancy category: D in second and third trimesters.
Class side effects: Hypotension, dizziness, nasal congestion, muscle cramps;
    rare: cough, angioedema.
Class contraindications: Hypersensitivity to the medication.

IRBESARTAN

Avapro
Tabs: 75, 150, 300 mg
Angiotensin receptor blockers

NO   3   C/D

Indication: Hypertension
Initial dose: 150 mg PO daily
Max dose: 300 mg daily

Comments:
Drug/drug: In patients undergoing aggressive diuresis, halve initial dose.
Pregnancy category: D in second and third trimesters.
Class side effects: Hypotension, dizziness, nasal congestion, muscle cramps;
    rare: cough, angioedema.
Class contraindications: Hypersensitivity to the medication.

LOSARTAN

Cozaar
Tabs: 25, 50, 100 mg
Angiotensin receptor blockers

NO   3   C/D

Indication: Hypertension
Initial dose: 50 mg PO daily
Max dose: 100 mg daily

Comments:
Significant blood pressure lowering is seen in 1-2 wk; maximal blood pressure
    lowering is usually seen in 3-6 wk.
Divided dosage may be more effective in controlling blood pressure than same
    dose given once daily.
Drug/drug: In patients undergoing aggressive diuresis, halve initial dose.
Dosage increment 25 mg q1-2 mo.
Pregnancy category: D in second and third trimesters.
Class side effects: Hypotension, dizziness, nasal congestion, muscle cramps;
    rare: cough, angioedema.
Class contraindications: Hypersensitivity to the medication.

TELMISARTAN
Micardis
Tabs: 40, 80 mg
Angiotensin receptor blockers

NO   3   C/D

 Indication: Hypertension
Initial dose: 40 mg PO daily
Max dose: 80 mg daily

 Comments:
Significant blood pressure lowering seen in 2 wk; maximal blood pressure is
usually seen in 4 wk.
Drug/drug: In patients undergoing aggressive diuresis, halve initial dose.
Increased lithium levels may be seen with coadministration.
Use with caution in patients with biliary obstructive disorders or hepatic
insufficiency.
Pregnancy category: D in second and third trimesters.
Class side effects: Hypotension, dizziness, nasal congestion, muscle cramps;
rare: cough, angioedema.
Class contraindications: Hypersensitivity to the medication.

VALSARTAN
Diovan
Caps: 80, 160 mg
Angiotensin receptor blockers

NO   3   C/D

 Indication: Hypertension
Initial dose: 80 mg PO daily
Max dose: 320 mg daily

 Comments:
Significant blood pressure lowering seen in 2 wk, maximal blood pressure is
usually seen in 4 wk.
Drug/drug: In patients undergoing aggressive diuresis, halve initial dose.
Pregnancy category: D in second and third trimesters.
Class side effects: Hypotension, dizziness, nasal congestion, muscle cramps;
rare: cough, angioedema.
Class contraindications: Hypersensitivity to the medication.

Antiadrenergic
Peripherally Acting Agents

DOXAZOSIN

Cardura
Tabs, scored: 1, 2, 4, 8 mg
Antiadrenergic, peripherally acting agents

NO   X   B

Indication: Hypertension, benign prostatic hyperplasia
Initial dose: 1 mg PO qhs
Max dose: 16 mg daily

Adverse drug reaction: Somnolence.
Comments:
α-Blockers not recommended as monotherapy hypertensive agents.
Dosage increment q1-2 wk.
Orthostatic effects most likely to occur 2-6 hr after dose.
Doses exceeding 4 mg daily are associated with a greater incidence of postural effects.
Drug/herb: Butcher's broom, avoid use together.
Class side effects: First-dose syncope, headache, dizziness, nausea, hypotension.
Class contraindications: Hypersensitivity to the medication or other quinazoline derivatives.

PRAZOSIN

Minipress
Caps: 1, 2, 5 mg
Antiadrenergic, peripherally acting agents

NO   ?   C

Indication: Hypertension, benign prostatic hyperplasia
Initial dose: 1 mg PO bid or tid
Max dose: 20 mg daily

Adverse drug reaction: Palpitation.
Comments:
α-Blockers not recommended as monotherapy hypertensive agents.
Dosage increment q1-2 wk.
Drug/herb: Butcher's broom, avoid use together.
Drug/diagnostic: Causes increases in levels of urinary metabolite of norepinephrine and vanillylmandelic acid, altering results of screening for pheochromocytoma and giving a false positive result.
Class side effects: First-dose syncope, headache, dizziness, nausea, hypotension.
Class contraindications: Hypersensitivity to the medication or other quinazoline derivatives.

RESERPINE

YES ? C

Tabs: 0.1, 0.25 mg
Antiadrenergic, peripherally acting agents

Indication: Hypertension
Initial dose: 0.05-0.1 mg PO daily
Max dose: 0.25 mg daily
Renal dose: CrCl <10 mL/min: Avoid

Adverse drug reaction: Syncope, vomiting, diarrhea, gynecomastia,
  drowsiness, fatigue, depression (suicide), bradycardia; rare: extrapyramidal
  side effects
Comments:
Dosage increment every 1-2 months in general.
Contraindicated in depression (suicidal ideation), peptic ulcer disease,
  ulcerative colitis.
Class side effects: First-dose syncope, severe mental depression, headache,
  lethargy, bradycardia, dizziness, nausea, hypotension.
Class contraindications: Hypersensitivity to the medication or other quinazoline
  derivatives.

TERAZOSIN

NO ? C

Hytrin
Tabs and caps: 1, 2, 5, 10 mg
Antiadrenergic, peripherally acting agents

Indication: Hypertension
Initial dose: 1 mg PO qhs
Max dose: 20 mg daily

Adverse drug reaction: Asthenia, somnolence, palpitation, nasal congestion.
Comments:
α-Blockers not recommended as monotherapy hypertensive agents.
Dosage increment: Usual dosage range is 1 to 5 mg daily. May increase dose
  slowly, q2 wk to achieve blood pressure response.
Divided dosage may be more effective in controlling blood pressure than same
  dose given once daily.
Class side effects: First-dose syncope, headache, dizziness, nausea,
  hypotension.
Class contraindications: Hypersensitivity to the medication or other quinazoline
  derivatives.

For explanation of icons, see p. 1068.

Centrally Acting Agents

CLONIDINE

Catapres, Catapres TTS
Tabs, scored: 0.1, 0.2, 0.3 mg
Patch, transdermal: 0.1, 0.2, 0.3 mg/24 hr
Antiadrenergic, centrally acting agents

NO   ?   C

Indication: Hypertension
Initial dose: 0.1 mg PO bid/tid
  0.1 mg/24 hr q7 days (transdermal)
Max dose: 2.4 mg daily
  0.6 mg daily (patch)

Adverse drug reaction: Severe rebound hypertension, sedation, dry mouth, constipation, pruritus, dermatitis (patch).

Comments:

May need oral therapy during initiation of transdermal therapy.

Patches applied every 7 days to hairless intact skin. Blood pressure effects seen after 2-3 days. May increment dose every 1-2 wk.

Severe rebound hypertension with sudden discontinuation.

Dosage increment 0.1-0.2 mg PO at weekly intervals. Reduce dose gradually over 2-4 days.

Remove transdermal systems when attempting defibrillation.

Drug/drug interactions: Tricyclic antidepressants and monoamine oxidase inhibitors (avoid use together).

Drug/herb: Capsicum (may reduce antihypertensive effect).

Drug/laboratory: May decrease urinary excretion of vanillylmandelic acid and catecholamines; may cause a weakly positive Coombs' test.

Contraindicated in combination with or within 5 wk of discontinuation of monoamine oxidase inhibitor.

Class side effects: Dizziness, drowsiness, dry mouth, hypotension.

Class contraindications: Hypersensitivity to the medication.

METHYLDOPA
Aldomet
Tabs: 125, 250, 500 mg
Antiadrenergic, centrally acting agents

  YES 1 B/C

Indication: Hypertension
Initial dose: 250 mg PO bid/tid
Max dose: 3 g daily
Renal dose: CrCl 10-50 mL/min: divided bid/tid
CrCl <10 mL/min: daily or divided bid

Adverse drug reaction: Orthostatic hypotension, drug fever, nasal congestion, pancreatitis rare: hemolytic anemia, liver disorders.
Comments:
Monitor liver function tests, Coombs' test, erythrocyte count, hematocrit, weight at baseline and periodically.
Drug-drug: Lithium (increased lithium levels).
Drug-laboratory: May interfere with measurement of urinary uric acid, serum creatinine, urinary catecholamines.
Pregnancy category is B with oral administration, C with intravenous administration.
Contraindications: Active hepatic disease, hypersensitivity to this product, concomitant monoamine oxidase inhibitor therapy.
Class side effects: Dizziness, drowsiness, sedation, dry mouth.
Class contraindications: Hypersensitivity to the medication.

β-Blockers
β₁-Selective Agents

ACEBUTOLOL
Sectral
Caps: 200, 400 mg
β-blockers, selective agents

  YES 1 B

Indication: Hypertension, ventricular arrhythmias
Initial dose: 400 mg PO daily or divided bid
Max dose: 1.2 g daily
Renal dose: CrCl 10-50 mL/min: 50% dose
CrCl <10 mL/min: 30%-50% dose

Comments:
Dosage increment q1-2 mo, discontinue gradually over 2 wk; do not abruptly stop.
Contraindicated in second- or third-degree heart block.

Continued

FORMULARY

Cardiovascular—β-Blockers

For explanation of icons, see p. 1068.

ACEBUTOLOL *continued*

Class side effects: Fatigue, dizziness, bradycardia, hypotension, dyspnea; rare:
depression, bronchospasm, heart failure.

Class contraindications: Hypersensitivity to the medication, severe bradycardia,
second- or third-degree heart block with no pacer, overt cardiac failure,
cardiogenic shock.

ATENOLOL

Tenormin
Tabs, scored*: 25, 50*,100 mg
Inj: 5 mg/10 mL
β-*Blockers, selective agents*

YES   X   D

Indication: Hypertension, acute myocardial infarction, angina
Initial dose:
   Hypertension: 25-50 mg PO daily or divided bid
   Acute myocardial infarction: 2.5-5 mg IV over 2-5 min; repeat in 2-10 min
Max dose: 100 mg PO daily (clinical)
Renal dose: CrCl 10-50 mL/min: 50% dose q24h
            CrCl <10 mL/min: 30%-50% dose q96h

Adverse drug reaction: Agranulocytosis, thrombocytopenia purpura
Comments:
Dosage increment: Increase q1-2 wk intervals.
Doses up to 200 mg daily have been used for angina control.
IV atenolol may be given undiluted or diluted no more than 1 mg/min.
Do not abruptly discontinue.
Class side effects: Fatigue, dizziness, bradycardia, hypotension, dyspnea; rare:
depression, bronchospasm, heart failure.
Class contraindications: Hypersensitivity to the medication, severe bradycardia,
second- or third-degree heartblock with no pacer, overt cardiac failure,
cardiogenic shock.

BETAXOLOL

Kerlone
Tabs: 10, 20 mg
β-*Blockers, selective agents*

YES   ?   C/D

Indication: Hypertension, angina
Initial dose: 5-10 mg PO daily
Max dose: 20 mg daily
Renal dose: CrCl <10 mL/min: 50% dose

Continued

BETAXOLOL *continued*

Comments:
Dosage increment: Maximal blood pressure lowering seen after 7-14 days.
Do not abruptly discontinue.
Pregnancy category: D in second and third trimesters.
Class side effects: Fatigue, dizziness, bradycardia, hypotension, dyspnea; rare: depression, bronchospasm, heart failure.
Class contraindications: Hypersensitivity to the medication, severe bradycardia, second- or third-degree heart block with no pacer, overt cardiac failure, cardiogenic shock.

BISOPROLOL

Zebeta
Tabs, scored*: 5*, 10 mg
β-*Blockers, selective agents*

YES ? C/D

Indication: Hypertension
Initial dose: 2.5-5 mg PO daily
Max dose: 20 mg daily
Renal dose: CrCl 10-50 mL/min: 75% dose

Comments:
Do not stop medication abruptly.
Contraindicated in second- or third-degree heart block.
Pregnancy category: D in second and third trimesters.
Drug/drug: Other β-blockers, reserpine.
Class side effects: Fatigue, dizziness, bradycardia, hypotension, dyspnea; rare: depression, bronchospasm, heart failure.
Class contraindications: Hypersensitivity to the medication, severe bradycardia, second- or third-degree heart block with no pacer, overt cardiac failure, cardiogenic shock.

ESMOLOL

Brevibloc
Inj: 10 mg/mL (10 mL)
Inj, concentrate: 250 mg/mL (10 mL)
β-*Blockers, selective agents*

YES ? C/D

Indication: Supraventricular tachycardia
Initial dose: Load: 250-500 µg/kg × 1 min
Maintenance: 50-100 µg/kg/min × 4 min
Max dose: 200 µg/kg/min (clinical)

Continued

FORMULARY

Cardiovascular—β-Blockers

For explanation of icons, see p. 1068.

ESMOLOL *continued*

Adverse drug reaction: Hypotension.
Comments:
Monitor blood pressure, electrocardiogram, mean arterial pressure (goal is decrease <25% in 2 hr).
IV concentrations greater than 10 mg/mL may cause irritation.
IV not compatible with 5% sodium bicarbonate injection USP.
The 10 ml vial is ready to use.
The 2500 mg vial is not for direct IV injection. It must be diluted.
Pregnancy category: D in second and third trimesters.
Class side effects: Fatigue, dizziness, somnolence, bradycardia, hypotension, dyspnea; rare: depression, bronchospasm, heart failure.
Class contraindications: Hypersensitivity to the medication, severe bradycardia, second- or third-degree heart block with no pacer, overt cardiac failure, cardiogenic shock.

METOPROLOL

YES   ?   C/D

Lopressor, Toprol-XL
Tabs, scored: 50, 100 mg
Tabs, extended-release: 50, 100, 200 mg (Toprol-XL)
Inj: 1 mg/mL
β-*Blockers, selective agents*

Indication: Hypertension, angina, acute myocardial infarction
Initial dose:
  Hypertension: 25-50 mg PO bid
  Angina: 100 mg PO bid (extended-release)
  Acute myocardial infarction: 5 mg rapid IV injection q5 min if tolerated
                                                  50 mg PO q6h for 2 days, then 100 mg
                                                  PO bid
Max dose: 450 mg daily
                    400 mg daily (extended-release)
                    15 mg over 15 min

Comments:
Dosage increment weekly.
Do not stop medication abruptly.
Contraindicated in sick sinus syndrome with no pacer.
Pregnancy category: D in second and third trimesters.
Class side effects: Fatigue, dizziness, bradycardia, hypotension, dyspnea; rare: depression, bronchospasm, heart failure.
Class contraindications: Hypersensitivity to the medication, severe bradycardia, second- or third-degree heartblock with no pacer, overt cardiac failure, cardiogenic shock.

Nonselective Agents

CARVEDIOL
Coreg, Coreg tiltabs
Tabs, scored*: 3.125, 6.125*, 12.5*, 25* mg
β-*Blockers, nonselective agents*

 YES ? C/D

Indication: Heart failure, hypertension
Initial dose:
   Heart failure: 3.125 mg PO bid × 2 wk
   Hypertension: 6.25 mg PO bid
Max dose: 25 mg bid (<85 kg)
          50 mg bid (>85 kg)

Adverse drug reaction: Diarrhea; rare: atrioventricular block,
   thrombocytopenia.
Comments:
Stabilize patient with other therapy before starting Coreg in congestive heart
   failure.
Observe patient for 1 hr after dose in congestive heart failure, administer with
   food to decrease orthostasis
Taking drug with food minimizes orthostatic effects. Discontinue gradually over
   1-2 wk.
Decrease dose if heart rate <55 beats/min.
Drug/drug: Rifampin decreases Coreg levels by 70%.
Drug/food: Food delays rate of absorption, not extent of bioavailability.
Contraindicated in second- or third-degree heart block, New York Heart
   Association class IV decompensated heart failure requiring IV inotropic
   treatment, sick sinus syndrome with no pacer.
Pregnancy category: D in second and third trimesters.
Class side effects: Fatigue, dizziness, bradycardia, hypotension, heart failure;
   rare: depression, bronchospasm.
Class contraindications: Hypersensitivity to the medication, severe bradycardia,
   second- or third-degree heart block with no pacer, bronchial asthma, overt
   cardiac failure, cardiogenic shock.

LABETALOL

Normodyne, Trandate
Tabs, scored: 100, 200, 300 mg
Tabs: 300 mg (Normodyne)
Inj: 5 mg/mL (20, 40, 60 mL)
β-*Blockers, nonselective agents*

NO   1   C/D

Indication: Hypertension
Initial dose:
    Hypertension: 100 mg PO bid
    Hypertension emergency: 20-80 mg IV push over 2 min may repeat q10
                        min or 0.5-2 mg/min IV
Max dose: 2.4 g daily
        300 mg IV cumulative

Adverse drug reaction: Orthostatic hypotension; rare: ventricular arrhythmias
    without bradycardia.
Comments:
Dosage increment 100 mg q2-3 days.
Maximum hypotensive effect occurs in 5-15 min after each injection.
Do not mix IV with 5% sodium bicarbonate injection.
Contraindicated in prolonged hypotension.
Drug/laboratory: May falsely elevate levels of urinary catecholamines,
    vanillylmandelic acid, metanephrine. May produce a false positive test for
    amphetamine when urine is screened.
Pregnancy category: D in second and third trimesters.
Class side effects: Fatigue, dizziness, bradycardia, hypotension, heart failure;
    rare: depression, bronchospasm.
Class contraindications: Hypersensitivity to the medication, severe bradycardia,
    second- or third-degree heart block with no pacer, bronchial asthma, overt
    cardiac failure, cardiogenic shock.

NADOLOL

Corgard
Tabs, scored: 20, 40, 80, 120, 160 mg
β-*Blockers, nonselective agents*

YES   1   C/D

Indication: Hypertension, angina pectoris
Initial dose: 20-40 mg PO daily
Max dose: 320 mg daily
        Angina: 240 mg daily
Renal dose: CrCl <30 mL/min: q24-48h
             CrCl <10 mL/min: q40-60h

Continued

NADOLOL *continued*

Comments:
Dosage increment 40-80 mg q2-14 days.
Usual maintenance dosage is 40-80 mg daily.
Do not abruptly discontinue; gradually taper.
Pregnancy category: D in second and third trimesters.
Class side effects: Fatigue, dizziness, bradycardia, hypotension, heart failure;
rare: depression, bronchospasm.
Class contraindications: Hypersensitivity to the medication, severe bradycardia,
second- or third-degree heart block with no pacer, bronchial asthma, overt
cardiac failure, cardiogenic shock.

PINDOLOL

Visken
Tabs: 5, 10 mg
β-*Blockers, nonselective agents*

NO   1   B

Indication: Hypertension
Initial dose: 5 mg PO bid
Max dose: 60 mg daily

Adverse drug reaction: Insomnia, nervousness, muscle pain.
Comments:
Dosage increment 10 mg q3-4 wk.
Do not abruptly discontinue; gradually taper.
Class side effects: Fatigue, dizziness, bradycardia, hypotension, heart failure;
rare: depression, bronchospasm.
Class contraindications: Hypersensitivity to the medication, severe bradycardia,
second- or third-degree heart block with no pacer, bronchial asthma, overt
cardiac failure, cardiogenic shock.

For explanation of icons, see p. 1068.

PROPRANOLOL

Inderal, Inderal LA
Tabs, scored: 10, 20, 40, 60, 80 mg
Oral liquid: 20, 40 mg/5 mL
Oral liquid, concentrated: 80 mg/mL
Caps, extended-release: 60, 80, 120, 160 mg
Inj: 1 mg/mL
β-*Blockers, nonselective agents*

NO   1   C/D

Indication: Hypertension, angina pectoris
Initial dose:
   Hypertension: 20-40 mg PO bid
   Angina: 60-80 mg PO daily (extended-release)
Max dose: 640 mg daily

Adverse drug reaction: Rare: agranulocytosis.
Comments:
May increase at 3- to 7-day intervals.
Usual maintenance dose is 160-480 mg daily or 120-160 mg daily (extended release).
Do not abruptly discontinue; gradually taper.
Pregnancy category: D in second and third trimesters.
Drug/drug: Aluminum hydroxide antacids (decreased absorption), verapamil (depress contractility or atrioventricular conduction), cocaine (increased angina induction).
Drug/herb: Betel palm.
Class side effects: Fatigue, dizziness, bradycardia, hypotension, heart failure; rare: depression, bronchospasm.
Class contraindications: Hypersensitivity to the medication, severe bradycardia, second- or third-degree heart block with no pacer, bronchial asthma, overt cardiac failure, cardiogenic shock.

TIMOLOL

Blocadren
Tabs, scored*: 5, 10*, 20* mg
β-*Blockers, nonselective agents*

NO   1   C/D

Indication: Hypertension, post–myocardial infarction
Initial dose:
   Hypertension: 10 mg PO bid
   Post–myocardial infarction: Initiate within 1-4 wk of myocardial infarction
Max dose: 60 mg daily

Continued

Comments:
Contraindicated in chronic obstructive pulmonary disease, second- or third-degree atrioventricular block.
Pregnancy category: D in second and third trimesters.
Comments:
Do not abruptly discontinue; gradually taper.
Class side effects: Fatigue, dizziness, bradycardia, hypotension, heart failure; rare: depression, bronchospasm.
Class contraindications: Hypersensitivity to the medication, severe bradycardia, second- or third-degree heart block with no pacer, bronchial asthma, overt cardiac failure, cardiogenic shock.

Calcium Channel Blockers
Dihydropyridine Agents

AMLODIPINE
Norvasc
Tabs: 2.5, 5, 10 mg   NO   ?   C
Calcium channel blockers, dihydropyridine agents

Indication: Hypertension, angina pectoris
Initial dose:
  Hypertension: 2.5-5 mg PO daily
  Angina: 5-10 mg PO daily
Max dose: 10 mg daily

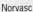
Comments:
Longest time to onset in class.
Maximum blood pressure lowering seen in 6-8 wk.
Class side effects: Pedal edema, headache, dizziness, flushing, lightheadedness, asthenia
Class contraindications: Hypersensitivity to the medication.

FELODIPINE
Plendil
Tabs, extended-release: 2.5, 5, 10 mg   NO   ?   C
Calcium channel blockers, dihydropyridine agents

Indication: Hypertension
Initial dose: 5 mg PO daily
Max dose: 20 mg daily

Continued

FELODIPINE *continued*

Comments:
Dosage increment at a minimum q2 wk; doses >10 mg increase potential for peripheral edema.
Class side effects: Pedal edema, headache, dizziness, flushing, lightheadedness, asthenia.
Class contraindications: Hypersensitivity to the medication.

ISRADIPINE

DynaCirc
Caps: 2.5, 5 mg
Calcium channel blockers, dihydropyridine agents

NO ? C

Indication: Hypertension
Initial dose: 2.5 mg PO bid
Max dose: 20 mg daily

Comments:
Dosage increment 5 mg q2-4 wk.
Class side effects: Pedal edema, headache, dizziness, flushing, lightheadedness, asthenia.
Class contraindications: Hypersensitivity to the medication.

NICARDIPINE

Cardene, Cardene SR
Caps: 20, 30 mg
Caps, extended-release: 30, 45, 60 mg
Inj: 2.5 mg/mL
Calcium channel blockers, dihydropyridine agents

NO ? C

Indication: Hypertension, angina, hypertension emergency
Initial dose:
    Hypertension: 30 mg PO bid (extended release)
    Angina: 20 mg PO tid
    Hypertension emergency: 5 mg/hr IV
Maintenance: 3 mg/hr IV

Oral dose	Equivalent IV infusion rate
20 mg PO tid	0.5 mg/hr IV
30 mg PO tid	1.2 mg/hr IV
40 mg PO tid	2.2 mg/hr IV

    Max dose: 120 mg daily
              15 mg/hr IV

Continued

NICARDIPINE *continued*

Comments:
Titrate 2.5 mg/hr IV q15 min for gradual reduction, q5 min for rapid reduction.
When used IV, change IV site every 12 hr to minimize venous irritation.
Contraindicated in advanced aortic stenosis.
Drug/drug: Cyclosporine (increased levels), digoxin (increased levels).
Drug/food: Grapefruit juice.
Class side effects: Peripheral edema, hypotension, headache, dizziness, flushing, lightheadedness, asthenia.
Class contraindications: Hypersensitivity to the medication.

NIFEDIPINE

NO   1   C

Adalat CC, Procardia XL
Tabs, extended-release: 30, 60, 90 mg
Calcium channel blockers, dihydropyridine agents

Indication: Hypertension, angina pectoris, vasospastic angina
Initial dose: 30-60 mg PO daily (extended release)
Max dose: 120 mg daily (extended release)

Adverse drug reaction: Weakness; rare: heart failure, pulmonary edema.
Comments:
Immediate-release SL administration associated with increased morbidity.
Dosage increment q7-14 days.
Procardia XL and Adalat CC are not therapeutically equivalent.
Drug/drug: Digoxin (may increase levels).
Drug/food: Grapefruit juice.
Class side effects: Peripheral edema, headache, hypotension, dizziness, flushing, lightheadedness, asthenia.
Class contraindications: Hypersensitivity to the medication.

NISOLDIPINE

NO   ?   C

Sular
Tabs, extended-release: 10, 20, 30, 40 mg
Calcium channel blockers, nondihydropyridine agents

Indication: Hypertension
Initial dose: 20 mg PO daily
Max dose: 60 mg daily

Continued

NISOLDIPINE *continued*

Comments:
Dosage increment 10 mg q1-2 wk.
Class side effects: Peripheral edema, headache, dizziness, flushing, lightheadedness, asthenia.
Comments:
Tablets should not be chewed, divided, or crushed.
Do not administer with a high-fat meal.
Drug/drug: Phenytoin (nisoldipine levels undetectable).
Drug/food: Grapefruit juice.
Class contraindications: Hypersensitivity to the medication.

Nondihydropyridine Agents

DILTIAZEM

Cardizem CD, Cardizem SR, Dilacor XR, Tiazac, Diltia XT
Tabs, scored*: 30, 60*, 90*, 120* mg   NO   1   C
Caps, sustained-release (bid): 60, 90, 120 mg (Cardizem SR)
Caps, extended-release (daily): 120, 180, 240, 300, 360 mg (Cardizem CD)
Caps, extended-release (daily): 120, 180, 240, 300, 360, 420 mg (Tiazac)
Caps, extended-release (daily): 120, 180, 240 mg (Dilacor XR, Diltia XT)
Caps, extended-release (daily): 120, 180, 240, 300 mg (Cartia XT)
Calcium channel blockers, nondihydropyridine agents

Indication: Hypertension, chronic stable angina, atrial fibrillation or atrial flutter (IV), paroxysmal supraventricular tachycardia (IV)
Initial dose:
    Angina: 30 mg PO qid
            120-180 mg PO daily (Cardizem CD, Diltia XT, Dilacor XR)
    Hypertension: 60-120 mg PO bid (Cardizem SR)
            180-240 mg PO daily (Tiazac)
Max dose: 360 mg daily (clinical)

Adverse drug reaction: Abnormal electrocardiogram, asthenia, edema.
Comments:
Initial dose IV: 0.25 mg/kg actual body weight as a bolus administered over 2 min.
Recommended infusion rate is 10 mg/hr; may be increased up to 15 mg/hr as needed.
Duration of infusion over 24 hr not recommended.
Drug/drug: Increases cyclosporin levels.
Contraindicated in acute myocardial infarction with pulmonary congestion.
Class side effects: Atrioventricular block, bradycardia, dizziness, headache, constipation, nausea.
Class contraindications: Hypersensitivity to the medication, sick sinus syndrome with no pacer, second- or third-degree heart block with no pacer, hypotension with systolic blood pressure <90 mm Hg.

VERAPAMIL

NO ? C

Calan SR, Covera-HS, Isoptin, Verelan PM
Tabs, scored: 40, 80, 120 mg
Tabs, extended-release: 120 mg (Calan SR, Isoptin SR)
Tabs, scored, extended-released: 180, 240 mg (Calan SR, Isoptin SR)
Caps, sustained-release: 120, 180, 240, 360 mg (Verelan PM)
Caps, extended-release: 180, 240 mg (Covera HS)
Tabs, extended-release: 100, 200, 300 mg (Verelan PM)
Inj: 2.5 mg/mL
Calcium channel blockers, nondihydropyridine agents

Indication: Hypertension, angina
Initial dose:
  Hypertension: 120-240 mg PO daily
                   >240 mg PO split dose bid (Isoptin, Calan SR)
                   180 mg PO qhs (Covera-HS)
  Angina: 40-80 mg PO tid/qid (immediate-release)
            200 mg PO qhs (Verelan PM)
Max dose: 480 mg daily
          400 mg daily (Verelan)

Adverse drug reaction: Rare: paralytic ileus.
Comments:
Avoid concomitant IV β-blocker use.
Discontinue disopyramide 48 hr before starting verapamil.
Drug/drug: Increases digoxin levels, flecainide, β-blockers, rifampin (decreased blood pressure effect)
Drug/herb: Black catechu, yerba mate.
Drug/food: Food increases absorption.
Contraindicated in cardiogenic shock, atrial flutter or fibrillation with accessory bypass tract, severe left ventricular dysfunction.
Class side effects: Atrioventricular block, bradycardia, dizziness, headache, constipation, nausea.
Class contraindications: Hypersensitivity to the medication, sick sinus syndrome with no pacer, second- or third-degree heart block with no pacer, hypotension with systolic blood pressure <90 mm Hg.

Cardiovascular—Calcium Channel Blockers FORMULARY

For explanation of icons, see p. 1068.

Renal and Genitourinary
Diuretics, Loop Agents

BUMETANIDE

Bumex
Tabs: 0.5, 1, 2 mg
Inj: 0.25 mg/mL
Renal and genitourinary, diuretics, loop agents

NO 3 D

Indication: Edema
Initial dose: 0.5-2 mg PO daily
0.5-1 mg IV, repeat q2-3h as needed
Max dose: 10 mg daily

Adverse drug reaction: Rare: thrombocytopenia, encephalopathy.
Comments:
Ototoxicity associated with rapid injection, concomitant ototoxic drugs,
impaired renal function (usually reversible).
Monitor fluid status and electrolytes closely with IV use.
Contraindicated in patients with hypersensitivity to sulfonamides or with hepatic
coma.
Class side effects: Ototoxicity dose related and increased in end-stage renal
disease.
Class contraindications: Hypersensitivity to the medication, anuria.

ETHACRYNIC ACID

Edecrin
Tabs, scored: 25, 50 mg
Inj: 50 mg
Renal and genitourinary, Diuretics, Loop agents

YES 3 D

Indication: Edema, ascites
Initial dose: Edema: 25-50 mg PO daily or divided bid
Ascites: 0.5-1 mg/kg IV (average adult = 50 mg) × 1; may repeat
Max dose: 400 mg daily
100 mg/dose IV
Renal dose: CrCl <10 mL/min: Avoid

Adverse drug reaction: Severe watery diarrhea, pancreatitis, agranulocytosis,
thrombocytopenia, electrolyte abnormalities.
Comments:
When administering second IV dose, change sites to avoid thrombophlebitis.
Ototoxicity associated with rapid injection, concomitant ototoxic drugs,
impaired renal function; usually reversible.

Continued

ETHACRYNIC ACID *continued*

Monitor fluid status and electrolytes closely with IV use.

Drug/drug: Aminoglycosides, cisplatin (increased risk of ototoxicity), steroid and amphotericin B (increased potassium loss), lithium (increased levels).

Class side effects: Ototoxicity dose related and increased in end-stage renal disease; hypotension.

Class contraindications: Hypersensitivity to the medication, anuria, administration to infants.

FUROSEMIDE

NO ? C

Lasix
Tabs, scored*: 20, 40*, 80 mg
Oral liquid: 10 mg/mL (Lasix, 11.5% ethyl alcohol)
Oral liquid: 40 mg/5 mL (generic)
Inj: 10 mg/mL
Renal and genitourinary, diuretics, loop agents

Indication: Edema
Initial dose: 20-80 mg PO/IV
Max dose: 600 mg daily

Adverse drug reaction: Tinnitus; rare: blood dyscrasias.

Comments:

Furosemide 40 mg IV/80 mg PO = Bumetanide 1 mg IV/2 mg PO = Torsemide 20 mg IV/PO.

Ototoxicity is associated with rapid injection, concomitant ototoxic drugs, and impaired renal function; it is usually reversible.

Monitor fluid status and electrolytes closely with IV use.

Dosage increment: Titrate by doubling dose q6-8h until desired response, then increase frequency as necessary. High doses are effective in end-stage renal disease.

Drug/drug: Ethacrynic acid, aminoglycosides and cisplatin (increased risk of ototoxicity), corticosteroids, amphotericin B, metolazone (increased risk of hypokalemia).

Drug/herb: Aloe.

Drug/lifestyle: Sun exposure increases risk of photosensitivity reactions.

Class side effects: Ototoxicity dose related and increased in end-stage renal disease; hypotension, volume depletion, pancreatitis, frequent urination, hematologic, headache, dizziness.

Class contraindications: Hypersensitivity to the medication, anuria.

For explanation of icons, see p. 1068.

TORSEMIDE

Demadex

NO   ?   B

Tabs, scored: 5, 10, 20, 100 mg
Inj: 10 mg/mL
Renal and genitourinary, diuretics, loop agents

Indication: Edema
Initial dose: 10-20 mg PO/IV daily
                40 mg IV/80 mg PO = 1 mg IV/2 mg PO = 20 mg IV/PO
Max dose: >200 mg daily; not studied

Adverse drug reaction: Headache.
Comments:
Ototoxicity is associated with rapid injection, concomitant ototoxic drugs, and
    impaired renal function; it is usually reversible.
Monitor fluid status and electrolytes closely with IV use.
High doses are effective in end-stage renal disease.
Contraindicated with hypersensitivity to sulfonylureas.
Class side effects: Ototoxicity dose related and increased in end-stage renal
    disease.
Class contraindications: Hypersensitivity to the medication, anuria.

Diuretics, Potassium-Sparing Agents

AMILORIDE

Midamor

YES   ?   B

Tabs: 5 mg
Renal and genitourinary, diuretics, potassium-sparing agents

Indication: Diuretic-induced hypokalemia, edema
Initial dose: 5 mg PO daily
Max dose: 10 mg daily
Renal dose: CrCl 10-50 mL/min: 50% dose
             CrCl <10 mL/min: Avoid

Adverse drug reaction: Nausea, vomiting, anorexia, diarrhea, headache.
Comments:
Rarely used alone, since weak diuretic and antihypertensive effects.
Contraindicated in patients taking potassium-sparing and potassium-
    supplementing agents and those with chronic renal insufficiency or diabetic
    nephropathy.
Class side effects: Hyperkalemia.
Class contraindications: Hypersensitivity to the medication, anuria,
    hyperkalemia (K^+ >5.5 mEq/L), acute renal insufficiency.

SPIRONOLACTONE
Aldactone
Tabs, scored*: 25, 50*, 100* mg
Renal and genitourinary, diuretics, potassium-sparing agents

YES 1 D

 Indication: Edema, hypertension
Initial dose: 25-100 mg PO daily or divided bid
Renal dose: CrCl 10-50 mL/min: q12-24h
CrCl <10 mL/min: Avoid

Adverse drug reaction: Gynecomastia, hyperchloremic acidosis
Comments:
Dosage increments 25 mg at 5 days for edema and 2-4 wk for hypertension.
Class side effects: Hyperkalemia.
Class contraindications: Hypersensitivity to the medication, anuria,
hyperkalemia (K+ >5.5 mEq/L), acute renal insufficiency.

Diuretics, Thiazide Agents

CHLOROTHIAZIDE
Diuril
Tabs, scored: 250, 500 mg
Oral liquid: 250 mg/5 mL
Inj: 500 mg (Diuril)
Renal and genitourinary, diuretics, thiazide agents

YES 1 D

Indication: Hypertension, edema
Initial dose:
  Hypertension: 125-500 mg PO bid
  Edema: 500-1000 mg PO/IV daily or divided bid
Max dose:
  Hypertension: 500 mg daily
  Edema: 2 g daily
Renal dose: CrCl <30 mL/min: Ineffective
CrCl <10 mL/min: Avoid

Comments:
Ototoxicity is associated with rapid injection, concomitant ototoxic drugs, and
  impaired renal function; it is usually reversible.
Monitor fluid status and electrolytes closely with IV use.
Contraindicated with sulfonamide-derived drugs.
Class side effects: Increase in uric acid, calcium, cholesterol, and glucose
  levels (transiently); decrease in potassium and magnesium levels.
Class contraindications: Hypersensitivity to the medication, anuria, renal
  decompensation.

Cardiovascular—Diuretics

For explanation of icons, see p. 1068.

CHLORTHALIDONE

Thalitone
Tabs: 15, 25, 50, 100 mg
Renal and genitourinary, diuretics, thiazide agents

YES   1   D

Indication: Hypertension, edema
Initial dose:
    Hypertension: 12.5-25 mg PO daily
                       15 mg PO daily (Thalitone)
    Edema: 50-100 mg PO daily
                  30-60 mg PO daily (Thalitone)
Max dose:
    Hypertension: 100 mg daily
                       50 mg daily (Thalitone)
    Edema: 200 mg daily
              120 mg daily (Thalitone)
Renal dose: CrCl <30 mL/min: Ineffective
                    CrCl <10 mL/min: Avoid

Comments:
Ototoxicity is associated with rapid injection, concomitant ototoxic drugs, and
    impaired renal function; it is usually reversible.
Monitor fluid status and electrolytes closely with IV use.
Thalitone has faster and better bioavailability.
Doses >50 mg daily are associated with higher side effects and decreased
    efficacy.
Dosage increments 12.5 mg at 2-4 wk.
Contraindicated with sulfonamide-derived drugs.
Class side effects: Increase in uric acid, calcium, cholesterol, and glucose
    levels (transiently and may not be clinically significant); decrease in
    potassium and magnesium levels.
Class contraindications: Hypersensitivity to the medication, anuria, renal
    decompensation.

HYDROCHLOROTHIAZIDE

Esidrix, HydroDIURIL, Microzide
Tabs, scored: 25, 50 mg (Esidrix, HydroDIURIL)
Caps: 12.5 mg (Microzide)
Oral liquid: 50 mg/5 mL
Renal and genitourinary, diuretics, thiazide agents

YES   1   D

Indication: Hypertension, edema
Initial dose:
    Hypertension: 12.5-25 mg PO daily
    Edema: 25-50 mg PO daily or divided bid

Continued

HYDROCHLOROTHIAZIDE *continued*

Max dose: 25-50 mg daily (clinical)
Renal dose: CrCl <30 mL/min: Ineffective
  CrCl <10 mL/min: Avoid

Comments:
Metabolic effects more commonly seen with doses above 25 mg daily.
Ototoxicity is associated with rapid injection, concomitant ototoxic drugs, and impaired renal function; it is usually reversible.
Monitor fluid status and electrolytes closely with IV use.
Class side effects: Increase in uric acid, calcium, cholesterol, and glucose levels (transiently and may not be clinically significant); decrease in potassium and magnesium levels.
Class contraindications: Hypersensitivity to the medication, anuria, renal decompensation.

INDAPAMIDE

YES 1 D

Lozol
Tabs: 1.25, 2.5 mg
Renal and genitourinary, diuretics, thiazide agents

Indication: Hypertension, edema
Initial dose:
  Hypertension: 1.25-5 mg PO daily
  Edema: 2.5-5 mg PO daily
Max dose: 5 mg daily (clinical)
Renal dose: CrCl <30 mL/min: Ineffective
  CrCl <10 mL/min: Avoid

Comments:
Ototoxicity is associated with rapid injection, concomitant ototoxic drugs, and impaired renal function; it is usually reversible.
Monitor fluid status and electrolytes closely with IV use.
Dosage increments to 5 mg at 1 wk (edema), to 2.5 mg daily at 1-2 months (hypertension).
Class side effects: Increase in uric acid, calcium, cholesterol, and glucose levels (transiently); decrease in potassium and magnesium levels, hypotension, headache, nervousness, volume depletion and dehydration, palpitations.
Drug/drug: Lithium (increased levels).
Class contraindications: Hypersensitivity to the medication and other sulfonamide-derived drugs, anuria, renal decompensation.

METOLOZONE

Mykrox, Zaroxolyn
Tabs: 0.5 mg (Mykrox)
2.5, 5, 10 mg (Zaroxyln)
Renal and genitourinary, diuretics, thiazide agents

YES   1   D

Indication: Hypertension, edema
Initial dose:
  Hypertension: 0.5 mg PO daily (Mykrox)
                  1.25-2.5 mg PO daily (Zaroxolyn)
  Edema: 5-10 mg PO daily (Zaroxolyn)
Max dose:
  Hypertension: 1 mg daily (Mykrox)
                  10 mg daily (Zaroxolyn)
  Edema: 20 mg daily (Zaroxolyn)
Renal dose: CrCl <10 mL/min: Use with caution

Adverse drug reaction: Hypotension, rapid hyponatremia, dizziness, pancreatitis, hepatitis, drowsiness, nausea.
Comments:
Used as an adjunct in furosemide-resistant edema.
Ototoxicity is associated with rapid injection, concomitant ototoxic drugs, and impaired renal function; it is usually reversible.
Monitor fluid status and electrolytes closely with IV use.
Mykrox and Zaroxolyn are not therapeutically equivalent.
High doses are effective in end-stage renal disease.
Contraindicated in hepatic coma.
Class side effects: Increase in uric acid, calcium, cholesterol, and glucose levels (transiently); decrease in potassium and magnesium levels.
Drug/drug: Lithium (increased levels), cholestyramine, colestipol (separate by 1 hr).
Drug/laboratory: Interferes with tests for parathyroid function; discontinue before testing.
Class contraindications: Hypersensitivity to the medication, anuria, renal decompensation.

Vasodilators
Nitrate Agents

ISOSORBIDE DINITRATE

Isordil, Sorbitrate, Dilatrate-SR
Tabs, scored: 5, 10, 20, 30 ,40 mg (Isordil, Sorbitrate)   NO   ?   C
Tab, extended-release: 40 mg
Tabs, sublingual: 2.5, 5, 10 mg
Caps, extended-release: 40 mg (Dilatrate-SR)
Renal and genitourinary, vasodilators, nitrate agents

Indication: Acute angina, angina
Initial dose:
    Acute angina: 2.5-5 mg PO q5-10 min (SL tabs)
                  5-40 mg PO bid/tid (7 AM, noon, 5 PM)
    Angina: 40-80 mg PO bid (sustained-release) (8 AM, 2 PM)
Max dose: 3 SL doses/30 min
            160 mg daily (Dilatrate)

Comments:
Allow a nitrate-free interval of 12-14 hr to avoid development of tolerance.
Do not stop abruptly.
Class side effects: Headache, flushing, orthostatic hypotension, rash,
    dizziness, ankle edema, cutaneous vasodilation; rare: hypersensitivity
    reactions.
Class contraindications: Hypersensitivity to the medication, other nitrates or
    nitrites.

ISOSORBIDE MONONITRATE

ISMO, Monoket, Imdur
Tabs, scored: 20 mg (ISMO)   NO   ?   C
Tabs, scored: 10, 20 mg (Monoket)
Tabs, scored, extended-release: 30, 60, 120 mg (Imdur)
Renal and genitourinary, vasodilators, nitrate agents

Indication: Angina
Initial dose: 20 mg PO bid (8 AM, 3 PM)
               30-60 mg PO daily (extended-release)
Max dose: 240 mg daily

Continued

For explanation of icons, see p. 1068.

ISOSORBIDE MONONITRATE *continued*

Comments:
Allow a nitrate-free interval of 12-14 hr to avoid development of tolerance.
Two doses must be taken 7 hr apart, with a gap of 17 hr between the second dose and the dose the following day.
Class side effects: Headache, hypotension, rash, dizziness; rare: hypersensitivity reactions.
Class contraindications: Hypersensitivity to the medication, other nitrates or nitrites, severe hypotension, acute myocardial infarction with low left ventricular filling pressure.

NITROGLYCERIN OINTMENT

Nitrol, Nitro-bid
Topical: 15 mg/inch   NO   ?   B
Renal and genitourinary, vasodilators, nitrate agents

Indication: Angina
Initial dose: 0.5 inch topical q8h
Max dose: 4 inches q4-6h

Comments:
Allow a nitrate-free interval of 12-14 hr to avoid development of tolerance.
Increase dose increments until headache occurs, then decrease to previous dose.
Drug/drug: Sildenafil, ergot alkaloids.
Class side effects: Headache, hypotension, rash, dizziness; rare: hypersensitivity reactions.
Class contraindications: Hypersensitivity to the medication, other nitrates or nitrites.

NITROGLYCERIN SPRAY

Nitrolingual
Inhalation, nasal: 0.4 mg/spray   NO   ?   B
Renal and genitourinary, vasodilators, nitrate agents

Indication: Acute angina
Initial dose: 1-2 sprays under tongue q3-5 min prn
Max dose: 3 sprays within a 15-min period

Continued

NITROGLYCERIN SPRAY *continued*

Comments:
Class side effects: Headache, hypotension, rash, dizziness; rare:
   hypersensitivity reactions.
Class contraindications: Hypersensitivity to the medication, other nitrates or
   nitrites.

NITROGLYCERIN SUBLINGUAL

Nitrostat, NitroQuick

NO   ?   B

Tabs, sublingual: 0.3, 0.4, 0.6 mg
Renal and genitourinary, vasodilators, nitrate agents

Indication: Acute angina
Initial dose: 0.4 mg SL, repeat dose q5 min prn
Max dose: 3 doses

Comments:
Dissolve under tongue or in the buccal pouch at onset of angina attack.
Ask patients about use of sildenafil before using nitrates.
Drug/drug: Sildenafil.
Class side effects: Headache, hypotension, rash, dizziness; rare:
   hypersensitivity reactions.
Class contraindications: Hypersensitivity to the medication, other nitrates or
   nitrites, early myocardial infarction, angle-closure glaucoma, severe anemia.

NITROGLYCERIN SUSTAINED-RELEASE

Nitroglyn

NO   ?   B

Caps, extended-release: 2.5, 6.5, 9 mg
Renal and genitourinary, vasodilators, nitrate agents

Indication: Angina
Initial dose: 2.5 mg PO bid/tid

Comments:
Allow a nitrate-free interval of 12-14 hr to avoid development of tolerance.
Drug/drug: Ergot alkaloids (may precipitate angina), sildenafil.
Class side effects: Headache, hypotension, rash, dizziness; rare:
   hypersensitivity reactions.
Class contraindications: Hypersensitivity to the medication, other nitrates or
   nitrites.

For explanation of icons, see p. 1068.

NITROGLYCERIN TRANSDERMAL

Deponit, Minitran, Nitro-Dur, Nitrodisc
Transdermal patch: 0.1, 0.2, 0.3, 0.4, 0.6, 0.8 mg/hr (Nitro-Dur)   NO   ?   B
0.1, 0.2, 0.4, 0.6 mg/hr (Minitran)
0.3, 0.4 mg/hr (Nitrodisc)
0.2, 0.4 mg/hr (Deponit)
Renal and genitourinary, vasodilators, nitrate agents

Indication: Angina
Initial dose: 1 transdermal patch worn 12-14 hr daily

Adverse drug reaction: Contact dermatitis.
Comments:
Allow a nitrate-free interval of 12-14 hr to avoid development of tolerance.
Drug/drug: Sildenafil.
Class side effects: Headache, hypotension, rash, dizziness; rare:
hypersensitivity reactions.
Class contraindications: Hypersensitivity to the medication, other nitrates or
nitrites.

NITROGLYCERIN IV

Tridil
Inj, solution: 100, 200, 400 µg/mL in D_5W NO   ?   B
Renal and genitourinary, vasodilators, nitrate agents

Indication: Acute angina, acute myocardial infarction, congestive heart failure
Initial dose: 10-20 µg/min IV
Max dose: Hypertension: 400 µg/min

Comments:
Dosage increment 5-10 µg/min IV q5-10 min until response.
Drug/drug: Sildenafil potentiates hypotension.
Class side effects: Headache, hypotension, rash, dizziness; rare:
hypersensitivity reactions.
Class contraindications: Hypersensitivity to the medication, other nitrates or
nitrites.

Peripheral Vasodilating Agents

EPOPROSTENOL

Flolan

Inj: 0.5, 1.5 mg/17 mL

M ? B

Renal and genitourinary, vasodilators, peripheral vasodilating agents

Indication: Primary pulmonary hypertension
Initial dose: 2 ng/kg/min IV

Adverse drug reaction: Bradycardia, anxiety.
Comments:
Initiation and titration should take place in a monitored setting.
Dosage increment 1-2 ng/kg/min IV q15 min.
Contraindicated for long-term use in severe heart failure; pulmonary edema has developed during initiation.
Class side effects: Flushing, headache, nausea, vomiting, dizziness, hypotension.
Class contraindications: Hypersensitivity to the medication.

HYDRALAZINE

Apresoline

Tabs: 10, 25, 50, 100 mg

NO 1 C

Inj: 20 mg/mL

Renal and genitourinary, vasodilators, peripheral vasodilating agents

Indication: Moderate to severe hypertension, heart failure
Initial dose: 10 mg PO qid × 4 days
5-10 mg IV q20-30 min, then titrate
10-50 mg IM
Max dose: 400 mg daily
200 mg daily in slow acetylators

Adverse drug reaction: Agranulocytosis, angina, palpitation, tachycardia, systemic lupus erythematosus–like syndrome at high doses.
Comments:
Dosage increment 25 mg PO qid rest of wk, 50 PO mg qid if needed.
Recommend complete blood count and antinuclear antibody titers at baseline and periodically during long-term therapy.
Advise patients to report symptoms of systemic lupus erythematosus (sore throat, fever, rash, muscle and joint pain).
Headache and palpitations usually occur within 2-4 hr of dose and then subside.
Contraindicated in coronary artery disease, rheumatic heart disease.
Drug/drug: Diazoxide, monoamine oxidase inhibitors (severe hypotension).
Class side effects: Flushing, headache, nausea, vomiting, dizziness, hypotension, sodium retention.
Class contraindications: Hypersensitivity to the medication.

MINOXIDIL
Loniten
Tabs, scored: 2.5, 10 mg
Renal and genitourinary, vasodilators, peripheral vasodilating agents

NO 1 C

Indication: Severe hypertension
Initial dose: 2.5-5 mg PO daily
Max dose: 100 mg daily

Adverse drug reaction: Hypertrichosis, sodium and water retention, tachycardia, breast tenderness; rare: Stevens-Johnson syndrome, pericardial effusion and tamponade.
Comments:
Consider concomitant diuretic and β-blocking agent.
Usual maintenance dosing range is 10-40 mg daily.
Rebound hypertension on discontinuation.
Contraindicated in patients with pheochromocytoma.
Class side effects: Flushing, headache, nausea, vomiting, dizziness, hypotension.
Class contraindications: Hypersensitivity to the medication.

NITROPRUSSIDE
Nitropress
Inj: 50 mg
Renal and genitourinary, vasodilators, peripheral vasodilating agents

NO ? C

Indication: Hypertension emergency
Initial dose: 0.25-0.3 µg/kg/min IV titrated q2 min
Max dose: 10 µg/kg/min

Adverse drug reaction: Profound hypotension, bradycardia, irritation at injection site, increased serum creatinine level, restlessness, ileus, muscle twitching, thiocyanate/cyanide accumulation (seizures, coma), methemoglobinemia, acidosis, increased intracranial pressure.
Comments:
Thiocyanate accumulation usually >2 µg/kg/min.
Contraindicated in patients with inadequate cerebral circulation, compensatory hypertension (atrioventricular shunt), congenital optic atrophy, tobacco-induced amblyopia.
Class side effects: Flushing, headache, nausea, vomiting, dizziness, hypotension.
Class contraindications: Hypersensitivity to the medication.

Miscellaneous
Vasopressor Agents

DOPAMINE

Intropin
Inj, solution: 0.8, 1.6, 3.2 mg/mL in D_5W
Inj, solution concentrated: 40, 60, 80, 160 mg/mL
Miscellaneous, vasopressor agents

NO ? C

Indication: Sympathomimetic
Initial dose: 2-5 µg/kg/min IV
  2.5-5 µg/kg/min IV (renal dose [dopaminergic])
  5-10 µg/kg/min IV (cardiac dose [dopaminergic/β_1])
  >10 µg/kg/min IV (dopaminergic/β_1/α_1)
Max dose: 50 µg/kg/min

Adverse drug reaction: Hypotension; rare: asthmatic episodes, anaphylactic reactions.
Comments:
Dosage increment 1-4 µg/kg/min at 10-min intervals; titrate off in a monitored setting to avoid severe hypotension.
Central vein preferred after extravasation; if extravasation occurs, stop drip and administer 5-10 mg phentolamine in 10 mL NS into site.
Contraindicated in uncorrected tachyarrhythmias, pheochromocytoma, ventricular fibrillation.
Class side effects: Tachycardia, chest pain, palpitations, increased blood pressure.
Class contraindications: Hypersensitivity to the medication, pheochromocytoma.

MIDODRINE

ProAmatine
Tabs, scored: 2.5, 5 mg
Miscellaneous, vasopressor agents

YES ? C

Indication: Orthostatic hypotension
Initial dose: 2.5 mg PO tid while awake
Max dose: 40 mg daily
Renal dose: CrCl 10-50 mg/min: 50% dose
  CrCl <10 mg/min: No data

Adverse drug reaction: Paresthesia, dysuria, pruritus, supine hypertension.
Comments:
Dosage increment 2.5 mg tid weekly.
Monitor standing and supine blood pressure.

Cardiovascular—Vasopressors

For explanation of icons, see p. 1068.

FORMULARY

Continued

MIDODRINE *continued*

Do not administer <4 hr before bedtime or if supine during the day for prolonged time.

Contraindicated in severe organic heart disease, urinary retention, thyrotoxicosis.

Class side effects: Tachycardia, chest pain, palpitations, increased blood pressure.

Class contraindications: Hypersensitivity to the medication, pheochromocytoma.

Inotropic Agents

DIGOXIN

Lanoxin, Lanoxicaps
Tabs: 0.125, 0.25, 0.5 mg
Oral liquid: 50 µg/mL (ethyl alcohol 10%)
Miscellaneous, inotropic agents

YES   1   C

Indication: Rate control, heart failure
Initial dose: Load: 1 mg PO/IV × 1 day divided tid
Maintenance: 0.125-0.25 mg PO daily
Renal dose: CrCl 10-50 mL/min: 50% dose q36 hr
    CrCl <10 mL/min: 10%-25% dose q48 hr

Adverse drug reaction: Vision changes, anorexia, nausea, fatigue, hallucinations, agitation, muscle weakness; rare: arrhythmias.

Comments:

Hypokalemia, hypercalcemia, and hypomagnesemia predispose patients to digoxin toxicity; may be life threatening.

Drug/drug: Amiodarone, diltiazem, and verapamil increase digoxin levels.

Antidote: Digibind: average 6 vials for adult; calculate dosage by whatever best means:

divide total body load by 0.5 (no. of vials required) or by 0.8 in acute ingestion; if unknown, 10-20 vials recommended.

Contraindicated in patients with ventricular fibrillation or tachycardia.

Class contraindications: Hypersensitivity to the medication.

MILRINONE

Primacor
Inj: 1 mg/mL (10, 20 mL)
Inj, solution: 200 µg/mL in 100 mL D₅W
Miscellaneous, inotropic agents

YES ? C

Indication: Heart failure
Initial dose: Load: 50 µg/kg IV over 10 min
Maintenance infusion: 0.375-0.75 µg/kg/min IV
Max dose: 1.13 mg/kg daily
Renal dose: CrCl <10 mL/min: 50%-75% dose

Adverse drug reaction: Ventricular arrhythmias, hypotension, headache.
Comments:
Monitor blood pressure and electrolytes.
Class contraindications: Hypersensitivity to the medication, acute phase of post–myocardial infarction.

DILTIAZEM

Cardizem
Inj: 5 mg/mL (25, 50 mL)
Miscellaneous, inotropic agents

NO ? C

Indication: Rate control, hypertension
Initial dose: Bolus: 0.25-0.35 mg/kg over 2 min
Maintenance infusion: 5-15 mg/hr

Adverse drug reaction: Abnormal electrocardiogram, asthenia, edema.
Comments:
Drug/drug: Increases cyclosporin levels.
Contraindicated in acute phase of myocardial infarction with pulmonary congestion, severe aortic or pulmonic valvular disease in place of surgical correction.
Class contraindications: Hypersensitivity to the medication.

NESIRITIDE
Natrecor
Inj, solution: 0.5 mg in 250 mL D_5W
Miscellaneous, inotropic agents

NO ? C

Indication: Acute decompensated heart failure
Initial dose: Load: 2 µg/kg
Maintenance infusion: 0.01 µg/kg/min
Max dose: 0.03 µg/kg/min

Adverse drug reaction: Hypotension, increased serum creatinine level, headache.
Comments:
Dosage increment 0.005 µg/kg/min q3h with 1 µg/kg bolus at each increase.
Drug/drug: avoid concomitant IV vasodilators
Contraindicated in patients with low cardiac filling pressures and as primary treatment for cardiogenic shock.
Class contraindications: Hypersensitivity to the medication.

Miscellaneous, Combinations

AMLODIPINE/BENAZEPRIL
Lotrel
Caps: 2.5/10, 5/10, 5/20 mg
Miscellaneous, combinations

Indication: Hypertension

CANDESARTAN/ HYDROCHLOROTHIAZIDE
Atacand HCT
Tabs: 16/12.5, 32/12.5 mg
Miscellaneous, combinations

Indication: Hypertension

ATENOLOL/CHLORTHALIDONE
Tenoretic
Tabs, scored*: 50/25*, 100/25 mg
Miscellaneous, combinations

 Indication: Hypertension

BENAZEPRIL/ HYDROCHLOROTHIAZIDE
Lotensin HCT
Tabs: 5/6.25, 10/12.5, 20/12.5, 20/25 mg
Miscellaneous, combinations

 Indication: Hypertension

BISOPROLOL/ HYDROCHLOROTHIAZIDE
Ziac
Tabs: 2.5/6.25, 5/6.25, 10/6.25 mg
Miscellaneous, combinations

 Indication: Hypertension

CLONIDINE/CHLORTHALIDONE
Combipres, Clorpres
Tabs, scored: 0.1/15, 0.2/15, 0.3/15 mg
Miscellaneous, combinations

 Indication: Hypertension

ENALAPRIL/FELODIPINE
Lexxel
Tabs, extended-release: 5/2.5, 5/5 mg
Miscellaneous, combinations

 Indication: Hypertension

ENALAPRIL/HYDROCHLOROTHIAZIDE
Vaseretic
Tabs: 5/12.5, 10/25 mg
Miscellaneous, combinations

 Indication: Hypertension

HYDRALAZINE/ HYDROCHLOROTHIAZIDE
Apresazide, Hydra-Zide
Caps: 25/25, 50/50, 100/50 mg
Miscellaneous, combinations

 Indication: Hypertension

HYDRALAZINE/ HYDROCHLOROTHIAZIDE/RESERPINE
Uni-Serp
Tabs: 25/15/0.1 mg
Miscellaneous, combinations

 Indication: Hypertension

IRBESARTAN/ HYDROCHLOROTHIAZIDE

Avalide
Tabs: 150/12.5, 300/12.5 mg
Miscellaneous, combinations

 Indication: Hypertension

LISINOPRIL/HYDROCHLOROTHIAZIDE

Prinizide, Zestoretic
Tabs: 10/12.5, 20/12.5, 20/25 mg
Miscellaneous, combinations

 Indication: Hypertension

LOSARTAN/HYDROCHLOROTHIAZIDE

Hyzaar
Tabs: 50/12.5, 100/25 mg
Miscellaneous, combinations

 Indication: Hypertension

METHYLDOPA/CHLOROTHIAZIDE

Aldoclor
Tabs: 250/250 mg
Miscellaneous, combinations

 Indication: Hypertension

For explanation of icons, see p. 1068.

METHYLDOPA/ HYDROCHLOROTHIAZIDE
Aldoril, Aldoril D
Tabs: 250/15, 250/25, 500/30, 500/50 mg
Miscellaneous, combinations

Indication: Hypertension

METOPROLOL/ HYDROCHLOROTHIAZIDE
Lopressor HCT
Tabs, scored: 50/25, 100/25, 100/50 mg
Miscellaneous, combinations

Indication: Hypertension

MOEXIPRIL/HYDROCHLOROTHIAZIDE
Uniretic
Tabs, scored: 7.5/12.5, 15/25 mg
Miscellaneous, combinations

Indication: Hypertension

NADOLOL/BENDROFLUMETHIAZIDE
Corzide
Tabs, scored: 40/5, 80/5 mg
Miscellaneous, combinations

Indication: Hypertension

PRAZOSIN/POLYTHIAZIDE

Minizide
Caps: 1/0.5, 2/0.5, 5/0.5 mg
Miscellaneous, combinations

 Indication: Hypertension

PROPRANOLOL/ HYDROCHLOROTHIAZIDE

Inderide, Inderide LA
Tabs, scored: 40/25, 80/25 mg
Caps, extended-release: 80/50, 120/50, 160/50 mg
Miscellaneous, combinations

 Indication: Hypertension

RESERPINE/HYDRALAZINE/ HYDROCHLOROTHIAZIDE

Uni-Serp
Tabs: 0.1/25/15 mg
Miscellaneous, combinations

 Indication: Hypertension

RESERPINE/HYDROFLUMETHIAZIDE

Salutensin Demi, Salutensin
Tabs: 0.125/25 mg (Demi)
　　　0.125/50 mg
Miscellaneous, combinations

 Indication: Hypertension

RESERPINE/METHYCLOTHIAZIDE

Diutensen-R
Tabs: 0.1/2.5 mg
Miscellaneous, combinations

Indication: Hypertension

TELMISARTAN/ HYDROCHLOROTHIAZIDE

Micardis HCT
Tabs: 40/12.5, 80/12.5 mg
Miscellaneous, combinations

Indication: Hypertension

TIMOLOL/HYDROCHLOROTHIAZIDE

Timolide
Tabs: 10/25 mg
Miscellaneous, combinations

Indication: Hypertension

TRANDOLAPRIL/VERAPAMIL

Tarka
Tabs, extended release: 1/240, 2/180, 2/240, 4/240 mg
Miscellaneous, combinations

Indication: Hypertension

VALSARTAN/HYDROCHLOROTHIAZIDE
Diovan HCT
Tabs: 80/12.5, 160/12.5 mg
Miscellaneous, combinations

 Indication: Hypertension

AMILORIDE/HYDROCHLOROTHIAZIDE
Moduretic
Tabs, scored: 5/50 mg
Miscellaneous, combinations

 Indication: Hypertension

SPIRONOLACTONE/ HYDROCHLOROTHIAZIDE
Aldactazide
Tabs, scored: 25/25, 50/50 mg
Miscellaneous, combinations

 Indication: Hypertension

TRIAMTERENE/ HYDROCHLOROTHIAZIDE
Dyazide, Maxzide
Tabs, scored: 37.5/25, 75/50 mg
Caps: 37.5/25, 50/25 mg
Miscellaneous, combinations

 Indication: Hypertension

Antilipemic Agents
HMG CoA Reductase Inhibitors

ATORVASTATIN

Lipitor
Tabs: 10, 20, 40, 80 mg
Antilipemic, HMG CoA reductase inhibitors

NO   3   X

Indication: Hypercholesterolemia
Initial dose: 10 mg PO daily
Max dose: 80 mg daily

Comments:
Comparison for ≈ 40% LDL reduction: atorvastatin 10 mg ≈ simvastatin
   20 mg ≈ lovastatin 80 mg ≈ pravastatin 40 mg ≈ fluvastatin 80 mg.
Monitor liver function tests at baseline and 4-6 wk or after a dosage change
   and periodically thereafter; discontinue drug if test results >3 times upper
   limit of normal. Creatine phosphokinase levels >10 times baseline may
   necessitate discontinuation.
Drug/drug: Increased risk of rhabdomyolysis with erythromycin, gemfibrozil,
   clofibrate, niacin, cyclosporine, azole antifungals.
Dosage increments: q3-4 wk (after checking fasting lipid profile).
Class side effects: Headache, constipation, diarrhea; rare: elevated liver
   enzyme levels, rhabdomyolysis, myopathy.
Class contraindications: Hypersensitivity to the medication, patients with unexplained persistent elevations in serum transaminases, active liver disease.

FLUVASTATIN

Lescol, Lescol XL
Caps: 20, 40 mg
Tabs, extended-release: 80 mg
Antilipemic, HMG CoA reductase inhibitors

NO   3   X

Indication: Hypercholesterolemia
Initial dose: 20-40 mg PO qhs
Max dose: 80 mg daily

Adverse drug reaction: Rare: thrombocytopenia, leukopenia, hemolytic anemia.
Comments:
Monitor liver function tests at baseline and 4-6 wk or after a dosage change
   and periodically thereafter; discontinue drug if test results >3 times upper
   limit of normal. Creatine phosphokinase levels >10 times baseline may
   necessitate discontinuation.

Continued

FLUVASTATIN *continued*

> Drug/drug: Increased risk of rhabdomyolysis with erythromycin, gemfibrozil.
> Dosage increments: q3-4 wk (after checking fasting lipid profile).
> Class side effects: Headache, constipation, diarrhea; rare: elevated liver enzyme levels, rhabdomyolysis, myopathy.
> Class contraindications: Hypersensitivity to the medication, patients with unexplained persistent elevations in serum transaminases, active liver disease.

LOVASTATIN

Mevacor
Tabs: 10, 20, 40 mg
Antilipemic, HMG CoA reductase inhibitors

NO 3 X

Indication: Hypercholesterolemia
Initial dose: 20-40 mg PO qhs
Max dose: 80 mg daily

Comments:
Monitor liver function tests at baseline and 4-6 wk; discontinue drug if test results >3 times upper limit of normal. Creatine phosphokinase levels >10 times baseline may necessitate discontinuation.
Drug/drug: Increased risk of rhabdomyolysis with erythromycin, gemfibrozil, clofibrate, niacin, cyclosporine, azole antifungals.
Dosage increments: q4-6 wk (after checking fasting lipid profile).
Class side effects: Headache, constipation, diarrhea; rare: elevated liver enzyme levels, rhabdomyolysis, myopathy.
Class contraindications: Hypersensitivity to the medication, patients with unexplained persistent elevations in serum transaminases, active liver disease.

PRAVASTATIN

Pravachol
Tabs: 10, 20, 40 mg
Antilipemic, HMG CoA reductase inhibitors

NO 3 X

Indication: Hypercholesterolemia
Initial dose: 10-20 mg PO qhs
Max dose: 40 mg daily

Comments:
Monitor liver function tests at baseline and 4-6 wk; discontinue drug if test results >3 times upper limit of normal. Creatine phosphokinase levels >10 times baseline may necessitate discontinuation.

Continued

For explanation of icons, see p. 1068.

Cardiovascular—Antilipemics

FORMULARY

PRAVASTATIN *continued*

Potentially less drug interaction than other HMG CoA reductase inhibitors because it is not metabolized by P450 3A4 or 2C9 pathway. Metabolism is through sulfation.

Drug/drug: Increased risk of rhabdomyolysis with erythromycin, gemfibrozil, clofibrate, niacin, cyclosporine, azole antifungals.

Dosage increments: q4-6 wk (after checking fasting lipid profile).

Class side effects: Headache, constipation, diarrhea; rare: elevated liver enzyme levels, rhabdomyolysis, myopathy.

Class contraindications: Hypersensitivity to the medication, patients with unexplained persistent elevations in serum transaminases, active liver disease.

SIMVASTATIN
Zocor
Tabs: 5, 10, 20, 40, 80 mg
Antilipemic, HMG CoA reductase inhibitors

NO   3   X

Indication: Hypercholesterolemia
Initial dose: 20 mg PO qhs
Max dose: 80 mg daily

Comments:

Monitor liver function tests at baseline and 4-6 wk; discontinue drug if test results >3 times upper limit of normal. Creatine phosphokinase levels >10 times baseline may necessitate discontinuation.

Drug/drug: Increased risk of rhabdomyolysis with erythromycin, gemfibrozil, clofibrate, niacin, cyclosporine, azole antifungals.

Dosage increments: q4-6 wk (after checking fasting lipid profile).

Class side effects: Headache, constipation, diarrhea; rare: elevated liver enzyme levels, rhabdomyolysis, myopathy.

Class contraindications: Hypersensitivity to the medication, patients with unexplained persistent elevations in serum transaminases, active liver disease.

Bile Acid Sequestrants

CHOLESTYRAMINE

Questran, Prevlite
Oral powder: 4 g resin/9 g powder
Antilipemic, bile acid sequestrants

NO   ?   C

Indication: Hypercholesterolemia
Initial dose: 4 g PO divided bid/qid before meals
Max dose: 36 g daily

Comments:
Dosage increment q1-2 months.
Should be taken within 1 hr of a meal.
Drugs whose absorption is reduced by cholestyramine should be given at least
   1-2 hr before or 6 hr after doses of the resins.
Drug/drug: Reduces absorption of numerous medications (corticosteroids,
   digoxin, thiazide diuretics, thyroid hormones, warfarin, acetaminophen).
Contraindicated in patients with complete biliary obstruction.
Class side effects: Constipation, flatulence, abdominal discomfort, nausea,
   vitamin A, D, E, K deficiencies; rare: fecal impaction.
Class contraindications: Hypersensitivity to the medication.

COLESTIPOL

Colestid
Tabs: 1 g
Oral granules: 5 g packet or 300, 500 g multidose
Antilipemic, bile acid sequestrants

NO   ?   C

Indication: Hypercholesterolemia
Initial dose: 2 g PO daily/bid
                  5 g PO daily/bid (granules)
Max dose: 16 g daily
              30 g daily (granules)

Comments:
Dosage increment 2 g q1-2 months.
Drugs whose absorption is reduced by cholestyramine should be given at least
   1-2 hr before or 6 hr after doses of the resins.
Drug/drug: Reduces absorption of numerous medications (corticosteroids,
   digoxin, thiazide diuretics, thyroid hormones, warfarin, acetaminophen).
Class side effects: Constipation, flatulence, abdominal discomfort, nausea,
   vitamin A, D, E, K deficiencies; rare: fecal impaction.
Class contraindications: Hypersensitivity to the medication.

For explanation of icons, see p. 1068.

COLESEVELAM
Welchol
Tabs: 625 mg
Antilipemic, bile acid sequestrants

NO ? B

Indication: Hypercholesterolemia
Initial dose: 3 tabs bid with meals or 6 tabs daily
Max dose: 7 tabs daily

Comments:
Contraindicated in bowel obstruction.
Class side effects: Constipation, flatulence, abdominal discomfort, nausea, vitamin A, D, E, K deficiencies; rare: fecal impaction.
Class contraindications: Hypersensitivity to the medication.

Fibric Acid Derivatives

FENOFIBRATE
TriCor
Caps: 67 mg
Antilipemic, fibric acid derivatives

NO X C

Indication: Hypertriglyceridemia
Initial dose: 67 mg PO daily
Max dose: 201 mg daily (3 caps)

Adverse drug reaction: Rare: arrhythmias.
Comments:
Dosage increment q6-8 wk.
Most useful for patients with high triglyceride levels.
Monitor liver function tests at baseline, 6 and 12 wk, then periodically.
Contraindicated in primary biliary cirrhosis, preexisting gallbladder disease, unexplained persistent elevations in serum transaminase levels.
Class side effects: Nausea, constipation, gastrointestinal symptoms, diarrhea, rash, increase in liver function test results, dyspepsia, vomiting; rare: fecal impaction.
Class contraindications: Hypersensitivity to the medication, hepatic or significant renal dysfunction.

GEMFIBROZIL

Lopid
Tabs: 600 mg
Caps: 300 mg
Antilipemic, fibric acid derivatives

NO ? C

Indication: Hypertriglyceridemia
Initial dose: 600 mg PO bid
Max dose: 600 mg PO bid

Adverse drug reaction: Rare: leukopenia, thrombocytopenia.
Comments:
Dosage increment q6-8 wk.
Monitor liver function tests at baseline, 6 and 12 wk, then periodically.
Contraindicated in patients with preexisting gallbladder disease.
Class side effects: Nausea, constipation, diarrhea, increase in liver function test
  results, dyspepsia, vomiting; rare: fecal impaction, skin reactions.
Class contraindications: Hypersensitivity to the medication, hepatic or
  significant renal dysfunction.

CLOFIBRATE

Atromid-S
Caps: 500 mg
Oral powder: 25 g
Antilipemic, fibric acid derivatives

YES ? C

Indication: Hypertriglyceridemia
Initial dose: 2 g PO divided bid/qid
Renal dose: CrCl 10-50 mL/min: q12-18h
           CrCl <10 mL/min: Avoid

Adverse drug reaction: Rare: thromboembolic events, leukopenia,
  thrombocytopenia, arrhythmias, cholelithiasis, cholecystitis.
Comments:
Monitor liver function tests at baseline, 6 and 12 wk, then periodically.
Dosage increment q6-8 wk.
Used infrequently because of long-term safety concerns.
Contraindicated in patients with primary biliary cirrhosis.
Class side effects: Nausea, constipation, diarrhea, increase in liver function test
  results, dyspepsia, vomiting; rare: fecal impaction, skin reactions.
Class contraindications: Hypersensitivity to the medication, hepatic or
  significant renal dysfunction.

For explanation of icons, see p. 1068.

Other Agents

NIACIN

Niaspan, Nicor

Tabs: 25, 50, 100, 125, 250, 400, 500 mg (OTC)
YES   ?   A/C

Caps: 500 mg

Tabs, timed released: 250, 500, 750 mg (OTC), 500, 750, 1000 mg

Caps, timed release: 125, 250, 300, 400, 500, 750 mg (OTC)

Oral liquid: 50 mg/5 mL

Antilipemic, other

Indication: Hypertriglyceridemia, niacin deficiency
Initial dose:
    Hypertriglyceridemia: 50-100 mg PO bid/tid
                      375 mg (timed released) PO qhs
    Niacin deficiency: 10-20 mg PO daily
  Max dose: 6 g daily
          2 g qhs (timed-release)
Renal dose: CrCl 10-50 mL/min: 50% dose
            CrCl <10 mL/min: 25% dose

Comments:

Flushing may be minimized by taking an aspirin 30 min before dose.

Dosage increment 300 mg daily q wk to goal of 2-3 g daily

Withhold therapy when short-term risk of renal dysfunction is high (use of IV dye, dehydration).

Pregnancy category: C if doses greater than recommended daily allowance.

Use with caution in patients with gout, peptic ulcer disease, inflammatory bowel disease, or diabetes mellitus.

Class side effects: Flushing, headache, bloating, flatulence, nausea, abnormalities in liver function tests, jaundice.

Class contraindications: Hypersensitivity to the medication, significant or unexplained hepatic dysfunction, active peptic ulcer disease, arterial bleeding

Combination Agents

LOVASTATIN/NIACIN

Advicor

Tabs: 500/20 mg, 750/20 mg, 1000/20 mg

Antilipemic, combination agents

Anticoagulation
Antiplatelet Agents

ANAGRELIDE

Agrylin
Caps: 0.5, 1 mg
Anticoagulation, antiplatelet agents

NO ? C

Indication: Essential thrombocythemia
Initial dose: 0.5 mg PO qid or 1 mg bid × 1 wk
Max dose: 10 mg daily or 2.5 mg/dose

Adverse drug reaction: Palpitations, diarrhea, edema, headache, nausea,
   hypotension, thrombocytopenia.
Comments:
Monitor blood counts, hepatic and renal function especially in first 2 wk.
Titrate to lowest effective dose 0.5 mg q wk, onset 7-14 days, max 4-12 wk.
Class contraindications: Hypersensitivity to the medication.

ASPIRIN

Ecotrin, Halfprin, Bayer, Aspergum
Tabs: 225, 325, 500, 650 mg (Bayer)
Chewing gum: 227 mg
Tabs, chewable: 81 mg
Tabs, delayed-release, enteric coated: 81, 162 mg (Halfprin)
Tabs, enteric coated: 81, 325, 500 mg (Ecotrin)
Suppository: 60, 120, 200, 325, 600 mg
Anticoagulation, antiplatelet agents

NO 3 C/D

Indication: Stroke, transient ischemic attack, myocardial infarction
Initial dose: 81-325 mg PO daily
Max dose: 4 g daily (arthritis)

Adverse drug reaction: Dypepsia, abdominal pain, nausea, bleeding, anemia.
Comments:
Withhold for 1 wk before surgery.
Avoid use in children with flu or chicken pox (Reye's syndrome).
Contraindicated in patients with a history of Reye's syndrome, triad of
   asthma–rhinitis–nasal polyps.
Pregnancy category: D in third trimester.
Class contraindications: Hypersensitivity to the medication.

CLOPIDOGREL
Plavix
Tabs: 75 mg
Anticoagulation, Antiplatelet Agents

NO ? B

 Initial dose: 75 mg PO daily

 Adverse drug reaction: Rash; rare: thrombotic thrombocytopenic purpura.
  Comments:
Withhold for 1 wk before surgery.
Usually used in patients intolerant to aspirin.
Contraindicated in patients with active pathological bleeding.
Drug/drug: Heparin, warfarin (use cautiously).
Drug/herb: Red clover.
Class contraindications: Hypersensitivity to the medication, pathological
  bleeding, such as peptic ulcer or intracranial hemorrhage.

DIPYRIDAMOLE
Persantine
Tabs: 25, 50, 75 mg
Anticoagulation, antiplatelet agents

NO 1 C

 Indication: Stroke, transient ischemic attack
Initial dose: 75-100 mg PO qid

Adverse drug reaction: Headache, dizziness, hypotension, nausea, blood
  pressure lability; rare: vomiting, flushing.
Drug/drug: Aminophylline.
Class contraindications: Hypersensitivity to the medication.

Glycoprotein IIb/IIIa Inhibitors

ABCIXIMAB
ReoPro
Inj: 2 mg/mL (5 mL)
Anticoagulation, glycoprotein IIb/IIIa inhibitors

NO ? C

Indication: Percutaneous coronary intervention, unstable angina, non-Q-wave
  myocardial infarction

Continued

ABCIXIMAB *continued*

Initial dose:
    Bolus: 0.25 mg/kg IV via separate infusion line before procedure
    Infusion: 0.125 µg/kg/min IV for 12 hr
Max dose: 10 µg/min

Comments:
Can use up to 24 hr max.
Drug/drug: Concomitant anticoagulant and thrombolytic additive effects.
Contraindicated in patients with cerebrovascular accident within previous 2 yr,
    thrombocytopenia <100,000/mm^3, intracranial neoplasm, arteriovenous
    malformation, aneurysm, severe uncontrolled hypertension, use of oral
    anticoagulant in which patient >1.2 × control level, hypersensitivity to murine
    proteins.
Class side effects: Bleeding, thrombocytopenia, nausea, hypotension,
    bradycardia.
Class contraindications: Hypersensitivity to the medication.

EPTIFIBATIDE

Integrilin
Inj: 0.75, 2 mg/mL (100 mL)
Anticoagulation, glycoprotein IIb/IIIa inhibitors

YES   ?   B

Indication: Acute coronary syndromes, percutaneous coronary intervention
Initial dose:
    Acute coronary syndromes:
        Bolus: 180 µg/kg IV
        Infusion: 2 µg/kg/min IV for 72 hr
    Percutaneous coronary intervention:
        Bolus: 180 µg/kg IV × 2 separated by 10 min
        Infusion: 1 µg/kg/min IV for 20-24 hr
Max dose: Weights >121 kg: same dose
Renal dose: Serum creatinine <2 mg/dL: bolus 180 µg/kg, maintenance
                2 µg/kg/min
                Serum creatinine >2-4 mg/dL: bolus 135 µg/kg, maintenance 0.5
                µg/kg/min

Comments:
Drug/drug: Concomitant anticoagulant and thrombolytic additive effects.
Contraindicated in patients with severe hypertension (>200/ >110 mm Hg),
    stroke within the previous 30 days, hemorrhagic stroke, platelet level
    <100,000/mm^3, serum creatinine level >4 mg/dL, hemodialysis.
Class side effects: Bleeding, thrombocytopenia, nausea, hypotension,
    bradycardia.
Class contraindications: Hypersensitivity to the medication.

For explanation of icons, see p. 1068.

TIROFIBAN

Aggrastat
Inj: 250 µg/mL (50 mL)
Inj, solution: 50 µg/mL (250, 500 mL NS)
Anticoagulation, glycoprotein IIb/IIIa inhibitors

YES   3   B

Indication: Acute coronary syndromes, percutaneous transluminal coronary angioplasty
Initial dose:
  Bolus: 0.4 µg/kg/min IV for 30 min
  Infusion: 0.1 µg/kg/min IV for 48-108 hr
Max dose: Weights >153 kg: same dose
Renal dose: Serum creatinine level <2 mg/dL: bolus 0.4 µg/kg, maintenance 0.1 µg/kg/min
  Serum creatinine level >2-4 mg/dL: bolus 0.2 µg/kg, maintenance 0.05 µg/kg/min

Comments:
Drug/drug: Concomitant anticoagulant and thrombolytic additive effects.
Contraindicated in patients with intracranial hemorrhage, intracranial neoplasm, arteriovenous malformation, aneurysm, stroke within previous 30 days, hemorrhagic stroke, aortic dissection, severe hypertension (>180/>110 mm Hg), acute pericarditis.
Class side effects: Bleeding, thrombocytopenia, nausea, hypotension, bradycardia.
Class contraindications: Hypersensitivity to the medication.

Heparin and Heparinoids

DALTEPARIN

Fragmin
Inj, prefilled syringe: 2500, 5000 anti–factor Xa IU/0.2 mL
Anticoagulation, heparin and heparinoids

YES   ?   B

Indication: Deep venous thrombosis (DVT) prophylaxis, abdominal and hip surgery, unstable angina, non-Q-wave myocardial infarction (NQWMI)
Initial dose:
  DVT prophylaxis, abdominal and hip surgery: 2500 (5000 high risk) IU SQ daily × 5-10 days
  Unstable angina, NQWMI: 120 units/kg SQ q12h (with ASA 75-165 mg daily)
Max dose: 10,000 units SQ q12h with ASA
Renal dose: Caution in renal insufficiency

Continued

DALTEPARIN *continued*

Comments:
Partial antidote is protamine 1% 1 mg for every 100 IU of anti–factor Xa.
Do not administer intramuscularly.
Perform complete blood cell count, platelet count, stool occult blood test
  periodically.
Contraindicated in patients with hypersensitivity to heparin, pork products.
Class side effects: Hemorrhage, ecchymoses, hematoma (SQ); rare:
  thrombocytopenia.
Class contraindications: Hypersensitivity to the medication, thrombocytopenia
  with positive antibody response to medication, active internal bleeding,
  recent major surgery, spinal puncture.

ENOXAPARIN

Lovenox
Inj, prefilled syringe: 30, 40, 60, 80, 100 mg
Anticoagulation, heparin and heparinoids

YES   ?   B

Indication: Deep venous thrombosis (DVT) prophylaxis (hip, knee, abdomen),
  outpatient DVT without pulmonary embolism (PE), inpatient DVT and
  PE, unstable angina, non-Q-wave myocardial infarction (NQWMI)
Initial dose:
  DVT prophylaxis (hip, knee, abdomen): 30 mg SQ q12h × 7-10 days
                                          40 mg SQ daily × 7-10 days
  Outpatient DVT without PE: 1 mg/kg SQ q12h until international
                                normalized ratio (INR) at goal
  Inpatient DVT and PE: 1 mg/kg SQ q12h or 1.5 mg/kg SQ q24h until INR
    at goal
  Unstable angina, NQWMI: 1 mg/kg SQ q12h (with ASA 75-325 mg daily) ×
    2-8 days
Max dose: Weights >150 kg not studied
Renal dose: CrCl <30 mL/min: Use with caution

Comments:
Partial antidote is protamine 1% 1 mg for every 1 mg enoxaparin.
Do not administer intramuscularly.
Perform complete blood cell count, platelet count, stool occult blood test
  periodically.
Contraindicated in patients with hypersensitivity to heparin, pork products.
Class side effects: Hemorrhage, ecchymoses, hematoma (SQ); rare:
  thrombocytopenia.
Class contraindications: Hypersensitivity to the medication, thrombocytopenia
  with positive antibody response to medication, active internal bleeding,
  recent major surgery, spinal puncture.

HEPARIN

Inj, solution: 100 units/mL (250 mL 0.45 NS)
Inj: 1000, 5000, 10000 units/mL
Anticoagulation, heparin and heparinoids

NO   1   C

Indication: Treatment, Prophylaxis
Initial dose: Bolus 80 units/kg IV
Infusion 18 units/kg/h IV (round to nearest 100 units)
5000 units sqq12h
Max dose: 1600 units/h initial

Comments:
Antidote is protamine 1% 100 heparin units.
Dosage increment based on activated partial thromboplastin time q4-6h.
Perform complete blood cell count, platelet count, stool occult blood test
periodically.
Contraindicated in patients with hypersensitivity to heparin, pork products.
Class side effects: Hemorrhage, ecchymoses, hematoma (SQ); rare:
thrombocytopenia.
Class contraindications: Hypersensitivity to the medication, thrombocytopenia
with positive antibody response to medication, active internal bleeding,
recent major surgery, spinal puncture.

TINZAPARIN

Innohep
Inj: 20,000 anti–factor Xa IU/mL (2 mL)
Anticoagulation, heparin and heparinoids

YES   ?   B

Indication: Deep venous thrombosis with or without pulmonary embolism
Initial dose: 175 anti–factor Xa IU/kg SQ daily until international normalized
ratio at goal
Max dose: Body mass index >40 kg/m² not studied
Weights >122 kg: Same dose
Renal dose: CrCl <30 mL/min: Use with caution

Comments:
Partial antidote is protamine 1% 1 mg for every 100 IU of anti–factor Xa.
Do not administer intramuscularly.
Perform complete blood cell count, platelet count, stool occult blood test
periodically.

Continued

TINZAPARIN continued

Contraindicated in patients with hypersensitivity to sulfites, pork products, benzyl alcohol.
Class side effects: Hemorrhage, ecchymoses, hematoma (SQ); rare: thrombocytopenia.
Class contraindications: Hypersensitivity to the medication, thrombocytopenia with positive antibody response to medication, active internal bleeding, recent major surgery, spinal puncture.

Combination Agents

DIPYRIDAMOLE/ACETYLSALICYLIC ACID
Aggrenox, Renox
Caps: 200/25 mg
Anticoagulation, combination

 Indication: Stroke, transient ischemic attack

Miscellaneous Anticoagulant Agents

WARFARIN
Coumadin
Tabs, scored: 1, 2, 2.5, 3, 4, 5, 6, 7.5, 10 mg
Anticoagulation, miscellaneous anticoagulant agents

 NO 1 X

 Indication: Deep venous thrombosis, pulmonary embolism, prosthetic heart valves, atrial fibrillation
Initial dose: 5 mg PO daily × 2 days

 Adverse drug reaction: Rare: warfarin-induced necrosis.
Comments:
Intensive education and close monitoring are suggested.
Antidote is vitamin K SQ or PO 2.5-10 mg depending on bleeding and international normalized ratio (INR).
Dosage increment: 10%-15% dose change; titrate to goal INR.
Drug/drug: Concomitant anticoagulant and thrombolytic additive effects.
Contraindicated in patients with active ulceration, blood dyscrasias, inadequate monitoring (or unsupervised patients with senility), spinal puncture.
Class side effects: Bleeding, bruising.
Class contraindications: Hypersensitivity to the medication.

For explanation of icons, see p. 1068.

DANAPAROID

Orgaran
Inj: 750 anti-factor Xa IU/0.6 mL
Anticoagulation, miscellaneous anticoagulant agents

NO   ?   B

Indication: Deep venous thrombosis prophylaxis, hip surgery
Initial dose: 750 anti-Xa units SQ bid × 7-10 days

Adverse drug reaction: Fever, nausea, constipation.
Comments:
No antidote is available.
Do not administer intramuscularly.
Drug/drug: Concomitant anticoagulant and thrombolytic additive effects.
Contraindicated in patients with hypersensitivity to pork products, severe
    hemorrhagic diathesis, type 2 thrombocytopenia, hemorrhagic stroke.
Class side effects: Bleeding, bruising.
Class contraindications: Hypersensitivity to the medication.

LEPIRUDIN

Refludan
Inj: 50 mg
Anticoagulation, miscellaneous anticoagulant agents

YES   3   B

Indication: Thromboembolism in heparin-induced thrombocytopenia
Initial dose:
    Bolus: 0.4 mg/kg IV
    Infusion: 0.15 mg/kg/hr IV
Max dose: Weight >110 kg: same dose
Renal dose: Decrease bolus 0.2 mg/kg
            CrCl 45-60 mL/min: 0.075 mg/kg/hr
            CrCl 30-44 mL/min: 0.045 mg/kg/hr
            CrCl 15-29 mL/min: 0.0225 mg/kg/hr
            CrCl <15 mL/min: Avoid

Adverse drug reaction: Abnormal liver function, allergic reaction.
Comments:
No antidote is available.
Drug/drug: Concomitant anticoagulant and thrombolytic additive effects.
Dosage increment based on activated partial thromboplastin time q4h; if above
    goal, withhold for 2 hr, then restart 50% original infusion; if below goal,
    increase steps 20%.
Class side effects: Bleeding, bruising.
Class contraindications: Hypersensitivity to the medication.

Antiarrhythmics
Class 1a

DISOPYRAMIDE

Norpace, Norpace CR
Caps, extended-release: 100, 150 mg
Caps: 100, 150 mg
Antiarrhythmics, Class 1a

YES 1 C

Indication: Atrial fibrillation, ventricular tachycardia
Initial dose: Bolus: 200 mg PO (<50 kg), 300 mg PO (>50 kg)
Maintenance: 100-150 mg PO q6h
200-300 mg PO q12h controlled release
Max dose: 400 mg q6h
Renal dose: CrCl >50 mL/min q8h
CrCl 10-50 mL/min q12-24h
CrCl <10 mL/min q24-48h

Adverse drug reaction: Dry mouth.
Comments:
Drug/drug: avoid drugs that prolong the QT interval.
Class side effects: QT prolongation, torsades de pointes.
Class contraindications: Second- or third-degree atrioventricular block,
cardiogenic shock, excessive baseline QT prolongation.

PROCAINAMIDE

Pronestyl, Procanbid
Caps/tabs: 250, 375, 500 mg (Pronestyl)
Tabs, extended-release: 250, 500, 1000 mg (Procanbid)
Inj: 100 mg/mL (10 mL), 500 mg/mL (2 mL)
Antiarrhythmics, class 1a

YES 1 C

Indication: Atrial fibrillation, ventricular tachycardia
Initial dose: 50 mg/kg PO daily
0.5-1 g IM q3-6h
Bolus: 100 mg IV q5 min
Maintenance:2-6 mg/min IV
Max dose: Bolus 1 g
IV continuous 2 g daily PO 4 g daily
Renal dose: CrCl >50 mL/min q4h
CrCl 10-50 mL/min q6-12h
CrCl <10 mL/min q8-24h

Continued

PROCAINAMIDE *continued*

Adverse drug reaction: Systemic lupus erythematosus, syndrome, seizures, nausea, vomiting, hypotension (IV); rare: severe hematological effects.

Comments:

For initial oral therapy use conventional capsules and tablets; use extended release tablets for maintenance therapy.

Monitoring of N-acetylprocainamide and procainamide levels is recommended, especially in patients with renal insufficiency.

Discontinue medication after QT prolongation and QRS intervals (≤50% widening).

Class side effects: QT prolongation, torsades de pointes.

Drug/drug: Cholinergic agents, neuromuscular blocking agents.

Drug/herb: Jimsonweed.

Drug/food: Licorice.

Class contraindications: Second- or third-degree atrioventricular block, cardiogenic shock, excessive baseline QT prolongation.

QUINIDINE

Cardioquin, Quinidex, Quinaglute

Tabs (sulfate): 200, 300 mg (Quinidex)   YES   1   C
Tabs, extended-release (sulfate): 300 mg (Quinidex)
Tabs, extended-release (gluconate): 324 mg (Quinaglute)
Tabs, scored (polygalacturonate): 275 mg (Cardioquin)
Antiarrhythmics, class 1a

Indication: Atrial fibrillation, ventricular tachycardia
Initial dose: Gluconate form: 324-660 mg PO q8h or 648 mg PO q12h
Max dose: 3-4 g daily
Renal dose: CrCl <10 mL/min: 75% dose

Adverse drug reaction: Nausea, vomiting, diarrhea, anorexia, abdominal pain, esophagitis, syncope, severe hypotension (IV).

Comments:

Drug/drug: Rifampin induces metabolism. Drug levels highly variable depending on assay, class and severity of arrhythmias, and sensitivity of the patient.

Class side effects: QT prolongation, torsades de pointes.

Class contraindications: Second- or third-degree atrioventricular block, cardiogenic shock, excessive baseline QT prolongation.

Class 1b

LIDOCAINE

Xylocaine
Inj, syringes: 10 mg/mL (10 mL)
Antiarrhythmics, class 1b

NO   1   C

Indication: Ventricular tachycardia, ventricular fibrillation
Initial dose: Bolus: 1-1.5 mg/kg IV over 2-3 min, may repeat 0.5-0.75 mg/kg
IV in 5-10 min
Continuous infusion: 1-4 mg/min
Max dose: Bolus 3 mg/kg

Adverse drug reaction: Rare: seizures, drowsiness, respiratory or
cardiovascular depression.
Comments:
Measure levels when signs of toxicity develop or duration is >24 hr; drowsiness
may be first sign of toxicity.
Class contraindications: Second- or third-degree atrioventricular block,
cardiogenic shock.

MEXILETENE

Mexitil
Caps: 150, 200, 250 mg
Antiarrhythmics, class 1b

YES   X   C

Indication: Ventricular tachycardia
Initial dose: Load: 400 mg PO if needed
Maintenance: 200 mg PO q8h
Max dose: 1.2 g daily
Renal dose: CrCl <10 mL/min: 50%-75% dose

Adverse drug reaction: Dizziness, tremor, nausea, vomiting, heartburn; rare:
seizures, leukopenia, thrombocytopenia, new or worsened arrhythmias.
Drug/drug: High-dose antacids, metoclopramide, phenobarbital, phenytoin,
rifampin.
Class contraindications: Second- or third-degree atrioventricular block,
cardiogenic shock.

Cardiovascular—Antiarrhythmics

For explanation of icons, see p. 1068.

TOCAINIDE
Tonocard
Tabs: 400, 600 mg
Antiarrhythmics, class 1b

YES   ?   C

Indication: Ventricular tachycardia
Initial dose: 400 mg PO q8h
Max dose: 2.4 g daily
Renal dose: CrCl <10 mL/min: 50% dose

Adverse drug reaction: Lightheadedness, vertigo, tremor, headache, nausea, vomiting, rash, paresthesia; rare: pulmonary fibrosis, agranulocytosis.
Comments:
Poor correlation between drug levels and toxic or therapeutic effects; tremor may indicate max dose.
Class contraindications: Second- or third-degree AV block, cardiogenic shock

Class 1c

FLECAINIDE
Tambocor
Tabs, scored*: 50, 100*, 150* mg
Antiarrhythmics, class 1c

YES   1   C

Indication: Life-threatening ventricular tachycardia, paroxysmal supraventricular tachycardia
Initial dose: 100 mg PO q12h
Max dose: 400 mg daily
Renal dose: CrCl <10 mL/min: 50%-75% dose

Adverse drug reaction: Visual disturbances, palpitations, dyspnea, chest pain.
Comments:
Dosage increments 50-100 mg q4 days.
Class side effects: Dizziness, headache, fatigue, nausea, arrhythmogenic.
Class contraindications: Hypersensitivity to the medication, cardiogenic shock, conduction disorders.

PROPAFENONE
Rythmol
Tabs, scored: 150, 225, 300 mg
Antiarrhythmics, class 1c

NO   ?   C

Indication: Ventricular tachycardia, paroxysmal supraventricular tachycardia
Initial dose: 150 mg PO q8h
Max dose: 900 mg daily

Adverse drug reaction: Vomiting, dysgeusia, constipation; rare: blood
  dyscrasias, bronchospasm.
Comments:
Drug/drug: Inhibits Coumadin metabolism.
Contraindicated in bronchospastic disorders, uncontrolled congestive heart
  failure, bradycardia.
Class side effects: Dizziness, headache, fatigue, nausea, arrhythmogenic.
Class contraindications: Hypersensitivity to the medication, cardiogenic shock,
  conduction disorders.

Class II

ESMOLOL
Brevibloc
Inj: 10 mg/mL (10 mL); 250 mg/mL (10 mL)
Antiarrhythmics, class II

YES   1   C/D

Indication: Supraventricular tachycardia
Initial dose: Bolus: 500 µg/kg IV over 1 min
Maintenance: 50-100 µg/kg/min IV
Max dose: 300 µg/kg/min

Adverse drug reaction: Symptomatic hypotension, diaphoresis, nausea,
  dizziness.
Comments:
If response inadequate, repeat bolus q4 min and increase maintenance dose.
Pregnancy category: D in second and third trimesters.
Drug/drug: IV morphine (increased esmolol levels), xanthines (decreased
  xanthine clearance).
Class side effects: Bradycardia, heart block, hypotension, bronchoconstriction,
  fatigue.
Class contraindications: Hypersensitivity to the medication, sinus bradycardia,
  second- or third-degree heartblock, acute congestive heart failure,
  cardiogenic shock.

Cardiovascular—Antiarrhythmics

For explanation of icons, see p. 1068.

PROPRANOLOL

Inderal, Inderal LA

Caps, extended-release: 60, 80, 120, 160 mg
Inj: 1 mg/mL (10 mL)
Tabs, scored: 10, 20, 40, 60, 80 mg
Antiarrhythmics, class II

YES   1   C/D

Indication: Supraventricular tachycardia, digoxin toxicity without atrioventricular block
Initial dose: 10-30 mg PO q6-8h, 1-3 mg IV; second dose in 2 min, third dose no sooner than q4h
Max dose: 16 mg/kg daily or 60 mg daily
3 mg IV at 1 mg/min
Renal dose: CrCl <10 mL/min: 25% dose

Adverse drug reaction: Erectile dysfunction.
Comments:
Taper off drug; rebound symptoms may occur after sudden discontinuation.
Contraindicated in pulmonary edema, hyperactive airway disease.
Pregnancy category: D in second and third trimesters.
Class side effects: Bradycardia, heart block, hypotension, bronchoconstriction, fatigue.
Class contraindications: Hypersensitivity to the medication, sinus bradycardia, second- or third-degree heartblock, acute congestive heart failure, cardiogenic shock.

Class III

AMIODARONE

Pacerone, Cordarone

Inj: 50 mg/mL (Cordarone)
Tabs, scored: 200 mg
Antiarrhythmics, class III

NO   X   C

Indication: Ventricular tachycardia (VT), atrial fibrillation and flutter, ventricular fibrillation (VF) and pulseless VT, breakthrough VF and pulseless VT
Initial dose:
VT, atrial fibrillation and flutter:
  Bolus: 800-1600 mg/day PO for 1-3 wks
  Maintenance: 600-800 mg/day PO for 4 wk, then 400 mg/day
VF and pulseless VT:
  Bolus: 300 mg IV push undiluted/unfiltered; may repeat bolus with 150 mg if needed
  Load: 1 mg/min IV × 6 hr
  After the first 6 hr: 0.5 mg/min IV

Continued

AMIODARONE *continued*

Breakthrough VF and pulseless VT: 150 mg IV push unfiltered/undiluted
Amiodarone conversion:

IV	PO
<1 wk IV infusion	800-1600 mg daily
1-3 wk IV infusion	600-800 mg daily
>3 wk IV infusion	400 mg daily

Adverse drug reaction: Thyroid function changes, nausea, vomiting, constipation, photosensitivity, anorexia, corneal microdeposits, pigment deposition, conduction delays, hypotension (IV); rare: hepatotoxicity, pneumonitis, liver function test abnormalities (elevations).

Comments:

Drug/drug: Inhibits procainamide and warfarin metabolism. Decrease digoxin dose 50%.

Avoid drugs that prolong Tc interval.

Dosage increment load in first 24 hr is approximately 1000 mg.

Contraindicated in severe sinus node dysfunction, second- or third-degree atrioventicular block.

Class side effects: QT prolongation, torsades de pointes, arrhythmogenic.

Class contraindications: Hypersensitivity to the medication.

DOFETILIDE

Tikosyn
Caps: 125, 250, 500 μg   YES   3   C
Antiarrhythmics, class III

Indication: Afib, Aflutter
Initial dose: 125-500 μg PO bid

Initial dose	Adjusted dose if QTc elevated
500 μg bid	250 μg bid
250 μg bid	125 μg bid
125 μg bid	125 μg daily

Renal dose: CrCl >60 mL/min: 500 μg bid
CrCl 40-60 mL/min: 250 μg bid
CrCl 20-39 mL/min: 125 μg bid
CrCl <20 mL/min: Avoid

Adverse drug reaction: Headache, chest pain, dizziness, dyspnea, nausea, diarrhea.

Comments:

Must monitor electrocardiogram, creatinine clearance (CrCl) for minimum 3 days.

Do not use if baseline CrCl is <20 mL/min or QTc interval is >440 msec.

Continued

DOFETILIDE *continued*

Check QTc 2-3 hr after dose; if >500 msec or >15% increase, discontinue drug.
Drug/drug: Megestrol/prochlorperazine inhibits elimination. Avoid use of drugs that prolong QT interval. Trimethoprim (Bactrim) increases maximum dofetilide concentration 93%.
Contraindicated in patients with long QT syndromes (QT >440 msec), severe renal impairment (CrCl <20 mL/min), baseline heart rate <50 beats/min, concurrent amiodarone use.
Class side effects: QT prolongation, torsades de pointes, arrhythmogenic.
Class contraindications: Hypersensitivity to the medication.

IBUTILIDE

Corvert
Inj: 0.1 mg/mL
Antiarrhythmics, class III

NO　3　C

Indication: Atrial fibrillation
Initial dose: Bolus: 0.01 mg/kg IV over 10 min (<60 kg)
　　　　　　1 mg IV over 10 min (>60 kg)

Adverse drug reaction: Ventricular tachycardia, nausea
Comments:
If no change in 10 min, repeat one time only.
Must monitor with electrocardiogram for 6 hr after administration (QT prolongation).
Contraindicated in patients with a history of polymorphic ventricular tachycardia.
Drug/drug: Avoid drugs that prolong the QT interval or cause hypokalemia or hypomagnesmia.
Class side effects: QT prolongation, torsades de pointes, arrhythmogenic.
Class contraindications: Hypersensitivity to the medication.

SOTALOL

Betapace, Betapace AF
Tabs, scored: 80, 120, 160, 320 mg (Betapace)
　　　　　　80, 120, 160 mg (Betapace AF)
Antiarrhythmics, class III

YES　1　B/D

Indication: Atrial fibrillation, ventricular tachycardia
Initial dose: 80 mg PO bid
Maintenance: 160-320 mg PO divided bid/tid

Continued

SOTALOL *continued*

> **Max dose:** 480-640 mg daily; atrial fibrillation: 160 mg bid
> **Renal dose:** CrCl 30-60 mL/min q24h
> CrCl 10-30 mL/min q36-48h
> CrCl <10 mL/min: Individualize dose
> CrCl <40 mL/min: Avoid use of Betapace AF

Adverse drug reaction: Bradycardia, fatigue, dizziness, dyspnea, nausea, vomiting, rash, visual disturbances, bronchospasm.
Comments:
Increase gradually over 2-3 days.
Drug/drug: Avoid drugs that prolong the QT interval.
Contraindicated in bronchial asthma, sinus bradycardia, second- and third-degree atrioventricular block, long QT syndromes, cardiogenic shock, congestive heart failure.
Pregnancy category: D in second and third trimesters
Class side effects: QT prolongation, torsades de pointes, arrhythmogenic.
Class contraindications: Hypersensitivity to the medication.

Class IV

DILTIAZEM

Cardizem
Inj: 5 mg/mL
Antiarrhythmics, class IV

NO   1   C

Indication: Atrial fibrillation, paroxysmal supraventricular tachycardia
Initial dose: Bolus 0.25 mg/kg (usually 20 mg) IV over 2 min; if necessary, repeat bolus as 0.35 mg/kg IV in 15 min.
Continuous infusion: 10-15 mg/hr IV prn
Max dose: 0.45 mg/kg/dose (clinical)
IV >24 hr or >15 mg/hr not recommended

Adverse drug reaction: Hypotension, asthenia.
Comments:
Contraindicated in severe hypotension, second- or third-degree heart block, sick sinus syndrome, pulmonary congestion.
Class side effects: Bradycardia, abnormal electrocardiogram, asthenia, first-degree atrioventricular block, headache, dizziness, constipation, nausea, rare: paralytic ileus.
Class contraindications: Hypersensitivity to the medication.

VERAPAMIL

Isoptin, Calan, Calan SR
Inj: 2.5 mg/mL
Tabs, scored: 40, 80, 120 mg
Tabs, extended-release: 120 mg (Calan SR, Isoptin SR)
Tabs, scored, extended-released: 180, 240 mg (Calan SR, Isoptin SR)
Antiarrhythmics, class IV

NO   1   C

Indication: Atrial fibrillation, supraventricular tachycardia
Initial dose:
    Digitalized patients: 240-320 mg/day PO divided bid/qid
    Nondigitalized patients: 240-480 mg/day PO divided bid/qid
        5-10 mg IV push over 2 min, may repeat after 30
        min with 5-10 mg IV over 2 min

Adverse drug reaction: Dyspepsia, lethargy, heart failure, pulmonary edema.
Comments:
In patients with sick sinus syndrome or an accessory bypass tract (ejection
    fraction <20), antiarrhythmic effects may be seen within 48 hr.
Drug/drug: May increase the area under the curve (AUC) of metoprolol by
    300%. May increase carbamazepine, cyclosporin A, and digoxin levels. Avoid
    use of IV verapamil with β-blockers.
Contraindicated in patients with sinus bradycardia, advanced heartblock,
    cardiogenic shock, and atrial fibrillation or flutter associated with accessory
    conduction pathways (Wolff-Parkinson-White syndrome).
Class side effects: Bradycardia, abnormal electrocardiogram, asthenia, first-
    degree atrioventricular block, headache, dizziness, constipation, nausea,
    rare: paralytic ileus.
Class contraindications: Hypersensitivity to the medication.

Miscellaneous Antiarrhythmics

ADENOSINE

Adenocard
Inj: 3 mg/mL
Antiarrhythmics, miscellaneous

NO   ?   C

Indication: Supraventricular tachycardia, paroxysmal supraventricular
    tachycardia
Initial dose: 6 mg IV push; if not effective, may repeat bolus with 12 mg after
    1-2 min
Max dose: 12 mg/dose

Continued

ADENOSINE *continued*

Adverse drug reaction: Facial flushing, dizziness, chest pain,
bronchoconstriction, temporary asystole.
Comments:
Rapid IV push over 1-2 sec via peripheral line, followed with rapid flush.
Drug/drug: Methylxanthines decrease effectiveness. Dipyridamole increases
effectiveness. Carbamazepine increases risk of heart block.
Class contraindications: Sick sinus syndrome, atrial fibrillation or flutter.

ANTINEOPLASTIC
Alkylating Agents

BUSULFAN
Myleran
Tabs, scored: 2 mg
Inj: 60 mg/10 mL
Alkylating agents

NO   X   D

Indication: Chronic myelogenous leukemia (CML)
Initial dose: CML: 4 mg PO daily for several wk
Max dose: 12 mg daily

Adverse drug reaction: Anemia, leukopenia, infection, neutropenia,
thrombocytopenia, hepatic venoocclusive disease, nausea, vomiting,
stomatitis; rare: pancytopenia, interstitial pulmonary fibrosis.
Comments:
Ensure adequate hydration.
Monitor complete blood count with differential: weekly for PO, daily for IV.
Contraindicated without a definitive diagnosis of chronic myelogenous leukemia.
Class contraindications: Hypersensitivity to the medication.

CISPLATIN
Platinol-AQ
Inj: 50, 100 mg
Alkylating agents

YES   X   D

Indication: Carcinoma of bladder, ovaries, testes, cervix, or lung
Initial dose: 100 mg/m^2 IV as single or divided dose over 2-5 days q3-4 wk
Max dose: 120 mg/m^2/cycle
Renal dose: CrCl 10-50 mL/min: 75% dose
CrCl <10 mL/min: 50% dose

Continued

For explanation of icons, see p. 1068.

CISPLATIN *continued*

Adverse drug reaction: Nephrotoxicity, nausea, vomiting, peripheral
neuropathies, ototoxicity, electrolyte abnormalities.
Comments:
Force fluids up to 2 L/day.
If medication is not used within 6 hr, use light protection.
Vesicant at high concentration or volume: Never administer SQ or IM at high
doses.
Monitor complete blood count, kidney function, uric acid, electrolytes.
Class contraindications: Hypersensitivity to the medication.

CYCLOPHOSPHAMIDE

Cytoxan
Tabs: 25, 50 mg
Inj: 100, 200, 500 mg, 1, 2 g
Alkylating agents

YES X D

Indication: Carcinoma of breast or ovaries, acute and chronic leukemia,
Hodgkin's and non-Hodgkin's lymphoma, as part of bone marrow or
stem cell transplantation conditioning regimen, cerebral vasculitis,
Wegener's granulomatosis

Initial dose:
Carcinoma of breast or ovaries: Various, e.g., 1-5 mg/kg/day PO
Leukemias and lymphomas: Various, e.g., 1.5 g/m² on day 1-4 in
multidrug regimen
Transplant: Various, e.g., 1 g/m³ for 3 days in multidrug conditioning
regimen
Wegener's granulomatosis: 2-5 mg/kg PO daily
Cerebral vasculitis: Various, e.g., 500-1000 mg/m² IV q1-3 months or 1-2
mg/kg PO daily
Max dose: 50 mg/kg IV divided 2-5 days
Renal dose: CrCl <10 mL/min: 75% dose

Adverse drug reaction: Amenorrhea, leukopenia, infection, cardiotoxicity,
syndrome of inappropriate antidiuretic hormone (SIADH)-like syndrome,
hemorrhagic cystitis, hyperuricemia, uric acid nephropathy, pneumonitis,
interstitial pulmonary fibrosis, thrombocytopenia, anemia, nausea, vomiting,
anorexia.
Comments:
Force fluids.
Monitor complete blood count with differential: baseline, nadir, and before next
course.
Contraindicated in patients with severely depressed bone marrow function, or
prior hypersensitivity to the medication.

LOMUSTINE
CeeNU
Caps: 10, 40, 100 mg
Alkylating agents

NO ? D

Indication: Hodgkin's lymphoma, brain tumors
Initial dose: 130 mg/m^2 PO q6 wk

Adverse drug reaction: Immunosuppression, leukopenia, infection, thrombocytopenia.
Comments:
Dosage increment: According to previous leukocyte nadir; see package insert.
Administer on empty stomach.
Monitor complete blood count with differential for at least 6 wk after each dose.
Class contraindications: Hypersensitivity to the medication.

TEMOZOLOMIDE
Temodar
Caps: 5, 20, 100, 250 mg
Alkylating agents

NO X D

Indication: Refractory anaplastic astrocytoma
Initial dose: 150 mg/m^2/day PO for 5 consecutive days per 28-day cycle

Adverse drug reaction: Amnesia, fever, hemiparesis or paresis, infection, leukopenia, neutropenia, peripheral edema, seizures, thrombocytopenia, nausea, vomiting, ataxia.
Comments:
Do not open capsules.
If baseline absolute neutrophil count (ANC) >1500/mm^3 or platelet count >100,000/mm^3, start drug.
Monitor complete blood count with differential at baseline, at 21 days after first dose, then weekly. Once the ANC >1500/mm^3 and platelet count >100,000/mm^3, start the next cycle of medication.
Dosage increment: If ANC <1000/mm^3 or platelet count <50,000/mm^3, decrease dose by 50 mg/m^2.
Class contraindications: Hypersensitivity to the medication or dacarbazine.

For explanation of icons, see p. 1068.

Antibiotics

BLEOMYCIN

Blenoxane
Inj: 15, 30 units
Antibiotics

YES   ?   D

Indication: Carcinoma of cervix, penis, larynx ,testes, head, neck, or skin,
Hodgkin's or non-Hodgkin's lymphoma
Initial dose: 10-20 units/m^2 IM, SQ, or IV once or twice/wk
Maintenance: 1 unit IM, SQ, or IV daily or 5 units IM, SQ, IV per wk (Hodgkin's
lymphoma)
Max dose: <400 units cumulative
Renal dose: CrCl 10-50 mL/min: 75% dose
CrCl <10 mL/min: 50% dose

Adverse drug reaction: Fever, chills, pneumonitis, stomatitis, interstitial
pulmonary fibrosis.
Comments:
Test dose of 2 units before therapeutic dose.
Monitor chest radiographs, white blood cell and platelet counts, and pulmonary
function tests.
Class contraindications: Hypersensitivity to the medication.

DAUNORUBICIN

Cerubidine
Inj: 20 mg
Antibiotics

YES   ?   D

Indication: Acute lymphoblastic leukemia, acute myelogenous leukemia, acute
monocytic leukemia, Kaposi's sarcoma
Initial dose: 30-60 mg/m^2 IV daily for 3-5 days q3-4 wk
Max dose: <550 mg/m^2 cumulative
<400 mg/m^2 cumulative plus radiation
Renal dose: Serum creatinine level 3 mg/dL: 50% dose
Hepatic dose: Bilirubin level 1.2-3 mg/dL: 75% dose
3 mg/dL:50% dose

Adverse drug reaction: Esophagitis, stomatitis, leukopenia, infection,
cardiotoxicity, vesicant, thrombocytopenia, alopecia, anemia, dose-related
cardiac failure.

Continued

DAUNORUBICIN *continued*

Comments:

Protect from sunlight.

Conventional daunorubicin is not interchangeable with the liposomal formulation.

Will cause red discoloration of the urine.

Monitor complete blood count with differential before each course of therapy.

Vesicant: Never administer SQ or IM.

Contraindicated in patients who have prior hypersensitivity to the medication or who received complete cumulative doses of other anthracyclines or anthracenes.

DOXORUBICIN

Adriamycin, Rubex

Inj: 10, 20, 50, 150 mg (Adriamycin)

    2 mg/mL (5, 10, 25, 100 mL) (Adriamycin)

    10, 50, 100 mg (Rubex)

Antibiotics

NO   X   D

Indication: Acute lymphoblastic leukemia, acute myelogenous leukemia, soft tissue and bone sarcomas, breast, thyroid, gastric, transitional cell, or bladder carcinoma, Hodgkin's disease

Initial dose: 60-75 mg/m^2 q21 days; 40-60 mg/m^2 q21-28 days as multidrug regimen

Max dose: <550 mg/m^2 cumulative

    <450 mg/m^2 cumulative + radiation

Hepatic dose: bilirubin level 1.2-3 mg/dL: 50% dose

    3.1-5 mg/dL: 25% dose

Adverse drug reaction: Leukopenia, infection, stomatitis, esophagitis, anemia, cardiotoxicity, vesicant, thrombocytopenia, alopecia.

Comments:

Conventional doxorubicin is not interchangeable with the liposomal formulation.

May give cardioprotectant dexrazoxane when 300 mg/m^2 lifetime dose of doxorubicin is reached.

Monitor complete blood count with differential before each course of therapy.

Vesicant: Never administer SQ or IM.

Contraindicated in patients who have prior hypersensitivity to the medication or who received complete cumulative doses of other anthracyclines or anthracenes.

For explanation of icons, see p. 1068.

Antimetabolites

CAPECITABINE

Xeloda
Tabs: 150, 500 mg
Antimetabolites

NO   X   D

Indication: Metastatic colorectal carcinoma, metastatic resistant breast carcinoma
Initial dose: 2500 mg/m^2/day PO in 2 divided doses for 14 days, then 7 days of rest
Renal dose: CrCl <30 mL/min: Avoid use

Adverse drug reaction: Abdominal pain, anemia, diarrhea, neutropenia, nausea or vomiting, hand and foot syndrome, stomatitis, thrombocytopenia, altered coagulation
Drug/drug: May elevate phenytoin levels. .
Class contraindications: Hypersensitivity to the medication.

CYTARABINE

Cytosar-U
Inj: 100, 500 mg, 1, 2 g
Inj: 20 mg/mL (5 mL)
Antimetabolites

NO   ?   D

Indication: Acute lymphoblastic leukemia, acute myelogenous leukemia, chronic lymphocytic leukemia, meningeal leukemia
Initial dose: Low-dose treatment: 200 mg/m^2 IV daily × 7 days

---

Adverse drug reaction: Leukopenia, infection, thrombocytopenia, stomatitis, anemia, ocular toxicity, cerebellar toxicity, rash.
Comments:
Contraindicated in active meningeal infection.
Conventional cytarabine is not interchangeable with the liposomal formulation.
Contraindicated in active meningeal infection or prior hypersensitivity to the medication.
Monitor with frequent leukocyte and platelet counts, liver and kidney function tests.

5-FLUOROURACIL

Adrucil, Efudex

NO ? D

Inj: 50 mg/mL (10, 50, 100 mL)
Topical, solution: 2%, 5%
Topical, cream: 5%
Antimetabolites

 Indication: Carcinoma of breast, colon, rectum, stomach, or pancreas, basal cell carcinoma, actinic or solar keratosis.

Initial dose:

Solid tumor: Various regimens, e.g., 12 mg/kg IV daily for 4 days; then if no toxicity, 6 mg/kg IV on days 6, 8, 10, 12.
Basal cell carcinoma: Use only 5% topical to affected areas bid.
Actinic/solar keratosis: Topical application to affected areas bid.
Max dose: 800 mg IV daily

 Adverse drug reaction: Nausea, vomiting, diarrhea, chest pain, dyspnea, esophagitis, leukopenia, infection, ulcerative stomatitis, hand and foot syndrome, anorexia, pruritic maculopapular rash.

Comments:

Avoid topical application to mucous membranes or irritated skin.

Monitor serum glucose level, renal and hepatic function tests, white blood cell count with differential, and platelet count.

Class contraindications: Hypersensitivity to the medication.

HYDROXYUREA

Hydrea, Droxia

YES X D

Caps: 500 mg (Hydrea)
200, 300, 400 mg (Droxia)
Antimetabolites

Indication: Head, neck, or ovarian carcinoma, chronic myelogenous leukemia, sickle cell anemia

Initial dose:

Cancer, leukemia: 20-30 mg/kg/day PO or 80 mg/kg PO q third day
Sickle cell anemia: 15 mg/kg daily
Renal dose: CrCl 10-50 mL/min: 50% dose
CrCl <10 mL/min: 20% dose

Adverse drug reaction: Anemia, leukopenia, thrombocytopenia; rare: hepatitis, pancreatitis, severe peripheral neuropathy.

Comments:

Monitor complete blood count with differential weekly.

Continued

For explanation of icons, see p. 1068.

FORMULARY

Antineoplastic—Antimetabolites

HYDROXYUREA *continued*

Contraindicated with marked bone marrow suppression (white blood cell count <2500/mm^3, platelet count <100,000/mm^3), severe anemia, or prior hypersensitivity to the medication.

MERCAPTOPURINE
Purinethol
Tabs, scored: 50 mg
Antimetabolites

NO   ?   D

Indication: Acute lymphoblastic leukemia, acute myelogenous leukemia, acute myelomonocytic leukemia
Initial dose: 2.5 mg/kg PO daily or 80-100 mg/m^2 PO daily; then adjust according to blood counts

Adverse drug reaction: Anemia, hepatotoxicity or biliary stasis, leukopenia, immunosuppression, infection, thrombocytopenia.
Comments:
Monitor complete blood count with differential, liver function tests weekly at initiation and monthly thereafter.
Drug/drug: Reduce dose 25%-33% when administered with allopurinol.
Contraindicated in prior hypersensitivity to the medication.

METHOTREXATE
Folex, Rheumatrex, Trexall
Tabs, scored: 2.5 mg (Rheumatrex)
Tabs: 5, 7.5, 10, 15 mg (Trexall)
Inj: 25, 50, 100, 250 mg (Folex)
Antimetabolites

YES   X   D

Indication: Acute leukemias, carcinoma of head, neck, lung, and breast, mycosis fungoides, lymphosarcoma, rheumatoid arthritis, psoriasis, meningeal leukemia.
Initial dose:
  Cancer, leukemia: Variable, e.g., 15-30 mg/day PO/IM for 5 days or 20-30 mg/m^2 PO/IM twice/wk
  Rheumatoid arthritis: 7.5 mg PO weekly
  Psoriasis: 10-25 mg PO/IM weekly
Renal dose: CrCl 10-50 mL/min: 50% dose
           CrCl <10 mL/min: Avoid
Hepatic dose: Bilirubin level 3.1-5 mg/dL: 75% dose

Continued

METHOTREXATE *continued*

Adverse drug reaction: Gastrointestinal ulceration, enteritis, intestinal perforation, leukopenia, bacterial infection, sepsis, thrombocytopenia, ulcerative stomatitis, nephrotoxicity.

Comments:

Use with caution in patients with "third spaces" (pleural effusions, ascites, etc.).

Person administering dose must be familiar with leucovorin rescue process.

Contraindicated in prior hypersensitivity to the medication, psoriasis and rheumatoid arthritis with concomitant alcoholism, alcoholic liver, chronic liver disease, immunodeficiency syndromes, or preexisting blood dyscrasias.

Biologicals

INTERFERON ALFA-2b, INTERFERON ALFA-2a

NO   ?   C

Intron A (2b), Roferon (2a)
Inj: 3, 5, 10, 18, 25, 50 million units (Intron)
Inj: 3, 6, 9, 18, 36 million units (Roferon)
Inj, prefilled pen: 3, 5, 10 million units (Intron)
Biologicals

Indication: Hairy cell leukemia, Kaposi's sarcoma, chronic hepatitis C, chronic myelogenous leukemia (2a only)

Initial dose:
   Leukemia: Various, e.g., 2-5 million units/m^2 SQ 3 daily
   Kaposi's sarcoma: 30 million units/m^2 IM/SQ 3 times/wk
   Chronic hepatitis C: 3 million units/m^2 IM/SQ 3 times/wk
Max dose: 36 million units daily

Adverse drug reaction: Neutropenia, thrombocytopenia, cardiotoxicity, thyroid changes, neurotoxicity, peripheral neuropathy, stomatitis, dry skin, leg cramps, rash, flulike symptoms, dry mouth, change in taste or vision, psychiatric symptoms.

Comments:

Ensure adequate hydration.

Class contraindications: Hypersensitivity to the medication.

For explanation of icons, see p. 1068.

Hormonal Agents

ANASTROZOLE

NO   ?   D

Arimidex
Tabs: 1 mg
Hormonal agents

Indication: Carcinoma of breast
Initial dose: 1 mg PO daily

Adverse drug reaction: Chest pain, dyspnea, peripheral edema, hot flushes, nausea, headache.
Comments: No glucocorticoid or mineral corticoid replacement treatment necessary.
Monitoring of complete blood count with differential, routine blood chemistry, liver function tests, and serum lipids is advised.
Class contraindications: Hypersensitivity to the medication.

BICALUTAMIDE

NO   X   X

Casodex
Tabs: 50 mg
Hormonal agents

Indication: Stage D_2 prostate cancer
Initial dose: 50 mg PO daily in combination with a luteinizing hormone–releasing hormone analog

Adverse drug reaction: Hot flashes, back pain, asthenia, headache, diarrhea, nausea, vomiting, anemia, peripheral edema, dizziness, dyspnea, gynecomastia; rare: liver injury.
Comments:
Class contraindications: Hypersensitivity to the medication.

FLUTAMIDE

Eulexin
Caps: 125 mg
Hormonal agents

NO   X   D

Indication: Carcinoma of prostate
Initial dose: 250 mg PO tid in combination with a luteinizing
hormone–releasing hormone analog

Adverse drug reaction: Hot flashes, gynecomastia, galactorrhea, back pain,
asthenia, headache, diarrhea, nausea, vomiting, anemia, peripheral edema,
dizziness, dyspnea; rare: hepatotoxicity.
Comments: Monitor serum transaminase levels at baseline and with symptoms
of liver dysfunction; discontinue if >2 times upper limit of normal.
Contraindicated in severe hepatic impairment, prior hypersensitivity to the
medication.

GOSERELIN

Zoladex
Inj, depot: 3.6, 10.8 mg
Hormonal agents

NO   X   X

Indication: Advanced carcinoma of prostate, endometriosis, breast cancer
Initial dose:
Endometriosis, breast cancer: 3.6 mg SQ implant q28 days
Prostate cancer: 3.6 mg SQ implant q28 days or 10.8 mg SQ implant q12 wk

Adverse drug reaction: Hot flashes, transient exacerbation of the tumor,
impotence, gynecomastia; rare: cardiac arrhythmias.
Comments:
Class contraindications: Hypersensitivity to the medication.

LETROZOLE

Femara
Tabs: 2.5 mg
Hormonal agents

YES   ?   D

Indication: Advanced carcinoma of breast
Initial dose: 2.5 mg PO daily
Renal dose: CrCl <10 mL/min: No data

Continued

LETROZOLE *continued*

Adverse drug reaction: Rare: chest pain, dyspnea, peripheral edema, hypertension, depression.
Comments:
Glucocorticoid replacement not required during letrozole administration.
Class contraindications: Hypersensitivity to the medication.

LEUPROLIDE

Lupron
Inj: 5 mg/mL
Inj, depot: 3.75, 7.5, 11.25, 22.5, 30 mg
Hormonal agents

NO   X   D

Indication: Carcinoma of prostate, endometriosis, uterine fibroids
Initial dose:
Carcinoma of prostate: 1 mg SQ daily, 7.5 mg IM depot q28 days, 22.5 mg IM depot q3 months, 30 mg IM depot q4 months
Endometriosis, uterine fibroids: 3.75 mg IM depot q28 days + iron, 11.25 mg IM depot q3 months + iron

Adverse drug reaction: Hot flashes, increased bone pain; rare: cardiac arrhythmias.
Comments:
Class contraindications: Hypersensitivity to the medication.

MEGESTROL

Megace
Oral liquid: 40 mg/mL (5 mL)
Tabs, scored: 20, 40 mg
Hormonal agents

NO   X   X

Indication: Breast or endometrial carcinoma; AIDS-associated cachexia
Initial dose:
Breast carcinoma: 160 mg PO divided q6h
Endometrial carcinoma: 40-320 mg/day PO in divided doses
Cachexia: 400-800 mg PO daily

Adverse drug reaction: Amenorrhea, menorrhagia, Cushing-like syndrome, hyperglycemia, carpal tunnel syndrome.
Comments:
Monitor for adrenal insufficiency if clinically warranted.
Class contraindications: Hypersensitivity to the medication.

NILUTAMIDE

Nilandron
Tabs: 50, 150 mg
Hormonal agents

NO ? C

Indication: Metastatic prostate carcinoma
Initial dose: 300 mg PO daily for 30 days, then 150 mg PO daily in
combination with a luteinizing hormone–releasing hormone analog

Adverse drug reaction: Anemia, dyspnea, edema, fever, infection, nausea,
diarrhea, hot flashes, constipation, gynecomastia, blurred vision.
Comments:
Start on the day after surgical castration.
Monitor serum transaminase levels at baseline and with symptoms of liver
dysfunction; discontinue if >2 times upper limit of normal; avoid concomitant
alcohol use.
Contraindicated in severe hepatic impairment, severe respiratory insufficiency,
or prior hypersensitivity to the medication.

TAMOXIFEN

Nolvadex
Tabs: 10, 20 mg
Hormonal agents

NO X D

Indication: Carcinoma of breast
Initial dose:
  Breast cancer: 20-40 mg PO daily
  Prophylaxis in high-risk patients: 20 mg PO daily for 5 yr
Max dose: >20 mg: Give divided bid

Adverse drug reaction: Rare: confusion, Stevens-Johnson syndrome,
hepatotoxicity, pulmonary embolism, thrombosis, vaginal discharge, uterine
sarcoma, endometrial cancer.
Comments:
Monitor complete blood count, calcium level, hepatic and renal function
periodically.
Contraindicated in women who require warfarin-type anticoagulant or have
history of deep venous thrombosis, pulmonary embolism, or hypersensitivity
to the medication.

For explanation of icons, see p. 1068.

TOREMIFENE

Fareston
Tabs: 60 mg
Hormonal agents

NO   ?   D

 Indication: Metastatic breast carcinoma
Initial dose: 60 mg PO daily

Comment:
Monitor complete blood count, calcium level, hepatic and renal function
periodically.
Adverse drug reaction: Nausea, vomiting, hot flashes; rare: hepatotoxicity,
hypercalcemia.
Class contraindications: Hypersensitivity to the medication.

Nitrogen Mustard Derivatives

CHLORAMBUCIL

Leukeran
Tabs: 2 mg
Nitrogen mustard derivatives

NO   ?   D

 Indication: Chronic lymphocytic leukemia, Hodgkin's and non-Hodgkin's
lymphoma
Initial dose: 0.1-0.2 mg/kg/day PO for 3-6 wk as required
0.4 mg/kg PO single-pulse dose, biweekly or monthly
Maintenance: 2-4 mg PO daily

Adverse drug reaction: Lymphopenia, leukopenia, neutropenia, infection,
immunosuppression, thrombocytopenia; rare: hepatotoxicity, pulmonary
fibrosis, peripheral neuropathy, seizures, Stevens-Johnson syndrome.
Comments:
Monitor complete blood count with differential.
Contraindicated with hypersensitivity to other alkylating agents or with prior
resistance to the medication.

MELPHALAN

Alkeran
Tabs, scored: 2 mg
Inj: 50 mg
Nitrogen mustard derivatives

YES ? D

Indication: Ovarian carcinoma; multiple myeloma
Initial dose:
  Ovarian carcinoma: 0.2 mg/kg/day PO for 5 days, repeat q4-5 wk
  Myeloma: 6 mg/day PO for 2-3 wk
      16 mg/m^2 IV q2 wk for 4 doses
      Repeat q4 wk
Renal dose: CrCl 10-50 mL/min: 70% dose
      CrCl <10 mL/min: 50% dose

Adverse drug reaction: Neutropenia, leukopenia, infection, thrombocytopenia, stomatitis.
Comments:
Must administer diluted solution within 60 minutes of preparation.
Monitor complete blood count with differential
Class contraindications: Hypersensitivity to the medication, prior resistance.

Plant Alkaloids

DOCETAXEL

Taxotere
Inj: 20, 80 mg (13% ethyl alcohol)
    40 mg/mL (0.5, 2 mL)
Plant alkaloids

NO X D

Indication: Resistant breast carcinoma; resistant non–small cell lung carcinoma
Initial dose:
  Breast carcinoma: 60-100 mg/m^2 IV q3 wk
  Lung carcinoma: 75 mg/m^2 q3 wk
Max dose: 100 mg/m^2

Adverse drug reaction: Severe neutropenia; anemia, fever, fluid retention, leukopenia, neutropenia, alopecia, nausea, vomiting , diarrhea, stomatitis, sensory neuropathy, hypersensitivity; rare; cardiotoxicity.
Comments:
Premedication with oral corticosteroids (dexamethasone 8 mg bid × 3 days) beginning 1 day before treatment.

Continued

DOCETAXEL *continued*

Monitor complete blood count with differential, liver and kidney function tests, serum electrolytes, electrocardiogram at baseline, then weekly.

Protect medication from light.

Dose increment: Do not administer the medication if the total bilirubin level is more than four times the upper limit of normal ($\times$ ULN) or if the transaminase levels are more than $1.5 \times$ ULN or the alkaline phosphatase level is more than $2.5 \times$ ULN.

Contraindicated in patients with prior hypersensitivity to polysorbate 80 or the medication or with neutrophil counts less than 1500 cells/mm^3.

PACLITAXEL

Taxol
Inj: 6 mg/mL (5, 16.7, 50 mL)
Plant alkaloids

NO   X   D

Indication: Ovarian, breast, non–small cell lung carcinoma, Kaposi's sarcoma
Initial dose:
Ovarian cancer: 135 mg/m^2 IV in combination with cisplatin, or 175 mg/m^2 IV q3 wk
Breast cancer: 175 mg/m^2 IV q3 wk
Non–small cell lung cancer: 135 mg/m^2 IV in combination with cisplatin
Kaposi's sarcoma: 135 mg/m^2 IV q3 wk or 100 mg/m^2 q2 wk

Adverse drug reaction: Anemia, hypersensitivity reaction, leukopenia, nausea or vomiting, thrombocytopenia, neutropenia, infection, peripheral neuropathy, hypotension, bradycardia.

Comments:

Infuse through 0.22 μm filter.

Monitor complete blood count with differential, liver and renal function, serum lipid levels, creatine phosphokinase level, blood pressure, and electrocardiogram periodically.

Pretreatment for hypersensitivity reaction with H$_2$ blocker, corticosteroid, and diphenhydramine required.

Vesicant: Never administer SQ or IM.

Contraindicated in patients with hypersensitivity to polyoxyethylated castor oil, baseline neutrophil count <1500/mm^3 or <1000/mm^3 in HIV-infected patients, or prior hypersensitivity to the medication.

VINCRISTINE

NO ? D

Oncovin, Vincasar PFS
Inj: 1 mg/mL (1, 2, 5 mL) (Oncovin, Vincasar PFS)
Plant alkaloids

Indication: Acute lymphoblastic leukemia, Hodgkin's or non-Hodgkin's
lymphoma
Initial dose: 1-2 mg/m^2 IV single dose q wk
Max dose: 2 mg/dose
Hepatic dose: Bilirubin level >3 mg/dL: 50% dose.

Adverse drug reaction: Constipation, painful or difficult urination, hyperuricemia,
uric acid nephropathy, progressive neurotoxicity.
Comments:
Monitor complete blood count with differential and liver function periodically.
Fatal if given intrathecally.
Vesicant: Never administer SQ or IM.
Contraindicated in patients with demyelinating form of Charcot-Marie-Tooth
syndrome or prior hypersensitivity to the medication.

Other Agents

PROCARBAZINE

NO X D

Matulane
Caps: 50 mg
Other Agents

Indication: Hodgkin's lymphoma
Initial dose: 2-4 mg/kg/day PO for 7 days, then 4-6 mg/kg/day PO until
maximum response
Maintenance: 1-2 mg/kg/day PO

Adverse drug reaction: Anemia, leukopenia, thrombocytopenia, central nervous
system stimulation, immunosuppression, infection, seizures, hemolytic
anemia, missed menstrual periods, pneumonitis, nausea, vomiting.
Comments:
Monitor complete blood count with differential and liver function.
No alcohol permitted because of disulfiram-like effect.
Drug/drug: Do not use with monoamine oxidase inhibitors or foods that have a
high tyramine content.
Contraindicated with inadequate marrow reserve demonstrated by bone
marrow aspiration or prior hypersensitivity to the medication.

Antineoplastic—Other Agents

For explanation of icons, see p. 1068.

THALIDOMIDE
Thalomid
Caps: 50, 100, 200 mg
Other Agents

NO ? X

Indication: Graft versus host disease (GVHD), erythema nodosum leprosum
Initial dose:
  GVHD: 800-1600 mg PO divided qid
  Erythema nodosum leprosum: 100-300 mg PO qhs until resolution of
           symptoms

Adverse drug reaction: Peripheral neuropathy, drowsiness, dizziness, rash, leukopenia, constipation.
Comments:
Monitor pregnancy test weekly in first month. Women must use two forms of contraception, men must use latex condoms during any sexual contact.
Follow STEPS program for drug procurement (phone: 1-888-423-5436).
Dosage increment: Adjust dose in GVHD to achieve minimum plasma levels 5 µg/mL (2 hr after dose).
Class contraindications: Hypersensitivity to the medication.

IMATINIB
Gleevec
Caps: 100 mg
Other Agents

NO X D

Indication: Chronic myelogenous leukemia
Initial dose:
  Accelerated/blast phase: 600-800 mg PO daily
  Chronic phase: 400 mg PO daily
Hepatic dose: Stop medication if liver function test (LFT) >5 times the upper limit of normal (× ULN) or bilirubin level >3 × ULN. Restart when LFT <2.5 × ULN or bilirubin level <1.5 × ULN.

Adverse drug reaction: Fluid retention, nausea, vomiting, neutropenia, thrombocytopenia, abdominal pain, diarrhea, muscle cramps.
Comments:
Drug/drug: Many cytochrome P450 drug interactions, such as carbamazepine, phenytoin, may increase drug levels; erythromycin and ketoconazole may decrease drug levels; levels of cyclosporine, simvastatin, and warfarin may be increased.
Class contraindications: Hypersensitivity to the medication.

ENDOCRINE
Thyroid
Thyroid Hormone Replacement Agents

LIOTHYRONINE

Cytomel, Triostat

NO ? A

Tabs: 5, 25, 50 µg
Thyroid, thyroid hormone replacement agents

Indication: Hypothyroidism, myxedema, T_3 suppression test
Initial dose:
  Hypothyroidism: 25 µg PO daily
  Myxedema: 5 µg PO daily
  T_3 suppression test: 75-100 µg PO daily × 7 days
Max dose: 100 µg daily

Comments:
Dosage increments 12.5-25 µg q1-2 wk.
Discontinue medication 7-10 days before radioactive iodine uptake study.
When switching from liothyronine to levothyroxine, initiate levothyroxine several
  days before stopping liothyronine.
Class side effects: Nervousness, insomnia, tremor, tachycardia; rare:
  arrhythmias, cardiac arrest.
Class contraindications: Hypersensitivity to the medication, untreated
  thyrotoxicosis, acute myocardial infarction, adrenal insufficiency.

THYROID, DESICCATED

Thyroid USP, Armour

NO ? A

Tabs: 15, 30, 60, 90, 120, 180, 240, 300 mg (Armour)
    15, 30, 60, 90, 120, 300 mg (Thyroid USP)
Thyroid, thyroid hormone replacement agents

Indication: Hypothyroidism
Initial dose: 30 mg PO daily
Max dose: 180 mg daily (clinical)

Comments:
Dosage increment 15 mg q2-3 wk.
Class side effects: Nervousness, insomnia, tremor, tachycardia; rare:
  arrhythmias, cardiac arrest.
Class contraindications: Hypersensitivity to the medication, untreated
  thyrotoxicosis, acute myocardial infarction, adrenal insufficiency.

LIOTRIX
Thyrolar

Tabs: 15, 30, 60, 120, 180 mg (thyroid equivalents)
Thyroid, thyroid hormone replacement agents

NO ? A

Indication: Hypothyroidism
Initial dose: 30 mg thyroid equivalents PO daily
Max dose: 180 mg daily (clinical)

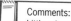

Comments:

Little advantage for this product (T_3/T_4 combination), since most patients convert T_4 to T_3 adequately and cost is not justified.

Dosage increment 15 mg q2-3 wk.

Class side effects: Nervousness, insomnia, tremor, tachycardia; rare: arrhythmias, cardiac arrest.

Class contraindications: Hypersensitivity to the medication, untreated thyrotoxicosis, acute myocardial infarction, adrenal insufficiency.

LEVOTHYROXINE
Levoxyl, Synthroid

Tabs: 25, 50, 75, 88, 100, 112, 125, 137, 150, 175, 200, 300 µg
Thyroid, thyroid hormone replacement agents

NO ? A

Indication: Hypothyroidism
Initial dose: 50-100 µg PO daily, 25 µg daily (coronary artery disease)
Max dose: 300 µg daily

Comments:

Dosage increment 25 µg.

Repeat measurement of thyroid-stimulating hormone 3-4 months after dosage change.

T_4 is treatment of choice in most cases (consistent potency, prolonged duration, restoration of normal balance between T_4 and T_3).

Class side effects: Nervousness, insomnia, tremor, tachycardia; rare: arrhythmias, cardiac arrest.

Drug/drug: Rifampin, carbamazepine, phenytoin (increase levothyroxine clearance), cholestyramine (do not administer together).

Class contraindications: Hypersensitivity to the medication, untreated thyrotoxicosis, acute myocardial infarction, adrenal insufficiency.

Antithyroid Agents

METHIMAZOLE

Tapazole
Tabs, scored: 5, 10 mg
Thyroid, antithyroid agents

NO   1   D

Indication: Hyperthyroidism
Initial dose: 15-60 mg PO daily divided tid depending on severity, until
euthyroid (15 mg daily if mild; 30-40 mg daily if moderate; 60 mg
daily if severe)
Maintenance: 5-15 mg PO daily

Comments:
Once the patient is euthyroid, start maintenance dose of 5-15 mg daily.
Adjust dosage after 4-8 weeks of therapy.
Drug/drug: Anti–vitamin K action potentiates warfarin. Additive effects with
hepatotoxic agents and bone marrow suppressants.
Monitor complete blood cell count and liver function tests if symptoms warrant;
doses >40 mg increase risk of agranulocytosis.
Lactation: Propylthiouracil preferred.
Class side effects: Rash, urticaria, fever, arthralgias, drowsiness; rare:
Agranulocytosis, leukopenia, thrombocytopenia, aplastic anemia, hepatitis,
vomiting.
Class contraindications: Hypersensitivity to the medication.

PROPYLTHIOURACIL

Tabs: 50 mg
Thyroid, antithyroid agents

NO   1   D

Indication: Hyperthyroidism
Initial dose: 300-450 mg daily divided tid
Maintenance: 100 mg PO daily divided tid

Comments:
Adjust dosage after 4-8 wk of therapy.
Drug/drug: Anti–vitamin K action potentiates warfarin. Additive effects with
hepatotoxic agents and bone marrow suppressants.
Monitor complete blood cell count and liver function tests if symptoms warrant;
doses >40 mg increase risk of agranulocytosis.
Class side effects: Anxiety, insomnia, nervousness, palpitations; rare:
Agranulocytosis, leukopenia, thrombocytopenia, aplastic anemia, hepatitis,
vomiting.
Class contraindications: Hypersensitivity to the medication.

For explanation of icons, see p. 1068.

Antirheumatic Agents
Nonsteroidal Antiinflammatory Drugs (NSAIDs), Cyclooxygenase 2 (Cox-2) Inhibitors

CELECOXIB

Celebrex
Caps: 100, 200 mg
Antirheumatic agents, NSAIDs, Cox-2 inhibitors

NO   3   C/D

Indication: Rheumatoid arthritis, osteoarthritis, familial adenomatous polyposis, pain (acute), primary dysmenorrhea.
Initial dose: 100-200 mg PO bid
Max dose: 400 mg

Adverse drug reaction: Headache, peripheral edema, dizziness, gastrointestinal effects (less likely than with NSAIDs).
Pregnancy category: D in third trimester.
Contraindicated in patients with allergy to sulfonamides.
Class contraindications: hypersensitivity to the medication, allergy to acetylsalicylic acid or NSAIDs.

ROFECOXIB

Vioxx
Tabs: 12.5, 25, 50 mg
Antirheumatic agents, NSAIDs, Cox-2 inhibitors

NO   3   C/D

Indication: Rheumatoid arthritis, osteoarthritis, dysmenorrhea, pain
Initial dose: 25 mg daily
           50 mg × 5 days (dysmenorrhea)
Max dose: 25 mg

Adverse drug reaction: Headache, peripheral edema, dizziness, gastrointestinal effects (less likely than with NSAIDs) , cardiovascular effects (VIGOR study).
Pregnancy category: D in third trimester.
Drug/drug: Aluminum and magnesium antacids (administer 1 hr apart).
Class contraindications: Hypersensitivity to the medication, allergy to acetylsalicylic acid or NSAIDs, advanced renal disease, severe hepatic insufficiency.

VALDECOXIB

Bextra
Tabs: 10, 20 mg
Antirheumatic agents, NSAIDs, Cox-2 inhibitors

NO   3   C/D

 Indication: Rheumatoid arthritis, osteoarthritis, dysmenorrhea
Initial dose: 10 mg daily
            20 mg bid prn (dysmenorrhea)
Max dose: 10 mg

Adverse drug reaction: Headache, peripheral edema, dizziness, gastrointestinal
    effects (less likely than with NSAIDs).
Pregnancy category: D in third trimester.
Drug/drug: Aluminum and magnesium antacids (administer 1 hr apart).
Class contraindications: Hypersensitivity to the medication, allergy to
    acetylsalicylic acid or NSAIDs, active peptic ulcer disease, advanced renal
    disease, severe hepatic insufficiency.

Disease-Modifying Arthritis Drugs

ETANERCEPT

Enbrel
Inj: 25 mg
Antirheumatic agents, disease-modifying arthritis drugs

NO   3   B

Indication: Rheumatoid arthritis, psoriatic arthritis
Initial dose: 25 mg single-use vial

Adverse drug reaction: Injection site reactions, increased risk of infections,
    development of autoantibodies, headache, rhinitis.
Comments:
Injection site reaction usually diminishes after first month.
Can be used in combination with methotrexate for patients who did not respond
    adequately.
Clinical responses seen in 2 wk to 3 months.
Contraindicated in patients with active infection (sepsis), concurrent live
    vaccinations.
Drug/herb: anakinra
Class contraindications: Hypersensitivity to the medication.

For explanation of icons, see p. 1068.

AZATHIOPRINE
Imuran
Tabs, scored: 50 mg
Antirheumatic agents, disease-modifying arthritis drugs

YES   ?   D

Indication: Rheumatoid arthritis
Initial dose: 1mg/kg PO daily or divided bid
Max dose: 2.5 mg/kg daily
Renal dose: CrCl 10-50 mL/min: 75% dose
               CrCl <10 mL/min: 50% dose

Adverse drug reaction: Severe leukopenia, nausea, vomiting; rare: bone
    marrow suppression, thrombocytopenia, hepatotoxicity, increased risk of
    infections and neoplasia, pancreatitis.
Comments:
Dosage increment 0.5 mg/kg daily after 8 and 12 wk, onset of action 6-8 wk.
Clinical efficacy may take up to 12 wk to see.
Monitoring: CBC and platelet count weekly × 1 month, twice monthly for second
    and third month, then monthly.
Drug/drug: When given with methotrexate, monitor complete blood cell count
    with platelets and liver function test monthly. Allopurinol inhibits metabolism;
    decrease azathioprine dose 33%-50%.
Class contraindications: Hypersensitivity to the medication, pregnancy.

CYCLOSPORINE
Neoral, Gengraf
Caps: 25, 100 mg
Oral solution: 100 mg/mL (50 mL)
Antirheumatic agents, disease-modifying arthritis drugs

NO   1   C

Indication: Rheumatoid arthritis
Initial dose: 2.5 mg/kg daily divided bid
Max dose: 4 mg/kg daily

Adverse drug reaction: Hypertension, nausea, vomiting, gum hyperplasia,
    tremor, headache, increased risk of infections; rare: seizures, nephrotoxicity,
    leukopenia, thrombocytopenia, anaphylaxis, hepatotoxicity.
Comments:
Dosage increment 0.5-0.75 mg/kg daily after 8 and 12 wk, onset of action 4-8
    wk, decrease 25%-50% to control side effects.
Drug/drug: Avoid nephrotoxic drugs, inhibitors and inducers of P450 3A4.
Drug/food: Grapefruit juice (increases trough levels).

Continued

CYCLOSPORINE *continued*

Monitor hepatic and renal function routinely.
Contraindicated in patients with rheumatoid arthritis, psoriasis, abnormal renal function, uncontrolled hypertension, malignancies.
Class contraindications: Hypersensitivity to the medication or to polyoxyethylated castor oil.

GOLD SODIUM THIOMALATE

Aurolate
Inj: 25 mg/mL, 50 mg/mL
Antirheumatic agents, disease-modifying arthritis drugs

YES   3   C

Indication: Rheumatoid arthritis
Initial dose: 10 mg IM wk 1, 25 mg wk 2
Max dose: 100 mg/dose
Renal dose: CrCl >50 mL/min: 50% of dose
CrCl <50 mL/min: Avoid use

Adverse drug reaction specific to medication: Itching, rash, stomatitis, urticaria, diarrhea, bradycardia, proteinuria, hematuria, metallic taste; rare: seizures, nephrotoxic syndrome, agranulocytosis, aplastic anemia, leukopenia, thrombocytopenia, anaphylaxis, hepatitis.
Comments:
Administer all gold salts intramuscularly, preferably intragluteally.
Normal color of drug is pale yellow.
Monitor complete blood cell count with differential and platelet count monthly; stop drug if platelet count <100,000/mm^3.
Urinalysis for protein before each injection.
Report of metallic taste usually predates stomatitis.
Dosage increment 10 mg IM q1-4 wk. If dosage reaches 1 g without effect, patient usually will not respond. Onset of action up to 3 mo.
Contraindicated in patients with severe debilitation, systemic lupus erythematosus, previous toxicity to gold products, hepatitis, exfoliative dermatitis, severe uncontrolled diabetes, renal disease, hepatic dysfunction, uncontrolled heart failure, severe hematological disorders, recent radiation therapy.
Drug/drug: Drugs known to cause blood dyscrasias.
Drug/lifestyle: Sun or ultraviolet light exposure.
Class contraindications: Hypersensitivity to the medication.

For explanation of icons, see p. 1068.

HYDROXYCHLOROQUINE

Plaquenil
Tabs: 200 mg (155 mg base)
Antirheumatic agents, disease-modifying arthritis drugs

NO   3   C

Indication: Rheumatoid arthritis, systemic lupus erythematosus
Initial dose: 400-600 mg (310-465 mg base) PO daily
400 mg (310 mg base) PO daily/bid
Maintenance: 200-400 mg PO daily

Adverse drug reaction: Muscle weakness; rare: agranulocytosis, leukopenia,
thrombocytopenia, hemolysis, aplastic anemia, seizures.
Comments:
Dosage increment reduced by half with response. Onset of action 4-12 wk.
Examine vision at baseline; monitor for changes.
Caution patient to avoid sun exposure.
Contraindicated with patients with hypersensitivity to 4-aminoquinoline
compounds, retinal or visual field changes, porphyria, severe gastrointestinal
and blood disorders.
Drug/drug: Monitor for digoxin toxicity.
Drug/laboratory: May cause inversion or depression of T wave or widening of
the QRS on the electrocardiogram.
Class contraindications: Hypersensitivity to the medication.

LEFLUNOMIDE

Arava
Tabs: 10, 20, 100 mg
Antirheumatic agents, disease-modifying arthritis drugs

NO   3   X

Indication: Rheumatoid arthritis
Initial dose: Load: 100 mg PO daily × 3 doses
Maintenance: 10-20 mg PO daily
Max dose: 20 mg daily

Adverse drug reaction: Diarrhea, respiratory infections, hypertension, alopecia,
rash; rare: allergic reaction.
Comments:
Monitor liver function tests at baseline and monthly until stable.
Men planning to father a child should discontinue drug therapy and follow
discontinuation protocol.

Continued

LEFLUNOMIDE *continued*

Guidelines for discontinuation: Alanine aminotransferase level >2 × upper limit of normal (ULN) = dosage reduction to 10 mg/day, >2 but <3 × ULN = liver biopsy recommended, >3 × ULN = discontinuation of leflunomide (protocol: cholestyramine 8 g tid for 11 days.)

Contraindicated in women who are or may become pregnant or who are breastfeeding, in patients with hepatic insufficiency, hepatitis B or C, severe immunodeficiency, or bone marrow dysplasia, and after vaccination with live vaccines.

Drug/drug: Methotrexate and other hepatotoxic drugs, rifampin (increased leflunomide levels).

Class contraindications: Hypersensitivity to the medication.

METHOTREXATE

Rheumatrex

Tabs, scored: 2.5 mg

Antirheumatic agents, disease-modifying arthritis drugs

YES   X   X

Indication: Rheumatoid arthritis
Initial dose: 7.5 mg PO weekly or
         7.5-15 mg IM once/wk
Max dose: 20 mg/wk PO
Renal dose: CrCl 10-50 mL/min: 50% dose
         CrCl <10 mL/min: Avoid use

Adverse drug reaction: Gastrointestinal intolerance, bone marrow toxicity, arachnoiditis (intrathecal), nausea, vomiting, tubular necrosis, rash, psoriatic lesions, urticaria, hyperpigmentation, photosensitivity, ecchymoses, pruritus; rare: neurotoxicity, necrotizing demyelinating leukoencephalopathy, seizures, renal failure, blood dyscrasias, hepatoxicity, pulmonary fibrosis, pneumonitis.

Comments:

Clinical response seen in 3-6 wk, maximum effect at 3 months.

Dosage increment by 2.5 mg every other wk to maximum of 20 mg weekly or response.

Baseline laboratory tests: complete blood count, platelet count, hepatic enzymes, renal function, and chest radiography.

Follow-up testing: hematological tests every month, renal and liver tests q1-2 months. May wish to monitor uric acid levels.

For prolonged use, perform baseline liver biopsy and repeat at each 1-1.5 g cumulative dose.

Consider folate supplementation, caution patient to avoid sunlight, force fluids (2-3 L/day).

Antidote is leucovorin administered within 1 hr.

Continued

METHOTREXATE *continued*

Contraindicated in patients with psoriasis or rheumatoid arthritis who have alcoholism, chronic liver disease, immunodeficiency syndromes, preexisting blood dyscrasias, and during pregnancy or breastfeeding.

Drug/drug: Avoid use of nonsteroidal antiinflammatory drugs with increased dosage regimens, probenecid (use lower dose of methotrexate), phenytoin (increased risk of seizures).

Drug/laboratory: May alter assay for folate.

Class contraindications: Hypersensitivity to the medication.

SULFASALAZINE

Azulfidine EN
Tabs, extended-release: 500 mg
Antirheumatic agents, disease-modifying arthritis drugs

NO 3 B

Indication: Rheumatoid arthritis
Initial dose: 500 mg PO daily wk 1, bid in wk 2
Max dose: 4 g daily

Adverse drug reaction: Nausea, vomiting, diarrhea, abdominal pain, anorexia, hypersensitivity reactions; rare: seizures, blood dyscrasias, erythema multiforme, Stevens-Johnson syndrome, exfoliative dermatitis, anaphylaxis.

Comments:

May turn body fluids or skin orange-yellow.

Dosage increment 500 mg q wk until 1 g bid. Onset of action 4-12 wk.

Most adverse reactions involve gastrointestinal tract (administer drug after food).

Contraindicated in patients with hypersensitivity to sulfonamides, salicylates, intestinal or urinary obstruction, porphyria, during pregnancy and at term, breastfeeding women.

Drug/drug: Antacids (increased absorption), antibiotics that alter intestinal flora (decreased efficacy), urine-acidifying agents (increased risk of crystalluria).

Drug/laboratory: May alter urine glucose tests.

Class contraindications: Hypersensitivity to the medication.

TUMOR NECROSIS FACTOR/ INFLIXAMAB

NO   X   C

Remicade
Inj: 100 mg/vial (20 mL)
Antirheumatic agents, disease-modifying arthritis drugs

Indication: Rheumatoid arthritis
Initial dose: 3 mg/kg at weeks 0, 2, 6, then q8 wk

Adverse drug reaction: Risk of infection, infusion-related reactions (dyspnea, flushing, headache, and rash), headache, nausea, fever, abdominal pain, antibody formation, lupuslike syndrome.
Comments:
Patient should receive tuberculin skin test before therapy.
If response inadequate, consider treating q4 wk or adjusting dose to 10 mg/kg.
Contraindicated in patients with hypersensitivity to murine proteins, active infection, concurrent live vaccination or New York Heart Association class III/IV congestive heart failure.
Class contraindications: Hypersensitivity to the medication.

Diabetes
Insulin Secretagogue Agents, First-Generation Sulfonylureas

CHLORPROPAMIDE

YES   3   C

Diabinese
Tabs, scored: 100, 250 mg
Diabetes, insulin secretagogue agents, first-generation sulfonylureas

Indication: Diabetes mellitus type 2
Initial dose: 250 mg PO daily
Max dose: 500 mg daily
Renal dose: CrCl <50 mL/min: Avoid use

Comments:
Avoid use in elderly because of long half-life.
Dosage increment 50-125 mg q5-7 wk.
Class side effects: Prolonged hypoglycemia, headache, gastrointestinal effects, weight gain, hyponatremia; rare: leukopenia, thrombocytopenia, aplastic anemia, agranulocytosis.
Drug/drug: β-Blockers mask and prolong hypoglycemia. Disulfiram-like effect.
Class contraindications: Hypersensitivity to the medication or other sulfonylureas, diabetes mellitus type 1 monotherapy, diabetic ketoacidosis with or without coma.

For explanation of icons, see p. 1068.

TOLAZAMIDE

Tolinase
Tabs, scored: 100, 250, 500 mg
Diabetes, insulin secretagogue agents, first-generation sulfonylureas

NO 3 C

Indication: Diabetes mellitus type 2
Initial dose: Fasting blood sugar >200 mg/dL: 250 mg PO daily
Fasting blood sugar <200 mg/dL: 100 mg PO daily
Max dose: 1 g daily

Comments:
Avoid use in elderly because of long half-life.
Dosage increment 50-125 mg q5-7 wk, >500 mg divided bid.
Drug/drug: β-Blockers mask and prolong hypoglycemia. Disulfiram-like effect.
Class side effects: Prolonged hypoglycemia, headache, gastrointestinal effects,
weight gain, hyponatremia; rare: leukopenia, thrombocytopenia, aplastic
anemia, agranulocytosis.
Class contraindications: Hypersensitivity to the medication or other
sulfonylureas, diabetes mellitus type 1 monotherapy, diabetic ketoacidosis
with or without coma.

TOLBUTAMIDE

Orinase
Tabs, scored: 500 mg
Diabetes, insulin secretagogue agents, first-generation sulfonylureas

NO 3 C

Indication: Diabetes mellitus type 2
Initial dose: 1 g PO daily or divided bid/tid
Max dose: 3 g daily

Comments:
Avoid use in elderly because of long half-life.
Drug/drug: β-Blockers mask and prolong hypoglycemia. Disulfiram-like effect.
Class side effects: Prolonged hypoglycemia, headache, gastrointestinal effects,
weight gain, hyponatremia; rare: leukopenia, thrombocytopenia, aplastic
anemia, agranulocytosis.
Class contraindications: Hypersensitivity to the medication or other
sulfonylureas, diabetes mellitus type 1 monotherapy, diabetic ketoacidosis
with or without coma.

FORMULARY

Insulin Secretagogue Agents, Second-Generation Sulfonylureas

GLIPIZIDE
Glucotrol, Glucotrol XR
Tabs, scored: 5, 10 mg
Tabs, extended-release: 2.5, 5, 10 mg
Insulin secretagogue agents, second-generation sulfonylureas

NO 3 C

Indication: Diabetes mellitus type 2
Initial dose: 5 mg PO daily
Max dose: 40 mg daily
20 mg XR daily

Adverse drug reaction: Asthenia.
Comments:
Dosage increment 2.5-5 mg q wk; ER formulation 5 mg q3 mo; >15 mg divided bid.
Drug/drug: β-Blockers mask and prolong hypoglycemia.
Class side effects: Hypoglycemia; rare: leukopenia, thrombocytopenia, aplastic anemia, agranulocytosis.
Class contraindications: Hypersensitivity to the medication, diabetic ketoacidosis with or without coma, diabetes mellitus type 1 monotherapy.

GLYBURIDE
DiaBeta, Glynase Pres-Tab, Micronase
Tabs, scored-micronized: 1.25, 2.5, 5 mg (DiaBeta, Micronase)
Tabs, scored: 1.5, 3, 6 mg (Pres-Tab)
Insulin secretagogue agents, second-generation sulfonylureas

YES 3 C

Indication: Diabetes mellitus type 2
Initial dose: 2.5-5 mg PO daily; 1.5-3 mg PO daily (micronized)
Max dose: 20 mg daily; 12 mg daily (micronized)
Renal dose: Use with caution

Adverse drug reaction: Rare: angioedema.
Comments:
Dosage increment 2.5 mg q wk; >10 mg divided bid.
Drug/drug: β-Blockers mask and prolong hypoglycemia.
Class side effects: Hypoglycemia; rare: leukopenia, thrombocytopenia, aplastic anemia, agranulocytosis.
Class contraindications: Hypersensitivity to the medication, diabetic ketoacidosis with or without coma, diabetes mellitus type 1 monotherapy.

Endocrine—Diabetes

For explanation of icons, see p. 1068.

GLIMEPIRIDE
Amaryl
Tabs: 1, 2, 4 mg
Insulin secretagogue agents, second-generation sulfonylureas

NO   3   C

Indication: Diabetes mellitus type 2
Initial dose: 1 mg PO daily
Max dose: 8 mg daily

Comments:
Dosage increment 1-2 mg q1-2 wk.
Drug/drug: β-Blockers mask and prolong hypoglycemia.
Secondary mechanisms include decreased basal gluconeogenesis, enhanced
   insulin sensitivity.
Class side effects: Hypoglycemia; rare: leukopenia, thrombocytopenia, aplastic
   anemia, agranulocytosis.
Class contraindications: Hypersensitivity to the medication, diabetic
   ketoacidosis with or without coma, diabetes mellitus type 1 monotherapy.

Insulin Secretagogue Agents, Meglitinides

REPAGLINIDE
Prandin
Tabs: 0.5, 1, 2 mg
Insulin secretagogue agents, meglitinides

NO   3   C

Indication: Diabetes mellitus type 2
Initial dose: 0.5 mg PO bid/qid depending on meal patterns
Max dose: 16 mg daily

Comments:
If the patient misses a meal, he or she should skip a dose.
Class side effects: Hypoglycemia, headache, nausea; rare: diarrhea, arthralgia.
Class contraindications: Hypersensitivity to the medication, diabetic
   ketoacidosis with or without coma, diabetes mellitus type 1 monotherapy.

NATEGLINIDE

Starlix
Tabs: 60, 120 mg
Insulin secretagogue agents, meglitinides

NO 3 C

 Indication: Diabetes mellitus type 2
Initial dose: 120 mg PO tid depending on meal patterns

 Comments:
If the patient misses a meal, he or she should skip a dose.
Class side effects: Hypoglycemia, headache, nausea; rare: diarrhea, arthralgia.
Class contraindications: Hypersensitivity to the medication, diabetic
    ketoacidosis with or without coma, diabetes mellitus type 1 monotherapy.

Insulin Sensitizing Agents, Biguanides

METFORMIN

Glucophage, Glucophage-XR
Tabs: 500, 850, 1000 mg
Tabs, extended-release: 500 mg
Insulin sensitizing agents, biguanides

YES ? B

Indication: Diabetes mellitus type 2
Initial dose: 500 mg PO with evening meal
Max dose: 2550 mg daily; 2 g ER
Renal dose: CrCl <50 mL/min: 50% dose
    CrCl 10-50 mL/min: 25% dose
    CrCl <10 mL/min: Avoid use

 Comments:
Dosage increment 500 mg q wk or 850 mg every other wk.
Withhold doses for hypoxemic patients, nothing by mouth (NPO) status, acute
    renal insufficiency, scheduled IV contrast studies.
Class side effects: Nausea, diarrhea, abdominal bloating and pain, weight loss,
    rash, urticaria; rare: megaloblastic anemia, lactic acidosis.
Class contraindications: Renal disease (serum creatinine level >1.5 mg/dL in
    males, >1.4 mg/dL in females), hepatic disease, congestive heart failure
    requiring drug therapy, acute or chronic metabolic acidosis, diabetic
    ketoacidosis with or without coma, contrast agents (stop at time of study;
    restart after 48 hr and normalization of serum creatinine level).

For explanation of icons, see p. 1068.

Insulin Sensitizing Agents, Thiazolidinediones

ROSIGLITAZONE

Avandia
Tabs: 2, 4, 8 mg
Insulin sensitizing agents, thiazolidinediones

NO   ?   C

Indication: Diabetes mellitus type 2
Initial dose: 4 mg PO daily or divided bid
Max dose: 8 mg daily

Comments:

Monitor alanine aminotransferase (ALT) level at baseline and every 2 mo for first yr, then periodically. Hemoglobin and hematocrit values may decrease during first 4-8 wk of therapy.

Lipid changes include increased levels of total cholesterol and low- and high-density lipoproteins.

Dosage increment 4 mg q12 wk.

Class side effects: Weight gain, headache, edema, anemia, liver function test abnormalities (increases), alterations in cholesterol.

Class contraindications: Hypersensitivity to the medication, active liver disease or ALT >2.5 × upper limit of normal, New York Heart Association class III or IV heart failure, diabetes mellitus type 1, diabetic ketoacidosis, history of jaundice while receiving medication.

PIOGLITAZONE

Actos
Tabs: 15, 30, 45 mg
Insulin sensitizing agents, thiazolidinediones

NO   ?   C

Indication: Diabetes mellitus type 2
Initial dose: 15 mg PO daily
Max dose: 45 mg daily

Comments:

Dosage increment 15 mg every 8-12 wk.

Favorable effect of lipid panel (decreases triglyceride, increases high-density lipoprotein).

Class side effects: Weight gain, headache, edema, anemia, liver function test abnormalities (increases), alterations in cholesterol.

Class contraindications: Hypersensitivity to the medication, active liver disease or alanine aminotransferase level >2.5 × upper limit of normal, New York Heart Association class III or IV heart failure, diabetes mellitus type 1, diabetic ketoacidosis, history of jaundice while receiving medication.

Other Diabetes Agents, α-Glucosidase Inhibitors

ACARBOSE

Precose
Tabs: 25, 50, 100 mg
Other diabetes agents, α-glucosidase inhibitors

YES ? B

Indication: Diabetes mellitus type 2
Initial dose: 25 mg PO tid with first bite of food
Max dose: 50 mg tid (<60 kg)
100 mg tid (>60 kg)
Renal dose: CrCl >50 mL/min: 50%-100% dose
CrCl <50 mL/min: Avoid use

Comments:
Dosage increment q4-8 wk.
Must take with first bite of each meal.
When used alone, does not cause hypoglycemia.
When used in combination, if hypoglycemia occurs, treat with oral glucose
(dextrose).
Monitor serum trasaminase levels q3 months during first year and then
periodically when using doses exceeding 50 mg tid.
Class side effects: Diarrhea, abdominal pain, flatulence, liver function test
abnormalities (increases).
Class contraindications: Hypersensitivity to the medication, diabetic
ketoacidosis, cirrhosis, irritable bowel disease, colonic ulceration, intestinal
obstruction, disorders of digestion or absorption.

MIGLITOL

Glyset
Tabs, scored*: 25, 50*, 100 mg
Other diabetes agents, α-glucosidase inhibitors

YES ? B

Indication: Diabetes mellitus type 2
Initial dose: 25 mg PO tid with first bite of food
Max dose: 100 mg tid
Renal dose: Serum creatine level >2 mg/dL: Avoid use

Comments:
Dosage increment q4-8 wk.
Class side effects: Diarrhea, abdominal pain, flatulence, liver function test
abnormalities (increases).
Class contraindications: Hypersensitivity to the medication, diabetic
ketoacidosis, cirrhosis, irritable bowel disease, colonic ulceration, intestinal
obstruction, disorders of digestion or absorption.

For explanation of icons, see p. 1068.

Other Diabetes Agents, Combination Agents

GLYBURIDE/METFORMIN

Glucovance
Tabs: 1.25/250, 2.5/500, 5/500 mg
Other diabetes agents, Combination agents

 Indication: Diabetes mellitus type 2

GLIPIZIDE/METFORMIN

Metaglip
Tabs: 2.5/500, 5/500 mg
Other Diabetes Agents, Combination Agents

 Indication: Diabetes mellitus type 2

METFORMIN/ROSIGLITAZONE

Avandamet
Tabs: 500/1, 500/2, 500/4 mg
Other Diabetes Agents, Combination Agents

 Indication: Diabetes mellitus type 2

Other Diabetic Agents, Insulin Agents

INSULIN LISPRO

Humalog
Other diabetic agents, insulin agents

YES 3 B

 Onset (hr): 0.5-1.5
Peak (hr): 0.5-1.5
Duration (hr): 6-8

 Class side effects: Hypoglycemia, weight gain; rare: lipoatrophy, lipohypertrophy.
Class contraindications: Hypoglycemia.

INSULIN REGULAR

Novolin R, Humulin R
Other diabetic agents, insulin agents

YES   3   B

 Onset (hr): 0.5-1
Peak (hr): 2-3
Duration (hr): 8-12

 Class side effects: Hypoglycemia, weight gain; rare: lipoatrophy, lipohypertrophy.
Class contraindications: Hypoglycemia.

INSULIN ASPARTATE

Novolog
Other diabetic agents, insulin agents

YES   3   C

 Onset (hr): 0.5
Peak (hr): 1-3
Duration (hr): 3-5

Class side effects: Hypoglycemia, weight gain; rare: lipoatrophy, lipohypertrophy.
Class contraindications: Hypoglycemia.

INSULIN ISOPHANE SUSPENSION, NPH

Novolin N, Humulin N
Other diabetic agents, insulin agents

YES   3   B

 Onset (hr): 1-1.5
Peak (hr): 4-12
Duration (hr): 24

 Class side effects: Hypoglycemia, weight gain; rare: lipoatrophy, lipohypertrophy.
Class contraindications: Hypoglycemia.

For explanation of icons, see p. 1068.

INSULIN ZINC SUSPENSION, LENTE

Novolin L, Humulin L
Other diabetic agents, insulin agents

YES 3 B

Onset (hr): 1-2.5
Peak (hr): 8-12
Duration (hr): 18-24

Class side effects: Hypoglycemia, weight gain; rare: lipoatrophy,
lipohypertrophy.
Class contraindications: Hypoglycemia.

INSULIN EXTENDED ZINC, ULTRALENTE

Humulin U
Other diabetic agents, insulin agents

YES 3 B

Onset (hr): 4-8
Peak (hr): 16-18
Duration (hr): >36

Class side effects: Hypoglycemia, weight gain; rare: lipoatrophy,
lipohypertrophy.
Class contraindications: Hypoglycemia.

INSULIN GLARGINE

Lantus
Other diabetic agents, insulin agents

YES 3 C

Duration (hr): 24

Comments:
Lantus must not be diluted or mixed with any other insulin.
Class side effects: Hypoglycemia, weight gain; rare: lipoatrophy,
lipohypertrophy.
Class contraindications: Hypoglycemia.

Other Diabetes Agents, Combination Products

ISOPHANE REGULAR
Humulin or Novolin 70/30: 50% regular + 50% NPH
Humulin or Novolin 70/30: 30% regular + 70% NPH
Other diabetes agents, combination products

Onset (hr): 0.5
Peak (hr): 2-12
Duration (hr): 24

LISPRO PROTAMINE/LISPRO

Humalog mix 50/50: 50% Lispro protamine + 50% Lispro
Humalog mix 75/25: 75% Lispro protamine + 25% Lispro
Other diabetes agents, combination products

GASTROINTESTINAL
H$_2$-Receptor Antagonists

CIMETIDINE
Tagamet
Tabs: 200, 300, 400, 800 mg
Oral liquid: 300 mg/5mL
Inj: 300 mg/2 mL
Solution, inj: 300 mg/50 mL in 0.9% NS
H$_2$-receptor antagonists

YES   1   B

Indication: Active duodenal or gastric ulcers, hypersecretory conditions, gastroesophageal reflux disease (GERD)
Initial dose:
  Ulcers, hypersecretory conditions: 400 mg PO bid or 800 mg PO qhs or 300 IM/IV q6-8h

  GERD: 800 mg PO bid
Max dose: 2.4 g PO/IV/IM daily
Renal dose: CrCl 10-50 mL/min: 50% dose
           CrCl <10 mL/min: 25% dose

Continued

For explanation of icons, see p. 1068.

CIMETIDINE *continued*

Adverse drug reaction: Mental status changes, diarrhea; rare: agranulocytosis, neutropenia, thrombocytopenia, aplastic anemia.

Comments:

Active treatment for 4-8 weeks.

Drug/drug: May decrease metabolism of phenytoin, benzodiazepines, disulfiram, metronidazole, warfarin. May affect absorption of medications that require low pH (e.g., ketoconazole).

Administer before meals for prevention of symptoms.

Class side effects: Headache; rare: somnolence, dizziness, liver function test abnormalities (increase), rash.

Class contraindications: Hypersensitivity to the medication.

FAMOTIDINE

Pepcid, Pepcid AC
Tabs: 10 (OTC), 20, 40 mg
Oral liquid: 40 mg/5mL
Inj: 10 mg/mL
H₂-receptor antagonists

YES   ?   B

Indication: Active duodenal or gastric ulcers, gastroesophageal reflux disease (GERD), hypersecretory conditions, heartburn

Initial dose:
  Ulcers, GERD: 40 mg PO qhs or 20 mg PO bid
  Hypersecretory conditions: 20 mg PO q6h
  Heartburn: (OTC) 10 mg PO daily/bid
Max dose: 160 mg q6h
Self-medication: 10 mg bid × 2 wk
Renal dose: CrCl 10-50 mL/min: 25% dose
            CrCl <10 mL/min: 10% dose

Comments:

Administer before meals for prevention of symptoms.

Drug/drug: May affect absorption of medications that require low pH (e.g., ketoconazole).

Lactation: Less concentrated in milk.

Class side effects: Headache; rare: somnolence, dizziness, liver function test abnormalities (increase), rash.

Class contraindications: Hypersensitivity to the medication.

NIZATIDINE
Axid, Axid AR
Tabs: 75 mg (OTC)
Caps: 150, 300 mg
H₂-receptor antagonists

YES ? B

Indication: Active duodenal or gastric ulcers, gastroesophageal reflux disease (GERD), heartburn
Initial dose:
  Ulcers, GERD: 300 mg PO qhs or 150 mg PO bid
  Heartburn: (OTC) 75 mg PO bid, 30-60 min before meals
Max dose: Self-medication: 2 tabs/day × 2 wk
Renal dose: CrCl 10-50 mL/min: 50% dose
       CrCl <10 mL/min: 25% dose

Adverse drug reaction: Rare: arrhythmias.
Comments:
Administer before meals for prevention of symptoms.
Drug/drug: May affect absorption of medications that require low pH (e.g., ketoconazole).
Lactation: Less concentrated in milk.
Class side effects: Headache; rare: somnolence, dizziness, liver function test abnormalities (increase), rash.
Class contraindications: Hypersensitivity to the medication.

RANITIDINE
Zantac
Tabs: 75, 150, 300 mg
Oral liquid: 75 mg/5 mL
Granules, effervescent: 150 mg
Solution, inj: 50 mg in 50 mL of 0.9% NS
H₂-receptor antagonists

YES ? B

Indication: Active duodenal or gastric ulcers, gastroesophageal reflux disease (GERD), hypersecretory conditions, erosive esophagitis
Initial dose:
  Ulcers: 150 mg PO bid or 300 mg PO qhs
  GERD, hypersecretory conditions, erosive esophagitis: 150 mg PO bid
  IV (intermittent or infusion): 50 mg IV/IM q6-8h
Max dose: 6 g daily
       Self-medication: 150 mg daily × 2 wk
Renal dose: CrCl 10-50 mL/min: 50% dose
       CrCl <10 mL/min: 25% dose

Continued

RANITIDINE *continued*

Adverse drug reaction: Rare: pancytopenia, granulocytopenia,
   thrombocytopenia, anaphylaxis.
Comments:
Administer before meals for prevention of symptoms.
Drug/drug: May affect absorption of medications that require low pH (e.g.,
   ketoconazole).
Contraindicated in patients with acute porphyria or prior hypersensitivity to the
   medication.
Class side effects: Headache; rare: somnolence, dizziness, liver function test
   abnormalities (increase), rash.

Proton Pump Inhibitors

OMEPRAZOLE

Prilosec
Caps, delayed-release: 10, 20 mg
Proton pump inhibitors

NO X C

Indication: Active duodenal ulcer, gastric ulcer, gastroesophageal reflux
            disease (GERD), hypersecretory conditions, erosive esophagitis,
            Helicobacter pylori
Initial dose:
   Active duodenal ulcer, GERD, erosive esophagitis: 20 mg PO daily
   Gastric ulcer: 40 mg PO daily
   H. pylori: 40 mg PO daily in multidrug regimen
   Hypersecretory conditions: 60 mg PO daily
Max dose: 120 mg tid (>80 mg: use divided dosing)

Comments:
Can be administered via a nasogastric tube; generic omeprazole now available
Drug/drug: may decrease metabolism of diazepam, phenytoin, propranolol,
   warfarin. May affect absorption of medications that require low pH (e.g.,
   ketoconazole).
Class side effects: Rare: headache, diarrhea, abdominal pain, rash,
   constipation, cough, dizziness.
Class contraindications: Hypersensitivity to the medication.

LANOPRAZOLE

NO   X   B

Prevacid
Caps, delayed-release: 15, 30 mg
Oral packet: 15 mg
Proton pump inhibitors

Indication: Active duodenal ulcer, gastric ulcer, gastroesophageal reflux disease (GERD), hypersecretory conditions, *Helicobacter pylori*, erosive esophagitis

Initial dose:
  Active duodenal ulcer, GERD: 15 mg PO daily
  Gastric ulcer: 30 mg PO daily
  H pylori: 30 mg bid in multidrug regimen
  Hypersecretory conditions: 60 mg PO daily
Max dose: No therapeutic benefit to 60-mg dose in ulcer/erosive esophagitis
  Hypersecretory conditions: >120 mg: use divided doses

Comments:
Can be administered via a nasogastric tube.
Drug/drug: May affect absorption of medications that require low pH (e.g., ketoconazole).
Class side effects: Rare: headache, diarrhea, abdominal pain, rash, constipation, cough, dizziness.
Class contraindications: Hypersensitivity to the medication.

PANTOPRAZOLE

NO   X   B

Protonix
Tabs, delayed-release: 20, 40 mg
Inj: 40 mg
Proton pump inhibitors

Indication: Gastroesophageal reflux disease (GERD), Zollinger-Ellison syndrome, acute nonvariceal upper gastrointestinal bleeding (GIB) (not FDA approved)

Initial dose:
  GERD: 40 mg PO daily
  Zollinger-Ellison syndrome: 80 mg IV q12h
  Acute variceal upper GIB:
  Load: 80 mg IV, then 8 mg/hr × 72 hr
  Maintenance: 40 mg PO daily (not approved)

Continued

PANTOPRAZOLE *continued*

Comments:
Drug/drug: May affect absorption of medications that require low pH (e.g., ketoconazole).
Class side effects: Rare: headache, diarrhea, abdominal pain, rash, constipation, cough, dizziness.
Class contraindications: Hypersensitivity to the medication.

RABEPRAZOLE
Aciphex
Tabs, delayed-release: 20 mg
Proton pump inhibitors

NO X B

Indication: Active duodenal ulcer, gastroesophageal reflux disease (GERD), hypersecretory conditions
Initial dose:
  Active duodenal ulcer, GERD: 20 mg PO daily
  Hypersecretory conditions: 60 mg PO daily
Max dose: 100 mg daily, or 60 mg bid

Comments:
Drug/drug: May affect absorption of medications that require low pH (e.g., ketoconazole).
Class side effects: Rare: headache, diarrhea, abdominal pain, rash, constipation, cough, dizziness.
Class contraindications: Hypersensitivity to the medication.

ESOMEPRAZOLE
Nexium
Tabs, delayed-release: 20, 40 mg
Proton pump inhibitors

NO X B

Indication: Gastroesophageal reflux disease, erosive esophagitis
Initial dose: 20-40 mg PO daily
Max dose: 40 mg daily

Comments:
Drug/drug: May affect absorption of medications that require low pH (e.g., ketoconazole).
Class side effects: Rare: headache, diarrhea, abdominal pain, rash, constipation, cough, dizziness.
Class contraindications: Hypersensitivity to the medication.

NEUROLOGY
Antiepileptic Agents

PHENYTOIN
Dilantin

NO 1 D

Caps, extended-release: 30, 100 mg
Caps: 100 mg
Tabs, chewable: 50 mg
Oral liquid: 125 mg/5 mL (5 mL, 240 mL)
Injection: 50 mg/mL (2 mL, 5 mL) (ethyl alcohol 10%, propylene glycol 40%)
Antiepileptic agents

Indication: Tonic-clonic seizures, status epilepticus, nonepileptic seizures
Initial dose:
    Tonic-clonic, status epilepticus, nonepileptic seizures:
        Load: 10-15 mg/kg IV daily or 1 g PO divided (400, 300, 300 mg) by 2 hr
        Maintenance: 200-300 mg PO daily (extended-release) or divided tid
    Max dose: 50 mg/min IV

Adverse drug reaction: Nystagmus, ataxia, slurred speech, diplopia, confusion, nausea, vomiting, toxic hepatitis, hirsutism, dizziness, osteomalacia, gingival hyperplasia; rare: Stevens-Johnson syndrome, peripheral neuropathy, toxic epidermal necrolysis, pancytopenia, thrombocytopenia, leukopenia, agranulocytosis

Comments:

Dosage increment 100 mg q2-4 wk, therapeutic level 10-20 µg/mL. Do not stop abruptly.

Avoid intramuscular administration.

Drug/drug: Allopurinol, amiodarone, diazepam, fluconazole, isoniazid may increase levels. Barbiturates, carbamazepine, rifampin may decrease levels. Phenytoin may decrease amiodarone, cyclosporine, meperidine levels.

Stop enteral feedings 2 hr before or after phenytoin dose.

Contraindicated in patients with prior hypersensitivity to the medication or in patients with sinus bradycardia, second- or third-degree atrioventricular block, or Adams-Stokes syndrome in patients using the IV formulation.

Class contraindications: Hypersensitivity to the medication.

For explanation of icons, see p. 1068.

CARBAMAZEPINE

Tegretol, Carbatrol, Epitol, Tegretol XR

Tabs, scored, chewable*: 100*, 200 mg (Epitol, Tegretol*)   NO   1   D
Tabs, extended-release: 100, 200, 400 mg (Tegretol XR)
Caps, extended-release: 200, 300 mg (Carbatrol)
Oral liquid: 100 mg/5 mL
Antiepileptic agents

Indication: Tonic-clonic seizures, partial with complex symptoms, mixed seizures, neuralgia (trigeminal, glossopharyngeal), resistant acute mania (not approved by Food and Drug Administration)

Initial dose:
  Seizures, mania: 200 mg PO bid or 100 mg PO qid (liquid)
  Neuralgia: 100 mg PO bid
Max dose: 1.2 g daily
Hepatic dose: Active liver disease—not recommended.

Adverse drug reaction: Drowsiness, dizziness, diplopia, ataxia, blurred vision, nausea, vomiting, increase in liver transaminases, rare: arrhythmia, atrioventricular block, aplastic anemia, agranulocytosis, thrombocytopenia, hyponatremia, leukopenia, Stevens-Johnson syndrome, peripheral neuropathy, water retention.

Comments:

Dosage increment 200 mg q wk, therapeutic level 4-12 μg/mL. Do not stop abruptly.

Convert from regular to sustained release using same daily dose.

Monitor complete blood count with reticulocytes, serum iron, renal and liver function: baseline and periodically.

Drug/drug: Autoinduction occurs during initial 3-5 weeks of therapy. Verapamil, fluoxetine, valproic acid, erythromycin may increase levels. Phenytoin, primidone, phenobarbital may decrease levels. Carbamazepine may decrease phenytoin, warfarin, haloperidol levels.

Contraindicated in patients with history of bone marrow suppression, prior hypersensitivity to tricyclic antidepressants, or for use in combination with or within 14 days of discontinuation of a monoamine oxidase inhibitor.

Class contraindications: Hypersensitivity to the medication.

OXCARBAZEPINE

Trileptal
Tabs, scored: 150, 300, 600 mg
Oral liquid: 300 mg/5 mL (250 mL)
Antiepileptic agents

YES ? C

Indication: Partial seizures
Initial dose: 600 mg PO daily
Max dose: 1.2-2.4 g PO daily
Renal dose: CrCl <30 mL/min: 50% initial dose

Adverse drug reaction: Hyponatremia, somnolence, dizziness, diplopia, fatigue,
ataxia, nausea, vomiting, abnormal vision, abdominal pain, tremor,
dyspepsia, cross-reaction with carbamazepine 25%.
Comments:
Monitor serum electrolytes frequently.
Dosage increment 300 q3 days. Do not stop abruptly. Target dose 1200 mg
daily.
Drug/drug: Verapamil, phenytoin, carbamazepine, phenobarbital may decrease
levels.
Monitor serum sodium levels. Use caution with other medications that lower
serum sodium levels.
Contraindicated with prior hypersensitivity to the medication.

PHENOBARBITAL

Tabs: 15, 16, 30, 32, 60, 65, 100 mg
Oral liquid: 20 mg/5 mL
Antiepileptic agents

YES X D

Indication: Tonic-clonic seizures, partial seizures
Initial dose: 60-250 mg PO qhs or 2-3 mg/kg/day
Max dose: 600 mg PO daily or 60 mg/min IV push
Renal dose: CrCl <10 mL/min: q12-16h

Adverse drug reaction: Sedation, dizziness; rare: peripheral neuropathy,
respiratory depression, apnea, angioedema, Stevens-Johnson syndrome.
Comments:
Monitor: Serum levels 15-40 µg/mL.
Dosage increment: Full anticonvulsant effect requires 2-3 wk. Do not stop
abruptly.

Continued

PHENOBARBITAL *continued*

> Drug/drug: Use caution with other central nervous system and respiratory depressant medication. Valproic acid, disulfiram decrease metabolism. Phenobarbital increases metabolism of estrogen, theophylline, corticosteroids, warfarin, clozepine, cyclosporine.
>
> Contraindicated in prior hypersensitivity to the medication or any of the barbiturates, marked impairment of liver function, porphyria.

PRIMIDONE

Mysoline
Tabs, scored*: 50, 250* mg
Tabs, chewable: 125 mg
Oral liquid: 250 mg/5 mL (240 mL)
Antiepileptic agents

YES   3   D

> **Indication:** Partial, complex, tonic-clonic seizures
> **Initial dose:** 100-125 mg PO qhs × 3-5 days
> **Max dose:** 2 g PO divided tid
> **Renal dose:** CrCl <10 mL/min: q12-24h

> Adverse drug reaction: Ataxia, drowsiness, vertigo, lethargy, anorexia, nausea, vomiting; rare: thrombocytopenia, megaloblastic anemia, granulocytopenia, systemic lupus erythematosus–like disease.
>
> Comments:
>
> Dosage increment 125 mg q5 days to goal 250 mg tid, therapeutic levels 5-12 μg/mL. Do not stop abruptly.
>
> Drug/drug: Use caution with other central nervous system and respiratory depressant medication. Valproic acid, disulfiram decrease metabolism. Phenobarbital increases metabolism of estrogen, theophylline, corticosteroids, warfarin, clozepine, cyclosporine.
>
> Twenty percent of drug is metabolized to phenobarbital.
>
> Contraindicated in patients with hypersensitivity to barbiturates or history of latent porphyria.

VALPROIC ACID

Depakote, Depakene, Depacon
Caps: 250 mg

NO 1 D

Oral liquid: 50 mg/mL (480 mL) (Depakene)
Caps, sprinkle: 125 mg (Depakote)
Tabs, delayed-release: 125, 250, 500 mg (Depakote)
Tabs, extended-release: 500 mg (Depakote ER)
Inj: 100 mg/mL (5 mL) (Depacon)
Antiepileptic agents

Indication: Absence seizures, atypical absence seizures, complex partial
seizures, mania, migraine headaches
Initial dose:
  Seizures: 10-15 mg/kg PO divided bid/tid
  Mania: 750 mg PO in divided doses
  Migraine: 250 mg PO bid or 500 mg extended release PO daily
Max dose: 60 mg/kg daily
Hepatic dose: Active liver disease—not recommended

Adverse drug reaction: Nausea, vomiting, indigestion, increased LFTs; rare:
  alopecia, hepatic failure, systemic lupus erythematosus, thrombocytopenia,
  leukopenia, bone marrow suppression, sedation, hyperammonemia,
  pancreatitis.
Comments:
Dosage increment: 5-10 mg/kg q wk, therapeutic levels 50-100 μg/mL.
Depakote has a bid dosage. Do not stop abruptly.
Monitor liver function tests and complete blood count: Baseline, then frequently
  for the first 6 mo.
Drug/drug: Rifampin induces metabolism.
Contraindicated in hepatic disease and prior hypersensitivity to the medication.

TOPIRAMATE

Topamax
Tabs: 25, 100, 200 mg

YES 1 D

Caps, sprinkle: 15, 25 mg
Antiepileptic agents

Indication: Adjunctive therapy in tonic-clonic and partial seizures, Lennox-
Gastaut syndrome.
Initial dose: 50 mg PO qhs
Max dose: 1.6 g PO daily
Renal dose: CrCl 10-50 mL/min: 50% dose
  CrCl <10 mL/min: 25% dose

Continued

For explanation of icons, see p. 1068.

TOPIRAMATE *continued*

Adverse drug reaction: Somnolence, ataxia, confusion, nervousness, nystagmus, paresthesia, speech disorders, psychomotor slowing, diplopia, nausea, fatigue, emotional lability, tremor; rare: leukopenia, suicide attempts, weight loss, kidney stones, acute myopia with secondary angle closure glaucoma.

Comments:

Maintain fluid intake (6-8 glasses daily) to minimize risk of kidney stones.

Dosage increment 50 mg daily; increase every other day until target dose of 200 mg bid. Do not stop abruptly.

Drug/drug: Phenytoin, carbamazepine, phenobarbital may decrease levels.

Contraindicated in prior hypersensitivity to the medication.

ZONISAMIDE

Zonegran
Caps: 100 mg
Antiepileptic agents

YES   ?   C

Indication: Partial seizures
Initial dose: 100 mg PO daily
Max dose: 600 mg PO daily
Renal dose: CrCl <50 mL/min: Avoid use
Hepatic dose: Use caution in patients with active liver disease.

Adverse drug reaction: Depression; rare: Stevens-Johnson syndrome, toxic epidermal necrolysis, aplastic anemia, agranulocytosis, hyperthermia, somnolence, fatigue, nephrolithiasis.

Comments:

Monitor liver and kidney function.

Drug-drug: Phenobarbital, phenytoin may decrease levels.

Dosage increment 100 mg daily q2 wk divided bid. Do not stop abruptly. Doses >400 mg have not been found to be more effective.

Maintain fluid intake (6-8 glasses daily) to minimize risk of kidney stones.

Contraindicated with prior hypersensitivity to the medication or other sulfonamides.

TIAGABINE
Gabitril
Tabs: 2, 4, 12, 16, 20 mg
Antiepileptic agents

NO ? C

Indication: Adjuvant treatment for partial seizures
Initial dose: 4 mg daily qhs for 1 wk
Max dose: 56 mg PO daily
Hepatic dose: Use caution in patients with active liver disease

Adverse drug reaction: Rare: dizziness, asthenia, somnolence, nervousness, nausea, difficulty thinking or concentrating, edema.
Comments: Dosage increment 4-8 mg daily q wk divided bid/qid. Do not stop abruptly.
Drug/drug: Phenytoin, carbamazepine, phenobarbital may decrease levels.
Contraindicated in prior hypersensitivity to the medication.

LAMOTRIGINE
Lamictal
Tabs, scored: 25, 100, 150, 200 mg
Tabs, chewable: 5, 25 mg
Antiepileptic agents

NO X C

Indication: Partial seizures, Lennox-Gastaut syndrome
Initial dose: 50 mg PO daily for 2 wk, then 50 mg PO bid for 2 wk (without valproic acid)
25 mg PO every other day for 2 wk, then 25 mg PO daily (with valproic acid)
Max dose: 500 mg (with inducing agent)
200 mg (with valproic acid alone)
Hepatic dose: Moderate dysfunction (Child-Pugh grade B) 50% dose, severe dysfunction (Child-Pugh grade C) 25% dose.

Adverse drug reaction: Rash, dizziness, ataxia, somnolence, headache, nausea, anorexia, dysmenorrhea, diplopia, blurred vision; rare: Stevens-Johnson syndrome, photosensitivity reactions.
Comments:
Dosage increment 100 mg daily q1-2 wk to a target dose of 300-500 mg daily without valproic acid or 100-400 mg daily with valproic acid. Do not stop abruptly.
Drug/drug: Phenytoin, carbamazepine, phenobarbital, primidone may decrease levels. Valproic acid increases levels.
Contraindicated in prior hypersensitivity to the medication.

FORMULARY

Neurology—Antiepileptic Agents

For explanation of icons, see p. 1068.

PSYCHIATRY
Antidepressants
Selective Serotonin Reuptake Inhibitors

CITALOPRAM

Celexa
Tabs, scored: 10, 20, 40 mg
Oral liquid: 10 mg/5 mL (120 mL)
Antidepressants, selective serotonin reuptake inhibitors

NO   ?   C

Indication: Major depression
Initial dose: 20 mg PO daily
Max dose: 60 mg daily

Adverse drug reaction: Insomnia; rare: atrioventricular block, bradycardia.
Comments:
Dosage increment 20 mg, onset of action 2-4 wk, adequate trial 6-8 wk
   (geriatric patients up to 12 wk). Most patients do not require dosage
   >40 mg.
Contraindicated in combination with or within 2 wk of discontinuation of
   monoamine oxidase inhibitor or with prior hypersensitivity to the medication.
Class side effects: Activation of mania, dizziness, syndrome of inappropriate
   secretion of antidiuretic hormone, drowsiness, tremor, anorexia,
   photosensitivity, ejaculatory disorder, sexual dysfunction, headache,
   diarrhea, constipation, nausea, jitteriness.

FLUOXETINE

Prozac, Sarafem
Caps: 10, 20 mg (Prozac, Sarafem) 40 mg (Prozac)
Caps, timed release: 90 mg
Oral liquid: 20 mg/5 mL (120 mL)
Antidepressants, selective serotonin reuptake inhibitors

NO   X   B

Indication: Depression, obsessive-compulsive disorder (OCD), bulimia nervosa,
   premenstrual dysphoric disorder (PMDD)
Initial dose:
   Depression, OCD, PMDD: 20 mg PO daily
   Bulimia nervosa: 60 mg PO daily
Max dose: 80 mg daily

Continued

FLUOXETINE *continued*

Adverse drug reaction: Rash, central nervous system stimulation, bradycardia, insomnia.
Comments:
Once weekly dose (90 mg PO q wk) available for stable patients.
Dosage increment: Onset 2-4 wk, adequate trial 6-8 wk, geriatric patients up to 12 wk.
Drug/drug: Potent P450 2D6 inhibitor; use caution when administering with β-blockers, antipsychotic agents, tricyclic antidepressants.
Contraindicated in combination with or within 5 weeks of discontinuation of monoamine oxidase inhibitor, or with prior hypersensitivity to the medication.
Class side effects: Activation of mania, dizziness, syndrome of inappropriate secretion of antidiuretic hormone, drowsiness, tremor, anorexia, photosensitivity, sexual dysfunction, headache, diarrhea, constipation, nausea, jitteriness.

FLUVOXAMINE

NO   ?   C

Luvox
Tabs, scored*: 25, 50*, 100* mg
Antidepressants, selective serotonin reuptake inhibitors

Indication: Obsessive-compulsive disorder
Initial dose: 25-50 mg PO daily, >150 mg PO divided bid
Max dose: 300 mg daily

Adverse drug reaction: Insomnia, withdrawal upon abrupt discontinuation.
Comments:
Drug/drug: Potent P450 1A2 inhibitor; use caution when administering with theophylline, olanzapine.
Dosage increment 50 mg, onset 2-4 wk, adequate trial 6-8 wk (geriatric patients up to 12 wk).
Class side effects: Activation of mania, dizziness, syndrome of inappropriate secretion of antidiuretic hormone, drowsiness, tremor, anorexia, photosensitivity, sexual dysfunction, headache, diarrhea, constipation, nausea, jitteriness.
Class contraindications: Hypersensitivity to the medication.

PAROXETINE

Paxil
Tabs, scored*: 10, 20*, 30, 40 mg
Oral liquid: 10 mg/5 mL (250 mL) orange
Antidepressants, selective serotonin reuptake inhibitors

YES ? B

Indication: Depression, obsessive-compulsive disorder, social anxiety disorder, panic disorder
Initial dose: 10-20 mg PO daily
Max dose: 60 mg daily
Renal dose: CrCl 10-50 mL/min: 50%-75% dose
CrCl <10 mL/min: 50% dose

Adverse drug reaction: Dry mouth, increased appetite, excessive sweating, drowsiness, withdrawal on abrupt discontinuation.
Comments:
Drug/drug: Potent P450 2D6 inhibitor; use caution when administering with β-blockers, antipsychotic agents, tricyclic antidepressants.
Dosage increment 10 mg, onset 2-4 wk, adequate trial 6-8 wk (geriatric patients up to 12 wk).
The only selective serotonin reuptake inhibitors with anticholinergic side effects.
Class side effects: Activation of mania, dizziness, syndrome of inappropriate secretion of antidiuretic hormone, drowsiness, tremor, anorexia, photosensitivity, sexual dysfunction, headache, diarrhea, constipation, nausea, jitteriness.
Class contraindications: Hypersensitivity to the medication.

SERTRALINE

Zoloft
Tabs, scored: 25, 50, 100 mg
Oral liquid: 20 mg/mL (60 mL), 12% ethyl alcohol
Antidepressants, selective serotonin reuptake inhibitors

NO ? C

Indication: Depression, panic disorder, obsessive-compulsive disorder (OCD), posttraumatic stress disorder (PTSD)
Initial dose:
  Depression, OCD: 50 mg PO daily
  Panic disorder, PTSD: 25 mg PO daily, after 1 wk increase to 50 mg
Max dose: 200 mg daily

Continued

SERTRALINE *continued*

Comments:
Dosage increment 50 mg, onset 2-4 wk, adequate trial 6-8 wk (geriatric patients up to 12 wk).
Contraindicated in combination with or within 2 wk of discontinuation of monoamine oxidase inhibitor or with prior hypersensitivity to the medication.
Class side effects: Activation of mania, dizziness, syndrome of inappropriate secretion of antidiuretic hormone, drowsiness, tremor, anorexia, photosensitivity, sexual dysfunction, headache, diarrhea, constipation, nausea, jitteriness.

Tricyclics

AMITRIPTYLINE

Elavil
Tabs: 12, 25, 50, 75, 100, 150 mg
Inj: 100 mg/10 mL
Antidepressants, tricyclics

NO   ?   D

Indication: Depression
Initial dose: 50-100 mg PO qhs or divided bid/tid
Max dose: 150 mg daily (outpatient)

Comments:
Dosage increment: 25-50 mg titrate dose after 3-5 wk based on drug levels (110-250 mg/mL). Monitor: Obtain baseline electrocardiogram.
Drug/drug: Avoid use with agents that can cause QT prolongation.
Contraindicated in acute recovery after myocardial infarction, with second and third atrioventricular block, in combination with or within 14 days of discontinuation of monoamine oxidase inhibitor or with prior hypersensitivity to the medication.
Class side effects: Seizures, sexual dysfunction, anticholinergic effects, somnolence, dizziness, photosensitivity, postural hypotension, conduction disturbances, blood dyscrasias, withdrawal on abrupt cessation.

CLOMIPRAMINE

Anafranil
Caps: 25, 50, 75 mg
Antidepressants, tricyclics

NO   1   C

Indication: Obsessive-compulsive disorder
Initial dose: 25 mg PO daily
Max dose: 250 mg daily

Continued

CLOMIPRAMINE *continued*

Adverse drug reaction: Seizures.
Comments:
Monitor: Obtain baseline electrocardiogram.
Dosage increment: 25 mg, titrate over first 2 wk to 100 mg/day in divided
doses. Once patient is stabilized, entire dose can be administered qhs.
Titrate dose after 3-5 wk based on drug levels (80-100 mg/mL).
Drug/drug: Can cause QT prolongation.
Contraindicated in acute recovery after myocardial infarction, with second or
third atrioventricular block, in combination with or within 14 days of
discontinuation of monoamine oxidase inhibitor, or with prior hypersensitivity
to the medication.
Class side effects: Seizures, sexual dysfunction, anticholinergic effects,
somnolence, dizziness, photosensitivity, postural hypotension, conduction
disturbances, blood dyscrasias, withdrawal on abrupt cessation.

DESIPRAMINE

Norpramin
Tabs: 10, 25, 50, 75, 100, 150 mg
Antidepressants, tricyclics

NO   ?   C

Indication: Depression
Initial dose: 75-150 mg PO daily or divided bid/tid
Max dose: 300 mg daily

Comments:
Monitor: Obtain baseline electrocardiogram.
Dosage increment: Titrate dose after 3-5 wk based on drug levels (125-300
mg/mL).
Drug/drug: Can cause QT prolongation. Once patient is stabilized, entire dose
can be administered qhs.
Contraindicated in acute recovery after myocardial infarction, with second or
third atrioventricular block, in combination with or within 14 days of
discontinuation of monoamine oxidase inhibitor, or with prior hypersensitivity
to the medication.
Class side effects: Seizures, sexual dysfunction, anticholinergic effects,
somnolence, dizziness, photosensitivity, postural hypotension, conduction
disturbances, blood dyscrasias, withdrawal on abrupt cessation.

DOXEPIN

Sinequan, Adapin
Caps: 10, 25, 50, 75, 100, 150 mg
Oral liquid: 10 mg/mL (120 mL)
Antidepressants, tricyclics

NO   ?   C

Indication: Depression, anxiety
Initial dose: 25-150 mg PO qhs
Max dose: 300 mg daily, 150 mg/dose

Comments:
Dosage increment: 150 mg; titrate dose after 3-5 wk based on drug levels (100-200 mg/mL).
Monitor: Obtain baseline electrocardiogram, complete blood count, liver function, blood pressure.
Drug/drug: Can cause QT prolongation.
Contraindicated in patients with glaucoma or urinary retention, in combination with or within 14 days of discontinuation of monoamine oxidase inhibitor, or with prior hypersensitivity to medication.
Class side effects: Seizures, ejaculatory dysfunction or priapism, anticholinergic effects, somnolence, dizziness, photosensitivity, postural hypotension, conduction disturbances, blood dyscrasias, withdrawal on abrupt cessation.

IMIPRAMINE

Tofranil, Tofranil PM
Tabs: 10, 25, 50 mg (Tofranil)
Caps: 75, 100, 125, 150 mg (Tofranil PM)
Antidepressants, tricyclics

NO   ?   D

Indication: Depression
Initial dose: 50-100 mg PO daily
Max dose: 200 mg daily (outpatient)

Comments:
Monitor: Obtain baseline electrocardiogram.
Dosage increment: Titrate dose after 3-5 wk based on drug levels (200-350 mg/mL). Once patient is stabilized, entire dose can be administered qhs.
Drug/drug: Can cause QT prolongation. No advantage between dosage forms.
Contraindicated in acute recovery after myocardial infarction, with second and third atrioventricular block, in combination with or within 14 days of discontinuation of monoamine oxidase inhibitor, or with prior hypersensitivity to the medication.

Continued

For explanation of icons, see p. 1068.

IMPRAMINE *continued*

Class side effects: Seizures, sexual dysfunction, anticholinergic effects, somnolence, dizziness, photosensitivity, postural hypotension, conduction disturbances, blood dyscrasias, withdrawal on abrupt cessation.

NORTRIPTYLINE

Pamelor
Caps: 10, 25, 50, 75 mg
Oral liquid: 10 mg/5 mL (480 mL)
Antidepressants, tricyclics

 NO ? D

Indication: Depression
Initial dose: 25-50 mg PO qhs
Max dose: 150 mg daily

Comments:
Monitor: Dosage increment 25 mg titrate dose to tid/qid gradually based on drug levels (50-150 mg/mL). Obtain baseline electrocardiogram.
Drug/drug: Can cause QT prolongation. Once patient is stabilized, entire dose can be administered qhs.
Contraindicated in acute recovery after myocardial infarction, with second and third atrioventricular block, in combination with or within 14 days of discontinuation of monoamine oxidase inhibitor, or with prior hypersensitivity to the medication.
Class side effects: Seizures, sexual dysfunction, anticholinergic effects, somnolence, dizziness photosensitivity, postural hypotension, conduction disturbances, blood dyscrasias, withdrawal on abrupt cessation.

Other Agents

VENLAFAXINE

Effexor, Effexor XR
Tabs, scored: 25, 37.5, 50, 75, 100 mg
Caps, extended-release: 37.5, 75, 150 mg
Antidepressants, other agents

 YES ? C

Indication: Depression, anxiety
Initial dose:
  Depression: 75 mg PO divided bid/tid
  Anxiety: 37.5-75 mg PO daily (extended-release)
Max dose: 375 mg daily, 225 mg daily ER formulation
Renal dose: CrCl 10-50 mL/min: 75% dose.

Continued

VENLAFAXINE *continued*

Adverse drug reaction: Nausea, vomiting, diarrhea, insomnia, jitteriness, syndrome of inappropriate secretion of antidiuretic hormone, withdrawal on abrupt discontinuation, sexual dysfunction; rare: systolic hypertension with doses >225 mg/day.
Comments:
No anticholinergic or histaminergic side effects.
Dosage increments 75 mg q4 day; taper dose 75 mg/wk over several wk to avoid withdrawal.
Contraindicated in combination with or within 14 days of discontinuation of monoamine oxidase inhibitor or with prior hypersensitivity to the medication.

BUPROPION

Wellbutrin, Wellbutrin SR, Zyban
Tabs: 75, 100 mg
Tabs sustained-release: 100, 150, 200 mg
Antidepressants, other agents

NO ? B

Indication: Depression, smoking cessation
Initial dose:
 Depression: 100 mg PO bid or 75 mg PO tid
 Smoking cessation: 150 mg SR PO daily for 3 days, then 150
Max dose: 450 mg daily (150 mg/dose)
 400 mg daily SR (200 mg/dose)
Hepatic dose: Severe hepatic cirrhosis 75 mg daily

Adverse drug reaction: Seizures (dose-related), arrhythmias, decreased appetite, hypertension, agitation, blurred vision, excessive sweating, insomnia.
Comments:
Not associated with sexual dysfunction.
Drug/drug: P450 2D6 inhibitor; use caution when administering with β-blockers, antipsychotic agents, tricyclic antidepressants.
To reach 25% quit rate, smoking cessation therapy must include intensive psychological support.
Attempt educational and behavioral interventions before drug therapy in pregnancy.
Dosage increment: Increase to 100 mg tid by day 4 (depression), max effect 4 wk.
Contraindicated in combination or within 14 days of discontinuation of monoamine oxidase inhibitor and in patients with history of bulimia, anorexia nervosa, seizure disorder, or prior hypersensitivity to the medication.

MIRTAZAPINE

Remeron, Remeron Soltab (Soltab)
Tabs, scored*: 15*, 30*, 45 mg
Tab, disintegrating: 15, 30, 45 mg orange
Antidepressants, other agents

YES   ?   C

Indication: Depression
Initial dose: 15 mg PO qhs
Max dose: 45 mg daily
Renal dose: CrCl <10 mL/min: 50% dose

Adverse drug reaction: Increased levels of cholesterol, triglycerides, and transaminases, increased appetite, central nervous system effects, sedation.
Comments:
Dosage increment 15 mg q2 wk.
Contraindicated with prior hypersensitivity to the medication.

NEFAZODONE

Serzone
Tabs, scored*: 50, 100*, 150*, 200, 250, mg
Antidepressants, Other

NO   ?   C

Indication: Depression
Initial dose: 100 mg PO bid
Max dose: 600 mg daily

Adverse drug reaction: Liver failure (black box warning), sedation, orthostatic hypotension.
Comments:
Drug/drug: P450 3A3/4 inhibitor. Cyclosporine, triazolam levels may rise. Increased risk of QT prolongation with terfenadine, astemizole, cisapride, or pimozide. Carbamazepine may induce metabolism of nefazodone.
Dosage increment: 100 mg bid q1-2 wk.
Contraindicated in patients hypersensitive to other phenylpiperazine antidepressants or with prior hypersensitivity to the medication.

TRAZODONE

Desyrel, Desyrel Dividose
Tabs: 50, 100 mg

NO   ?   C

Tabs, triple-scored: 150, 300 mg (Desyrel Dividose)
Antidepressants, other agents

Indication: Depression
Initial dose: 150 mg PO daily divided bid
Max dose: 400 mg daily (outpatient)

Adverse drug reaction: Drowsiness, dry mouth, hypotension, priapism.
Comments:
Not associated with sexual dysfunction.
Dosage increment 50 mg q3-4 days, peak effect 2-4 wk.
Contraindicated in acute recovery after myocardial infarction or with prior
hypersensitivity to the medication.

Antimanic Agents

LITHIUM

Eskalith, Lithobid, Lithonate CIBAlith-S
Caps: 150, 300, 600 mg (Eskalith, Lithonate)

YES   X   D

Tabs, scored: 300 mg (Eskalith)
Tabs, extended-release: 300 mg (Lithobid), 450 mg (Duralith, Eskalith CR)
Oral liquid: 300 mg/5 mL (480 mL) (CIBAlith-S)
Antimanic

Indication: Mania
Initial dose: 300 mg PO bid
Max dose: 2.4 g daily
Renal dose: CrCl 10-50 mL/min: 50%-75% dose
CrCl <10 mL/min: 25%-50% dose

Adverse drug reaction: Leukocytosis, headache, sedation, weight gain,
confusion, impaired memory, fine tremor, nausea, vomiting, diarrhea,
nephrogenic diabetes insipidus, hypothyroidism, polyuria, polydipsia.
Comments:
Monitor renal function, thyroid function tests q3 months, drug levels q2 months
(normal 0.2-1.2 mEq/L).
Drug/drug: Nonsteroidal antiinflammatory drugs, Cox-2 inhibitors, angiotensin
receptor blockers, loop diuretics, angiotensin-converting enzyme inhibitors
increase lithium levels.
Contraindicated in patients unavailable for follow-up or with prior
hypersensitivity to the medication.

For explanation of icons, see p. 1068.

Antipsychotics
Dopamine Antagonists

CHLORPROMAZINE

NO   ?   C

Thorazine
Tabs: 10, 25, 50, 100, 200 mg
Oral liquid, concentrate: 30, 100 mg/mL (120, 240 mL)
Caps, extended-release: 30, 75, 150 mg (Thorazine Spansule)
Oral liquid: 10 mg/5 mL (120 mL)
Suppositories: 25, 100 mg
Inj: 25 mg/mL
Antipsychotics, dopamine antagonists

Indication: Schizophrenia, hiccups, emesis
Initial dose:
    Schizophrenia: 25-50 mg PO divided bid/tid
    Hiccups: 25-50 mg PO tid-qid for 2-3 days
    Emesis: 10-25 mg IM q4-6h prn
            25 mg IM, may repeat in 1 hr, then bid/tid
Max dose: 800 mg (outpatient)
              1 g daily (clinical)
              400 mg IM q4-6h

Adverse drug reaction: Cutaneous pigmentation and photosensitivity changes.
Comments:
Dosage increment: 20-50 mg semiweekly, max effect weeks-months.
Switch to oral therapy as soon as feasible. IV administration is very irritating
   and not recommended for routine use.
Monitor: Liver function, complete blood counts q6 months.
Drug/drug: Use caution with other central nervous system depressants.
Contraindicated in patients with hypersensitivity to phenothiazines, comatose
   states, bone marrow depression.
Class side effects: Extrapyramidal symptoms (akathisia, dystonia,
   pseudoparkinsonian), tardive dyskinesia, drowsiness, anticholinergic effects,
   hypotension, tachycardia, leukopenia, ocular changes, increased prolactin,
   erectile dysfunction, cholestatic jaundice, neuromuscular malignant
   syndrome, QT prolongation.

FLUPHENAZINE

NO ? C

Prolixin, Permitil
Tabs, scored: 1, 2.5*, 5*, 10* mg
Oral liquid: 2.5 mg/5 mL (473 mL) (Prolixin 14% ethyl alcohol)
Oral liquid, concentrate: 5 mg/mL (120 mL) (Permitil, Prolixin 14% ethyl alcohol)
Inj: 2.5 mg/mL (HCL)
Inj: 25 mg/mL (Enthanoate, Decanoate)
Antipsychotics, dopamine antagonists

Indication: Schizophrenia
Initial dose: 0.5-10 mg PO daily divided tid/qid
1.25 mg HCL IM then 2.5-10 mg IM divided q6-8 hr
Depot Enthanoate 25 mg IM q2 wk
Depot Decanoate 12.5 mg IM q3 wk
Max dose: 40 mg PO daily, 100 mg IM q2-6 wk

Comments:
Dosage increment 12.5 mg IM; use caution with oral doses >20 mg; 12.5 mg IM decanoate q3 wk = 10 mg PO daily.
Oral should replace intramuscular administration as soon as feasible.
Avoid mixing oral concentrate with caffeinated products, tea, apple juice.
Contraindicated in patients with hypersensitivity to phenothiazines, subcortical brain damage, blood dyscrasias, liver damage, comatose states, prior hypersensitivity to the medication.
Class side effects: Extrapyramidal symptoms (akathisia, dystonia, pseudoparkinsonian), tardive dyskinesia, drowsiness, anticholinergic effects, hypotension, tachycardia, leukopenia, ocular changes, increased prolactin, erectile dysfunction, cholestatic jaundice, neuromuscular malignant syndrome, QT prolongation.

HALOPERIDOL

NO ? C

Haldol
Tabs, scored: 0.5, 1, 2, 5, 10, 20 mg
Oral liquid: 2 mg/mL (15, 120 mL)
Inj: 5 mg/mL
Inj, depot: 50, 100 mg/mL (Decanoate)
Antipsychotics, dopamine antagonists

Indication: Acute psychosis, schizophrenia, Tourette's syndrome
Initial dose: 0.5-5 mg PO bid-tid
2-5 mg IM, then q4-8h
Depot 10-15 mg times PO dose, not >100 mg initially
Max dose: 40 mg PO daily
450 mg daily (Decanoate)

Continued

HALOPERIDOL *continued*

Comments:
Dosage increment: Adjust rapidly according to clinical situation; adverse side effects significantly increase above 40 mg PO.

Monitor: Liver function, complete blood counts q6 months; assess extrapyramidal symptoms q3 months.

Once the patient's condition is controlled with intramuscular administration, switch to oral doses.

Contraindicated in severe toxic central nervous system depression, Parkinson disease, comatose states, or prior hypersensitivity to the medication.

Class side effects: Extrapyramidal symptoms (akathisia, dystonia, pseudoparkinsonian), tardive dyskinesia, drowsiness, anticholinergic effects, hypotension, tachycardia, leukopenia, ocular changes, increased prolactin, erectile dysfunction, cholestatic jaundice, neuromuscular malignant syndrome, QT prolongation.

LOXAPINE

NO ? C

Loxitane, Loxitane C, Loxitane IM
Caps: 5, 10, 25, 50 mg
Oral liquid: 25 mg/mL (120 mL) (Loxitane C)
Inj: 50 mg/mL (Loxitane IM)
Antipsychotics, Dopamine antagonists

Indication: Schizophrenia
Initial dose: 10 mg PO bid
    12.5-50 mg IM q4-6h
Max dose: 250 mg daily

Adverse drug reaction: Initial transient drowsiness.
Comments:
Monitor: Liver function, complete blood counts q6 months; assess extrapyramidal symptoms q3 months.

Contraindicated with hypersensitivity to dibenzoxazepine derivatives, severe drug-induced depressed states, comatose states, or prior hypersensitivity to the medication.

Class side effects: Extrapyramidal symptoms (akathisia, dystonia, pseudoparkinsonian), tardive dyskinesia, drowsiness, anticholinergic effects, hypotension, tachycardia, leukopenia, ocular changes, increased prolactin, erectile dysfunction, cholestatic jaundice, neuromuscular malignant syndrome, QT prolongation.

MOLINDONE

NO   ?   C

Moban
Tabs: 5, 10, 25, 50, 100 mg
Oral liquid: 20 mg/mL (120 mL) cherry
Antipsychotics, dopamine antagonists

Indication: Schizophrenia
Initial dose: 50-75 mg PO daily divided tid/qid
Maintenance dose: 5-25 mg PO tid/qid
Max dose: 225 mg daily

Adverse drug reaction: Initial transient drowsiness.
Comments:
Dosage increment: q3-4 days
Monitor: Liver function, complete blood count
Contraindicated in severe toxic central nervous system depression, comatose states, or prior hypersensitivity to the medication.
Class side effects: Extrapyramidal symptoms (akathisia, dystonia, pseudoparkinsonian), tardive dyskinesia, drowsiness, anticholinergic effects, hypotension, tachycardia, leukopenia, ocular changes, increased prolactin, erectile dysfunction, cholestatic jaundice, neuromuscular malignant syndrome, QT prolongation.

THIORIDAZINE

NO   ?   C

Mellaril, Mellaril-S
Tabs: 10, 15, 25, 50, 100, 150, 200 mg
Oral liquid: 30, 100 mg/mL
Oral liquid: 50, 20 mg/mL (1 pint) (Mellaril-S)
Antipsychotics, dopamine antagonists

Indication: Schizophrenia
Initial dose: 50-100 mg PO tid
Max dose: 800 mg daily

Adverse drug reaction: QT prolongation (black box warning, dose related), sudden death, torsades de pointes.
Comments:
Monitor: Baseline electrocardiogram and potassium; abnormal involuntary movement scale (AIMS), liver function, complete blood counts q6 months; assess extrapyramidal symptoms q3 months.
Drug/drug: Avoid use with drugs that prolong the QT interval.
Highest risk in class for QT prolongation.

Continued

For explanation of icons, see p. 1068.

THIORIDAZINE *continued*

Contraindicated in severe toxic central nervous system depression, comatose states, QT interval >450 µsec, prior cardiac arrhythmias, or prior hypersensitivity to the medication.

Class side effects: Extrapyramidal symptoms (akathisia, dystonia, pseudoparkinsonian), tardive dyskinesia, drowsiness, anticholinergic effects, hypotension, tachycardia, leukopenia, ocular changes, increased prolactin, erectile dysfunction, cholestatic jaundice, neuromuscular malignant syndrome, QT prolongation.

DROPERIDOL

Inapsine
Inj: 2.5 mg/mL
Antipsychotics, dopamine antagonists

NO   ?   C

Indication: Postoperative emesis.
Initial dose: 2.5-10 mg IM prn for agitation
Maintenance: 1.25-2.5 IV

Adverse drug reaction: QT prolongation (black box warning), drowsiness; rare: extrapyramidal symptoms, hypotension.
Comments:
Monitor: Baseline electrocardiogram, then q2-3h until treatment completed.
Administer 30-60 minutes before procedure.
Drug/drug: Additive effects with other central nervous system depressants.
Contraindicated in patients with history of cardiac arrhythmias, comatose states, QT interval >440 µsec in males and >450 µsec in females, prior cardiac arrhythmias, or prior hypersensitivity to the medication.
Class side effects: Extrapyramidal symptoms (akathisia, dystonia, pseudoparkinsonian), tardive dyskinesia, drowsiness, anticholinergic effects, hypotension, tachycardia, leukopenia, ocular changes, increased prolactin, erectile dysfunction, cholestatic jaundice, neuromuscular malignant syndrome, QT prolongation.

Serotonin Dopamine Receptor Antagonists

CLOZAPINE

Clozaril

Tabs, scored: 25, 100 mg

Antipsychotics, serotonin dopamine receptor antagonists

NO   X   B

Indication: Refractory schizophrenia
Initial dose: 12.5 mg PO daily or divided bid
Max dose: 900 mg daily

Adverse drug reaction: Agranulocytosis (black box warning), myocarditis (black box warning), urinary incontinence, hyperlipidemia, sialorrhea, seizures, hypotension, tachycardia, hyperglycemia, anticholinergic effects.

Comments:

Monitor: White blood cell count q wk × 6 months then q2 wk.

Dosage increment: 25-50 mg, target 300-450 mg per day by wk 2. If >2 days are missed, restart at 12.5 mg bid.

Must obtain rechallenge number before first dose from Clozaril Patient Management System.

Drug/drug: Use caution with other drugs that lower seizure threshold and cause blood dyscrasias or both.

Lowest risk in class of extrapyramidal symptoms.

Contraindicated in patients with severe toxic central nervous system depression, comatose states, myeloproliferative disorders, uncontrolled epilepsy, history of clozapine-induced agranulocytosis or granulocytopenia, or prior hypersensitivity to the medication.

Class side effects: Sedation, weight gain, orthostatic hypotension.

OLANZAPINE

Zyprexa, Zyprexa Zydis

Tabs: 2.5, 5, 7.5, 10, 15, 20 mg (Zyprexa)

Tabs, disintegrating: 5, 10, 15, 20 mg (Zyprexa Zydis)

Antipsychotics, serotonin dopamine receptor antagonists

NO   X   C

Indication: Acute manic episodes, schizophrenia
Initial dose: 5-10 mg PO daily
Max dose: 40 mg daily

Adverse drug reaction: Hyperglycemia, hyperlipidemia, liver function test abnormalities (increase), anticholinergic effects, dizziness, asthenia.

Comments:

Dosage increment: 5 mg q wk.

Class side effects: Sedation, weight gain, orthostatic hypotension.

Class contraindications: Hypersensitivity to the medication.

QUETIAPINE

Seroquel
Tabs: 25, 100, 200, 300 mg
Antipsychotics, serotonin dopamine receptor antagonists

NO   ?   C

Indication: Schizophrenia
Initial dose: 25 mg PO bid
Max dose: 800 mg PO daily

Adverse drug reaction: Anticholinergic effects, agitation, headache, dizziness, asthenia.
Comments:
Low risk of extrapyramidal symptoms.
Dosage increment: 25-50 mg bid; initial target is 300-400 mg divided bid/tid by day 4 as tolerated.
Class side effects: Sedation, weight gain, orthostatic hypotension.
Contraindicated with prior hypersensitivity to the medication.

RISPERIDONE

Risperdal
Tabs: 0.25, 0.5, 1, 2, 3, 4 mg
Oral liquid: 1 mg/mL (100 mL)
Antipsychotics, serotonin dopamine receptor antagonists

NO   ?   C

Indication: Schizophrenia
Initial dose: 1 mg PO bid
Max dose: 8 mg daily

Comments: Highest risk in class of extrapyramidal symptoms (occur with >6 mg/day).
Dosage increment 1 mg bid q wk; initial target is 3 mg bid by day 3 as tolerated.
Class side effects: Sedation, weight gain, orthostatic hypotension.
Class contraindications: Hypersensitivity to the medication.

Other Agents

ZIPRASIDONE

Geodon
Caps: 20, 40, 60, 80 mg
Inj: 20 mg/mL
Antipsychotics, other agents

NO   ?   C

Indication: Schizophrenia
Initial dose: 20 mg PO bid
    10 mg IM q2h or 20 mg IM q4h
Max dose: 100 mg PO daily
    40 mg IM per day

Adverse drug reaction: Orthostatic hypotension, somnolence, insomnia, agitation, QT prolongation, weight gain, nausea.
Comments:
Weight-neutral antidepressant.
Drug/drug: Avoid use with drugs that can cause QT prolongation or are central nervous system depressants.
Dosage increment: 20 mg, max effect 2 wk.
Contraindicated in history of QT prolongation, recent acute myocardial infarction, uncompensated heart failure, or hypersensitivity to the medication.

Anxiolytics and Hypnotics
Benzodiazepines

ALPRAZOLAM

Xanax
Tabs, scored: 0.25, 0.5, 1, 2 mg
Anxiolytics and hypnotics, benzodiazepines

NO   X   D

Indication: Anxiety, panic disorder
Initial dose: 0.25-0.5 mg PO tid
Max dose: 4 mg daily
Hepatic dose: Initial 0.25 mg PO bid, titrate to effect

Comments:
Drug/drug: Additive to central nervous system depressants, no major active metabolite.
Dosage increment q3-4 days, avoid abrupt discontinuation, taper 0.5 mg q 3 days.

Continued

ALPRAZOLAM *continued*

Class side effects: Dose-dependent central nervous system effects
(anterograde amnesia, sedation, ataxia, confusion, delirium), respiratory
depression, nystagmus.

Contraindicated with prior hypersensitivity to the medication or other
benzodiazepines, acute narrow-angle glaucoma, or concomitant use of
ketoconazole or itraconazole.

CHLORDIAZEPOXIDE

Librium, Libritabs
Caps: 5, 10, 20 mg (Librium)   YES   X   D
Tabs, scored: 5, 10. 20 mg (Libritabs)
Inj: 100 mg (propylene glycol 20%)
Anxiolytics and hypnotics, benzodiazepines

Indication: Mild and severe anxiety, preoperative anxiety, alcohol withdrawal
Initial dose:
    Mild anxiety: 5-10 mg PO tid/qid
    Severe anxiety: 20-25 mg PO tid/qid
    Preoperative anxiety: 50-100 mg IM 1 hr before surgery
    Alcohol withdrawal: 50-100 mg PO/IM/IV prn
Max dose: 300 mg daily
Renal dose: CrCl <10 mL/min: 50% dose

Comments:
Drug/drug: Additive to central nervous system depressants.
Class side effects: Dose-dependent central nervous system effects
(anterograde amnesia, sedation, ataxia, confusion, delirium), respiratory
depression, nystagmus.
Class contraindications: Hypersensitivity to the medication or other
benzodiazepines, acute narrow angle glaucoma.

CLONAZEPAM

Klonopin
Tabs, scored: 0.5, 1, 2 mg   NO   ?   C
Anxiolytics and hypnotics, benzodiazepines

Indication: Panic disorder, seizures
Initial dose:
    Panic: 0.25 mg PO bid
    Seizures: 1.5 mg PO divided tid
Max dose: 4 mg daily (panic), 20 mg daily (seizures)

Continued

CLONAZEPAM *continued*

Adverse drug reaction: Ataxia, hypotonia, behavioral disturbances.
Comments:
Drug/drug: Additive to central nervous system depressants.
Dosage increment: Avoid abrupt discontinuation, increase 0.5-1 mg q3 days
  until controlled.
Contraindicated in significant liver disease, acute narrow-angle glaucoma, or
  prior hypersensitivity to the medication or other benzodiazepines.
Class side effects: Dose-dependent central nervous system effects
  (anterograde amnesia, sedation, ataxia, confusion, delirium), respiratory
  depression, nystagmus.

DIAZEPAM

Valium, Diastat, Diazepam Intensol, Q-PAM, Valcaps
Tabs, scored: 2, 5, 10 mg (Q-PAM, Valcaps)   NO   ?   D
Tabs: 2, 5, 10 mg (Valium)
Oral liquid: 5 mg/5 mL
Oral liquid, concentrate: 5 mg (Diazepam Intensol 19% ethyl alcohol)
Rectal gel: 2.5, 5, 10, 15, 20 mg (Diastat 10% ethyl alcohol)
Inj: 5 mg/mL (Valium 19% alcohol, propylene glycol 40%)
Anxiolytics and hypnotics, benzodiazepines

Indication: Anxiety, alcohol withdrawal, seizures
Initial dose:
  Anxiety: 2-10 mg PO/IV/rectal bid-qid
  Alcohol withdrawal: 10 mg PO/IV tid-qid for 1 day, then reduce to 5 mg
Max dose: 30 mg/8 hr PO, 5 mg/min IV

Adverse drug reaction: Hypotension, blood dyscrasias
Comments:
Drug/drug: Additive to central nervous system depressants.
Dosage increment: Avoid abrupt discontinuation.
Contraindicated in acute narrow-angle glaucoma or with prior hypersensitivity to
  the medication or other benzodiazepines.
Class side effects: Dose-dependent central nervous system effects
  (anterograde amnesia, sedation, ataxia, confusion, delirium), respiratory
  depression, nystagmus.

LORAZEPAM

Ativan
Tabs, scored: 0.5, 1, 2 mg   NO ? D
Oral liquid: 2 mg/mL
Inj: 2, 4 mg/mL (propylene glycol vehicle)
Anxiolytics and hypnotics, benzodiazepines

Indication: Anxiety, preoperative anxiety, status epilepticus
Initial dose:
    Anxiety: 2-3 mg PO daily divided bid/tid
    Preoperative anxiety: 0.044 mg/kg (up to 2 mg) IV 15-20 min before
                 surgery
    Status epilepticus: 4 mg slowly over 2 min, repeat × 1 after 10-15 min.
    Max dose: 8 mg total dose IV

Comments:
Drug/drug: Additive to central nervous system depressants.
Avoid abrupt discontinuation.
Polyethylene glycol vehicle can cause toxicity with IV dosage form.
Contraindicated in sleep apnea, severe respiratory insufficiency, intraarterial
    administration, acute narrow-angle glaucoma, or prior hypersensitivity to the
    medication or other benzodiazepines.
Class side effects: Dose-dependent central nervous system effects
    (anterograde amnesia, sedation, ataxia, confusion, delirium), respiratory
    depression, nystagmus.

OXAZEPAM

Serax
Caps: 10, 15, 30 mg   NO ? D
Tabs: 15 mg
Anxiolytics and hypnotics, benzodiazepines

Indication: Mild and severe anxiety, alcohol detoxification
Initial dose:
    Mild anxiety: 10-15 mg PO tid/qid
    Severe anxiety, alcohol detoxification: 15-30 mg PO tid/qid

Comments:
Drug/drug: Additive to central nervous system depressants.
Class side effects: Dose-dependent central nervous system effects
    (anterograde amnesia, sedation, ataxia, confusion, delirium), respiratory
    depression, nystagmus.
Class contraindications: Hypersensitivity to the medication or other
    benzodiazepines, acute narrow angle glaucoma.

TEMAZEPAM
Restoril
Caps: 7.5, 15, 30 mg
Anxiolytics and hypnotics, benzodiazepines

NO   ?   D

 Indication: Insomnia
Initial dose: 7.5-15 mg PO qhs

 Comments:
Drug/drug: Additive to central nervous system depressants.
Avoid abrupt discontinuation.
Contraindicated in uncontrolled severe pain.
Class side effects: Dose-dependent central nervous system effects
  (anterograde amnesia, sedation, ataxia, confusion, delirium), respiratory
  depression, nystagmus.
Class contraindications: Hypersensitivity to the medication or other
  benzodiazepines, acute narrow angle glaucoma.

Other Agents

BUSPIRONE
BuSpar
Tabs, scored: 5, 10, 15, 30 mg
Anxiolytics and hypnotics, other agents

NO   ?   B

 Indication: Anxiety
Initial dose: 10-15 mg PO daily divided bid/tid
Max dose: 60 mg daily

 Adverse drug reaction: Dizziness, drowsiness, headache, nausea.
Comments:
Dosage increment 5 mg q2-3 days.
Class contraindications: Hypersensitivity to the medication.

CHLORAL HYDRATE

Aquachloral Supprettes
Caps: 500 mg
Oral liquid: 500 mg/5 mL
Suppositories: 324, 648 mg (Aquachloral Supprettes), 500 mg
Anxiolytics and hypnotics, other agents

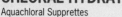

YES   1   C

Indication: Insomnia, sedation
Initial dose:
  Insomnia: 500-1000 mg PO qhs
  Sedation: 250 mg PO tid
Max dose: 2000 mg daily
Renal dose: CrCl <50 mL/min: Avoid use

Adverse drug reaction: Nausea, vomiting, diarrhea, acute intermittent
  porphyria (rare).
Comments:
Short-term use only.
Contraindicated in severe hepatic disease.
Class contraindications: Hypersensitivity to the medication.

ZALEPLON

Sonata
Caps: 5, 10 mg
Anxiolytics and hypnotics, other agents

NO   ?   C

Indication: Insomnia
Initial dose: 10 mg PO qhs
Max dose: 20 mg daily

Adverse drug reaction: Headache, dizziness, nausea, dyspepsia,
  depersonalization, anterograde amnesia.
Comments:
Avoid abrupt discontinuation.
Class contraindications: Hypersensitivity to the medication.

ZOLPIDEM

Ambien
Tabs: 5, 10 mg
Anxiolytics and hypnotics, other agents

NO   X   B

Indication: Insomnia
Initial dose: 10 mg PO qhs
Max dose: 10 mg daily

Adverse drug reaction: Headache, drowsiness, dizziness, dyspepsia, diarrhea.
Comments:
Avoid abrupt discontinuation.
Class contraindications: Hypersensitivity to the medication.

Drug Dependence Treatment

NICOTINE GUM

Nicorette, Nicorette DS
Oral gum: 2, 4 mg
Drug dependence treatment

NO   3   D

Indication: Smoking cessation
Initial dose: For 6 wk: 1 piece q1-2h
　　　　　　　 For 3 wk: 1 piece q2-4h
　　　　　　　 For 3 wk: 1 piece q4-8h
Max dose: 24 pieces (4 mg gum = 96 mg nicotine)

Adverse drug reaction: Nausea, vomiting, tachycardia, dizziness, headache,
　　jaw pain.
Comments:
To reach 25% quit rate, smoking cessation therapy must include intensive
　　psychological support.
Not chewing gum. Chew until peppery taste develops, then park in gums for 10
　　minutes, repeat until peppery taste is gone.
Attempt educational and behavioral interventions before drug therapy in
　　pregnancy.
Contraindicated with concurrent smoking, pregnant or nursing women, severe
　　angina, life-threatening arrhythmias, immediately after myocardial infarction.

For explanation of icons, see p. 1068.

NICOTINE INHALATION SYSTEM

Nicotrol Inhaler
Inhaler: 10 mg/cartridge (4 mg delivered)
Drug dependence treatment

NO   3   D

Indication: Smoking cessation
Initial dose: 6-16 cartridges per day first 6 wk, taper over next 6-12 wk

Adverse drug reaction: Headache, dyspepsia, nausea, diarrhea, hiccups.
Comments:

To reach 25% quit rate, smoking cessation therapy must include intensive
psychological support.

Attempt educational and behavioral interventions before drug therapy in
pregnancy.

Contraindicated with concurrent smoking, pregnant or nursing women, severe
angina, life-threatening arrhythmias, immediately after myocardial infarction.

NICOTINE NASAL SPRAY

Nicotrol NS
Inhaler, nasal: 0.5 mg/spray
Drug dependence treatment

NO   3   D

Indication: Smoking cessation
Initial dose: 1-2 doses/hr
Max dose: 40 doses daily

Adverse drug reaction: Sinus irritation, headache, facial flushing.
Comments:

To reach 25% quit rate, smoking cessation therapy must include intensive
psychological support.

1 dose = 1 (0.5 mg) spray in each nostril/hr.

Attempt educational and behavioral interventions before drug therapy in
pregnancy.

Contraindicated with concurrent smoking, pregnant or nursing women, severe
angina, life-threatening arrhythmias, immediately after myocardial infarction.

NICOTINE PATCHES

Nicoderm, Nicotrol, Habitrol
Patch, transdermal: 7, 14, 21 mg/24 hr (Nicoderm CQ-OTC)
15 mg/16 hr (Nicotrol-OTC)
Drug dependence treatment

NO   3   D

Indication: Smoking cessation
Initial dose: 6 wk 21 mg patch (>10 cigarettes/day) (Nicoderm, Habitrol)
2 wk 14 mg patch
2 wk 7 mg patch
6 wk 14 mg patch (<10 cigarettes/day) (Nicoderm, Habitrol)
2 wk 7 mg patch
6 wk 15 mg patch worn for 16 hr/day (Nicotrol)

Adverse drug reaction: Contact hypersensitivity, nightmares
Comments:
To reach 25% quit rate, smoking cessation therapy must include intensive
psychological support.
Caution patients *not to smoke* while using this product.
Attempt educational and behavioral interventions before drug therapy in
pregnancy.
Contraindicated with concurrent smoking, pregnant or nursing women, severe
angina, life-threatening arrhythmias, immediately after myocardial infarction.

NALOXONE

Narcan
Drug dependence treatment

NO   3   B

Indication: Opioid depression
Initial dose: 0.4-2 mg IV/IM/SQ, repeat q2-3 min
Max dose: 10 mg; reevaluate if no response
Inj: 0.4, 1 mg/mL

Adverse drug reaction: Consistent with narcotic reversal.
Comments:
Dosage increment: Multiple doses are usually needed because of short half-life.
Contraindicated with prior hypersensitivity to the medication.

For explanation of icons, see p. 1068.

DISULFIRAM
Antabuse
Tabs: 250, 500 mg
Drug dependence treatment

NO   3   C

Indication: Alcohol deterrent
Initial dose: 500 mg PO daily × 1-2 wk
Max dose: 500 mg daily

Adverse drug reaction: Peripheral neuropathy, psychosis, hepatitis, blood
    dyscrasias, symptoms of reaction (nausea, throbbing headache, nausea,
    copious vomiting, chest pain, palpitations, confusion, syncope).
Comments:
Warn patient of symptoms of reaction.
Dosage increment: Discontinue medication if liver transaminase levels are >3
    times the upper limit of normal
Monitor complete blood cell count, serum chemistry q3 months.
Most fatal reactions occur with >500 mg doses and >2 drinks (some have
    occurred with 1 drink).
Contraindicated in severe myocardial disease, psychosis, hypersensitivity to
    thiuram derivatives used in pesticides and rubber vulcanization, ethyl alcohol
    intoxication, psychoses, cardiovascular disease.

FLUMAZENIL
Romazicon
Inj: 0.1 mg/mL
Drug dependence treatment

NO   3   C

Indication: Benzodiazepine overdose
Initial dose: 0.2 mg IV over 15 sec
               Repeat bolus at 1-min intervals
Max dose: 1 mg/dose or 3 mg/hr

Adverse drug reaction: Seizures, withdrawal symptoms
Comments: Use with caution in benzodiazepine-dependent patients.
Dosage increment: Multiple doses usually needed because of short half-life.
Contraindicated when using a benzodiazepine to treat a life-threatening
    condition, or in serious tricyclic antidepressant overdose.

PULMONARY
β₂-Agonists

ALBUTEROL

Ventolin, Proventil, Proventil HFA, Nebule, Airet

NO   1   C

Tabs, scored: 2, 4 mg
Tabs, extended-release: 4, 8 mg
Solution, nebulization: 0.5% solution (2.5 mL) (Proventil), 0.021%, 0.042% solution (Accuneb) 0.083% (Airet, Proventil)
Inhaler, dry powder: 200 μg/inhalation (Rotahaler)
Oral liquid: 2 mg/5 mL
Inhaler: 90 μg/actuation (120 actuations) (Proventil, Proventil HFA, Ventolin)

β₂-*Agonists*

Indication: Bronchospasm, exercise induced, asthma
Initial dose: 2 puffs q4-6h prn
         2-4 mg PO tid-qid
         4-8 mg extended release PO bid
         0.5 mL of 0.5% solution (2.5 mg) nebulized q3-4h
         200-400 μg (1-2 caps) inhaled q4-6h (dry powder)
         90-180 μg (1-2 puffs) inhaled q4-6h
Max dose: 12 puffs daily
         32 mg PO daily 5 mg q4h (nebulization)

Adverse drug reaction: Palpitations, vomiting, tremor, nervousness, nausea; rare: hypertension, central nervous system stimulation, dizziness, diaphoresis, upper respiratory tract infection.
Comments:
Drug/drug: Additive cardiovascular effects with monoamine oxidase inhibitors and tricyclic antidepressants.
Drug/drug: β-Blockers may antagonize effect.
Reinforce technique at each interaction with health care team.
Class side effects: Rare: tachycardia, coughing, bronchospasm, hypersensitivity reaction.
Contraindicated in prior hypersensitivity to the medication.

For explanation of icons, see p. 1068.

LEVALBUTEROL

Xopenex
Solution, nebulization: 0.63, 1.25 mg
β₂-*Agonists*

NO 3 C

Indication: Asthma
Initial dose: 0.63 mg nebulized q6-8h

Adverse drug reaction: Rhinitis; rare: hypertension, dizziness, tremor.
Comments:
Dosage increment: May be increased to 1.25 mg tid for nonresponders.
Drug/drug: Additive cardiovascular effects with monoamine oxidase inhibitors
   and tricyclic antidepressants. β-Blockers may antagonize effect.
Contraindicated in patients with hypersensitivity to racemic albuterol.
Class side effects: Rare: tachycardia, coughing, bronchospasm,
   hypersensitivity reaction.
Contraindicated in prior hypersensitivity to the medication.

SALMETEROL XINAFOATE

Serevent, Serevent Discus
Inhaler: 21 µg/actuation (60, 120 actuations)
Inhaler, dry powder: 50 µg/inhalation (25, 60 blisters) (Diskus)
β₂-*Agonists*

NO 3 C

Indication: Bronchospasm (exercise induced), asthma, chronic obstructive
            pulmonary disease
Initial dose: 2 puffs bid (42 µg)
Max dose: 2 puffs bid

Adverse drug reaction: Headache, pharyngitis, upper respiratory tract infection;
   rare: palpitations, ventricular arrhythmias.
Comments:
Monitor blood pressure, heart rate, peak expiratory flow rate: periodically.
Drug/drug: Additive cardiovascular effects with monoamine oxidase inhibitors
   and tricyclic antidepressants. β-Blockers may antagonize effect.
Reinforce technique at each interaction with health care team.
Dry powder inhalers use fast deep inhalation, whereas metered dose inhaler
   uses slower deep inhalation. Do not exhale into dry powder device; must be
   used from a horizontal and level position.
Contraindicated in acutely deteriorating asthma or with prior hypersensitivity to
   the medication.
Class side effects: Rare: tachycardia, coughing, bronchospasm,
   hypersensitivity reaction.

Inhaled Steroids

BECLOMETHASONE DIPROPIONATE

NO   ?   C

Beclovent, Vanceril, Vanceril DS, Beconase, Vancenase,
Beconase AQ, Vancenase AQ
Inhaler, nasal: 42 µg/nasal inhalation (Beconase, Vancenase)
Inhaler, nasal: 42, 84 µg/nasal spray (Beconase AQ, Vancenase AQ)
Inhaler, oral: 42 µg/actuation (Beclovent), 42, 84 µg/actuation (Vanceril)
Inhaled steroids

Indication: Asthma, allergic rhinitis
Initial dose:
  Asthma:
    2 puffs tid/qid or 4 puffs bid (Beclovent, Vanceril)
    2 puffs bid (Vanceril DS)
  Rhinitis:
    1 nasal inhalation each nostril bid/qid (Beconase,
      Vancenase)
    1-2 sprays each nostril bid or daily (Beconase AQ, Vancenase AQ)
Max dose: 20 puffs daily (10 puffs DS)

Adverse drug reaction: Rare: bronchospasm, angioedema, adrenal insufficiency.
Comments:
Spacer devices can decrease risk of local infection and dysphonia and improve
  technique.
Rinse out mouth after each use to prevent local infection.
Deaths have been documented in patients abruptly switched from oral to
  inhaled steroids. Overlapping is recommended.
Reinforce technique at each interaction with health care team.
Contraindicated in patients with status asthmaticus (oral) or prior
  hypersensitivity to the medication.
Class side effects: Rare: oral fungal infection (oral), irritation or burning nasal
  mucosa (nasal), cough, dysphonia, epistaxis (nasal), cataracts, glaucoma,
  bone loss (high dose).

For explanation of icons, see p. 1068.

BUDESONIDE

Pulmicort Pulmicort respules, Rhinocort Aqua
Inhaler, dry powder: 200 µg/actuation (Pulmicort), 250,
500 µg/actuation (Pulmicort respules)
Inhaler, nasal: 32 µg/spray (Rhinocort Aqua)
Inhaled steroids

NO   ?   C

Indication: Asthma, rhinitis
Initial dose:
   Asthma: 1-2 puffs bid
   Rhinitis: 2 sprays each nostril bid or 4 sprays each nostril daily
Max dose: 256 µg (4 sprays) per nostril daily

Adverse drug reaction: Headache, pharyngitis, sinusitis; rare: hypersensitivity
   reactions.
Comments:
Dry powder inhalers use fast deep inhalation, whereas metered dose inhaler
   uses slower deep inhalation.
Spacer devices can decrease risk of local infection and improve technique.
Rinse out mouth after each use to prevent local infection.
Deaths have been documented in patients abruptly switched from oral to
   inhaled steroids. Overlapping is recommended.
Reinforce technique at each interaction with health care team.
Contraindicated in patients with recent septal ulcer (nasal), nasal surgery,
   trauma, or prior hypersensitivity to the medication.
Class side effects: Rare: oral fungal infection (oral), irritation or burning nasal
   mucosa (nasal), cough, dysphonia, epistaxis (nasal), cataracts, glaucoma,
   bone loss (high dose).

FLUNISOLIDE

AeroBid, AeroBid-M, Nasalide, Nasarel
Inhaler, oral: 250 µg/actuation (100 actuations)
Solution: 250 µg/dose
Inhaler, nasal: 25 µg/spray (200 sprays) (Nasalide, Nasarel)
Inhaled steroids

NO   ?   C

Indication: Asthma, allergic rhinitis
Initial dose:
   Asthma: 2-4 puffs bid
   Rhinitis: 2 sprays each nostril bid
Max dose: 8 puffs (2 mg) daily
              2 sprays/nostril tid

Continued

FLUNISOLIDE *continued*

Adverse drug reaction: Nausea, vomiting, diarrhea, upper respiratory tract
infection.
Comments:
Spacer devices can decrease risk of local infection and improve technique.
Rinse out mouth after each use to prevent local infection.
Deaths have been documented in patients abruptly switched from oral to
inhaled steroids. Overlapping is recommended.
Reinforce technique at each interaction with health care team.
Contraindicated in status asthmaticus (oral), respiratory infections, untreated
localized nasal infection (nasal), or prior hypersensitivity to the medication.
Class side effects: Rare: oral fungal infection (oral), irritation or burning nasal
mucosa (nasal), cough, dysphonia, epistaxis (nasal), cataracts, glaucoma,
bone loss (high dose).

FLUTICASONE

Flovent, Flovent Rotadisk, Flonase, Cutivate
Inhaler, oral: 44, 110, 220 µg/actuation (60, 120 actuations) NO ? C
Inhaler, dry powder: 50, 100, 250 µg/actuation (60 actuations) (Rotadisk)
Inhaler, nasal: 50 µg/spray (Flonase)
Topical, ointment: 0.0005% (15, 30, 60 g tube) (Cutivate)
Topical, cream: 0.05% (15, 30, 60 g tube) (Cutivate)
Inhaled steroids

Indication: Asthma, allergic rhinitis, atopic dermatitis, eczema, psoriasis
Initial dose:
    Asthma: 1-2 puffs (110-220 µg) bid
           1 inhalation (100 µg) bid
    Rhinitis: 2 sprays each nostril daily or 1 spray bid
    Dermatitis, eczema, psoriasis: Applied to affected areas daily-bid.
    Max dose: 440 µg bid
             500 µg powder bid
             2 sprays per nostril daily

Adverse drug reaction: Rare: bronchospasm, adrenal insufficiency.
Comments:
Dry powder inhalers use fast deep inhalation, whereas metered dose inhaler
uses slower deep inhalation.
Spacer devices can decrease risk of local infection and improve technique.
Rinse out mouth after each use to prevent local infection.
Deaths have been documented in patients abruptly switched from oral to
inhaled steroids. Overlapping is recommended.
Reinforce technique at each interaction with health care team.

Continued

FLUTICASONE *continued*

Contraindicated as primary agent in acute settings or with prior hypersensitivity to the medication.

Class side effects: Rare: oral fungal infection (oral), irritation or burning nasal mucosa (nasal), cough, dysphonia, epistaxis (nasal), cataracts, glaucoma, bone loss (high dose).

TRIAMCINOLONE ACETONIDE

Azmacort, Nasacort, Aristocort
Inhaler, oral: 100 µg/actuation (240 actuations)   NO   ?   C
Inhaler, nasal: 55 µg/spray (Nasacort)
Topical, cream: 0.025%, 0.1%, 0.5% (15 and/or 60 g tubes) (Aristocort)
Topical, ointment: 0.1%, 0.5% (15 and/or 60 g tubes) (Aristocort)
Inhaled steroids

Indication: Asthma, allergic rhinitis, atopic dermatitis, eczema, psoriasis, lichen planus
Initial dose:
  Asthma: 2 puffs tid/qid
  Allergic rhinitis: 2 sprays each nostril daily or 1 spray bid
  Allergic rhinitis: 2 sprays each nostril daily or 1 spray bid
  Dermatitis, eczema, psoriasis, lichen planus: Applied to affected areas bid-qid (0.025%), or bid-tid (0.1%, 0.5%)

Max dose: 16 puffs daily
        4 sprays/nostril daily

Comments:
Dosage increment: May administer 4 puffs bid as maintenance.
Built-in spacer devices can decrease risk of local infection and improve technique.
Rinse out mouth after each use to prevent local infection.
Deaths have been documented in patients abruptly switched from oral to inhaled steroids. Overlapping is recommended.
Reinforce technique at each interaction with health care team.
Contraindicated in status asthmaticus (oral), untreated localized nasal infection (nasal), or prior hypersensitivity to the medication.
Class side effects: Rare: oral fungal infection (oral), irritation or burning nasal mucosa (nasal), cough, dysphonia, epistaxis (nasal), cataracts, glaucoma, bone loss (high dose).

Leukotriene Inhibitors

MONTELUKAST

Singulair
Tabs: 10 mg
Tabs, chewable: 4, 5 mg
Leukotriene inhibitors

NO ? B

Indication: Asthma
Initial dose: 10 mg PO qhs
Max dose: 10 mg daily

Comments:
Drug/drug: Rifampin increases metabolism.
Class side effects: Headache; rare: increased alanine aminotransferase levels,
    dizziness, insomnia, abdominal pain.
Contraindicated in prior hypersensitivity to the medication, status asthmaticus.

ZAFIRLUKAST

Accolate
Tabs: 10, 20 mg
Leukotriene inhibitors

NO X B

Indication: Asthma
Initial dose: 20 mg PO bid
Max dose: 40 mg daily

Comments:
Drug/drug: May increase warfarin levels.
Class side effects: Headache; rare: increased alanine aminotransferase levels,
    dizziness, insomnia, abdominal pain.
Contraindicated in prior hypersensitivity to the medication, status asthmaticus.

ZILEUTON

Zyflo Filmtab
Tabs, scored: 600 mg
Leukotriene inhibitors

NO ? C

Indication: Asthma
Initial dose: 600 mg PO qid
Max dose: 2.4 g daily

Continued

For explanation of icons, see p. 1068.

Adverse drug reaction: Headache; rare: leukopenia.
Comments:
Monitor liver function tests (LFTs): Baseline, q month for 3 months, q2-3 months for the first year, then periodically.
Drug/drug: β-Blockers, ergot derivates, pimozide, theophylline, warfarin may increase levels.
Contraindicated in patients with acute hepatic disease, LFT result >3 times upper limit of normal, prior hypersensitivity to the medication, or status asthmaticus.
Class side effects: Headache; rare: increased alanine aminotransferase levels, dizziness, insomnia, abdominal pain.

Other Agents

CROMOLYN SODIUM

Intal, Nasalcrom
Inhaler, oral: 800 μg/actuation
Solution, inhalation: 10 mg/mL (2 mL)
Inhaler, nasal: 5.2 mg/spray (100, 200 metered sprays)
Other Agents

NO   ?   B

Indication: Asthma, allergic rhinitis
Initial dose:
    Asthma: 2 puffs qid
             1 (20 mg) nebulized qid
    Allergic rhinitis: 1 spray (5.2 mg) each nostril tid/qid
Max dose: 6 sprays daily

Adverse drug reaction: Unpleasant taste, coughing; rare: angioedema, bronchospasm.
Comments:
Dosage increment: Max effect seen at 2-4 wk. Once the patient is stabilized, the frequency may be titrated down to tid and then bid according to patient's tolerance.
Reinforce technique at each interaction with health care team.
Contraindicated in patients with status asthmaticus or prior hypersensitivity to the medication.

DORNASE ALFA

Pulmozyme
Solution, inhalation: 1 mg/mL (2.5 mL)
Other Agents

NO 3 B

Indication: Cystic fibrosis
Initial dose: 2.5 mg nebulized daily
Max dose: 20 mg inhaled for up to 6 days

Adverse drug reaction: Rare: pharyngitis, voice alteration, chest pain, rash, conjunctivitis, cough, dyspnea.
Comments:
Dosage increment: Older patients (>21 yr) or those with forced vital capacity >85% may benefit from bid doses.
Contraindicated in patients with hypersensitivity to dornase, Chinese hamster ovary cell products (epoetin alfa).

IPRATROPIUM

Atrovent
Inhaler: 18 µg/actuation (200 actuations)
Solution, nebulization: 0.02% (500 µg/vial) (2.5 mL)
Inhaler, nasal: 0.03%, 0.06% (21, 42 µg/metered spray)
Other Agents

NO ? B

Indication: Bronchospasm in chronic bronchitis, emphysema
Initial dose: 2 puffs qid
      1 (500 µg) nebulization q6-8h
      2 sprays each nostril bid/tid
Max dose: 12 puffs daily
      500 µg q6h

Adverse drug reaction: Rare: dizziness, fatigue, headache, nervousness, nausea, cough, palpitations, insomnia.
Comments:
Poorly absorbed, so systemic effects are rare.
Drug/drug: Antimuscarinic agents have additive effects.
Reinforce technique at each interaction with health care team.
Contraindicated in patients with hypersensitivity to the medication, atropine or its derivatives, lecithin, soybeans, or peanuts.

For explanation of icons, see p. 1068.

NEDOCROMIL

Tilade
Inhaler: 1.75 mg/actuation (112 actuations)
Other Agents

NO ? B

Indication: Asthma
Initial dose: 2 puffs qid
Max dose: 14 mg daily

Adverse drug reaction: Unpleasant taste; rare: chest pain, dizziness, dysphonia, headache, rash, diarrhea, dyspepsia.
Comments:
Reinforce technique at each interaction with health care team.
Contraindicated in patients with acute asthma flare or prior hypersensitivity to the medication.

THEOPHYLLINE

Theo-24, Theo-Dur, Slo-Bid, Gyrocaps, Uni-Dur, Theolair
Caps, extended-release: 75, 100, 125, 200, 300, 400 mg
(Slo-Bid, Theo-24)
Oral liquid: 27, 50 mg/5 mL
Tabs, scored: 100, 125, 200, 250, 300, mg (various)
Tabs, extended-release, scored: 100, 200, 300, 400, 450, 600 mg (various)
Other Agents

NO 1 C

Indication: Asthma, chronic obstructive pulmonary disease
Initial dose: 10 mg/kg/day (max 300 mg daily) for 3 days, then 13 mg/kg/day for 3 days
Max dose: 13 mg/kg or 900 mg daily without measuring levels
Hepatic dose: Monitor levels more frequently and adjust dose accordingly

Adverse drug reaction: Nausea, vomiting, diarrhea, abdominal pain, nervousness, restlessness, headache, insomnia, agitation, palpitations, extrasystoles, tachycardia, dizziness; rare: seizures, arrhythmias, respiratory arrest.
Comments:
Monitor: Electrocardiogram in toxic ingestions.
Dosage increment: Based on previous levels and lean body weight, each 0.5 mg/kg PO/IV loading dose increases levels by 1 µg/mL. Convert to once daily formulation by adding up the previous total daily dose.
Level <10 µg/mL = increase 25%, recheck in 3 days
Level 10-20 µg/mL = recheck q6-12 months

Continued

THEOPHYLLINE *continued*

Level > 20 µg/mL = decrease 10%, recheck in 3 days

Level >30 µg/mL = skip 2 doses, then decrease 50% recheck in 3 days

Drug/drug: Allopurinol, erythromycin, propranolol, ciprofloxacin, cimetidine may increase levels. Theophylline is a competitive antagonist at the adenosine receptor; may need to increase the dose of adenosine. Theophylline decreases benzodiazepine levels. Barbiturates, ketoconazole, phenytoin, rifampin, smoking may decrease levels.

Contraindicated in patients with uncontrolled arrhythmias, hyperthyroidism, peptic ulcers, uncontrolled seizure disorders, hypersensitivity to the medication or other methyl xanthines.

Combination Agents

ALBUTEROL/ATROVENT

Combivent
Inhaler: 90/18 µg
Combination agents

 Indication: Chronic obstructive pulmonary disease

SALMETEROL/FLUTICASONE PROPIONATE

Advair
Inhaler, dry powder: 50/100, 250, 500 µg
Combination agents

 Indication: Asthma

PART IV

Rapid References

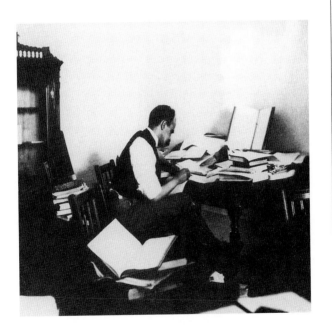

Rapid References

Chrishonda M. Curry, Erica A. Kaiser, Shin Lin, Jennifer Meuchel,
Daniel Mudrick, Matthew Pipeling, Rita Rastogi, and Abe Shaikh

Cardiology

EQUATIONS
Fick principle

$$\text{Cardiac output (L/min)} = \frac{O_2 \text{ consumption (mL/min)}}{\text{Arteriovenous } O_2 \text{ difference (mL/L)}}$$

$$\text{SVR} = \frac{80(\text{MAP} - \text{RA})}{\text{CO}}$$

where
SVR = systemic vascular resistance [(dyne·sec)/cm^5]
MAP = mean arterial pressure (mm Hg)
RA = right atrial pressure (mm Hg)
CO = cardiac output (L/min)
80 = for conversion of dimensions

$$\text{PVR} = \frac{80(\text{PA} - \text{PCW or LA})}{\text{CO}}$$

where
PVR = pulmonary vascular resistance [(dyne·sec)/cm^5]
PA = pulmonary artery mean pressure (mm Hg)
PCW = pulmonary capillary wedge mean pressure (mm Hg)
LA = left atrial mean pressure (mm Hg)
CO = cardiac output (L/min)

$$A = \frac{\text{Flow}}{[K\sqrt{(\Delta P)}]} \quad \text{(Gorlin formula)}$$

where
A = valve orifice area (cm^2)
Flow = blood flow across valve (mL/sec) measured as cardiac output/flow
   time × heart rate
ΔP = mean pressure gradient (mm Hg)
K = constant (K = 44.3 for aortic valve and 37.7 for mitral valve)

SUPPLEMENTAL ELECTROCARDIOGRAPHIC FEATURES
1. **Arrhythmias.**
a. Atrial rhythms.
   (1) Sinus arrhythmia.
      (a) Normal P wave morphology and axis.
      (b) Gradual phasic change in PP interval (may be abrupt).

(c) Longest and shortest PP interval vary by >0.16 sec or 10%.

(2) Ectopic atrial rhythm.
   (a) P wave axis or morphology different from sinus node.
   (b) Rate <100 beats/min.
   (c) PR >0.11 sec.
   (d) With inverted P in II, III, and aVF and PR >0.11 sec suggests a low atrial rhythm.
   (e) With inverted P in II, III, and aVF but PR <0.11 sec suggests atrioventricular (AV) junctional rhythm.

(3) Wandering atrial pacemaker.
   (a) P waves with three or more morphologies.
   (b) Rate <100 beats/min (rate >100 beats/min is called multifocal atrial tachycardia).
   (c) Varying PR, RR, and RP intervals.
   (d) No dominant P wave morphology, in contradistinction to sinus rhythm with multifocal atrial premature complexes.
   (e) Distinct isoelectric baseline, in contradistinction to atrial fibrillation and flutter with a moderate ventricular response.

(4) Atrial flutter.
   (a) F waves (rapid regular atrial undulations) at 240 to 350 per minute (faster in children, slower in those taking antiarrhythmic drugs [type IA, IC, III] and with massively dilated atria).
   (b) Typical atrial flutter morphology.
      i. Picket fence or sawtooth appearance (inverted F waves without isoelectric baseline) in II, III, and aVF.
      ii. Small positive deflections with a distinct isoelectric baseline in V_1.
   (c) Rate and regularity of QRS depend on AV conduction sequence.
      i. AV conduction ratio (flutter waves to QRS) is usually fixed but may vary.
         (1) If ≥4:1, consider concomitant AV conduction disease.
         (2) Complete heart block with a junctional or ventricular escape rhythm may be present.
   (d) With complete heart block and junctional tachycardia, consider digitalis toxicity (see 8j).
   (e) Flutter waves can deform QRS, ST, or T to mimic intraventricular conduction delay or myocardial ischemia.
   (f) With wide QRS, consider Wolff-Parkinson-White (WPW) syndrome.

(5) Atrial fibrillation.
   (a) P wave absent.
   (b) Irregular atrial activity represented by fibrillatory (f) waves of varying amplitude, duration, and morphology, causing random oscillation of the baseline best seen in V_1, V_2, and inferior leads.
   (c) Ventricular rhythm is irregularly irregular.
      i. If RR interval is regular, third-degree AV block is present.

ii. Digoxin toxicity may result in regularization of QRS because of complete heart block with junctional tachycardia.
(d) Ventricular rate is 100 to 180 beats/min in absence of drugs.
    i. If the rate without AV blocking drugs is less than 100 beats/min, AV conduction system disease is likely to be present.
(e) With wide QRS and ventricular rate >200 beats/min, consider WPW syndrome.
(6) Sinus arrest.
  (a) PP interval (pause) >6 to 2.0 sec.
  (b) Resumption of sinus rhythm that is not a multiple of the basic sinus PP rhythm.
(7) Sinoatrial block.
  (a) First degree.
    i. Not detectable on surface ECG.
  (b) Second degree.
    i. Type I (Mobitz I).
      (1) P wave morphology and axis consistent with sinus node origin.
      (2) "Group beating" with PP shortening leading to a pause, constant PR, and PP pause less than twice the normal PP interval.
    ii. Type II (Mobitz II).
      (1) Constant PP followed by a pause that is a multiple of the normal PP.
  (c) Third degree.
    i. Cannot be differentiated from sinus arrest
(8) Atrial tachycardia with block.
  (a) Abnormal P wave axis and morphology.
  (b) Atrial rate: 150 to 240 beats/min.
  (c) Isoelectric intervals between P waves in all leads.
  (d) Second- or third-degree AV block.
  (e) Regular atrial rhythm.
  (f) Has distinct isoelectric baseline between P waves in contradistinction to atrial flutter (except in V_1 for atrial flutter).
b. Ventricular rhythms.
  (1) Ventricular premature complexes (VPC). Require all of the following.
    (a) A wide, notched, or slurred QRS that is premature relative to the normal RR interval and not preceded by a P wave.
    (b) Secondary ST and T wave changes in direction opposite to the major deflection of the QRS.
    (c) Coupling interval (relation of VPCs to the preceding QRS) is constant or varies by <0.08 sec.
    (d) Morphology of VPCs in any given lead is uniform.
  (2) Ventricular tachycardia (VT).
    (a) Rapid succession of three or more premature ventricular beats at a rate >100 beats/min.

      (b) RR interval is usually regular but may be irregular.

      (c) Abrupt onset and termination of arrhythmia are evident.

      (d) AV dissociation is common.

      (e) Retrograde atrial activation (inverted P waves in leads II, III, and aVF) and capture occur.

   (3) Ventricular fibrillation (VF).

      (a) Extremely rapid and irregular ventricular rhythm demonstrating chaotic and irregular deflections of varying amplitude and contour, *and*

      (b) Absence of distinct P waves, QRS complexes, or T waves.

2. **AV conduction abnormalities.**

a. Short PR interval (with sinus rhythm and normal QRS duration).

   (1) Normal P wave axis and morphology.

   (2) PR <0.12 sec.

   (3) No delta wave (QRS <0.11 sec).

   (4) No sinus rhythm with AV dissociation.

b. Wolff-Parkinson-White (WPW) pattern.

   (1) Normal P wave axis and morphology.

   (2) PR <0.12 sec.

   (3) Delta wave (initial slurring of QRS) resulting in a wide QRS (>0.10 sec).

   (4) Secondary ST and T wave changes (opposite in direction to main deflection of QRS).

   (5) PJ interval (beginning of P wave to end of QRS complex) is constant and ≤0.26 sec.

3. **Intraventricular conduction disturbances (IVCDs).**

a. Right bundle branch block (RBBB), incomplete.

   (1) rSR' in V_1 with QRS duration between 0.09 and 0.12 sec.

      (a) Differential diagnosis should include normal variant, right ventricular hypertrophy, posterior wall myocardial infarction (MI), incorrect lead placement, and skeletal deformities (e.g., pectus excavatum).

b. RBBB, complete.

   (1) Prolonged QRS (≤0.12 sec).

   (2) rsR' or rSR' in V_1 and V_2.

   (3) Delayed onset of intrinsicoid deflection (beginning of QRS to peak of R wave ≥0.05 sec) in V_1 and V_2.

   (4) Secondary ST and T wave changes (downsloping ST segment, T wave inversion) in V_1 and V_2.

   (5) Wide slurred S wave in I, V_5, and V_6.

c. Left anterior fascicular block.

   (1) Left axis deviation with mean QRS axis between −45° and −90°.

   (2) qR or R in I and aVL.

   (3) Normal or slightly prolonged QRS duration (0.08-0.10 sec).

   (4) Exclusion of other causes of left axis deviation (left ventricular hypertrophy [6a], inferior wall MI, chronic lung disease [8f], LBBB [3e], atrial septal defect primum [8e], severe hyperkalemia [8m]).

    (5) Poor R wave progression.

  d. Left posterior fascicular block

    (1) Right axis deviation with mean QRS axis between +100° and +180°.

    (2) S_1Q_3 (deep S wave in I and Q wave in III).

    (3) Normal or slightly prolonged QRS duration (0.08-0.10 sec).

    (4) Exclusion of other causes of right axis deviation (right ventricular hypertrophy [RVH] [6b], vertical heart, chronic lung disease [8f], pulmonary embolism, lateral wall MI, dextrocardia [8h], lead reversal, and WPW syndrome [2b]).

  e. Left bundle branch block (LBBB), complete.

    (1) Prolonged QRS duration (≥0.12 sec).

    (2) Delayed onset of intrinsicoid deflection (beginning of QRS to peak of R wave ≥0.05 sec) in I, V_5, and V_6.

    (3) Broad monophasic R in I, V_5, and V_6 that is usually notched or slurred.

    (4) Secondary ST and T wave changes opposite in direction to the major QRS deflection (i.e., ST depression and T wave inversion in I, V_5, and V_6; ST elevation and upright T wave in leads V_1 and V_2).

    (5) rS or QS complexes in right precordial leads.

    (6) Left axis deviation may be present.

  f. LBBB, intermittent.

    (1) Features of complete LBBB seen during tachycardia (but maybe bradycardia as well).

4. P wave aberrancies.

  a. Right atrial abnormality.

    (1) Upright P wave.

      (a) >2.5 mm in II, III, and aVF (P-pulmonale) *or*

      (b) >1.5 mm in leads V_1 or V_2.

    (2) P wave axis shifted rightward (i.e., axis ≥70°).

    (3) Substantial minority of P-pulmonale may actually represent left atrial enlargement. Suspect this possibility when features of left atrial abnormality (4b) are present in lead V_1.

  b. Left atrial abnormality.

    (1) Notched P wave ≥0.12 sec in II, III, or AVF (P-mitrale) *or*

    (2) Terminal negative portion of the P wave in V_1 ≥1 mm deep and ≥0.04 sec in duration.

  c. Biatrial enlargement suggested by the following.

    (1) Large biphasic P wave in V_1 ≤0.04 sec with the following.

      (a) An initial positive amplitude >1.5 mm, *and*

      (b) A terminal negative amplitude ≤1 mm.

    (2) Tall peaked P waves (>1.5 mm) in the right precordial leads (V_1-V_3) and wide notched P waves in the left precordial leads (V_5-V_6).

    (3) P wave amplitude ≥2.5 mm in the limb leads with a duration ≥0.12 sec.

5. QRS voltage or axis abnormalities.

  a. Low voltage, limb leads only (differential diagnosis includes chronic lung disease [8f], pericardial effusion [8s], myxedema [8e], obesity, pleural effusion, restrictive or infiltrative cardiomyopathies, and diffuse coronary disease).

    (1) R+S <5 mm in all limb leads.

b. Low voltage, limb and precordial leads (differential diagnosis as above).

    (1) R+S <10 mm in each precordial lead and R+S <5 mm in all leads.

c. Left axis deviation (differential diagnosis includes left anterior fascicular block [axis <−45°; see 3c]; inferior wall MI; LBBB [3e]; LVH [6a]; atrial septal defect [ASD] primum [8e]; chronic obstructive pulmonary disease [COPD] [8f], hyperkalemia [8m]).

    (1) Mean QRS axis between −30° and −106°.

d. Right axis deviation (differential diagnosis includes RVH [6b]; vertical heart; COPD [8f]; pulmonary embolism; left posterior fascicular block [3d]; lateral wall MI; dextrocardia [8h]; lead reversal; and ASD secundum [8d]).

    (1) Mean QRS axis between 101° and 254°.

e. Electrical alternans (differential diagnosis includes pericardial effusion [8s], severe left ventricular failure, hypertension, coronary artery disease, rheumatic heart disease, supraventricular or ventricular tachycardia, and deep respirations).

    (1) Alternation in the amplitude or direction of P, QRS, and T waves.

6. Ventricular hypertrophy.

a. Left ventricular hypertrophy (LVH).

    (1) Voltage.

        (a) Cornell criteria: R wave in aVL + S wave in V_3 >24 mm in men or >20 mm in women.

        (b) Precordial leads.

            i. S wave in V_1 + R wave in V_5 or V_6.

                (1) >35 mm if age >30 years.

                (2) >40 mm if age between 20 and 30 years.

                (3) >60 mm if age between 16 and 19 years.

            ii. Maximum R wave + S wave in precordial leads >45 mm.

            iii. R wave in V_5 >26 mm.

            iv. R wave in V_6 >20 mm.

        (c) Limb leads.

            i. R wave in I + S wave in II ≥26 mm.

            ii. R wave in lead I ≥14 mm.

            iii. S wave in aVR ≥15 mm.

            iv. R wave in aVL ≥12 mm (highly specific).

            v. R wave in aVF ≥21 mm.

    (2) ST-T segment abnormalities.

        (a) ST and T wave deviation opposite in direction to the major QRS deflection.

        (b) ST depression in I, aVL, III, aVF, or V_4-V_6.

        (c) Slight ST elevation (<1-2 mm) in leads V_1-V_3.

        (d) Inverted T waves in leads I, aVL, and V_4-V_6.

        (e) Prominent or inverted U waves.

   (3) Other features.
      (a) Left atrial abnormality (see 4b).
      (b) Left axis deviation.
      (c) Nonspecific intraventricular conduction delay.
      (d) Delayed onset of intrinsicoid deflection (beginning of QRS to peak of R wave >0.05 sec).
      (e) Low anterior forces (small or absent R waves in V_1-V_3).
      (f) Absent Q waves in I, V_5, and V_6.
      (g) Abnormal Q waves in leads II, III, and aVF (from left axis deviation).
      (h) Prominent U waves (see 7f).
b. Right ventricular hypertrophy (RVH) (for feature in the setting of chronic lung disease, see 8f).
   (1) Right axis deviation with mean QRS axis ≥+100°.
   (2) Dominant R wave.
      (a) R/S ratio in V_1 or V_{3R} >1. Alternatively, R/S ratio in V_5 or V_6 ≤1.
      (b) R wave in V_1 ≥7 mm.
      (c) R wave in V_1 + S wave in V_5 or V_6 >10.5 mm.
      (d) rSR′ in V_1 with R′ >10 mm.
      (e) qR complex in V_1.
   (3) Downsloping ST depression or T wave inversion in right precordial leads.
   (4) Right atrial abnormality (see 4a).
   (5) Onset of intrinsicoid deflection in V_1 between 0.035 and 0.055 sec.
c. Combined ventricular hypertrophy.
   (1) Meets criteria for both LVH and RVH.
   (2) Precordial leads show LVH but right axis deviation.
   (3) LVH (see 6a), R wave > Q wave in aVR, S wave > R wave in V_5, and T wave inversion in V_1.
   (4) Katz-Wachtel phenomenon (large amplitude, equiphasic [R = S] complexes in V_3 and V_4).
   (5) Right atrial abnormality (see 4a) with LVH pattern (see 6a) in precordial leads.

7. ST, T, and U wave aberrancies.
a. Early repolarization (normal variant most common in young healthy individuals).
   (1) elevated take-off of J point (the junction between the QRS and ST).
   (2) Concave upward ST elevation ending with a symmetrical upright T wave.
   (3) Notch or slur on downstroke of R wave.
   (4) Features found in V_2-V_5 and sometimes in II, III, and aVF.
   (5) No reciprocal ST segment depression.
b. Nonspecific ST or T wave abnormalities (may be normal, but differential diagnosis includes organic heart disease, drugs, electrolyte disorders, hyperventilation, hypothyroidism [see 8r], stress, pancreatitis, pericarditis, CNS disorders, LVH [6a], RVH [6b], BBB).

       (1) Slight ST depression or elevation (<1 mm).

       (2) T wave flat or slightly inverted.

  c. ST or T wave abnormalities suggesting acute pericarditis.

     (1) Classic evolutionary pattern.

       (a) Stage 1: upwardly concave ST elevation in almost all leads except aVR, in which there may be reciprocal ST depression.

       (b) Stage 2: J point returns to baseline and T wave amplitude decreases.

       (c) Stage 3: T waves invert.

       (d) Stage 4: ECG returns to baseline.

     (2) Other suggestive features include sinus tachycardia, PR depression early (elevation in aVR), low voltage QRS (see 5a and 5b), and electrical alternans (see 5e) if pericardial effusion is present (see 8s).

  d. J point (the junction between the QRS and ST) depression (most frequently seen in exercise testing).

     (1) ST depression ≥1 mm and lasting ≥0.08 sec at the J point.

  e. Peaked T waves (differential diagnosis includes normal variant, acute MI, hyperkalemia [8m], intracranial bleeding, LVH [6a], and LBBB [3e]).

     (1) T wave >6 mm in limb leads *or*

     (2) T wave >10 mm in precordial leads.

  f. Prominent U waves (differential diagnosis includes hypokalemia [8n], bradyarrhythmias, hypothermia [8p], LVH [6a], organic heart disease, drugs [e.g., digitalis, quinidine, amiodarone, isoproterenol]).

     (1) Amplitude ≥1.5 mm.

8. Miscellaneous.

a. Acute cor pulmonale (features are often transient).

   (1) Sinus tachycardia.

   (2) Features of right ventricular pressure overload.

     (a) Right atrial abnormality (see 4b).

     (b) Inverted T waves in V_1-V_3.

     (c) Right axis deviation.

     (d) S_1Q_3 (deep S wave in I and Q wave in III) or $S_1Q_3T_3$ (prominence of S wave in I, Q wave in III, and T wave inversion in III).

     (e) Pseudoinfarct pattern in inferior leads.

     (f) Incomplete or complete RBBB.

     (g) Supraventricular tachyarrhythmias.

b. Antiarrhythmic drug effect.

   (1) Prolonged QT.

   (2) Prominent U waves.

   (3) ST or T wave changes.

   (4) Atrial flutter rate decrease.

c. Antiarrhythmic drug toxicity.

   (1) Prolonged QT.

   (2) Ventricular arrhythmias including torsade de pointes.

   (3) Wide QRS.

      (4) Any degree of AV block.

      (5) Marked sinus bradycardia, sinus arrest (see 1a[6]), or sinoatrial (SA) block (see 1a[7]).

d. Atrial septal defect (ASD) secundum.

      (1) Typical RSR' or rSR' complex in V_1 with QRS <0.11 sec.

      (2) RBBB, incomplete (see 3a).

      (3) Right axis deviation ± RVH (see 6b).

      (4) Right atrial abnormality (see 4a) in some cases.

      (5) First-degree AV block in some cases.

e. ASD primum.

      (1) RSR' complex in V_1.

      (2) Left axis deviation.

      (3) First-degree AV block in some cases.

      (4) Biventricular hypertrophy (see 6c) in advanced cases.

f. Chronic lung disease.

      (1) RVH.

         (a) Rightward shift of QRS.

         (b) Inverted T wave in V_1 and V_2.

         (c) ST depression in II, III, and aVF.

         (d) Transient RBBB.

         (e) RSR' or QR complex in V_1.

      (2) Right axis deviation.

      (3) Right atrial abnormality (see 4a).

      (4) Poor R wave progression.

      (5) Low voltage QRS (see 5a and 5b).

      (6) Pseudo–anteroseptal infarct pattern.

      (7) S waves in I, II, and III (S_1, S_2, S_3 pattern).

      (8) Sinus tachycardia, junctional rhythm, various degrees of AV block, intraventricular conduction delay (IVCD).

g. CNS disorder.

      (1) Classic changes are large or deeply inverted T waves, marked prolongation of QT, and prominent U waves in the precordial leads.

      (2) T wave notching with loss of amplitude.

      (3) Diffuse ST elevation (as in acute pericarditis [see 7c]) *or* focal ST elevation (as in acute myocardial injury) *or* ST depression.

      (4) Q waves (as in MI).

      (5) Almost any arrhythmia.

h. Dextrocardia (mirror image).

      (1) P-QRS-T in I and aVL are upside down.

      (2) Reverse R wave progression in precordial leads (if [1] without [2], think lead reversal).

i. Digitalis effect.

      (1) PR lengthening.

      (2) Sagging ST depression with upward concavity.

      (3) QT shortening.

      (4) Flat, inverted, or biphasic T wave.

      (5) Increased U wave amplitude.

j. Digitalis toxicity: any dysrhythmia or conduction disturbance except BBB, including most commonly the following.
  (1) Paroxysmal atrial tachycardia (PAT) with block (see 1a[8]).
  (2) Atrial fibrillation (see 1a[5]) with complete heart block (regular RR).
  (3) Second- or third-degree AV block.
  (4) Complete heart block with accelerated junctional rhythm or accelerated idioventricular rhythm.
    (a) Accelerated junctional rhythm.
      i. Regular QRS rhythm at rate >60 beats min.
      ii. P wave proceeds, is buried in, or follows QRS.
      iii. QRS is usually narrow but may be wide if aberrant or preexisting IVCD and BBB.
      iv. Variation in atrial and ventricular rates.
    (b) Accelerated idioventricular rhythm.
      i. Regular or slightly irregular ventricular rhythm.
      ii. Rate: 60 to 110 beats/min.
      iii. QRS morphology similar to that seen in VPCs (see 1b[1]).
        (1) Wide, notched, or slurred QRS that is premature relative to the normal RR and not preceded by a P wave.
        (2) Secondary ST and T wave changes opposite to QRS deflection.
        (3) Coupling interval (relation of VPCs to the preceding QRS) is constant or varies by <0.08 sec.
        (4) Uniform VPC morphology in a given lead.
      iv. AV dissociation common.
        (1) Atrial and ventricular rhythms are independent.
        (2) Ventricular rate greater than or equal to atrial rate.
      v. Fusion beats common.
        (1) QRS complex intermediate in morphology between QRS of two simultaneously activated sources.
  (5) Supraventricular tachycardia with alternating BBB.

k. Hypercalcemia.
  (1) QTc shortening.
  (2) PR prolongation occasionally.

l. Hypocalcemia.
  (1) QTc prolongation.
  (2) T wave flattening, peaking, or inversion.

m. Hyperkalemia. Note: any ECG change may occur at any abnormal level of potassium; ECG changes do not necessarily move in an orderly fashion as potassium increases (i.e., a patient may progress from peaked T waves to ventricular fibrillation).
  (1) [K$^+$] = 5.5 to 6.5 mEq/L.
    (a) Narrow-based, tall, peaked T waves.
    (b) QT shortening.
    (c) Reversible left anterior fascicular block (see 3c) or left posterior fascicular block (see 3d).

(2) [K⁺] = 6.5 to 7.5 mEq/L.
    (a) First-degree AV block.
    (b) P wave flattening and widening.
    (c) ST depression.
    (d) QRS widening.
(3) [K⁺] >7.5 mEq/L.
    (a) P wave disappearance.
    (b) LBBB (see 3e), RBBB (see 3b), or markedly widened and diffuse intraventricular conduction delay resembling a sine-wave pattern.
(4) Arrhythmias and conduction disturbances, including VT (see 1b[2]), VF (see 1b[3]), idioventricular rhythm, asystole.

n. Hypokalemia.
  (1) Prominent U waves.
  (2) T wave flattening.
  (3) P wave amplitude and duration increase.
  (4) Sometimes QT prolongation.
    (a) Arrhythmias and conduction disturbances including PAT with block (see 1a[8]); first-degree AV block; second-degree AV block, type I; AV dissociation; VPCs (see 1b[1]); VT (see 1b[2]); and VF (see 1b[3]).

o. Hypertrophic cardiomyopathy.
  (1) Left atrial abnormality (see 4b) common, right atrial abnormality (see 4a) sometimes.
  (2) Large amplitude QRS.
  (3) Large abnormal Q waves (pseudoinfarct pattern in precordial and inferior leads).
  (4) Tall R wave with inverted T wave in V_1 (as in RVH [see 6b]).
  (5) ST and T wave abnormalities.
  (6) If T wave inversions in V_4-V_6, think apical variant of hypertrophic cardiomyopathy.
  (7) Left axis deviation sometimes.

p. Hypothermia.
  (1) Sinus bradycardia.
  (2) Prolonged PR, QRS, and QT.
  (3) Osborne ("J") wave (late upright terminal deflection of QRS complex): amplitude increases as temperature declines.
  (4) Atrial fibrillation (see 1a[5]) often.
  (5) Other arrhythmias including AV junctional rhythm, VT (see 1b[2]), and VF (see 1b[3]).
  (6) Ventricular fibrillation risk exists during rewarming.

q. Mitral valve disease.
  (1) Mitral stenosis.
    (a) Suggested by RVH (see 6b) and left atrial abnormality (see 4b).
  (2) Mitral valve prolapse.
    (a) Flattened or inverted T waves in leads II, III, and aVF ± ST segment depression sometimes in left precordial leads.

    (b) Prominent U waves.

    (c) Prolonged QT.

  r. Myxedema (hypothyroidism).

    (1) Low QRS voltage.

    (2) Sinus bradycardia.

    (3) Flattened or inverted T wave.

    (4) Prolonged PR sometimes.

    (5) Features of pericardial effusion (see 8s).

    (6) Electrical alternans (see 5e) sometimes.

  s. Pericardial effusion.

    (1) Low-voltage QRS.

    (2) Electrical alternans (see 5e).

    (3) Features of acute pericarditis (see 7c).

  t. Sick sinus syndrome.

    (1) Marked sinus bradycardia.

    (2) Sinus arrest (see 1a[6]) or SA exit block (see 1a[7]).

    (3) Tachycardia alternating with bradycardia.

    (4) Atrial fibrillation (see 1a[5]) with slow ventricular response preceded or followed by sinus bradycardia, sinus arrest, or SA exit block.

    (5) Prolonged sinus node recovery time after atrial premature complex or atrial tachyarrhythmias.

    (6) AV junctional escape rhythm.

    (7) Conduction system disease, including AV block, IVCD, and BBB.

NORMAL VALUES*

Heart rate (HR)	60-100 beats/min
Cardiac output (CO)	4-8 L/min

$$CO = SV \times HR$$

$$\text{Fick principle: } CO = \frac{\text{Rate of } O_2 \text{ consumption}}{\text{Arterial } O_2 \text{ content} - \text{Venous } O_2 \text{ content}}$$

Systolic blood pressure (SBP)	120 mm Hg
Diastolic blood pressure (DBP)	80 mm Hg
Pulse pressure (PP) = SBP − DBP	40 mm Hg
Mean arterial pressure (MAP)	70-105 mm Hg

$$MAP = CO \times \text{Total peripheral resistance (TPR)}$$
$$= DBP + 1/3\ PP$$

Body surface area (BSA)	1.73 m^2 (average 70-kg man)
Stroke volume (SV)	60-100 mL/beat

$$SV = CO/HR$$

End diastolic volume (EDV)	70 mL/m^2
Ejection fraction (EF)	55%-65%

$$EF = \frac{(EDV - ESV)}{EDV} = \frac{SV}{EDV}$$

Right atrial pressure (RAP)	0-8 mm Hg
Central venous pressure (CVP)	0-8 mm Hg
Pulmonary artery pressure (PAP)	

Pulmonary artery systolic pressure (PAS)	15-30 mm Hg
Pulmonary artery diastolic pressure (PAD)	5-12 mm Hg
Mean pulmonary artery pressure (PAP)	10-15 mm Hg
Pulmonary capillary wedge pressure (PCWP)	5-12 mm Hg
Coronary perfusion pressure (CPP)	60-70 mm Hg

$$\text{Resistance} = \frac{\text{Driving pressure } (\Delta P)}{\text{Flow } (Q)} = \frac{8\eta(\text{Viscosity}) \times \text{Length}}{\pi r^4}$$

HEART SOUNDS*

S_1: mitral and tricuspid valves closing
S_2: aortic and pulmonic valves closing
S_3: end of rapid ventricular filling (seen in decompensated heart failure)
S_4: atrial systole and stiff ventricle ("atrial kick," associated with reduced LV compliance)

MURMURS*

Aortic regurgitation: diastolic, high-pitched "blowing" murmur with wide pulse pressure
Aortic stenosis: systolic ejection, crescendo-decrescendo murmur
Mitral regurgitation: holosystolic, high-pitched "blowing" murmur
Mitral stenosis: late diastolic, rumbling murmur with opening snap
Mitral prolapse: systolic murmur with midsystolic click

BARORECEPTORS*

Aortic arch: responds to increase in blood pressure via vagus nerve transmission
Carotid sinus: responds to increase or decrease in blood pressure via glossopharyngeal nerve transmission

CHEMORECEPTORS*

Carotid and aortic bodies: both respond to PO_2 <60 mm Hg, increased PCO_2, and decreased pH
Central receptors: respond to changes in pH and PCO_2 of cerebrospinal fluid, which is determined by arterial CO_2

AUTOREGULATION OF BLOOD FLOW*

Organ	Respond(s) to
Brain	CO_2, pH, local metabolites
Heart	O_2, NO, adenosine, local metabolites
Lungs	Hypoxia induces vasoconstriction
Skeletal muscles	Lactate, adenosine, K^+, local metabolites

CAPILLARY FLUID EXCHANGE*

Starling forces:
P_c = Capillary pressure

P_i = Interstitial fluid pressure

π_c = Plasma colloid osmotic pressure

π_i = Interstitial fluid colloid osmotic pressure

σ = protein reflection coefficient

Net filtration pressure = $P_{net} = (P_c - P_i) - \alpha(\pi_c - \pi_i)$

Net fluid flow = $P_{net} \times K_f$

DIAGNOSIS OF MYOCARDIAL INFARCTION*

Electrocardiogram	First 6 hours
Troponin I	First 4 hours up to 7-10 days
Creatinine kinase (CK)-MB	First 24 hours
Lactate dehydrogenase (LDH)	Elevated from 2-7 days
Aspartate aminotransferase (AST)	Peaks 24-48 hours; nonspecific (found in heart, liver, skeletal muscles)

ADRENERGIC AND SYMPATHOMIMETIC DRUG ACTIONS*

Dopa	Vasodilation
α	Vasoconstrict arterioles
β_1	Increase chronotropy
	Increase inotropy
	Increase AV conduction
β_2	Increase chronotropy
	Vasodilation
	Bronchodilation

TEMPORARY PACEMAKERS*

Cathode (negative pole)	Bipolar: distal tip
	Unipolar: heart contact
	Electrons flow from
Anode (positive pole)	Bipolar: proximal tip
	Unipolar: ground/pulse generator
	Electrons flow toward

(*Data from Rollings RC. Facts and formulas. Savannah, Ga: Facts and Formulas; 1998; and Tao L et al. First aid for the USMLE Step 1: 2001. New York: McGraw-Hill; 2001.)

Endocrinology

FREE THYROXINE INDEX

The free thyroxine index (FTI) corrects for thyroxine abnormalities caused by protein binding.

$$FTI = \frac{T_4 \times T_3RU}{100} \text{ (Normal = 1-4)}$$

where

T_4 = thyroxine

T_3RU = triiodothyronine resin uptake

REGULAR INSULIN SLIDING SCALE

Use of this sliding scale to determine regular insulin dosage is appropriate when the blood glucose level is between 200 and 450 mg/dL.

$$Dose = \left(\frac{Glucose}{25}\right) - 6 \text{ units}$$

Gastroenterology

RANSON'S CRITERIA FOR PANCREATITIS*

One point is given for each of the factors below:

Admission	Initial 48 hours
Age >55 years	Decrease in hematocrit >10% with hydration
White blood cell count >16,000/μL	Increase in blood urea nitrogen >5 mg/dL
Serum lactate dehydrogenase >350 IU/L	Serum calcium <8 mg/dL
Aspartate aminotransferase >250 IU/L	Arterial Po$_2$ <60 mm Hg
Blood glucose >200 mg/dL	Fluid deficit >6 L
	Base deficit >4 mEq/dL

Ranson's score of 0-2: <5% mortality
Ranson's score of 3-4: 10%-20% mortality
Ranson's score of 5-6: ~40% mortality
Ranson's score of >7: ~100% mortality
(*Data from Ranson JHC et al. Surg Gynecol Obstet 1974; 139:69.)

CHILD-TURCOTTE CLASSIFICATION*

The Child-Turcotte classification is used for evaluation of patients with liver disease.

	A	B	C
Bilirubin (mg/dL)	<2.3	2.3-2.9	>2.9
Albumin (g/dL)	>3.5	3.0-3.5	<3.0
Ascites	None	Easily controlled	Poorly controlled
Nutrition	Excellent	Good	Fair
Encephalopathy	None	Mild	Advanced

Prognosis worsens from A to C.
(*Data from Child CG, Turcotte JG. Surgery and portal hypertension. In Child CG, ed. The liver and portal hypertension. Philadelphia: WB Saunders; 1964.)

CHILD-PUGH CLASSIFICATION*

The Child-Pugh classification is used for evaluation of patients with liver disease.

Points Assigned	Bilirubin (mg/dL)	Albumin (g/dL)	Prothrombin Time (sec)	Ascites	Encephalopathy
1	<2	>3.5	1-3	None	None
2	2-3	2.8-3.5	4-6	Mild	Grade 1-2
3	>3	<2.8	>6	Moderate	Grade 3-4

Point total of 5-6 = class A; point total of 7-9 = class B; point total of >9 = class C.
(*Data from Pugh RN et al. Br J Surg 1973; 60:646.)

HEPATITIS DISCRIMINANT FUNCTION (MADDREY SCORE)*

The Maddrey Score is used to evaluate the severity of alcoholic hepatitis. Patients with scores higher than 32 have a high short-term mortality.

$$\text{Maddrey Score} = 4.6 \times (\text{Prothrombin time} - \text{Control prothrombin time}) + \text{Serum bilirubin (mg/dL)}$$

(*Data from Carithers RL Jr et al. Ann Intern Med 1989; 110:685.)

FRIEDEWALD FORMULA FOR TOTAL CHOLESTEROL*

$$\text{Total cholesterol} = \text{LDL} + \text{HDL} + \frac{\text{Triglycerides}}{5}$$

All values are in plasma or serum (mg/dL). This formula is invalid if the triglyceride level is greater than 400 mg/dL (4.52 mmol/L). Desirable cholesterol level is less than 200 mg/dL (5.2 mmol/L), borderline is 200 to 239 mg/dL (5.2-6.19 mmol/L), and high is 240 mg/dL or more (≥6.2 mmol/L).

(*Data from Friedewald WT et al. Clin Chem 1972; 18:499.)

Hematology and Oncology

HEMATOLOGICAL INDICES*

Hematocrit (Hct): Packed cell volume. Volume percentage of red blood cells (RBCs) in plasma.

Mean corpuscular volume (MCV): Average RBC volume, directly measured by automatic cell counters, in femtoliters (10^{-15} L).

Mean corpuscular hemoglobin (MCH): Average quantity of hemoglobin per RBC, in picograms (10^{-12} g).

Mean corpuscular hemoglobin concentration (MCHC): Grams of hemoglobin per 100 mL packed RBCs.

Red cell distribution width (RDW): Coefficient of variation in RBC size. Increased in anisocytosis, reticulocytosis, iron deficiency, and hemolysis.

Reticulocyte count: Reticulocytes are young RBCs with remnants of cytoplasmic RNA.

Corrected reticulocyte count (CRC): Indicator of erythropoietic activity, corrected for differences in Hct. CRC greater than 1.5 suggests increased RBC production as a result of hemolysis or blood loss.

$$\text{CRC} = \% \text{ Reticulocytes} \times \frac{\text{Patient Hct}}{\text{Normal Hct}}$$

Reticulocyte distribution index: Allows assessment of reticulocyte response for degree of anemia.*

$$\text{Index} = \frac{\text{Measured Hct/Normal Hct} \times \text{Reticulocyte count}}{\text{Maturation factor}}$$

Maturation factor (MF) equals 1 if patient's Hct = 45; each 10-point drop in patient's Hct increases MF by 0.5.

In anemia, index <2 is inadequate, 2-3 is borderline, >3 is normal.

(*Data from Hillman RS, Finch CA. Br J Haematol 1969; 17:313.)

CLASSIFICATION OF ANEMIA

Reticulocyte Count	Microcytic Anemia	Normocytic Anemia	Macrocytic Anemia
Low	Iron deficiency; lead poisoning; chronic disease; aluminum toxicity; copper deficiency; protein malnutrition	Chronic disease; RBC aplasia (infection, drug induced); malignancy; endocrinopathies; renal failure	Folate deficiency; vitamin B_{12} deficiency; aplastic anemia; congenital bone marrow dysfunction; drug induced; hypothyroidism
Normal	Thalassemia trait; sideroblastic anemia	Acute bleeding; hypersplenism; dyserythropoietic anemia type II	
High	Thalassemia syndromes; hemoglobin C disorders	Antibody-mediated hemolysis; hypersplenism; microangiopathy (HUS, TTP, DIC); membranopathies (spherocytosis, elliptocytosis); enzyme disorders (G6PD, pyruvate kinase); hemoglobinopathies	Dyserythropoietic anemia types I, III; active hemolysis

DIC, Disseminated intravascular coagulation; *G6PD,* glucose 6-phosphate dehydrogenase deficiency; *HUS,* hemolytic-uremic syndrome; *RBC,* red blood cell; *TTP,* thrombotic thrombocytopenic purpura.

COMMON CAUSES OF MICROCYTIC ANEMIA

	Iron Deficiency	β-Thalassemia Trait	Chronic Inflammation
Reticulocyte count	↓	↔ to ↑	↔
RDW	↑	↓	↔
Ferritin	↓	↔ to ↑	↔ to ↑
FEP	↑	↔	↑
Iron	↓	↔	↓
TIBC	↑	↔	↓
Electrophoresis	Normal	↑ HbA_2	Normal
ESR	↔	↔	↑
Smear	Hypochromic, target cells, microcytic, fine basophilic stippling	Normochromic, microcytic, coarse basophilic stippling	Variable

ESR, Erythrocyte sedimentation rate; *FEP,* free erythrocyte protoporphyrin; *Hb,* hemoglobin; *RDW,* red blood cell distribution width; *TIBC,* total iron-binding capacity.

ABSOLUTE NEUTROPHIL COUNT

Neutropenia is defined as an absolute neutrophil count (ANC) less than 1000/mm^3. African-Americans may normally have an ANC as low as 1200/mm^3.

$$ANC \text{ (per mm}^3) = WBC \times (\% \text{ PMNs}/100 + \% \text{ Band cells}/100)$$

where
WBC = white blood cell count (per mm^3)
PMNs = polymorphonuclear cells

WEIGHT-BASED HEPARIN DOSAGE NOMOGRAM*

Initial heparin dose is 80 U/kg bolus, followed by 18 U/kg per hour. Determine activated partial thromboplastin time (aPTT) 6 hours after bolus dose and repeat measurement 6 to 8 hours after every dose adjustment. Repeat daily during stable dosage period. Check platelet count every third day until heparin is discontinued.

aPTT (sec)	Control Ratio	Heparin Dose Adjustment
<35	<1.2 × control	80 U/kg bolus, then 4 U/kg per hour increase
35-45	1.2-1.5 × control	40 U/kg bolus, then 2 U/kg per hour increase
46-70	1.5-2.3 × control	No change
71-90	2.3-3.0 × control	Decrease infusion by 2 U/kg per hour
>90	>3.0 × control	Hold infusion for 1 hour, then decrease infusion rate by 3 U/kg per hour

Data from Raschke RA, et al. Ann Intern Med 1993; 119:874.

In a randomized, controlled trial of 115 patients requiring heparin treatment for thrombosis or unstable angina, the weight-based nomogram was superior to the "standard care" (5000-U bolus, 1000 U/hr) group. In the weight-based group, 60/62 (97%) achieved therapeutic aPTT in 24 hours compared with 37/48 (77%) in the standard care group (p <.002). Only one major bleed occurred, and it was in the standard care group.

WARFARIN DOSAGE*

A 5-mg initial dose produced less excess anticoagulation (international normalized ratio [INR] >2.0) in the first 24 hours after administration than did a 10-mg initial dose. The excess anticoagulation achieved by the 10-mg dose was due to decreases in factor VII, which does not reflect the anticoagulant effect of warfarin (determined by factor II levels). The 5-mg dose also avoids the potential hypercoagulable state caused by decreases in protein C levels during the first 36 hours of warfarin use.
(*Data from Harrison L et al. Ann Intern Med 1997; 126:133.)

TARGET INTERNATIONAL NORMALIZED RATIO RANGES FOR WARFARIN ANTICOAGULATION

Clinical Indication	INR
Venous thrombosis	
Treatment	2.0-3.0
Prevention	1.5-2.5
Atrial fibrillation	2.0-3.0
Lupuslike anticoagulants	3.0-4.0
Mechanical heart valves	See Chapter 18
Cardiomyopathy	2.0-3.0

INR, International normalized ratio, such that INR = $(PT_{patient}/PT_{normal})^{ISI}$, where PT = prothrombin time.

BLOOD PRODUCTS FOR TRANSFUSIONS*

Blood Product	Volume (mL)	Components	Clinical Response
PRBCs	180-200	RBCs with variable leukocyte content, small amount of plasma	Hemoglobin level increases 1 g/dL and hematocrit increases 3%
Platelets	50-70	5.5×10^{10}/RD unit	↑ Platelet count increases 5000-10,000/mm³
Platelets	200-400	$>3.0 \times 10^{11}$/SDAP product	CCI $>10 \times 10^9$/L within 1 hr and $> 7.5 \times 10$/L within 24 hr
FFP	200-250	Plasma proteins (coagulation factors, proteins C and S, antithrombin)	Coagulation factors increase approximately 2%

CCI, Corrected count increment; *FFP*, fresh frozen plasma; *PRBCs*, packed red blood cells; *RBC*, red blood cell; *RD*, random donor; *SDAP*, single-donor apheresis platelets.

CORRECTED COUNT INCREMENT*

Corrected count increment (CCI) is used to evaluate effectiveness of platelet transfusion. At 1 hour after transfusion, CCI of 10×10^9/L is considered acceptable. At 18 to 24 hours after transfusion, CCI of 7.5×10^9/L is acceptable.

(*Data from Braunwald E et al. Harrison's principles of internal medicine, 15th ed. New York: McGraw-Hill; 2001.)

GLUCOSE 6-PHOSPHATE DEHYDROGENASE DEFICIENCY*

Glucose 6-phosphate dehydrogenase (G6PD) deficiency is an X-linked disorder, although heterozygous females may have 50% affected red blood cells. In the majority of patients acute hemolysis develops in response to infections, metabolic stress, or drugs.

Drugs Considered Safe in G6PD Deficiency	Drugs Unsafe in G6PD Deficiency
Acetaminophen, ascorbic acid, aspirin, chloramphenicol, chloroquine; colchicine, diphenhydramine, isoniazid, L-dopa, PABA, phenacetin, phenytoin, probenecid, procainamide, pyrimethamine, quinidine, quinine, streptomycin, sulfisoxazole, trimethoprim, vitamin K	Antimalarials: primaquine, pamaquine, dapsone Sulfonamides: sulfamethoxazole (Bactrim) Nitrofurantoin Analgesics: acetanilide Others: vitamin K, doxorubicin, methylene blue, nalidixic acid, naphthalene (mothballs)

PABA, Paraaminobenzoic acid.
(*Data from Beutler E. N Engl J Med 1991; 324[3]:170; and Beutler E. Blood 1994; 84:3613.)

ORGANISMS LIKELY TO CAUSE INFECTIONS IN GRANULOCYTOPENIC PATIENTS*

Gram-positive cocci
  Staphylococcus epidermidis
  Staphylococcus aureus
  Viridans *Streptococcus*
  Enterococcus faecalis
  Streptococcus pneumoniae
Gram-negative bacilli
  Escherichia coli
  Klebsiella spp.
  Pseudomonas aeruginosa
  Non-*aeruginosa Pseudomonas* spp.
  Enterobacter spp.
  Serratia spp.
  Acinetobacter spp.
  Citrobacter spp.
Gram-positive bacilli
  Diphtheroids
  Corynebacterium jeikeium
Fungi
  Candida spp.
  Aspergillus spp.

(*Data from Braunwald E et al. Harrison's principles of internal medicine, 15th ed. New York: McGraw-Hill; 2001.)

Nutrition

BODY MASS INDEX*

Body mass index (BMI) is highly correlated with direct measures of body fat in most populations.

$$BMI = \frac{\text{Weight in kg}}{(\text{Height in meters})^2}$$

BMI 25-29.9: overweight

BMI ≥30: obese

(*Data from Calle EE et al. N Engl J Med 1999; 341:1097; and Keys A et al. J Chron Dis 1972; 25:329.)

BODY MASS INDEX CLASSIFICATIONS

BMI (kg/m^2)	Classification
<18.5	Underweight
18.5-24.9	Normal
25.0-29.9	Overweight
30.0-34.9	Obese
35.0-39.9	Severely obese
≥40.0	Morbidly obese

IDEAL BODY WEIGHT

Ideal body weight (IBW) (male) = 50 kg + 2.3 kg for each inch over 5 feet

IBW (female) = 45.5 kg + 2.3 kg for each inch over 5 feet

Alternative formulas*:

IBW (male) (kg) = 51.65 + (1.85 × [Height in inches − 60])

IBW (female) (kg) = 48.67 + (1.65 × [Height in inches − 60])

(*Data from the Metropolitan Life Insurance Company height and weight tables. In Robinson JD et al. Am J Hosp Pharm 1983; 40:1016.)

BASAL ENERGY EXPENDITURE: HARRIS-BENEDICT FORMULA*

Basal energy expenditure (BEE) (in kcal/day at rest) is typically multiplied by a stress factor (1.1-2.0) to obtain a nutritional goal.

BEE (male) = 66 + [13.7 × Weight (kg)] + [5 × Height (cm)] − [6.8 × Age (years)]

BEE (female) = 655 + [9.6 × Weight (kg)] + [1.8 × Height (cm)] − [4.7 × Age (years)]

For BMI >30 , adjust weight.

$$Adjusted\ weight = IBW + [(ABW − IBW) × 0.25]$$

where

BMI = body mass index

IBW = ideal body weight

ABW = actual body weight

Easy estimate of BEE:

$$BEE = 25\text{-}30\ kcal/kg$$

(*Data from Harris J, Benedict F. A biometric study of basal metabolism in man. Washington, DC: Carnegie Institute of Washington; 1919.)

CALCULATED CALORIC REQUIREMENT

Calculated caloric requirement (CCR) = BEE × Activity factor × Injury factor

Activity factor: bed rest = 1.2
ambulatory = 1.3
Injury factor: minor surgery = 1.2
trauma = 1.35
sepsis = 1.6
severe burn = 2.1

CALCULATED PROTEIN REQUIREMENT
Maintenance calculated protein requirement (CPR):

Normal CPR = 0.8 g protein/kg IBW/day
CPR with moderate stress = 1.0-1.5 (elective surgery, severe infection, <30% burn)
CPR with severe stress = 2.0-2.6 (multiple traumas, >40% burn)

CPR in renal failure:

With creatinine clearance >20 mL/min, CPR = 0.5-0.8 g protein/kg IBW/day
With creatinine clearance 10-20 mL/min, CPR = 0.5 g protein/kg IBW/day
With hemodialysis, CPR = 1.0-1.2 g protein/kg IBW/day
With peritoneal dialysis, CPR = 1.2-1.5 g protein/kg IBW/day

NITROGEN BALANCE
This equation is not accurate for patients with burns, fistulae, draining wounds, or renal failure; add 1 g for each 500 mL of fistula drainage or diarrhea.

$$\text{Grams of protein} = 6.25 \text{ g nitrogen}$$

$$\text{Nitrogen balance} = \frac{\text{Total protein intake (g)}}{6.25} - (\text{UUN} + 4 \text{ g})$$

where
UUN = urinary urine nitrogen in g/24-hour collection
= UUN (g/L) × L of urine

Zero balance: normal; may be maximum attainable in severe stress
Negative balance: continuing deficit in protein compartments
Positive balance: growth and repair

CONTENT OF COMMON INTRAVENOUS FLUIDS

IVF Solution	Na$^+$ (mEq/L)	K$^+$ (mEq/L)	Cl$^-$ (mEq/L)	HCO$_3^-$ (mEq/L)	Dextrose (mOsm/L)	Dextrose (g/L)	Dextrose (kcal/L)
D$_5$W					278	50	170
D$_{10}$W					556	100	340
D$_{20}$W					1112	200	680
D$_{70}$W					3892	700	2380
½ NS	77		77		143		0
NS	154		154		286		0
3% saline	513		513		1026		0
5% saline	855		855		1710		0
D$_5$ ¼ NS	39		39		350	50	170
D$_5$ ½ NS	77		77		421	50	170
D$_5$ NS	154		154		564	50	170
LR	130	4	109	28	272	50	170
D$_5$ LR	130	4	109	28	524	50	170

D, Dextrose; *IVF*, intravenous fluid; *LR*, lactated Ringer's solution; *NS*, normal saline solution; *W*, water.

WATER DEFICIT

This equation is used to estimate body water deficit in hypovolemic hypernatremia. Rapid correction may cause cerebral edema. Sodium should be corrected at a rate of less than 0.5 mEq/L/hr (1 mEq/L/hr if patient is symptomatic).

$$\text{Free water deficit} = \frac{\text{Corr. factor} \times \text{wt (kg)} \times (\text{Patient's [Na]} - \text{Normal [Na]})}{\text{Normal [Na]}}$$

Males: Correction factor = 0.6
Females: Correction factor = 0.5

Normal volumes:

Total body water (TBW):
  Males (L): TBW = 0.6 × Lean body weight (kg)
  Females (L): TBW = 0.5 × Lean body weight (kg)
Intracellular body water = 0.4 × Weight (kg)
Extracellular body water = 0.2 × Weight (kg)
  Interstitial fluid volume = 0.15 × Weight (kg)
  Plasma volume: estimated 50 mL/kg
  Blood volume: estimated 75 mL/kg

Pulmonary

ALVEOLAR-ARTERIAL OXYGEN GRADIENT

A-a gradient (sea level, 37° C) = PA$_{O_2}$ − Pa$_{O_2}$
= [FI$_{O_2}$(P$_{atm}$ − P$_{H_2O}$) − Pa$_{CO_2}$/RQ] − Pa$_{O_2}$
≈ [713 × FI$_{O_2}$ − (1.25 × Pa$_{CO_2}$)] − Pa$_{O_2}$
≈ 150 − (Pa$_{CO_2}$/0.8)
Normal value ≤ [Age/4] + 4

DEAD SPACE

$$V_D = V_T \times (PA_{CO_2} - PE_{CO_2})/(PA_{CO_2})$$
Should be ~2.2 mL/kg

COMPLIANCE

Compliance is $\Delta V/\Delta P$, where V = volume and P = pressure.

$$C_{RS} = \frac{V_T}{P_{plateau} - PEEP}$$

where
C_{RS} = Respiratory system compliance
$P_{plateau}$ = Inspiratory plateau pressure
PEEP = Positive end-expiratory pressure

LUNG VENTILATION-PERFUSION ZONES

Zone I:
$$P_A > P_a > P_v$$

Zone II:
$$P_a > P_A > P_v$$

Zone III:
$$P_a > P_v > P_A$$

Where
P = pressure
a = arterial
A = alveolar
v = venous

SHUNT FRACTION

$$QS/QT\ (\%) = (C_{CO_2} - C_{aO_2})/(C_{CO_2} - C_{vO_2})$$

where
QS/QT = shunt fraction
C_{CO_2} = end-capillary oxygen content, derived from PA_{O_2} and O_2 dissociation curve
C_{aO_2} = arterial oxygen content
C_{vO_2} = mixed venous oxygen content

STATIC LUNG VOLUMES

Total lung capacity (TLC)	Vital capacity (VC)	Inspiratory capacity (IC)	Inspiratory reserve volume (IRV)
			Tidal volume (TV)
		Functional residual capacity (FRC)	Expiratory reserve volume (ERV)
	Residual volume (RV)		Residual volume (RV)

PULMONARY FUNCTION TESTS

	Pulmonary Function Test Parameters					
Lung Impairment	FEV$_1$	FVC	FEV$_1$/FVC	RV	TLC	DL$_{CO}$
Obstructive	↓	↓/nl	↓	↑/nl	↑/nl	↓/nl
Restrictive, intrinsic	↓/nl	↓	↑/nl	↓/nl	↓	nl
Restrictive, extrinsic	↓/nl	↓	↑/nl	↓/nl	↓	↓
Combined obstructive and restrictive	↓	↓	↓	↓/nl	↓	↓/nl

Arrow, Increase or decrease; *bold arrow*, marked decrease; *DLCO*, Diffusing capacity of lung for carbon monoxide; *FEV$_1$*, forced expiratory volume in 1 second; *FVC*, forced vital capacity; *nl*, normal; *RV*, residual volume; *TLC*, total lung capacity.

PREDICTED PEAK FLOW*
Males

$$PPF(L/min) = e^{0.544 \times ln(Age) - (0.0151 \times Age) - (29.4/Height) + 5.48}$$

	Height (inches)				
Age (years)	60	65	70	75	80
20	554	576	594	611	627
25	580	603	622	640	656
30	594	617	637	655	672
35	599	622	643	661	677
40	597	620	641	659	675
45	591	613	634	652	668
50	580	602	622	640	656
55	567	588	608	625	640
60	551	572	591	607	623
65	533	554	572	588	603
70	515	535	552	568	582

Females: PPF (L/min) = $e^{0.376 \times ln(Age) - (0.0120 \times Age) - (23.1/Height) + 5.63}$

	Height (inches)				
Age (years)	55	60	65	70	75
20	444	460	474	486	497
25	455	471	485	498	509
30	459	475	490	502	513
35	458	474	489	501	512
40	454	470	484	496	507
45	446	462	476	488	499
50	437	453	467	479	489
55	427	442	455	467	478
60	415	430	443	455	465
65	403	418	430	441	451
70	391	404	417	427	437

(*Data from Nunn AJ, Gregg I. Br Med J 1989; 298:1068.)

OXYGEN CONTENT

Arterial oxygen content:

$$Cao_2 \text{ (mL } O_2/\text{mL blood)} = 1.36 \times Hgb \times Sao_2 + 0.003 \times Pao_2$$

Mixed venous oxygen content:

$$Cvo_2 \text{ (mL } O_2/\text{mL blood)} = 1.36 \times Hgb \times Svo_2 + 0.003 \times Pvo_2$$

OXYGEN SUPPORT

Oxygen Source	Flow Rate (L/min)	Fio_2	Pao_2 at Sea Level (mm Hg)
Room air		0.21	100
Nasal cannula	1-6	↑ by 0.04/L/min	≥227
Venturi mask	1-4	≥0.5	≥300
Face mask	6-15	≥0.6	≥370
Partial rebreather	5-7	≥0.8	≥512
Nonrebreather	≥15	≥1.0 (actual ~0.9)	≥655

OXYHEMOGLOBIN DISSOCIATION CURVE*

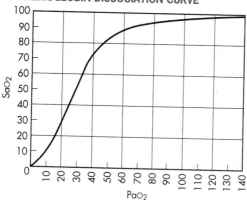

(*Data from www.rnceus.com/abgs/abgcurve.html.)

SHIFT OF OXYHEMOGLOBIN DISSOCIATION CURVE

Left shift (higher affinity of hemoglobin for oxygen):
  Alkalosis
  Hypothermia
  Decreased 2,3-diphosphoglycerate (DPG)
  Fetal hemoglobin
Right shift (lower affinity of hemoglobin for oxygen):
  Acidosis
  Hyperthermia
  Increased 2,3-DPG

COMMUNITY ACQUIRED PNEUMONIA: PORT PREDICTION RULE*

Characteristic	Points
Age	
Men	Age (years)
Women	Age–10 (years)
Nursing home resident?	10
Coexisting illnesses	
Neoplasm	30
Liver disease	20
Congestive heart failure	10
Cerebrovascular disease	10
Renal disease	10
Examination findings	
Altered mental status	20
Respirations ≥30/min	20
Systolic blood pressure <90 mm Hg	20
Temperature ≥40° C, <35° C1	5
Heart rate ≥125 beats/min	10
Laboratory and radiographic findings	
Arterial pH <7.35	30
Blood urea nitrogen ≥30 mg/dL	20
Sodium <130 mmol/L	20
Glucose ≥250 mg/dL	10
Hematocrit <30%	10
Pao_2 <60 mm Hg	10
Pleural effusion	10

Class	Definition	Mortality (%)	Recommendation
I	Age <50, no points for underlying illness or examination findings	<0.5	Outpatient
II	≤70 points	<1	Outpatient; consider observation
III	71-90 points	<4	Observation; consider outpatient
IV	91-130 points	4-10	Inpatient
V	>130 points	>10	Inpatient

(*Data from Fine MJ et al. N Engl J Med 1997; 336:243.)

PULMONARY EMBOLISM PROBABILITY*

RESULTS OF PIOPED STUDY: FREQUENCY OF PULMONARY EMBOLISM BY PULMONARY ANGIOGRAM, GIVEN V̇/Q̇ SCAN RESULTS AND PRETEST CLINICAL SUSPICION

	Clinical Probability (%)			
V̇/Q̇ Interpretation	>80	20-79	<20	Total (%)
High probability	96	88	56	87
Intermediate probability	66	28	16	30

PIOPED, Prospective Investigation of Pulmonary Embolism Diagnosis; *V̇/Q̇*, ventilation-perfusion ratio.
(*Data from JAMA 263:2753, 1990.)

Continued

PULMONARY EMBOLISM PROBABILITY*—cont'd
RESULTS OF PIOPED STUDY: FREQUENCY OF PULMONARY EMBOLISM BY PULMONARY ANGIOGRAM, GIVEN $\dot{V}/\dot{Q}$ SCAN RESULTS AND PRETEST CLINICAL SUSPICION

$\dot{V}/\dot{Q}$ Interpretation	Clinical Probability (%)			Total (%)
	>80	20-79	<20	
Low probability	40	16	4	14
Near normal	0	6	2	4
Total	68	30	9	28

PLEURAL EFFUSION: TRANSUDATE VERSUS EXUDATE*
The effusion is an exudate if any one of the following is true:
Pleural fluid protein/serum protein ratio greater than 0.5
Pleural fluid lactate dehydrogenase (LDH)/serum LDH ratio greater than 0.6
Pleural fluid LDH more than two thirds the upper limits of normal serum LDH
(*Data from Light RW et al. Ann Intern Med 1972; 77:507.)

ADULT RESPIRATORY DISTRESS SYNDROME CRITERIA
Bilateral pulmonary infiltrates
Pao_2/Fio_2 <200 mm Hg
PCWP <18 mm Hg (noncardiogenic)

ACID-BASE BALANCE
1. Verify: Real result or laboratory error?
   Henderson-Hasselbalch equation:

$$H^+ = \frac{24 \times Pco_2}{HCO_3^-}$$

pH	7.7	7.6	7.5	7.45	7.4	7.35	7.3	7.25	7.2	7.1	7.0	6.9
$[H^+]$	20	25	32	35	40	44	50	56	63	80	100	125

   If the equation does not hold, suspect laboratory error.
2. Identify primary disorder.
   Acidosis (pH <7.35) or alkalosis (pH >7.45)
   Metabolic (CO_2 shifted in same direction as pH) or respiratory (CO_2 shifted in opposite direction)
3. Identify secondary disorder: expected compensation.
   Metabolic acidosis:

$$Pco_2 = 1.5 \times [HCO_3^-] + 8 \pm 2 \text{ (Winters' formula)}$$
$$\Delta Pco_2 = \Delta HCO_3^- \times 1.2$$

   Metabolic alkalosis:

$$Pco_2 = 0.9 \times [HCO_3^-] + 9 \pm 2$$
$$\Delta Pco_2 = \Delta HCO_3^- \times 0.7$$

Respiratory acidosis:

Acute: $\Delta HCO_3^- = \Delta Pco_2 \times 0.1$
Chronic: $\Delta HCO_3^- = \Delta Pco_2 \times 0.2$ to $\Delta Pco_2 \times 0.35$

Respiratory alkalosis:

Acute: $\Delta HCO_3^- = \Delta Pco_2 \times 0.2$
Chronic: $\Delta HCO_3^- = \Delta Pco_2 \times 0.4$

4. **Metabolic acidosis differential.**
   Check for anion gap acidosis:

   $$[Na^+] - ([Cl^-] + [HCO_3^-]) = \text{Anion gap}$$
   $$\text{Normal} = 12 \; (+/- \; 2)$$

   Adjust for albumin: For each g/dL of albumin less than normal (4 g/dL), expected AG increases by 2.5-3.

   Adjust for pH:
      Acidotic: Expected AG decreases by 1-3
      Alkalotic: Expected AG increases by 3-5

   Anion gap acidosis: Check for mixed metabolic disorder
      Delta gap = $\Delta AG/\Delta HCO_3$ (change from normal)
         >2 = metabolic alkalosis plus AG acidosis
         1-2 = pure AG acidosis
         <1 = non-AG acidosis plus AG acidosis

   Differential diagnosis for anion gap acidosis: MUDPILES (methanol, uremia, diabetic ketoacidosis, paraldehyde, ischemia, lactate, ethylene glycol, salicylates or starvation)
   Differential diagnosis for non–anion gap acidosis: DURHAM (diarrhea, ureteral diversion, renal tubular acidosis, hyperalimentation, acetazolamide or ammonium chloride, miscellaneous [chloridorrhea, amphotericin B, others])

   Non–anion gap acidosis: renal or not?
      Urine anion gap = $[Na^+] + [K^+] - [Cl^-]$
         <0 = Non–renal tubular acidosis
         >0 = Renal tubular acidosis

5. **Differential diagnosis for metabolic alkalosis:**
   Urine chloride level <15 mEq/L: gastrointestinal loss (nasogastric suctioning, vomiting), hypovolemia (diuretics), post hypercapnia
   Urine chloride level >15 mEq/L: mineralocorticoids, renal artery stenosis, hypomagnesemia, severe hypokalemia, Bartter's syndrome, $NaHCO_3$ administration, licorice ingestion, milk alkali syndrome

6. **Differential diagnosis for respiratory acidosis.**
   Chest cavity: muscle disorders, nerve disorders, severe kyphoscoliosis, pleural effusion, pneumothorax

Central: sedation, decreased respiratory center function (infection, ischemia)

Lung and airways: pneumonia, pulmonary edema, bronchospasm, laryngospasm, chronic obstructive pulmonary disease, mechanical obstruction (foreign body, tumor)

7. **Differential diagnosis for respiratory alkalosis.**

Systemic: sepsis, salicylates, liver failure, hyperthyroid, pregnancy

Central: ischemia, cerebrovascular accident, tumor, infection, progesterone, anxiety

Pulmonary: pulmonary embolus, restrictive lung disease, hypoxemia (pneumonia, pulmonary edema)

RENAL

ESTIMATED SERUM OSMOLALITY

$$\text{Calculated osmolality} = 2 \times Na + BUN/2.8 + Glucose/18$$
$$= 275 - 290 \text{ mOsm/kg}$$

Osmolal gap = Measured Osm − Calculated Osm
= <10 (high osmolar gap suggests presence of osmotically active agent such as alcohol, isopropyl alcohol, mannitol, or radiocontrast dye)

CREATININE CLEARANCE

$$\text{Normal (male)} = 100 - 125 \text{ mL/min/1.73 m}^2$$

$$\text{Normal (female)} = 85 - 105 \text{ mL/min/1.73 m}^2$$

$$\text{Measured} = \frac{Ucreat \text{ (mg/dL)}}{Pcreat \text{ (mg/dL)}} \times \frac{Uvolume \text{ (mL/day)}}{(1440 \text{ min/1 day})} = \frac{Ucreat \text{ (mg/day)}}{[Pcreat](mg/dL)} \times 0.07$$

$$\text{Estimate} = \frac{140 - Age}{Pcreat} \times \frac{Weight \text{ (kg)}}{72} (\times 0.85 \text{ Female})$$

FRACTIONAL EXCRETION OF SODIUM

FE_{Na} = % Filtered sodium load excreted

$$= \frac{Urine\ Na}{Ucreat} \times \frac{Pcreat}{Plasma\ Na} \times 100$$

= <1% in normal urine and prerenal azotemia (most helpful in oliguric patient [see below])

FRACTIONAL EXCRETION OF UREA

$$FE_{urea} = \frac{Uurea}{BUN} \times \frac{Pcreat}{Ucreat} \times 100$$

= <35% in prerenal conditions, even if diuretics have been given

OLIGURIA

Urine volume = <500 mL/day or <20 mL/hr

LABORATORY FINDINGS IN PRERENAL AND INTRARENAL RENAL FAILURE

Finding	Prerenal	Intrarenal (ATN)
BUN/creatinine ratio	≥20	10-20
FENa (%)	<1	>2
Urine Na$^+$ (mEq/L)	<20	>40
Specific gravity	≥1.02	≅1.01
Urine osmolality (mOsm/kg)	≥500	<350
Sediment	Normal	Granular casts, epithelial cell casts

ATN, Acute tubular necrosis; *BUN*, blood urea nitrogen; *FENa*, fractional excretion of sodium.

URINE ANION GAP

Value for urine anion gap (UAG) is negative if ammonium ion exertion is high. Value is positive if patient has a distal tubular problem suggesting difficulty acidifying urine via ammonium excretion.

$$UAG = [Na^+] + [K^+] - [Cl^-]$$

RENAL TUBULAR ACIDOSIS

	Type 1 (Distal)	Type 2 (Proximal)	Type 4 (Hypoaldosteronism)
Defect	Decreased distal acidification	Decreased proximal HCO$_3$ reabsorption	Aldosterone decrease or resistance
Urine pH	>5.3	Variable	<5.3
Plasma K$^+$	Low	Low	High
Urine NH$_4$	Low	Normal	Low
UAG	>0	Negative	>0

TRANSTUBULAR POTASSIUM GRADIENT

Transtubular potassium (K$^+$) gradient (TTKG):

$$TTKG = \frac{Urine\ K^+ \times Plasma\ osmoles}{Plasma\ K^+ \times Plasma\ osmoles} = 4\text{-}14\ (normal—varies\ with\ diet)$$

With hyperkalemia:
    TTKG <6: renal (decreased aldosterone effect)
    TTKG >10: nonrenal hyperkalemia (normal aldosterone effect)
With hypokalemia:
    TTKG <2: gastrointestinal loss
    TTKG >4: renal loss (excess aldosterone)

FLUID COMPARTMENTS

Intracellular fluid (ICF) = Total body water (TBW) − Extracellular fluid (ECF)
TBW in males = 0.6 × Lean body weight (kg)

$$\text{TBW in females} = 0.5 \times \text{Lean body weight (kg)}$$
$$\text{ICF} = 0.4 \times \text{Lean body weight (kg)}$$
$$\text{ECF} = 0.2 \times \text{Lean body weight (kg)}$$
$$\text{Interstitial volume} = 0.15 \times \text{Lean body weight (kg)}$$
$$\text{Plasma volume} = 0.05 \times \text{Lean body weight (kg)}$$

COMPOSITION OF TOTAL BODY WEIGHT AND TOTAL BODY WATER

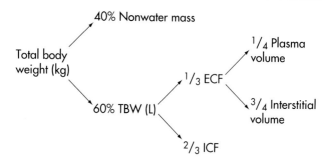

where
TBW = total body water
ECF = extracellular fluid
ICF = intracellular fluid

WATER DEFICIT

$$\text{Water deficit} = 0.6 \times \text{Lean body weight (kg)} \times \frac{(\text{Plasma sodium[mg/dL]} - 1)}{140}$$

SODIUM DEFICIT

$$\text{Sodium deficit} = 0.6 \times \text{Lean body weight (kg)} \times (140 - \text{Measured Na [mg/dL]}) + (140 \times \text{Volume deficit [L]})$$

CORRECTIONS TO PLASMA VALUES

$$\text{Corrected serum sodium} = 0.016 (\text{Measured glucose} - 100) + \text{Measured Na}$$
$$\text{Corrected serum calcium} = (4 - \text{Albumin}) \times 0.8 + \text{Measured serum calcium}$$

Miscellaneous

BODY SURFACE AREA (BSA)

$$\text{BSA} = \sqrt{\frac{\text{Height (cm)} \times \text{Weight (kg)}}{60}}$$

BODY WATER DEFICIT

$$\text{Body water deficit (L)} = \frac{0.6 \times \text{Weight (kg)} \times (\text{Na[mg/dL]} - 140)}{140}$$

Or

$$\text{Body water deficit (L)} = \text{Weight (kg)} \times 0.6 \times \left(1 - \frac{\text{Normal osm}}{\text{Observed osm}}\right)$$

(Body weight used should be ideal body weight)

MAINTENANCE FLUIDS

For a 24-hour period:
  100 mL/day/kg for first 10 kg
  Add 50 mL/day/kg for second 10 kg
  Add 20 mL/day/kg for each additional kg

  Divide by 24 to obtain the hourly rate

Example: For a 70-kg man,
  100 mL/day/kg × 10 kg = 1000 mL/day
  50 mL/day/kg × 10 kg = 500 mL/day
  20 mL/day/kg × 50 kg = 1000 mL/day
  Total = 2500 mL/day

  Divided by 24 = 104 mL/hr maintenance rate

For an hourly rate:
  4 mL/hr/kg for first 10 kg
  Add 2 mL/hr/kg for second 10 kg
  Add 1 mL/hr/kg for each additional kg
Example: For a 70 kg man,
  4 mL/hr/kg × 10 kg = 40 mL/hr
  2 mL/hr/kg × 10 kg = 20 mL/hr
  1 mL/hr/kg × 50 kg = 50 mL/hr
  Total = 110 mL/hr maintenance rate

CORRECTED TOTAL CALCIUM (CONCENTRATIONS IN mg/dL)

$$\text{Corrected calcium} = [\text{Ca}] + 3.6 - (0.8 \times \text{Albumin})$$

SERUM SODIUM FORMULAS

Serum Na correction in hyperglycemia (Na increases by 1.6 mmol/L per 100 mg/dL of serum glucose above 100 mg/dL)*

$$\text{Corrected [Na] (mmol/L)} = \text{measured Na (mmol/L)} + [1.6 \times [[\text{glucose (mg/dL)} - 100]/100]]$$

Serum Na correction in hyperlipidemia (Na increases by 1.0 mmol/L for each 500 mg/dL of plasma lipid (triglyceride and cholesterol)*

Corrected Na$^+$ (mmol/L) = Na$^+$ measured (mmol/L) + [0.002 × Lipids (mg/dL)]

Serum Na correction in hyperproteinemia (Na increases by 1.0 mmol/L for each 4.0 g/dL of plasma protein above 8.0 g/dL)*

Decrease (mEq/L) in serum Na in hyperproteinemia = Increase of total protein >8 g/dL × 0.25

Estimated Na excess in hypernatremia†

Na excess (mEq/L) = 0.6 Body weight (kg) × (Current plasma [Na] − 140)

Estimated Na deficit in hyponatremia†

Na deficit (mEq) = 0.6 × Body weight × (Desired plasma [Na] − Current plasma [Na])

(*Data from Roberts JR, Hedges JR, eds. Clinical procedures in emergency medicine, 3rd ed, Philadelphia: WB Saunders; 1998. †Data from Adrogué HJ, Madias NE. N Engl J Med 2000; 342[21]:1581.)

OSMOLALITY FORMULAS
Calculated osmolality (concentrations in mg/dL)

$$\text{Calculated osmolality} = 2([Na] + [K]) + \frac{\text{Glucose}}{18} + \frac{\text{BUN}}{2.8}$$

Effective osmolality (concentrations in mg/dL)

$$\text{Effective osmolality} = 2([Na]) + \frac{\text{Glucose}}{18}$$

Osmolal gap

Osmolal gap = Measured osmolality − Calculated osmolality

Stool osmolal gap (concentrations in mg/dL)

Osmotic gap (stool) = Plasma osmolality − 2 × (Stool [Na] + Stool [K])

CALORIC REQUIREMENT

Caloric requirement = BEE × (1 + Activity factor + Injury factor)

Activity factor:
Bed rest = 0.2
Ambulatory = 0.25
Injury factor:
None = 0
Low stress = 0.5
Moderate stress = 0.6
Normotensive sepsis = 0.7

Severe stress = 1
Severe burns >40% BSA, normotensive = 1.5

SENSITIVITY, SPECIFICITY, AND PREDICTIVE VALUE

Disease

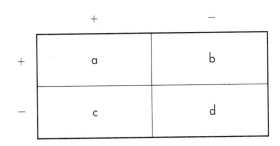

$$\text{Sensitivity} = \frac{a}{a + c}$$

$$\text{Specificity} = \frac{d}{b + d}$$

$$\text{Positive predictive value} = \frac{a}{a + b}$$

$$\text{Negative predictive value} = \frac{d}{c + d}$$

GENERAL CONVERSIONS

Weight

$$1 \text{ lb} = 0.454 \text{ kg}$$
$$1 \text{ kg} = 2.2 \text{ lb}$$
$$70 \text{ kg} = 154 \text{ lb}$$

Temperature

$$°C = (°F - 32)/1.8$$
$$°F = (°C \times 1.8) + 32$$

Length

$$1 \text{ in} = 2.54 \text{ cm}$$
$$1 \text{ cm} = 0.394 \text{ in}$$

Volume

$$1 \text{ L} = 1000 \text{ ml} = 0.264 \text{ gal} = 1.06 \text{ qt} = 33.81 \text{ oz}$$

RAPID REFERENCES

Index

A

AAI(R) mode pacing, 253
Abdomen
  in hypotension and shock, 238t
  inadequate nutrition and, 841t-842t
Abdominal aortic aneurysm, ruptured,
    402
Abdominal pain, 399-412
Ablation
  for atrial flutter, 146
  atrioventricular node, for atrial fibrilla-
    tion, 142-143
  pulmonary vein radiofrequency, for atrial
    fibrillation, 143
Abciximab, formulary, 1168
Abscess, 636-638
Absence seizure, 829
Absolute neutrophil count, 1294
Abuse
  alcohol, 1055-1063
  drug, 776
Acarbose, formulary, 1219
Acebutolol, 105t
  formulary, 1123
Acetaminophen
  for fever, 59
  in hyperthyroidism, 394
  overdose of, 414, 419-421
    risk stratification in, 425
  in sickle cell anemia, 509t
Acetazolamide in tumor lysis syndrome,
    549-550
Acidosis
  diabetic ketoacidosis and, 383
  metabolic
    hyperkalemia and, 801
    renal failure with, 767
  renal tubular, 512
Activated partial thromboplastin time
  in gastrointestinal hemorrhage, 480
  in thromboembolism, 963
Acute coronary syndrome, 72-78
  non-ST segment elevation, 96-110
    risk stratification of, 102, 103t, 104
  ST elevation with, 111-120. *See also*
    ST segment elevation
Acute interstitial pneumonia, 927, 930
Acute meningitis
  aseptic, 665
  bacterial, 665-681. *See also*
    Meningitis
Acute renal failure, 763-772. *See also*
  Renal failure
Acute respiratory failure, 1001-1010.
  See also Respiratory failure
Acute tubular necrosis, renal failure *versus*,
    765t

Acyclovir
  formulary, 1073
  for genital herpes, 701, 702
  for herpes zoster, 330t
Addison's disease, 365-378
Adenitis, mesenteric, 411
Adenosine, formulary, 1184
Adjusted body weight, 846
Adrenal failure, 390
Adrenal insufficiency, 365-378
Adrenergic drug actions, 1290
Adult respiratory distress, 948
Advanced cardiovascular life support,
    4f-5f
AFASAK trial, 132t-134t, 135
Age
  community-acquired pneumonia and,
    661
  cystic fibrosis and, 900
AIDS. *See* Human immunodeficiency virus
    infection
Air bubble in blood gas analysis, 993
Air embolism, parenteral nutrition and,
    860t-864t
Airway
  in cystic fibrosis, 904
  in obstructive sleep apnea, 1011-1012
Alanine aminotransferase, 795
Albumin, 845t
  in ascites, 445
Albuterol
  for asthma, 875
  formulary, 1263
Albuterol/atrovent, formulary, 1273
Alcohol
  hypomagnesemia and, 776
  obstructive sleep apnea and, 1019
Alcohol withdrawal, 1055-1063
  benzodiazepines in, 1058-1059,
    1060-1061, 1062t
Alkaline phosphatase, 795
Allen test, 43
Allergic bronchopulmonary aspergillosis,
    877-878
  cystic fibrosis and, 907-908
Allergy
  asthma and, 875
  in hemodialysis, 788
Allopurinol
  for gout, 1036
  for tumor lysis syndrome, 549
  tumor lysis syndrome and, 549
Alpha$_1$-antitrypsin deficiency
  in chronic obstructive pulmonary
    disease, 882
  screening for, 884

INDEX